Dynamic Electrocardiography

EDITED BY

Professor Marek Malik MSc, PhD, MD, DSc, DSc (Med), FACC, FESC

Professor of Cardiac Electrophysiology,
Department of Cardiac and Vascular Sciences,
St. George's Hospital Medical School,
London SW17 0RE, United Kingdom

AND

Professor A. John Camm QHP, BSc, MD, FRCP, FESC, FACC, FAHA, FCGC, CStJ

Professor of Clinical Cardiology,
Department of Cardiac and Vascular Sciences,
St George's Hospital Medical School,
London SW17 0RE, United Kingdom

Blackwell Futura

To Kate and Joy

Published by Futura, an imprint of Blackwell Publishing
Blackwell Publishing, Inc./Futura Division, 3 West Main Street, Elmsford, New York 10523, USA
Blackwell Publishing, Inc., 350 Main Street, Malden, Massachusetts 02148-5020, USA
Blackwell Publishing Ltd, 9600 Garsington Road, Oxford OX4 2DQ, UK
Blackwell Science Asia Pty Ltd, 550 Swanston Street, Carlton, Victoria 3053, Australia

04 05 06 07 5 4 3 2 1

ISBN: 0-4051-1960-8

Library of Congress Cataloging-in-Publication Data

Dynamic electrocardiography / [edited by] Marek Malik, A. John Camm. – 1st ed.
p. ; cm.
Includes bibliographical references and index.
ISBN 1-405-11960-8
1. Electrocardiography.
[DNLM: 1. Electrocardiography. WG 140 D9974 2004] I. Malik, Marek. II. Camm, A. John.
RC683.5.E5D966 2004
616.1′207547 – dc22

2003023262

A catalogue record for this title is available from the British Library

Acquisitions: Steve Korn
Production: Fiona Pattison and Deirdre Prinsen
Typesetter: SNP Best-set Typesetter Ltd., Hong Kong
Printed and bound by CPI Bath, Bath, UK

For further information on Blackwell Publishing, visit our website: www.futuraco.com

Contents

Contributors

Solange Akselrod, PhD
Professor Head of Medical Physics
Abramson Center for Medical Physics
School of Physics and Astronomy
Tel-Aviv University
Ramat-Aviv, 69978
Israel
solange@post.tau.ac.il

Maurits A. Allessie, MD, PhD
Professor of Physiology
Chairman of the Department of Physiology
Department of Physiology
University Maastricht
PO Box 616
6200 MD Maastricht
The Netherlands
m.allessie@fys.unimaas.nl

Kelley P. Anderson, MD, FACC
Cardiologist
Department of Cardiology 2D2
Marshfield Clinic
1000 North Oak Avenue
Marshfield, WI 54449-5777
USA
kpand@att.net

Charles Antzelevitch, PhD, FACC, FAHA
Executive Director/Director of Research
Gordon K Moe Scholar and Professor of Pharmacology
Masonic Medical Research Laboratory
2150 Bleecker Street
Utica, NY 13501-1787
USA
ca@mmrl.edu

Vico Baier, DIng
Research Assistant
Department of Medical Engineering
University of Applied Sciences Jena
Carl-Zeiss-Promenade 2
07745 Jena
Germany
vico.baier@fh-jena.de

Gust H. Bardy, MD, FACC
Clinical Professor of Medicine
University of Washington
Box 356422: Suite 300
7900 East Greenlake Drive
Seattle, WA 98103
USA
gbardy@u.washington.edu

Petra Barthel, MD
Senior Resident
Deutsches Herzzentrum München
Technische Universität München
Arbacherstrasse 10
81371 Munich
Germany
barthel@med1.med.tum.de

Giuseppe Baselli, MS
Professor in Biomedical Engineering
Department of Bioengineering
Polytechnic University in Milano
Piazza Leonardo da Vinci 32
20133 Milano
Italy
baselli@biomed.polimi.it

Velislav N. Batchvarov, MD
Senior Research Fellow
Department of Cardiac and Vascular Sciences
St. George's Hospital Medical School
Cranmer Terrace
London SW17 0RE
United Kingdom
vbatchva@sghms.ac.uk

Axel Bauer, MD
Resident
Deutsches Herzzentrum München
Technische Universität München
Arbacherstrasse 10
81371 Munich
Germany
bauer.de@web.de

Antoni Bayés de Luna, MD, PhD, FESC, FACC
Professor of Cardiology
Chief of Institute of Cardiology
Hospital de Sant Pau i Santa Creu
St Antoni Ma Claret 167
08025 Barcelona
Spain
Abayesluna@hsp.santpau.es

Antoni Bayés Genis, MD, PhD, FESC
Assistant Professor
Heart Failure Unit Coordinator
Institute of Cardiology
Hospital de Sant Pau i Santa Creu
St Antoni Ma Claret 167
08025 Barcelona
Spain
Abayesgenis@hsp.santpau.es

Elijah Behr, MA, MBBS, MRCP
Specialist Registrar
Department of Cardiac and Vascular Sciences
St George's Hospital Medical School
Cranmer Terrace
London SW17 0RE
United Kingdom
ebehr@sghms.ac.uk

Gary G. Berntson, PhD
Professor of Psychology, Psychiatry & Pediatrics
Department of Psychology
The Ohio State University
1885 Neil Avenue
Columbus, OH 43210
USA
berntson@osu.edu

Anna M. Bianchi, MS
Assistant Professor
Department of Bioengineering
Polytechnic University in Milano
Piazza Leonardo da Vinci 32
20133 Milano
Italy
annamaria.bianchi@polimi.it

Christoph Bode, MD, FESC
Professor of Medicine and Chairman
Universitätsklinikum Freiburg
Innere Medizin III, Kardilogie und Angiologie
Hugstetterstrasse 55
D-79106 Freiburg
Germany
bode@mm31.ukl.uni-freiburg.de

Annie Britton, PhD
Lecturer in Epidemiology and Public Health
International Centre for Health and Society
Department of Epidemiology and Public Health
University College London
1-19 Torrington Place
London WC1E 6BT
United Kingdom
a.britton@ucl.ac.uk

Konrad Brockmeier, MD
Professor of Pediatrics
Head of Pediatric Cardiology
University of Cologne
Joseph-Stelzmann-Strasse 9
50924 Köln
Germany
k.brockmeier@uni-koeln.de

Josep Brugada, MD, PhD
Director, Arrhythmia Unit
Cardiovascular Institute
Hospital Clinic
University of Barcelona
Villarrael 170, 08036
Spain
jepbrugada@grn.es

Pedro Brugada, MD, PhD, FESC, FAHA
Professor of Medicine
Director, Arrhythmia Unit
OLV Hospital, Cardiovascular Center Aalst
9300 Aalst
Belgium
p.brugada@planetinternet.be

Ramon Brugada, MD
Director, Molecular Genetics Program
Masonic Medical Research Laboratory
2150 Bleecker Street
Utica, NY 13501-1787
USA
rbrugada@mmrl.edu

A. John Camm, QHP, BSc, MD, FRCP, FESC, FACC, FAHA, FCGC, CStJ
British Heart Foundation Professor of Clinical Cardiology
Department of Cardiac and Vascular Sciences
St. Georges Hospital Medical School
Cranmer Terrace
London SW17 0RE
United Kingdom
jcamm@sghms.ac.uk

John T. Cacioppo, PhD
Tiffany and Margaret Blake Distinguished Service Professor
Department of Psychology
The University of Chicago
5848 South University Avenue
Chicago, IL 60637
USA
cacioppo@uchicago.edu

Alessandro Capucci, MD, FESC, FACC
Director of Department of Cardiology
Guglielmo da Saliceto General Hospital
Cantone del Cristo
29100 Piacenza
Italy
progettovita@hotmail.com

Barbara Casadei, MD, DPhil, FESC, FRCP
Reader in Cardiovascular Medicine
University Department of Cardiovascular Medicine
John Radcliffe Hospital
Oxford OX3 9DU
United Kingdom
barbara.casadei@cardiov.ox.ac.uk

Sergio Cerutti, MS, FIEEE, FIAMBE
Professor and Head of the Department of Bioengineering
Polytechnic University in Milano
Piazza Leonardo da Vinci 32
20133 Milano
Italy
cerutti@biomed.polimi.it

Rory W. Childers, MD
Professor of Medicine/Director, Heart Station
Cardiology Section
Department of Medicine
University of Chicago Medical Center
5758 South Maryland Avenue MC 9024
Chicago, IL 60637
USA
rchilder@medicine.bsd.uchicago.edu

Andrea Colella, MD
Senior Physician
Department of Medical and Surgical Critical Care
Section of Internal Medicine and Cardiology
University of Firenze
v. le Morgagni, 85
50134 Firenze
Italy
elettrofisiologia@dfc.unifi.it

Xavier Copie, MD, PhD
Consultant Cardiologist
Centre Cardiologique du Nord
32-36 rue des Moulins Gémeaux
93200 Saint-Denis
France
x.copie@ccncardio.com

Otto Costantini, MD
Assistant Professor of Medicine
Director, Arrhythmia Prevention Center
Case Western Reserve University @ MetroHealth Medical Center
Heart & Vascular Center H-334
2500 MetroHealth Drive
Cleveland, OH 44109
USA
ocostantini@metrohealth.org

Philippe Coumel, MD, FESC
Consultant Cardiologist
Department of Cardiology
Lariboisière Hospital
2, rue Ambroise-Paré
75010 Paris
France
philippe.coumel@lrb.ap-hop-paris.fr

Iwona Cygankiewicz, MD, PhD
Fellow of Cardiology
Institute of Cardiology
Hospital de Sant Pau i Santa Creu
St Antoni Ma Claret 167
08025 Barcelona
Spain
Icygankiewicz@hsp.santpau.es

Polychronis E. Dilaveris, MD, FESC
Research Registrar
Department of Cardiology
University of Athens Medical School
22 Miltiadou Str
155 61 Holargos
Athens
Greece
hrodil@yahoo.com

Dwain L. Eckberg, MD
Professor, Medicine and Physiology
Medical College of Virginia at Virginia Commonwealth University
4614 Riverside Drive
Richmond, VA 23225
USA
deckberg@ekholmen.com

Paul J. Erlinger, BSEE
Field Clinical Engineer
Cameron Health Inc.
905 Calle Amanecer
Suite 300
San Clemente, CA 92673
USA
perlinger@cameronhealth.com

Ernest L. Fallen, MD FRCP(C)
Professor Emeritus, Department of Medicine
McMaster University Faculty of Health Sciences
McMaster University Medical Center, Rm 3U8
1200 Main St. West
Hamilton
Ontario L8N 3Z5
Canada
fallene@mcmaster.ca

Shlomo Feldman, MD, FACC
Senior Lecturer in Cardiology
Tel Aviv University.
Past Director of the Pacemaker and Electrophysiology Unit
Heart Institute
Sheba Medical Center
Tel Hashomer Hospital
Ramat Gan
Israel 52621
shlomofeldman@hotmail.com

Michael R. Franz, MD, PhD, FACC
Professor of Medicine and Pharmacology
George Town University Medical Center
Director, Clinical and Experimental Electrophysiology
VA Medical Center
50 Irving St. NW
Washington, DC 20422
USA
michael.r.franz@verizon.net

J. Lee Garvey, MD
Medical Director, Chest Pain Evaluation Center
Department of Emergency Medicine
Carolinas Medical Center
1000 Blythe Blvd
Charlotte, NC 28203
USA
lgarvey@carolinas.org

Peter Geelen, MD, PhD
Co-director, Arrhythmia Unit
OLV Hospital, Cardiovascular Center Aalst
164, Moorselbaan
9300 Aalst
Belgium
peter.geelen@olvz-aalst.be

Gian Franco Gensini, MD
Professor of Internal Medicine
Department of Medical and Surgical Critical Care
Section of Internal Medicine and Cardiology
University of Firenze
v. le Morgagni, 85
50134 Firenze,
Italy
g.gensini@dfc.unifi.it

John E. Gialafos, MD, FESC, FACC
Professor of Cardiology
Department of Cardiology
University of Athens Medical School
37 Ipsilantou Street
106 76 Athens
Greece
gialaf@yahoo.com

Andreas Grom, MD
Research Fellow
Universitätsklinikum Freiburg
Innere Medizin III, Kardilogie und Angiologie
Hugstetterstrasse 55
D-79106 Freiburg
Germany
grom@med1.ukl.uni-freiburg.de

Roger Hainsworth, MB, ChB, PhD, DSc
Professor of Applied Physiology and Honorary Consultant
Clinical Physiologist
Institute for Cardiovascular Research
University of Leeds
Leeds LS2 9JT
United Kingdom
medrh@leeds.ac.uk

Juha E. K. Hartikainen, MD, PhD
Senior Consultant Cardiologist
Department of Medicine
Kuopio University Hospital
Box 1777
70211 Kuopio
Finland
juha.hartikainen@kuh.fi

Harry Hemingway, MRCP
Reader in Clinical Epidemiology
International Centre for Health and Society
Department of Epidemiology and Public Health
University College London
1-19 Torrington Place
London WC1E 6BT
United Kingdom
h.heminway@ucl.ac.uk

Katerina Hnatkova, MSc, PhD, FESC
Senior Research Fellow
Department of Cardiac and Vascular Sciences
St George's Hospital Medical School
Cranmer Terrace
London SW17 0RE
United Kingdom
k.hnatkova@sghms.ac.uk

Stefan H. Hohnloser, MD, FACC, FESC
Professor of Medicine
Department of Medicine
Division of Electrophysiology
Theodor-Stern-Kai 7
60590 Frankfurt
Germany
Hohnloser@em.uni-frankfurt.de

B. Milan Horacek, PhD
Professor of Biophysics
Department of Physiology & Biophysics
Dalhousie University
Sir Charles Tupper Medical Building
5859 University Avenue
Halifax, Nova Scotia B3H 4H7
Canada
milan.horacek@dal.ca

Richard P.M. Houben, BSc
Principal Design Engineer
Advanced Concepts
Medtronic Bakken Research Center
Endepolsdomein 5
6229 GW Maastricht
The Netherlands
richard.houben@medtronic.com

Heikki Huikuri, MD, PhD, FACC, FESC
Professor in Medicine
Department of Internal Medicine
Division of Cardiology
Oulu University Hospital, Oulu
PO Box 20
FIN-90029 OYS
Finland
heikki.huikuri@oulu.fi

Bogdan G. Ionescu, MD
Fellow in Cardiology
Institute of Cardiology
Hospital de Sant Pau i Santa Creu
St Antoni Ma Claret 167
08025 Barcelona
Spain
bionescu@hsp.santpau.es

Juan Carlos Kaski, MD, DSc, FRCP, FACC, FESC
Professor of Cardiovascular Science
Department of Cardiac and Vascular Sciences
St George's Hospital Medical School
Cranmer Terrace
London SW17 0RE
United Kingdom
jkaski@sghms.ac.uk

Josef Kautzner, MD, PhD, FESC
Head, Department of Cardiology
Institute for Clinical and Experimental Medicine
Videnska 800
140 21 Prague 4
Czech Republic
josef.kautzner@medicon.cz

Milos Kesek, MD
Consultant Cardiologist
Department of Cardiology
Norrland University Hospital
901 85 Umea
Sweden
milos.kesek@comhem.se

Robert E. Kleiger, MD, FACC
Professor of Medicine
Cardiovascular Division
Washington University School of Medicine
660 S. Euclid Ave
Campus Box 8086
St. Louis, MO 63110
USA
mleaders@im.wustl.edu

Paul Kligfield, MD, FACC
Professor of Medicine
Division of Cardiology
Weill Medical College of Cornell University
1300 York Avenue
New York, NY 10021
USA
pkligfi@med.cornell.edu

Maria Teresa La Rovere, MD, FESC
Director Autonomic Laboratories
Department of Cardiology
Fondazione 'Salvatore Maugeri', IRCCS
Istituto Scientifico di Montescano
27040 Montescano (Pavia)
Italy
mtlarovere@fsm.it

Uwe Leder, MD
Cardiologist
Department of Cardiology
Clinic of Internal Medicine III
University of Jena
Erlanger Allee 101
07740 Jena
Germany
uwe.leder@uni-jena.de

Jean-Yves Le Heuzey, MD
Professor of Medicine
Department of Cardiology
Hôpital Européen Georges Pompidou
20 rue Leblanc
75015 Paris
France
Jean-yves.le-heuzey@egp.ap-hop-paris.fr

Samuel Lévy, MD, FACC, FESC
Professor
Hopital Nord Cardiologie
13015 Marseille
France
samuel@samuel-levy.com

Fred W. Lindemans, PhD
General Manager
Medtronic Bakken Research Center
Endepolsdomein 5
6229 GW Maastricht
The Netherlands
fred.lindemans@medtronic.com

Federico Lombardi, MD, FESC
Associate Professor of Cardiology
Cardiologia, Dip. di Medicina, Chirurgia e Odontoiatria
Ospedale San Paolo, University of Milan
Via A. di rudinì 8
20142 Milan
Italy
Federico.Lombardi@unimi.it

Robert L. Lux, PhD
Professor of Medicine
CVRTI/Bldg 500
University of Utah
95 South 2000 East
Salt Lake City, UT 84112-2000
USA
lux@cvrti.utah.edu

Luca T. Mainardi, MS, PhD
Assistant Professor
Department of Bioengineering
Polytechnic University in Milano
Piazza Leonardo da Vinci 32
20133 Milano
Italy
mainardi@biomed.polimi.it

Timo Mäkikallio, MD, PhD
Associate Professor of Experimental Cardiology
Department of Internal Medicine
Division of Cardiology
Oulu University Hospital, Oulu
PO Box 20
FIN-90029 OYS
Finland
timo.makikallio@oulu.fi

Marek Malik, MSc, PhD, MD, DSc, DSc(Med), FACC, FESC
Professor of Cardiac Electrophysiology
Department of Cardiac and Vascular Sciences
St. George's Hospital Medical School
Cranmer Terrace
London SW17 0RE
United Kingdom
m.malik@sghms.ac.uk

Alberto Malliani, MD
Head of Department
Dipartimento di Scienze Cliniche 'Luigi Sacco'
Ospedale Sacco
Via GB Grassi 74
20157 Milano
Italy
alberto.malliani@unimi.it

Rahul Mehra, PhD
Senior Director, Atrial Fibrillation Research
Medtronic, Inc.
7000 Central Avenue N.E
Minneapolis, MN 55432,
USA
rahul.mehra@medtronic.com

Carl J. Meurling, MD, PhD, FESC
Consultant Cardiologist
Department of Cardiology
University Hospital of Lund
SE-221 85 Lund
Sweden
carl.meurling@kard.lu.se

Antonio Michelucci, MD
Associate Professor of Cardiology
Department of Medical and Surgical Critical Care
Section of Internal Medicine and Cardiology
University of Firenze
v. le Morgagni, 85
50134 Firenze
Italy
michelucci@unifi.it

Nicola Montano, PhD, MD
Assistant Professor of Medicine
Dipartimento di Scienze Cliniche "Luigi Sacco"
Ospedale Sacco
Via GB Grassi 74
20157 Milano
Italy
nicola.montano@unimi.it

Roger Moore, BSc (Hons), MBChB, MRCP
Cardiology Specialist Registrar
Cardiothoracic Centre
Liverpool L14 3PE
United Kingdom
moore@roger.go-legend.net

James Nolan, MBChB, FRCP, MD
Consultant Cardiologist and Honorary Senior Lecturer
University Hospital
578 Newcastle Road, Stoke-on-Trent
North Staffordshire ST4 6QG
United Kingdom
nolanjim@hotmail.com

Peter M. Okin, MD, FACC
Professor of Medicine
Division of Cardiology
Weill Medical College of Cornell University
1300 York Avenue
New York 10021
USA
pokin@med.cornell.edu

Walter H. Olson, PhD
Senior Director
Implantable Defibrillators
Medtronic, Inc. B173
7000 Central Avenue N.E
Minneapolis, MN 55432-3576,
USA
walt.olson@medtronic.com

S. Bertil Olsson, MD, PhD, FESC, FAHA, RPhS
Professor of Cardiology
Department of Cardiology
University Hospital of Lund
SE-221 85 Lund
Sweden
Bertil.Olsson@kard.lu.se

Luigi Padeletti, MD
Associate Professor of Cardiology
Department of Medical and Surgical Critical Care
Section of Internal Medicine and Cardiology
University of Firenze
v. le Morgagni, 85
50134 Firenze
Italy
elettrofisiologia@dfc.unifi.it

Sundip J. Patel, MBBCh, MRCP
Specialist Registrar in Cardiology
Department of Cardiology
6th Floor, East Wing
St Thomas' Hospital
Lambeth Palace Road
London SE1 7EH
United Kingdom
sundip.patel@gstt.sthames.nhs.uk

Divaka Perera, MA, MBBChir, MRCP
Specialist Registrar in Cardiology
Department of Cardiology
6th Floor, East Wing
St Thomas' Hospital
Lambeth Palace Road
London SE1 7EH
United Kingdom
divaka.perera@gstt.sthames.nhs.uk

Juha Perkiömäki, MD, PhD
Senior Lecturer in Internal Medicine
Department of Internal Medicine, Division of Cardiology
Oulu University Hospital,
Oulu
PO Box 20
FIN-90029 OYS
Finland
juha.perkiomaki@oulu.fi

Massimo F. Piepoli, MD, PhD, FESC
Consultant Cardiologist
Cardiology Department
Guglielmo da Saliceto General Hospital
Cantone del Cristo
29100 Piacenza
Italy
m.piepoli@ic.ac.uk

Paolo Pieragnoli, MD
Senior Physician
Department of Medical and Surgical Critical Care
Section of Internal Medicine and Cardiology
University of Firenze
v. le Morgagni, 85
50134 Firenze
Italy
elettrofisiologia@dfc.unifi.it

Alberto Porta, MS, PhD
Research Fellow
LITA-Vialba, Department of Pre-Clinical Sciences
University in Milano
via G.B. Grassi 74
20157 Milano
Italy
alberto.porta@unimi.it

Esther Pueyo, BSc
Lecturer in Biomedical Engineering
Department of Electronic Engineering and Communications
University of Zaragoza
Maria de Luna 1
50018 Zaragoza
Spain
epueyo@unizar.es

Simon R. Redwood, MBBS, MD, FRCP, FACC
Consultant Cardiologist
Department of Cardiology
6th Floor, East Wing
St Thomas' Hospital
Lambeth Palace Road
London SE1 7EH
United Kingdom
simon.redwood@gstt.sthames.nhs.uk

David Ritscher, MS
Principal Scientist,
Atrial Fibrillation Research
Medtronic, Inc.
7000 Central Avenue N.E.
Mailstop B170
Minneapolis, MN 55432
USA
david.ritscher@medtronic.com

Maximo Rivero-Ayerza, MD
Clinical Fellow, Electrophysiology
Arrhythmia Unit
OLV Hospital Aalst, Cardiovascular Center
9300 Aalst
Belgium
mriveroayerza@yahoo.com.ar

Marten Rosenqvist, MD, PhD
Professor of Cardiology
Karolinska Institutet,
Stockholm Söder Hospital
Department of Cardiology
118 83 Stockholm
Sweden
marten.rosenqvist@sos.sll.se

Juan Cosin Sales, MD
Research Fellow
Department of Cardiac and Vascular Sciences
St George's Hospital Medical School
Cranmer Terrace
London SW17 0RE
United Kingdom
jcosin@sghms.ac.uk

Alexander Schirdewan, MD
Cardiologist
Head of the Department of Electrophysiology
Franz-Volhard-Clinic Berlin
Humboldt University Berlin
Wiltbergstrasse 50
13125 Berlin
Germany
schirdewan@fvk.charite-buch.de

Georg Schmidt, MD
Professor of Medicine
1. Medizinische Klinik
Technische Universität München
Munich
Germany
gschmidt@med1.med.tum.de

Raphael Schneider, Dipl. Ing. (FH)
Software Engineer
1. Medizinische Klinik
Technische Universität München
Munich
Germany
rasch@med1.med.tum.de

Ulrich Schotten, MD, PhD
Assistant Professor of Physiology
Department of Physiology
University Maastricht
PO Box 616
6200 MD Maastricht
The Netherlands
schotten@fys.unimaas.nl

Paul Schweitzer, MD, FACC
Director, Cardiac Arrhythmia Services
Professor of Medicine
Albert Einstein College of Medicine
Beth Israel Medical Center
Milton and Carroll Petrie Division
First Avenue at 16th Street
New York, NY 10003
USA
pschweit@bethisraelny.org

Peter Smetana, MD
Cardiologist
Wilhelminenspital der Stadt Wien
Department of Cardiology
Montleartstrasse 37
1160 Vienna
Austria
psmetana@hotmail.com

Leif Sörnmo, MSEE, PhD
Professor of Electrical Engineering
Department of Electroscience
Lund University
Box 118
SE-221 00 Lund
Sweden
leif.sornmo@es.lth.se

Phyllis K. Stein, PhD
Director, Heart Rate Variability Laboratory
Cardiovascular Division
Washington University School of Medicine
4625 Lindell Blvd, Suite 402
St Louis, MO 63108
USA
pstein@im.wustl.edu

Shlomo Stern, MD, FACC, FAHA, FESC
Professor Emeritus of Medicine
Hebrew University
Department of Cardiology
Bikur Cholim Hospital
PO Box 492
Jerusalem 91004
Israel
sh_stern@netvision.net.il

Martin Stridh, MSEE, PhD
Researcher
Department of Electroscience
Lund University
Box 118
SE-221 00 Lund
Sweden
martin.stridh@es.lth.se

Aneesh Tolat, MD
Clinical Cardiac Electrophysiology Fellow
Beth Israel Deaconess Medical Center
Department of Medicine, Division of Cardiology
330 Brookline Avenue, W/BA-4
Boston, MA 02215
USA
atolat@bidmc.harvard.edu

Marion VanDyck, MD, FACC
Director, Cardiology Outpatient Services
Clinical Instructor of Medicine
Beth Israel Medical Center
Milton and Carroll Petrie Division
First Avenue at 16th Street
New York, NY10003
USA
mvandyck@bethisraelny.org

Richard L. Verrier, PhD, FACC
Associate Professor of Medicine,
Harvard Medical School
Beth Israel Deaconess Medical Center
Harvard Institutes of Medicine
4 Blackfan Circle, Room 223
Boston, MA 02115
USA
rverrier@bidmc.harvard.edu

Giovanni Q. Villani, MD
Consultant Cardiology, EP Laboratory
Cardiology Department
Guglielmo da Saliceto General Hospital
Cantone del Cristo
29100 Piacenza
Italy
gqvillani@hotmail.com

Xavier Viñolas, MD
Chief of Electrophysiology Laboratory
Institute of Cardiology
Hospital de Sant Pau i Santa Creu
St Antoni Ma Claret 167
08025 Barcelona
Spain
xvinolas@hsp.santpau.es

Andreas Voss, PhD
Professor of Medical Informatics and Biosignal Analysis
Department of Medical Engineering
University of Applied Sciences Jena
Carl-Zeiss-Promenade 2
07745 Jena
Germany
voss@fh-jena.de

Galen S. Wagner, MD
Associate Professor of Medicine
Department of Medicine
Duke University Medical Center
2400 Pratt St., Room 0306
Durham, NC 27705
USA
wagne004@mc.duke.edu

Mari A. Watanabe, MD, PhD
Postdoctoral Research Associate
Institute of Biomedical Life Sciences
Glasgow University
Glasgow G12 8QQ
United Kingdom
maw16h@udcf.gla.ac.uk

Dan Wichterle, MD
Clinical Electrocardiologist
2nd Department of Internal Medicine
1st Medical School, Charles University
U nemocnice 2
128 08 Prague 2
Czech Republic
wichterle@hotmail.com

Shamil Yusuf, BSc (Hons), MbChB (Hons), MCOptom, MRCP
Research Fellow in Cardiology
Department of Cardiac and Vascular Sciences
St. Georges Hospital Medical School
Cranmer Terrace
London SW17 0RE
United Kingdom
syusuf@sghms.ac.uk

Markus Zabel, MD
Director of Electrophysiology
Division of Cardiology
Charité - Campus Benjamin Franklin
Hindenburgdamm 30
12200 Berlin
Germany
mzabel@compuserve.com

Manfred Zehender, MD, MBA, FESC
Professor of Medicine
Universitätsklinikum Freiburg
Innere Medizin III, Kardilogie und Angiologie
Hugstetterstrasse 55
D-79106 Freiburg
Germany
zehender@medizin.ukl.uni-freiburg.de

Foreword

The mysteries of the electrocardiogram unfold in the encyclopaedic tome, *Dynamic Electrocardiography*, edited by Marek Malik and John Camm. Since the first published human electrocardiogram was recorded in 1887 by Augustus Waller (*Journal of Physiology* 1887; **8**: 229–234), our understanding of cardiac arrhythmias and the electrical manifestations of cardiac diseases has burgeoned. Over the last several decades, advanced signal analysis and processing techniques have been applied to the electrocardiographic signal to extract increasingly important information regarding cardiac physiology. These techniques and their clinical importance are highlighted in *Dynamic Electrocardiography*.

The editors have been extensively involved in setting the standards in many of the areas discussed in the book. They fortunately provide their expertise as both authors and editors. Drs Malik and Camm have also assembled an outstanding group of contributors, many of whom are the leading experts in their field. As with all new developments, there are many applications and misapplications of these techniques. The editors have synthesized the topics so that the reader may focus on the technical details of how the techniques are performed, how they are properly applied, and what they might mean to the clinician. This compendium therefore serves as an important resource to the clinician and researcher. To our knowledge, there is no book that has the breadth of topics and the breadth of appeal.

The book opens with a section on heart rate variability. This section describes the multiple techniques that are used to measure heart rate variability and puts into context how these measurements are to be interpreted. The ability to extract information regarding autonomic modulation of the heart rate from detailed signal processing techniques focused on characterizing small changes in heart rhythm has opened up many areas of study. Because heart rate variability measurements can be made noninvasively, much effort has been expended to better understand what it means physiologically and prognostically. The ability of these measurements of heart rate variability to provide prognostic information regarding mortality, particularly in patients with cardiac disease, has been an important contribution. The role of the autonomic nervous system in modulating cardiac electrophysiology underlies its pathophysiologic link to sudden cardiac death. Further work in this area will better define this link. Ongoing and future studies will provide the information necessary on how to use these techniques to better treat patients and improve their survival.

Section II deals with measurement of baroreflex sensitivity and heart rate turbulence. These techniques are used to measure the responsiveness of the autonomic nervous system to a perturbation, via the arterial baroreflex. Once again, the physiology, techniques, and clinical utility of these tests are described in this section. These measurements have been shown to be independent powerful predictors of mortality, even when compared to standard heart rate variability measurements. Just as the exercise electrocardiogram is a more useful test for the detection of myocardial ischaemia than the resting electrocardiogram, so too these provocative manoeuvres may provide additional information not obtained by resting measurements of autonomic modulation.

Section III is devoted to evaluation of the ST segment for detection of myocardial ischaemia with review of the underlying basic electrophysiology and clinical methods. Though ST segment changes as a manifestation of myocardial ischaemia have long been recognized, this represents a crucial area of electrocardiography with important implications in patients with ischaemic heart disease.

Section IV highlights the developments made in understanding ventricular repolarization and their impact on patients with cardiac disease.

The complexities of ventricular repolarization become apparent with the multiple ways that exist to characterize it: the QT/RR relationship; circadian variation; QT dispersion; T wave morphology; and T wave alternans. The improved understanding from the cellular to the tissue level has led to the advanced application of these techniques. The chapters are very well organized to help guide the reader through the multidimensional approach to ventricular repolarization.

Sections V, VI, and VII deal with atrial fibrillation, ventricular arrhythmias, and recordings from implanted devices. These sections include selected topics regarding electrocardiographic techniques with a specific focus on newer techniques.

This book will serve the reader as an important reference for this broad array of topics. As the chapters are succinct and to the point, they will provide the reader the most readily accessible information in an easy to read format. Congratulation to Drs Malik and Camm on a superb effort.

Jeffrey Goldberger, MD
Melvin Scheinman, MD

Preface

Compared to many clinical methods and procedures, electrocardiography is not particularly new. The first human electrocardiogram was recorded by Dr Augustus Desiré Waller in 1887. Since that time, the development of electrocardiography was not uniform. Several waves of advancement of the physiologic understanding and clinical utility of the electrocardiogram can be traced throughout the past century. After the very first human recording, it took about 20 years for more precise equipment to be developed that allowed recordings to be made with sufficient fidelity for meaningful biological interpretation. Another two decades elapsed before the very core and principal rhythm abnormalities were appreciated and classified; it took some further decades to understand the ischaemic patterns in details; and so on.

The most recent wave of electrocardiographic advances resulted from the observations that not only the static snapshots of cardiac electrical activity but also their temporal development carry physiologically important and clinically useful information. In many aspects, the investigation of this dynamicity of electrocardiographic recordings was not only facilitated but directly allowed by modern electronic and computing technologies. Indeed, it is inconceivable to imagine a modern electrocardiograph without substantial electronic and computer components aimed not only at recording the tiny electrical potentials at the body surface but also at their processing and detailed elaboration. Meaningful and important electrocardiographic measurements and valuable clinical diagnoses reached in this way frequently go far beyond the 'classical' visual interpretation of the recorded images.

Because of the research and clinical importance of this new window of electrocardiography, we were very pleased when asked by Futura/Blackwell to edit a comprehensive book aimed at summarizing the most recent advances in electrocardiography, concentrating primarily but not exclusively on the dynamicity of the recordings. The field of modern dynamic electrocardiography is obviously rather broad. Therefore, we have divided the book into seven sections dealing with heart rate variability, baro-reflexes, dynamicity of ischaemic patterns, electrocardiography of ventricular repolarization, atrial fibrillation, ventricular arrhythmias, and finally the recordings made by an implanted device.

As with any other multi-author book, we faced the usual editorial dilemma between having the book tightly cross-referenced and having the individual chapters suitable for stand-alone reading. We eventually felt that a volume of this size should also serve as a reference textbook and that having individual chapters as stand-alone reviews is therefore preferable. Consequently, we are happy to recommend the reader to select separate chapters according to his/her particular needs. Needless to say, reading the book in its entirety will provide a more comprehensive insight into the recent advances in dynamic electrocardiography. In some areas of the field, the rapid development in dynamic electrocardiography leads to occasional controversies. In such cases, we tried to offer the reader the possibility of learning and comparing the different views.

With a book of this broad spectrum, we of course needed to rely on the help of others. Our sincere thanks therefore go to all the contributors who helped us by writing individual chapters. We truly appreciate their efforts – without their enthusiasms and kind involvement in the project, the book would never have been written. We are also grateful to the publisher for careful technical editing of the text and for their understanding and flexibility. Finally, our deep thanks go to Mrs Pam Fernandes who helped us with running the editorial office of the book. It would have been extremely difficult to organise the whole volume without her meticulous involvement.

Marek Malik
A. John Camm
October 2003

SECTION I
Heart Rate Variability

CHAPTER 1

Physiological Background of Heart Rate Variability

Roger Hainsworth

Introduction

Heart rate shows variations which are related, amongst other things to breathing, circadian rhythm and exercise. Resting heart rates can be very different in different subjects, with some having rates of 100 beats/min and others only 50 beats/min for no obvious reason. Highly trained endurance athletes may have resting rates of only 40–50 beats/min with very large stroke volumes to compensate. The maximum rate is partly age-dependent with older subjects achieving maxima during heavy exercise of 20–30 beats/min less than those achieved by younger individuals.

The rate of the heart and its beat-to-beat variations are dependent on the rate of discharge of the pacemaker, normally the sinu-atrial node. The sinu-atrial node in turn is influenced by activity in the two main divisions of autonomic nerves, which are controlled in a complex way by a variety of reflexes as well as by cortical factors.

This chapter will consider in turn the effects on the heart of the autonomic nerves, the control of autonomic activity by various reflexes, and the interaction of these reflexes during some more complex events.

Effects of the autonomic nerves

In the absence of activity in sympathetic or parasympathetic nerves and with low levels of circulating hormones, particularly catecholamines, the heart will beat at its intrinsic rate of 100–120 beats/min. The rate at any particular time is determined by the balance between vagal activity, which slows it, and sympathetic activity, which accelerates it (Levy & Martin 1979). Generally, if the rate is lower than the intrinsic rate of the pacemaker, it implies predominant vagal activity, whereas high heart rates are achieved by increased sympathetic drive.

Vagal responses

The cell bodies of the vagal neurones lie in the dorsal motor nucleus and the nucleus ambiguus. The vagi run down the neck alongside the carotid arteries into the thorax. These nerves carry not only the nerve fibres which control heart rate but many other efferent nerves including those to the bronchi and the gastrointestinal tract. They also contain vast numbers of both myelinated and nonmyelinated afferent nerves innervating thoracic and abdominal viscera. Activity in the vagal branches innervating the sinu-atrial node determines heart rate. Activity in nerves to the conducting mechanism reduces its conduction velocity and high levels of vagal activity may completely block atrioventricular conduction. The question of vagal efferent activity on ventricular contractility remains controversial. Earlier work indicated that in mammalian hearts inotropic responses occurred only in atrial and not in ventricular muscle (Furnival *et al.* 1973). Confusion has arisen due to the depressed atrial contractility causing reduced ventricular filling. Recent work, however, does point to the existence of a small vagally mediated negative inotropic effect in the human ventricular myocardium (Casadei 2001).

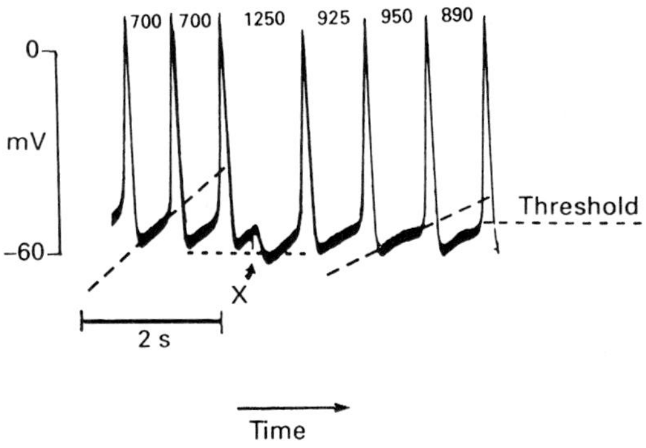

Fig. 1.1 Effects of vagal stimulation on pacemaker potential. Note that there is an almost immediate hyperpolarization and a slower rate of depolarization.

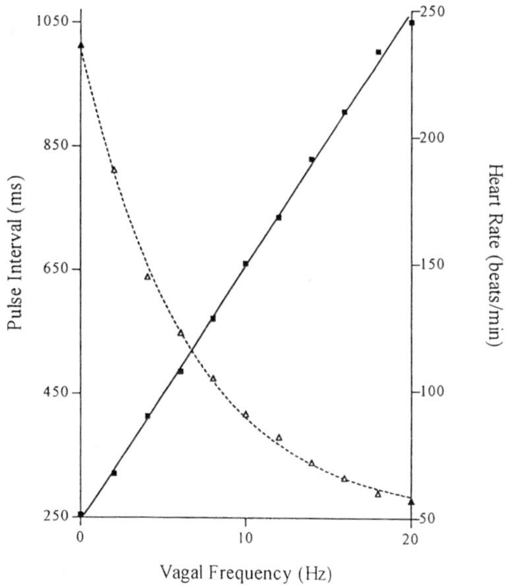

Fig. 1.2 Effects of graded stimulation of efferent vagal nerve in the rabbit. Responses shown as heart rate (-■-■-■-) having a hyperbolic relationship with stimulus frequency and as pulse interval (-△--△--△-) with a linear relationship. (Results obtained from data of Parker *et al.* 1984, with permission.)

Electrical stimulation of either vagus nerve results in slowing of the heart, and high frequencies of stimulation may result in asystole and this may last several seconds. Often during prolonged atrial asystole 'escape' beats may originate from other parts of the conducting mechanism. In animals at least, stimulation of the right vagus nerve seems to have a larger chronotropic effect than that from left vagal stimulation (Hamlin & Smith 1968). Stimulation of the left nerve has been reported to have a greater effect on A-V conduction and high frequencies cause A-V conduction block.

The relationship between vagal stimulation frequency and the resulting change in heart rate is hyperbolic, with changes in frequency at low heart rates having a much greater effect than when the rate is high. However, vagal activity does not directly control heart rate but rather it acts to regulate the interval between successive beats. If therefore, instead of plotting heart rate, we plot pulse interval against vagal stimulation, we see that the relationship becomes linear instead of hyperbolic (Fig. 1.2). The choice between pulse interval and heart rate is largely influenced by the interpretation that is required. If it is intended to be used to calculate cardiac output, then clearly heart rate is the appropriate variable. If, however, we wish to quantitate a vagal response, for example to a baroreceptor stimulus, then pulse interval should be used. The effect of this can be seen if, for example, a change in vagal activity induces a prolongation of pulse interval of 333 ms. At a heart rate of 90 beats/min this would correspond to a rate change of 30 beats/min, but at 180 beats/min the change in rate would be three times as much at 90 beats/min.

Sympathetic responses

The effect of vagal stimulation is very rapid. A single pulse has been reported to induce a maximal effect in only 400 ms (Levy *et al.* 1970). The significance of this is that heart rate can be controlled through changes in vagal activity, on a beat-to-beat basis. The effect of vagal stimulation is to release the neurotransmitter acetylcholine and this has two effects on the pacemaker potentials. Firstly, the cells become hyperpolarized and secondly, their rate of depolarization is decreased. Both effects prolong the interval before the critical depolarizing threshold is reached (Fig. 1.1)

Cardiac sympathetic preganglionic nerve fibres originate in the lateral grey horn of the upper thoracic region, synapse in the sympathetic ganglia, then form a plexus together with parasympathetic fibres over the mediastinum, before supplying all parts of the heart. Increasing the activity in cardiac sympathetic nerves is the principal way by which heart rate is

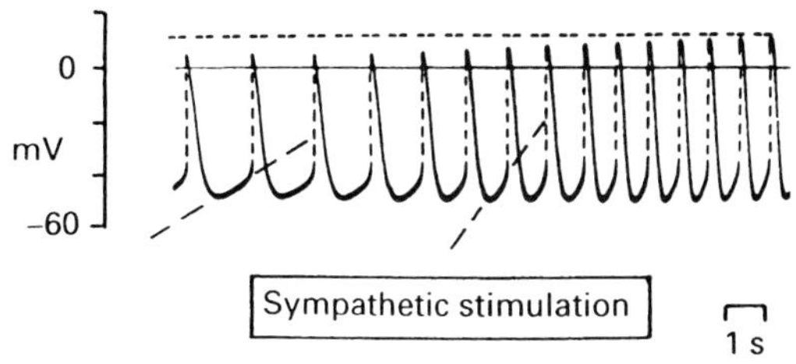

Fig. 1.3 Effect of sympathetic stimulation on pacemaker potential. Note the gradual increase in rate of depolorization and in rate of impulse generation.

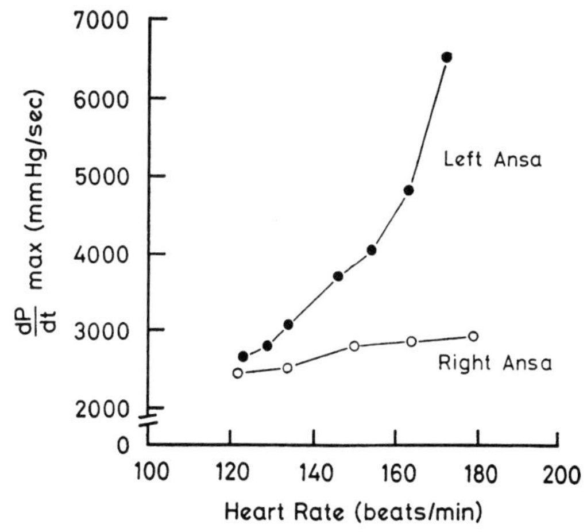

Fig. 1.4 Comparison of the relative responses of heart rate and inotropic state (d*P*/d*t* max) to graded stimulation of right and left sympathetic nerves. Note the relatively larger effect on heart rate from the right nerves. (Reproduced from Furnival *et al.* 1973, with permission.)

increased above its intrinsic level. This is achieved by causing an increase in the rate of depolarization of the pacemaker cells, causing the critical depolarization of the pacemaker cells to be reached more rapidly (Fig. 1.3). Sympathetic activity, therefore, acts in a similar way to vagal activity in that it directly regulates the pulse interval rather than the heart rate. The responses differ from those to vagal stimulation in that they develop much more slowly. Following the start of stimulation, there is a latency of up to 5s and then heart rate gradually increases to reach a new steady level in 20–30 s. This is clearly of significance when considering heart rate variability and reflex responses. If a change occurs in response to a stimulation within 5 s of its application the efferent mechanism can only be vagally mediated. Responses with longer latencies are likely to be mainly sympathetic.

In addition to its effect on the sinu-atrial node, sympathetic fibres also influence the conducting mechanism and the ventricular myocardium. The right sympathetic nerves, at least in dogs, have a greater effect on heart rate whereas the left nerves have a relatively greater inotropic effect (Fig. 1.4). It should be noted, however, that the high levels of heart rate reached through sympathetic activity can only be achieved because sympathetic activity also shortens the duration of ventricular systole. At rest, ventricular systole lasts about 300 ms in a cardiac cycle of 800 ms. At high heart rates, when the entire cardiac cycle shortens to 300 ms, systolic time must be reduced to allow time for filling.

Reflex control of heart rate

The efferent activity in both vagal and sympathetic nerves is regulated by the central nervous system in response to excitatory and inhibitory reflex inputs. Table 1.1 lists some reflexes responsible for decreasing or increasing the heart rate. The body, however, is influenced by many diverse inputs and the overall effect is dependent on often complex interactions as well as cortical influences.

Table 1.1 Reflex control of heart rate

Reflexes increasing heart rate	*Reflexes decreasing heart rate*
Atrial receptors	Baroreceptors
Pulmonary stretch receptors	Chemoreceptors
Muscle metaboreceptors	Ventricular chemosensitive afferents
Pain receptors	Pulmonary 'J' receptors
	Trigeminal afferents (diving)

Baroreceptors

Arterial baroreceptors exist in many regions of the body. Owing to their accessibility those in the carotid sinuses have been most extensively studied, and in humans these are the only receptors capable of being selectively stimulated. Animal studies, however, have established potentially important baroreceptors in the aortic arch

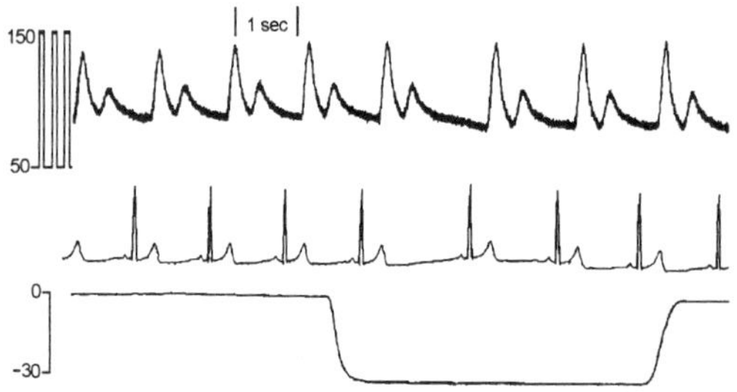

Fig. 1.5 Responses of cardiac interval to stimulation of carotid baroreceptors in humans by neck suction. A negative pressure applied to a lead chamber fitted over the subject's neck distends carotid baroreceptors and causes an immediate prolongation of the interval.

(Hainsworth *et al.* 1970), the coronary arteries (Drinkhill *et al.* 1993) and in the abdominal circulation (Doe *et al.* 1996; Drinkhill *et al.* 1997). Baroreceptors are stretch receptors which respond to changes in vessel transmural pressure. An important characteristic is their response to changes in pulsatility. This enables them to respond to changes in cardiac stroke volume caused by changes in venous return which may be too small to be detected as changes in pressure (Taylor *et al.* 1995). Baroreceptors are effective at 'buffering' short-term changes in blood pressure. They are less effective in long-term pressure control due to their property of resetting (Chapleau & Abboud, 1993).

Baroreceptors control blood pressure by their effects on the heart and blood vessels. The immediate cardiac response is vagally mediated and occurs very rapidly (Fig. 1.5). Eckberg (1978) applied brief stimuli to carotid baroreceptors by means of a neck suction device that increased carotid transmural pressure. He observed that maximal effects were obtained when a stimulus was applied 750 ms before a subsequent anticipated P wave. Baroreceptors, therefore, can control heart period on a beat-to-beat basis. Variations in heart rate mediated through the baroreflex can occur at relatively high frequencies. The actual frequency is dependent rather on the variations in the stimulus than on latency of the reflex.

Baroreceptor reflex stimulus–response relationships have a limited range of linearity. The nonlinearity may be a feature of the effector mechanism. For example in resting conditions where sympathetic activity is low baroreceptor stimulation has little effect on vascular resistance, whereas unloading can cause an increase in resistance (Vukasovic *et al.* 1990). Cardiac responses have different constraints. Stimulation at rest causes interval prolongation and unloading causes interval shortening. During exercise or orthostatic stress, if little vagal activity is present baroreceptor unloading would be expected to have a smaller effect.

It seems likely that the various baroreceptor groups operate over different ranges of pressures. Coronary artery baroreceptors have been shown in the dog to have very low operating ranges and therefore are suited to protect against hypotension. (McMahon *et al.* 1996). Carotid and aortic receptors have higher operating ranges and can, therefore, stabilize both increases and decreases in pressure.

Chemoreceptors

Peripheral chemoreceptors are situated in carotid and aortic bodies and are stimulated by asphyxia, i.e. hypoxia, hypercapnia and acidaemia, as well as by severe hypotension. Under most conditions their level of stimulation is low and it is only during severe hypoxia or hypotension that they become strongly stimulated. The most obvious response to chemoreceptor stimulation is an increase in breathing. Their effects on the cardiovascular system are complicated by the effect on respiration. These effects are mediated mainly through pulmonary stretch receptors and, if this secondary modulation is prevented, carotid chemoreceptor stimulation leads to a cardiac slowing (Fig. 1.6).

Trigeminal afferents: the diving reflex

Immersion of the face or stimulation of trigeminal receptors by application of cold packs to the face elicits a diving reflex. This is very pronounced and of great importance to diving mammals. A response can also be seen in humans (Daly 1985). This comprises apnoea, hypertension and bradycardia. The respiratory arrest leads to asphyxial changes which stimulates chemoreceptors and further augments the bradycardia and vasoconstriction.

Cardiac and pulmonary nonmyelinated afferents

The various cardiac chambers are extensively innervated with nonmyelinated vagal afferents

(Hainsworth, 1991a). Similar innervation extends to the lungs, the so-called J receptors (Paintal 1995). The most effective stimuli to any of these nerves is injection of various noxious chemicals such as veratridine, capsaicin and phenyldiguanide. The most sensitive intrathoracic region for chemical stimulation is the left coronary artery and minute injections of stimulating chemicals there can lead to a profound bradycardia and hypotension (Fig. 1.7). Excitation of these cardiac and pulmonary reflexes may occur in humans following intravenous drug administration or injection of radio-opaque dyes (Perez-Gomez & Garcia-Aguado, 1977).

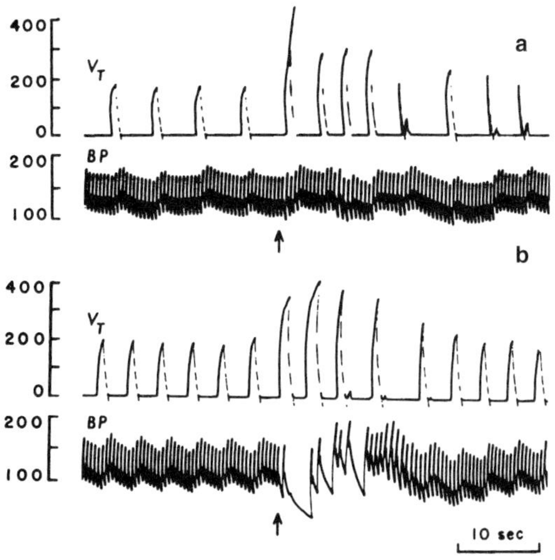

Fig. 1.6 Responses to stimulation of carotid chemoreceptors in the dog by injection of 10 μg nicotine bitartrate into common carotid artery: (a) with lung innervation intact; (b) following lung denervation. Note the unmasking of the primary reflex bradycardia to chemoreceptor stimulation following lung denervation. (Reproduced from Hainsworth *et al.* 1973, with permission.)

The normal physiological role of cardiac and pulmonary nonmyelinated afferents seems to be relatively minor. Large changes in ventricular pressure may cause a transient stimulation of ventricular afferents, but pressures need to be beyond those normally encountered (Drinkhill *et al.* 1993), and changes in coronary arterial pressure cause much larger responses. Similarly pulmonary nonmyelinated afferents are only excited by chemical stimulation, pulmonary congestion or gross overdistension (Coleridge & Coleridge 1991). It is hard to disagree with the proposition that, although cardiac and pulmonary nonmyelinated afferents may be involved in disease processes, they do not have an important regulatory role.

Atrial receptors

Complex unencapsulated nerve endings of myelinated nerve fibres are located mainly near the junctions between the venae cava and the pulmonary veins with the atria (Nonidez, 1937). They are responsible for what was originally known as the Bainbridge reflex. They are stretch receptors and their discharge is linearly related to atrial volume and pressure. Because atrial filling is dependent, amongst other things, on blood volume they are often thought of as volume receptors.

Stimulation of atrial receptors induces an unusual pattern of responses (Linden &

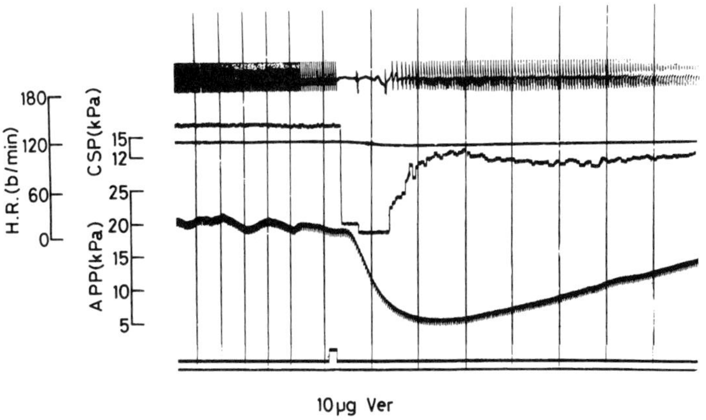

Fig. 1.7 The Bezold–Jarisch reflex. Veratridine (10 μg) was injected into the aortic root of an anaesthetized dog. This almost immediately caused profound bradycardia and vasodilatation, seen as a fall in perfusion pressure to a hind limb. (Modified from McGregor *et al.* 1986, with permission.)

Kappagoda 1982; Hainsworth 1991b). Heart rate increases, but atrial receptors have little or no effect on vascular resistance in most regions. They do, however, target the kidney and increase salt and water excretion through a reduction in renal nerve activity and central inhibition of vasopressin. In this way an increase in cardiac filling leads to a diuresis and a natriuresis. Note that these responses are reflexly mediated in that nervous pathways are involved. They should not be confused with the diuresis and natriuresis resulting from the release of atrial natriuretic peptide. This occurs in response to stretching of cardiac myocytes and its physiological significance is uncertain.

Atrial receptors are likely to have an important role in circulatory control. However, the time course of any change needs to be considered in relation to its possible role in influencing heart rate variability. Because responses are mediated through sympathetic efferents, following stimulation a period of 20–30 s is required for a maximal response. Atrial receptors, therefore, are unlikely to be important in mediating or modulating high frequency heart rate oscillations.

Heart rate changes during complex events

The foregoing has considered the effects of changes in stimuli to single discrete reflexogenic areas. This is of importance in analysing the mechanisms which are involved but normal daily activities, including breathing, straining, changes in body position and various forms of physical exercise, result in changes in the stimulation of many diverse reflex mechanisms. This section is concerned with some of the more common activities which can affect the heart rate.

Sinus arrhythmia

Sinus arrhythmia is caused by variations in cardiac vagal efferent activity. Vagal activity occurs only during expiration, being inhibited during the inspiratory phase (Fig. 1.9). Several mechanisms seem to contribute. Reflexes from the low threshold pulmonary stretch receptors, which are also responsible for the Hering–Breuer reflex, almost certainly play a part (Hainsworth 1974). However, sinus arrhythmia can be seen to some extent in paralysed animals in absence of breathing movements and this has been attributed to central connections between the respiratory centres and the vagal nuclei (Anrep *et al.* 1936). Baroreceptors are also likely to be involved as the variations in heart rate are also associated with variations in blood pressure. It has been proposed that there is a central 'gating' mechanism whereby during inspiration the baroreflex is inhibited (Spyer & Jordan 1987). This concept is supported by the findings of Eckberg *et al.* (1980) who applied brief stimuli to the carotid baroreceptors in humans and observed maximal prolongation of pulse interval during expiration and almost complete inhibition of the reflex in early inspiration (Fig. 1.10).

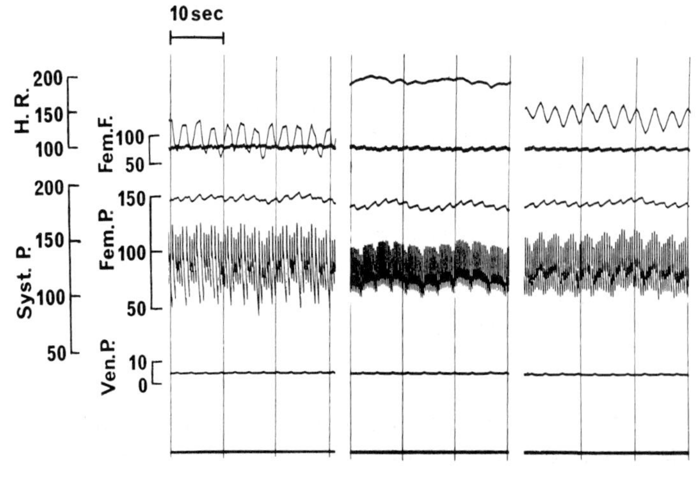

Fig. 1.8 Responses to stimulation of atrial receptors. Receptors at the pulmonary vein–atrial junctions in anaesthetized dogs were stimulated using small balloons. This resulted in tachycardia (heart rate increased by nearly 100 beats/min) but no peripheral vascular responses (no change in pefusion pressure to perfused limb or in mean arterial blood pressure). (Reproduced from Carswell *et al.* 1970, with permission.)

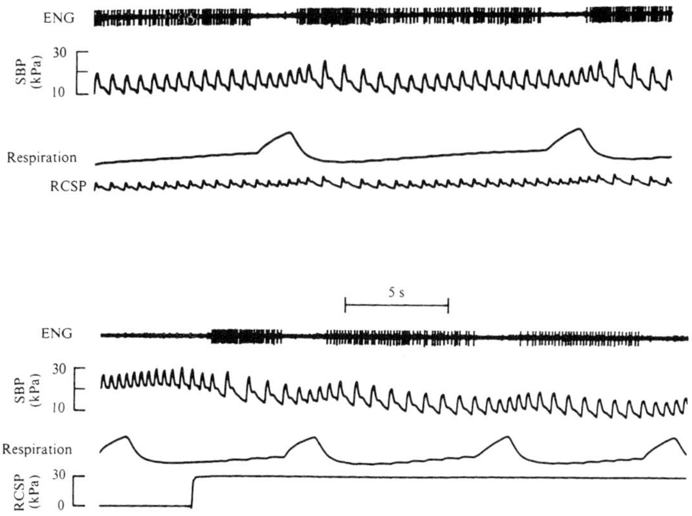

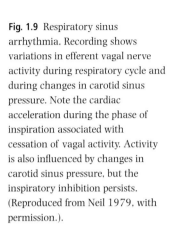

Fig. 1.9 Respiratory sinus arrhythmia. Recording shows variations in efferent vagal nerve activity during respiratory cycle and during changes in carotid sinus pressure. Note the cardiac acceleration during the phase of inspiration associated with cessation of vagal activity. Activity is also influenced by changes in carotid sinus pressure, but the inspiratory inhibition persists. (Reproduced from Neil 1979, with permission.).

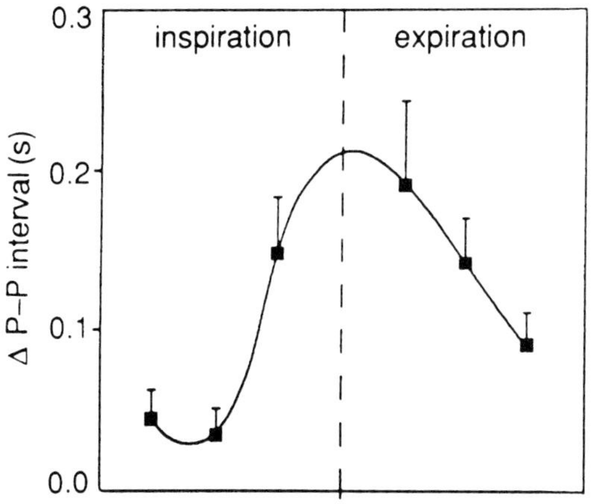

Fig. 1.10 Influence of the phase of the respiratory cycle on the cardiac response to brief stimulation of the carotid baroreceptors in humans using neck suction. Note the almost complete loss of the response during early inspiration. (Reproduced from Eckberg *et al.* 1980, with permission.)

Sinus arrhythmia occurs with a period of about 4 s which is too fast for variations in sympathetic activity to be of major importance; it is therefore not unreasonable to consider the efferent limb of this response to be mainly if not entirely vagal in origin (Eckberg 1983; Fouad *et al.* 1984).

Postural changes

In humans moving from supine to motionless standing results not only in displacement of blood into dependent capacitance vessels but also in a progressive transudation of plasma fluid across dependent capillaries (Hainsworth 1999). This inevitably results in decreases in venous return and in pulse pressure. This and the altered position of carotid baroreceptors leads to compensatory reflex vasoconstriction and tachycardia. Because of the exquisite sensitivity of baroreceptors to changes in pulsatility mean blood pressure in the upright position is maintained close to or even above that in the supine position. If the orthostatic stress becomes too great, and in susceptible individuals this can happen with relatively minor stresses, the vasoconstriction and tachycardia abruptly reverse to become vasodilatation and bradycardia (Fig. 1.11). This was described by Lewis (1932) as a vasovagal reaction indicating vasodilatation and a vagally mediated bradycardia. Occasionally, the bradycardia may extend to several seconds of asystole. The mechanism switching off the sympathetic activity and turning on vagal activity is unknown. It was formerly thought to be the result of a paradoxical stimulation of the ventricular receptor but this has now been shown not to be the case (see Hainsworth 2003).

Valsalva

The Valsalva manoeuvre involves straining against either a closed glottis or an external resistance. Pressures within the thorax and abdomen are greatly increased, impeding the inflow of

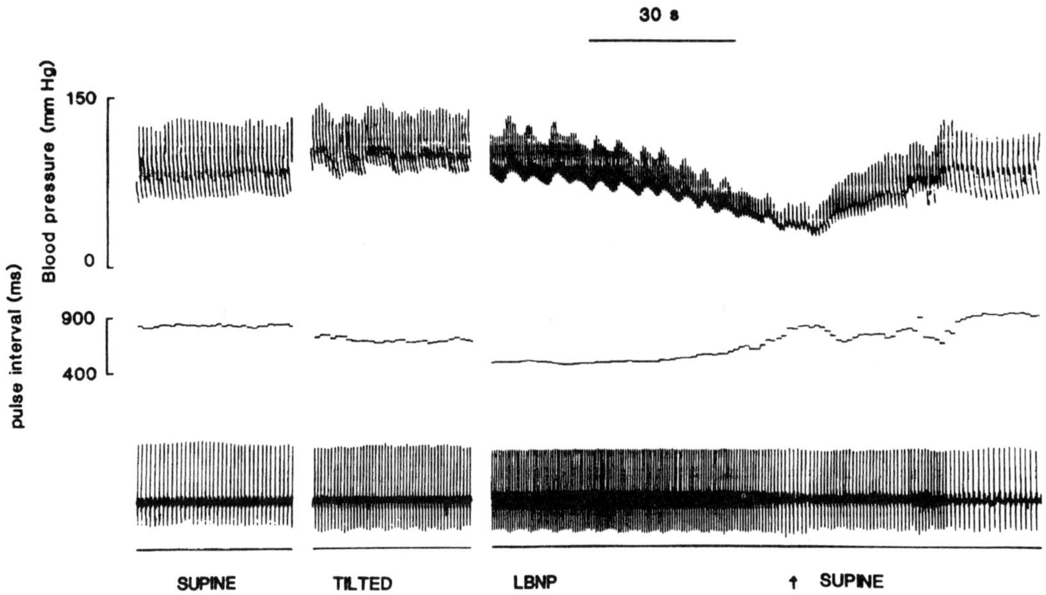

Fig. 1.11 Effects of orthostatic stress and the vasovagal reaction in a healthy human. During head-up tilting and particularly during application of lower body negative pressure, there is a marked increase in heart rate with little change in blood pressure. Eventually, however, blood pressure falls and heart rate slows. (Reproduced from El-Bedawi & Hainsworth 1994, with permission.)

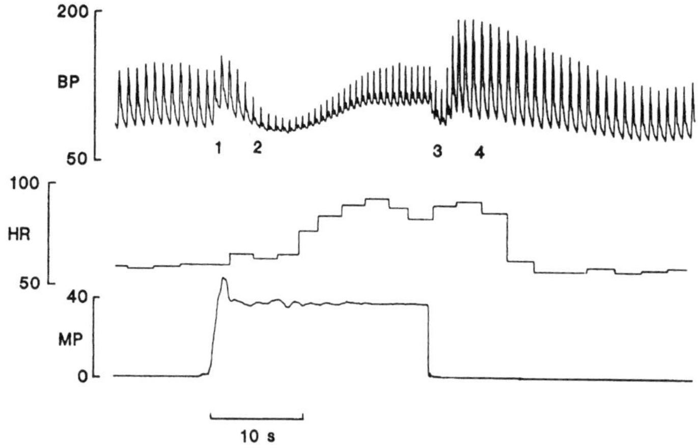

Fig. 1.12 The Valsalva manoeuvre. The four phases are seen: initial transient increase in blood pressure; fall in pressure followed by recovery with tachycardia; transient fall in pressure at the end of the strain; pressure overshoot and cardiac slowing.

blood from outside these regions. It is important to note that, unlike positive pressure ventilation, blood does not pool in the abdomen. Fig.1.12 shows effects of a controlled Valsalva and illustrates the various phases. Firstly, the raised intrathoracic and intra-abdominal pressures compress the major vessels causing an abrupt transient pressure rise. Secondly, the reduced venous return leads to a fall in cardiac output and blood pressure. The pressure fall is compensated by reflex vaso-constriction and tachycardia. On releasing the Valsalva, the intrathoracic and intraabdominal pressures fall again decompressing the vessels and causing a transient fall in arterial pressure. The previously impeded blood flows rapidly into the heart, and is pumped out into a constricted circulation resulting in an overshoot of blood pressure and, often, bradycardia.

The Valsalva manoeuvre provides a test of the integrity of the autonomic nerves and of the baroreceptor reflex. Deficient reflexes result in failure of compensation of heart rate and blood pressure in the second phase, and absence of the overshoot in pressure in the final phase.

Exercise

Heavy physical exercise induces large increases in cardiac output effected by increases in both stroke volume and heart rate. Physical training results in larger stroke volumes, both at rest and during exercise. Resting heart rate is lower but the maximal rate is unchanged so that the actual change in heart rate is much greater in trained subjects. Isometric exercise causes much more modest changes in cardiac output although heart rate increases. Because vascular resistance decreases with dynamic exercise, only systolic pressure increases. During static (isometric) exercise there are increases in both systolic and diastolic pressures.

Heart rate increases immediately at the start of exercise and this is attributed to a decrease in vagal tone mediated by 'central command'. Subsequently muscle mechanoreceptors and metaboreceptors become stimulated resulting in a further and sustained heart rate increase.

The mechanisms involved in exercise are very complex and the reader is referred to more extensive reviews (Saltin *et al.* 1968; Mitchell & Schmidt 1983; Coote 1995).

References

Anrep, G.V., Pascual, W. & Rossler, R. (1936) Respiratory variations of the heart. The reflex mechanisms of the respiratory arrhythmia. *Proceedings of the Royal Society of London B Biological Science*, **119**, 191–217.

Carswell, F., Hainsworth, R. & Ledsome, J.R. (1970) The effect of distension of the pulmonary vein–atrial junctions upon peripheral vascular resistance. *Journal of Physiology*, **207**, 1–14.

Casadei, B. (2001) Vagal control of myocardial contractility in humans. *Experimental Physiology*, **86**, 817–823.

Chapleau, M.W. & Abboud, F.M. (1993) Mechanisms of adaptation and resetting of the baroreceptor reflex. In: *Cardiovascular Reflex Control in Health and Disease* (eds R. Hainsworth, & A. L. Mark), pp. 165–194. Saunders, London.

Coleridge, H.M. & Coleridge, J.C.G. (1991) Afferent innervation of lungs, airways and pulmonary artery. In: *Reflex Control of the Circulation* (eds I. H. Zucker & J. P. Gilmore), pp. 579–608. CRC Press, Boca Raton, FL.

Coote, J.H. (1995) Cardiovascular responses to exercise: central and reflex contributions. In: *Cardiovascular Regulation* (eds D. Jordan & J. M. Marshall), pp. 93–112. Portland Press, London.

Daly, M. de B. (1985) Interactions between respiration and circulation. In: *Handbook of Physiology*, Section III, Vol. 2, Part II (eds N. S. Cherniak & J. G. Widdicombe), pp. 529–594. American Physiological Society, Bethesda, MD.

Doe, C.P.A, Drinkhill, M.J., Myers, D.S., Self, D.A. & Hainsworth, R. (1996) Reflex vascular responses to abdominal venous distension in the anesthetized dog. *American Journal of Physiology*, **271**, H1049–H1056.

Drinkhill, M.J., Doe, C.P.A., Myers, D.S., Self, D.A. & Hainsworth R. (1997) Reflex vascular responses to alterations in abdominal arterial pressure and flow in anaesthetized dogs. *Experimental Physiology*, **82**, 995–1005.

Drinkhill, M.J., Moore, J. & Hainsworth, R. (1993) Afferent discharges from coronary arterial and ventricular receptors in anaesthetized dogs. *Journal of Physiology*, **472**, 785–800.

Eckberg, D.L. (1978) Temporal response patterns of the human sinus node to brief carotid baroreceptor stimuli. *Journal of Physiology*, **258**, 769–782.

Eckberg, D.L., Kifle, Y.T. & Roberts, V.L. (1980) Phase relationship between normal human respiration and baroreflex responsiveness. *Journal of Physiology*, **54**, 489–502.

Eckberg, D.L. (1983) Human sinus arrhythmia as an index of vagal cardiac outflow. *Journal of Applied Physiology*, **54**, 961–966.

El-Bedawi, K.M. & Hainsworth, R. (1994) Combined head-up tilt and lower body suction: a test of orthostatic tolerance. *Clinical Autonomic Research*, **4**, 41–47

Furnival, C.M., Linden, R.J. & Snow, H.M. (1973) Chronotopic and inotropic effects on the dog heart of stimulating the efferent cardiac sympathetic nerves. *Journal of Physiology*, **230**, 137–153.

Fouad, F.M., Tazazi, R.C., Ferrario, C.M., Fighaly, S. & Alicandri, C. (1984) Assessment of parasympathetic control of heart rate by a noninvasive method. *American Journal of Physiology*, **246**, H838-H842.

Hainsworth, R. (1974) Circulatory responses from lung inflation in anesthetized dogs. *American Journal of Physiology*, **226**, 247–255

Hainsworth, R. (1991a) Reflexes from the heart. *Physiological Reviews*, **71**, 617–658.

Hainsworth, R. (1991b) Atrial receptors. In: *Reflex Control of the Circulation* (eds I. H. Zucker, & J. P. Gilmore), pp. 273–436. CRC Press, Boca Raton, FL.

Hainsworth, R. (1999) Syncope and fainting: classification and pathophysiological basis. In: *Autonomic Failure* (eds C. J. Matthias & R. Bannister), pp. 428–436. Oxford University Press, Oxford.

Hainsworth, R. (2003) Syncope: what is the trigger? *Heart*, **89**, 123–124 (editorial).

Hainsworth, R., Jacobs, L. & Comroe, J.H., Jr (1973) Afferent lung denervation by brief inhalation of steam. *Journal of Applied Physiology*, **34**, 708–714.

Hainsworth, R., Ledsome, J.R. & Carswell, F. (1970) Reflex responses from aortic baroreceptors. *American Journal of Physiology*, **218**, 423–429.

Hamlin, R.L. & Smith, C.R. (1968) Effects of vagal stimulation on S-A and A-V nodes. *American Journal of Physiology*, **215**, 560–568.

Levy, M.N. & Martin, P.J. (1979) Neural control of the heart. In: *Handbook of Physiology* (ed. R. M. Berne), pp. 581–620. American Physiological Society, Bethesda, MD.

Levy, M.N., Martin, P.J, Iano, T. & Zieske, H. (1970) Effects of single vagal stimuli on the heart rate and atrioventricular conduction. *American Journal of Physiology*, **218**, 1256–1262.

Lewis, T. (1932) Vasovagal syncope and the carotid sinus mechanism. *British Medical Journal*, **1**, 873–876.

Linden, R.J. & Kappagoda, C.T. (1982) *Atrial Receptors*. Cambridge University Press, Cambridge.

McGregor, K.H. Hainsworth, R. & Ford, R. (1986) Hind-limb vascular responses in anaesthetized dogs to aortic root injections of veratridine. *Quarterly Journal of Experimental Physiology*, **71**, 577–587.

McMahon, N.C., Drinkhill, M.J. & Hainsworth, R. (1996) Reflex vascular responses from aortic arch, carotid sinus and coronary baroreceptors in the anaesthetized dog. *Experimental Physiology*, **81**, 969–981.

Mitchell, J.H. & Schmidt, R.F. (1983) Cardiovascular reflex control by afferent fibres from skeletal muscle receptors. In: *Handbook of Physiology. The Cardiovascular System*, Vol. 3 (eds J. T. Shepherd & F. M. Aboud), pp. 623–658. American Physiological Society, Bethesda, MD.

Neil, E. (1979) Cardiac vagal efferent activity. In: *Cardiac Receptors* (eds R. Hainsworth, C. Kidd & R. J. Linden), p. 365. Cambridge University Press, Cambridge.

Nonidez, J.F. (1937) Identification of the receptor areas in the venae cavae and the pulmonary veins which initiate reflex cardiac acceleration (Bainbridge's reflex). *American Journal Anatomy*, **61**, 203–231.

Paintal, A.S. (1995) Some recent advances in studies on J receptors. In: *Control of the Cardiovascular and Respiratory Systems in Health and Disease* (eds C. T. Kappagoda & M. P. Kaufman), pp. 15–26. Plenum Press, New York.

Parker, P., Celler, B.G, Potter, E.K. & McCloskey, D.I. (1984) Vagal stimulation and cardiac slowing. *Journal of the Autonomic Nervous System*, **11**, 226–231.

Perez-Gomez, F. & Garcia-Aguado, A. (1977) Origin of ventricular reflexes caused by coronary arteriography. *British Heart Journal*, **39**, 967–973.

Saltin, B., Blomquist, G., Mitchell, J.H., Johnson, R.L., Jr, Wildenthal, K. & Chapman, C.B. (1968) Response to exercise after bed rest and after training. *Circulation*, **37** (Suppl. 7), 1–78.

Spyer, K.M. & Jordan, D. (1987) Electrophysiology of the nucleus ambigus. In: *Cardiogenic Reflexes* (eds R. Hainsworth, P. N. McWilliam, & D. A. S. G. Mary), pp. 237–249. Oxford University Press, Oxford.

Taylor, J.A., Halliwill, J.R., Brown, T. E., Hayano, J. & Eckberg, D. L. (1995) Non-hypotensive hypovolaemia reduces ascending aortic dimensions in humans. *Journal of Physiology*, **483**, 289–298.

Vukasovic, J.L., Al-Timman, J.K.A. & Hainsworth, R. (1990) The effect of lower body negative pressure on baroreceptor responses in humans. *Experimental Physiology*, **75**, 81–89.

CHAPTER 2

Standard Measurement of Heart Rate Variability

Marek Malik

Introduction

The seminal report suggesting a clinical utility of the assessment of heart rate variability (HRV) was published almost quarter of a century ago (Wolf *et al.* 1978). Since that time, the subject of regulations, modulations, and physiological variability of cardiac cycles has been researched very extensively. Presently, the evaluation of HRV is an established tool for the assessment of cardiac autonomic status. Recognizing the need of standardization, two major task forces have been established in the past decade and their reports (ESC/NASPE Task Force 1996; Berntson *et al.* 1997) offer general guidelines and suggestions both for experimental and clinical applications and for further research.

This chapter summarizes the standard methods for measurement of HRV. In addition to the standard methods discussed here, several novel approaches have been proposed more recently. Their principles and utility are discussed elsewhere in the book. This chapter is meant as the basic introduction into the methodology of HRV measurement.

Although the term HRV suggests that it is the variability of heart rate which is being measured, the variability of individual cardiac cycles is being investigated in most instances. Still, the term HRV became used so broadly and universally that it is generally adopted also when dealing with variability of cardiac periods. Variability of heart rate, usually computed over short time windows, was used in some early studies but presently, variability of cardiac periods is used almost exclusively. Because of the nonlinear inverse relationship between heart rate and cardiac periods, some complex measures of HRV, e.g. proportion of spectral components, derived from cardiac periods do not parallel those derived from heart rate samples. In this text, the term HRV refers solely to the variability of cardiac cycles.

Electrocardiogram processing

Having measured individual *RR* intervals, HRV can in principle be assessed in any electrocardiogram (ECG) of sufficient duration. However, the following rules have to be observed.

1 The signal to noise ratio of the ECG should allow all QRS complexes to be properly identified (Bailey *et al.* 1990).

2 The digital sampling of the ECG signal must be regular and sufficiently robust algorithms must be used to localize the fiducial points of individual QRS complexes. In particular this means that when recording the ECG on an analogue medium (e.g. a magnetic tape), the signal must be accompanied by a time track record that is used by the analysing equipment.

3 The morphology and rhythm characteristics of all QRS complexes should be classified to distinguish between cardiac cycles of sinus rhythm and other origin.

4 Only *RR* intervals between normal sinus rhythm beats (the so-called normal-to-normal or *NN* intervals) should be considered and no such intervals should be excluded. This means that coupling intervals of atrial and ventricular ectopics as well as their compensatory pauses are excluded but all other *NN* intervals are used, including those immediately preceding a coupling interval of an ectopic beat or following its compensatory pause (ESC/NASPE Task Force 1996).

The sequence of *NN* intervals can be analysed in many different ways. Usually, the so-called time-domain, frequency-domain, and non-linear methods for the assessment of HRV are distinguished.

Time-domain methods

The time-domain methods treat the *NN* interval sequence as an unordered set of intervals (or pairs of intervals) measurement and employ different ways to express the variance of such data. Numerous approaches have been proposed to estimate the variance the *NN* interval data and its surrogates. As many of these methods lead to practically equivalent results, only selected methods have been proposed as 'gold standard' time-domain approaches (ESC/NASPE Task Force 1996). These include three so-called statistical methods which are based on the formula of standard deviation and provide results in units of time.

The SDNN measure is the standard deviation of the durations of all *NN* intervals, the SDANN measure is the standard deviation of the durations of *NN* intervals averaged over all non-overlapping subsections of the original ECG (although different subsections can be considered, 5 min segments are used as a standard), and the RMSSD measure is the root of the averaged squares of differences between neighbouring *NN* intervals (which is a surrogate of the standard deviation of the differences between neighbouring *NN* intervals). In assessing HRV from long-term ECGs, such as 24-h Holter recordings, the contribution of longer periodic and nonperiodic variations overwhelms the short-term variations, such as respiratory arrhythmia, and there is only little difference between SDNN and SDANN values (Fig. 2.1). The RMSSD measure is practically equivalent to the frequently used measure pNN50 which is the percentage of *NN* intervals differing by > 50 ms from the immediately preceding *NN* interval. In turn, pNN50 method is fairly equivalent to the NN50 method that expresses the absolute count of *NN* intervals that differ by > 50 ms from the immediately preceding interval (Fig. 2.2). Compared to pNN50 and NN50, the RMSSD values have better statistical properties.

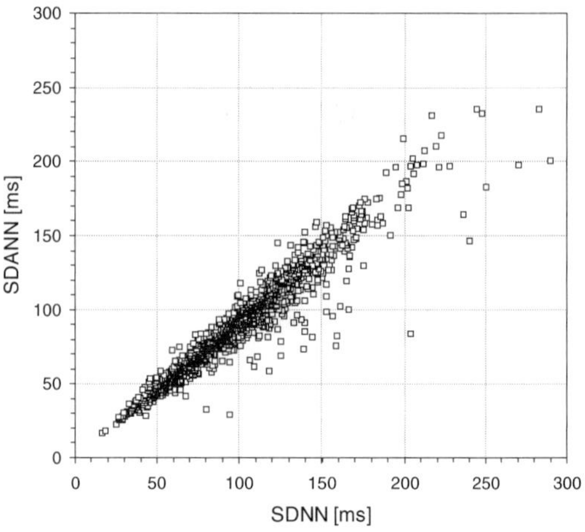

Fig. 2.1 Correspondence between SDNN and SDANN values derived from 24-h recordings of survivors of acute myocardial infarction.

While the SDNN and RMSSD methods can be applied to practically any electrocardiogram, the SDANN method is usually used only with long-term (e.g. 24-h) ECG recordings. However, the length of the ECG recording is an important determinant of the HRV. With increasing length of ECG recording, SDNN and RMSSD (as well as SDANN) values increase. It is therefore inappropriate to compare HRV data obtained from ECG recordings of different durations.

All these statistical methods depend crucially on the quality of the data of the *NN* intervals (Malik *et al.* 1993). Achieving high-quality *NN* intervals is not usually difficult with short-term ECGs, where automatic analysis can be visually verified to include the localization and morphological and rhythm classification of each single QRS complex. It is frequently problematic, however, to achieve a high quality *NN* interval sequence derived from long-term electrocardiograms. This is especially true with recordings obtained in standard clinical environments and when resources do not allow the careful verification by the ECG analysing technician of all *NN* intervals found by the automatic equipment. Even with advanced Holter systems, a precise analysis of a long-term ECG can involve time-consuming operator involvement when some low-voltage QRS patterns are not automatically identified and/or when tall T waves and recording artefacts are misidentified as QRS complexes. When such long-term recordings are only

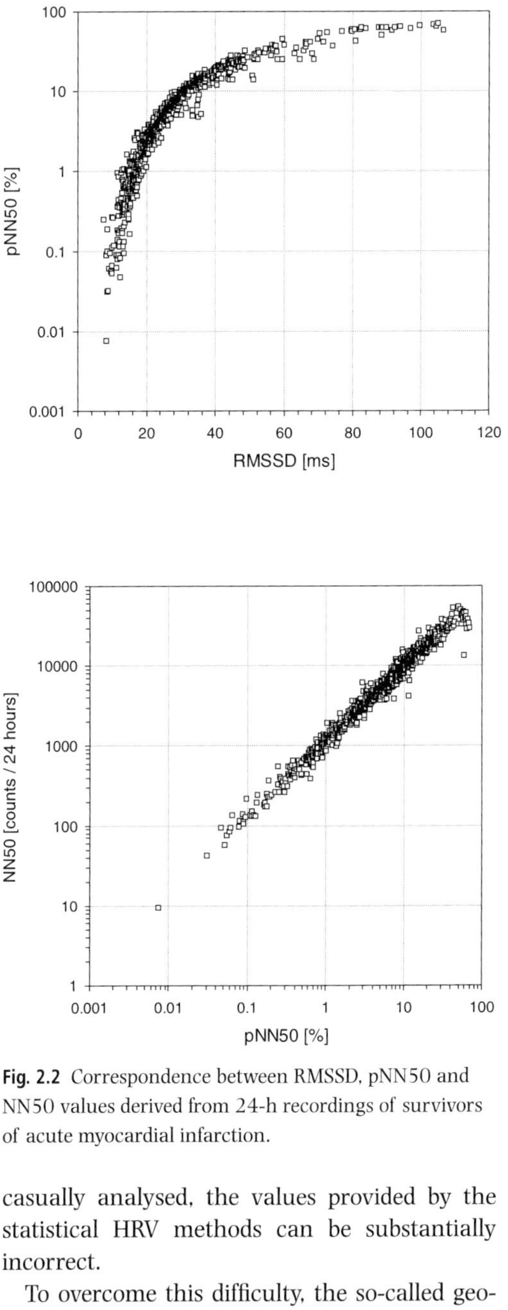

Fig. 2.2 Correspondence between RMSSD, pNN50 and NN50 values derived from 24-h recordings of survivors of acute myocardial infarction.

casually analysed, the values provided by the statistical HRV methods can be substantially incorrect.

To overcome this difficulty, the so-called geometrical methods for HRV assessment have been proposed. These methods use the *NN* interval sequence to construct a geometrical form and express HRV by assessing a certain parameter or shape of that form. As the incorrect *NN* intervals are usually outliers of the geometrical form, they can be easily excluded from the HRV assessment. Of these methods, most experience exists with the so-called HRV triangular index method (Malik *et al.* 1989) which constructs the sample density histogram of all *NN* intervals and approximates its baseline width (a surrogate of the standard deviation of *NN* intervals) by computing the proportion between total number of *NN* intervals (that is the 'area' of the histogram) and the number of intervals of modal durations (that is the 'height' of the histogram; Fig. 2.3). This method, which has also been proposed as one of the 'gold standard' approaches to the analysis of long-term electrocardiograms (ESC/NASPE Task Force 1996) depends crucially on the size of the bins used to construct the histogram. When used with the bins of 1/128 s (⊕ 7.8 ms) which correspond to the usual sampling rate of Holter equipment and when applied to properly edited *NN* interval sequence, the method provides results fairly corresponding to SDNN (1 unit of HRV triangular index ~2.5 ms of SDNN).

Frequency-domain methods

Power spectral density analysis (Kay *et al.* 1981) provides the basic information of how power (i.e. variance) distributes as a function of frequency. Independently of the method employed, only an estimate of the true spectral density of the signal can be obtained.

Methods for the calculation of power spectral density may be generally classified as nonparametric and parametric. In most instances, both methods provide comparable results (Fig. 2.5). The advantages of the nonparametric methods are the simplicity of the algorithms used (usually fast Fourier transform – FFT) and the high processing speed, whilst the advantages of parametric methods are smoother spectral components which can be distinguished independently of preselected frequency bands, easy postprocessing of the spectrum with an automatic calculation of low and high frequency power components with an easy identification of the central frequency of each component, and an accurate estimation of power spectral density even on a small number of samples on which the signal is supposed to maintain stationarity. The basic disadvantage of parametric methods is the need of verification of the suitability of the chosen model and of its complexity (i.e. the order of the model).

Three main spectral components are distinguished in a spectrum calculated from short-

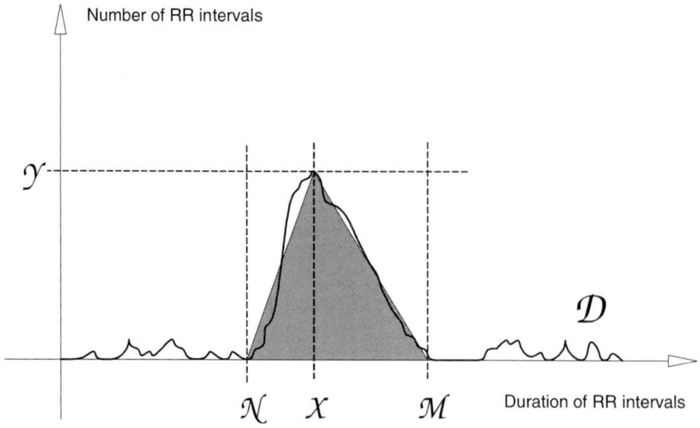

Fig. 2.3 Concept of the so-called HRV triangular index method. A sample density histogram *D* is constructed from the sequence of measured *RR* intervals. The number total of *RR* intervals is divided by the height *Y* of the histogram, that is by the modal number of the distribution which is the sample frequency of the most frequent *RR* interval duration *X*. The result corresponds to the baseline width ($N - M$) of a triangle ([*N*,0], [*M*,0],[*X*,*Y*]) which has the same area as the area under the histogram *D*. Outliers in the *RR* (or *NN*) interval sequence owing to ECG noise and recognition artefact are effectively filtered out.

term recordings of at least 2 min (Sayers 1973; Akselrod *et al.* 1981; Hirsh *et al.* 1981; Pomeranz *et al.* 1985; Pagani *et al.* 1986; Malliani *et al.* 1991). These are the very low frequency (VLF) below 0.04 Hz, low frequency (LF) 0.04–0.15 Hz, and high frequency (HF) 0.15–0.4 Hz components. The distribution of the power and the central frequency of LF and HF are not fixed but may vary in relation to changes in autonomic modulations of heart period. The nonharmonic component which does not have coherent properties and which is affected by algorithms of baseline or trend removal is commonly accepted as a major constituent of VLF. Thus VLF assessed from short-term recordings is a rather dubious measure. The measurement of VLF, LF and HF power components is usually made in absolute values of power (ms^2). LF and HF may also be measured in normalized units (Pagani *et al.* 1986; Malliani *et al.* 1991), which represent the relative value of each power component in proportion to the total power minus the VLF component. The representation of LF and HF in normalized units has been proposed to emphasize the balanced behaviour of the two branches of the autonomic nervous system. Moreover, the normalization tends to minimize the effect of changes in total power on the values of LF and HF components. Nevertheless, normalized units should always be quoted with absolute values of the LF and HF power in order to describe completely the distribution of power in spectral components.

Spectral analysis may also be used to analyse the sequence of *NN* intervals of the entire 24-h period. The result then includes an ultra-low frequency component (ULF) below 0.0033 Hz, in addition to VLF, LF and HF components. The slope of the 24-h spectrum can also be assessed on a log–log scale by linear fitting the spectral values (Fig. 2.6).

The problem of stationarity should be carefully considered with long-term recordings (Furlan *et al.* 1990). If mechanisms responsible for heart period modulations of a certain frequency remain unchanged during the whole period of recording, the corresponding frequency component of HRV may be used as a measure of these modulations. If the modulations are not stable, the interpretation of the results of frequency analysis is less well defined. In particular, physiological mechanisms of heart period modulations responsible for LF and HF power components cannot be considered stationary during the 24-h period. Thus spectral analysis performed on entire 24-h period as well as spectral results obtained from shorter segments averaged over the entire 24-h period provide averages of the modulations attributable to the LF and HF components. Such averages

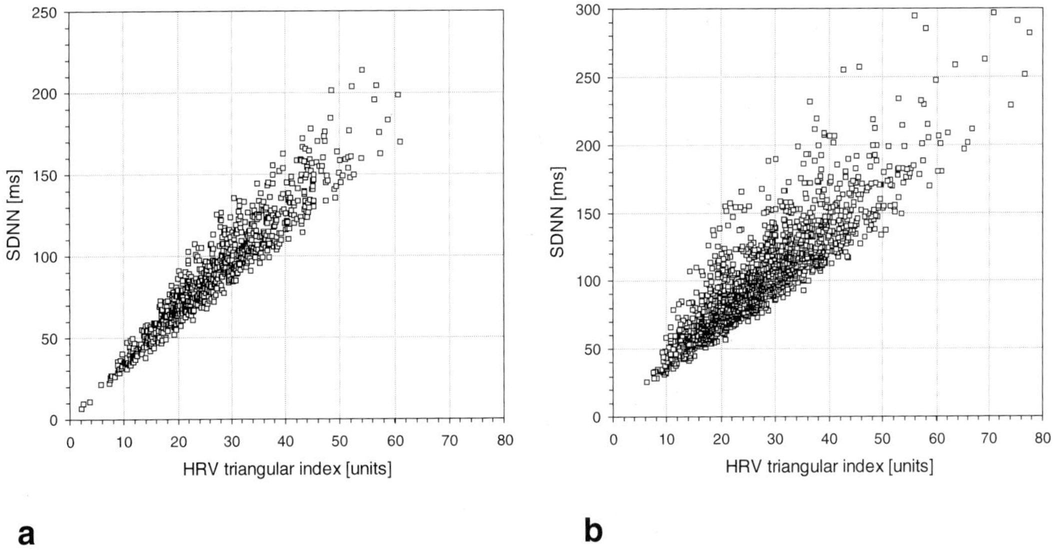

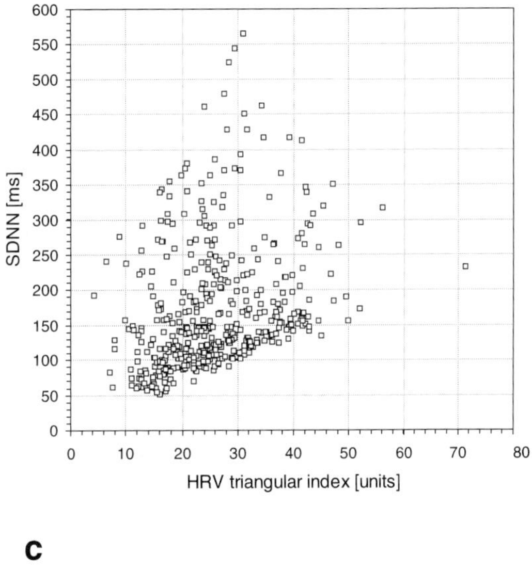

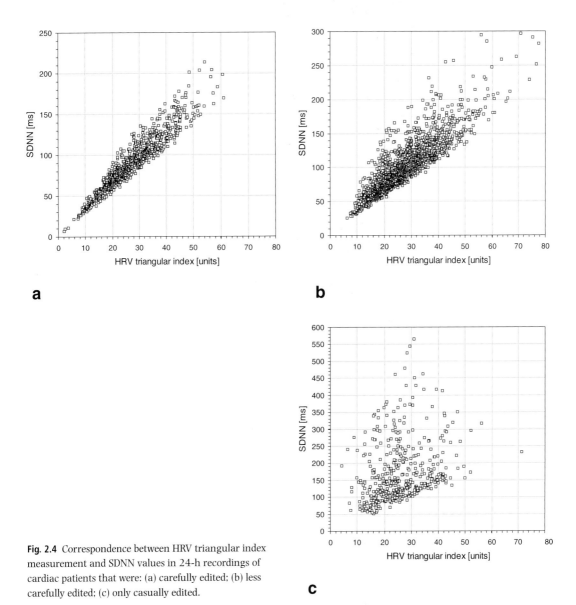

Fig. 2.4 Correspondence between HRV triangular index measurement and SDNN values in 24-h recordings of cardiac patients that were: (a) carefully edited; (b) less carefully edited; (c) only casually edited.

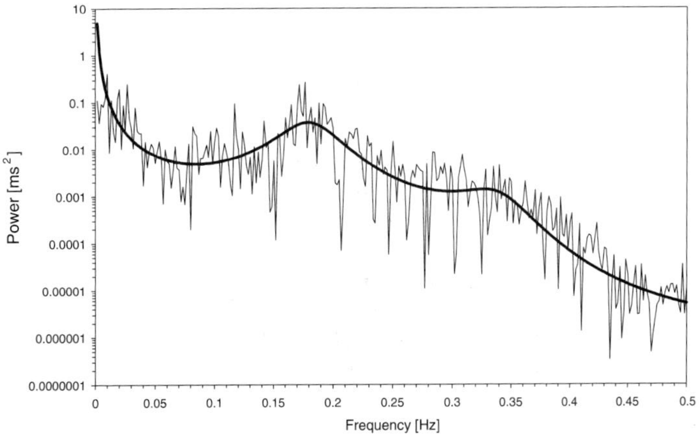

Fig. 2.5 Example of power spectral density estimation of the same sequence of *NN* intervals provided by a nonparametric FFT method (fine line) and parametric autoregressive modelling (bold line).

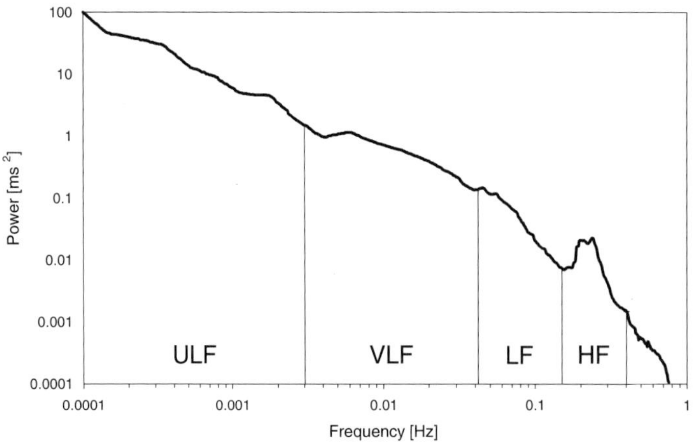

Fig. 2.6 Typical result of a spectral analysis of 24-h *NN* interval sequence. Spectral components of ultra-low (ULF), very low (VLF), low (LF) and high (HF) frequency component are distinguished. Although the HF and LF components parallel the physiological models of the short-term HRV assessment, the distinction between VLF and ULF components does not correspond to any real physiological mechanisms.

obscure the detailed information about autonomic modulation of *RR* intervals that is available in shorter recordings (see next section). It should be remembered that the components of HRV provide measurement of the degree of autonomic modulations rather than of the level of autonomic tone and averages of modulations do not represent an averaged level of tone (Malik & Camm 1993).

Nonlinear analyses

Nonlinear phenomena are certainly involved in the genesis of HRV. They are determined by complex interactions of haemodynamic, electrophysiological and humoral variables, as well as by the autonomic and central nervous regulations. It has been repeatedly proposed that analysis of HRV based on the methods of nonlinear dynamics might elicit valuable information for physiological interpretation of HRV. The parameters which have been used to measure nonlinear properties of HRV include $1/f$ scaling of Fourier spectra (Kobayashi & Musha 1982; Saul *et al.* 1988), H scaling exponent, and coarse graining spectral analysis (Yamamoto & Hughson 1991). For data representation, Poincaré sections, low-dimension attractor plots, singular value decomposition, and attractor trajectories have been proposed. For other quantitative descriptions, the D_2 correlation dimension, Lyapunov exponents, and Kolmogorov entropy have been used (Babloyantz & Destexhe 1988). Some encouraging results have also been obtained using differential (Morfill *et al.* 1994; Schmidt & Monfill 1995), rather than integral complexity measures, but no systematic study has been conducted to investigate large patient populations using these methods.

The Poincaré plots, that is maps of dots with coordinates corresponding to durations of pairs of successive *NN* intervals, have attracted some attention among clinical investigators (Woo *et al.*

Fig. 2.7 Examples of Poincaré plots (maps showing dots of co-ordinates given by R_iR_{i+1} and $R_{i+1}R_{i+2}$ interval durations) used to assess the quality of the normal-to-normal *RR* interval sequence in 24-h recordings: (a) – (c) properly edited *RR* interval sequences in three congestive heart failure patients in sinus rhythm with increasing heart rate variability; (d) and (e) recordings in which the ectopic activity was not properly edited; (f) intermittent atrial bigeminy in which short and long cycles alternate; (g) generated by an automatic system which fails to recognize some QRS complexes and provides measurement of *RR* intervals which are actually composed of two or more cardiac cycles; (h) generated by a Holter system which analysed a magnetic tape without phase-locked time track – the measured *RR* intervals are distorted by irregularities in tape revolution, this is combined with irregularities of fiducial point localization – different QRS complexes are detected at different moments of ventricular depolarization; (i) a similar problem combined with poor editing of the recording; (j) very poorly edited Holter recording with frequent artefacts and ectopic beats; (k) and (l) Holter tape with episodes of paroxysmal atrial fibrillation; (m) and (n) chronic atrial fibrillation; (o) recordings of chronic atrial fibrillation in which tall T waves were mistaken for QRS complexes by the automatic Holter system and not properly edited.

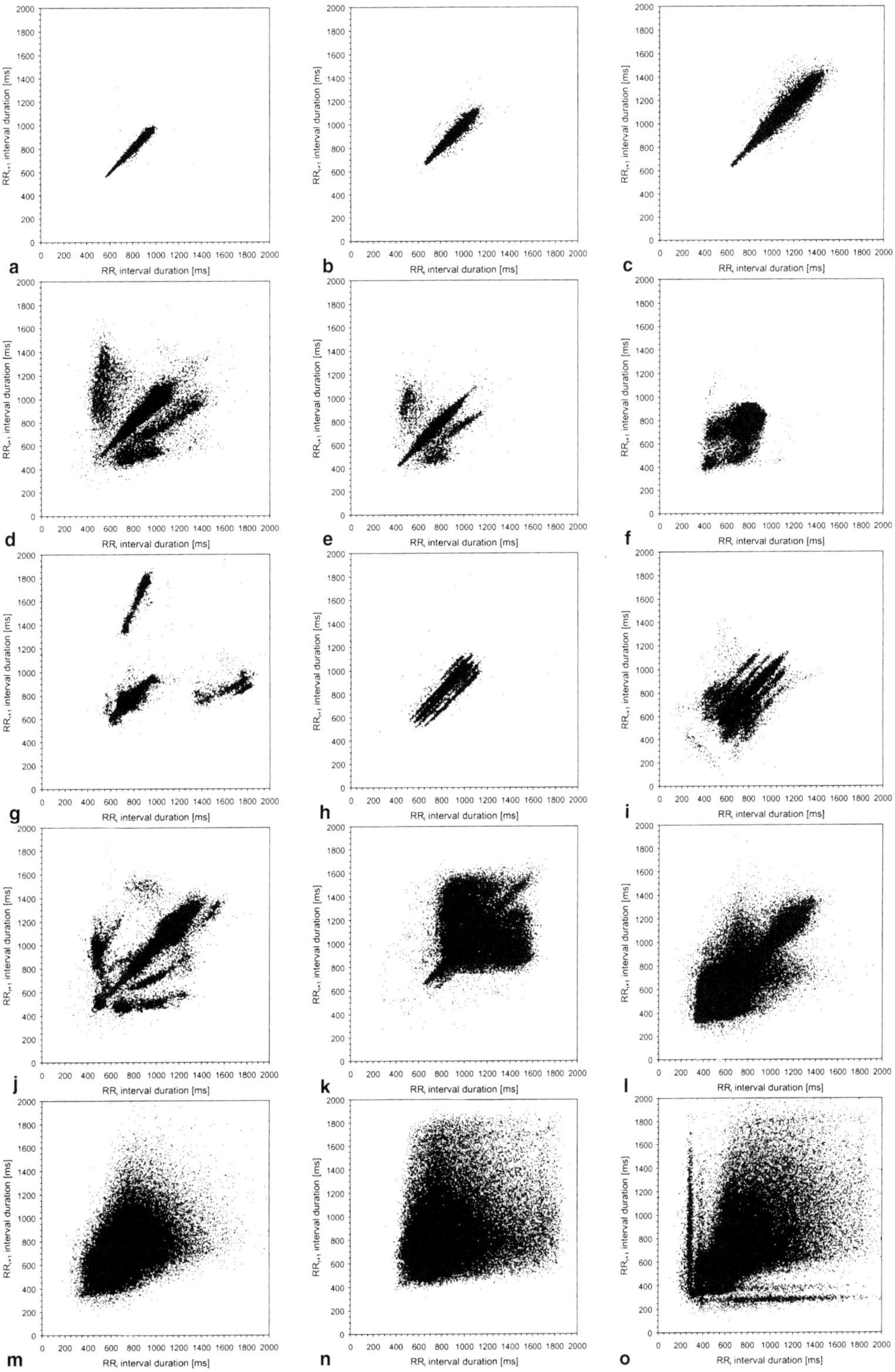
RR$_{i+1}$ interval duration [ms]
RR$_i$ interval duration [ms]
0 200 400 600 800 1000 1200 1400 1600 1800 2000
a
b
c
d
e
f
g
h
i
j
k
l
m
n
o

1994; Kamen & Tonkin, 1995; Copie *et al.* 1996) possibly because of the supposed easiness of the classification of the patterns of the plots. Some authors propose classifications based on categories from a 'torpedo' or 'cigar' shape to the 'comet' and 'butterfly' shape of the plot. However, such a classification is highly subjective (Hnatkova *et al.* 1995) and has never been tested in a truly blinded prospective fashion. Thus the practical utility of Poincaré plots is probably restricted only to the assessment of the quality of *NN* interval sequence. The plots usually make outliers and artefacts very visible (Fig. 2.7).

Optimum modes for HRV analysis

Standardization of the HRV assessment is particularly needed in respect of the duration of analysed ECG recordings and of the conditions under which the recordings are obtained. The measurements provided by the time-domain methods increase with the duration of the recordings (Saul *et al.* 1988) and the physiological relevance of the LF and HF spectral components depends on the stationarity of underlying autonomic modulations. Recognizing this, standards of two different analytical modes have been proposed (ESC/NASPE Task Force 1996) that should be adopted unless some special reasons dictate to the contrary.

Studies of physiological details of autonomic status of the heart are best served by spectral analysis of short, preferably 5-min, ECG recordings that are obtained under stationary conditions, i.e. conditions during which the physiological processes regulating heart rate remain in a steady state.

On the contrary, optimum assessment of cardiac autonomic 'responsiveness' to the surrounding environment is based on nominal 24-h ECG recordings, that is recordings obtained over 24 h that contain at least 18 h of analysable data including representative proportions of both day and night ECGs. These long-term recordings should preferably be analysed by time-domain methods. Although the *NN* interval sequences from long-term ECGs can be processed by frequency-domain methods, the stationarity of the underlying regulatory mechanisms cannot be maintained over a prolonged period. Thus physiological interpretation of individual spectral components obtained from long-term recordings is questionable and frequency-domain analysis of long-term recordings offers only the same information that can be more easily obtained by time-domain methods.

In both situations, the conditions of the recording significantly influence the mechanisms regulating heart rate and should therefore be carefully controlled and/or monitored. For instance, it is inappropriate to compare spectral HRV components in short-term recordings obtained in a group of seated subjects with those from standing subjects. Similarly, it is inappropriate to compare 24-h measures of HRV obtained from patients within a hospital setting with those obtained in fully mobile control subjects.

References

Akselrod, S., Gordon, D., Ubel, F.A. *et al.* (1981) Power spectrum analysis of heart rate fluctuation: a quantitative probe of beat to beat cardiovascular control. *Science*, **213**, 220–222.

Babloyantz A. & Destexhe A. (1988) Is the normal heart a periodic oscillator? *Biological Cybernetics*, **58**, 203–211.

Bailey, J.J., Berson, A.S., Garson, A., Jr *et al.* (1990) Recommendations for standardization and specifications in automated electrocardiography. *Circulation*, **81**, 730–739.

Berntson, G.G., Bigger, J.T., Jr, Eckberg, D.L. *et al.* (1997) Heart rate variability: origins, methods, and interpretative caveats. *Psychphysiology*, **34**, 623–648.

Copie, X., Le Heuzey, J.Y., Iliou, M.C. *et al.* (1996) Correlation between time-domain measures of heart rate variability and scatterplots in postinfarction patients. *PACE (Pacing and Clinical Electrophysiology)*, **19**, 342–347.

ESC/NASPE (European Society of Cardiology/North American Society of Pacing and Electrophysiology) Task Force (1996) Heart rate variability. Standards of measurement, physiological interpretation, and clinical use. *Circulation*, **93**, 1043–1065.

Furlan, R., Guzetti, S., Crivellaro, W. *et al.* (1990) Continuous 24-h assessment of the neural regulation of systemic arterial pressure and RR variabilities in ambulant subjects. *Circulation*, **81**, 537–547.

Hirsh, J.A. & Bishop, B. (1981) Respiratory sinus arrhythmia in humans, how breathing pattern modulates heart rate. *American Journal of Physiology*, **241**, H620–H629.

Hnatkova, K., Copie, X., Staunton. A. & Malik, M. (1995) Numeric processing of Lorenz plots of *RR* intervals from long-term ECGs. Comparison with time-domain measures of heart rate variability for risk stratification after myocardial infarction. *Journal of Electrocardiology*, **28**, 74–80.

Kamen, P.W. & Tonkin, A.M. (1995) Application of the Poincaré plot to heart rate variability: a new measure of functional status in heart failure. *Australian and New Zealand Journal of Medicine*, **25**,18–26.

Kay, S.M. & Marple, S.L (1981) Spectrum analysis: a modern perspective. *Proceedings of the IEEE (Institute of Electrical and Electronics Engineers)*, **69**, 1380–1419.

Kobayashi, M. & Musha, T. (1982) 1/*f* fluctuation of heart beat period. *IEEE (Institute of Electrical and Electronics Engineers) Transactions on Biomedical Engineering*, **29**, 456–457.

Malik, M. & Camm, A.J. (1993) Components of heart rate variability – what they really mean and what we really measure. *American Journal of Cardiology*, **72**, 821–822.

Malik, M., Farrell, T., Cripps, T. *et al.* (1989) Heart rate variability in relation to prognosis after myocardial infarction: selection of optimal processing techniques. *European Heart Journal*, **10**, 1060–1074.

Malik, M., Xia, R., Odemuyiwa, O. *et al.* (1993) Influence of the recognition artefact in the automatic analysis of long-term electrocardiograms on time-domain measurement of heart rate variability. *Medical & Biological Engineering & Computing*, **31**, 539–544.

Malliani, A., Pagani. M., Lombardi, F. *et al.* (1991) Cardiovascular neural regulation explored in the frequency-domain. *Circulation*, **84**, 1482–1492.

Morfill, G.E., Demmel, V. & Schmidt, G. (1994) Der plötzliche Herztod: Neue Erkenntnisse durch die Anwendung komplexer Diagnoseverfahren. *Bioscope*, **2**, 11–19.

Pagani, M., Lombardi, F., Guzzetti, S. *et al.* (1986) Power spectral analysis of heart rate and arterial pressure variabilities as a marker of sympatho-vagal interaction in man and conscious dog. *Circulation, Research*, **59**, 178–193.

Pomeranz, M., Macaulay, R.J.B., Caudill, M.A. *et al.* (1985) Assessment of autonomic function in humans by heart rate spectral analysis. *American Journal of Physiology*, **248**, H151–H153.

Saul, J.P., Albrecht, P., Berger, R.D. *et al.* (1988) Analysis of long-term heart rate variability: methods, 1/*f* scaling and implications. In: *Computers in Cardiology 1987*, pp. 419–422. IEEE Computer Society Press, Washington, DC.

Sayers, B.M. (1973) Analysis of heart rate variability. *Ergonomics*, **16**, 17–32.

Schmidt, G. & Monfill, G.E. (1995) Nonlinear methods for heart rate variability assessment. In: *Heart Rate Variability* (eds M. Malik, & A. J. Camm), pp. 87–98. Futura, Armonk, NY.

Wolf, M.M., Varigos, G.A., Hunt, D. *et al.* (1978) Sinus arrhythmia in acute myocardial infarction. *Medical Journal of Australia*, **2**, 52–55.

Woo, M.A., Stevenson, W.G., Moserm, D.K. *et al.* (1994) Complex heart rate variability and serum noradrenaline levels in patients with advanced heart failure. *Journal of the American College of Cardiology*, **23**, 565–569.

Yamamoto, Y. & Hughson, R.L. (1991) Coarse-graining spectral analysis: new method for studying heart rate variability. *Journal of Applied Physiology*, **71**, 1143–1150.

CHAPTER 3

Nonlinear Dynamics of *RR* intervals

Timo H. Mäkikallio, Juha S. Perkiömäki
and Heikki V. Huikuri

Introduction

Conventionally, heart rate variability has been analysed with time- and frequency-domain methods, which measure the overall magnitude of *RR* interval fluctuation around its mean value, or the magnitude of fluctuations in some predetermined frequencies (ESC/NASPE Task Force 1996). These measures have been used to detect alterations of autonomic cardiovascular regulation in many physiological conditions and disease states (ESC/NASPE Task Force 1996). For uncovering new additive alterations and abnormalities in heart rate dynamics that cannot be detected by traditional analysis techniques, methods based on the nonlinear system theory have been constantly developed (Saul *et al.* 1987; Yamamoto & Hughson, 1991; Skinner *et al.* 1993; Pincus & Goldberger, 1994; Peng *et al.* 1995).

In an analysis of *RR* interval time series, only one quantity (*RR* interval) is obtained and the purpose is to explain the characteristics of the continuous fluctuations in successive *RR* intervals over time. In addition to specific spectral peaks, the power spectrum of heart rate time series also reveals more or less periodic frequency components and frequency spans showing noise-like, irregular variability, particularly in 'free-running' conditions when respiration and other external conditions are not standardized (Pagani *et al.* 1986; ESC/NASPE Task Force 1996; Eckberg 1997; Persson 1997). This suggests that the mechanisms involved in cardiovascular regulation probably interact with each other in a nonlinear way, and therefore theoretically nonlinear techniques may detect alterations in heart rate dynamics that are not detectable by conventional techniques. The fundamental problem in selecting a valid mathematical model for the analysis of heart rate dynamics is that we deal with a system in which we cannot record all the effecting variables and in which the total number of degrees of freedom is not exactly known. Therefore, for diagnostic and clinical purposes, the applicability of different methods should be tested in specific populations. A review of the literature suggests that semantic differences concerning claims of classifications of observed dynamics are far from settled in this research field. Because concepts are more important than semantics, in this chapter we have focused on reviewing the methods that are most widely used and tested in clinical settings.

Methods of nonlinear *RR* interval dynamics

Numerous algorithms have been developed to describe the dynamic fluctuations of heart rate, and a variety of different nonlinear methods have been used for the analysis of *RR* interval dynamics in different clinical conditions. Geometrical analyses, several types of different fractal scaling measures, power-law analyses, different complexity measures and various symbolic measures have been tested in various patient populations. However, we focus here on discussing briefly on the methods that are best studied in clinical settings.

Methods of analysing the fractal-like scaling properties of time series data have been commonly used in heart rate fluctuation analysis among patient populations with cardiovascular disorders. These analysis methods differ from the traditional measures of heart rate variability, because they are not designed to assess the magnitude of variability, but rather quality properties of the signal. The word 'fractal' refers to one of the fundamental properties of a specific structure: self-scaling similarity over a wide range of scales. The normal heart rate time series is 'fractal-like' and seems to display the fractal property of self-similarity over various time scales and obey $1/f$ fluctuation. Furthermore, heart beat values vary with their short- and long-term history in a fractal manner (Goldberger 1990; Goldberger 1996). The origin of $1/f$ fluctuation is largely unknown, but model simulations suggest that relatively simple processes may be responsible for this puzzling behaviour. Nevertheless, analysis based on the notion of $1/f$ characteristics of heart rate time series has provided valuable information in various patient populations (Bigger *et al.* 1996; Mäkikallio *et al.* 1997, 1998, 1999; Huikuri *et al.* 1998, 2000). The breakdown of this scale-invariant, fractal organization could lead to either uncorrelated randomness or highly predictable (single-scale) behaviour, both of which may result in a less adaptable system. Thus, changes from $1/f$ scale-invariant behaviour toward behaviour resembling either random fluctuations or toward more highly correlated behaviour with less complexity might be physiologically deleterious (Bigger *et al.* 1996; Goldberger 1996; Lombardi *et al.* 1996; Mäkikallio *et al.* 1997, 1998, 1999; Pikkujämsä *et al.* 1999; Huikuri *et al.* 1998, 2000).

Power-law heart rate variability analysis

A plot of spectral power and frequency on a bilogarithmic scale and the slope of this relation provides an index for the long-term scaling characteristics of heart rate data. The slope is typically calculated for very low frequencies. This slope has been found to be altered amongst patients with cardiovascular disorders (Bigger *et al.* 1996; Huikuri *et al.* 2000). In normal subjects the power-law slope is equal to −1 and becomes more steeper, for example, after myocardial infarction (Bigger *et al.* 1996). Analysis of the spectral inverse power-law slope has provided prognostic information beyond the traditional heart rate variability measures not only among patients with myocardial infarction, but also among the elderly population in general (Huikuri *et al.* 1998). The notion that qualitative scaling properties may provide more powerful prognostic information than conventional heart rate variability measures has encouraged investigators to search for new methods that could be useful in heart rate variability analyses.

Detrended fluctuation analysis

Some of these newer methods have already provided valuable information in relation to heart disease (Lombardi *et al.* 1996; Ho *et al.* 1997; Mäkikallio *et al.* 1997, 1998, 1999, 2001a, b; Huikuri *et al.* 2000). The detrended fluctuation analysis technique is one such measure. It quantifies the presence or absence of the fractal correlation properties of *RR* intervals and has been validated for time series data. It was developed to characterize fluctuations on scales of multiple lengths. The self-similarity occurring over a large range of time scales can be defined for a selected time scale with this method. The details of this method have been described by Peng *et al.* (1995). This measure is partly related to changes in the spectral characteristics of heart rate behaviour. The ratio of the low- to high-frequency spectral components correlates with the short-term scaling exponent of detrended fluctuation analysis, particularly when breathing is controlled. But when recordings are carried out in 'free running' conditions, such as 24-h Holter recordings, the association is weak. Therefore, fractal correlation properties may be more suitable than simple spectral ratios for detecting subtle alterations in heart rate dynamics.

Complexity measures

The Lyapunov exponent is a quantitative nonlinear measure to evaluate how chaotic the system is (Eckmann & Ruelle 1985). The feasibility of this method is limited in heart rate variability analysis because it requires large data sets and systems to remain stable over the recording time, which biological systems rarely do. The complexity of the system can be measured by the Haussdorff correlation dimension D, but this measure has limited value in heart rate variability analysis owing to large errors of estimation. Therefore, it is more convenient to evaluate the correlation dimension D_2 from a heart rate time series (Eckman & Ruelle 1985; Grassberger & Procaccia 1983b). The pointwise correlation dimension (Skinner *et al.* 1993) is a measure which overcomes the requirement of large data sets by allowing operations with short and nonstationary data. This measure has also provided valuable clinical information (Skinner *et al.* 1993).

Another quantity of the characterization of deterministic chaotic activity is Kolmogorov entropy *K*, which refers to system randomness and predictability (Grassberger & Procaccia 1983a). It can be estimated only from large data sets, and therefore approximate entropy is commonly used as an alternative approach for classifying complex systems in relatively short data sets (Pincus & Goldberger 1994)

Approximate entropy

Approximate entropy measures the regularity and complexity of time series data by quantifying the likelihood that runs of patterns that are close remain close on next incremental comparisons. The larger the value of approximate entropy, the greater the unpredictability in the *RR* interval time series. The input variables m and r must be fixed to compute approximate entropy. The variable m determines the length of compared runs of *RR* interval data, and the variable r sets the tolerance for the comparison of these runs. Although approximate entropy can be calculated from relatively short data sets, the amount of data points has an influence on the approximate entropy. However, the measure is commonly used in various heart rate variability analyses and it has provided some valuable clinical information in different patient populations (Pincus & Viscarello 1992; Pincus & Goldberger 1994; Mäkikallio *et al.* 1996; Hogue *et al.* 1998; Pikkujämsä *et al.* 1999).

Return maps

The two-dimensional Poincaré plots method (also called return maps) is a geometrical method, which provides a beat-to-beat visual and quantitative analysis of *RR* intervals (Woo *et al.* 1994; Huikuri *et al.* 1996). This quantitative method of heart rate variability analysis is based on the notion of different temporal effects of changes in the vagal and sympathetic modulation of heart rate on the subsequent *RR* intervals without a requirement for a stationary quality of the data. The shape of the plot can be used to classify the signal into one of several classes (Woo *et al.* 1994; Huikuri *et al.* 1996), and the irregular shapes quantified from Poincaré plots may then be classified as nonlinear. In quantitative analysis, short-term *RR* interval variability and long-term *RR* interval variability of the plot can be quantified separately (Fig. 3.1).

Methodological considerations

Whether the various nonlinear methods detect nonlinear behaviour is an important scientific issue, but from the physician's practical point of view, it is important to know whether they are applicable for clinical purposes. Concepts of nonlinear dynamics, fractals, inverse power-law, entropy and other terms used in the context with newer analysis methods of heart rate variability refer more to mathematics than to medicine, and may be received with some scepticism by clinicians. Since these measures become more familiar to clinicians, it can be noticed that understanding of the methodology of analysis of scaling behaviour of heart rate dynamics may not require the knowledge of advanced mathematics. There is increasing evidence from multiple studies to support the utility of the analysis methods of heart rate variability that are based on nonlinear dynamics (Perkiömäki *et al.* 2000). Some of the nonlinear measures of heart rate variability, such as the short-term scaling exponent obtained by the detrended fluctuation analysis technique, have some advantages over the traditional measures of heart rate variability when considering risk stratification purposes: less dependency on heart rate, less interindividual variation (Perkiömäki *et al.* 2001a; Pikkujämsä *et al.* 2001), smaller relative changes of individual values over time after an acute myocardial infarction (Perkiömäki *et al.* 2001), and relatively good comparability of individual values between long-term and short-term electrocardiographic recordings (Perkiömäki *et al.* 2001). Sophisticated nonlinear techniques seem to be helpful for analysing complex mechanisms involved in cardiovascular regulation. The utility of these methods in different clinical settings is discussed below.

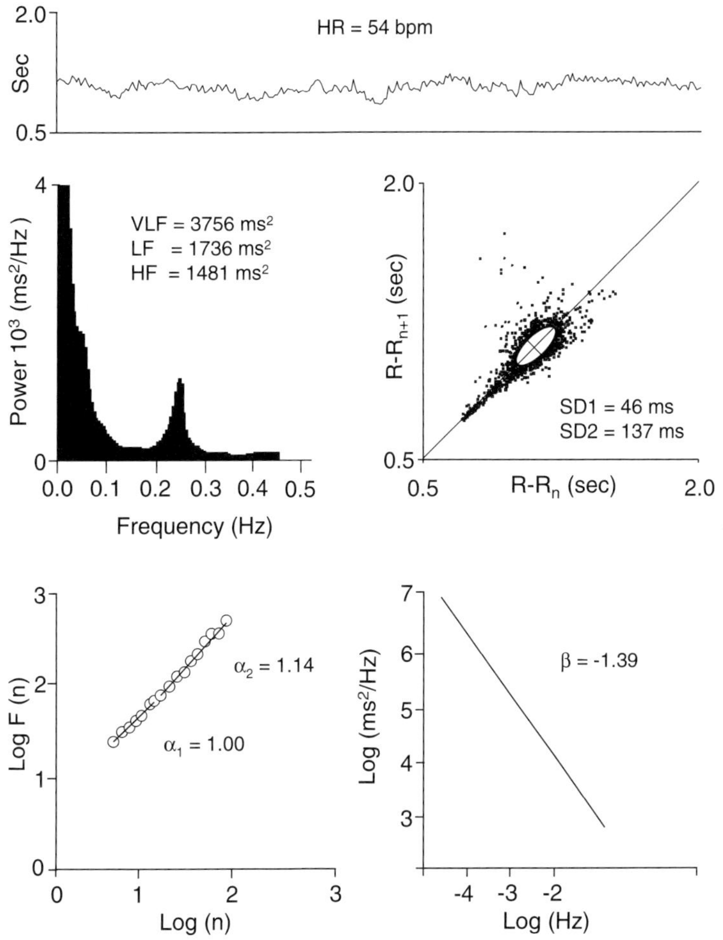

Fig. 3.1 Representative examples of *RR* interval tachogram (upper panel), power spectra (middle panel, left side), two-dimensional vector analyses of Poincaré plot (middle panel, right side), detrended fluctuation analysis (DFA) (lower panel, left side), and a scaling slope of long-term fluctuations of heart rate variability (lower panel, right side). The *RR* interval tachogram is derived from 5 min recording at night and the spectrum, Poincaré plot and DFA analysis are derived from 1 h portion at night in a healthy subject. The long-term scaling slope is derived from entire 24 h recording. HR, heart rate; VLF, very-low-frequency spectral component; LF, low-frequency spectral component; HF, high frequency spectral component; SD1, short-term beat-to-beat *RR* interval variability from Poincaré plot; SD2, long-term *RR* interval variability from Poincaré plot; α_1, the short-term fractal scaling exponent (from 4 to 11 beats) derived by the DFA method; α_2, the intermediate-term fractal scaling exponent (>11 beats) derived by the DFA method; β, the long-term scaling slope for entire 24 h recording.

Clinical studies using methods based on nonlinear heart rate dynamics

In late 1980s, the landmark study by Kleiger *et al.* (1987) attested to the value of low heart rate variability measured by time-domain indices for predicting mortality after a myocardial infarction. Later, numerous reports have also shown a decrease in heart rate variability after a myocardial infarction (Huikuri *et al.* 1999). Although altered approximate entropy, fractal and scaling values have been observed among patients with various cardiac disorders, the prognostic power of the methods based on nonlinear dynamics has not been tested in large-scale studies until recently.

Long-term power-law slope

The ability of spectral scaling properties of long-term fluctuations of heart rate to predict death after myocardial infarction was first reported by

Bigger and coworkers (1996). They studied 715 patients with myocardial infarction, 274 healthy persons and 19 patients with heart transplants. A steep power-law slope was a powerful predictor of all-cause mortality or arrhythmic death and predicted these outcomes better than the traditional power spectral bands. In addition to patients with myocardial infarction, long-term scaling properties have been observed to predict mortality among randomly selected general populations of the elderly (Huikuri *et al.* 1998). The steep slope of heart rate variability predicted both cardiac and cerebrovascular death suggesting that altered long-term behaviour of heart rate implies an increased risk for vascular causes of death rather than being a marker of any disease or frailty leading to death.

Detrended fluctuation analysis

Recently, altered short-term fractal properties of heart rate fluctuations have shown superior prognostic power compared to conventional measures among patients with acute myocardial infarction and depressed left ventricular function (Mäkikallio *et al.* 1997; Huikuri *et al.* 2000). Initially, short-term fractal-like correlation properties of *RR* intervals were studied in 159 patients with an acute myocardial infarction and left ventricular ejection fraction of <35%. The patients were followed-up for 4 years. Among analysed variables, the reduced short-term scaling exponent was the best predictor of mortality. The study showed that reduction in fractal correlation properties implies more random short-term heart rate dynamics in patients with increased risk of death after acute myocardial infarction (Mäkikallio *et al.* 1997). More recently, in a large population of 446 survivors of acute myocardial infarction with a left ventricular ejection fraction of <35%, reduced short-term fractal exponent was the most powerful heart rate variability measure that predicted all-cause mortality. A reduced short-term fractal exponent predicted both arrhythmic death and nonarrhythmic cardiac death. It yielded more powerful prognostic information than the traditional measures of heart rate variability (Fig. 3.2) (Huikuri *et al.* 2000). Recently, the prognostic power of the short-term fractal scaling index has also been demonstrated among a general population of patients with myocardial infarction and broad variation in their left ventricular systolic function (Tapanainen *et al.* 2002).

Patients with chronic heart failure have also shown altered fractal organization in heartbeat dynamics (Peng *et al.* 1995). Furthermore, altered fractal correlation properties of heart rate have been observed to be related to mortality among patients with chronic congestive heart failure (Ho *et al.* 1997). Fractal scaling properties

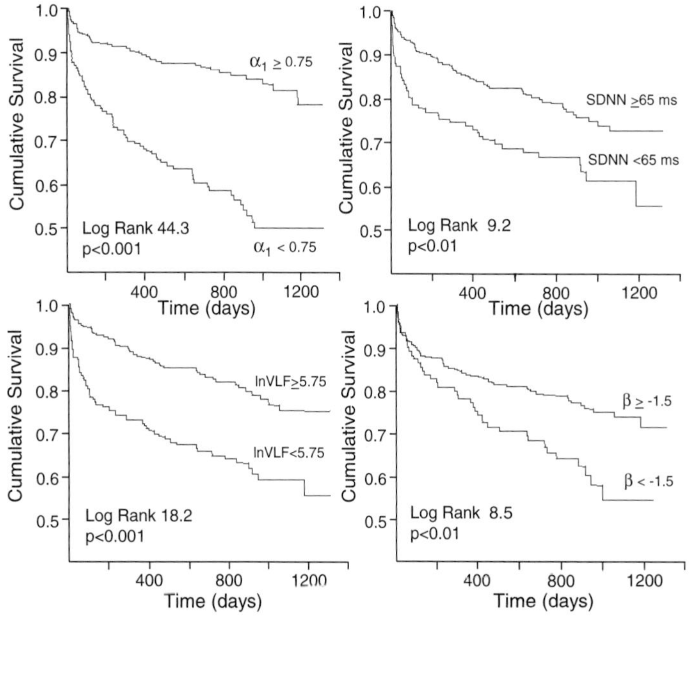

Fig. 3.2 Kaplan–Meier survival curves for the patients with the short-term fractal-like scaling exponent (α_1) ≥ 0.75 or α_1 < 0.75 (upper left), patients with standard deviation of all normal-to-normal (*NN*) intervals (SDNN) ≥ 65 ms and < 65 ms (upper right), patients with natural logarithm of very-low-frequency spectral component (ln VLF) ≥ 5.75 and < 5.75 (lower left), and patients with scaling exponent (≥ −1.5 and < −1.5 (lower right) included in the DIAMOND study. Short-term scaling exponent was a better predictor of mortality than standard deviation of all *NN* intervals in these postinfarction patients. (Modified from Huikuri *et al.* 2000, with permission.)

predicted survival over a mean follow-up period of 1.9 years among patients with chronic congestive heart failure. This suggests that nonlinear heart rate variability indices may contribute a prognostic value that complements traditional heart rate variability measures also in patients with chronic congestive heart failure. More recently, the predictive power of an altered short-term scaling exponent has also been observed in a large heart failure population who had undergone 24-h electrocardiographic recordings (Mäkikallio *et al.* 2001a). In addition to patient populations with advanced cardiovascular disease, the short-term scaling exponent has been shown to be a powerful predictor of cardiac mortality among the general elderly population (Mäkikallio *et al.* 2001a).

Two specific features characterize the heart rate dynamics in patients with complicated ischaemic coronary artery disease and congestive heart failure. First, the low frequency oscillation of heart rate is typically reduced or even absent among those patients with congestive heart failure (Lombardi *et al.* 1996; Van de Borne *et al.* 1997). Secondly, the high frequency oscillation is not reduced but may even be increased among high risk patients (Mäkikallio *et al.* 1997). This erratic increase in beat-to-beat heart rate dynamics seems not to be respiratory related (Tulppo *et al.* 1998, 2001). These changes cause a lack of a prominent spectral spike in high- and low-frequency areas and contribute to low short-term fractal values indicating increased short-term randomness.

Approximate entropy

In addition to life-threatening arrhythmias, altered nonlinear dynamics have also been observed before the spontaneous onset of atrial fibrillation among patients without structural heart disease (Vikman *et al.* 1999). When heart rate variability indices were analysed in 20-min intervals before 92 episodes of spontaneous, paroxysmal atrial fibrillation in 22 patients without structural heart disease, traditional measures showed no significant changes before the onset of atrial fibrillation. However, a progressive decrease occurred both in approximate entropy and the short-term fractal exponent before the onset of atrial fibrillation episodes, showing that changes in the complexity and fractal properties of heart rate precede the spontaneous onset of atrial fibrillation in patients with no structural heart disease. These values before the onset of atrial fibrillation were also lower than values obtained from matched healthy control subjects. Reduced approximate entropy values indicating larger predictability in heart rate dynamics have also been reported to precede spontaneous episodes of atrial fibrillation after coronary artery bypass surgery (Hogue *et al.* 1998). Patients with postoperative complications after cardiac surgery have also been shown to have reduced complexity in heart rate dynamics (Fleisher *et al.* 1993).

Physiological background of altered nonlinear measures

A specific abnormality in cardiovascular regulation may explain the breakdown of short-term fractal scaling and its association with a risk of dying. Recent observations have shown that noradrenaline infusion causes abrupt temporal changes in *RR* interval dynamics, which result in reduction of short-term correlation properties of heart rate dynamics. These results suggest that elevated levels of circulating catecholamines may explain the breakdown of fractal-like behaviour of heart rate dynamics (Tulppo *et al.* 1998, 2001). Similarly, erratic beat-to-beat heart rate dynamics have also been shown to be associated with high levels of noradrenaline in patients with heart failure (Woo *et al.* 1994). The analysis of the short-term fractal scaling exponent from Holter recordings seems to partially reflect the levels of circulating catecholamines over a 24-h period. In alignment with this notion, recent data suggest that the beta blocker therapy increases the short-term scaling exponent in patients with heart failure indicating the reversal of the deteriorated heart rate scaling behaviour (Lin *et al.* 2001; Ridha *et al.* 2002). Recent observations in healthy subjects have shown that parasympathetic blocking by atropine increases the short-term scaling exponent (Tulppo *et al.* 2001; Perkiömäki *et al.* 2002); however, vagal tone seems not to be a major determinant of approximate entropy (Perkiömäki *et al.* 2002). In general, the physiological background of nonlinear indices of heart rate dynamics is not well established.

Future perspectives

Research on heart rate variability has increased exponentially during the last decade (Huikuri *et al.* 1999). Methods derived from nonlinear system theory have shown new insights into the abnormalities in heart rate behaviour in various pathological conditions, providing additional prognostic information as compared to traditional measures of heart rate variability, and clearly complementing conventional analysis methods. Furthermore, new risk variable concepts describing alterations in heart rate response have been introduced recently (Schmidt *et al.* 1999). Despite statistical data that suggest the predictive power of the various conventional and newer risk markers describing heart rate behaviour, none of these markers are widely used in clinical practice to guide the preventive therapy of individual patients, because no trial has adequately linked the reliability of any of these variables to clinical outcome with an intervention. Therefore, more clinical studies using the new methods and concepts will be needed, before the clinical applicability of these methods can be definitively established. Although the concepts of chaos theory, fractal mathematics and complexity measures in relation to the untoward cardiac events are still far removed from clinical medicine, they are obviously a fruitful area for future research to expand our knowledge concerning the initiation and perpetuation of life-threatening arrhythmias or other adverse cardiac events.

References

Bigger, J.T., Jr, Steinman, R.C., Rolnitzky, L.M. *et al.* (1996) Power law behaviour of *RR*-interval variability in healthy middle-aged persons, patients with recent acute myocardial infarction, and patients with heart transplants. *Circulation*, **93**, 2142–2151.

Eckberg, D.L. (1997) Sympatho-vagal balance; a critical appraisal. *Circulation*, **96**, 3224–3227.

Eckmann, J.P. & Ruelle, D. (1985) Ergodic theory of chaos and strange attractors. *Reviews of Model Physics*, **57**, 617–656.

ESC/NASPE (European Society of Cardiology/ North American Society of Pacing and Electrophysiology) Task Force (1996) Heart rate variability. Standards of measurement, physiological interpretation, and clinical use. *Circulation*, **93**, 1043–1065.

Fleisher, L.A., Pincus, S.M. & Rosenbaum, S.H. (1993) Approximate entropy of heart rate as a correlate of postoperative ventricular dysfunction. *Anesthesiology*, **78**, 683–692.

Goldberger, A.L. (1990) Nonlinear dynamics, fractals and chaos: applications to cardiac electrophysiology. *Annals of Biomedical Engineering*, **18** 195–198.

Goldberger, A.L. (1996) Non-linear dynamics for clinicians: chaos theory, fractals, and complexity at the bedside. *Lancet*, **347**, 1312–1314.

Grassberger, P. & Procaccia, I. (1983a) Estimation of the Kolmogorov entropy from a chaotic signal. *Physics Review A*, **28**, 2591–93

Grassberger, P. & Procaccia, I. (1983b) Measuring the strangeness of strange attractors. *Physica*, **9D**, 189–208.

Ho, K.K.L., Moody, G.B., Peng, C.K. *et al.* (1997) Predicting survival in heart failure cases and controls using fully automated methods for deriving nonlinear and conventional indices of heart rate dynamics. *Circulation*, **96**, 842–848.

Hogue, C.W., Jr, Domitrovich, P.P., Stein, P.K. *et al.* (1998) *RR* interval dynamics before atrial fibrillation in patients after coronary artery bypass graft surgery. *Circulation*, **98**, 429–434.

Huikuri, H.V., Mäkikallio, T., Airaksinen, K.E.J. *et al.* (1999) Measurement of heart rate variability: a clinical tool or a research toy? *Journal of the American College of Cardiology*, **34**, 1878–1883.

Huikuri, H.V., Mäkikallio, T.H., Airaksinen, K.E.J. *et al.* (1998) Power-law relationship of heart rate variability as a predictor of mortality in the elderly. *Circulation*, **97**, 2031–2036.

Huikuri, H.V., Mäkikallio, T.H., Peng, C.K. *et al.* for the DIAMOND Study Group (2000) Fractal correlation properties of *RR* interval dynamics and mortality in patients with depressed left ventricular function after an acute myocardial infarction. *Circulation*, **101**, 47–54.

Huikuri, H.V., Seppänen, T., Koistinen, M.J. *et al.* (1996) Abnormalities in beat-to-beat dynamics of heart rate before the spontaneous onset of life-threatening ventricular tachyarrhythmias in patients with prior myocardial infarction. *Circulation*, **93**, 1836–1844.

Kleiger, R.E., Miller, J.P., Bigger, J.T., Jr *et al.* the Multicentre Post-Infarction Research Group (1987) Decreased heart rate variability and its association with increased mortality after acute myocardial infarction. *American Journal of Cardiology*, **59**, 256–262.

Lin, L.Y., Lin, J.L., Du, C.C. *et al.* (2001) Reversal of deteriorated fractal behaviour of heart rate variability by beta blocker therapy in patients with advanced congestive heart failure. *Journal of Cardiovascular Electrophysiology*, **12**, 26–32.

Lombardi, F., Sandrone, G., Mortara, A. *et al.* (1996) Linear and nonlinear dynamics of heart rate variability after acute myocardial infarction with normal and reduced left ventricular ejection fraction. *American Journal of Cardiology*, **77**, 1283–1288.

Mäkikallio, T.H., Høber, S., Køber, L. *et al.* for the Trace Investigators (1999) Fractal analysis of heart rate dynamics as a predictor of mortality in patients with depressed left ventricular function after acute myocardial infarction. *American Journal of Cardiology*, **83**, 836–839.

Mäkikallio, T.H., Huikuri, H.V., Hintze, U. *et al.* (2001a) Fractal analysis and time and frequency domain measures of heart rate variability as predictors of mortality in patients with heart failure. *American Journal of Cardiology*, **87**, 178–182.

Mäkikallio, T.H., Huikuri, H.V., Mäkikallio, A. *et al.* (2001b) Prediction of sudden cardiac death by fractal analysis of heart rate variability in elderly subjects. *Journal of the American College of Cardiology*, **37**, 1395–1402.

Mäkikallio, T.H., Ristimäe, T., Airaksinen, K.E.J. *et al.* (1998) Heart rate dynamics in patients with stable angina pectoris and utility of fractal and complexity measures. *American Journal of Cardiology*, **81**, 27–31.

Mäkikallio, T.H., Seppänen, T., Airaksinen, K.E.J. *et al.* (1997) Dynamic analysis of heart rate may predict subsequent ventricular tachycardia after myocardial infarction. *American Journal of Cardiology*, **80**, 779–783.

Mäkikallio, T.H., Seppänen, T., Niemelä, M. *et al.* (1996) Abnormalities in beat-to-beat complexity of heart rate dynamics in patients with a prior myocardial infarction. *Journal of the American College of Cardiology*, **28**, 1005–1011.

Pagani, M., Lombardi, F., Guzzetti, S. *et al.* (1986) Power spectral analysis of heart rate and arterial blood pressure variabilities as a marker of sympatho-vagal interaction in man and conscious dog. *Circulation, Research*, **59**, 178–193.

Peng, C.K., Havlin, S., Stanley, H.E. *et al.* (1995) Quantification of scaling exponents and crossover phenomena in nonstationary heartbeat time series. *Chaos*, **5**, 82–87.

Perkiömäki, J.S., Mäkikallio, T.H. & Huikuri, H.V. (2000) Nonlinear analysis of heart rate variability: fractal and complexity measures of heart rate behaviour. *Annals of Noninvasive Electrocardiology*, **5**, 179–187.

Perkiömäki, J.S., Zareba, W., Badilini, F. *et al.* (2002) Influence of atropine on fractal and complexity measures of heart rate variability. *Annals of Noninvasive Electrocardiology*, **7**, 326–331.

Perkiömäki, J.S., Zareba, W., Kalaria, V.G. *et al.* (2001a) Comparability of nonlinear measures of heart rate variability between long- and short-term electrocardiographic recordings. *American Journal of Cardiology*, **87**, 905–908.

Perkiömäki, J.S., Zareba, W., Ruta, J. *et al.* for the IDEAL Investigators (2001b) Fractal and complexity measures of heart rate dynamics after acute myocardial infarction. *American Journal of Cardiology*, **88**, 777–781.

Persson, P.B. (1997) Spectrum analysis of cardiovascular time series. *American Journal of Physiology*, **273**, R1201–R1210.

Pikkujämsä, S.M., Airaksinen, K.E.J., Mäkikallio, T.H. *et al.* (2001) Determinants and interindividual variation of *RR* interval dynamics in middle-aged subjects. *American Journal of Physiology*, **280**, H1400–H1406.

Pikkujämsä, S.M., Mäkikallio, T.H., Sourander, L.B. *et al.* (1999) Cardiac interbeat interval dynamics from childhood to senescence: comparison of conventional and new measures based on fractals and chaos theory. *Circulation*, **100**, 393–399.

Pincus, S.M. & Goldberger, A.L. (1994) Physiological time-series analysis: what does regularity quantify? *American Journal of Physiology*, **226**, H1643–H1656.

Pincus, S.M. & Viscarello, R.R. (1992) Approximate entropy: a regularity statistic for fetal heart rate analysis. *Obstetrics and Gynecology*, **79**, 249–255.

Ridha, M., Mäkikallio, T.H., Lopera, G. *et al.* (2002) Effects of carvedilol on heart rate dynamics in patients with congestive heart failure. *Annals of Noninvasive Electrocardiology*, **7**, 133–138.

Saul, J.P., Albrecht, P., Berger, R.D. *et al.* (1987) Analysis of long-term heart rate variability: methods, $1/f$ scaling and implications. In: *Computers in Cardiology*, pp. 419–422. IEEE Computer Society Press, Silver Spring, MD.

Schmidt, G., Malik, M., Barthel, P. *et al.* (1999) Heart-rate turbulence after ventricular premature beats as a predictor of mortality after acute myocardial infarction. *Lancet*, **353**, 1390–1396.

Skinner, J.E., Pratt, C.M. & Vybiral, T. (1993) A reduction in the correlation dimension of heartbeat intervals precedes imminent ventricular fibrillation in human subjects. *American Heart Journal*, **125**, 731–743.

Tapanainen, J.M., Thomsen, P.E., Kober, L. *et al.* (2002) Fractal analysis of heart rate variability and mortality after an acute myocardial infarction. *American Journal of Cardiology*, **90**, 347–352.

Tulppo, M.P., Mäkikallio, T.H., Seppänen, T. *et al.* (1998) Heart rate dynamics during accentuated sympatho-vagal interaction. *American Journal of Physiology*, **274**, H810–H816.

Tulppo, M.P., Mäkikallio, T.H., Seppänen, T. *et al.* (2001) Effects of pharmacological adrenergic and vagal modulation on fractal heart rate dynamics. *Clinical Physiology*, **21**, 515–523.

Van de Borne, P., Montano, N., Pagani, M. *et al.* (1997) Absence of low-frequency variability of sympathetic activity in severe heart failure. *Circulation*, **95**, 1449–1454.

Vikman, S., Mäkikallio, T.H., Yli-Mäyry, S. *et al.* (1999) Altered complexity and correlation properties of *RR* interval dynamics before the spontaneous onset of paroxysmal atrial fibrillation. *Circulation*, **100**, 2079–2084.

Woo, M.A., Stevenson, W.G., Moser, D.K. & Middlekauff, H.R. (1994) Complex heart rate variability and serum noradrenaline levels in patients with advanced heart failure. *Journal of the American College of Cardiology*, **23**, 565–569.

Yamamoto, Y. & Hughson, R.L. (1991) Coarse-graining spectral analysis: new method for studying heart rate variability. *Journal of Applied Physiology*, **71**, 1143–1150.

CHAPTER 4

Correlations Among Heart Rate Variability Components and Autonomic Mechanisms

Dwain L. Eckberg

Introduction

In this chapter the physiological bases that underlie human autonomic and cardiovascular rhythms are explored. The arguments are based on the notions that simple interventions and careful analysis can yield important insights into neurophysiological mechanisms. The discussion is organized according to the methods available for the study of humans, in ascending order of intrusiveness and complexity.

Simple resting recordings

Arguably, the most straightforward approach to study of human rhythms is simply to record and analyse them, with no intervention whatever. Figure 4.1 shows a recording obtained from a healthy, resting supine subject breathing at 0.25 Hz (or, once every 4 s), and corresponding power spectra (derived from 3-min recordings). The dashed vertical lines in the spectra (lowest three panels, right) indicate the imposed breathing frequency. Cursory perusal of the time series on the left indicates that even with fixed-rate breathing, human autonomic and haemodynamic outflow is not constant – these panels indicate beyond argument, that healthy humans are always changing, and that changes may be conspicuous, over periods as short as 1 min.

Figure 4.1 indicates also that not only are the signals changing continuously, but they are also changing in complex ways. For example, it is obvious that *RR* interval and systolic pressure fluctuations occur rapidly (with breathing), and that these rapid fluctuations are superimposed upon slower rhythms. The power spectra are not pretty and smooth – they are jagged and irregular. The right panels document important spectral power at frequencies below that of respiration. The power spectra also suggest that respiration influences all of the outflows depicted. Although all signals have peaks at the breathing frequency, however, power at that frequency, and the distribution of power over the entire 0.0–0.3 Hz frequency range are not identical for all signals. Muscle sympathetic nerve activity and systolic pressures are little influenced, and *RR* intervals are strongly influenced by breathing.

The data shown in Fig. 4.1 point toward change and instability, not 'stationarity'. Such observations (and others) led my group to propose that humans are not stationary – stationarity is a construct that does not apply to neurophysiological data from (healthy) humans (Badra *et al.* 2001). This conclusion illustrates an inherent problem with simple spectral analyses – they lump all fluctuations together into one spectrum, which is an average for the entire recording period. Therefore, a single power spectrum can provide no information regarding how a signal might be changing during the recording period – if fluctuations are present and ongoing, the spectrum provides no way to know what they are. In this context, the jagged appearance of the spectra shown in Fig. 4.1 may signify episodic change, and therefore, may not merely reflect noise.

The spectra in Fig. 4.1 point to a pervasive influence of respiration. However, the mere presence of spectral peaks at the respiratory-frequency does not inform the mechanisms responsible for the associations between breath-

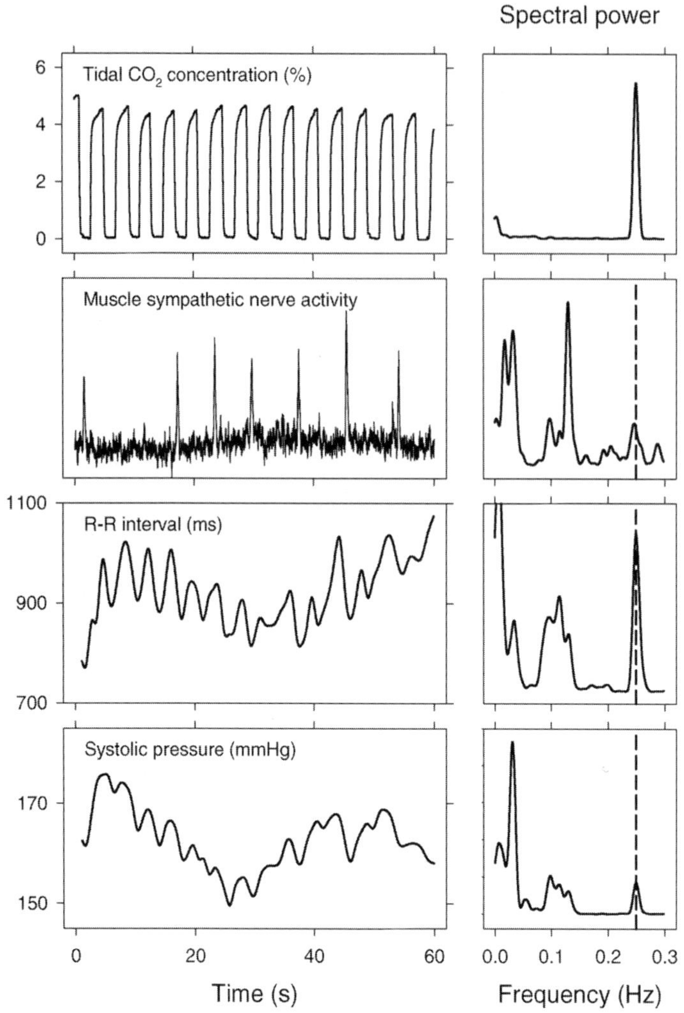

Fig. 4.1 Time series and power spectra from one healthy supine subject breathing at 0.25 Hz.

ing and other measurements. One well documented mechanism is the 'respiratory gate' (Lopes & Palmer 1976). [Respiratory gating of human autonomic and haemodynamic outflows was the subject of a recent review by Eckberg (2003).] Respiratory activity phasically reduces responsiveness of vagal and sympathetic motoneurones to autonomic sensory inputs and thereby modulates their firing (Eckberg & Orshan 1977; Eckberg *et al.* 1980, 1985). Does respiratory gating explain all fluctuations occurring at respiratory frequencies? Not necessarily. A second candidate was proposed by De Boer *et al.* (1985) and by Pagani *et al.* (1988), Baselli *et al.* (1994) and their coworkers, who suggested that respiration triggers a cascade of events, such that (1) breathing provokes rhythmic arterial pressure fluctuations, and (2) arterial pressure fluctuations provoke parallel *RR* interval fluctuations, by means of simple baroreflex physiology.

We tested this baroreflex hypothesis with partial coherence analysis. Partialization is a mathematical treatment used to evaluate interrelations among *three* signals (Kocsis *et al.* 1993). First, fluctuations occurring in one signal are removed from the other two signals, and then residual coherence between the two remaining signals is sought. In her study, Badra *et al.* (2001), removed the influence of respiration with partialization, and then measured residual correlations between systolic pressures and *RR* intervals. Figure 4.2 shows an example of partialization derived from a 5-min recording made with a supine subject breathing spontaneously.

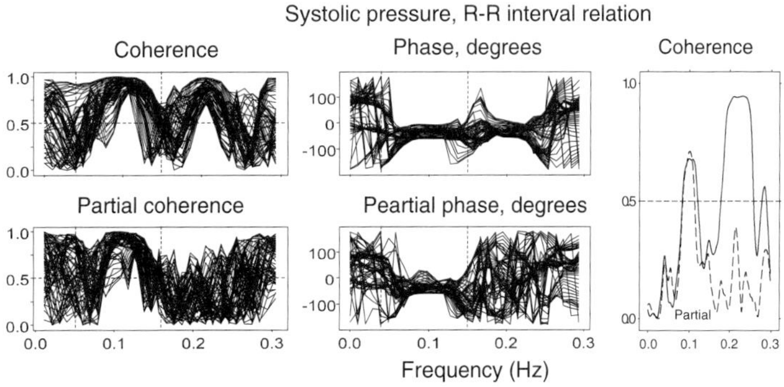

Fig. 4.2 Sliding cross-spectra and coherence before and after partialization. (Adapted from Bodra *et al.* 2001, with permission.)

(For this analysis, correlations and phase angles between systolic pressures and *RR* intervals were measured in a 90-s window and plotted. Then the 90-s window was advanced 3 s, the analysis was repeated, and the result was plotted over the first. This iterative process was continued until the 90-s window had moved through the entire 300 s of data.) Before partialization (upper two upper left panels), there was strong coherence (approaching perfect coherence of 1.0) at low, ~0.12 Hz, and respiratory, ~0.22 Hz, frequencies. After partialization (two lower left panels), low frequency coherence and phase were intact and unchanged, and respiratory-frequency coherence and phase were abolished. The great reduction of coherence by partialization is documented by the average coherence values plotted at right. This analysis, and other evidence marshalled elsewhere (Eckberg 2003), suggest that the strong correlations that exist between systolic pressures and *RR* intervals at respiratory frequencies reflect direct respiratory influences on those outflows, and not baroreflex physiology.

Physiological interventions

Since humans can cooperate as research subjects, they can alter their physiology in ways that might yield insights into mechanisms only hinted at by baseline resting recordings. One simple intervention is breathing: motivated healthy human volunteers can control their breathing exquisitely.

One intervention Badra *et al.* (2001) used to tease out the influence of breathing was to make measurements in the absence of breathing. Badra instructed subjects to hyperventilate while breathing 100% oxygen, and then hold their breaths in inspiration, for as long as they could. In her study, all subjects were able to maintain apnoea for at least 3 min, a duration sufficiently long to register spectral power over frequencies as low as ~0.05 Hz. Figure 4.3 shows horizontal sections made through sliding fast Fourier transforms of *RR* intervals (60-s data segments, moved in 2-s steps, through a 3-min recording), during uncontrolled breathing (top) and apnoea (bottom). (In the left panels, the frequency of the signals is indicated on the horizontal axis, and the spectral power is indicated by the numbers of concentric lines.)

The simple intervention of breath holding yields several insights into mechanisms responsible for the signal fluctuations present in Fig. 4.1. First, the sliding fast Fourier transformations (left panels) indicate that the jagged appearances of the power spectra in Fig. 4.1 do not represent noise. During these 3-min recordings, both the frequencies and intensities of *RR* interval oscillations changed continuously. Changing frequencies are shown to particular advantage by high frequency *RR* interval fluctuations (upper left panel, right), which reflect an ongoing quasiperiodic oscillation of breathing frequency. This observation is not new; it is well recognized that fluctuations of human respiratory rates can be large (Lenfant 1967). An obvious corollary of the sliding fast Fourier transformations is that when spectra are filtered with mathematical smoothing or autoregressive modelling, physiological information is lost.

Second, Fig. 4.3 suggests, and Badra's study (2001) proves, that respiratory-frequency *RR* interval fluctuations (as well as those of systolic pressure and muscle sympathetic nerve activity, not shown) are secondary to breathing – they are

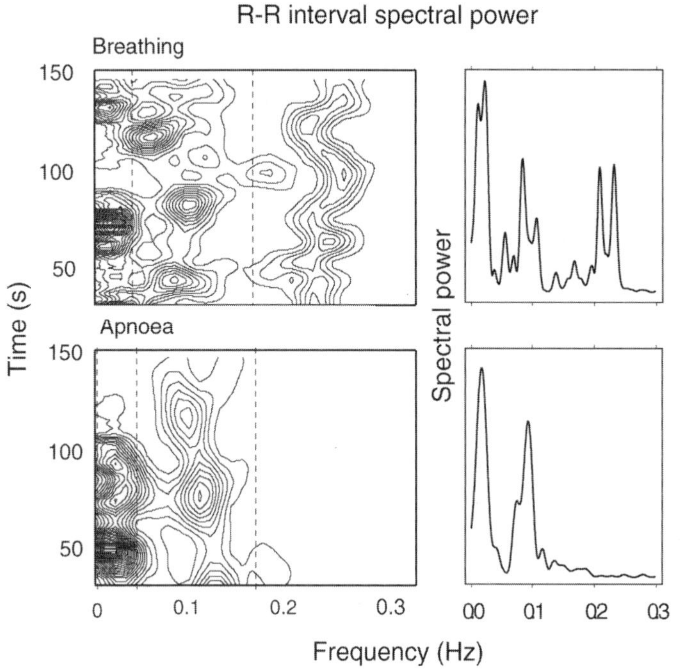

Fig. 4.3 Contour map from sliding fast Fourier transformations, and power spectra from one subject during uncontrolled breathing and apnoea. (Adapted from Eckberg 2003, with permission.)

not present in the absence of breathing. Therefore, such rapid fluctuations are not attributable to some other oscillator or pacemaker, which also drives breathing. Third, Fig. 4.3 indicates that in resting humans, *RR* intervals oscillate importantly at low frequencies. In Badra's study (2001), no breathing modality (including uncontrolled breathing, fixed-frequency breathing, hyperventilation, and apnoea) altered the intensity of low frequency *RR* interval, systolic pressure, and muscle sympathetic nerve fluctuations. Thus, although breathing is a prerequisite for the occurrence of respiratory-frequency oscillations in these outflows, breathing exerts no influence on low-frequency oscillations.

Figure 4.4 shows average *RR* interval power spectra recorded in nine supine subjects who were asked to breathe at seven different frequencies (Brown *et al.* 1993). The simple expedient of breathing at different rates provoked profound differences of *RR* interval spectral power: when subjects breathed at 7.5 breaths/min (0.125 Hz), *RR* interval spectral power was about 10-fold greater than when subjects breathed at 24 breaths/min (0.4 Hz). In spontaneously breathing dogs, respiratory-frequency fluctuations of *RR* intervals are linear functions of vagus nerve traffic to the heart (Katona & Jih 1975). Therefore, the spectra depicted in Fig. 4.4 suggest that slow breathing increases vagal-cardiac nerve traffic. However, in this study, mean *RR* intervals (not shown) were the same across all breathing

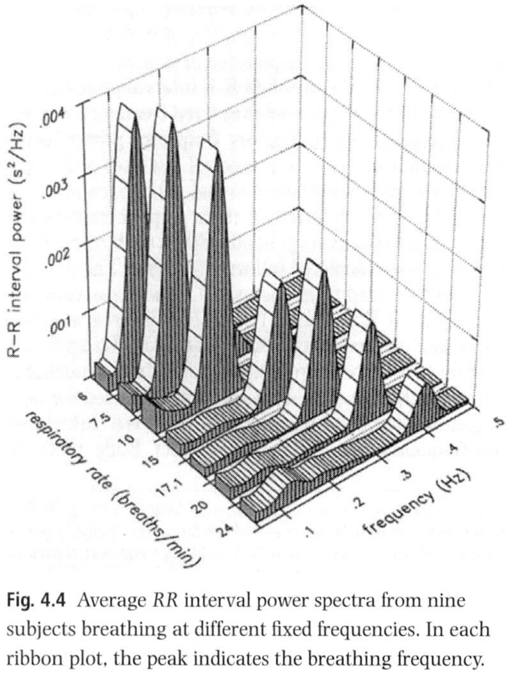

Fig. 4.4 Average *RR* interval power spectra from nine subjects breathing at different fixed frequencies. In each ribbon plot, the peak indicates the breathing frequency. (Adapted from Brown *et al.* 1993, with permission.)

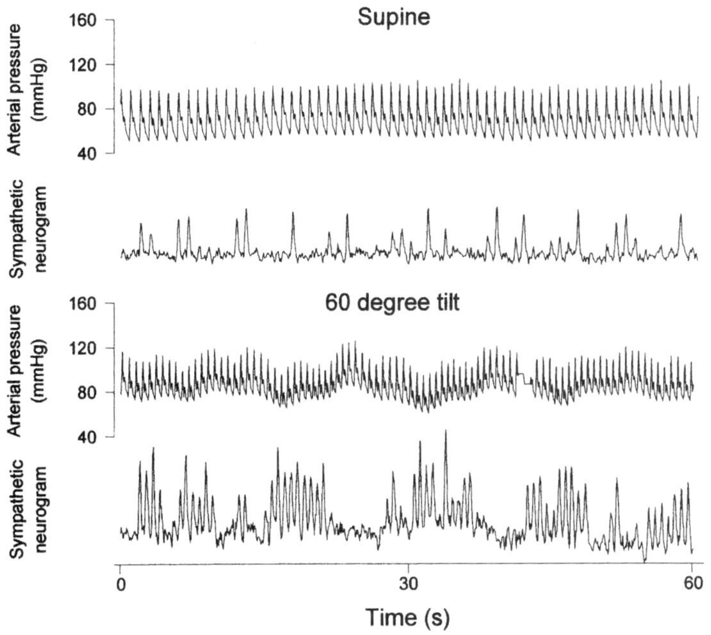

Fig. 4.5 Recording from one subject in supine and upright tilt positions. (Adapted from Cooke *et al.* 1999, with permission.)

frequencies. Since in dogs, both mean *RR* intervals *and* peak minus valley respiratory *RR* interval differences during breathing are related linearly to vagal-cardiac nerve activity (Katona *et al.* 1970), the *RR* interval spectra shown in Fig. 4.4 and the constant average *RR* interval support internally inconsistent conclusions. Because of this conflict, the simple intervention of asking subjects to breathe at different rates is not sufficient to determine if breathing rate affects net vagal traffic to the heart.

Passive upright tilt provides a means to reduce the level of afferent baroreceptor nerve activity systematically and physiologically. Figure 4.5 depicts recordings of photoplethysmographic finger arterial pressure (Imholz *et al.* 1998) and muscle sympathetic nerve activity in supine and upright tilt positions (Cooke *et al.* 1999). The arterial pressure recording provided no evidence that baroreceptor input was reduced by tilt; as observed previously (Borst *et al.* 1984; Morillo *et al.* 1997), arterial pressure may be higher in tilted than supine positions. Also, fluctuations of arterial pressure were greater in tilted than supine positions. Muscle sympathetic nerve burst size and frequency increased greatly in the tilted position, with a ~0.1 Hz periodicity.

Figure 4.6 shows average muscle sympathetic nerve spectral power, measured in nine healthy young volunteers during graded, passive upright tilt (Cooke *et al.* 1999). Iwase *et al.* (1987) showed that human muscle sympathetic nerve activity increases linearly with the sine of the tilt angle. The data shown in Fig. 4.6 extend Iwase's observations by showing that fluctuations of muscle sympathetic nerve activity also increase with the angle of tilt, both at low and respiratory frequencies (lower panel).

Respiration rhythmically modulates responsiveness of muscle sympathetic, as well as vagal-cardiac motoneurones (see below) (Eckberg *et al.* 1985), but in an opposite way. Progressive reductions of baroreceptor stimulation lead to progressive increases of sympathetic activity. However, Fig. 4.7 shows that increasing levels of sympathetic stimulation progressively reduce respiratory gating of sympathetic motoneurone responsiveness. Therefore, the ability of respiration to gate responses to stimulation of sympathetic motoneurones is finite, and can be overcome.

Figure 4.8 shows average *RR* interval power spectra from nine subjects during tilt (Cooke *et al.* 1999). These data indicate that upright tilt progressively reduces respiratory-frequency *RR* interval fluctuations – respiratory sinus arrhythmia. Although postural changes alter physiology by means other than baroreflex mechanisms

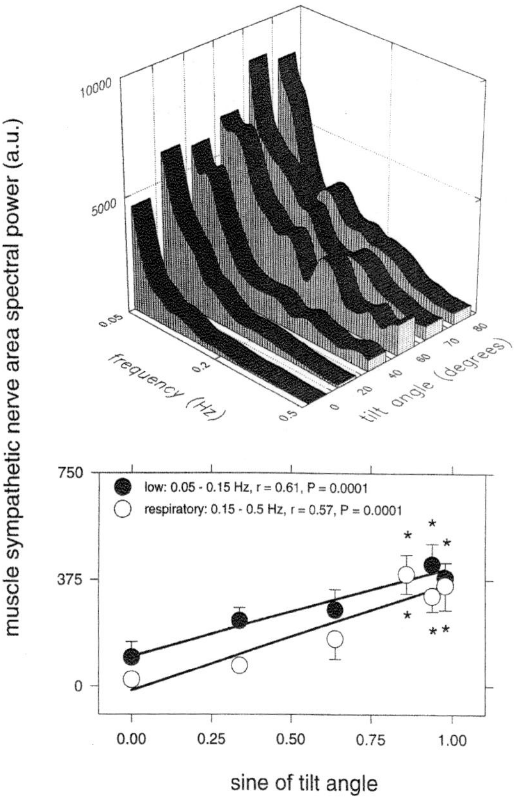

Fig. 4.6 Average muscle sympathetic nerve power spectra from nine subjects tilted passively at different degrees. Lower panel depicts results of linear regression. * *P* ″ 0.05 vs. supine. (Adapted from Cooke *et al.* 1999, with permission.)

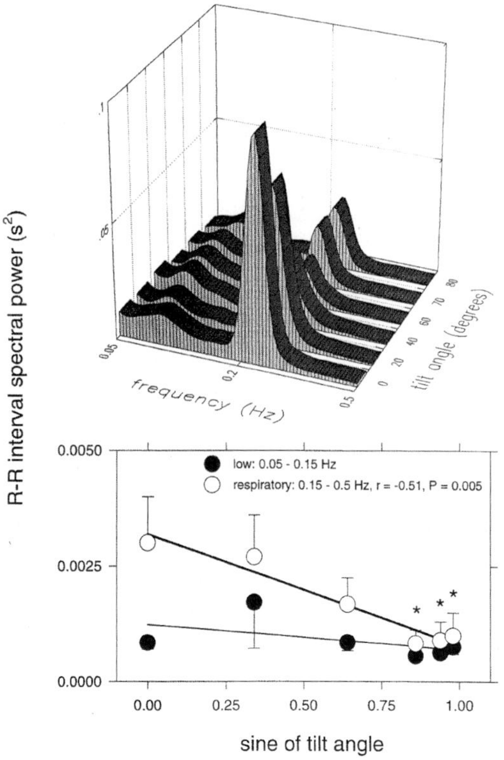

Fig. 4.8 Average *RR* interval power spectra from nine subjects tilted passively at different degrees. (Adapted from Cooke *et al.* 1999, with permission.)

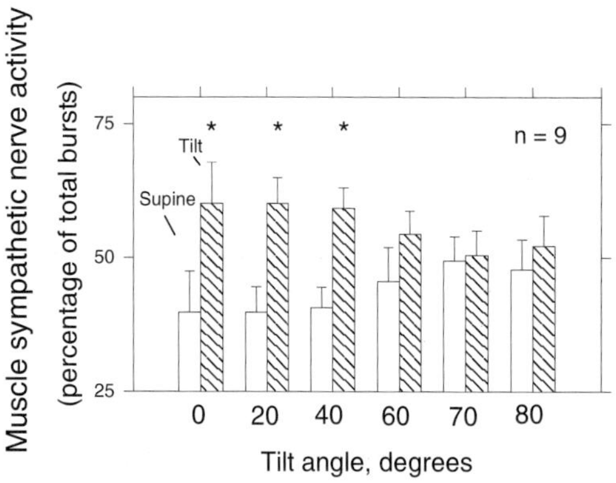

Fig. 4.7 Average inspiratory (clear bars) and expiratory muscle sympathetic nerve activity of nine subjects at various angles of upright tilt. * *P* ″ 0.05, supine vs. tilt. (Adapted from Cooke *et al.* 1999, with permission.)

(Yates & Miller 1994), reductions of respiratory sinus arrhythmia in response to tilt, are consistent with simple baroreflex physiology. As mentioned, respiration rhythmically modulates the susceptibility of vagal motoneurones to baroreceptor stimulation (Eckberg & Orshan 1977; Eckberg *et al.* 1980, 1985; Gilbey *et al.* 1984). The reductions of respiratory sinus arrhythmia with tilt shown in Fig. 4.8, may reflect simply the reductions of baroreceptor stimulation that occur.

Reduction of respiratory sinus arrhythmia with reduction of baroreceptor stimulation was documented originally in 1936 by Anrep, Pascual & Rössler, who reported that the magnitude of vagally mediated peak minus valley *RR* interval fluctuations depends critically on the level of arterial pressure, and that reductions of arterial pressure reduce respiratory-frequency *RR* interval fluctuations. Their study also made an important point that is not illustrated by Fig. 4.8, that the ability of respiration to gate responsiveness of vagal-cardiac motoneurones is finite, such that increases of baroreceptor stimulation to high levels also abolish respiratory sinus arrhythmia. We confirmed this observation in humans, by showing that vagal responses to intense baroreceptor stimulation with neck suction (Eckberg & Orshan 1977) are equal in inspiration and expiration. Goldberger *et al.* (1994) also confirmed Anrep's observations in humans with pharmacological arterial pressure elevations.

Figure 4.8 also illustrates *RR* interval fluctuations at low (~0.10 Hz) frequencies. Low frequency power did not change significantly in proportion to the angle of tilt. This result was surprising, and was even counter-intuitive. Low-frequency *RR* interval changes are thought to reflect baroreflex physiology importantly (Parlow *et al.* 1995; Parati *et al.* 1995). The net level of arterial baroreceptor stimulation declines progressively during tilt. If upright tilt carries subjects from the linear to the threshold portions of their sigmoid baroreceptor–cardiac reflex relations (Eckberg 1980), vagal baroreflex gain and low-frequency *RR* interval fluctuations should diminish.

Absolute levels (Iwase *et al.* 1987), however, and fluctuations (Cooke *et al.* 1999) of sympathetic nerve activity increase progressively with upright tilt. Since sympathetic stimulation opposes vagal inhibition (Taylor *et al.* 2001), vagally mediated *RR* interval fluctuations could be reduced. On the other hand, episodic sympathetic stimulation could directly (and periodically, Fig. 4.5) stimulate the sinoatrial node and thereby increase low frequency *RR* interval fluctuations. These two factors may neutralize each other during tilt, with the net result that progressive upright tilt provokes no change of *RR* interval spectral power (Fig. 4.8, lower panel). A third possible explanation for absence of change of low frequency *RR* interval spectral power is that *RR* interval fluctuations do not necessarily reflect vagal and sympathetic influences equally. In 1935, Samaan reported that vagal activity is prepotent in modulating sinus node function; the presence of any vagal activity neutralizes sympathetic influences. One practical implication of responses to upright tilt is that (absolute) low-frequency *RR* interval fluctuations cannot be taken as simple quantitative indicators of sympathetic activity. It is only when low-frequency spectral power is divided by respiratory-frequency spectral power that low- ('normalized') frequency spectral power becomes an index of sympathetic nerve traffic (Pagani *et al.* 1988). The propriety of this mathematical treatment has been challenged (Eckberg 1997).

Pharmacological blockade

It is an utterly simple matter to give human volunteers drugs that block the effects of released neurotransmitters or circulating hormones. That said, drugs exert complex effects, which are understood imperfectly. In this chapter, I take a simple approach to changes provoked by autonomic drugs. I assume that β-adrenergic blockade opposes adrenergic receptor responses to β-adrenergic stimulation. Cholinergic blockade with atropine sulphate is more complex. Vagal-cardiac nerve traffic increases in proportion to increasing doses of atropine (Katona *et al.* 1977). However, the central vagal-cardiac motoneurone stimulating effects of atropine are seen only at low doses; at high doses, the peripheral blocking effects override the central stimulating effects and cause tachycardia. Cardioacceleration depends on the presence of vagal-cardiac nerve traffic, since intravenous atropine does not alter the sinoatrial rate of transplanted human hearts (Epstein *et al.* 1990). Therefore, I assume simply that large dose atropine blocks the effects of neurally released acetylcholine on the sinoatrial node.

Taylor *et al.* (2001) gave injections of saline, the hydrophilic β-adrenergic receptor blocker, atenolol, and the muscarinic-blocker, atropine sulphate, to supine healthy subjects who breathed at a wide range of controlled frequencies. Average measurements are shown in Fig. 4.9. This figure illustrates several important features of human rhythms. First, as discussed, breathing frequency influences the degree of *RR* interval fluctuations. Respiratory fluctuations are small at the most rapid breathing, 0.25 Hz (one breath every 4 s), and large at slower breathing frequencies. Cholinergic blockade with atropine nearly abolished all fluctuations. β-Adrenergic receptor blockade [the cross-hatched area indicates the difference between control

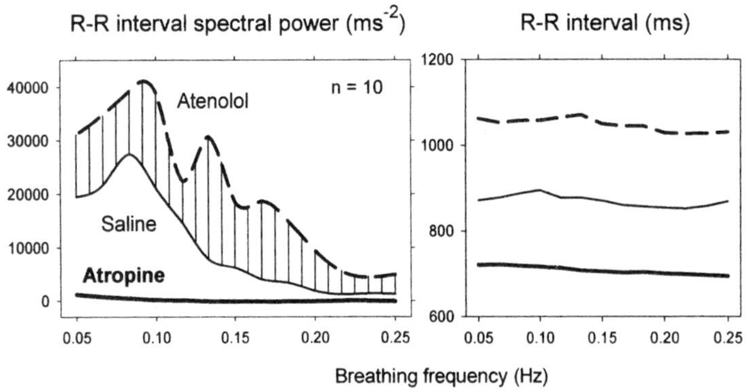

Fig. 4.9 Average *RR* interval power spectra from 10 subjects after saline, atenolol, and atrophine infusions. The stippled area indicates the increase of spectral power provoked by atenolol.

measurements (saline) and measurements after atenolol] augmented *RR* interval fluctuations. The right panel of Fig. 4.9 reinforces the observation (Seals *et al.* 1990; Brown *et al.* 1993) that breathing frequency does not alter net autonomic traffic to the human heart.

The data shown in Fig. 4.9 document a generally unrecognized aspect of human autonomic regulation, namely that sympathetic stimulation opposes vagal responses at all breathing frequencies, rapid as well as slow. There are at least three corollaries of this. First, rapid, respiratory-frequency rhythms are not the exclusive preserve of vagal fluctuations; their absolute level also reflects the degree of sympathetic damping. Second, the degree of sympathetic damping of vagal responses depends on the frequency of breathing. Damping is small at rapid breathing frequencies, and large at slower breathing frequencies, which allow more time for decay of sinus node responses to sympathetic stimulation (Wallin & Nerhed 1982). Third, measured (absolute) low-frequency *RR* interval fluctuations cannot be taken as indexes of sympathetic outflow; on the contrary, blockade of sympathetic effects augments and does not reduce low-frequency oscillations.

Conclusions

This review treats fluctuations of *RR* intervals, systolic pressures, and muscle sympathetic nerve activity, as they are altered by breathing, upright tilt, and autonomic blockade. *RR* interval fluctuations measured during brief recording periods, reflect primarily vagal-cardiac nerve traffic fluctuations, which are opposed by sympathetic stimulation at all breathing frequencies. Respiratory-frequency *RR* interval, systolic pressure, and muscle sympathetic nerve fluctuations derive from breathing; they are absent during apnoea. Respiratory activity does not alter low-frequency fluctuations of autonomic and haemodynamic outflows. The magnitude of *RR* interval fluctuations depends on breathing frequency: spectral power is low at rapid, and high at slow breathing frequencies. However, breathing rate over a wide range of breathing frequencies, does not influence net vagal-cardiac or sympathetic-muscle nerve traffic. Upright tilt, which reduces the level of baroreceptor stimulation, systematically decreases mean levels and fluctuations of *RR* intervals, and increases mean levels and fluctuations of muscle sympathetic nerve activity. Upright tilt does not alter low-frequency *RR* interval fluctuations. Simple recordings of human *RR* intervals, systolic pressure, and muscle sympathetic nerve activity, interpreted judiciously, provide important information regarding human neurophysiological mechanisms.

References

Anrep, G.V., Pascual, W. & Rössler, R. (1936) Respiratory variations of the heart rate. I – The reflex mechanism of the respiratory arrhythmia. *Proceedings of the Royal Society of London B Biological Sciences*, **119**, 191–217.

Badra, L.J., Cooke, W.H., Hoag, J.B. *et al.* (2001) Respiratory modulation of human autonomic rhythms. *American Journal of Physiology*, **280**, H2674–H2688.

Baselli, G., Cerutti, S., Badilini, F. *et al.* (1994) Model for the assessment of heart period and arterial pressure variability interactions and respiration influences. *Medical & Biological Enginering & Computing*, **32**, 143–152.

Borst, C., van Brederode, J.F.M., Wieling, W. *et al.* (1984) Mechanisms of initial blood pressure response to postural change. *Clinical Science*, **67**, 321–327.

Brown, T.E., Beightol, L.A., Koh, J. *et al.* (1993) Important influence of respiration on human *RR* interval power spectra is largely ignored. *Journal of Applied Physiology*, **75**, 2310–2317.

Cooke, W.H., Hoag, J.B., Crossman, A.A. *et al.* (1999) Human responses to upright tilt: a window on central autonomic integration. *Journal of Physiology*, **517**, 617–628.

De Boer, R.W., Karemaker, J.M. & Strackee, J. (1985) Relationships between short-term blood-pressure fluctuations and heart-rate variability in resting subjects 1: a spectral analysis approach. *Medical & Biological Engineering & Computing*, **23**, 352–358.

Eckberg, D.L. (1980) Nonlinearities of the human carotid baroreceptor-cardiac reflex. *Circulation Research*, **47**, 208–216.

Eckberg, D.L. (1997) Sympathovagal balance. A critical appraisal. *Circulation*, **96**, 3224–3232.

Eckberg, D.L. (2003) The human respiratory gate. *Journal of Physiology*, **548**, 339–352.

Eckberg, D.L., Kifle, Y.T. & Roberts, V.L. (1980) Phase relationship between normal human respiration and baroreflex responsiveness. *Journal of Physiology*, **304**, 489–502.

Eckberg, D.L., Nerhed, C. & Wallin, B.G. (1985) Respiratory modulation of muscle sympathetic and vagal cardiac outflow in man. *Journal of Physiology*, **365**, 181–196.

Eckberg, D.L. & Orshan, C.R. (1977) Respiratory and baroreceptor reflex interactions in man. *Journal of Clinical Investigation*, **59**, 780–785.

Epstein, A.E., Hirschowitz, B.I., Kirklin, J.K. *et al.* (1990) Evidence for a central site of action to explain the negative chronotropic effect of atropine: studies on the human transplanted heart. *Journal of the American College of Cardiology*, **15**, 1610–1617.

Gilbey, M.P., Jordan, D., Richter, D.W. *et al.* (1984) Synaptic mechanisms involved in the inspiratory modulation of vagal cardio-inhibitory neurones in the cat. *Journal of Physiology*, **356**, 65–78.

Goldberger, J.J., Ahmed, M.W., Parker, M.A. *et al.* (1994) Dissociation of heart rate variability from parasympathetic tone. *American Journal of Physiology*, **266**, H2152-H2157.

Imholz, B.P.M., Wieling, W., van Montfrans, G.A. *et al.* (1998) Fifteen years experience with finger arterial pressure monitoring: assessment of the technology. *Cardiovascular Research*, **38**, 605–616.

Iwase, S., Mano, T. & Saito, M. (1987) Effects of graded head-up tilting on muscle sympathetic activities in man. *The Physiologist*, **30** (Suppl.), S62–S65.

Katona, P.G. & Jih, F. (1975) Respiratory sinus arrhythmia: noninvasive measure of parasympathetic cardiac control. *Journal of Applied Physiology*, **39**, 801–805.

Katona, P.G., Lipson, D. & Dauchot, P.J. (1977) Opposing central and peripheral effects of atropine on parasympathetic cardiac control. *American Journal of Physiology*, **232**, H146-H151.

Katona, P.G., Poitras, J.W., Barnett, G.O. *et al.* (1970) Cardiac vagal efferent activity and heart period in the carotid sinus reflex. *American Journal of Physiology*, **218**, 1030–1037.

Kocsis, B., Fedina, L., Gyimesi-Pelczer, K. *et al.* (1993) Differential sympathetic reactions during cerebral ischaemia in cats: the role of the desynchronised nerve discharge. *Journal of Physiology*, **469**, 37–50.

Lenfant, C. (1967) Time-dependent variations of pulmonary gas exchange in normal man at rest. *Journal of Applied Physiology*, **22**, 675–684.

Lopes, O.U. & Palmer, J.F. (1976) Proposed respiratory 'gating' mechanism for cardiac slowing. *Nature (London)* **264**, 454–456.

Morillo, C.A., Eckberg, D.L., Ellenbogen, K.A. *et al.* (1997) Vagal and sympathetic mechanisms in patients with orthostatic vasovagal syncope. *Circulation*, **96**, 2509–2513.

Pagani, M., Somers, V., Furlan, R. *et al.* (1988) Changes in autonomic regulation induced by physical training in mild hypertension. *Hypertension*, **12**, 600–610.

Parati, G., Saul, J.P., DiRienzo, M. *et al.* (1995) Spectral analysis of blood pressure and heart rate variability in evaluating cardiovascular regulation. A critical appraisal. *Hypertension*, **25**, 1276–1286.

Parlow, J., Viale, J.-P., Annat, G. *et al.* (1995) Spontaneous cardiac baroreflex in humans. Comparison with drug-induced responses. *Hypertension*, **25**, 1058–1068.

Samaan, A. (1935) The antagonistic cardiac nerves and heart rate. *Journal of Physiology*, **83**, 332–340.

Seals, D.R., Suwarno, N.O. & Dempsey, J.A. (1990) Influence of lung volume on sympathetic nerve discharge in normal humans. *Circulation Research*, **67**, 130–141.

Taylor, J.A., Myers, C.W., Halliwill, J.R. *et al.* (2001) Sympathetic restraint of respiratory sinus arrhythmia: implications for assessment of vagal-cardiac tone in humans. *American Journal of Physiology*, **280**, H2808–H2814.

Wallin, B.G. & Nerhed, C. (1982) Relationship between spontaneous variations of muscle sympathetic activity and succeeding changes of blood pressure in man. *Journal of the Autonomic Nervous System*, **6**, 293–302.

Yates, B.J. & Miller, A.D. (1994) Properties of sympathetic reflexes elicited by natural vestibular stimulation: implications for cardiovascular control. *Journal of Neurophysiology*, **71**, 2087–2092.

CHAPTER 5

Physiological Understanding of HRV Components

Federico Lombardi

Introduction

Heart rate variability (HRV) analysis is a noninvasive technique that can provide an evaluation of autonomic modulation of sinus node in normal subjects and in patients with different cardiac and noncardiac diseases. It can also facilitate the identification of patients at risk for an increased cardiac mortality (Malik & Camm 1995; Camm *et al.* 1996).

Since the initial report of Wolf and co-workers (1978), many computation modalities have been developed to extract information from the variability signal and nowadays we have the possibility to select a variety of options ranging from simple statistical descriptors to complex nonlinear mathematical parameters (Malik & Camm 1995; Camm *et al.* 1996).

A comprehensive review of the literature reveals, however, that in spite of a solid evidence regarding the prognostic value of almost all time, frequency and nonlinear parameters of HRV as predictors of arrhythmic and total cardiac mortality (Wolf *et al.* 1978; Kleiger *et al.* 1987; Bigger *et al.*1988; Farrel *et al.* 1991; Malliani *et al.* 1991; Malik & Camm 1995; Camm *et al.* 1996; Fauchier *et al.* 1997; La Rovere *et al.* 1998; Nolan *et al.* 1998), our understanding of the physiological significance of HRV components is far from being complete. Several factors have been identified as possible confounders. The complexity of the relationship between neural input, neurotransmitter release and sinus node pacemaking properties; the differences in results obtained in normal healthy subjects in comparison to patients with left ventricular dysfunction; the different interpretation of parameters measured on short-term recordings obtained under controlled condition in comparison to those obtained when considering 24-h ambulatory recordings; and the modest effects on HRV parameters of those pharmacological intervention known to affect autonomic modulation of sinus node, are, in my opinion the most relevant and will be briefly discussed.

Time-domain and geometrical parameters

It is generally accepted that overall variability is substantially dependent on vagal modulation, with respiratory arrhythmia and nocturnal slowing of the heart beat being two of the major determinants of HRV magnitude (Malik & Camm 1995; Camm *et al.* 1996). As a consequence, a reduction of SDNN (but the same concept is applicable to the interpretation of reduction in the geometrical triangular index) has been considered to reflect an alteration of the physiological balance between sympathetic and vagal activities consisting in a diminished vagal and an increased sympathetic modulation of sinus node (Wolf *et al.* 1978; Kleiger *et al.* 1987; Bigger *et al.* 1988; Farrel *et al.* 1991; Malliani *et al.* 1991; Malik & Camm 1995; Camm *et al.* 1996; Fauchier *et al.* 1997; La Rovere *et al.* 1998; Nolan *et al.* 1998). This interpretation is well in keeping not only with the experimental evidence indicating a proarrhythmic effect of sympathoexcitation (Lown & Verrier 1976, Schwartz *et al.* 1992) but also with the findings that a reduction of these parameters is capable of identifying patients with an increased cardiac mortality

(Malik & Camm 1995; Camm *et al.* 1996; Kleiger *et al.* 1987; Bigger *et al.*1988; Farrel *et al.* 1991, Fauchier *et al.* 1997; Nolan *et al.* 1998; La Rovere *et al.* 1998). The finding (Camm *et al.* 1996) that time-domain parameters were inversely correlated with ejection fraction, made clear that the causes of reduction of HRV indices and the interpretation of their predictive value were more complex than predicted and involved additional non-neural mechanisms.

One of the principal elements of support of the concept that a reduced HRV reflected a diminished vagal tone was the supposed linearity of the input–output relationship (neural discharge–cycle length) at sinus node level (Rocchetti *et al.* 2000; Zaza & Lombardi 2001). According to this hypothesis, a reduction in HRV had to be expected whenever vagal activity decreased. The effects of changes in sympathetic activation on cycle length variability were instead, less predictable and required a more complex explanation. Recent experimental findings (Rocchetti *et al.* 2000; Zaza & Lombardi 2001), however, indicate that neural modulation of cycle length is probably not linear, with, for example, a greater effect of acetylcholine at longer cardiac cycle. As a result time-domain parameters may exhibit an intrinsic rate dependency that complicates the assessment of autonomic tone particularly when comparing HRV parameters of subjects without considering their heart rate values.

The issue is further confounded because several non-neural factors could directly affect cycle length variability therefore mimicking or masking changes in autonomic activity (Zaza & Lombardi 2001). The faster kinetics of acetylcholine-mediated effects in comparison to noradrenaline, the direct effect of cycle length prolongation and the drug-induced changes on sinus node cell depolarization threshold, are only a few examples.

The interpretation of time-domain HRV parameters is even more complicated in patients with marked depression of ventricular function and clinical and humoral evidence of a persistent adrenergic activation. The extreme reduction in SDNN or triangular index in patients is likely to reflect both an abnormal autonomic modulation and an alteration of the transduction properties at sinus node level (Lombardi & Mortara 1998).

An additional aspect related to the significance of HRV parameters that deserves consideration is the finding that in most studies, time-domain measures of HRV have been effective in predicting, to a similar extent, arrhythmic and nonarrhythmic mortality of patients with coronary artery disease or heart failure. It is self evident that neural and non-neural mechanisms play a different role for deaths resulting from ventricular fibrillation or pump failure, but patients at high risk present similar HRV patterns.

Nevertheless, in the clinical setting time-domain parameters provide a suitable broad evaluation of the integrity of autonomic control mechanisms and evaluate more precisely the physiological responsiveness of the sinus node to autonomic modulation. Cut-off values of <70 ms for SDNN and of <20 u. for the triangular index are commonly used and proven to be effective for identifying patients at risk (Malik & Camm 1995; Camm *et al.* 1996).

Frequency-domain parameters

The possibility of identifying periodic oscillations in the HRV signal and correlating these oscillatory patterns to the neural discharge of sympathetic and vagal fibres directed to the heart has promoted the application of spectral techniques to HRV analysis (Akselrod *et al.* 1981; Pagani *et al.* 1986; Malliani *et al.* 1991; Malik & Camm 1995; Camm *et al.* 1996). It is generally accepted that two major oscillatory components corresponding to respiratory arrhythmia (high frequency (HF) component; ~0.25 Hz) and to a lower frequency (LF) rhythm (~0.10 Hz) are detectable in normal subjects under controlled conditions. The HF component is considered to directly reflect the vagally mediated respiratory effects on cycle length. This is easily demonstrated by shifting the central frequency of this component to the left or right by reducing or increasing the respiratory rate, respectively. Respiration, however, also affects cardiovascular dynamics that in turn may produce non-neural effects on sinus node function. The interpretation of LF as an index of sympathetic modulation is more complex as the power and centre frequency of LF is sensitive to various factors that complicate its physiological interpretation (Pagani *et al.* 1986; Malliani *et al.* 1991; Malik & Camm 1995;

Camm *et al.* 1996). In normal subjects under control conditions, the increase in LF component can be correlated with the extent of the reflex sympathetic activation induced by progressive augmentation of the tilting angle (Montano *et al.* 1994). In contrast, during physical exercise an increase in LF component can be detected only in the initial phases, while during strenuous exercise at fast heart rates, the characteristic constituents of the autospectrum are a drastic reduction of total power, a relatively predominant respiration related HF component and an important very low frequency (VLF) component (Pagani *et al.* 1986; Furlan *et al.* 1993; Malik & Camm 1995; Camm *et al.* 1996).

It is important to recall, however, that a LF rhythmicity can be recorded in the pattern of discharge of sympathetic fibres both in humans and in experimental animals. Using microneurographic techniques it has been possible to record muscle sympathetic activity and to correlate the LF component of neural discharge with the LF component of *RR* interval and systolic arterial pressure variability (Furlan *et al.* 2000). In cats, we reported (Montano *et al.* 1992) the presence of LF and HF rhythmicity in the pattern of discharge of both sympathetic and vagal fibres directed to the heart and observed a correlation between changes in the amplitude of the LF component of sympathetic discharge and the LF component of *RR* interval variability during experimental interventions capable of a reflex increase or reduction of sympathetic discharge.

The interpretation of the LF component as an index of sympathetic modulation is even more complex when considering the spectral analysis of short-term recordings in patients with an acute myocardial infarction (Lombardi *et al.* 1987;.Malik & Camm 1995; Camm *et al.* 1996; Lombardi *et al.* 1996a). In subjects with a preserved ventricular function, a predominant LF component is commonly observed (Lombardi *et al.* 1987, 1996c). In patients with a complicated myocardial infarction and signs of left ventricular dysfunction, the spectral profile is markedly different, being characterized by a reduction of total power, a fast heart rate, a small or even undetectable LF, a partially preserved HF and a predominant VLF component. In these patients, a fast resting heart rate and several clinical signs indicate the presence of sympatho-excitation (Lombardi *et al.* 1996a).

All the above findings suggest that the LF component cannot be considered an absolute measure of sympathetic activity as the amount of oscillation within this frequency band is the result of several neural and non-neural factors that may vary in individual patients and within specific cardiac and noncardiac disease. The same concept may apply to the interpretation of the HF component. This point is even more important when considering spectral analysis of 24 h recording, where LF and HF components account for <10% of total power and where changes in the power of individual bands parallel changes in total power and SDNN rather than reflecting a distinct alteration in autonomic control (Malik & Camm 1995; Camm *et al.* 1996).

To facilitate an appraisal of autonomic modulation based on the analysis of the reciprocal balance between LF and HF power independently of their absolute value, the ratio between LF and HF as an index of sympatho-vagal interaction has been proposed (Pagani *et al.* 1986; Malliani *et al.* 1991). This parameter is appropriate for exploring autonomic control of the sinus node during experimental interventions that are also capable of producing reflex sympathetic or vagal activation in the presence of significant changes in the variability signals. It was also effective for studying autonomic control in those clinical conditions associated with an increased sympathetic and reduced vagal modulation of sinus node such as, for example, the acute phase of myocardial infarction (Lombardi *et al.* 1987; Lombardi *et al.* 1996a,b) or the initial phases of heart failure (Malliani *et al.* 1991; Malik & Camm 1995; Camm *et al.* 1996; Lombardi & Mortara 1998). In these patients, values of LF/HF ratio >2 were considered to reflect a shift of sympatho-vagal balance toward a sympathetic predominance, whereas values <2 were considered to reflect a more physiological condition. Also, for LF/HF ratio, as for LF and HF components, however, it was evident that the physiological interpretation was progressively more problematic when moving from short-term to 24-h recordings or from normal subjects under controlled conditions to patients with a marked depression of ventricular function and tachycardia. In most of these subjects, in spite of clinical signs of sympathetic activation, a reduction rather than an increase in LF/HF ratio could be observed, and, of note, it was possible to correlate the reduction in LF/HF ratio with an increased cardiac mortality (Malik & Camm 1995; Camm *et al.* 1996; Lombardi & Mortara 1998). The mechanisms responsible for such a finding are not established and different factors, including an altered central pattern of discharge at vasomotor centres, a loss of rhythmicity in the excited sympathetic outflow, a reduced responsiveness of sinus node to neural inputs, have been advocated without, however, definitive data (Lombardi 2002).

It is interesting to note that, when considering spectral analysis of 24-h recording of healthy subjects and patients with different levels of severity of cardiac disease, a progressive increase in the relative power of VLF becomes evident. We therefore advanced the hypothesis of a shift toward the left of the energy spectral distribution within the frequency axis along with the progression of the disease, i.e. that the central frequencies of the sympathetic related component LF might shift toward the VLF frequency band. Even though the mechanisms responsible for such a change cannot be defined, it is reasonable to presume that a decrease in the frequencies of oscillations of autonomic modulatory activities during a process of deterioration of cardiac function and a diminished responsiveness of sinus node pace-making properties might contribute to this phenomenon. Preliminary observations (Milicevic & Lombardi, unpublished data) in patients with different levels of clinical and humeral signs of sympathetic activation seem to support this hypothesis: a leftward shift of spectral energy distribution was correlated with lower ejection fraction and SDNN values.

A careful review of the different parameters used to analyse sympatho-vagal balance in the clinical setting, has been recently published by J. J. Goldberger (1999) who evaluated heart rate, HRV and a new index termed vagal-sympathetic effect (VSE), which was defined as the ratio of the *RR* interval to the intrinsic *RR* interval. In normal subjects, the performance of *RR* interval and VSE was superior to traditional spectral parameters to reflect the changes in expected directions with parasympathetic and sympathetic stimulation and blockade. The difficulty of obtaining VSE in the clinical setting and in particular in large patients' populations made the author to conclude that *RR* interval had to be still considered the most suitable index of sympatho-vagal balance.

In conclusion, spectral analysis of HRV must be restricted to short-term recordings under controlled conditions in order to measure more correctly and to interpret more safely LF and HF components. When associated with continuous recording of arterial pressure and of respiratory activity (Pagani *et al.* 1986; Parati *et al.* 1988; Camm *et al.* 1996; Lombardi & Parati 2000), spectral analysis offers the unique opportunity of evaluating the effects of arterial pressure changes on heart period as well as of heart period changes on arterial pressure under either control conditions or selective activation of reflexogenic areas. Unfortunately, such methodologies cannot be implemented in the general clinical practice as they require not only the development of adequate analysis programs but also the expertise of careful investigators.

For the moment, in order to better extract all the information contained in a 24-h Holter recording, it is recommended to start with a 15 min period of rest under controlled conditions followed by a normal recording procedure. The first segment will be suitable for an appropriate computation of LF and HF components and of LF/HF ratio, thus allowing a characterization of sympatho-vagal balance, the remaining long-term period could be analysed with traditional time-domain parameters for risk stratification.

Nonlinear dynamics

The appraisal of the complexity of the different neural and non-neural mechanisms impacting on the sinus node and determining HRV has stimulated the search for novel indexes capable of describing the complexity and the correlation properties of the *RR* interval signal rather than the magnitude of its variability (Saul *et al.* 1987; Malik & Camm 1995; Peng *et al.* 1995; Bigger *et al.* 1996; Camm *et al.* 1996; A. L. Goldberger 1996; Lombardi 2000).

Indices such as the exponent β (of $1/f$ slope) for long-term analysis (Saul *et al.* 1987; A. L.

Goldberger 1996) or the scaling exponent α for short-term recordings (Peng *et al.* 1995; A. L. Goldberger 1996) provide measures of presence or absence of fractal correlation properties of *RR* intervals at different time scales. Thus, changes in these parameters cannot be interpreted as a result of specific variations of the activity of the autonomic nervous system, but rather reflect the characteristics of heart rate behaviour and, in particular, its complexity which is dependent on the functional integrity of autonomic control mechanisms (A. L. Goldberger 1996; Lombardi 2000). In normal subjects the power-law slope is equal to −1 whereas in post myocardial infarction patients the slope becomes more steeper and therefore more negative (Malik & Camm 1995; Bigger *et al.* 1996; Camm *et al.* 1996; A. L. Goldberger 1996; Lombardi *et al.* 1996c; Lombardi 2000). The detrended fluctuation analysis technique quantifies the relations of heart rate fluctuations at different time scales. Values <1 correspond to dynamics where magnitude of short and long-term variability are similar, whereas values >1 indicate greater long-term variability (Peng *et al.* 1995).

These new indices and in particular the scaling exponent have been particularly effective in identifying patients at risk for sudden cardiac death (Huikuri *et al.* 2000). Recently, analysis of short-term fractal properties of HRV has been demonstrated as superior to conventional HRV measures in terms of prognostic value in predicting both arrhythmic and nonarrhythmic cardiac death in postmyocardial infarction patients (Lombardi *et al.* 2001).

In patients with an implantable cardioverter defibrillator, analysis of the storage electrograms revealed a further reduction of power-law slope of slow fluctuations in the minute preceding the onset of ventricular tachycardia in comparison to control conditions (Lombardi *et al.* 2000). In these patients a reduction in total power as well as an increase in LF component of HRV was also detectable. Thus, the minutes preceding the onset of ventricular tachycardia or fibrillation seems to be characterized not only by signs of sympathetic activation but also by a loss of the fractal-like characteristics of the variability signal. A reduction of fractal correlation properties has also been observed to precede ventricular fibrillation onset among patients who experienced this arrhythmia during Holter recordings (Makikallio *et al.* 1999).

Thus, the analysis of the nonlinear dynamics of HRV seems to provide important prognostic information that is not based on a specific autonomic pattern but on the final effects of the complex interaction between neural and non-neural factors and sinus node transduction properties. Also, if the role of autonomic modulation in determining the fractal-like characteristics of HRV is difficult to assess, the integrity of the physiological neural modulation of sinus node, which at spectral analysis is reflected by the presence of well detectable LF and HF, seems to be necessary to observe a high degree of complexity in the variability signal. In contrast, in patients with left ventricular dysfunction, faster heart rate and reduced HRV, the complexity of the variability signal tends to decrease with more negative values of both $1/f$ slope and fractal scaling exponent α.

Effects of pharmacological interventions

Among the factors that have limited a more comprehensive interpretation of the physiological meanings of HRV parameters, are the small effects of pharmacological interventions such as, for example, β-adrenergic receptor blockade (Malik & Camm 1995; Camm *et al.* 1996). In spite of numerous reports (Malik & Camm 1995; Camm *et al.* 1996) that have indicated group differences in relation to drug administration, it is impossible to evaluate the effects of pharmacological interventions on autonomic control by analysing the drug-induced changes in time or frequency domain parameters of HRV. The changes are often small and usually attributable to the rate dependence of most HRV parameters. Also in antiarrhythmic therapy the drug-induced changes are too small to be used to guide patients' management and are likely to reflect the complex interaction between drug effect on ventricular function, arterial pressure and pacemaking properties rather than a distinct change in sympatho-vagal interaction. This may explain why in general clinical practice the effects of drugs on HRV are not taken into consideration to determine pharmacological therapy.

A final aspect for discussion is the interpretation of HRV signals in patients with frequent premature ventricular contractions. The analysis of these recordings to obtain a *RR* interval time series suitable for a satisfactory analysis is often time consuming. In some instances, however, the selection of data is based on empirical and inadequately defined criteria. It is well known that premature ventricular or atrial beats affect computation of both time-domain parameters by increasing overall variability and LF and HF components by augmenting power in the high frequency range (Malik & Camm 1995; Camm *et al.* 1996; Lombardi 2002). However, it must be recalled that the compensatory pause following a premature ventricular beat is associated with a marked reflex activation of sympathetic outflow to the heart (Lombardi *et al.* 1989) that may exert its effect also in the adjacent sinus cycles. This phenomenon has recently been of interest and a new methodology called 'heart rate turbulence' (Schmidt *et al.* 1999) has been developed to analyse the pattern of changes of the sinus cycles that follow a compensatory pause. This methodology has been proven effective in identifying patients with an increased cardiac mortality after a myocardial infarction (Schmidt *et al.* 1999). It is therefore possible that the removal of those intervals adjacent to premature ventricular contraction might obscure some of the effects of autonomic modulation on *RR* interval time series thus limiting our appraisal of sympatho-excitation.

Conclusions

The incomplete understanding of the physiological meaning of HRV parameters is largely the result of the complexity of the autonomic modulation of the sinus node. The concept of sympatho-vagal balance is difficult to define specifically as it involves a variety of neural and non-neural factors impinging upon sinus node pace-making properties. Indeed both sympathetic and parasympathetic neural activities directed to the sinus node may be characterized by the number of impulses for each cardiac cycle and by the modulation of this activity by the excitatory or inhibitory influences of different cardiovascular reflexogenic areas.

Nevertheless, a reduction in HRV parameters and in particular of SDNN or the triangular index has been consistently proven effective in identifying patients with increased mortality in various cardiovascular diseases including coronary artery disease, hypertension and congestive heart failure. When considering short-term recording under controlled conditions, the LF/HF ratio is likely to reflect sympatho-vagal interaction without defining, however, the individual contribution of each of the two limbs of the autonomic nervous system. For example, it should be of great interest to know whether in a patients with fast heart rate and a reduced SDNN the sympathetic predominance were the result of a marked sympatho-excitation with a relatively normal parasympathetic tone or of a persistent inhibition of parasympathetic activity.

In conclusions, time-domain parameters should have a primary role as noninvasive stratifiers of patients with increased mortality. LF and HF components and LF/HF ratio measured on short-term recordings may be used as indices of autonomic modulation of sinus node, whereas nonlinear dynamics parameters may be considered the best noninvasive predictors of sudden cardiac death.

References

Akselrod, S., Gordon, D., Ubel, F.A., Shannon, D.C., Barger, A.C. & Cohen, R.J. (1981) Power spectrum analysis of heart rate fluctuation: a quantitative probe of beat-to-beat cardiovascular control. *Science*, **213**, 220–222.

Bigger, J.T., Jr, Kleiger, R.E., Fleiss, J.L., Rolnitzky, L.M., Steinman, R.C., Miller, J.P. & the Multicentre Pot-Infarction Research Group (1988) Components of heart rate variability measured during healing of acute myocardial infarction. *American Journal of Cardiology*, **61**, 208–215.

Bigger, J.T., Steinman, R.C., Rolnitzky, L., Fleiss, J.L., Albrecttht, P. & Cohen, R.J. (1996) Power law behaviour of *RR*-interval variability in healthy middle-aged persons, patients with recent acute myocardial infarction, and patients with heart transplants. *Circulation*, **21**, 2142–2151.

Camm, A.J., Malik, M., Bigger, J.T. *et al.* (1996) Task Force of the European Society of Cardiology and the North American Society of Pacing and Electrophysiology. Heart rate variability. Standards of measurement, physiological interpretation, and clinical use. *Circulation*, **93**, 1043–1065.

Farrell, T.G., Bashir, Y., Cripps, T. *et al.* (1991) Risk stratification for arrhythmic events in postinfarction patients based on heart rate variability, ambulatory electrocardiographic variables and signal averaged electrocardiogram. *Journal of the American College of Cardiology*, **18**, 687–697.

Fauchier, L., Babutj, D., Cosnay, P., Autret, M.L. & Fauchier, J.P. (1997) Heart rate variability in idiopathic dilated cardiomyopathy characteristics and prognostic value. *Journal of the American College of Cardiology*, **30**, 1009–1014.

Furlan, R., Piazza, S., Dell'Orto, S. *et al.* (1993) Early and late effects of exercise and athletic training on neural mechanisms controlling heart rate. *Cardiovascular Research*, **27**, 482–488.

Furlan, R., Porta, A., Costa, F. *et al.* (2000) Oscillatory patterns in sympathetic neural discharge and cardiovascular variables during orthostatic stimulus. *Circulation*, **10**, 886–892.

Goldberger, A.L. (1996) Non-linear dynamics for clinicians: chaos theory, fractals, and complexity at the bedside. *Lancet*, **347**, 1312–1314.

Goldberger, J.J. (1999) Sympatho-vagal balance: how should we measure it? *American Journal of Physiology*, **276**, H1273–H1280.

Huikuri, H.V., Makikallio, T.H., Peng, C.K., Golberger, A.L., Hintze, U. & Moller, M. for the Diamond Study Group (2000) Fractal correlation properties of *RR* interval dynamics and mortality in patients with depressed left ventricular function after an acute myocardial infarction. *Circulation*, **101**, 47–53.

Kleiger, R.E., Miller, J.P., Bigger, J.T., Moss, A.R & the Multicentre Post-Infarction Research Group (1987) Decreased heart rate variability and its association with increased mortality after acute myocardial infarction. *American Journal of Cardiology*, **59**, 256–262.

La Rovere, M.T., Bigger, J.T., Jr, Marcus, F.I., Mortara, A. & Schwartz, P.J. (1998) Baroreflex sensitivity and heart rate variability in prediction of total cardiac mortality after myocardial infarction. ATRAMI (Autonomic Tone and Reflexes After Myocardial Infarction) Investigators. *Lancet*, **351**, 478–84.

Lombardi, F. (2000) Chaos theory, heart rate variability and arrhythmic mortality. *Circulation*, **101**, 8–10.

Lombardi, F. (2002) Clinical implications of present physiological understanding of HRV components. *Cardiac Electrophysiology Review*, **6**, 245–249.

Lombardi, F., Gnecchi Ruscone, T. & Malliani, A. (1989) Premature ventricular contractions and reflex sympathetic activation in cats. *Cardiovascular Research*, **23**, 205–212.

Lombardi, F., Makikallio, T.H., Myerburg, R.J. & Huikuri, H.V. (2001) Sudden cardiac death: role of heart rate variability to identify patients at risk. *Cardiovascular Research*, **50**, 210–217.

Lombardi, F., Malliani, A., Pagani, M. & Cerutti, S. (1996a) Heart rate variability and its sympatho-vagal modulation. *Cardiovascular Research*, **32**, 208–216.

Lombardi, F. & Mortara, A.(1998) Heart rate variability and heart failure. *Heart*, **80**, 213–214.

Lombardi, F. & Parati G. (2000) Cardiovascular and respiratory changes during sleep in normal and hypertensive subjects. *Cardiovascular Research*, **45**, 200–211.

Lombardi, F., Porta, A., Marzegalli, M. *et al.*(2000) Heart rate variability patterns before ventricular tachycardia onset in patients with implantable cardioverter defibrillator. *American Journal Cardiology*, **86**, 959–963.

Lombardi, F., Sandrone, G., Mortara, A. *et al.* (1996b) Linear and nonlinear dynamics of heart rate variability after acute myocardial infarction with normal and reduced left ventricular ejection fraction. *American Journal of Cardiology*, **77**, 1283–1288.

Lombardi, F., Sandrone, G., Pernpruner S. *et al.* (1987) Heart rate variability as an index of sympatho-vagal interaction after acute myocardial infarction. *American Journal of Cardiology*, **60**, 1239–1245.

Lombardi, F., Sandrone, G., Spinnler, M.T. *et al.* (1996) Heart rate variability in the early hours of an acute myocardial infarction. *American Journal of Cardiology*, **77**, 1037–1044.

Lown, B. & Verrier, R.L. (1976) Neural activity and ventricular fibrillation. *New England Journal of Medicine*, **294**, 1165–1176.

Makikallio, T.H., Koistinen, J., Jordaens, L. *et al.* (1999) Heart rate dynamics before spontaneous onset of ventricular fibrillation in patients with healed myocardial infarcts. *American Journal of Cardiology*, **83**, 880–884.

Malik, M. & Camm, A.J. (eds) (1995) *Heart Rate Variability*. Futura, Armonk, NY.

Malliani, A., Pagani, M., Lombardi, F. & Cerutti, S. (1991) Cardiovascular neural regulation explored in the frequency domain. *Circulation*, **84**, 482–492.

Montano, N., Gnecchi Ruscone, T., Porta, A., Lombardi, F., Pagani, M. & Malliani A. (1992) Power spectrum analysis of heart rate variability to assess the changes in sympatho-vagal balance during graded orthostatic tilt. *Circulation*, **90**, 1826–1831.

Nolan, J., Batin, P.D., Andrews, R. *et al.* (1998) Prospective study of heart rate variability and mortality in chronic heart failure. Results of the United Kingdom Heart Failure Evaluation and Assessment of Risk Trial (UK-Heart). *Circulation*, **98**, 1510–1516.

Pagani, M., Lombardi, F., Guzzetti, S. *et al.* (1986) Power spectral analysis of heart rate and arterial pressure variabilities as a marker of sympatho-vagal interaction in man and conscious dog. *Circulation Research*, **59**, 178–193.

Parati, G., Di Rienzo, M., Bertinieri, G. *et al.* (1988) Evaluation of the baroreceptor heart rate reflex by 24 h intra-arterial blood pressure monitoring in humans. *Hypertension*, **12**, 214–222.

Peng, C.K., Havlin, S., Stanley, H.E. & Goldberger, A.L.

(1995) Quantification of scaling exponents and crossover phenomena in nonstationary heartbeat time series. *Chaos*, **5**, 82–87.

Rocchetti, M., Malfatto, G., Lombardi, F. & Zaza, A. (2000). Role of the input/output relation of sinoatrial myocites in cholinergic modulation of heart rate variability. *Journal of Cardiovascular Electrophysiology*, **11**, 522–530.

Saul, J.P., Albrecht, P., Berger, R.D. & Cohen, R.J. (1987) Analysis of long-term heart rate variability: methods, 1/*f* scaling and implications. In: *Computers in Cardiology*, pp. 419–422. IEEE Computer Society Press, Silver Spring, MD.

Schmidt, G., Malik, M. & Barthel, P.(1999) Heart rate turbulence after ventricular premature beats as a predictor of mortality after acute myocardial infarction. *Lancet*, **353**, 1390–1396.

Schwartz, P.J., La Rovere, M.T. & Vanoli, E. (1992) Autonomic nervous system and sudden cardiac death: experimental basis and clinical observations for post-myocardial infarction risk stratification. *Circulation*, **85**, I77–I91.

Wolf, M.M., Varigos, G.A., Hunt, D. & Sloman, J.G. (1978) Sinus arrhythmia in acute myocardial infarction. *Medical Journal of Australia*, **2**, 52–53.

Zaza, A. & Lombardi, F. (2001) Autonomic indexes based on the analysis of heart rate variability: a view from the sinus node. *Cardiovascular Research*, **50**, 434–442.

CHAPTER 6

Autonomic Balance

Alberto Malliani and Nicola Montano

Introduction

General concepts are often quite useful in biology, although sometimes rather broad and difficult to quantify. It is the case of homeostasis (Cannon 1932) that proposing stability as an attribute of life ignores its continuous relationship with instability which, in a given range, is as necessary to develop various behaviours. In the field of cardiovascular neural regulation the concept of sympatho-vagal balance, or autonomic balance, may also appear quite elusive. Conversely it is the purpose of this chapter to summarize some experimental evidence that may support the view that this general concept is a tool useful for thinking and for investigating (Malliani 1999; Malliani 2000).

The balance

The neural regulation of circulatory function is mainly effected through the interplay of the sympathetic and vagal outflows. In most physiological conditions, the activation of either sympathetic or vagal outflow is accompanied by the inhibition of the other (therefore the concept of balance, as a horizontal beam pivoted at its centre). This is true for reflexes arising predominantly not only from the arterial baroreceptive areas but also from the heart. For instance, the stimulation of cardiac sympathetic afferents induces reflex sympathetic excitation and vagal inhibition, whereas the opposite effect is elicited by stimulating cardiac vagal afferents; this reciprocal reflex organization, alluding to a synergistic design, was demonstrated by recording the activity of single sympathetic or vagal efferent fibres isolated from the same mixed nerve impinging upon the heart (Schwartz *et al.* 1973). However, the most persuasive argument in favour of the concept of sympatho-vagal balance is the fact that sympathetic excitation and simultaneous vagal inhibition, or vice versa, are both presumed to contribute to the increase or decrease of cardiac performance to implement various behaviours.

The sympatho-vagal balance is tonically and phasically modulated by the interaction of at least three major factors: central neural integration, peripheral inhibitory reflex mechanisms (with negative feedback characteristics), and peripheral excitatory reflex mechanisms (with positive feedback characteristics) (Malliani *et al.* 1991; Fig. 6.1). Some dialectic interaction of opposite mechanisms appears indeed as another general principle in biology. It is the case of coagulation and anticoagulation, of endocrine interactions, and quite evidently, of flexor and extensor tonic or phasic actions. The point is that any regulated variable can be better modulated with two opposing mechanisms rather than with a single one (as in the traditional view of only negative feedback mechanisms regulating the circulatory function) (Malliani 2000). This concept of reciprocity has furnished us the key to interpret part of the complex features characterizing the analysis of heart rate variability (HRV) in the frequency domain. We believe, on the other hand, that the heuristic value of this approach has been fully demonstrated by the results that we briefly summarize in this chapter.

Experimental findings

The power spectrum of HRV of a normal subject in supine resting conditions is always characterized by three components. In the case represented in the left part of Fig. 6.2, obtained with an autoregressive algorithm (Pagani *et al.* 1986; Malliani *et al.* 1991) from a time series of 200

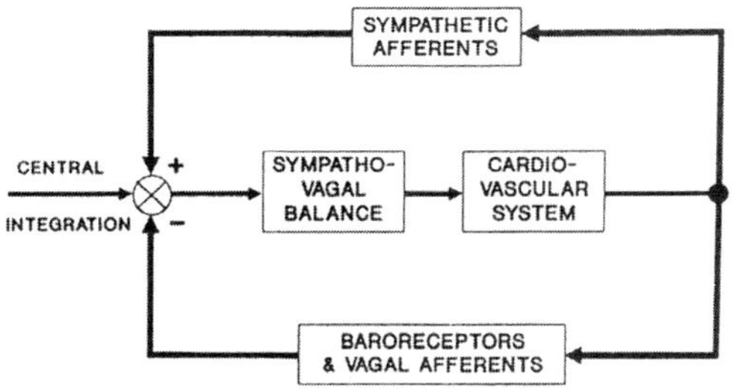

Fig. 6.1 Schematic representation of opposing feedback mechanisms that, in addition to central integration, subserve neural control of the cardiovascular system. Baroreceptive and vagal afferent fibres from the cardiopulmonary region mediate negative feedback mechanisms (exciting the vagal outflow and inhibiting the sympathetic outflow), whereas positive feedback mechanisms are mediated by sympathetic afferent fibres (exciting the sympathetic outflow and inhibiting the vagal outflow). (From Malliani *et al.* 1991, with permission.)

beats, three components are evident: a high frequency (HF) at 0.33 Hz, corresponding to respiratory activity, a low frequency (LF) at 0.09 Hz, usually corresponding to vasomotor waves, and a very low frequency (VLF) around 0 Hz. Under normal conditions, the VLF component cannot be properly assessed with short time series but only with longer periods of uninterrupted data. In the upright position (right part of Fig. 6.2), obtained with either active standing or passive up-tilt manoeuvre, the spectral profile is drastically modified as a rule, leading to a predominance or increasing the predominance of LF. Since our initial observations (Brovelli *et al.* 1983) we hypothesized that this change in spectral profile was alluding to a similar shift likely to occur in the *sympatho*-vagal balance. To test this hypothesis, however, the first crucial step was that of quantifying the spectral components in an appropriate way. In the case of Fig. 6.2, the upright position is accompanied by a marked predominance of LF which is, however, decreased in its absolute value as a result of the simultaneous drastic reduction of variance. Therefore, because the absolute values of spec-

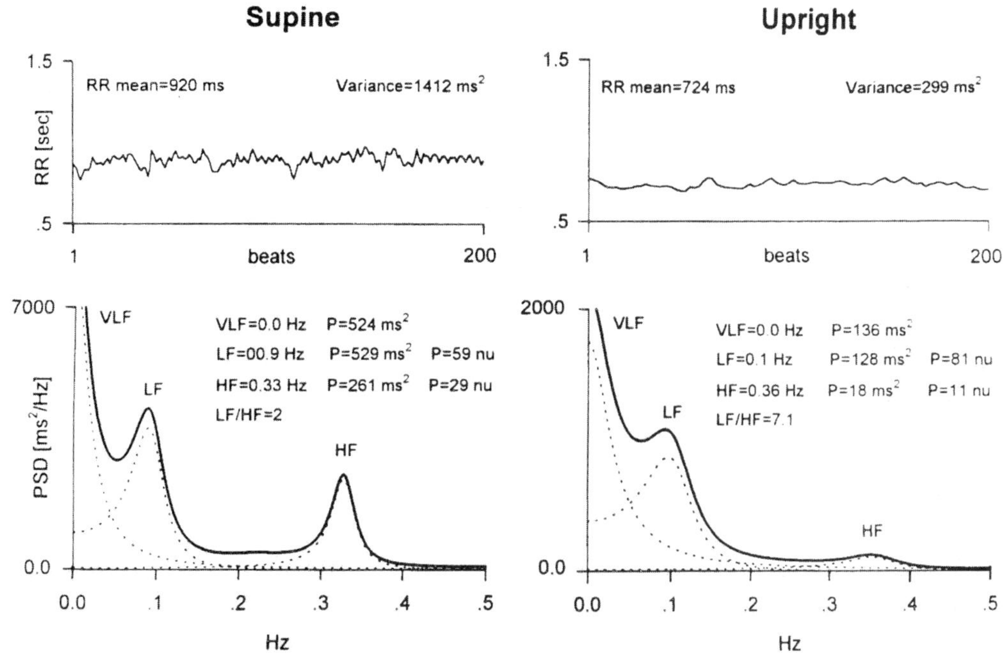

Fig. 6.2 Top: *RR* interval series (tachogram) of a healthy subject in supine and upright (passive 90° tilt) positions. Bottom: power spectrum autoregressive analysis (note 2 different scales). The power of each component (spectral decomposition) is indicated by dotted lines. PSD, power spectral density; VLF, very low frequency; LF, low frequency; HF, high frequency. For other details, see text. (From Malliani *et al.* 1997, with permission.)

tral components are highly correlated to variance (corresponding to total power), some further indexes focusing mainly on the fractional, or relative, distribution of power and independent of the absolute values of variance also seemed to be necessary. This was accomplished by calculating the LF/HF ratio or LF and HF in normalized units (nu) (Pagani *et al.* 1986; Malliani *et al.* 1991). Normalized units are obtained dividing LF or HF components by the total power from which the VLF has been subtracted (to minimize the influence of noise and slow trends affecting mainly the VLF) and multiplying by 100. Although the sum of LF_{nu} and HF_{nu} should approximate 100 nu, it usually falls short of this value (Fig. 6.2) because of the presence of smaller components. With this procedure the prevalence of LF component in the upright position of Fig. 6.2 is clearly expressed by its value in nu or by the LF/HF ratio.

In general, it is widely accepted that HF component of HRV can be considered as a marker of vagal modulation (Akselrod *et al.* 1981; Pagani *et al.* 1986). In the case of vagal excitation, the increase in HF can be appreciated both in absolute and normalized units because vagal excitation is usually associated with increased variance in HRV. Conversely, we advanced the hypothesis that the LF component of HRV is a marker of sympathetic modulation only when expressed in nu (Pagani *et al.* 1986; Malliani *et al.* 1991). In addition, the LF/HF ratio could be considered as another index of the balance. We also proposed the LF component of systolic arterial pressure variability (LF_{sap}) as a marker of sympathetic vasomotor modulation (Pagani *et al.* 1986), a proposal now widely accepted. Since arterial pressure variability does not decrease during sympathetic excitations, LF_{sap} can be evaluated both in absolute or normalized units.

In the most various experimental conditions, involving in addition to cardiovascular signals also neural recordings, the LF component of sympathetic discharge variability was increased whenever sympathetic excitation occurred: the sympathetic activity was recorded in animals from nerves directed to the heart (Montano *et al.* 1992) and in humans from muscle sympathetic nerve activity (MSNA) (Pagani *et al.* 1997; Furlan *et al.* 2000). These data suggest that when a shift occurs in HRV spectral profile, leading to a prevalence of LF over HF, this usually corresponds to a more general pattern characterized by an increase in the LF component present in arterial pressure and sympathetic discharge variability. This pattern is clearly evident in Fig. 6.3 displaying the recordings, in a normal subject, of ECG, arterial pressure, MSNA and respiratory movements. It is clear that during tilt, the spectral profile of respiration is unaffected, while a large predominance of LF component characterizes the other three spectral profiles.

This hypothesis does not imply that LF and HF components should be confined to sympathetic and vagal activities, respectively: actually, the opposite is true, because they are simultaneously present in the discharge of both autonomic outflows (Malliani *et al.* 1991). However, a rhythm, being a flexible and dynamic property of neural networks, should not necessarily be restricted to one specific neural pathway to carry a functional significance (as in the case of different electroencephalogram patterns). Our view is rather based on the redundancy of neural mechanisms and on the widespread distribution of neural rhythms. LF and HF rhythms were found, in experiments on cats, in the discharge variability of thalamic somatosensory neurones of conscious animals (Massimini *et al.* 2000), of medullar neurones recorded in animals deprived of sinoaortic afferents (Montano *et al.* 1996), as well as in the cardiac sympathetic discharge of decerebrate (Montano *et al.* 1992) or spinal animals (Montano *et al.* 2000). Thus numerous findings point to their widespread encephalic and spinal representation. Obviously, in closed-loop conditions, central and peripheral circuits have the potential to reinforce this rhythmicity throughout appropriate reflex actions and central integration.

The core of what we propose (Malliani *et al.* 1991; Montano *et al.* 1998; Malliani 2000) is that two main rhythms, one a marker of excitation and intrinsic in sympathetic activation (LF) and the other a marker of inhibition and quiescence and linked to vagal predominance (HF), would be organized, in physiological conditions, in a reciprocal manner. This could also be viewed as a widespread neural code signalling the balance between excitation and inhibition. We hypothesized that, if this is true, a similar oscillatory pattern should also be detectable in the

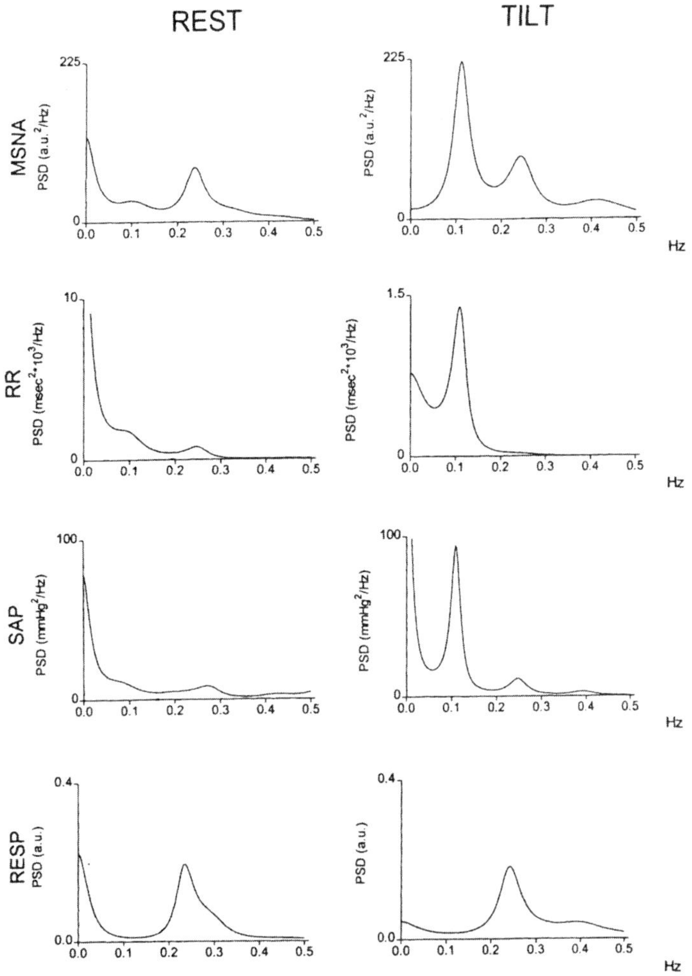

Fig. 6.3 Effects produced by tilt on power spectra of MSNA, *RR* interval (*RR*), SAP variability, and respiratory activity (RESP). At rest, two oscillatory components characterize spectra of MSNA, *RR* interval, and SAP variability. During sympathetic activation induced by tilt, LF component of MSNA increases, thus resembling changes obtained in the same oscillatory component of *RR* interval and SAP variability. Although HF_{MSNA} amplitude is unaffected by passive orthostatism, its relative power is reduced during tilt. Differences in *y*-axis scales between rest and tilt in power spectrum density (PSD) of *RR* interval variability reflect marked reduction of total *RR* interval variance induced by orthostatic stress. a.u., arbitrary units. (From Furlan *et al.* 2000, with permission.)

variability of the discharge of vagal efferent fibres. In preliminary ongoing experiments (Montano *et al.* unpublished observations) in which we recorded cardiovascular efferent vagal activity in anaesthetized rats, we observed an increase in LF nu and a decrease in HF nu in the vagal discharge variability during a hypotensive manoeuvre despite the reduction in the average vagal activity accompanying sympathetic excitation; conversely an increase in vagal discharge accompanying sympathetic inhibition, induced by a hypertensive manoeuvre was characterized by a decrease in LF nu and an increase in HF nu. These data seem to strongly support the hypothesis that in such a neural code of information, the relative increase in LF corresponds to a state of excitation and the relative increase of HF to a state of quiescence, independently of the specific variability signal (sympathetic or vagal) providing the time series.

Concerning the heuristic value of this approach we would like to stress that the study of complexity is more advisable on the basis of what occurs rather than how it may occur. With an observational approach, it was founded that a graded tilt angle was positively and highly correlated with LF_{nu} and LF/HF ratio and negatively with HF (Montano *et al.* 1994). Hence, spectral analysis of HRV was found to be capable of providing a noninvasive, quantitative evaluation of the presumed graded changes simultaneously occurring in sympatho-vagal balance.

As to the possibility of shifting the sympatho-vagal balance toward vagal predominance, this can be easily obtained by baroreceptor stimulation in animals (Montano *et al.* 1992) or by con-

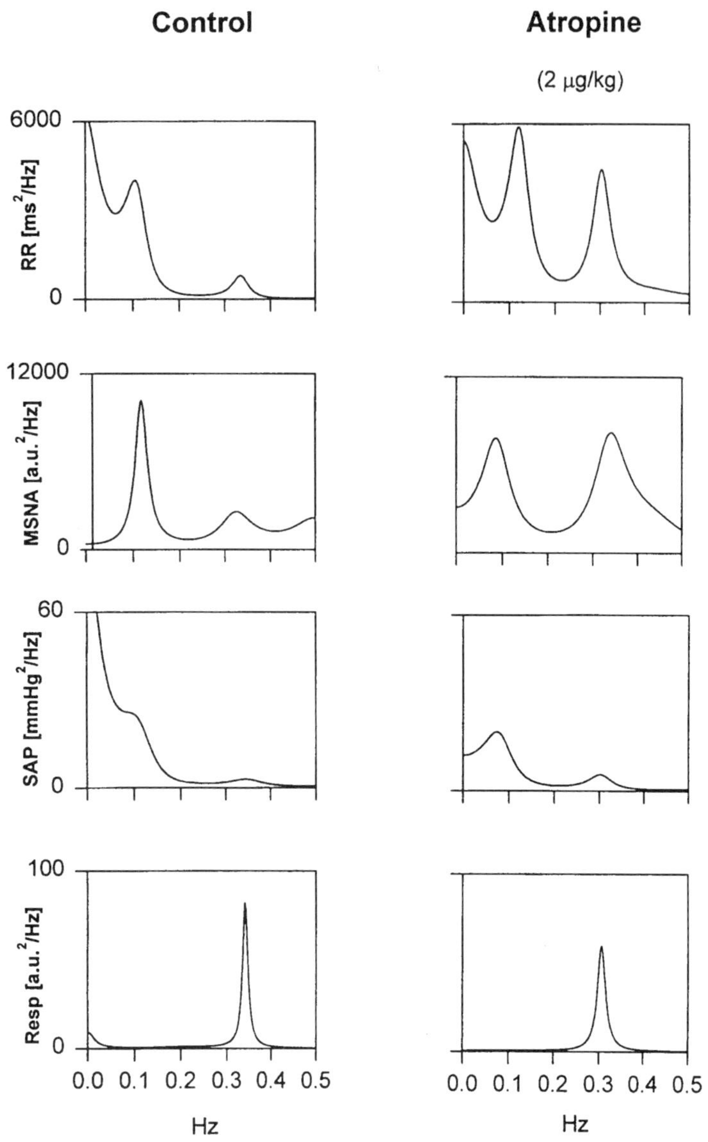

Fig. 6.4 Spectral oscillations of *RR* interval, MSNA, SAP, and respiration in a normal subject during control measurements and after low-dose atropine (2 μg/kg). After low-dose atropine, there is an increase in relative dominance of HF component of *RR* interval and MSNA. (From Montano *et al.* 1998, with permission.)

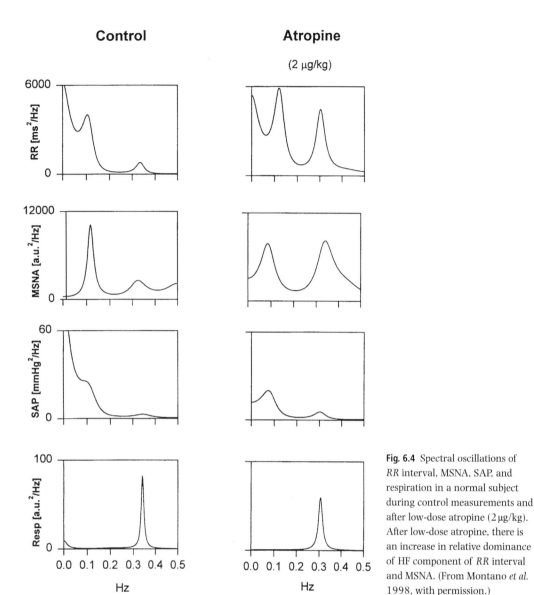

trolled respiration in man, at frequencies within the resting physiological range (Pagani *et al.* 1986; Malliani *et al.* 1991). The increase in vagal modulation obviously does not occur at all possible metronome frequencies, especially when the manoeuver tends to be stressful. It might be worthwhile to recall that in the oriental tradition the control of respiration, mastered to its furthest possibilities, is associated with the intention of reducing what we would refer to as sympathetic tone. Electrical or mechanical stimulation of the oesophagus (Tougas *et al.* 1997), richly innervated by vagal afferents, represent another manoeuvre capable of inducing a prevalence of vagal modulation and hence of HF_{nu} component. Low doses of atropine, known to exert a central vagotonic effect, have been used to induce a pattern of vagal predominance exemplified in Fig. 6.4. This pattern is, in a sense, the reciprocal of that illustrated in Fig. 6.3 corresponding to a sympathetic excitation. In the case of Fig. 6.4, however, the spectral profile of systolic arterial pressure is unmodified by the increased central vagal modulation.

A more direct appraisal of sympatho-vagal balance oscillation is also possible. Figure 6.5 is

Fig. 6.5 Time–frequency analysis of heart rate variability of a healthy subject in supine position followed by passive tilt at 90°. Metronome breathing at 0.25 Hz. Amplitude of oscillations was obtained by finite impulse response filtering. Top to bottom: HF and LF amplitude (ms), *RR* interval (ms), and instant centre frequency (in Hz) of whole spectral power (ICF) and of LF (ICF LF). Tilt between 7 and 8 min. (Modified from Jasson *et al.* 1997, with permission.)

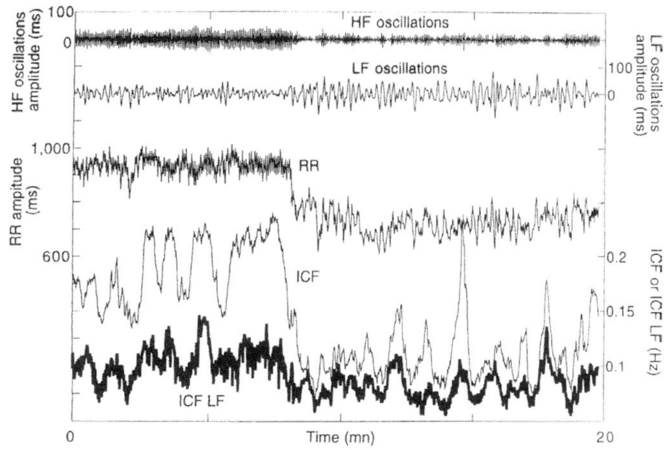

taken from the paper by Jasson *et al.* (1997), utilizing an algorithm (smoothed pseudo-Wigner Ville transform) capable of detecting transients and of displaying a frequency-domain analysis over time. In spite of its technical complexity, the biological interpretation of Fig. 6.5 is quite simple. In the top two tracings, the HF and LF oscillations can be appreciated in both their frequency and amplitude characteristics. The third tracing is the usual tachogram (*RR*), and the fourth tracing represents the instant centre frequency (ICF) of the whole spectrum, i.e. the median frequency of the whole power distribution. The bottom tracing is a similar instant centre frequency calculated for the LF component (ICF LF). These recordings were obtained from a normal subject who, after an initial period in a resting horizontal position, was passively tilted to an upright position at 90° (between the seventh and eighth min). During tilt the following simultaneous changes occurred and were maintained throughout its duration: the amplitude of HF decreased; that of LF increased; heart period also decreased indicating a tachycardia response; and ICF underwent a decrease, indicating that spectral power was redistributed toward the lower frequencies. In short, all the changes indicated a shift in sympatho-vagal balance toward sympathetic excitation and vagal inhibition. Thus the central push–pull organization of LF and HF oscillations is self-evident and is independent of a normalization procedure. This aspect is quite important because the use of normalized units has been criticized (Eckberg 1997) in view of its inherent mathematical simplicity; instead, we think that this simplicity adequately reflects a basic biological strategy characterizing antagonistic subsystems. Moreover, we think that the normalization procedure reinforces the hypothesis from which it was generated by proving its capability in extracting an information content that otherwise would remain undetected (Pagani & Malliani 2000).

However, the most indisputable proof of the pragmatic value of both the concept of sympatho-vagal balance and the corollary normalization procedure has been furnished by a study (Malliani *et al.* 1997), the protocol of which included 350 healthy subjects from whom ECG and respiratory recordings were obtained in controlled laboratory conditions. Each subject was studied both in supine and upright positions. Individual data were ordered consecutively in their historical sequence, and, subsequently, odd and even rank positions were assigned to a training or test set, respectively. Hence, the training and test sets each held 350 patterns characterized by 10 power-spectrum variables (those reported in Fig. 6.2) belonging to 175 subjects studied both in supine and upright positions. The features related to both postures were considered as independent. A forecasting linear method concentrated the information distributed in the various spectral variables into a normalized activation index (AI) (ranging from −1 for supine to +1 for upright posture). During the training set the algorithm had to match the target, i.e. the posture, which was classified by the experimenter, with the information that could be extracted from the interaction of the variables of

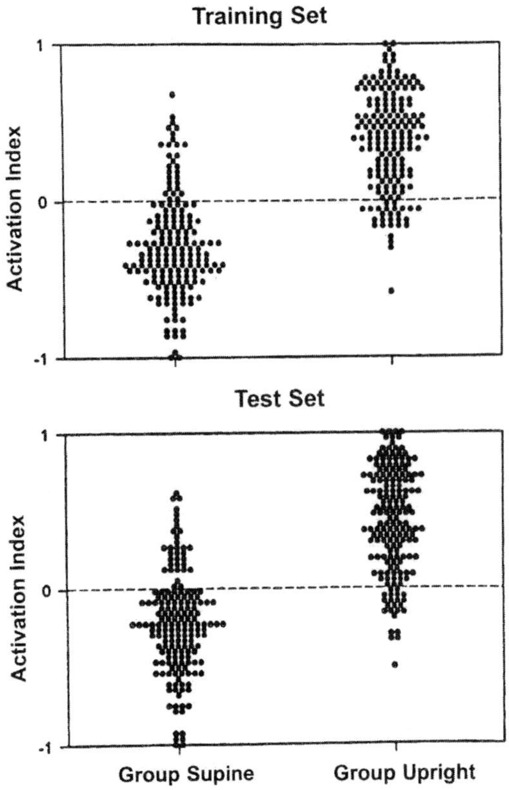

Fig. 6.6 Activation index (AI) of each individual feature belonging to either the training or the test set. Negative AI were normalized for supine posture between 0 and −1, and positive AI were normalized for upright posture between 0 and +1. Three variables (*RR* and LF and HF in normalized units) were used for discrimination and recognition rates. In the test set, 33 features were unrecognized in the supine group and 23 in the upright group, whereas all others were correctly assigned. (From Malliani *et al.* 1997, with permission.)

interest. A pattern was correctly discriminated when the supine position corresponded to an AI between 0 and −1 and the upright position to an AI between 0 and +1. During the Test set, as well, a negative value of the AI was intended to recognize the supine and a positive value the upright position. Such a blind forecasting on the Test set was capable of correctly assigning 83.4% (146 of 175) of features to the supine group and 86.3% (151 of 175) to the upright group, when 10 variables were evaluated simultaneously. Three variables (*RR*, LF_{nu} and HF_{nu}) were found to hold almost all the information content and could recognize an overall 84.0% of patterns, with a comparably good performance in both supine and upright groups (Fig. 6.6). When one of these three variables was not considered, the forecasting provided inconsistent results. Supine and upright postures, as an example of well-reproducible physiological conditions, are known to engender distinct levels of sympathetic activity and hence of sympatho-vagal balance. It was reported, for the first time, that a physiological noninvasive recording such as the ECG contains intrinsic information that can be used to recognize, individual by individual, the two different autonomic profiles related to posture. In addition to *RR* interval, the most powerful variables for both discrimination and recognition rates appear to be LF_{nu} and HF_{nu}, according to our hypothesis. The sympatho-vagal balance can also be studied along the 24 h. In this case as well LF_{nu} and HF_{nu} underwent the expected changes according to a sympathetic predominance during the day and a vagal predominance during the night (Furlan *et al.* 1990).

Alterations in the balance and its responsiveness

As already mentioned, it is clear that the LF and HF rhythmicity can be detected from the variability of various cardiovascular and neural signals. In the case of HRV, however, this approach needs an adequate responsiveness of sinus node pace-maker cells. When this responsiveness is lost, such as during the advanced phases of congestive heart failure (Guzzetti *et al.* 1995; van De Borne *et al.* 1997) this approach cannot offer any longer an estimate of the *autonomic balance*. However, in the case of CHF, the progressive decrease and the disappearance of an LF component from HRV can become a strong predictor of a poor prognosis (Mortara *et al.* 1997; La Rovere *et al.* 2003).

The sympatho-vagal balance is altered in the resting conditions of numerous pathophysiological processes. It is the case of essential arterial hypertension (Guzzetti *et al.* 1988), even in the presence of arterial pressure values still in the high normal range (Lucini *et al.* 2002), of patients after myocardial infarction (Lombardi *et al.* 1987) and of other abnormal states that have been summarized elsewhere (Malliani *et al.* 1991; Malliani 2000; Malliani & Montano

2002). However, it is important to point out that it is the reduced responsiveness of sympatho-vagal balance to an excitatory stimulus, such as the upright position, that most often adequately reflects the pathophysiological impairment. It is quite obvious that in physiology, given the finalistic design of a cardiovascular neural regulation, its possible marked oscillations are essential to subserve well-defined behavioural patterns. Conversely, a progressive reduction in the responsiveness of sympatho-vagal balance is practically a rule in the course of various abnormal conditions involving autonomic regulation (Malliani 2000; Malliani and Montano 2002).

Conclusions

Whatever may be the limitations of the proposed methodology, we think that it has the merit of being so far the only one available to evaluate simultaneously both sympathetic and vagal modulations, according to the reality of their continuous interaction. It is also relevant to point out that this approach can be totally non-invasive and applied to either short-term or long-term recordings (Malliani *et al.* 1991; Malliani 2000). The concept of sympatho-vagal balance intends to be neither a simple paradigm nor the proposal that its operation is linear throughout its range. It also does not suggest that the sympathetic and vagal outflows are both homogeneous functional entities. However, given all these limitations, the concept of balance has helped in extracting information that otherwise would have remained embedded in the original records.

References

Akselrod, S., Gordon, D., Ubel, F.A., Shannon, D.C., Barger, A.C. & Cohen, R.J. (1981) Power spectrum analysis of heart rate fluctuation: a quantitative probe of beat-to-beat cardiovascular control. *Science*, **213**, 220–222.

van de Borne, P., Montano, N., Pagani, M., Oren, R. & Somers, V.K. (1997) Absence of low-frequency variability of sympathetic nerve activity in severe heart failure. *Circulation*, **95**, 1449–1454.

Brovelli, M., Baselli, G., Cerutti, S. *et al.* (1983) Computerized analysis for an experimental validation of neurophysiological models of heart rate control. *Computerized Cardiology*, 205–208.

Cannon, W.B. (1932) *The Wisdom of the Body*. W.W. Norton, New York.

Eckberg, D.L. (1997) Sympatho-vagal balance: a critical appraisal. *Circulation*, **96**, 3224–3232.

Furlan, R., Guzzetti, S., Crivellaro *et al.* (1990) Continuous 24-h assessment of the neural regulation of systemic arterial pressure and *RR* variabilities in ambulant subjects. *Circulation*, **81**, 537–547.

Furlan, R., Porta, A., Costa, F. *et al.* (2000) Oscillatory patterns in sympathetic neural discharge and cardiovascular variables during orthostatic stimulus. *Circulation*, **101**, 886–892.

Guzzetti, S., Cogliati, C., Turiel, M., Crema, C., Lombardi, F. & Malliani, A. (1995) Sympathetic predominance followed by functional denervation in the progression of chronic heart failure. *European Heart Journal*, **16**, 1100–1107.

Guzzetti, S., Piccaluga, E., Casati, R. *et al.* (1988) Sympathetic predominance in essential hypertension: a study employing spectral analysis of heart rate variability. *Journal of Hypertension*, **6**, 711–717.

Jasson, S., Médigue, C., Maison-Blanche, P. *et al.* (1997) Instant power spectrum analysis of heart rate variability during orthostatic tilt using a time-/frequency-domain method. *Circulation*, **96**, 3521–3526.

La Rovere, M.T., Pinna, G.D., Maestri, R. *et al.* (2003) Short-term heart rate variability strongly predicts sudden cardiac death in chronic heart failure patients. *Circulation*, **107**, 565–570.

Lombardi, F., Sandrone, G., Pernpruner, S., Sala, R., Garimoldi, M., Cerutti, S., Baselli, G., Pagani, M., Malliani, A. (1987) Heart rate variability as an index of sympatho-vagal interaction after acute myocardial infarction. *American Journal Cardiology*, **60**, 1239–1245.

Lucini, D., Mela, G.S., Malliani, A. & Pagani, M. (2002) Impairment in cardiac autonomic regulation preceding arterial hypertension in humans: insight from spectral analysis of beat-by-beat cardiovascular variability. *Circulation*, **106**, 2673–2679.

Malliani, A. (1999) The pattern of sympatho-vagal balance explored in the frequency domain. *News in Physiological Sciences*, **14**, 111–117.

Malliani, A. (2000) *Principles of Cardiovascular Neural Regulation in Health and Disease*. Kluwer Academic Publishers, Dordrecht.

Malliani, A. & Montano, N. (2002) Heart rate variability as a clinical tool. *Italian Heart Journal*, **3**, 439–445.

Malliani, A., Pagani, M., Furlan, R. *et al.* (1997) Individual recognition by heart rate variability of two different autonomic profiles related to posture. *Circulation*, **96**, 4143–4145.

Malliani, A., Pagani, M., Lombardi, F. & Cerutti, S. (1991) Cardiovascular neural regulation explored in the frequency domain. *Research Advances Series, Circulation*, **84**, 482–492.

Massimini, M., Porta, A., Mariotti, M., Malliani, A. & Montano, N. (2000) Heart rate variability is encoded in the spontaneous discharge of thalamic somatosensory neurones in cat. *Journal of Physiology*, **526**(2), 387–396.

Montano, N, Cogliati, C., Porta, A. *et al.* (1998) Central vagotonic effects of atropine modulate spectral oscillations of sympathetic nerve activity. *Circulation*, **98**, 1394–1399.

Montano, N., Cogliati, C., Dias da Silva, V.J. *et al.* (2000) Effects of spinal section and of positive-feedback excitatory reflex on sympathetic and heart rate variability. *Hypertension*, **36**, 1029–1034.

Montano, N., Gnecchi-Ruscone, T., Porta, A., Lombardi, F., Pagani, M. & Malliani, A. (1994) Power spectrum analysis of heart rate variability to assess the changes in sympatho-vagal balance during graded orthostatic tilt. *Circulation*, **90**, 1826–1831.

Montano, N., Gnecchi-Ruscone, T., Porta, A., Lombardi, F., Malliani, A. & Barman, S.M. (1996) Presence of vasomotor and respiratory rhythms in the discharge of single medullary neurones involved in the regulation of cardiovascular system. *Journal of the Autonomic Nervous System*, **57**, 116–122.

Montano, N., Lombardi, F., Gnecchi-Ruscone, T. *et al.* (1992) Spectral analysis of sympathetic discharge, *RR* interval and systolic arterial pressure in decerebrate cats. *Journal of the Autonomic Nervous System*, **40**, 21–32.

Mortara, A., Sleight, P., Pinna, G.D. *et al.* (1997) Abnormal awake respiratory patterns are common in chronic heart failure and may prevent evaluation of autonomic tone by measures of heart rate variability. *Circulation*, **96**, 246–252.

Pagani, M., Lombardi, F., Guzzetti, S. *et al.* (1986) Power spectral analysis of heart rate and arterial pressure variabilities as a marker of sympatho-vagal interaction in man and conscious dog. *Circulation, Research*, **58**, 178–193.

Pagani, M. & Malliani, A. (2000) Interpreting oscillations of muscle sympathetic nerve activity and heart rate variability. *Journal of Hypertension*, **18**, 1709–1719.

Pagani, M., Montano, N., Porta, A. *et al.* (1997) Relationship between spectral components of cardiovascular variabilities and direct measures of muscle sympathetic nerve activity in humans. *Circulation*, **95**, 1441–1448.

Schwartz, P.J., Pagani, M., Lombardi, F., Malliani, A. & Brown, A.M. (1973) A cardiocardiac sympatho-vagal reflex in the cat. *Circulation, Research*,**32**, 215–220.

Tougas, G., Kamath, M., Watteel, G. *et al.* (1997) Modulation of neurocardiac function by oesophageal stimulation in humans. *Clinical Science* 92, 167–174.

CHAPTER 7

Heart Rate Variability: Stress and Psychiatric Conditions

Gary G. Berntson and John T. Cacioppo

Introduction

Psychological states and processes can impact dramatically on dynamic autonomic control of the heart. The literature in this area is far from simple, however, as the effects of stress states and psychiatric conditions on heart rate variability can be diverse. The present chapter will highlight selected aspects of this literature, and consider conceptual approaches that may help organize the diverse findings in this area. Clearly, this is an issue that requires interdisciplinary approaches across multiple levels of analysis, ranging from the psychological to the biological (Cacioppo *et al.* 2000).

Central origins of psychological influences on autonomic function

Brain mechanisms for somatomotor control and coordination have been extensively studied, and the complex, multilevel, hierarchical structure of central somatic motor systems is well recognized. As early as the 19th century, the notable English neurologist John Hughlings Jackson emphasized the continuous evolutionary layering and re-representation of motor systems at progressively higher levels of the neuraxis (Jackson 1958). Although spinal and brainstem reflexes organize primitive motor acts and provide important postural support for more complex activities, it is the higher levels in central motor systems that allow for flexibility and adaptability in motor control and underlie the awesome, graceful movements of an accomplished ballerina.

Historically, research and theory concerning autonomic regulation often focused on the lowest levels of central control. Although Walter Cannon clearly articulated the impact of emotion and other psychological processes on autonomic states (Cannon 1928), he viewed the autonomic nervous system largely as a homeostatic regulatory mechanism (Cannon 1929). Recent research, however, has revealed a re-representation and layering of autonomic functions from the spinal cord to rostral brain networks sufficiently similar to those for somatomotor control that they suggest a common evolutionary heritage.

Homeostatic functions of the autonomic nervous system are illustrated by the baroreceptor-heart rate reflex, through which a perturbation in blood pressure triggers a tightly coupled, reciprocal change in the activities of the autonomic branches. Postural hypotension, for example, results in a reflexive decrease in parasympathetic control of the heart, together with a reciprocal withdrawal of sympathetic cardiac control, which synergistically increase heart rate (and contractility). Together with vascular components, these changes serve to compensate for the hypotensive perturbation and normalize blood pressure (e.g. Cacioppo *et al.* 1994). Baroreceptor reflexes are prototypic homeostatic mechanisms and are organized largely within lower central autonomic substrates at brainstem levels. Through evolutionary development of rostral brain systems, however, these lower autonomic circuits become integrated with higher neural networks (Berntson & Cacioppo 2000).

Limbic and forebrain areas implicated in behavioural processes, including the hypothalamus, amygdala and medial prefrontal cortex, have been shown to issue monosynaptic projections to brainstem reflex networks as well as to autonomic source nuclei in the brainstem and spinal cord (for review see Berntson & Cacioppo 2000). Through these projections, higher neural processes can modulate or even bypass reflex networks and powerfully alter autonomic outflows. It is now clear that stressors, even as mild as mental arithmetic, can lead to an inhibition and/or a shift in set point of baroreceptor reflexes (Ditto & France 1990; Steptoe & Sawada 1989). Such effects reflect complex modulatory influences of rostral neural systems on lower autonomic substrates and have necessitated expansion of the simple negative-feedback homeostatic model of autonomic control.

Autonomic space and cardiac chronotropic control

As considered above, brainstem baroreceptor reflexes have highly specific afferent (baroreceptor) inputs and exert a rather rigid pattern of reciprocal control over the two autonomic branches, such that an increase in activity of one branch is associated with decreased activity in the other. This is apparent in the highly correlated cardiac chronotropic control exerted by the two autonomic branches during orthostatic stress (Berntson *et al.* 1994). Similarly, respiratory sinus arrhythmia is associated with reciprocal changes in the activities of the autonomic branches, which are approximately 180° out of phase. Based on findings such as these, autonomic control has often been considered to lie along a continuum with parasympathetic activation at one end and sympathetic activation at the other (see Fig. 7.1).

In contrast to this linear-continuum model of autonomic control, however, descending influences from higher neural systems are not so constrained. Rather, psychological states and processes associated with rostral neural networks can evoke reciprocal, independent, or even coactive changes in the autonomic branches (Berntson *et al.* 1991, 1993; Koizumi & Kollai 1992). The flexible nature of rostral autonomic control mandates an expansion of the linear model to a bivariate representation of autonomic space, as illustrated in Fig. 7.1.

Even in cases where rostral neural influences foster a generally reciprocal mode of autonomic control, there remain important differences from the pattern of control exerted by baroreceptor reflexes (Fig. 7.2). Selective pharmacological blockades of the autonomic branches revealed that an orthostatic challenge (change from sitting to standing) and standard psychological stressors (mental arithmetic, speech stress and a reaction time task) yield a similar pattern of reciprocal sympathetic activation and vagal withdrawal in human subjects, when considered at the group level (Berntson *et al.* 1994). The response to orthostatic stress displayed minimal individual variation, and the reciprocal changes in the autonomic branches were highly corre-

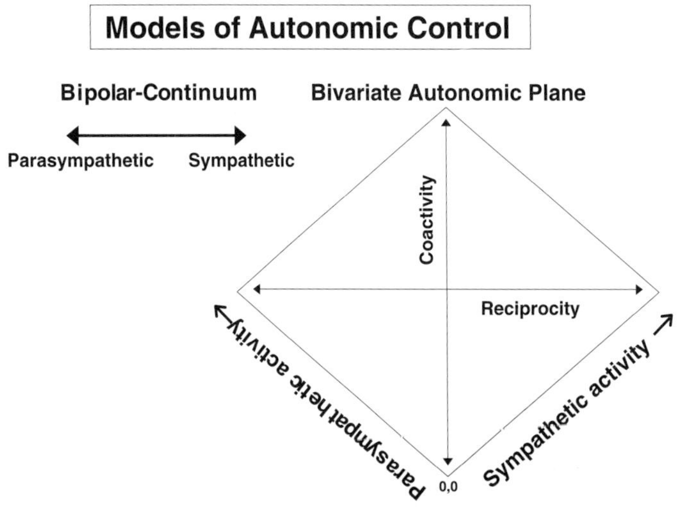

Fig. 7.1 Bivariate model of autonomic space (right), contrasted with the reciprocal bipolar-continuum model of autonomic control (left).

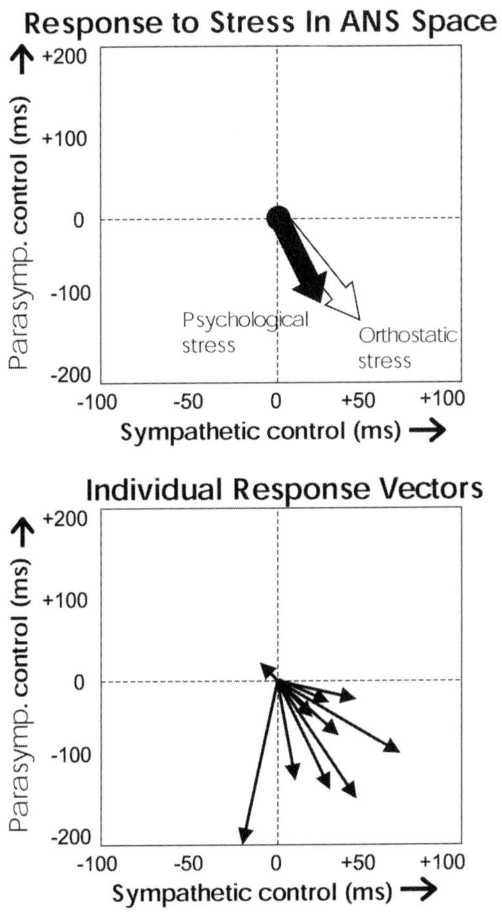

Fig. 7.2 Sympathetically and parasympathetically mediated changes in heart period in response to stress. Top panel: overall group responses to orthostatic and psychological stress. Bottom panel: in contrast to orthostatic stress, there were considerable individual differences in the response to psychological stressors, ranging from largely sympathetic activation to predominantly parasympathetic withdrawal. Arrows represent group (top) and individual (bottom) response vectors from pre-stress baseline, depicted at the intersection of the horizontal and vertical dotted lines. Response vectors were derived from single and dual pharmacological blockades of the autonomic branches (see Berntson *et al.* 1994).

lated across subjects. In contrast, psychological stressors, typical of those encountered in daily life, yielded wide individual differences in the mode of response, with some subjects consistently showing largely sympathetic activation, others primarily vagal withdrawal, and still others a reciprocal pattern of autonomic response (see Fig. 7.2). Hence, there was no significant correlation between the responses of the autonomic branches to psychological stress. This difference was not attributable to greater error variance in the response to psychological stress, as individual response patterns were highly stable across tasks. Rather, these findings reveal that people differ in how they respond to psychological stressors (individual response uniqueness) and that these differences are relatively stable across time (individual response consistency). In contrast, these individual differences are not apparent when the stressor engages predominantly brainstem systems (e.g. orthostatic stress). This is also documented by the finding that hostility is highly correlated with the autonomic response to cognitive stressors, but not the autonomic responses to tilt (Sloan *et al.* 2001).

The complexities of rostral influences on autonomic control probably underlie the disparate literature on autonomic function in stress, anxiety, and psychiatric conditions. This should not be surprising, as behavioural manifestations also vary widely across these conditions, even among subjects within a given condition. Consequently, it may be unrealistic to expect a simple pattern of altered autonomic control in various psychological and psychiatric states. Indeed, in addition to the individual differences outlined above, there are also differences in how people respond to distinct psychological tasks (stimulus response specificity). The tasks discussed above involve active cognitive processing and response (e.g. mental arithmetic, reaction time) and are generally associated with varied degrees of parasympathetic withdrawal and sympathetic activation. In contrast, more passive cognitive tasks, such as perceptual illusions, focused attention, or response inhibition may be accompanied by parasympathetic activation or coactivation of both the parasympathetic and sympathetic branches (Somsen *et al.* 1991; Berntson *et al.* 1996; Campbell *et al.* 1997; Jennings & Van der Molen 2002)

A meaningful understanding of the relationships between autonomic functions and cognitive processes, stress, and psychiatric conditions will depend on a greater appreciation of the role and complexity of rostral neurobehavioural systems. It is the complexity of rostral influences on autonomic control that likely contributes to the diversity in autonomic functions in stress, anxiety, and psychiatric conditions. The task confronting investigators is to identify the moderator variables underlying this diversity and to understand their interactions and functional implications. Such moderator variables can derive from three general sources: (1) contextual variables (types of tasks and their context, related to stimulus response specificity); (2) appraisal variables (how individuals appraise or interpret the condition, associated with individual response uniqueness); (3) individual differences in neural, neurochemical, and physiological variables associated with autonomic control (also related to individual response uniqueness).

Effects of stress on heart rate variability

Stressors are often associated with an increase in sympathetic cardiac control, a decrease in parasympathetic control, or both. Associated with these reactions is a frequently reported increase in low frequency (LF, centred around 0.1 Hz) heart rate variability, a decrease in high frequency (HF, 0.12 or 0.15–0.4 Hz) power, and/or an increase in the LF/HF ratio. Aspects of this general response pattern have been reported for: (a) acute laboratory psychological/cognitive stressors such as mental arithmetic, reaction time tasks, Stroop interference task, or speech stress (Berntson *et al.* 1994; Friedman *et al.* 1996; Delaney & Brodie, 2000; Hughes & Stoney 2000; Jain *et al.* 2001); (b) real-life acute stressors such as college examinations (Lucini *et al.* 2002), earthquakes (Lin *et al.* 2001), as well as typical day-to-day hassles (Sloan *et al.* 1994); and even (c) the level of chronic perceived stress associated with trait anxiety (Dishman *et al.* 2000). The Berntson *et al.* (1994) study on the autonomic effects of acute laboratory stressors, for example, reported a stress-related decrease in HF heart rate variability (LF was not quantified), associated with a significant reduction in parasympathetic cardiac control and an increase in sympathetic control, as revealed by selective pharmacological blockades of the autonomic branches.

Exceptions to this pattern include the forehead cold pressor manipulation (Hughes & Stoney 2000), water immersion and diving (Schipke & Pelzer 2001), and some attentional paradigms (e.g. Berntson *et al.* 1996), during which HF power may increase in both absolute and relative units. The increase in HF power in the cold pressor and immersion conditions may reflect a concurrent evocation of the dive reflex (see Gooden 1994), superimposed on a mild stress response (Friedman *et al.* 1996). In others cases, including attentional tasks, autonomic coactivation may represent an integrated response to specific cognitive reactions such as the orienting response (Quigley & Berntson 1990).

The relation of specific behavioural and psychological states to distinct patterns of autonomic control is an especially important issue for further investigation, from both the clinical and neuroscientific perspective. The construct of stress, however, is exceedingly broad and poorly defined. It is clear that no single pattern of autonomic adjustments, and associated changes in heart rate variability, will apply universally across distinct stressors. Of particular importance in future research will be a refinement in our conceptualization of stress, as well as the cognitive and behavioural responses individuals display to those stressors.

Heart rate variability in psychiatric conditions

Because psychiatric conditions derive from or impact on psychological processes, many of the issues and caveats raised above apply also to these conditions. The involvement of higher cerebral systems in psychopathological states predicts a considerable degree of complexity in the pattern of autonomic control. Space precludes a thorough consideration of autonomic function across the wide array of psychiatric states, so we limit our focus on anxiety disorders and depression, as illustrative of the impact of psychiatric states on autonomic control.

Anxiety

There is now an extensive literature on anxiety and autonomic control that documents complex links between behavioural and cardiovascular systems. Although some anxiety disorders, such as panic disorders and specific phobias, may be associated with enhanced autonomic activity or reactivity to threat-related cues, anxiety states such as generalized anxiety disorder may also be characterized by an overall diminished autonomic lability for non-threat cues (for review see Berntson *et al.* 1998). A similar diminished lability has been reported even for trauma-related material in post-traumatic stress disorder (Cohen *et al.* 2000).

A rather common finding in the literature on anxiety and autonomic control is diminished heart rate variability in anxiety disorders, especially in the HF band (Thayer *et al.* 1996; Friedman & Thayer 1998; Cohen *et al.* 2000), which is associated with vagal control (ESC/NASPE Task Force 1996; Berntson *et al.* 1997). This has been considered to reflect a reduction in vagal control and an associated loss of autonomic 'flexibility' (Friedman & Thayer 1998; Monk *et al.* 2001). The reduction in HF variability may be reflected in diminished total heart rate variability, despite a potential selective increase in LF variability (Yeragani *et al.* 1998).

The specific origins of anxiety-related effects on autonomic function remain to be clarified, but likely relate to alterations in higher neurobehavioural systems (Hugdahl 1996; Berntson *et al.* 1998). Although simple conditioned fears can be established and maintained largely by subcortical structures (including the amygdala; LeDoux 2000), more generalized anxiety states entail an attentional focus on threat-related cues together with a response bias that likely depend on higher-level cortical/cognitive processes (for review see Berntson *et al.* 1998). In this regard, cortical regions, such as the medial prefrontal cortex, that have been implicated in anxiety are the very areas that have been shown to have direct monosynaptic projections to brainstem autonomic centres and source nuclei (see Berntson *et al.* 1998).

The specific psychological origins of the autonomic features of anxiety states remain unclear. There is considerable overlap between autonomic characteristics of anxiety and those associated with stress, which raises the possibility that some of the autonomic accompaniments of anxiety may represent features of a stress response. A salient aspect of anxiety is the attentional focus on threat-related cues, which might be expected to trigger a stress reaction. In this regard, part of the complexity in the literature may be attributable to individual differences in stress reactions as discussed above (individual response uniqueness), as well as the existence of distinct categories of anxiety disorders that may be associated with different patterns of autonomic function (stimulus response specificity). We will consider below some general research strategies for addressing these issues.

Depression

Depression has often, but not universally, been reported to be associated with an overall reduction in total heart rate variability (Krittayaphong *et al.* 1997; Gorman & Sloan 2000; Carney *et al.* 2001; Agelink *et al.* 2002; Yeragani *et al.* 2002). This has generally been characterized by reduced HF variability, as well as other measures of vagal control of the heart (Watkins *et al.* 1999; Agelink *et al.* 2002; Yeragani *et al.* 2002), but these results also have not always been uniform (Carney *et al.* 2001).

Relations between depression and autonomic function are potentially important clinically, because depression is an independent risk factor for cardiovascular disease and for cardiac morbidity and mortality after myocardial infarction (for reviews see Gorman & Sloan 2000; Sheps & Sheffield 2001; Rugulies 2002). Moreover, decreased heart rate variability and vagal control of the heart are negative predictors of outcome after myocardial infarction (ESC/NASPE Task Force 1996; Malik 1998; La Rovere *et al.* 2001), which raises the possibility that the autonomic correlates of depression (decreased vagal and increased sympathetic control) may mediate in part the relation between depression and cardiovascular disease. Although the current picture is somewhat more complex than this, heart rate variability remains a important predictor of cardiac risk (Lombardi 2002). Conversely, HF heart rate variability is a predictor of outcome in major depressive disorders (Rottenberg *et al.* 2002).

In addition to the physiological mechanisms that underlie the relation between depression and cardiac function, which are addressed elsewhere in this volume, an important question arises as to the origin of the link between depression and heart rate variability. Depression is not a monolithic psychological state, and the relevant psychological dimensions that impact the pattern of heart rate variability have not been clearly established. A depressed mood, in and of itself, may not be the critical determinant, as depressed mood (indexed by the Beck Depression Inventory) is not necessarily accompanied by a significant decrease in basal HF heart rate variability, although it has been reported to be associated with an enhanced HF reduction to stress (Hughes & Stoney, 2000). In this regard, a recent meta-analysis revealed that clinical depression is a stronger predictor of coronary heart disease than is merely a depressed mood (Rugulies 2002). Although the distinction between clinical depression and depressed mood may be one of magnitude or degree, they may also reflect other associated behavioural factors, such as diet, sleep patterns, or activity levels.

Alternatively, the relations between depression and heart rate variability may be mediated by other psychological factors. Anxiety, for example is a common accompaniment of depression, and Watkins *et al.* (1999) report that the level of anxiety in a depressive sample correlated with reduced vagal regulation of the heart as indexed by baroreflex cardiac control, whereas the level of depression was not predictive of either baroreflex control or HF variability. Moreover, anxiety itself is a predictor of coronary heart disease (Kubzansky *et al.* 1998) and may contribute to the relation between depression and health. In this regard, the reduced heart rate variability in depression may represent a chronic, consolidated anxiety-related response to everyday hassles and aggravations. This could have substantial health implications, to the extent to which such a response fosters a suboptimal pattern of cardiac control. There are a number of alternative routes by which psychological or behavioural factors can impact health status (e.g. see Cacioppo *et al.* 2002), and this is an exceedingly important issue for further interdisciplinary research.

Directions for further research

The relations between behavioural/psychological processes and autonomic control are intricate and complex, as the neurobehavioural systems that give rise to these relationships represent some of the most sophisticated processing systems of the brain. Psychophysiology has advanced considerably over the decades, from a relatively limited focus on peripheral end-organ responses (heart rate, skin conductance, etc.) to its current appreciation of the interactions between central systems and peripheral organs and the impact of cognitive and emotional process on these interactions.

Further progress in this area will benefit from increased interdisciplinary research, which entails an integration of multiple levels of analysis ranging from the psychological to the organ system to the cellular. One impediment to such research is what has been referred to as the category error, or the lack of one-to-one mapping between the terms, constructs and theories of the distinct levels of analysis. This is likely a contributor to the lack of isomorphism between constructs such as anxiety and depression on the one hand, and physiological functions on the other. Important in future efforts will be a refinement in the constructs at each level of analysis, as they are illuminated by information derived from alternative levels of analysis. This will provide for a progressive reduction of category errors, and allow for an alignment or calibration of information across levels of analysis. Of particular importance in these studies will be the elucidation of the physiological and cellular mechanisms underlying psychophysiological relations.

The studies outlined above highlight the need for a more comprehensive and realistic framework for models of central autonomic control. Especially important will be the elucidation of the interactions between these central autonomic substrates and neurobehavioural, neuroendocrine, and immune systems. Of additional importance will be a recognition of the multiple, interacting levels of functional representation in central substrates that may underlie distinct aspects of psychophysiological relations. The benefit of such interdisciplinary, multilevel analyses will be a more comprehensive understanding of the relations between the mind and body, their health significance, and methods of intervention.

References

Agelink, M.W., Boz, C., Ullrich, H. & Andrich, J. (2002) Relationship between major depression and heart rate variability. Clinical consequences and implications for antidepressive treatment. *Psychiatry Research*, **113**, 139–149.

Berntson, G.G., Bigger, J.T., Eckberg, D.L. *et al.* (1997) Heart rate variability: origins, methods, and interpretive caveats. *Psychophysiology*, **34**, 623–648.

Berntson, G.G. & Cacioppo, J.T. (2000) From homeostasis to allodynamic regulation. In: *Handbook of Psychophysiology* (eds J. T. Cacioppo, L. G. Tassinary & G. G. Berntson), pp. 459–481. Cambridge University Press, Cambridge.

Berntson, G.G., Cacioppo, J T., Binkley, P.F., Uchino, B.N., Quigley, K.S. & Fieldstone, A. (1994). Autonomic cardiac control: III. Psychological stress and cardiac response in autonomic space as revealed by pharmacological blockades. *Psychophysiology*, **31**, 599–608.

Berntson, G.G., Cacioppo, J.T. & Fieldstone, A. (1996) Illusions, arithmetic, and the bidirectional modulation of vagal control of the heart. *Biological Psychology*, **44**, 1–17.

Berntson, G.G., Cacioppo, J.T. & Quigley, K.S. (1991) Autonomic determinism: the modes of autonomic control, the doctrine of autonomic space, and the laws of autonomic constraint. *Psychological Reviews*, **98**, 459–487.

Berntson, G.G., Cacioppo, J.T. & Quigley, K.S. (1993) Cardiac psychophysiology and autonomic space in humans: empirical perspectives and conceptual implications. *Psychological Bulletin*, **114**, 296–322.

Berntson, G.G., Sarter, M. & Cacioppo, J.T. (1998) Anxiety and cardiovascular reactivity: the basal forebrain cholinergic link. *Behavioural Brain Research*, **94**, 225–248.

Cacioppo, J.T., Berntson, G.G., Binkley, P.F., Quigley, K.S., Uchino, B.N. & Fieldstone, A. (1994) Autonomic cardiac control. II. Basal response, noninvasive indices, and autonomic space as revealed by autonomic blockades. *Psychophysiology*, **31**, 586–598.

Cacioppo, J.T., Berntson, G.G., Sheridan, J.F. & McClintock, M.K. (2000) Multi-level integrative analyses of human behaviour: the complementing nature of social and biological approaches. *Psychological Bulletin*, **126**, 829–843.

Cacioppo, J.T., Hawkley, L.C., Crawford, L.E. *et al.* (2002) Loneliness and health: potential mechanisms. *Psychosomatic Medicine*, **64**, 407–417.

Campbell, B.A., Wood, G. & McBride, T. (1997) Origins of orienting and defensive responses: an evolutionary perspective. In: *Attention and orienting: Sensory and Motivational Processes* (eds P. J. Lang, R. F. Simons & M. T. Balaban), pp. 41–68. Erlbaum, Hillsdale, NJ

Cannon, W.B. (1928) The mechanism of emotional disturbance of bodily functions. *New England Journal of Medicine*, **198**, 877–884.

Cannon, W.B. (1929) Organization for physiological homeostasis. *Physiological Reviews*, **9**, 399–431.

Carney, R.M., Blumenthal, J.A., Stein, P.K. *et al.* (2001) Depression, heart rate variability, and acute myocardial infarction. *Circulation*, **104**, 2024–2028.

Cohen, H., Benjamin, J., Geva, A.B., Matar, M.A., Kaplan, Z. & Kotler, M (2000) Autonomic dysregulation in panic disorder and in post-traumatic stress disorder: application of power spectrum analysis of heart rate variability at rest and in response to recollection of trauma or panic attacks. *Psychiatry Research*, **96**, 1–13.

Delaney, J.P. & Brodie, D.A. (2000) Effects of short-term psychological stress on the time and frequency domains of heart-rate variability. *Perceptual and Motor Skills*, **91**, 515–524.

Dishman, R.K., Nakamura, Y., Garcia, M.E., Thompson, R.W., Dunn, A.L. & Blair, S.N. (2000) Heart rate variability, trait anxiety, and perceived stress among physically fit men and women. *International Journal of Psychophysiology*, **37**, 121–133.

Ditto, B. & France, C. (1990) Carotid baroreflex sensitivity at rest and during psychological stress in offspring of hypertensives and non-twin sibling pairs. *Psychosomatic Medicine*, **52**, 610–620.

ESC/NASPE (European Society of Cardiology/North American Society of Pacing and Electrophysiology) Task Force (1996) Heart rate variability: standards of measurements, physiological interpretation, and clinical use. *Circulation*, **93**, 1043–1065.

Friedman, B.H. & Thayer, J.F. (1998) Anxiety and autonomic flexibility: a cardiovascular approach. *Biological Psychology*, **47**, 243–263.

Friedman, B.H., Thayer, J.F. & Tyrrell, R.A. (1996) Spectral characteristics of heart period variability during cold face stress and shock avoidance in normal subjects. *Clinical Autonomic Research*, **6**, 147–152.

Gooden, B.A. (1994) Mechanism of the human diving response. *Integrative Physiological and Behavioural Science*, **29**, 6–16.

Gorman, J.M. & Sloan, R.P. (2000) Heart rate variability in depressive and anxiety disorders. *American Heart Journal*, **140**, 77–83.

Hugdahl, K. (1996) Cognitive influences on human autonomic nervous system function. *Current Opinion in Neurobiology*, **6**, 252–258.

Hughes, J.W. & Stoney, C.M. (2000) Depressed mood is related to high-frequency heart rate variability during stressors. *Psychosomatic Medicine*, **62**, 796–803.

Jackson, J.H. (1958) Evolution and dissolution of the nervous system (Croonian Lectures). In: *Selected writings of John Hughlings Jackson*, Vol. 2 (ed. J. Taylor), pp. 45–63. Basic Books, New York [original work published in 1884].

Jain, D., Joska, T., Lee, F.A., Burg, M., Lampert, R. & Zaret, B.L. (2001) Day-to-day-reproducibility of mental stress-induced abnormal left ventricular function

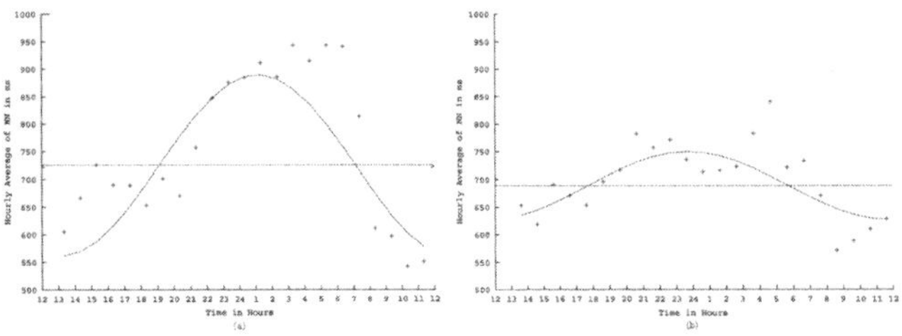

Fig. 8.1 Average hourly *NN* (normal-to-normal) intervals in a healthy elderly subject (a) and in a patient with clinical cardiovascular disease (b).

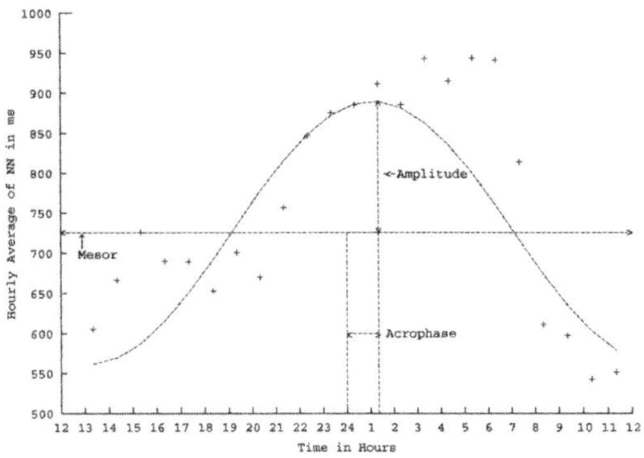

Fig. 8.2 The measures used in cosinor analysis are illustrated using the plot of average *NN* intervals for the healthy subject shown in Fig. 8.1.

the circadian rhythm, since the acrophase of the average *NN* interval is after 01.00 hours, but the lowest heart rates (highest average *NN*) actually occur at 05.00 and 06.00 hours.

Circadian patterns in healthy populations

Several investigators have explored circadian patterns of heart rate and HRV in healthy populations. Mølgaard *et al.* (1991) compared hourly values and day–night differences for SDNN, pNN50 (per cent *NN* intervals > 50 ms different from the prior one) and pNN6% (per cent *NN* intervals > 6% of local average *NN* difference from the prior one) in 140 healthy subjects aged 40–77 years. Night-time was the period of lowest heart rate, i.e. sleep time. Hourly SDNN decreased at night, while hourly pNN50 and pNN6% increased and peaked at about 05.00 hours. Values for 24-h SDNN reported to be associated with high risk in post-MI patients were not seen, but extremely low values for pNN50 and pNN6% and a lack of diurnal variation in pNN50 or pNN6% were seen in the healthy population. The highest values for HRV and lowest heart rates during sleep were seen in those with a high level of physical training. Yamasaki *et al.* (1996) investigated the effect of age and sex on diurnal HRV patterns in healthy adults. A consistent increase in HF power during the 00.00–06.00 period was seen in both women and men, independent of age. Normalized LF was higher for males and showed a different circadian pattern by gender. Highest values for normalized LF were seen between 08.00 and 12.00 hours in males and between 12.00 and 24.00 hours in females. Hartikainen *et al.* (1993) showed that circadian rhythms of HF power and SDNN persisted during 24-h of bed rest in healthy men.

Shift workers offer a naturalistic experiment in the effect of changing circadian activity patterns on the circadian rhythm of HRV. Results of small studies are generally consistent, suggesting that HRV while awake at work, awake not at work, and asleep is primarily determined by activity rather than time of day (Freitas *et al.* 1997; Ito *et al.* 2001). Furlan *et al.* (2000), however, in a slightly larger study (22 subjects compared with 12 and 10 subjects, respectively), reported decreased normalized LF and LF/HF ratio during night-time compared with morning and evening shifts, suggesting that this might be associated with diminished alertness during night-time shifts.

Circadian patterns of cardiovascular events

As mentioned, one of the first applications of circadian patterns of HRV was to compare the circadian cycle of cardiac events with the circadian rhythm of HRV. Thus, the well-known increase in cardiovascular events in the early morning clearly corresponds with a sharp increase in heart rate and a drop in parasympathetically-modulated HRV. Of interest are populations where the circadian pattern of cardiovascular events is unusual. An example is depressed post-MI patients who tend to have their events during the night (Carney *et al.* 1991). Consistent with other studies, nondepressed patients in the same study had their events in the morning. Whether this represents a difference in circadian autonomic rhythms or an adverse effect of sleep-disordered breathing in depressed cardiac patients remains to be determined. Marchant *et al.* (1994) compared patterns of myocardial ischaemia in early post-MI patients and patients with stable angina. In stable angina patients, ischaemic events had a circadian rhythm with a daytime peak, while no circadian pattern was seen among the post-MI patients. Both groups had a circadian rhythm in LF and HF, with a less pronounced rhythm in the post-MI patients, but only the stable angina group had a daytime peak in LF/HF. Although these differences may be a function of the fact that the post-MI patients were hospitalized, the principal finding was that the lack of circadian rhythm in LF/HF was associated with a lack of circadian rhythm in ischaemic episodes. The morning peak in cardiovascular events is also not seen among diabetics, although an evening peak has been reported. Aronson *et al.* (1999) compared parasympathetically mediated HRV between 06.00 and 10.00 hours vs. 22.00 and 06.00 hours in 22 type I subjects with diabetes and cardiac autonomic neuropathy. There was no day–night difference in either pNN50 or HF power, although rMSSD was slightly greater during the night-time. The authors conclude that patients with diabetes lack the normal night-time parasympathetic predominance, implying that the loss of parasympathetic predominance in the morning hours per se is part of the causal pathway for excess morning events.

The ICD has facilitated more detailed studies of the circadian rhythm of cardiovascular events. Recently, Fries *et al.* (2002) studied 20 consecutive ICD patients each of whom had received at least three spontaneous and appropriate shocks for ventricular tachyarrhythmias during a mean follow-up of 56 months. Circadian variation of events was determined as the frequency of events during four 6-h periods beginning at midnight. Patients were grouped as having ($n = 10$) or not having most of their arrhythmias in the morning ($n = 10$). HRV was determined for the first 5-min of each hour. Results, in apparent contradiction to those cited above among diabetics, suggest that the normal physiological increase of parasympathetically modulated HRV during sleep was present only in those patients without morning events, i.e. that increased parasympathetic modulation of heart rate at night is cardioprotective for morning events.

Circadian rhythms in coronary artery disease

There is a significant body of literature comparing circadian patterns of heart rate and HRV in cardiovascular clinical populations and healthy controls. A comparison of HRV in patients with CAD but no history of MI and normal controls was performed by Huikuri *et al.* (1994). Significantly, 24-h HRV indices were not different between groups. However, whilst healthy subjects had a significant circadian rhythm of normalized LF, normalized HF and the LF/HF ratio, measured using cosinor analysis, this rhythm was not seen in patients. This finding suggests a potential utility of these measures for screening patients. Also, the significant change in the LF/HF ratio upon awakening, seen in the healthy subjects, was absent in patients, although the change in HRV upon becoming upright was the same between groups.

Circadian rhythms post-MI

Total HRV has been well studied in post-MI patients, but fewer investigators have specifically considered circadian rhythms of HRV post-MI. Lombardi *et al.* (1992) compared 20 patients and 20 control subjects 4 weeks after an uncomplicated MI. HRV was, of course, significantly lower in the post-MI subjects. Day–night differences in HRV were seen in both groups and the maximal day–night difference in *RR* interval duration was similar between groups. When HRV was compared in 6-h segments, post-MI patients had a reduced daytime (06.00–24.00) and increased night-time variance in *RR* intervals. Although not addressed in the manuscript, we hypothesize that this increased night-time variance could be associated with a greater prevalence of sleep-disordered breathing. Post-MI patients also had higher values for normalized LF and lower values for normalized HF power, with a smaller circadian increase in HF power at night. The acrophase for HF power was also different for the post-MI patients, probably because they were hospitalized at the time of the recording. Malik *et al.* (1990) in an early case-control study of post-MI patients ($n = 20$ with and $n = 20$ without complications during 6-month follow-up), found that low-risk patients had a more marked diurnal rhythm of HRV than high-risk patients and suggested that longer-term HRV components must be included in risk stratification to capture this variation. Interestingly though, results of this small study suggested that the greatest separation of those with and without complications was found for HRV measured between 06.00 and 14.00 hours.

Circadian rhythms in sudden death survivors

Sudden death survivors have markedly decreased HRV. Huikuri *et al.* (1992) compared circadian rhythms in 22 survivors of sudden death not associated with acute myocardial infarction and in 22 matched controls. A significant circadian rhythm was observed in both groups and, despite reduced HRV in those who had experienced sudden death, no difference in the amplitude of the circadian rhythm using single cosinor analysis. However, the reduced HRV in the sudden death survivors in combination with the preserved circadian rhythm of HRV suggested the HRV in this group would be extremely low in the higher-risk early morning hours, potentially putting them at even higher risk for events. Burr *et al.* (1994) attempted to reproduce Huikuri *et al.*'s (1992) findings in groups of male and female normal subjects, sudden death survivors with an old MI and sudden death survivors with no current or prior MI. Results were generally consistent with the prior study, except that Burr *et al.* identified a group of female sudden death survivors with no cardiac history in whom very distinct 24-h HRV patterns associated with a *rise*, rather than the normal fall, in pNN50 during the daytime, suggesting that sudden death may be a more heterogeneous phenomenon than generally believed. Klingenhaben *et al.* (1995) compared circadian rhythms of HRV between 14 post-MI patients who had survived at least one out-of-hospital sudden death cardiac arrest and 14 matched post-MI patients without a history of malignant arrhythmias. Comparisons were based on averages of mean values for daytime and night-time and on hourly means. No circadian rhythm for parasympathetically mediated HRV was observed among sudden death survivors, but circadian rhythms were preserved among those without malignant arrhythmias. Circadian rhythms of LF power were comparable between groups. Differences in parasympathetic modulation of HRV was especially great during 16.00–19.00 hours. These results suggest that the absence of circadian patterns of HF power could be of prognostic significance, although, as previously mentioned, Mølgaard *et al.* (1991) found a lack of diurnal variation in parasympathetically mediated HRV in a healthy population.

Circadian rhythms in angina and diabetes

Angina patients and those with diabetes have been the subject of several studies of circadian patterns of HRV. Burger *et al.* (1999) compared daytime (8.00–24.00) and night-time (24.00–08.00) time- and frequency-domain HRV in 12 normal subjects, 23 patients with chronic angina and 23 patients with type I diabetes. All time-domain HRV except SDNNIDX (the average standard deviation of NNs over 5 min) and all frequency-domain HRV were significantly different between daytime and night-time, with the greatest difference among normal subjects, less among patients with angina and the least difference among those patients with diabetes. The differences among the groups reflected the greater reduction in night-time vagal modulation of heart rate among patients, especially among those with diabetes. In contrast to the results reported by Aronson *et al.* (1999) and cited above, a preserved circadian rhythm of HRV among patients with diabetes was reported by Malpas & Purdie (1990). HRV was evaluated every 30 min by cosinor analysis in 11 healthy subjects, 12 insulin-dependent patients and 7 patients with alcoholism and vagal neuropathy. Although patients had decreased HRV, circadian rhythms of heart rate and SDSD (the standard deviation of the differences between successive NNs) were preserved.

Hourly frequency-domain HRV was compared among drug-free angina patients ($n = 65$) and age-matched healthy controls ($n = 33$) (Wennerblom *et al.* 2001). Daytime (8.00–20.00) and night-time (24.00–05.00) HRV was also compared. To capture detailed differences in circadian patterns more accurately, the hourly maximum and minimum HRV, differences in the maximum and minimum (gradient), rate of change/h between the maximum and minimum (velocity) and largest difference between two consecutive hours (maximum velocity) were also measured between 00.00 and 10.00 hours (night-time and early morning). Healthy controls had a faster HF velocity and a higher HF gradient than angina patients, implying that faster vagal withdrawal in the morning is association with cardiac autonomic health. In another study of circadian HRV in angina patients, Watanabe *et al.* (2001) compared day–night differences in HRV among patients with vasospastic angina (single or multivessel) provoked by intracoronary acetylcholine administration, patients with effort angina and normal controls. Circadian rhythm of HF power was attenuated in both the multivessel spasm and effort angina patients, but not in those with single vessel spasm. Circadian variation in the LF/HF ratio was less in both groups with vasospastic angina. Thus, patients with multivessel vasospasm appear to have abnormal rhythms for both HF (reflecting vagal modulation of heart rate) and the LF/HF ratio (considered to reflect sympatho-vagal balance) whereas those with single vessel vasospasms may have abnormal rhythms for vagal modulation of heart rate only.

Decreased HRV is well-known among patients with congestive heart failure. Kim & Yum (2000) examined the circadian rhythm of standard and nonlinear HRV indices among 16 CHF patients compared with 20 normal controls. Despite the reduced HRV in CHF, circadian rhythm in heart rate and many HRV indices was preserved. However, circadian rhythms of HF power and of nonlinear (complexity) measures were lost in the CHF group.

Circadian rhythms in other cardiovascular patient populations

The relationship of circadian rhythms of blood pressure and outcome among patients with hypertension has been investigated in numerous studies. Chakko *et al.* (1993) investigated circadian patterns of HRV among 22 treated hypertensive patients, with left ventricular hypertrophy (LVH) but without coronary artery disease, and 11 healthy age-matched controls. Hourly values for HRV were compared using *t*-tests, and averaged values during wake (9.00–21.00) and sleep (23.00–07.00) were compared as well. SDNN (calculated as the average of hourly SDNN), pNN50, total, low and high frequency power were all significant lower among those with LVH. SDNN was decreased for each hour, and the morning rise in SDNN, seen in healthy subjects, was blunted in patients. Indeed SDNN remained relatively constant over the 24-h period in the LVH group. PNN50 was reported to be higher at night among the patients with LVH. We suspect this was related to the heart rate effects of undetected sleep-disordered breathing. Little circadian rhythm of LF power was seen in patients, whereas LF decreased during the night-time and increased during the morning hours in controls. Verdecchia *et al.* (1998) reported that a blunted circadian rhythm of heart rate was an independent predictor of mortality in essential hypertension. A 10% decrease in day–night difference was associated with a 1.3 relative risk of mortality after follow-up averaging 3.6 years. Moreover, day–night differences in heart rate correlated directly with day–night differences in systolic blood pressure.

Circadian rhythms of HRV in patients with nonsustained VT were investigated by Ooie *et al.* (1998). Patients were divided into two groups, HF+ patients who had a significant circadian rhythm in HF power and a night-time acrophase by cosinor analysis and HF– patients who lacked a significant circadian rhythm. Serial changes in HRV before episodes of NSVT were significantly different between the HF+ and HF– groups, with increasing HF before NSVT in the HF+ and decreasing HF in the HF– group. Serial changes in the LF/HF ratio did not differ between groups.

Effect of pharmacological interventions on circadian rhythms

The effect of interventions on the circadian rhythm of heart rate and HRV has also been studied. Beta blockers have been shown to reduce mortality in the post-MI period and to have an especially significant effect on morning events (Peters 1990). Mølgaard *et al.* (1993) described the effect of 4 weeks of treatment with metoprolol in male patients surviving their first MI. HRV was compared during the daytime and night-time (defined as the period of lowest heart rate). Beta-blockade did not affect total SDNN, but both daytime and night-time SDNN increased. Sandrone *et al.* (1994) also reported on the effect of 4 weeks of treatment with beta blockers (either metoprolol or atenolol) on heart rate and HRV post-MI. Treatment decreased normalized LF power and increased normalized HF power, with a more pronounced effect during the daytime. Significantly, the circadian rhythm of normalized LF power was decreased so that the early morning increase was no longer seen. No differences were seen in the effects of atenolol compared to metoprolol. An increase in 24-h values for vagally-modulated HRV indices, but no effect on the amplitude of the circadian rhythm of HRV after treatment with beta blockers, was reported by Niemela *et al.* (1994). The morning decrease in HF power, however, was blunted. The effect of metoprolol on circadian HRV in chronic stable angina patients compared to normal subjects was examined by Burger *et al.* (1999). Circadian rhythms were preserved, although smaller in angina patients before therapy. Beta blockade significantly improved, but did not normalize, daytime time-domain HRV, night-time pNN50 and rMSSD, and daytime values for total and high frequency power, but decreased day–night differences. When angina patients in the Wennerblom *et al.* (2001) study cited previously were given isosorbide (n = 30), the HF power gradient (difference between the maximum and minimum HRV between 00.00 and 10.00 hours) was increased. When patients (n = 33) were given metoprolol, the heart rate gradient and the maximum heart rate velocity also increased. With metoprolol treatment, the LF/HF gradient, velocity and maximum velocity were decreased. Finally, Sarma *et al.* (1994) evaluated the effect of treatment with the beta blocker nadolol on circadian patterns of HRV. Treatment significantly reduced mean heart rate intervals, with the greatest effect during the daytime. As a result cosinor amplitude of heart rate decreased significantly. Cosinor amplitude of LF power was unaffected and, consistent with other studies, HF power increased during the night.

The circadian effects of 30 days of treatment with quinapril or metoprolol was compared among post-MI patients (Kontopoulos *et al.* 1999). Pretreatment recordings were obtained 5 days after acute MI. Quinapril increased parasympathetic modulation of heart rate (quantified as normalized HF power) and decreased 'sympathetic' indices (quantified as normalized LF power or the LF/HF ratio). The maximum effect was reported to occur between 02.00 and 04.00, 08.00 and 11.00 and from 19.00 to 22.00 hours. Metoprolol also increased normalized HF and decreased normalized LF and LF/HF ratio, mainly between 08.00 and 12.00 and from 19.00 to 22.00 hours. There were no changes in the placebo group. Kontopoulos *et al.* concluded that quinapril and metoprolol had similar effects, but that the effect for quinapril was greater.

The long-term effect of quinapril in patients with diabetic autononopathy was studied by Athyros *et al.* (1998). Normalized LF, HF and the LF/HF ratio were measured at baseline and after 1 year of therapy in 60 patients of whom 30 received quinapril and 30 placebo. Thirty normal patients and 30 diabetic patients without diabetic neuropathy served as controls. In contrast to some previously cited studies, Athyros *et al.* reported no circadian rhythm of normalized power in those with diabetic autononopathy and a markedly higher LF/HF ratio. After 1 year of therapy, HF had increased, LF had decreased and the LF/HF ratio had improved, both when assessed in the morning (07.00–05.00) and night (23.00–07.00), with the greatest effect seen at night.

Finally, Yee *et al.* (2001), in a cross-over study of 28 CHF patients, reported that 4 weeks of spironolactone treatment improved HRV during the morning hours only.

Conclusions

As can be appreciated from the diverse collection of studies presented here, detailed analysis of circadian rhythms of heart rate and HRV has the potential to yield additional insights about HRV in high risk patients and about the effects of interventions. Results so far suggest that heart rate and HRV patterns in the early morning period are of special interest, at least in the usual cardiac patient population. The presence of high risk populations in which circadian rhythms of heart rate and HRV are abnormal bears further study. Little is known about circadian rhythms of nonlinear HRV measures or of newer measures like heart rate turbulence. A consensus among researchers that could standardize methodology and permit comparisons between studies is sorely needed. Circadian patterns of HRV could be examined for any of the many Holter datasets including MPIP, ATRAMI or EMIAT and the potential utility of circadian measures for risk stratification could be explored. In addition, circadian patterns of HRV could potentially be useful in individualizing therapy and assessing treatment response.

References

Aronson, D., Weinrauch, L.F., Elia, J.A., Tofler, G.H. & Burger, A.J. (1999) Circadian patterns of heart rate variability, fibrinolytic activity, and hemostatic factors in type I diabetes mellitus with cardiac autonomic neuropathy. *American Journal of Cardiology*, **84**, 449–453.

Athyros, V.G., Didangelos, T.P., Karamitsos, D.T., Papageorgiou, A.A., Boudoulas, H. & Kontopoulos, A.G. (1998) Long-term effect of converting enzyme inhibition on circadian sympathetic and parasympathetic modulation in patients with diabetic autonomic neuropathy. *Acta Cardiologica*, **53**, 201–209.

Burger, A.J.& Kamalesh, M. (1999) Effect of beta-adrenergic blocker therapy on the circadian rhythm of heart rate variability in patients with chronic stable angina pectoris. *American Journal of Cardiology*, **83**, 596–598.

Burger, A.J., Charlamb, M. & Sherman, H.B. (1999) Circadian patterns of heart rate variability in normals, chronic stable angina and diabetes mellitus. *International Journal of Cardiology*, **77**, 41–48.

Burr, R., Hamilton, P., Cowan, M. *et al.* (1994) Nycthemeral profile of nonspectral heart rate variability meanures in women and men. Description of a normal sample and two sudden cardiac arrest subsamples. *Journal of Electrocardiology*, **27**, 54–61.

Carney, R.M., Freedland, K.E. & Jaffe, A.S. (1991) Altered circadian variation of acute myocardial infarction in patients with depression. *Coronary Artery Disease*, **2**, 61–65.

Chakko, S., Mulingtapang, R.F., Hurikuri, H.V., Kessler, K.M., Materson, B.J. & Myerburg, R.J. (1993) Alterations in heart rate variability and its circadian rhythm in hypertensive patients with left ventricular hypertrophy free of coronary artery disease. *American Heart Journal*, **126**, 1364–1372.

Freitas, J., Lago, P., Puig, J., Carvalho, M.J., Costa, O. & De Freitas, A.F. (1997) Circadian heart rate variability rhythm in shift workers. *Journal of Electrocardiology*, **30**, 39–44

Fries, R., Hein, S. & Konig, J. (2002) Reversed circadian rhythms of heart rate variability and morning peak occurrence of sustained ventricular tachyarrhythmias in patients with implanted cardioverter defibrillator. *Medical Science Monitor*, **8**, 751–756.

Furlan, R., Barbic, F., Piazza, S., Tinelli, M., Seghizzi, P. & Malliani, A. (2000) Modification of cardiac autonomic profile associated with a shift schedule of work. *Circulation*, **102** 1912–1916.

Hartikainen, J., Tarkiainen, I., Tahvanainen, K., Mantysaari, M., Lansimies, E. & Pyorala, K. (1993) Circadian variation of cardiac autonomic regulation during 24-h bed rest. *Clinical Physiology*, **13**,185–196.

Huikuri, H.V., Niemela, M.J., Ojala, S., Rantala, A., Ikaheimo, M.J. & Airaksinen, K.E. (1994) Circadian rhythms of frequency-domain measures of heart rate variability in healthy subjects and patients with coronary artery disease. Effects of arousal and upright posture. *Circulation*, **90**, 121–126.

Huikuri, H.V., Linnaluoto, M.K., Seppanen, T. *et al.* (1992) Circadian rhythm of heart rate variability in survivors of cardiac arrest. *American Journal of Cardiology*, **70**, 610–615.

Ito, H., Nozaki, M., Maruyama, T., Kaji, Y. & Tsuda, Y. (2001) Shift work modifies the circadian patterns of heart rate variability in nurses. *International Journal of Cardiology*, **79**, 231–236.

Kim, S.G. & Yum, M.K. (2000) Decreased *RR* interval complexity and loss of circadian rhythm in patients with congestive heart failure. *Japanese Circulation Journal*, 64, 39–45.

Klingenhaben, T., Rapp, U. & Honhloser, S. (1995) Circadian variation of heart rate variability in postinfarction patients with and without life-threatening tachyarrhythmias. *Journal of Cardiovascular Electrophysiology*, **6**, 357–364.

Kontopoulos, A.G., Athyros, V.G., Papageorgiou, A.A. & Boudoulas, H. (1999) Effect of quinapril or metoprolol on circadian sympathetic and parasympathetic modulation after acute myocardial infarction. *American Journal of Cardiology*, **84**, 1164–1169.

Lombardi, F., Sadrone, G., Mortata, A. *et al.* (1992) Circadian variation of spectral indices of heart rate variability after myocardial infarction. *American Heart Journal*, **123**, 1521–1529.

Malik, M., Farrell, T. & Camm, A.J. (1990) Circadian rhythm of heart rate variability after acute myocardial infarction and its influence on the prognostic value of heart rate variability. *American Journal of Cardiology*, **66**, 1049–1054.

Malpas, S.C. & Purdie, G.L. (1990) Circadian variation of heart rate variability. *Cardiovascular Research*, **24**, 210–213.

Marchant, B., Stevenson, R., Vaishnav, S., Wilkinson, P., Ranjadayalan, K. & Timmis, A.D. (1994) Influence of the autonomic nervous system on circadian patterns of myocardial ischaemia: comparison of stable angina with the early postinfarction period. *British Heart Journal*, **71**, 329–333.

Mølgaard, H., Mickley, H., Pless, P., Bjerregaard, P. & Moller, M. (1993) Effects of metoprolol on heart rate variability in survivors of acute myocardial infarction. *American Journal of Cardiology*, **71**, 1357–1359.

Mølgaard, H., Sørensen, K.I., Pjerregaard, P. (1991) Circadian variation and influence of risk factors on heart rate variability in healthy subjects. *American Journal of Cardiology*, **68**, 777–784.

Muller, J.E., Ludmer, P.L., Willich, S.N. *et al.* (1987) Circadian variation in the frequency of sudden cardiac death. *Circulation*, **75**, 131–138.

Niemela, M.J., Airaksinen, K.E. & Huikuri, H.V. (1994) Effect of beta-blockade on heart rate variability in patients with coronary artery disease. *Journal of the American College of Cardiology*, **23**, 1370–1377.

Ooie, T., Saikawa, T., Hara, M., Takakura, T., Sato, Y. & Sakata, T. (1998) Role of circadian rhythmicity in the heart rate variability preceding non-sustained ventricular tachycardia. *Japanese Circulation, Journal*, **62**, 887–892.

Peters, R.M. (1990) Propranolol and the morning increase in sudden cardiac death (the Beta blocker Heart Attack Trial experience). *American Journal of Cardiology*, **63**, 1518–1520.

Sandrone, G., Mortara, A., Torzillo, D., La Rovere, M.T., Malliani, A. & Lombardi, F. (1994) Effects of beta blockers (atenolol or metoprolol) on heart rate variability after acute myocardial infarction. *American Journal of Cardiology*, **74**, 340–345.

Sarma,J.S., Singh, N., Schoenbaum, M.P., Venkataraman, K. & Singh, B.N. (1994) Circadian and power spectral changes of *RR* and *QT* intervals during treatment of patients with angina pectoris with nadolol providing evidence for differential autonomic modulation of heart rate and ventricular repolarization. *American Journal of Cardiology*, **74**, 131–136.

Verdecchia, P., Schillaci, G., Borgioni, C., Ciucci, A. *et al.* (1998) Adverse prognostic value of a blunted circadian rhythm of heart rate in essential hypertension. *Journal of Hypertension*, **16**, 1335–1343.

Watanabe, T., Kim, S., Akishita, M. *et al.* (2001) Circadian variation of autonomic nervous activity in patients with multivessel coronary spasm. *Japanese Circulation, Journal*, **65**, 593–598.

Wennerblom, B., Lurje, L., Karlsson, T., Tygesen, H., Vahisale, R. & Hjalmarson, A. (2001) Circadian variation of heart rate variability and the rate of autonomic change in the morning hours in healthy subjects and angina patients. *International Journal of Cardiology*, **79**, 61–69.

Yamasaki, Y., Kodama, M., Matsuhisa, M. *et al.* (1996) Diurnal heart rate variability in healthy subjects: effects of aging and sex difference. *American Journal of Cardiology*, **271**, H303–H310.

Yee, K.M., Pringle, S.D. & Struthers, A.D. (2001) Circadian variation in the effects of aldosterone blockade on heart rate variability and QT dispersion in congestive heart failure. *Journal of the American College of Cardiology*, **37**,1800–1807.

CHAPTER 9

Time–Frequency Analysis of Heart Rate Variability Under Autonomic Provocations

Solange Akselrod

Introduction

The electrocardiogram (ECG), including its dynamical changes as a function of time, in response to physical activity, or as a result of treatment, is perhaps the most basic and important clinical tool available to the cardiologist. Among others, it allows to diagnose abnormalities in cardiac electrical activity and propagation, in blood perfusion to the myocardium, and in neural control to the sinoatrial (SA) node.

The waveform of the ECG signal provides a wealth of information about electrical conduction in the myocardium. An even more basic measure, directly reflecting the autonomic control of the cardiovascular system, can be obtained from the time series of the interbeat intervals, typically expressed by either the instantaneous heart rate (*HR*), or the beat-to-beat *RR* intervals. This beat-to-beat time series discloses a host of dependent and independent data, concerning:

- the existence and features of cardiac arrhythmia;
- the existence and features of the normal sinus rhythm, disclosing the modulation of *HR* by neural and hormonal control mechanisms.

In this chapter, we will focus on the vast amount of information, which can be revealed by these *HR* fluctuations under conditions of sinus rhythm, both in steady-state and in transient-state conditions. Indeed, as changes in the ECG waveform reflect dynamics in electrical propagation, so do changes in the pattern of *HR* fluctuations disclose dynamics in the various cardiovascular control mechanisms.

Based on a large number of studies (Akselrod *et al.* 1981, 1985; Malliani *et al.* 1991), it is currently well accepted that the *HR* time series represents a rich, quantitative source of knowledge (Persson 1997). *HR* variability reflects the sympathetic and parasympathetic control of the heart, their mutual balance, the degree of peripheral fluctuations in vasomotor tone and therefore the resulting effect on blood pressure (*BP*) fluctuations (Akselrod 1995; Malik & Camm 1995).

The basic features of *HR* variability and their physiological significance are presented in detail in previous chapters.

An adequate analysis of *HR* fluctuations discloses the ability of the *HR* control mechanisms to help maintaining all cardiovascular fluctuations within a normal range, not too high, not too low, fulfilling the basic requirements of homeostasis (Hainsworth 1998).

However, it is well known that the ECG waveform, which may look perfectly benign in baseline conditions, may reveal existing problems only when some kind of challenge (such as an exercise test) is imposed to the cardiovascular system. Similarly, the *HR* fluctuations may unmask existing abnormalities, in one or several control mechanisms, only when an autonomic provocation is imposed (Keselbrener & Akselrod 1998; Malik 1998).

Indeed, for example, only when challenged to compensate for a drop in *BP* during an active transition from supine to standing position, will the changes in *HR* and *BP* as well as the changes in the pattern of their fluctuations, disclose abnormalities related to early hypertension. They will indicate whether both the sympathetic and parasympathetic branches respond efficiently, at the right timing and at the adequate intensity (Akselrod *et al.* 1997; Davrath *et al.* 2003).

Or, when considering an even more pathological condition, such as acute MI, the time-dependent pattern of *HR* fluctuations, may reveal whether some change (above a certain threshold) has occurred in the neural control of the SA node. If the observed change is in excess of a previously defined threshold, it may indicate a change in myocardial perfusion, and (perhaps) become a marker for successful reperfusion by thrombolysis (Toledo *et al.* 2003).

These examples, as well as many other widespread clinical conditions or provocations (such as ischaemia, exercise test, angina, tilt test, syncope, effects of medication) are all by definition 'non-steady' states. Therefore they do require a special signal processing approach (Cerutti *et al.* 2001).

Need for time–frequency (*t–f*) analysis

The features of *HR* variability (HRV) under steady-state conditions (or typically under the assumption that the conditions are close enough to steady state) have been extensively investigated and discussed in previous research (Malik & Camm 1995).

The earliest studies have focused on time-domain measures of *HR* fluctuations (such as mean, variance, standardized) and a set of modifications of these parameters (Kleiger *et al.* 1987; Coumel *et al.* 1991). Later studies have shown that specific control mechanisms express themselves in specific frequency bands, thus suiting ideally the transition to the frequency-domain (Oppenheim & Schafer 1975). Therefore, a preferred way to consider these fluctuations in *RR* or *HR*, in blood pressure (*BP*), in respiration or blood flow, is to perform spectral analysis, typically by fast Fourier transform (FFT) or autoregression (Akselrod *et al.* 1981; Malliani *et al.* 1991; Persson 1997).

However, a strict requirement necessitated by this 'classical' approach is that the signals have to clearly reflect steady-state conditions (Oppenheim & Schafer 1975), otherwise the spectral information will be artefactual and invalid (see Fig. 9.1).

From Fig. 9.1, it is clear that with the 'classical' PS of a non-steady trace, the time resolution is lost, it is impossible to know if and when a change has occurred in the frequency content, and the spectral decomposition lo longer reflects the true information. In such cases as Fig. 1c or 1f, or in any combination of such sudden changes, in frequency and/or amplitude, a time-dependent frequency decomposition becomes necessary.

In order to take optimal care of longer and more 'realistic' (not necessarily steady) *HR* time series, which obviously may undergo time-dependent changes in their spectral content, we need a sensitive and reliable way to perform *t–f* analysis, and to obtain a time-dependent power spectrum. To overcome the non-physiological assumption of stationarity, or in other words to deal with non-stationarity, new mathematical methods have been developed.

The implementation of these tools for the investigation of the cardiovascular system, results in the quantitative display of *t–f* spectral decomposition of the simultaneous *HR*, *BP*, blood flow and/or respiratory signals, whether steady or not.

Initial approach for *t–f* analysis: the STFT

A sequential estimation of power spectra, such as the use of a time-shifted short time Fourier transform (STFT) (Nawab & Quatieri 1988; Marchesi *et al.* 1991), is perhaps the most straightforward attempt to overcome the stationarity requirement (see Fig. 9.2). Yet the STFT suffers from the intrinsic compromise, which involves the absence of time resolution within the power spectrum of each subtrace, as well as a severe limitation regarding the minimal frequency it can focus on. Shortening the overlapping subtraces (reducing their duration *T*) would improve the time resolution; yet it would shift to higher frequencies the minimal frequency that can be investigated ($f_{min} > 1/T$), thus limiting the ability to quantify low frequency rhythms in the data. (see Fig. 9.2). For physiological information, this is an extremely important drawback.

Several remarks are imperative regarding the STFT.

- Although time-dependent spectral changes are displayed by subsequent subtraces, time

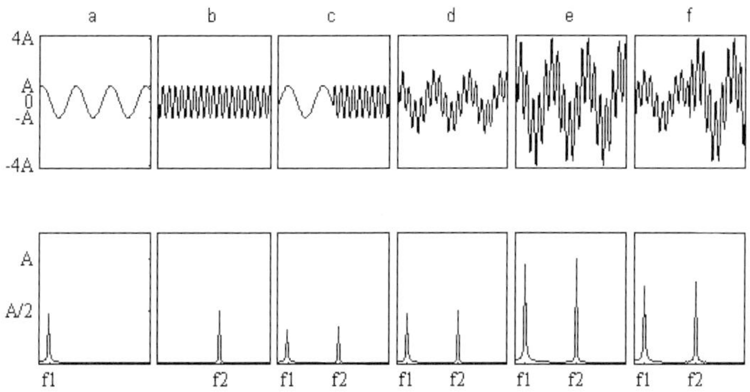

Fig. 9.1 Displays six different time-dependent signals (top) and their corresponding power spectrum (PS, bottom). All traces contain only one or two sinusoidal components, at frequency *f*1 and/or *f*2, while the amplitude of these components is either A or 2A. Four of the traces (a, b, d, e) are steady state traces, namely frequency content and amplitudes are constant all along each trace. (a) The signal contains a single sinus wave, of amplitude A, at frequency *f*1. Its PS displays accordingly a single peak at *f*1. (b) The signal contains a single sinus wave, of amplitude A, at frequency *f*2. Its PS displays accordingly a single peak at *f*2, of same amplitude as in (a). (d) The signal contains two sinus waves, each of amplitude A, at frequencies *f*1 and *f*2. Its PS displays accordingly two peaks, at *f*1 and *f*2, of same amplitude as in (a) and (b). (e) The signal contains two sinus waves, each of amplitude 2A, at frequencies *f*1 and *f*2. Its PS displays accordingly 2 peaks, at *f*1 and *f*2, of twice the amplitude in (d). Two traces, (c) and (f), are not steady. (c) The signal contains a single frequency component that suddenly switches from *f*1 to *f*2 in the middle of the trace. The PS does not display this sudden change. Instead, it provides an 'erroneous' frequency decomposition, averaged over the entire trace length: as if, the two frequency components *f*1 and *f*2 were active all along the trace, at an amplitude that is about half of their true amplitude. (f) The signal contains two frequency components, the amplitude of which switches suddenly from A to 2A, in the middle of the trace. Again the regular PS provides averaged, 'erroneous' information, as if the two frequency components were consistently at the same amplitude, about the average value between the initial amplitude A and the final amplitude 2A.

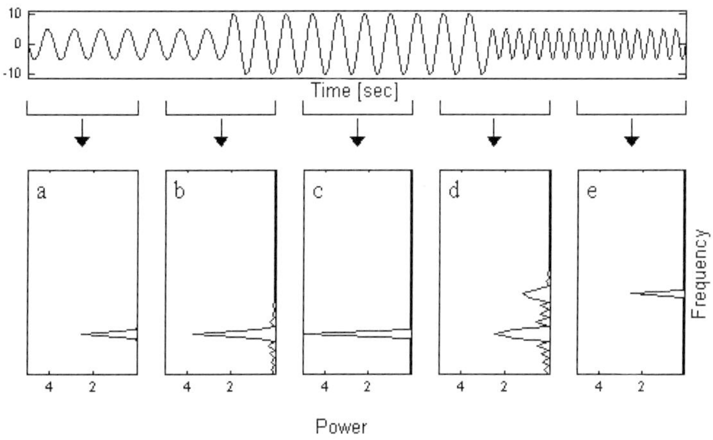

Fig. 9.2 Displays a non-steady signal (top), with first, a sudden increase in amplitude, and then, a sudden change in frequency together with a return to its initial amplitude. Five subsequent, nonoverlapping subtraces (of duration *T*) are indicated, and their corresponding, short-term power spectra are shown (bottom, a–e). The STFT approach typically displays the subtraces' power spectra as a function of time (for partially overlapping subtraces), as a 3D graph (power as function of *f* and *t*). Subtraces (a), (c) and (e) are steady, and therefore their corresponding short-term power spectra reliably reflect their frequency content. Subtraces (b) and (d) undergo sudden and marked changes in frequency and/or amplitude. Obviously the power spectra of these subtraces, and of other partially overlapping subtraces (not shown), do not allow a good time resolution.

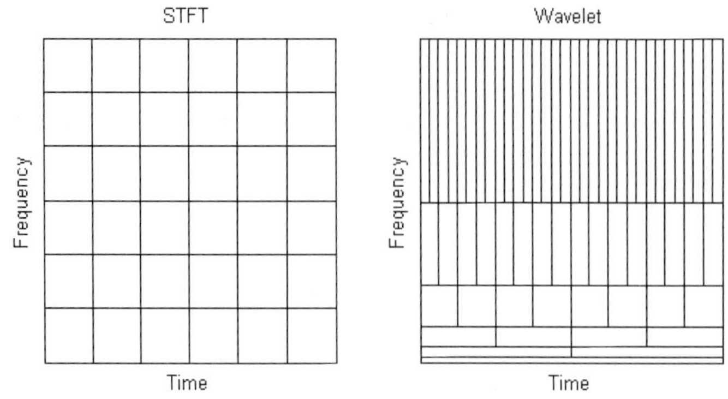

Fig. 9.3 Time–frequency plane for the STFT algorithm (left) is based on constant resolution of the *t–f* plane: at any time and frequency in the plane, the frequency and time resolution are equal (all subtraces are of the same duration *T*). Algorithms such as wavelet, SDA or continuous wavelet transform (left), are based on an unequal subdivision of the *t–f* plane: for each frequency, the duration of the considered time window is proportional to 1/*f*. At low frequencies the time window is longer, causing the time resolution to be reduced yet improving the frequency resolution; at higher frequencies the time resolution improves while the frequency resolution is reduced. The result is an unequal, optimal resolution of the *t–f* plane for each time and frequency.

resolution is significantly impaired (see Fig. 9.2b,d), as a result of the subtrace duration *T*.

• *T* is predetermined and remains constant in each subtrace, all along the analysed data. This fixes both the minimal frequency (f_{min}) that can be evaluated, as well as the time resolution. The sampling rate determines the maximal frequency (f_{max}), that can be evaluated for each subtrace, according to the Nyquist principle.

• At each time and frequency in the *t–f* plane, the time and frequency resolution remain constant. The entire *t–f* plane is thus equally divided (see Fig. 9.3, left).

• Trying to shorten *T* of the STFT, in order to improve the time resolution for the high frequency components, would impair the ability to investigate low frequency components. The STFT is therefore a rough compromise between time and frequency resolution

More sophisticated approaches for *t–f* analysis

Various more sophisticated approaches have been recently developed to overcome these limitations (see reviews by Cohen 1989; Daubechies 1990).

Some of the *t–f* approaches applied to cardiovascular signals include: the selective discrete algorithm (SDA) (Keselbrener *et al.* 1994, 1996; Keselbrener & Akselrod 1996), various enhanced versions of the Wigner–Ville transform (such as the SPWV applied by Novak & Novak 1993, and by Medigue *et al.* 2001, as well as the Modified WV developed by Maor *et al.* 2002), the time-dependent autoregression (Bianchi *et al.* 1993; Cerutti *et al.* 2001), wavelets (Calgagnini *et al.* 1998), and the continuous wavelet transform (Toledo *et al.* 2001, 2003).

The above algorithms have been primarily aimed at investigating autonomic activity (in steady and non-steady conditions) using the analysis of variability of cardiovascular signals. Typically, the investigations focus on specific disease conditions, such as: heart transplant (Toledo *et al.* 2002), hypertension (Akselrod *et al.* 1997; Maor *et al.* 2002; Davrath *et al.* 2003), tilt test for the diagnosis of recurrent syncope (Kenny *et al.* 1989; Akselrod *et al.* 2001; Cerutti *et al.* 2001), or thrombolysis during acute myocardial infarction (Toledo *et al.* 2003). The studies are then primarily directed at investigating the dynamic pathophysiology of the control mechanisms involved, by means of time-dependent spectral analysis of cardiovascular fluctuations.

The goal of these investigations was usually, first to characterize the diseased cardiovascular control, then to try and understand the autonomic dysfunction with its existing or developing compensatory mechanisms. The important next step, however, was to try and design some quantitative practical criteria that may have a clear clinical application. For instance, this step may lead to the development of a noninvasive clinical procedure for the early detection of hypertension or to differentiate the mechanism responsible for recurrent syncope. It may allow us to define a specific threshold quantifying the changes in *HR* variability, which would confirm reperfusion by thrombolysis or detect possible reocclusion.

The physiological signals (*HR*, *BP*, etc.) acquired during the experimental protocols of the abovementioned studies and similar ones, can be typically divided into two very different types of subtraces of these signals:

- steady-state conditions: e.g. supine rest, or steady standing;
- non-steady state: transitional conditions, in response to an autonomic perturbation such as a head-up tilt, an active change in posture, a handgrip manoeuvre, a Valsalva manoeuvre, a thermal trigger, as well as in response to a clear clinical change such as the occurrence of syncope, or a successful myocardial reperfusion.

Signals from the steady-state conditions may be analysed by the 'classical' spectral analysis approach, providing as output a single power spectrum reflecting cardiovascular control all along the recorded trace (see Fig. 9.1a–e for steady, simulated signals)

The quantitative investigation of the unsteady, transient conditions (such as Fig. 9.1c,f) requires the careful use of time–frequency analysis. Its output should reflect the spectral content that changes as a function of time, along the various, consecutive subtraces of the recorded signal, reflecting the time-dependent changes in cardiac autonomic control. A basic expectation from such a *t–f* algorithm is to optimize both time and frequency resolution.

Brief description of algorithms for *t–f* analysis

The essence of our initial SDA algorithm (Keselbrener & Akselrod 1996) and of its more advanced version, the closely related continuous wavelet transform (CWT) (Toledo *et al.* 2003), is derived from the basic rule, that, in order to estimate the power of a high frequency fluctuation, only a short string of data is required, while a low frequency fluctuation demands a much wider time window. In these algorithms, the window length is variable: at each time of interest, the optimal window is inversely related to the frequency of interest (Fig. 9.3, right).

The SDA and the CWT algorithms both deal with the time-frequency (*t–f*) plane, by choosing for each time of interest and for each frequency of interest, the minimal time-window over the relevant digitized signal (Keselbrener & Akselrod 1996). In both algorithms, the basis functions of the transform are closely related to a simple oscillatory function (sinus wave or complex exponent at the frequency of interest), for which the variable window length is defined by a constant number of periods and thus proportional to $1/f$ (see Fig. 9.3).

As a result, the instantaneous power content is obtained as a 3D surface (power as function of time and frequency) with a non-homogeneous t and f resolution, thus achieving the optimal time-resolution for each frequency (see Fig. 9.4).

Examples of *t–f* analysis of simulated and physiological signals

- Example 1. Non-steady simulated signal is displayed in Fig. 9.4, together with its corresponding *t–f* spectrum, computed with the CWT algorithm (Toledo *et al.* 2003). The simulated data undergoes a strong change in amplitude, as expressed both by the power in the 3D *t–f* transform, and by the time dependence of the two integrals of interest, over the low- (LF) and high-frequency (HF) ranges. We clearly observe that (in agreement with Fig. 9.3), the frequency resolution for LF is higher (narrower peak in the *t–f* plane), while time resolution is better for HF (narrower transition time at the sudden change in amplitude).
- Example 2. Non-steady traces of true physiological data are displayed, together with their corresponding *t–f* spectrum computed with the CWT algorithm. Instantaneous *HR* and *BP* (Figs 9.5 and 9.6) are shown during a change in position (CP) as autonomic challenge, in a young adult. The 3D *t–f* decomposition shows clearly the sudden change in frequency content evoked

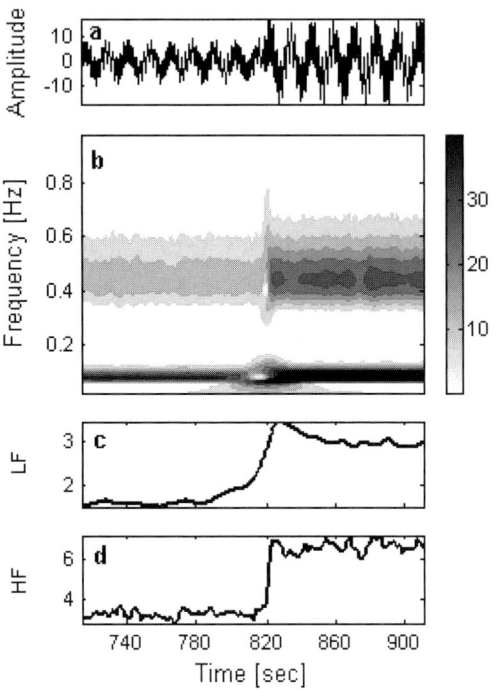

Fig. 9.4 Time–frequency decomposition, by CWT, of a simulated non-steady signal. (a) A signal which is a superposition of two sinus waves of different frequencies (low and high). At t = 820 s a sudden increase in the amplitude of both components occurs (see also Fig. 1f). (b) 3D output of the *t–f* transform of the signal in (a). The unequal *t* and *f* resolution of the plane is apparent. In the LF range, the peak as a function of time is much narrower than in the HF range. Frequency resolution is better at lower frequencies. The time resolution, however, is better in the HF range; indeed the rise time of the HF peak at the transition in amplitude, is much shorter than for the LF peak. (c) Integral of LF range as function of time, displays slow increase (reduced time resolution) at transition. (d) Integral of HF range as function of time, displays fast increase (enhanced time resolution).

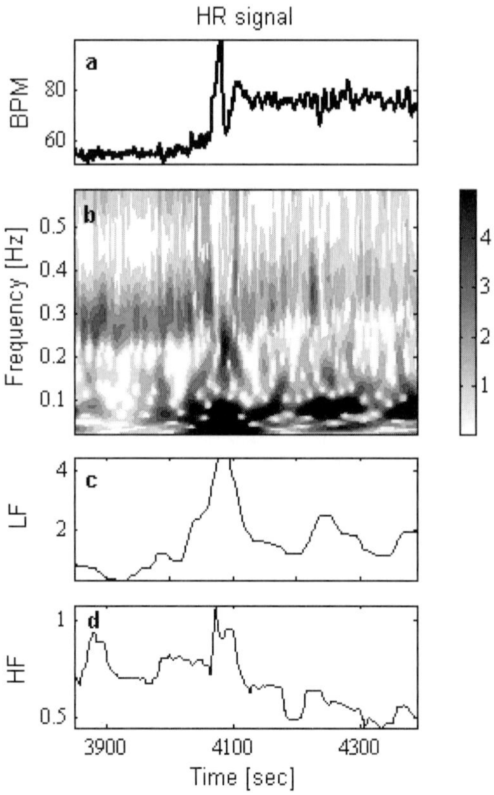

Fig. 9.5 Effect of active change in posture on *HR* fluctuations. (a) *HR* as function of time. CP causes a clear increase in mean *HR* and a change in the pattern of *HR* fluctuations. (b) 3D *t–f* decomposition of the *HR* fluctuations. CP causes a strong increase in LF power, and a marked decrease in HF power. (c) Integral of LF power as function of time. Note the strong yet slow increase at CP. (d) Integral of HF power as function of time. Note the marked decrease at CP, much faster than for LF. This reflects the enhanced time resolution at higher frequencies.

by the related autonomic perturbation. Indeed at CP a sudden reduction in HF and a slightly slower increase in LF are observed in the *t–f* transform of *HR* (Fig. 9.5), while the *t–f* transform of *BP* (Fig. 9.6) displays a strong, also slower increase in the LF range. These typical changes reflect the sudden alteration in sympatho-vagal balance during an active CP, as well as a simultaneous increase in vasomotor sympathetic activation.

From Figs 9.5 and 9.6, it is clear that this variable window approach for *t–f* analysis of non-steady state signals has the ability to disclose sudden changes in frequency or amplitude of *HR* and *BP* fluctuations elicited by an autonomic perturbation.

Extensive validation procedures (Keselbrener & Akselrod 1996) have confirmed this conclusion, and make the *t–f* transform an important tool for estimation of autonomic activity in true clinical conditions.

More details about the *t–f* algorithms (SDA, modified to CWT) developed in our laboratory at Tel-Aviv University, can be found in Keselbrener & Akselrod (1996) and Toledo *et al.* (2003) (see also Figs 9.3–9.6).

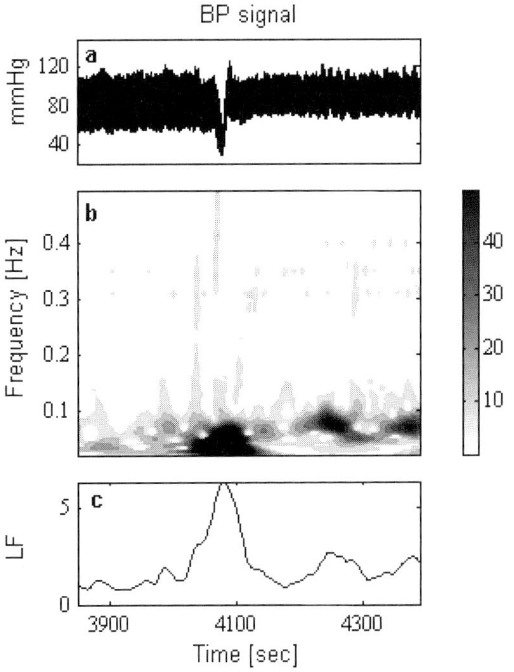

Fig. 9.6 Effect of active change in posture on *BP* fluctuations. (a) *BP* as function of time. CP causes a clear increase in mean *BP* and a change in the pattern of *BP* fluctuations. (b) 3D *t–f* decomposition of *BP* fluctuations. CP causes a strong increase in LF power. (c) Integral of LF power of *BP* fluctuations as function of time. Note the strong yet slow increase at CP. This increase can be used as a marker for hypertension: indeed it is extremely damped in mild hypertensive subjects (Akselrod *et al.* 1997).

Implementation of *t–f* analysis in clinical conditions

Hypertension

Hypertension affects approximately 25% of adults in industrialized countries; it contributes significantly to morbidity and mortality from stroke, heart failure, coronary heart disease and renal failure. Early identification of individuals prone to hypertension, may allow for early interference such as: lifestyle modifications, regular exercise and weight loss, targeted at reducing the risk factors for hypertension, and reducing sympathetic nervous system activation.

Since several studies have shown that essential hypertension is linked to basic alterations in cardiovascular autonomic control, our basic hypothesis was that challenging the autonomic system may unveil specific abnormalities already present at a very early stage of the disease, perhaps even before any sign of increased *BP* can be observed.

This hypothesis was based on our earlier work in spontaneously hypertensive rats (SHR), where we had shown that autonomic imbalance can be detected very early, well before the onset of overt hypertension (Akselrod *et al.* 1987; Oz *et al.* 1995). This imbalance was revealed by focusing on the *HR* and *BP* fluctuations of the rats, under steady state as well as in response to several perturbations. In the SHR rats, *BP* fluctuations were a more sensitive indicator of abnormal cardiovascular control than HRV.

Previous studies in hypertensive humans, which mainly focused on steady-state conditions, have led to controversial results, suggesting that a well-controlled autonomic challenge may be necessary to unveil the differences in cardiovascular control between normotensive and future hypertensive subjects.

Since prehypertensive subjects may be even more difficult to discriminate, because of the unpredictability of the genetics and the variability in the disease itself, we investigated the effect of an autonomic perturbation in two different experimental set-ups:

- Experiment 1 was performed in mild-hypertensive subjects, immediately after detection of the disease and before initiation of treatment, and compared to age-matched normotensive subjects (Akselrod *et al.* 1997).
- Experiment 2 was performed in young adult, normotensive offspring of one hypertensive parent (pre-hypertensive population with high probability to develop hypertension), and compared to normotensive offspring of two normotensive parents (Davrath *et al.* 2002a,b,c; Maor *et al.* 2002, Davrath *et al.*, 2003).

In both protocols, the autonomic challenge applied was, after supine rest, an active CP, typically lasting 5 s, followed by steady standing, in order to uncover autonomic alterations related to an early predisposition for hypertension. The continuously recorded signals were: ECG, blood pressure, and respiration. The entire traces, including baseline, CP and standing, were submitted to *t–f* analysis by SDA with individual time scales for optimal alignment (for experiment 1), and by CWT (for experiment 2). Spectral integrals were computed as a function of time; LF and HF ranges were carefully chosen according to the contour plot of the *t–f* spectra (see Figs 9.5 and 9.6).

• Results of experiment 1. In the mild-hypertensive compared to normotensive humans, the time-dependent changes in the LF integral in *BP*, disclosed the most impressive differences between the groups. Indeed, normotensive subjects displayed a very strong response (about 10-fold increase) in the LF fluctuations in *BP* during the CP challenge (see Fig. 9.6). The mild-hypertensive subjects displayed a marked reduction (by about a factor of 3) in the rise of LF *BP* fluctuations immediately following CP. This dampened response reflects an inadequate sympathetic response (Akselrod *et al.* 1997). This damping is so clear that we believe it could be used as an individual indicator of developing hypertension (still mild), or as independent confirmation of an early diagnosis.

• Results of experiment 2. This later study involved the comparison of young adult, normotensive offspring of one hypertensive parent (KHT) with young, normotensive offspring of two normotensive parents (YN). Our goal was to test whether an even earlier detection of essential hypertension by *t–f* analysis is feasible, well before any overt sign of hypertension has been observed

During the transition to stand, a significantly different response was observed between KHT and YN in the LF range of Heart Rate fluctuations, indicating enhanced sympathetic involvement in the *HR* response to active standing in KHT compared to YN. The CP provocation was required to unmask differences in autonomic behaviour between these groups, which were not at all evident during the steady-state rest (Davrath *et al.* 2002a,b,c; Maor *et al.* 2002; Davrath *et al.* 2003).

We thus observed a sympathetic exacerbation in the *HR* control of the group prone to hypertension (experiment 2), which seems to be present well before the development of any overt sign of hypertension, and before other autonomic abnormalities are observed, such as in the mild hypertensive subjects (experiment 1), where a strong damping in LF increase in *BP* fluctuations with standing was observed.

Our conclusion from both studies (experiment 1 and experiment 2) is that by applying CP as an autonomic challenge and performing *t–f* analysis of *HR* and *BP* around the transition to standing may help disclose hypertension at its earliest stage.

Perhaps this simple noninvasive test, leading to an enhanced LF *HR* response to standing, may be used in the future to identify individuals prone to hypertension before observable signs are evident. Other subjects, who already display some early, yet mild and inconsistent signs of hypertension, may possibly be diagnosed by the same procedure, according to their LF *BP* response to CP. Early diagnosis of hypertension has the enormous advantage that the patients can modify their lifestyle and effectively control or avoid the development of the disease.

Myocardial reperfusion

Myocardial infarction (MI) is one of the most critical cardiac conditions, and requires immediate treatment to minimize resultant damage. Patients, who reach the ICU in the acute stage, are often submitted to thrombolysis in order to restore cardiac perfusion. The *t–f* analysis of the instantaneous *HR* signal could become a crucial clinical application, if it had the ability to determine with a high degree of reliability whether myocardial reperfusion was induced and when.

Indeed, it is well known that acute MI does elicit a strong activation of the autonomic system. More specifically the type of activation is strongly related to the location of the infarct. Inferior MI is known to cause vagal enhancement, while anterior MI is know to promote sympathetic activation to the SA-node.

In our effort to develop a reliable marker of reperfusion, we assumed that the occurrence of reperfusion would cause an autonomic response in the opposite direction, again dependent on the location of the infarct (Toledo *et al.* 1998; Toledo *et al.*, 2003), and expressed by changes in the pattern of *HR* fluctuations

Our study involved the recording of ECG in two groups of acute MI patients (anterior and inferior), all undergoing thrombolytic therapy. Since these are obviously non-steady conditions, the *HR* fluctuations were analysed all along the procedure by a *t–f* transform (CWT algorithm). This analysis provides time-dependent versions of

HRV parameters such as: the LF and HF integrals, as well as of the LF/*HR* ratio (expressing the instantaneous sympatho-vagal balance).

- Marked alterations in at least one of these HRV parameters were observed during each of the reperfusions events.
- Significant changes in HRV parameters, compatible with a shift towards sympathetic preponderance were found in all cases (100%) of reperfusion in inferior MI patients.
- Significant changes in HRV parameters, in the opposite direction, compatible with relative vagal enhancement were found in 66% of the reperfusions in anterior MI patients
- Significant time-dependent changes were observed in the several cases of reocclusion.

These shifts reflect clear changes in autonomic activity, occurring at the time of reperfusion, the direction of which (towards more sympathetic, or more vagal) are closely linked to the infarct location, in agreement with our hypothesis.

Time–frequency analysis of *HR* fluctuations thus has the ability to reveal the occurrence of changes in myocardial perfusion (reperfusion, reocclusion). Careful design of a sensitive thresholding procedure, to be applied continuously to the time-dependent HRV parameters (*LF*(t), *HF*(t), *LF*(t)/*HF*(t)), may thus lead to a sensitive, on-line, independent marker of myocardial reperfusion by thrombolysis.

Conclusion

Chronic cardiovascular disease often involves abnormal autonomic control, which may be disclosed only by performing some kind of autonomic provocation. On the other hand, acute clinical conditions may involve strong and sudden alterations in cardiovascular control, which may be used as an indicator for a change in the patient's condition. In both situations there is an obvious need to consider dynamic, transient, non-steady physiological conditions.

The time intervals of greatest physiological interest are usually the dynamic periods The resulting, non-steady cardiovascular signals have thus to undergo one of the various procedures for time-dependent frequency decomposition.

The *t–f* analysis of cardiovascular signal, as a new investigation approach and as a clinical tool, enables a more flexible, custom made, subject-dependent and challenge-dependent approach to be applied during clinical and physiological studies.

Our hope is that these *t–f* studies will lead to the design of sensitive, noninvasive diagnostic tools which may contribute directly to the treatment, follow-up and recovery of patients.

References

Akselrod, S. (1995) Components of heart rate variability – basic studies. In: *Heart Rate Variability* (eds M. Malik & A. J. Camm). Futura Publishing, Armonk, NY.

Akselrod, S., Barak, Y., Ben-Dov, Y., Keselbrener, L. & Baharav, A. (2001) Estimation of autonomic response based on individually determined time axis. *Autonomic Neuroscience: Basic and Clinical*, **90**, 13–23.

Akselrod, S., Eliash, S., Oz, O. & Cohen, S. (1987) Hemodynamic regulation in the spontaneously hypertensive rat: investigation by spectral analysis. *American Journal of Physiology*, **253**, H176–H183.

Akselrod, S., Gordon, D., Madwed, J.B., Snidman, N.C., Shannon, D.C. & Cohen, R.J. (1985) Hemodynamic regulation: investigation by spectral analysis. *American Journal of Physiology*, **249**, H867–H875.

Akselrod, S., Gordon, D., Ubel, F.A., Shannon, D.C., Barger, A.C. & Cohen, R.J. (1981) Power spectrum analysis of heart rate fluctuations: a quantitative probe of beat-to-beat cardiovascular control. *Science*, **213**, 220–222.

Akselrod, S., Oz, O., Grinberg, M. & Keselbrener, L. (1997) Autonomic response to change of posture among normal and mild-hypertensive adults: investigated by time-dependent spectral analysis. *Journal of the Autonomic Nervous System*, **64**, 33–43.

Bianchi, A.M., Mainardi, L., Perucci, E., Signorini, M.G., Mainardi, M. & Cerutti, S. (1993) Time-variant power spectrum analysis for the detection of transient episodes in HRV signals. *IEEE (Institute of Electrical and Electronic Engineers) Transactions on Biomedical Engineering*, **40**, 136–144.

Calcagnini, G., Censi, F., Cesarini, A., Lino, S. & Cerutti, S. (1998) Self-similar properties of long term heart rate variability assessed by discrete wavelet transform. *IEEE (Institute of Electrical and Electronic Engineers) Computers in Cardiology*, **25**, 333–336.

Cerutti, S., Bianchi, A. & Mainardi, L.T. (2001) Advanced spectral methods for detecting dynamic behaviour. *Autonomic Neuroscience: Basic and Clinical*, **90**, 3–12.

Cohen, L.(1989) Time-frequency distributions – a review. *Proceedings of the IEEE (Institute of Electrical and Electronic Engineers)*, **77**, 7,941–7,981.

Coumel, Ph., Hermida, J.S., Wennerblom, B. *et al.* (1991) Heart rate variability in myocardial hypertrophy and heart failure and the effects of beta blocking therapy. *European Heart Journal*, **12**, 412–422.

Daubechies, I. (1990) The wavelet transform, time frequency localization and signal analysis. *IEEE (Institute of Electrical and Electronic Engineers) Transactions on Information Theory*, **36**, 961–1005

Davrath, L.R., Goren, Y., Pinhas, I. & Akselrod, S. (2003) Early autonomic malfunction in normotensive individuals with a genetic predisposition to essential hypertension. (*Submitted for publication*).

Davrath, L.R., Goren, Y., Pinhas, I., David, D. & Akselrod, S. (2002a) Investigation and early detection of essential hypertension by time–frequency analysis. *FASEB*, New Orleans, April 2002.

Davrath, L.R., Goren, Y., Pinhas, I., David, D. & Akselrod, S. (2002b) Early detection of essential hypertension by time–frequency analysis. *IEEE (Institute of Electrical and Electronic Engineers) Transactions on Computers in Cardiology* (in press).

Davrath, L.R., Goren, Y., Pinhas, I., David, D. & Akselrod, S. (2002c) Investigation and early detection of essential hypertension by time–frequency analysis of heart rate variability. *Experimental Biology*, 20–24 April 2002, New Orleans, Louisiana, USA.

Hainsworth, R. (1998) Physiology of the cardiac autonomic system. In: *Clinical Guide to Cardiac Autonomic Tests* (ed. M. Malik), pp. 3–28. Kluwer Academic Publishers, Dordrecht.

Kenny, R.A., Ingram, A., Bayless, J. & Sutton, R. (1989) Head up tilt: a useful test for investigating unexplained syncope. *Lancet*, **1**, 1352–1355.

Keselbrener, L. & Akselrod, S. (1996) Selective discrete Fourier transform algorithm – SDA – for time–frequency analysis: method and application on simulated and cardiovascular signals. *IEEE (Institute of Electrical and Electronic Engineers) Transactions on Biomedical Engineering*, **43**, 789–802.

Keselbrener, L. & Akselrod, S. (1998) Autonomic responses to blockades and provocations. In: *Clinical Guide to Autonomic Tests* (ed. M. Malik). Kluwer Academic Publishers, Dordrecht.

Keselbrener, L., Baharav, A. & Akselrod, S. (1994) Selective windowed time–frequency analysis for the quantitative evaluation of non-stationary cardiovascular signals. *IEEE (Institute of Electrical and Electronic Engineers) Computers in Cardiology*, **22**, 5–8.

Keselbrener, L., Baharav, A. & Akselrod, S. (1996) Estimation of fast vagal response by time-dependent analysis of heart rate variability in normal subjects. *Clinical Autonomic Research*, **6**, 321–327.

Kleiger, R.E., Miller, J.P., Bigger, J.T., Jr. & Moss, A.J. (1987) Decreased heart rate variability and its association with increased mortality after acute myocardial infarction. *American Journal of Cardiology*, **59**, 256–262.

Malliani, A., Pagani, M., Lombardi, F. & Cerutti, S. (1991) Cardiovascular neural regulation explored in the frequency domain. *Circulation*, **84** (2), 482–492.

Malik, M. (ed.) (1998) *Clinical Guide to Cardiac Autonomic Tests*. Kluwer Academic Publishers, Dordrecht.

Malik, M. & Camm, A.J. (eds) (1995) *Heart Rate Variability*. Futura, New York.

Maor, G., Davrath, L., Goren, Y. & Akselrod, S. (2002) A modified Wigner Ville transformation as a tool for hypertension detection. *2nd ESCGO meeting*, Sienna.

Marchesi, C., Venturi, M., Pola, S. *et al.* (1991) Sequential estimation of the power spectrum for the analysis of variability of non-stationary cardiovascular signals. *Proceedings of IEEE (Institute of Electrical and Electronic Engineers)* **13**, 578–579.

Medigue, C., Girard, A., Laude, D., Monti, A., Wargon, M. & Elghozi, J.L. (2001) Relationship between pulse interval and respiratory sinus arrhythmia: a time and frequency-domain analysis of the effects of atropine. *Pfluegers Archiv*, **441**, 650–655.

Nawab, S.H. & Quatieri, T.F. (1988). Short-time Fourier transform. In: *Advanced Topics in Signal Processing* (eds Lim & Oppenheim), pp. 289–337. Prentice Hall, Englewood Cliffs, NJ.

Novak, P. & Novak, V. (1993) Time-frequency mapping of the heart rate, blood pressure and respiratory signals. *Medical & Biological Engineering & Computing*, **31**, 103–110.

Oppenheim, A.V. & Shafer, R.W. (1985) *Digital Signal Processing*. Prentice Hall, Englewood Cliffs, NJ.

Oz, O., Eliash, S., Cohen, S. & Akselrod, S. (1995). Insight into blood-pressure control in SHR via the response to acute hemorrhage: a spectral analysis approach. *Journal of the Autonomic Nervous System*, **55**, 146–154.

Persson, P.B. (1997) Spectrum analysis of cardiovascular time series. *American Journal of Physiology*, **273** (*Regulatory Integrative and Comparative Physiology* **42**), R1201–R1210.

Toledo, E., Gurevitz, O., Hod, H., Eldar, M. & Akselrod, S. (1998). The use of a wavelet transform for the analysis of non-stationary heart rate variability signal during thrombolytic therapy as a marker of reperfusion. *IEEE (Institute of Electrical and Electronic Engineers) Transactions on Computers in Cardiology*, **25**, 609–612.

Toledo E., Gurevitz O., Hod H., Eldar M. & Akselrod, S. (2003) Wavelet analysis of instantaneous heart rate: a study of autonomic control during thrombolysis. *American Journal of Physiology (Regulatory Integrative and Comparative Physiology)*, (In press).

Toledo, E., Pinhas, I., Almog, Y., Aravot, D. & Akselrod, S. (2002) Functional restitution of cardiac control in heart transplant patients. *American Journal of Physiology (Regulatory Integrative and Comparative Physiology)*, **282**(3), R900–R908.

CHAPTER 10

Effects of Drugs

Xavier Copie and Jean-Yves Le Heuzey

Introduction

Heart rate variability results from complex interactions between the heart and the autonomic nervous system. Cardiovascular and also non-cardiovascular drugs may modify heart rate variability as a result of a direct effect on the autonomic nervous system, or as a consequence of their effect on the heart or the vessels eliciting a feed-back response.

Understanding the effect of drugs on heart rate variability is important from several points of view. In an experimental setting, pharmacological treatment was used to understand the effects of the components of the autonomic nervous system on heart rate variability (Akselrod *et al.* 1985; Pagani *et al.* 1986). Conversely, heart rate variability was subsequently used to understand the effects of various treatments on the control of the heart by the autonomic nervous system (Niemela *et al.* 1994; Copie *et al.* 1996b; Pousset *et al.* 1996). It is also important to understand the effects of drugs on the predictive value of heart rate variability in situations such as postmyocardial infarction, or heart failure.

Finally, one should be aware that the effects of drugs on heart rate variability differ profoundly according to the autonomic status of the patient. The same course of treatment may have different effects on healthy volunteers with elevated basal vagal tone when compared with heart failure patients with increased sympathetic tone.

Effects of beta blockers on heart rate variability

As heart rate and heart rate variability are closely related (Coumel *et al.* 1994; Copie *et al.* 1996a), the effects of beta blockers on heart rate variability are the subject of controversies.

In experimental conditions, in dogs or healthy volunteers, acute β-adrenergic blockade increased the high frequency component of heart rate variability (Akselrod *et al.* 1981; Coker *et al.* 1984; Pomeranz *et al.* 1985; Pagani *et al.* 1986). In the same experiments, there was no significant effect of acute β-blockade on the low frequency component of heart rate variability at rest, but a decrease after activation of the sympathetic system by tilt or standing. Consequently, in healthy volunteers, acute β-blockade is associated with a decrease in the low to high frequency ratio. However, a high level of parasympathetic tone at rest may challenge this result. In the study by Ahmed and co-workers, intravenous administration of propranolol in healthy volunteers had no effect on heart rate, nor on heart rate variability (Ahmed *et al.* 1994). In the study by Pagani and co-workers, chronic β-blockade was responsible for more important changes in heart rate variability than acute β-blockade (Pagani *et al.* 1986).

Chronic treatment with beta blockers results in an increase in beat-to-beat heart rate variability (pNN50, RMSSD) in healthy volunteers (Cook *et al.* 1991). In this study, no significant difference in global heart rate variability (SDNN) was evidenced between the placebo and atenolol period. The decrease in the night/day difference in heart rate was responsible for this lack of increase in SDNN despite an increase in beat-to-beat heart rate variability. Therefore, in healthy volunteers, the most prominent effect of chronic β-adrenergic blockade is to increase the measures of heart rate variability dependent on parasympathetic tone. Using a specific approach, Coumel *et al.* found a decrease in all components of heart rate variability (short, medium, and long oscillations) in healthy volunteers treated with acebutolol (Coumel *et al.* 1994). This change in heart rate variability was associated with a decrease in the long to short oscillations ratio (which can be assimilated to the low to high frequency ratio of the power spectra).

In patients with coronary artery disease and no recent myocardial infarction, Niemela and co-workers compared the effects of metoprolol, atenolol, and placebo on heart rate variability measured during 24-h Holter recordings (Niemela *et al.* 1994). Both beta blockers significantly increased all components of heart rate variability, but the low frequency power. A difference in baseline heart rate variability may explain the discrepancy between this study and studies in healthy volunteers.

In patients with a recent myocardial infarction, care should be taken to include a control group in all studies as heart rate variability changes rapidly in the weeks (Copie *et al.* 1995), and months (Bigger *et al.* 1991) following myocardial infarction. Several studies have addressed the effect of beta blockers on heart rate variability in patients with a recent myocardial infarction (Bekheit *et al.* 1990; Kontopoulos *et al.* 1996; Keeley *et al.* 1997) (Fig. 10.1). The most consistent effect of beta blockers demonstrated in these studies are a decrease in heart rate and an increase in beat-to-beat heart rate variability. An increase in global heart rate variability (SDNN or SDANN) was not evidenced in all studies.

The effects of beta blockers were also studied in patients with heart failure (Coumel *et al.* 1991; Copie *et al.* 1996b; Pousset *et al.* 1996; Piccirillo *et al.* 2000; Ridha *et al.* 2002). In these studies, beta blockers have a significant effect on heart rate and increase global and beat-to-beat heart rate variability (Fig. 10.2, Fig. 10.3). This effect of beta blockers may reflect a trend towards normalisation of impaired cardiovascular neural regulation in patients with heart failure.

In patients with frequent ventricular arrhythmias treated with sotalol, Hohnloser and co-workers found an increase in global and beat-to-beat heart rate variability (Hohnloser *et al.* 1993).

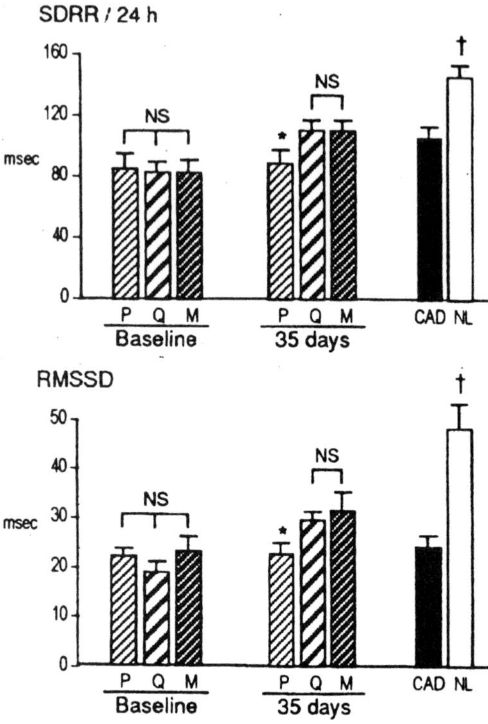

Fig. 10.1 Comparison of the effect of metoprolol (M) and quinapril (Q) on heart rate variability in post-myocardial infarction patients. After 35 days of treatment, metoprolol and quinapril significantly increased heart rate variability as compared to placebo (P). There was no significant difference in heart rate variability between patients receiving metoprolol and quinapril. These patients had a heart rate variability similar to patients with stable coronary artery disease (CAD). NL: normal volunteers, * $P < 0.05$ compared with quinapril and metoprolol, † $P < 0.05$ compared with stable CAD. (From Kontopoulos *et al.* 1996, with permission.)

Effects of renin–angiotensin modulators

In her landmark study, Akselrod and co-workers demonstrated a marked effect of converting enzyme inhibition on the power spectrum of heart rate fluctuations in conscious dogs (Akselrod *et al.* 1981). Converting enzyme inhibition had little or no effect on heart rate or blood pressure, but was associated with a marked increase in the area under the low frequency peak of heart rate fluctuations. This effect of ACE inhibitors was subsequently demonstrated in patients with a recent myocardial infarction

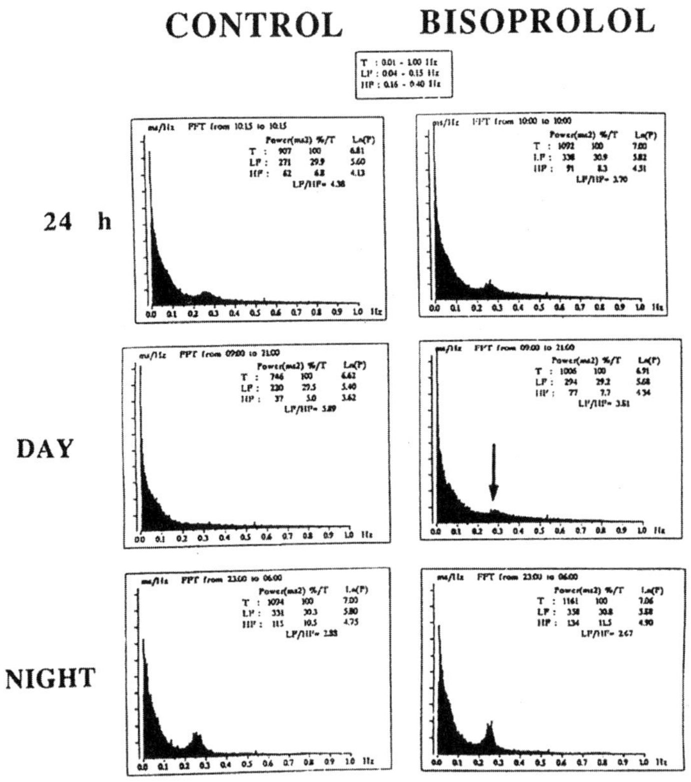

Fig. 10.2 Effect of bisoprolol on heart rate variability in patients with heart failure. Left panel, 24 h, day, and night power spectrum at baseline. Right panel, Left panel, 24 h, day, and night power spectrum after two months treatment with bisoprolol. Bisoprolol increased the daytime high frequency power and decreased the LF/HF ratio. (From Pousset *et al.* 1996, with permission.)

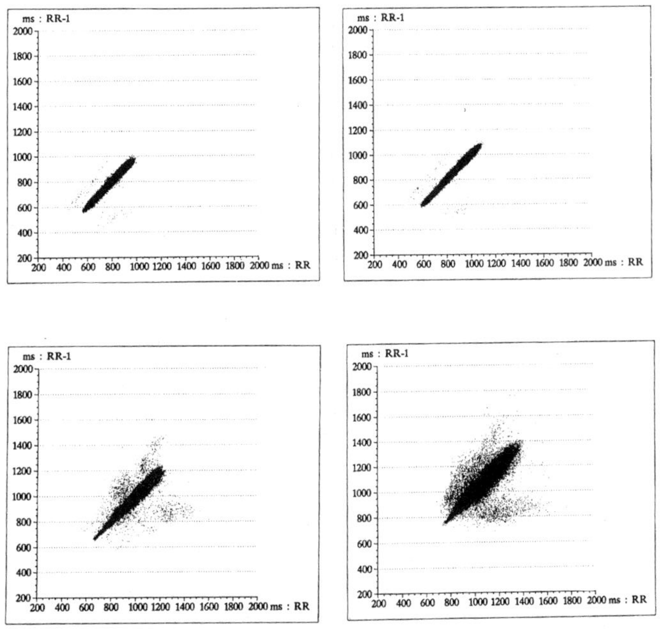

Fig. 10.3 Effect of bisoprolol on heart rate variability in patients with heart failure. Scatterplot evolution in a patient who received placebo (top) and a patient who received bisoprolol (bottom). (From Copie *et al.* 1996b, with permission.)

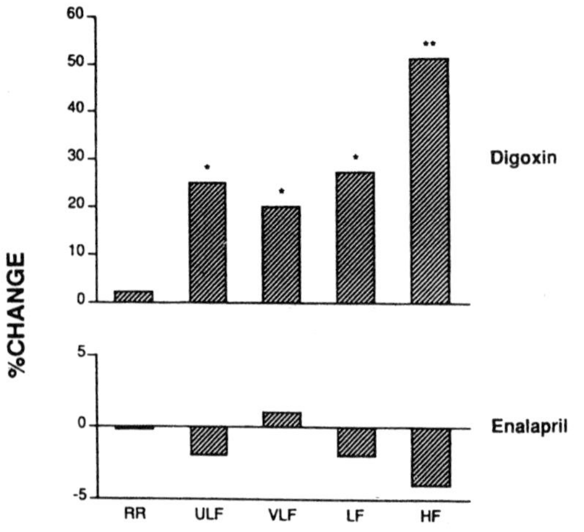

Fig. 10.4 Comparative effect of digoxin and enalapril on heart rate and heart rate variability in healthy volunteers. Digoxin significantly increased heart rate variability, while enalapril did not. *RR*, mean *RR* interval; ULF, ultra low frequency; VLF, very low frequency; LF, low frequency; HF, high frequency; * $P < 0.01$, ** $P < 0.001$. (From Kaufman *et al.* 1993, with permission.)

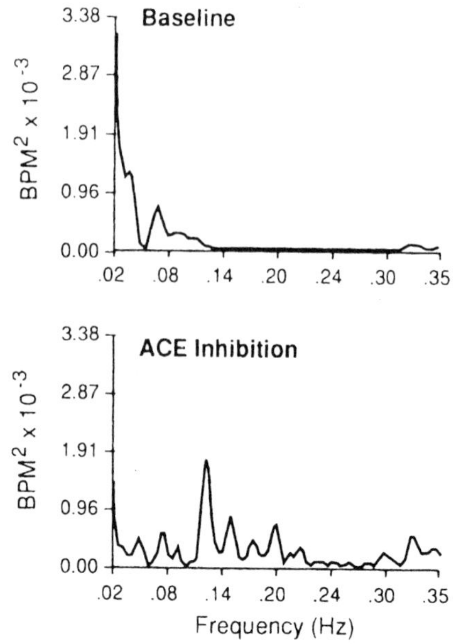

Fig. 10.5 Power spectral density of heart rate variability recorded in a patient with congestive heart failure at baseline (top) and after 12 weeks of therapy with zofenopril (bottom). There is marked augmentation of heart rate variability after therapy with angiotensin-converting enzyme inhibitor. (From Binkley *et al.* 1993, with permission.)

(Kontopoulos *et al.* 1996; Bonaduce *et al.* 1994) and in patients with heart failure (Flapan *et al.* 1992, Binkley *et al.* 1993). A study in healthy volunteers did not find a significant effect of enalapril on heart rate variability (Kaufman *et al.* 1993) (Fig. 10.4).

ACE-inhibitors have a different effect on beat-to-beat heart rate variability depending on the population studied. In healthy dogs (Akselrod *et al.* 1981), healthy volunteers (Kaufman *et al.* 1993), and patients with a recent myocardial infarction (Bonaduce *et al.* 1994), no change in beat-to-beat heart rate variability was evidenced. However, in patients with heart failure receiving zofenopril, Binkley and co-workers found an increase in the high frequency heart rate variability (Binkley *et al.* 1993) (Fig. 10.5). A careful monitoring substantiated the fact that changes in respiratory rates were not responsible for this increase in high frequency heart rate variability.

The effects of angiotensin 1-receptor antagonist irbesartan on heart rate variability was compared with the effect of an ACE-inhibitor, trandolapril, by Franchi and co-workers (Franchi *et al.* 2002). Their data demonstrate that in mild and uncomplicated essential hypertension, the chronic low-dose combination therapy with an ACE-inhibitor and an AT(1)-antagonist is more effective than the recommended full-dose monotherapy with either drug in reducing the LF component of the power spectrum of heart rate variability and the LF/HF ratio.

Effects of digitalis

The effect of digoxin on heart rate variability was studied both in healthy volunteers (Kaufman *et al.* 1993) and in patients with heart failure (Krum *et al.* 1995). In healthy volunteers, digoxin increased all components of heart rate variability. The magnitude of the effect was particularly important for the high frequency component of heart rate variability, corroborated by a similar increase in time-domain components of heart rate variability (RMSSD and pNN50). In patients with heart failure, Krum and co-workers found a significant decrease in mean *RR* interval and an increase in all spectral components of heart rate variability.

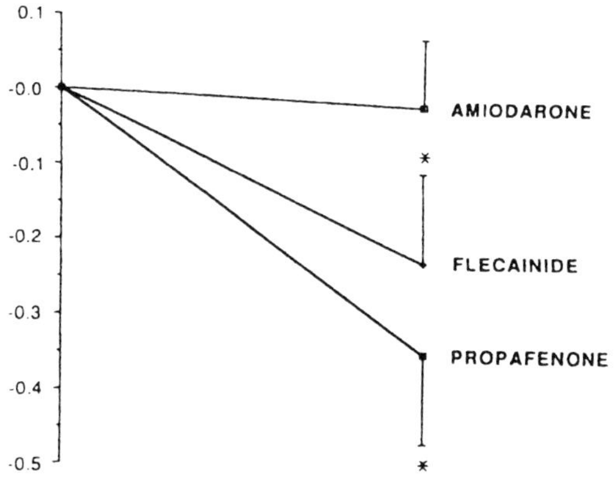

Fig. 10.6 Effect of three antiarrhythmic agents on heart rate variability, expressed as changes from baseline. (From Zuanetti *et al.* 1991, with permission.)

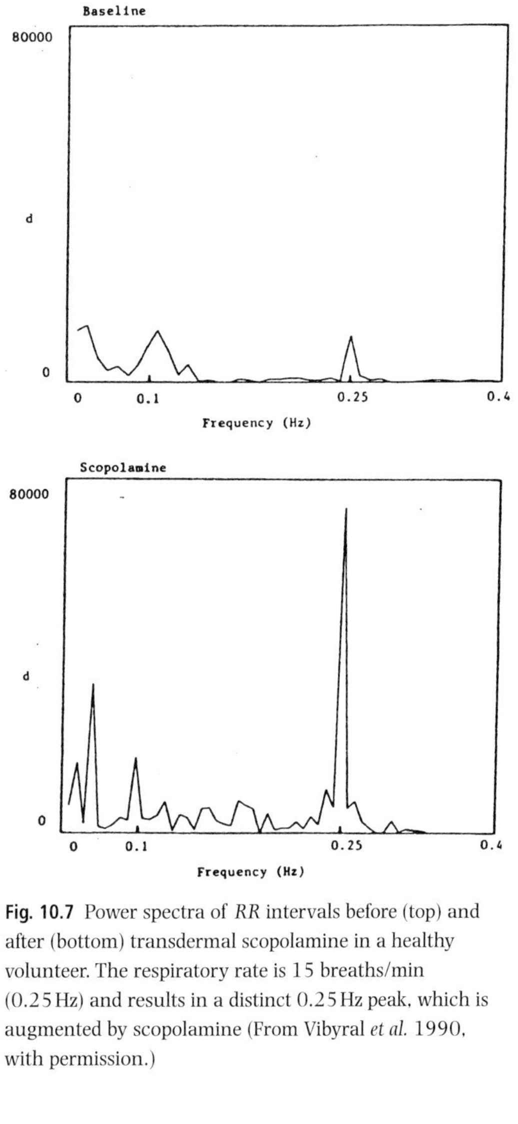

Fig. 10.7 Power spectra of *RR* intervals before (top) and after (bottom) transdermal scopolamine in a healthy volunteer. The respiratory rate is 15 breaths/min (0.25 Hz) and results in a distinct 0.25 Hz peak, which is augmented by scopolamine (From Vibyral *et al.* 1990, with permission.)

Effects of antiarrhythmic therapy

In a study comparing the effects of three antiarrhythmic drugs (amiodarone, flecainide, and propafenone) on heart rate variability, Zuanetti and co-workers found a decrease in beat-to-beat heart rate variability, as assessed by NN50, with flecainide and propafenone, whereas amiodarone did not change heart rate variability (Zuanetti *et al.* 1991) (Fig. 10.6). Changes in heart rate variability with propafenone were also evidenced by Lombardi and co-workers (Lombardi *et al.* 1992). Propafenone was responsible for an increase in the high frequency component and a decrease in the low frequency component of heart rate variability.

Effects of calcium channel blockers

In healthy volunteers, Cook and co-workers did not find any significant effect of diltiazem on heart rate and heart rate variability measured on 24-h Holter recordings (Cook *et al.* 1991). In patients with stable angina, lercanidipine, a novel dihydropyridine agent, did not change heart rate variability neither measured on a 24-h Holter recording nor from spectral analysis of short-term recordings (Acanfora *et al.* 2002). A similar result was obtained by Bekheit and co-workers with nifedipine in patients with a recent myocardial infarction, whereas diltiazem was responsible for a decrease in the low frequency power during tilt (Bekheit *et al.* 1990).

Effects of antimuscarinic agents

Antimuscarinic agents are most often used for their anticholinergic properties. However, low doses of these agents can increase vagal tone, an effect that is thought to result from a central action on inhibitory fibres. In addition to central actions, peripheral mechanisms, such as the presynaptic muscarinic modulation of acetylcholine release may contribute to the effect of low doses of antimuscarinic agents.

Several studies have addressed the effects of treatment with low dose antimuscarinic agents on indices of vagal activity in animal models (Hull *et al.* 1995), healthy volunteers (Vybiral *et al.* 1990) (Fig. 10.7), patients with myocardial infarction (Casadei *et al.* 1993), or heart failure (La Rovere *et al.* 1994). In all these studies, indices of vagal activity assessed by heart rate variability increase with low dose antimuscarinic agents.

Other agents

The effect on heart rate variability of several noncardiovascular drugs, mainly agents influencing the central nervous system, have been studied.

A decrease in heart rate variability was evidenced during treatment with imipramine (Yeragani *et al.* 1992), paroxetine and nortriptyline (Yeragani *et al.* 2002), amitriptyline (Siepmann *et al.* 2002) and clozapine (Eschweiler *et al.* 2002). As compared with amitriptyline, St John's wort extract did not affect heart rate variability (Siepmann *et al.* 2002).

Conclusion

Heart rate variability is a useful tool to study the effect of drugs on the autonomic nervous system. Treatments increasing heart rate variability have generally a favourable effect on mortality in patients with heart disease. However, care should be taken not to extrapolate too readily an effect on heart rate variability to morbidity and mortality outcome.

References

Acanfora, D., Trojano, L., Gheorghiade, M. *et al.* (2002) A randomised, double-blind comparison of 10 and 20 mg lercanidipine in patients with stable effort angina: effects on myocardial ischaemia and heart rate variability. *American Journal of Therapy*, **9**, 444–453.

Ahmed, M.W., Kadish, A.H., Parker, M.A. *et al.* (1994) Effect of physiological and pharmacologic adrenergic stimulation on heart rate variability. *Journal of the American College of Cardiology*, **24**, 1082–1090.

Akselrod, S., Gordon, D., Ubel, F.A. *et al.* (1981) Power spectrum analysis of heart rate fluctuations: a quantitative probe of beat-to-beat cardiovascular control. *Science*, **213**, 220–222.

Akselrod, S., Gordon, D., Madwed, J.B. *et al.* (1985) Hemodynamic regulation: investigation by spectral analysis. *American Journal of Physiology*, **249**, H867–H875.

Bonaduce, D., Marciano, F., Petretta, M. *et al.* (1994) Effects of converting enzyme inhibition on heart period variability in patients with acute myocardial infarction. *Circulation*, **90**, 108–113.

Bekheit, S., Tangella, M., el-Sakr, A. *et al.* (1990) Use of heart rate spectral analysis to study the effects of calcium channel blockers on sympathetic activity after myocardial infarction. *American Heart Journal*, **119**, 79–85.

Bigger, J.T., Fleiss,J.L., Rolnitzky, L.M. *et al.* (1991) Time course recovery of heart period variability after myocardial infarction. *Journal of the American College of Cardiology*, **18**, 1643–1649.

Binkley, P.F., Haas, J.G., Starling, R.C. *et al.* (1993) Sustained augmentation of parasympathetic tone with angiotensin-converting enzyme inhibition in patients with congestive heart failure. *Journal of the American College of Cardiology*, **21**, 655–661.

Casadei, B., Pipilis, A., Sessa, F. *et al.* (1993) Low doses scopolamine increase vagal tone in the acute phase of myocardial infarction. *Circulation*, **88**, 353–357.

Coker, R., Koziell, A., Oliver, C. *et al.* (1984) Does the sympathetic nervous system influence sinus arrhythmia in man? Evidence from combined autonomic blockade. *Journal of Physiology*, **356**, 459–464.

Cook, J.R., Bigger, J.T., Kleiger, R.E. *et al.* (1991) Effect of atenolol and diltiazem on heart period variability in normal persons. *Journal of the American College of Cardiology*, **17**, 480–484.

Copie, X., Le Heuzey, J.Y., Iliou, M.C. *et al.* (1995) Evolution de la variabilité de la fréquence cardiaque après infarctus du myocarde. Apport du diagramme de Poincaré. *Archives des Maladies du Cœur et Vaisseaux*, **88**, 1621–1626.

Copie, X., Hnatkova, K., Staunton, A. *et al.* (1996a) Predictive power of increased heart rate versus depressed left ventricular ejection fraction and heart rate variability for risk stratification after myocardial infarction. A two-year follow-up study. *Journal of the American College of Cardiology*, **27**, 270–276.

Copie, X., Pousset, F., Lechat, P. *et al.* (1996b) Effects of β-blockade with bisoprolol on heart rate variability in patients with advanced heart failure: analysis of scatterplots of *RR* intervals at selected heart rates. *American Heart Journal*, **132**, 369–375.

Coumel, P., Hermida, J.S., Wennerblöm, B. *et al.* (1991) Heart rate variability in myocardial hypertrophy and heart failure, and effects of beta-blocking therapy: a non-spectral analysis of heart rate oscillations. *European Heart Journal*, **65**, 1345–1350.

Coumel, P., Maison-Blanche, P., Catuli, D. (1994) Heart rate and heart rate variability in normal young adults. *Journal of Cardiovascular Electrophysiology*, **5**, 899–911.

Flapan, A.D., Nolan, J., Neilson, J.M.M. *et al.* (1992) Effect of captopril on parasympathetic activity in chronic cardiac failure secondary to coronary artery disease. *American Journal of Cardiology*, **69**, 532–535.

Franchi, F., Lazzeri, C., Foschi, M. *et al.* (2002) Cardiac autonomic tone during trandolapril–irbesartan low-dose combined therapy in hypertension: a pilot project. *Journal of Human Hypertension*, **16**, 597–604.

Hohnloser, S.H., Klingenheben, T., Zabel, M. *et al.* (1993) Effect of sotalol on heart rate variability assessed by Holter monitoring in patients with ventricular arrhythmias. *American Journal of Cardiology*, **72**, 67A–71A.

Hull, S.S., Vanoli, E., Adamson, P.B. *et al.* (1995) Do increases in markers of vagal activity imply protection from sudden death? The case of scopolamine. *Circulation*, **91**, 2516–2519.

Kaufman, E.S., Bosner, M.S., Bigger, J.T. *et al.* (1993) Effects of digoxin and enalapril on heart period variability and response to head-up tilt test in normal subjects. *American Journal of Cardiology*, **72**, 95–99.

Keeley, E.C., Lange, R.A., Hillis, D. *et al.* (1997) Correlation between time-domain measures of heart rate variability and scatterplots in patients with healed myocardial infarcts and the influence of metoprolol. *American Journal of Cardiology*, **79**, 412–414.

Kontopoulos, A.G., Athyros, V.G., Papageorgiou, A.A. *et al.* (1996) Effect of quinapril or metoprolol on heart rate variability in post-myocardial infarction patients. *American Journal of Cardiology*, **77**, 242–246.

Krum, H., Bigger, J.T., Goldsmith, R.L. *et al.* (1995) Effect of long-term digoxin therapy on autonomic function in patients with chronic heart failure. *Journal of the American College of Cardiology*, **25**, 289–294.

La Rovere, M.T., Mortara, A., Pantaleo, P. *et al.* (1994) Scopolamine improves autonomic balance in advanced congestive heart failure. *Circulation*, **90**, 838–843.

Lombardi, F., Torzillo, D., Sandrone, G. *et al.* (1992) Beta-blocking effect of propafenone based on spectral analysis of heart rate variability. *American Journal of Cardiology*, **70**, 1028–1034.

Niemela, M.J., Airaksinen, K.E.J. & Huikuri, H.V. (1994) Effect of β-blockade on heart rate variability in patients with coronary artery disease. *Journal of the American College of Cardiology*, **23**, 1370–1377.

Pagani, M., Lombardi, F., Guzzetti, S. *et al.* (1986) Power spectral analysis of heart rate and arterial pressure variabilities as a marker of sympatho-vagal interaction in man and conscious dog. *Circulation Research*, **59**, 178–193.

Piccirillo, G., Luparini, R.L., Celli, V. *et al.* (2000) Effects of carvedilol on heart rate and blood pressure variability in subjects with chronic heart failure. *American Journal of Cardiology*, **86**, 1392–1395.

Pomeranz, B., Macaulay, R.J.B., Caudill, M.A. *et al.* (1985) Assessment of autonomic function in man by heart rate analysis. *American Journal of Physiology*, **248**, H151–153.

Pousset, F., Copie, X., Lechat, P. *et al.* (1996) Effects of bisoprolol on heart rate variability in heart failure. *American Journal of Cardiology*, **77**, 612–617.

Ridha, M., Makikallio, T.H., Lopera, G. *et al.* (2002) Effects of carvedilol on heart rate dynamics in patients with congestive heart failure. *Annals of Noninvasive Electrocardiology*, **7**, 133–138.

Siepmann, M., Krause, S., Joraschky, P. *et al.* (2002) The effects of St John's wort extract on heart rate variability, cognitive function and quantitative EEG: a comparison with amitriptyline and placebo in healthy men. *British Journal of Clinical Pharmacology*, **54**, 277–282.

Vibyral, T., Bryg, R.J., Maddens, M.E. *et al.* (1990) Effects of transdermal scopolamine on heart rate variability in normal subjects. *American Journal of Cardiology*, **65**, 604–608.

Yeragani, V.K., Pohl, R., Balon, R. *et al.* (1992) Effect of imipramine treatment on heart rate variability measures. *Neuropsychobiology*, **26**, 27–32.

Yeragani, V.K., Pesce, V., Jayaraman, A. *et al.* (2002) Major depression with ischaemic heart disease: effects of paroxetine and nortriptyline on long-term heart rate variability measures. *Biol Psychiatry*, **52**, 418.

Zuanetti, G., Latini, R., Neilson, J.M.N. *et al.* (1991) Heart rate variability in patients with ventricular arrhythmias: effect of antiarrhythmic drugs. *Journal of the American College of Cardiology*, **17**, 604–612.

CHAPTER 11

Heart Rate Variability in Healthy Populations: Correlates and Consequences

Annie Britton and Harry Hemingway

Introduction

While attention has focused on measuring heart rate (*HR*) and heart rate variability (HRV) in patients with coronary disease, there is growing interest in the determinants and consequences of HRV in the general population. HRV, a measure of cardiac autonomic function, is determined by the interaction of cardiac sympathetic and parasympathetic activity, which causes changes in the beat-to-beat intervals and changes in the frequency components of the heart rate. In healthy populations, it is unclear how *HR* and HRV are correlated with conventional risk factors and clinical outcomes. The objective of this chapter is to review the literature on correlates (demographic, behavioural, biological, psychosocial) and consequences (mortality and morbidity) of *HR* and HRV in healthy populations. This review is restricted to literature published since 1990.

Cardiac autonomic function is associated with the prognosis of coronary patients; high resting heart rates (*HR*) and low heart rate variability (HRV) are associated with an increased risk of all-cause mortality and sudden death (Kleiger *et al.* 1987; Farrell *et al.* 1991; Bigger *et al.* 1992). While much of the initial research focused on patients with established coronary disease, more recent investigation of cardiac autonomic function has extended into the general population. Understanding the relationship between HRV and risk factors in healthy populations is crucial in determining whether the effects of HRV on clinical outcomes is aetiological. We carried out a literature review to address the four key questions outlined in the list below.

The autonomic nervous system determines HRV and *HR* and is an indicator of the interaction between cardiac sympathetic and parasympathetic activity, which causes changes in the beat-to-beat intervals and changes in the frequency components of the heart rate. Short-term variations in the beat-to-beat interval (measured as the standard deviation in normal-to-normal intervals; SDNN) are reduced by decreased parasympathetic activity or sympathetic overstimulation. High frequency (HF) power (typically 0.15–0.4 Hz) is a marker of parasympathetic activity; low levels of HF power indicate lower responsiveness to parasympathetic activity. Low frequency (LF) power (typically 0.04–0.15 Hz) reflects a combination of both parasympathetic and sympathetic modulations; low levels of LF power indicate lower parasympathetic activity, higher sympathetic activity or both. Some investigators have used the ratio of low- to high-frequency spectra as an index of parasympathetic–sympathetic balance.

1 How are *HR* and HRV associated with age and sex? Autonomic function declines with age and there are shifts in balance between sympathetic and parasympathetic components (O'Brien *et al.* 1986). It is not well documented whether measures of *HR* and HRV decline at the same point in the life course and at the same rate. Middle-aged women have higher resting heart rates than men, but the impact on HRV at different ages, for example, before and after the menopause, is unclear.

2 How are *HR* and HRV related to behavioural and biological risk factors? In order to understand the relationship between *HR* and HRV with clinical outcomes in the general population, it is important to explore how *HR* and HRV are related to conventional risk factors, which may confound or mediate any observed association. Do the associations follow predicted risk, i.e. are high *HR* and low HRV associated with adverse biological and behavioural risk factors? Are the effects consistent for both time and frequency domains of HRV?

3 How are *HR* and HRV related to social and psychosocial risk factors? The inverse social gradient in cardiovascular disease (CVD) is well established, but the relationship between measures of social position and HRV remains unclear. Exploring these relationships may elucidate pathways mediating the relationship between social position and CVD. Physiological systems fluctuate to meet the demands of external forces and this ability may be diminished by chronic activation of the sympathetic nervous system or chronic suppression of the parasympathetic system. The function of the autonomic nervous system is to respond to external stimuli, as shown in laboratory experiments; what is the evidence that *HR* and HRV correlate with real life stressors?

4 How are *HR* and HRV related to clinical outcome in healthy populations? Finally, a clear understanding of *HR* and HRV as predictors of risk in the general population is lacking. Which health outcomes are associated with impaired autonomic function? Are the time and frequency domains of HRV equally important? To what extent are these associations independent of conventional risk factors? What is the magnitude of difference in HRV which shows an effect on outcome?

Age and heart rate/heart rate variability (Table 11.1)

Heart rate

HR and age were not associated in the majority of the studies reviewed (Korkushko *et al.* 1991; Ryan *et al.* 1994; Jensen-Urstad *et al.* 1997; Greenland *et al.* 1999; Agelink *et al.* 2001). Those that did report an association were not consistent in the direction of the relationship. Stein *et al.* (1997) compared males aged 26–43 years with males aged 64–76 years and found that the older group had significantly higher *HR* than the younger cohort, whereas Ramaekers *et al.* (1998) and Umetani *et al.* (1998) reported that *HR* was negatively correlated with age in women.

HRV

Tsuji *et al.* (1996b) reported age to be the main determinant of HRV, accounting for 22–39% of the variance in SDNN, LF and HF power. Time-domain measures of HRV declined over the life course, in all studies. Umetani *et al.* (1998) suggested that SDNN decreased gradually with age, reaching 60% of baseline by 90 years. HF declined from age 20 years, whereas LF declines were not observed until 40 years of age (Korkushko *et al.* 1991). The relationship between the ratio of LF and HF frequency and age was less clear, with most studies reporting no association (Liao *et al.* 1995; Liao *et al.* 1997; Ramaekers *et al.* 1998; Agelink *et al.* 2001), and others reporting a decline in LF:HF with age (Sinnreich *et al.* 1998; Kuo *et al.* 1999). The magnitude of the decline was estimated to be around 15% in HF and LF power for every 10-year increase in age (Mølgaard *et al.* 1994).

Cross-sectional changes are not the same as within-person change

All except one of the studies reviewed was cross sectional. Tasaki *et al.* (2000) followed 15 elderly persons (mean age 70 years) for 15 years and reported a significant increase in heart rate and significant declines in SDNN, LF power and the LF/HF ratio. There was no significant change in the HF component with ageing. This study is broadly in agreement with the cross-sectional studies, but further longitudinal studies are needed in which HRV and *HR* are measured at several time points among the same cohort.

What explains lower HRV with older age?

The different components of HRV decline at different rates, suggesting a shift in balance between the parasympathetic and sympathetic pathways in autonomic control. In infancy sympathetic activity is dominant, followed by parasympathetic dominance. Early falls in the HF component suggest that the parasympathetic division declines first and by about age 50 years, the sympathetic division, whilst also exhibiting declines, is once more the dominant pathway in autonomic nervous control. Age and disease progression may have a similar influence on heart rate control, but before middle age, disease is unlikely to explain the entire decline in HRV measures. Most studies reviewed here removed

Table 11.1 Influence of age and gender on heart rate and heart rate variability in healthy populations*

Author, year, country	*Total sample (% women)*	*Age*	*Study group*	*Heart rate*	*Length of HRV recording*	*Time-domain SDNN*	*Frequency-domain LF*	*HF*	*HF/LF*
Korkushko *et al.* 1991 USSR	354 (50%)	3 months to 89 years	Population based (CVD excluded)	↓ age in early life → from 20 years	4 min	·	↑ age to 25–30 ↓ age 40+	↑ age to 15–19 ↓ age 20+	·
Mølgaard *et al.* 1994 Denmark	104 (38%)	40–77 years	Healthy volunteers (CVD excluded)	·	24 h	·	↓ age W < M	↓ age	·
Ryan *et al.* 1994 USA	67 (40%)	20–90 years	Healthy volunteers (CVD excluded)	→ age W = M	8 min	·	↓ age W < M	↓ age W > M	W > M
Liao *et al.* 1995 USA	1,984 (54%)	45–64 years	Selection from ARIC cohort (inc some with atherosclerosis)	·	2 min	·	↓ age W < M	↓ age W ≈ M	→ age W > M
Bigger *et al.* 1995 USA	274 (26%)	40–69 years	Healthy volunteers (CVD excluded)	·	24 h	·	↓ age W ≈ M	↓ age W ≈ M	·
Tsuji *et al.* 1996 USA	2,722 (55%)	21–93 years	Framingham offspring (CVD excluded)	·	2 h	↓ age W < M	↓ age W < M	↓ age W > M	·
Huikuri *et al.* 1996 Finland	374 (50%)	40–60 years	Population based (CVD excluded)	·	30 min	W < M	W < M	W > M	W < M
Yamasaki *et al.* 1996 Japan	105 (40%)	20–78 years	Mainly office workers (CVD excluded)	·	24 h	·	↓ age W < M	↓ age W ≈ M 20–49 years W > M 50+ years	·

Jensen-Urstad *et al.* 1997 Sweden	101 (51%)	20–69 years	Healthy volunteers (CVD excluded)	→ age W > M	24 h	↓ age W < M	↓ age W < M	↓ age W < M < 40 years W > M > 40 years	W < M
Liao *et al.* 1997 USA	2,252 (55%)	45–64 years	Healthy sample from ARIC (CVD excluded)	·	2 min	↓ age W < M	↓ age W < M	↓ age W > M	→ age W > M
Stein *et al.* 1997 USA	60 (50%)	26–43 years 64–76 years	Database of HRV recordings (CVD excluded)	↑ age in men W > M in younger group	24 h	↓ age W < M in young group W ≈ M in older group	↓ age W < M in young group W ≈ M in older group	↓ age W < M in young group W ≈ M in older group	·
Ramaekers *et al.* 1998 Belgium	276 (49%)	18–71 years	Healthy volunteers (CVD excluded)	↓ age in women W > M < 40 years W ≈ M > 40 years	24 h	↓ age in men W < M < 40 years W ≈ M > 40 years	↓ age W < M < 40 years W ≈ M > 40 years	↓ age W ≈ M	→ age W < M < 40 years W ≈ M > 40 years
Sinnreich *et al.* 1998 Israel	(i) 70 (54%) (ii) 294 (50%)	(i) 31–67 years (ii) 35–65 years	Samples from general population	W ≈ M	5 min	↓ age W ≈ M	↓ age W < M	↓ age W ≈ M	↓ age W < M
Umetani *et al.* 1998 USA	260 (57%)	10–99 years	Healthy volunteers, outpatients for routine evaluation (CVD excluded)	↓ age in women W > M < 50 years W ≈ M > 50 years	24 h	↓ age W < M < 30 W ≈ M > 50 years	·	·	·
Fagard *et al.* 1999 Belgium	424 (52%)	25–89 years	Population study (CVD excluded)	→ age W > M	15 min	↓ age W < M	↓ age W < M	↓ age (steeper in women) W ≈ M	W < M at younger ages

Table 11.1 *Continued*

Author, year, country	*Total sample (% women)*	*Age*	*Study group*	*Heart rate*	*Length of HRV recording*	*Time-domain SDNN*	*Frequency-domain LF*	*HF*	*HF/LF*
Kuo *et al.* 1999 Taiwan	1,070 (55.9%)	40–79 years	Healthy volunteers (CVD excluded)	·	5 min	↓ age W ≈ M	↓ age W ≈ M	↓ age W > M 40–49 W ≈ M > 60	↓ age W < M 40–59 W ≈ M > 60
Greenland *et al.* 1999 USA	33,781 (44%)	18–74 years	Employees	→ age W > M < 60 years	·	·	·	·	·
Dishman *et al.* 2000 USA	92 (43%)	20–59 years	Healthy volunteers (CVD excluded)	·	5 min	W < M	W < M	W ≈ M	·
Tasaki *et al.* 2000 Japan	15 (66%)	64–80 years baseline	Healthy elderly followed for 15 years	↑ age	5 h	↓ age	↓ age	→ age	↓ age
Agelink *et al.* 2001 Germany	309 (51%)	18–77 years	Healthy volunteers from hospital employees (CVD excluded)	→ age	5 min	·	↓ age W < M	↓ age W ≈ M	→ age W < M
Kuch *et al.* 2001 Germany	286 (48%)	56 years mean	Population study	·	5 min	·	↓ age W < M	↓ age W > M	·
Silvetti *et al.* 2001 Italy	103 (45%)	1–20 years	Healthy volunteers	·	24 h	↓ age W < M	·	·	·
Smetana *et al.* 2002 UK	51 (50%)	18–49 years	Healthy healthcare professional (CVD excluded)	W > M	24 h	·	·	·	·

* ↓ Inverse relationship; → no relationship; ↑ direct relationship; W > M, women have higher levels than men; W ≈ M, no difference between men and women. Frequency domain: LF, low frequency; HF, high frequency; HF/LF, ratio of high frequency to low frequency. Time domain: SDNN, standard deviation in normal-to-normal intervals.

people with clinically manifest disease from the analyses (Table 11.1) and still observed HRV declines with age. However, it is not possible to exclude the possibility that HRV declines are the result of subclinical disease.

Gender and heart rate/heart rate variability (Table 11.1)

Heart rate

Women had higher heart rates than men, particularly at younger ages (Jensen-Urstad *et al.* 1997; Stein *et al.* 1997; Ramaekers *et al.* 1998; Umetani *et al.* 1998; Fagard *et al.* 1999; Greenland *et al.* 1999; Smetana *et al.* 2002). There was evidence that the differences between the genders tailed off from about age 40–50 years. Ramaekers *et al.* (1998) estimated the difference between the genders to be in the order of 5 beats/min. whilst Umetani *et al.* (1998) estimated the difference to be around 7 beats/min among those aged 10–29 years.

HRV – time domain

SDNN was consistently shown to be lower in women than men, although this gender difference diminished at older ages. In a group of men and women aged 26 to 43 years, Stein *et al.* (1997) found men had a mean daytime SDNN of 153 ± 51 ms and women 97 ± 24 ms. There was no significant gender difference in the group aged 64–76 years.

HRV – frequency domain

Women tended to have lower LF but higher HF than men. There was no consistency in gender differences in the ratio of LF to HF power. In terms of the magnitude of the gender differences, Liao *et al.* (1995) reported in the Atherosclerosis Risk in Communities (ARIC) study that middle aged women had a geometric mean LF power of 3.12 ms^2 compared to a male geometric mean of 4.10 ms^2 ($P < 0.01$, adjusted for age and ethnicity). In a study of people aged 20–90 years, Ryan *et al.* (1994) reported that women had a mean HF power of 4.5 ms^2 compared to a mean HF of 3.3 ms^2 among men ($P < 0.05$). Yamasaki *et al.* (1996) suggested that the gender differences may not be consistent throughout the day, as men's peak LF was between 08.00 and 12.00 hours and women's LF peak was between 12.00 and 14.00 hours.

Age–sex interactions

Several authors suggested that gender differences diminished at older ages. In a comparison of two age groups: 26- to 43-year-olds and 64- to 76-year-olds, power spectral analyses revealed gender differences only among the younger cohort (log mean LF 7.6 ms^2 for younger men, 7.3 ms^2 for younger women $P < 0.05$) and not the older group (Stein *et al.* 1997). Likewise, in Ramaekers *et al.*'s (1998) study of 276 healthy volunteers aged 18–71 years, there were no gender differences in power spectral analyses after the age of 40 years. Kuo *et al.* (1999) reported that the gender differences diminished later at 60 years and above. Gender differences in the time components of HRV also weakened with age, perhaps as young as 30 years (Umetani *et al.* 1998).

What explains gender differences in HRV?

Men typically showed higher LF power than women, suggesting that they may have higher sympathetic activity. Conversely women had higher HF power, indicating higher parasympathetic tone. The gender differences were not simply confounded by behavioural factors (Huikuri *et al.* 1996). Gender differences declined around the time of the menopause, suggesting that there may be a hormonal explanation. This is supported by the finding that women undergo marked autonomic changes during the menstrual cycle. Sato *et al.* (1995) observed that LF power was higher and HF power was lower during the luteal phase than during the follicular phase, suggesting that sympathetic nervous activities are predominant in the luteal phase as compared with follicular phase. Also, Huikuri *et al.* (1996) explored the consequences of taking hormone replacement therapy among 40- to 60-year-old women and found increases in SDNN, HF and LF power, but no association with *HR*. It is not known whether declines in oestrogen levels are associated with a decline in HRV.

Behavioural/biological factors and heart rate/heart rate variability (Table 11.2)

In general, the pattern of these relationships followed risk, so that high *HR* and low HRV were associated with adverse conventional risk factors. A possible exception to this was with HF

Table 11.2 Behavioural and biological correlates of heart rate and heart rate variability in healthy populations*

Author, year, country	n *(% women) age*	*Population*	*Measurement (length of recording)*	*Exercise*	*Smoking and alcohol*	*Height, weight, BMI/obesity*	*SBP, DBP*	*Total cholesterol (TC), HDL, LDL cholesterol, triglycerides (TG)*	*Miscellaneous incl. diet and carbohydrate metabolism*
Mølgaard *et al.* 1991 Denmark	140 (36%) 40–77 years	Healthy volunteers	HRV (24 h)	SDNN ↑	SDNN ↓ smoking	·	·	·	·
Gillum 1992 USA	6,197 (54%) 25–74 years	NHANES-1	*HR*	*HR* ↓	*HR* ↑ smoking *HR* → alcohol	*HR* ↓ height *HR* ↓ weight *HR* U-shaped BMI	*HR* ↑	*HR* → TC	*HR* ↑ Hb, ↑ uric acid ↑ white cell count *HR* → coffee *HR* → tea
Bønaa & Arnesen 1992 Norway	19,152 (49%) 12–59 years	Healthy volunteers	*HR*	*HR* ↓	*HR* ↑ smoking	*HR* ↓ height *HR* U-shaped BMI	·	*HR* ↑ TC, *HR* ↓ HDL *HR* ↑ TG	·
Kupari *et al.* 1993 Finland	88 (53%) not stated	Healthy volunteers	HRV (10 min)	HF →	HF → smoking HF ↑ alcohol (women)	HF → BMI		HF → LDL HF → HDL	HF → coffee
Shaper *et al.* 1993 UK	7,735 (0%) 40–59 years	BRHS	*HR*	*HR* ↓	*HR* ↑ smoking *HR* ↑ alcohol	·	*HR* ↑	*HR* ↑ TC *HR* → HDL *HR* ↑ TG	*HR* ↑ glucose (not diabetes)
Koskinen *et al.* 1994 Finland	12 (0%) 24 mean	Healthy volunteers	HRV (5 min)	·	HF ↓ alcohol	·	·	·	·
Mølgaard *et al.* 1994 Denmark	104 (38%) 40–77 years	Healthy volunteers	HRV (24 h)	LF ↑ HF ↑	LF ↓ smoking HF ↓ smoking	·	·	·	·
Tsuji *et al.* 1996 USA	2,722 (55) 21–93 years	Fram'ham offspring	HRV (2 h)	·	SDNN ↓ smoking LF ↓ smoking SDNN ↑ alcohol LF ↑ alcohol	·	SDNN ↓ LF ↓ HF ↓	·	SDNN ↑ coffee LF ↑ coffee HF → coffee

Liao *et al.* 1997 USA	2,252 (55%) 45–64 years	Healthy random sample from ARIC	HRV (2 min)	·	SDNN ↓ smoking LF ↓ smoking HF→ smoking HF/LF → smoking	SDNN → BMI LF → BMI HF → BMI HF/LF → BMI	·	SDNN ↓ TC LF → TC HF → TC HF/LF → TC	·
Van de Borne *et al.* 1997 USA	16 (0) 26 mean	Healthy volunteers	*HR* and HRV after 1 g/kg alcohol	·	*HR* ↑ alcohol LF/HF ↑ alcohol	·	·	·	·
Kageyama *et al.* 1997 Japan	282 (0) 21–49 years	Male white collar workers	HRV (3 min)	·	LF → smoking HF → smoking LF → alcohol HF → alcohol	LF → obesity HF ↓ obesity	·	·	·
Liao *et al.* 1998 USA	2,359 (54%) 45–64 years	Random selection from ARIC cohort	HRV (2 min)	·	·	·	SDNN ↓ hypertension HF ↓ hypertension LF ↓ hypertension LF/HF → hypertension	SDNN → dyslipidemia HF → dyslipidemia LF → dyslipidemia LF/HF → dyslipidemia	SDNN ↓ diabetes HF ↓ diabetes LF ↓ diabetes LF/HF → diabetes SDNN ↓ fasting insulin HF ↓ fasting insulin LF ↓ fasting insulin LF/HF → fasting insulin
Fagard *et al.* 1999 Belgium	424 (52) 25–89 years	Healthy volunteers	*HR* and HRV (15 min)	*HR* ↓ men only HF ↑ LF/HF ↓	LF ↓ smoking HF ↑ smoking (women) LF/HF ↓ smoking *HR* → alcohol LF → alcohol HF → alcohol LF/HF → alcohol	HF ↑ BMI	·	·	·
Greenland *et al.* 1999 USA	33,781 (44%) 18–74 years	Employees	*HR*	·	*HR* ↑ smoking	*HR* ↑ obesity (young men)	*HR* ↑	*HR* → TC	·

Table 11.2 *Continued*

Author, year, country	*n (% women) age*	*Population*	*Measurement (length of recording)*	*Exercise*	*Smoking and alcohol*	*Height, weight, BMI/obesity*	*SBP, DBP*	*Total cholesterol (TC), HDL, LDL cholesterol, triglycerides (TG)*	*Miscellaneous incl. diet and carbohydrate metabolism*
Horsten *et al.* 1999 Sweden	300 (100) 31–65 years	General population	HRV (24 h)	SDNN ↑ LF ↑ HF → LF/HF ↑	SDNN ↓ smoking LF ↓ smoking HF → smoking LF/HF ↓ smoking	SDNN ↓ obesity LF ↓ obesity HF ↓ obesity LF/HF ↓ obesity	SDNN ↓ LF ↓ HF ↓ LF/HF →	·	·
Morcet *et al.* 1999 France	100,000 (32) 45 years mean	General population	*HR*	*HR* ↓	*HR* ↑ smoking men *HR* ↓ smoking women	*HR* ↓ height	*HR* ↑	*HR* ↑ TC (men only) *HR* ↑ TG	
Palatini *et al.* 1999 Italy	1,938 (61) 65+ years	Elderly population	*HR*	·	·	*HR* ↑ BMI	*HR* ↑	*HR* → TC *HR* → HDL *HR* ↑ TG (men only)	*HR* ↑ uric acid men *HR* ↑ uric acid women
Zhang & Kesteloot 1999 Belgium	9,177 (45%) 25–74 years	General population	*HR*	·	*HR* ↑ smoking	*HR* ↓ height	*HR* ↑	·	·
Dekker *et al.* 2000 USA	856 (55%) 40–65 years	ARIC	HRV (2 min)	·	SDNN → current smoking SDNN ↓ smoking years	SDNN ↓ BMI	·	SDNN ↑ HDL SDNN ↓ LDL SDNN ↓ TG	SDNN ↓ IMT
Flanagan *et al.* 2002 UK	21 (33) 21–41 yrs	Healthy volunteers	HRV (5 min)	·	*HR* → alcohol LF ↓ alcohol HF ↑ alcohol LF/HF ↑ alcohol	·	·	·	·
Minami *et al.* 2002 Japan	33 (0) 37 years mean	Habitual drinkers	*HR* and HRV (24 h)	·	*HR* ↑ alcohol HF ↓ alcohol LF/HF ↑ alcohol	·	·	·	·

* ↓ Inverse relationship; → no relationship; ↑ direct relationship. Frequency domain: LF, low frequency; HF, high frequency; HF/LF, ratio of high frequency to low frequency. Time domain: SDNN, standard deviation in normal-to-normal intervals; IMT, intima-media thickness.

power for which there was a lack of association with exercise and smoking.

Exercise

Exercise was found to be associated with a decrease in heart rate and an increase in measures of HRV (Mølgaard *et al.* 1991; Gillum 1992; Bønaa & Arnesen 1992; Shaper *et al.* 1993; Mølgaard *et al.* 1994; Fagard *et al.* 1999; Horsten *et al.* 1999; Morcet *et al.* 1999). For example, in a study of 300 Swedish subjects aged 31–65 years, Horsten *et al.* (1999) reported that those with a sedentary lifestyle had a mean LF power of 286.3 ms^2 compared to those who reported some forms of exercise with a mean LF power of 382.4 ms^2 ($P = 0.03$). HF power was not associated with exercise in two studies (Kupari *et al.* 1993: Horsten *et al.* 1999).

Smoking

Smoking was consistently associated with an increase in *HR* (Gillum 1992; Bønaa & Arnesen 1992; Shaper *et al.* 1993; Greenland *et al.* 1999; Zhang & Kesteloot 1999), although one study reported a decrease in *HR* among women smokers (Morcet *et al.* 1999). In terms of the size of effect, Gillum (1992) reported that the mean *HR* was about 2.9 beats/min higher in male smokers and 1.4 beats/min higher in women smokers than among ex- or never-smokers (adjusted $P < 0.01$). *HR* was also positively correlated with the number of cigarettes smoked per day. HRV measures, both time and frequency domains, showed decreases with smoking (Mølgaard *et al.* 1991; Kupari *et al.* 1993; Koskinen *et al.* 1994; Mølgaard *et al.* 1994; Tsuji *et al.* 1996b; Liao *et al.* 1997; Horsten *et al.* 1999). However, some studies suggested that the HF component might not be associated with smoking (Kupari *et al.* 1993; Liao *et al.* 1997; Kageyam *et al.* 1997; Horsten *et al.* 1999). Dekker *et al.* (2000) suggested that whilst current smoking is not associated with HRV, they found smoking years to be inversely related to SDNN.

Alcohol

The relationship between alcohol consumption and *HR* and HRV is more complex. An equal number of studies reported that alcohol did not affect *HR* (Gillum 1992; Fagard *et al.* 1999; Flanagan *et al.* 2002) as reported that alcohol (both usual intake and experimental intake) was associated with an increase in *HR* (Shaper *et al.* 1993; Van de Borne *et al.* 1997; Minami *et al.* 2002). In an experiment on 16 healthy volunteers Van de Borne *et al.* (1997) reported that 45 min after a dose of alcohol (1g/kg body weight) the resting heart rate increased on average from 59 beats/min to 65 beats/min. The effect of alcohol on HRV measures was not clear from these studies, as some reported an increase (Kupari *et al.* 1993;Tsuji *et al.* 1996b; Van de Borne *et al.* 1997; Flanagan 2002) and some reported a decrease (Koskinen *et al.* 1994) and yet others showed no association (Kageyama *et al.* 1997; Fagard *et al.* 1999). Further investigation is required to explore the effect of volume, frequency and type of alcohol consumption on cardiac autonomic function and to determine whether it mirrors the pattern of coronary risk.

Coffee

The few papers that explored the consequences of coffee intake were not consistent. Gillum reported no relationship between coffee or tea and heart rate (Gillum 1992). Tsuji *et al.* (1996b) reported an increase in HRV (SDNN and LF power, but not HF power) whilst Kupari *et al.* (1993) found no association between coffee and HF power.

Anthropometry

Height was consistently found to be inversely related to *HR* (Gillum 1992; Bønaa & Arnesen 1992; Morcet *et al.* 1999; Zhang & Kesteloot 1999). There was evidence of a U-shaped relationship between body mass index and *HR* (Gillum 1992; Bønaa & Arnesen 1992). HRV measures were either reduced with obesity (Horsten *et al.* 1999; Dekker *et al.* 2000) or were unrelated (Liao *et al.* 1997).

Blood pressure

Increasing blood pressure was associated with an increase in *HR* (Gillum 1992; Shaper *et al.* 1993; Greenland *et al.* 1999; Morcet *et al.* 1999; Palatini *et al.* 1999; Zhang & Kesteloot. 1999) and generally a decrease in HRV measures (Tsuji *et al.* 1996b; Liao *et al.* 1998; Horsten *et al.* 1999).

Lipids

Higher *HR* was associated with raised levels of total cholesterol, low density lipoproteins (LDL) and with triglycerides, but with decreases (Bønaa & Arnesen 1992) or no relationship (Shaper *et al.* 1993; Palatini *et al.* 1999) with raised levels of high density lipoproteins (HDL). Bønaa & Arnesen (1992) reported that men with heart rates > 89 beats/min had a 14.5% higher non-HDL cholesterol and 36.3% higher triglyceride levels than men with heart rates <60 beats/min (the corresponding differences in women were 12.5% and 22.2%). Decreases in heart rate variability were found with increases in total cholesterol and LDL (Kupari *et al.* 1993; Liao *et al.* 1997; Dekker *et al.* 2000) and some evidence of increases in SDNN with higher levels of HDL (Dekker *et al.* 2000).

Carbohydrate metabolism

Liao *et al.* (1998) reported that mean levels of HRV indices were lower among those with diabetes (SDNN mean 35 ms, LF mean 2.62 beats/min^2, HF mean 1.01 beats/min^2) compared to those without (SDNN mean 40 ms, LF mean 3.51 beats/min^2, HF mean 1.34 beats/min^2). In the same study higher levels of fasting insulin were associated with a higher likelihood of low HRV indices. The influence of each of the individual components of the metabolic syndrome on HRV was not investigated in any of the studies reviewed.

Psychosocial and social factors and heart rate/heart rate variability (Table 11.3)

Social factors

Although five papers reported the relationship between *HR* and HRV and social positiion, but in none was it the focus. In a study of 33 781 employees in the United States, Greenland *et al.* (1999) reported that education attainment was inversely correlated with heart rate in both men and women aged 18–59 years (unadjusted $P < 0.01$). This was consistent with the finding from the first National Health and Nutrition Examination Survey that resting pulse rate was raised among those with family incomes <$4000 (Gillum 1992). Other reports found no associations of resting heart rate with education (Gillum 1992) or with social class (Shaper *et al.* 1993). Using data from the ARIC study, Liao *et al.* (1997) reported that a greater proportion of people with high LF power had attained at least a high school education. Horsten *et al.* (1999) reported that education among women was not associated with any HRV measures.

Psychosocial factors

Among the investigators that explored the psychosocial correlates of *HR* and HRV some focused on short-term acute stressors, such as giving a presentation or inducing anger, whilst others investigated more chronic traits such as anxiety disorders, job stress and personality types. The studies tended to be small, in the order of 100 or fewer participants.

Heart rate was either found to increase with adverse psychosocial factors (Kawachi *et al.* 1995; Vrijkotte *et al.* 2000; Sloan *et al.* 2001; Laederach-Hofmann *et al.* 2002) or was unrelated to psychosocial factors (Kamada *et al.* 1992; Sato *et al.* 1998; Vrijkotte *et al.* 2000; Lampert *et al.* 2002). Using data from the Normative Aging Study, an inverse linear relationship was found with HRV. When categorized into four anxiety groups; scores 0–1 (low anxiety), 2, 3, ≥ 4., SDNN was respectively 3.54, 3.37, 3.35, 3.11 after adjustment for age, *HR* and body mass index (Kawachi *et al.* 1995). De Meersman *et al.* (1996) examined the effects of a real life stressor – research students giving a presentation in the setting of a (critical) audience and without an audience. There was higher LF and lower HF power in the 'with audience' recordings. In a population-based study of healthy women, Horsten *et al.* (1999) found that social isolation was associated with low HRV (SDNN, LF and LF/HF ratio, but not HF power) and an inability to relieve anger by talking to others was associated with decreases in SDNN and LF power (all analyses were adjusted for age, menopausal status, exercise, smoking, history of hypertension and body mass index). Depressive symptoms were unrelated to HRV. In a study of 70 office workers, the need for control was associated with a decrease in HF power. However, effort and rewards and effort–reward imbalance were not associated with HRV (Hanson *et al.* 2001).

HR and HRV and outcomes (Table 11.4)

Heart rate

In the review of longitudinal studies, higher *HR*s were associated with all cause mortality

Table 11.3 Influence of social and psychosocial factors on heart rate and heart rate variability in healthy populations*

Author, year, country	n (*% women) age*	*Study group*	*Design*	*Psychosocial factor A = acute, C = chronic*	*Social factor*	*Length of HRV recording*	HR	*SDNN*	*LF*	*HF*	*LF/HF ratio*
Gillum 1992 USA	6,197 (54) 25–74 years	NHANES-1	·	·	Education Income	·	→ education ↓ income	·	·	·	·
Kamada *et al.* 1992 Japan	19 (0) 21 years mean	Healthy students	Laboratory stressor	C: Type A and Type B	·	5 min	→	·	↑ more type A	↑ more type B	↑ among type A
Shaper *et al.* 1993 UK	7,735 (0) 40–59 years	BRHS	Cross sectional	·	Social class	·	→	·	·	·	·
Sloan *et al.* 1994 USA	35 (13) 36 yrs mean	Healthy volunteers	Normal daily activities	C: hostility	·	24 h	·	·	·	↓ among <40 years	↑ among <40 years
Kawachi *et al.* 1995 USA	581 (0) 47–86 years	Normative Aging study	Cross sectional	C: phobic anxiety	·	1 min	↑	↓	·	·	·
McCraty *et al.* 1995 USA	24 (63) 24–47 years	Healthy volunteers	Randomised trial	A: appreciation or anger	·	5 min	·	·	↑ anger ↑ appreciation	↑ anger → appreciation	·
De Meersman *et al.* 1996 USA	15 (73) 23–48 years	Healthy volunteers	Real life stressor (giving presentation)	A: anticipation of presentation with/without audience	·	30 min	·	·	↑ with audience	↓ with audience	↑ with audience
Liao *et al.* 1997 USA	2,252 (55) 54 years	ARIC	Cross sectional	·	Education	2 min	·	→ education	↑ education	→ education	→ education

Table 11.4 *Continued*

Author, year, country	n *(% women) age*	*Population*	*Follow-up*	*Outcome type (n events)*	*Length of HRV recording*	*Adjustments*	HR	*SDNN*	*LF*	*HF*	*LF/HF ratio*
Palatini *et al.* 1999 Italy	1,938 (61) 65+ years	Elderly population	12 years	All cause mortality	·	men only: age, BMI, hypertension, diabetes, angina, previous MI, medication, lipids, smoking, alcohol	↑ ACM men → ACM women ↑ CVD mort men	·	·	·	·
Dekker *et al.* 2000 USA	856 (55) 45–65 years	ARIC	6 years max	All cause mortality, CVD mortality, CHD incidence, cancer mortality	2 min	age, sex, race, smoking, triglycerides, HDL, diabetes, hypertension, BMI, WHR, IMT	↑ ACM ↑ CVD mort ↑ CHD incidence ↑ cancer mort	↓ ACM ↓ CVD mortality → CHD incidence → cancer	·	·	
Makikallio *et al.* 2001 Finland	325 (47) 65+ years	Elderly population	10 years	All cause mortality Cardiac/noncardiac death	24 h	age, sex, heart failure, angina, functional class, MI, medication, ventricular premature beats	·	→ ACM → cardiac death → sudden cardiac death → noncardiac death	·	·	·
Carnethon *et al.* 2002 USA	9,267 (60) 45–64 years	ARIC	10 years	MI, fatal CHD, non-CHD mortality	2 min	Age, race, gender, medication, heart rate	·	↓ MI → fatal CHD ↓ non-CHD mort	·	↓ MI → fatal CHD ↓ non-CHD	·

* ↓ Inverse relationship; → no relationship; ↑ direct relationship. *HR*, Heart rate; ACM, all cause mortality; CVD, cardiovascular disease; CHD, coronary heart disease; BMI, body mass index; TC, total cholesterol; MI, myocardial infarction; SBP, systolic blood pressure; DBP, diastolic blood pressure; WHR, waist hip ratio; IMT, carotid intima-media thickness.

(Mensink & Hoffmeister 1997; Benetos *et al.* 1999; Palatini *et al.* 1999; Dekker *et al.* 2000), coronary heart disease (Shaper *et al.* 1993; Mensink & Hoffmeister 1997; Benetos *et al.* 1999; Palantini *et al.* 1999; Dekker *et al.* 2000) and sudden cardiac death (Shaper *et al.* 1993). The Atherosclerosis Risk in Communities (ARIC) Study also found higher *HR* to be associated with an increased risk of cancer mortality (Dekker *et al.* 2000), but this was not supported by others (Mensink & Hoffmeister 1997; Greenland *et al.* 1999).

HRV

Only two studies – Framingham and ARIC – investigated the association of frequency-domain measures or HRV and subsequent clinical outcomes in initially healthy populations. Low HRV was associated with adverse outcomes in the majority of the studies, independent of conventional behavioural and biological risk factors. In a 4-year follow-up of participants in the Framingham study, Tsuji *et al.* reported that low SDNN, LF and HF (but not LF/HF ratio) increased the risk of cardiac events. The hazard ratios for subsequent cardiac events per 1 standard deviation decrement in SDNN, ln LF and ln HF were 1.45 (95% CI 1.13–1.85), 1.38 (95% CI 1.02–1.85), 1.38 (95% CI 1.03–1.84), respectively (adjusted for age, sex, cholesterol, HDL, smoking, diabetes, SBP, left ventricular hypertrophy, diuretic use and cardiac medication) (Tsuji *et al.* 1996a). In the ARIC study low HRV was associated with an increased risk of incident CHD (Liao *et al.* 1997). The adjusted relative risk for the lowest quartile of SDNN compared to the upper three quartiles was 1.39 (95% CL 0.94–2.04), for LF 1.09 (95% CI 0.72–1.64) and HF 1.72 (95% CI 1.17–2.51). In a study of referrals for HRV, those with low SDNN had more than twofold risk of sudden death than those with high SDNN after adjustment for age, cardiac dysfunction and myocardial infarction (Algra *et al.* 1993).

In a 4-year follow-up of over 5000 people aged over 55 years, de Bruyne *et al.* (1999) reported that participants in the lowest quartile of SDNN relative to those in the third quartile had an 80% age- and sex-adjusted increased risk for cardiac mortality (hazard ratio 1.8; 95% CI 1.0–1.3). The corresponding hazard ratios for noncardiac mortality and all cause mortality were 1.3 (95% CI 0.9–1.8) and 1.4 (95% CI 1.0–1.8) respectively. Interestingly, for subjects in the highest quartile of SDNN compared with those in the third quartile, an even more pronounced risk for cardiac mortality was found (hazard ratio 2.3; 95% CI 1.3–4.0). This elevated risk for high HRV has not been reported previously and further research is required to corroborate this finding.

What explains the associations between high heart rate and low HRV and mortality?

Physiologically rigid systems with less variability may be more vulnerable to adverse outcome. Experimental evidence from primates suggests that high heart rate may accelerate atherosclerosis (Beere *et al.* 1984) and in humans coronary artery by-pass patients with low HRV showed increased progression of coronary atherosclerosis (Huikuri *et al.* 1999a). In addition, high *HR*s increase pulsatile flow and alter local haemodynamic effects at the arterial walls, possibly influencing the distribution of lesions. Sympathetic predominance lowers the ventricular fibrillation threshold and has been suggested to be an important factor underlying the risk of sudden death in people with low HRV (Schwartz *et al.* 1992; Dekker *et al.* 1997).

Summary

All HRV measures declined with age, with high frequency (HF) power declining earliest at around age 20 years, signalling a fall in parasympathetic control. *HR* was not consistently related to age. Women had lower standard deviation in normal-to-normal intervals (SDNN) and low frequency power (LF), but higher HF power and higher *HR* than men. Gender differences diminished around the age of menopause, suggesting a possible hormonal influence in cardiac autonomic control. High *HR* and low HRV (SDNN and LF power) were associated with adverse behavioural and biological risk factors. HF was less consistently related to biological factors; some studies showed no HF relationship with smoking and exercise. The psychosocial studies tended to be small, but the two largest showed that *HR* was increased and HRV reduced in response to acute and chronic psychosocial factors. In most studies of healthy populations high *HR* and low HRV (SDNN, LF and HF power) were predictors of increased all-cause mortality and coronary morbidity, independent of conventional risk factors. However, only two healthy population studies – Framingham and ARIC – have reported frequency-domain measures of HRV in relation to clinical outcomes.

Conclusion

In healthy populations, high *HR* and low HRV tended to be associated with adverse risk factors and, independently, with adverse clinical outcomes. These relationships were not uniform across all measures of heart rate variability. Further prospective studies are required investigating mortality and morbidity in relation to specific components of HRV.

References

Agelink, M.W., Malessa, R., Baumann, B. *et al.* (2001) Standardized tests of heart rate variability: normal ranges obtained from 309 healthy humans, and effects of age, gender, and heart rate. *Clinical Autonomic Research*, **11**, 99–108.

Algra, A., Tijssen, J.G.P., Roelandt, J.R.T.C., Pool, J. & Lubsen, J. (1993) Electrophysiology: heart rate variability from 24 h electrocardiography and the 2-year risk for sudden death. *Circulation*, **88**, 180–185.

Beere, P.A., Glagov, S. & Zarins, C.K. (1984) Retarding effect of lowered heart rate on coronary atherosclerosis. *Science*, **226**, 180–182.

Benetos, A., Rudnichi, A., Thomas, F., Safar, M. & Guize, L. (1999) Influence of heart rate on mortality in a French population. Role of age, gender and blood pressure. *Hypertension*, **33**, 44–52.

Bernardi, L., Sleight, P., Bandinelli, G. *et al.* (2001) Effect of rosary prayer and yoga mantras on autonomic cardiovascular rhythms: comparative study. *British Medical Journal*, **323**, 1446–1449.

Bigger, J.T., Fleiss, J.L., Steinmann, R.C., Rolnitzky, L.M., Kleiger, R.E. & Rottman, J.N. (1992) Frequency domain measures after myocardial infarction. *Circulation*, **85**, 164–171.

Bigger, J.T., Fleiss, J.L., Steinmann, R.C., Rolnitzky, L.M., Schneider, W.J. & Stein, P.K. (1995) *RR* variability in healthy, middle-aged persons compared with patients with chronic coronary heart disease or recent acute myocardial infarction. *Circulation*, **91**, 1936–1943.

Bønaa, K.H. & Arnesen, E. (1992) Association between heart rate and atherogenic blood lipid fractions in a population. The Tromsø Study. *Circulation*, **86**, 394–405.

van de Borne, P., Mark, A.L., Montano, N., Mion, D. & Somers, V.K. (1997) Effects of alcohol on sympathetic activity, hemodynamics, and chemoreflex sensitivity. *Hypertension*, **29**, 1278–1283.

Carnethon, M.R., Liao, D., Evans, G.W. *et al.* (2002) Does the cardiac autonomic response to postural change predict incident coronary heart disease and mortality? The ARIC Study. *American Journal of Epidemiology*, **155**, 48–56.

Dekker, J.M., Crow, R.S., Folsom, A.R. *et al.* (2000) Low heart rate variability in a 2-min rhythm strip predicts risk of coronary heart disease and mortality from several causes. The ARIC Study. *Circulation*, **102**, 1239–1244.

Dekker, J.M, Schouten, E.G., Klootwijk, P., Pool, J., Swenne, C.A. & Kromhout, D. (1997) Heart rate variability from short electrocardiographic recordings predicts mortality from all causes in middle-aged and elderly men. The Zutphen Study. *American Journal of Epidemiology*, **145**, 899–908.

De Bruyne, M.C., Kors, J.A., Hoes, A.W. *et al.* (1999) Both decreased and increased heart rate variability on the standard 10-second electrocardiogram predict cardiac mortality in the elderly. The Rotterdam Study. *American Journal of Epidemiology*, **150**, 1282–1289.

De Meersman, R., Reisman, S., Daum, M. & Zorowitz, R. (1996) Vagal withdrawal as a function of audience. *American Journal of Physiology*, **270**, H1381–H1383.

Dishman, R.K., Nakamura, Y., Garcia, M.E., Thompson, R.W., Dunn, A.L. & Blair, S.N. (2000) Heart rate variability, trait anxiety, and perceived stress among physically fit men and women. *International Journal of Psychophysiology*, **37**, 121–133.

Fagard, R.H., Pardaens, K. & Staessen, J.A. (1999) Influence of demographic, anthropometric and life-style characteristics on heart rate and its variability in the population. *Journal of Hypertension*, **17**, 1589–1599.

Farrell, T.G., Bashir, Y., Cripps, T *et al.* (1991) Risk stratification for arrhythmic events in postinfarction patients based on heart rate variability, ambulatory electrocardiographic variables and the signal averaged electrocardiogram. *Journal of the American College of Cardiology*, **18**, 786–797.

Flanagan, D.E.H., Pratt, E., Murphy, J. *et al.* (2002) Alcohol consumption alters insulin secretion and cardiac autonomic activity. *European Journal of Clinical Investigation*, **32**, 187–192.

Gillum, R.F. (1992) Epidemiology of resting pulse rate of persons ages 25–74 – data from NHANES 1971–74. *Public Health Reports*, **107**, 193–201.

Greenland, P., Daviglus, M.L., Dyer, A.R. *et al.* (1999) Resting heart rate is a risk factor for cardiovascular and noncardiovascular mortality. The Chicago Heart Association Detection Project in Industry. *American Journal of Epidemiology*, **149**, 853–862.

Hanson, E.K.S., Godaert, G.L.R., Maas, C.J.M. & Meijman, T.F. (2001) Vagal cardiac control throughout the day: the relative importance of effort-reward imbalance and within-day measurements of mood, demand and satisfaction. *Biological Psychology*, **56**, 23–44.

Horsten, M., Ericson, M., Perski, A., Wamala, S.P., Schenck-Gutafsson, K. & Orth-Gomer, K. (1999) Psychosocial factors and heart rate variability in healthy women. *Psychosomatic Medicine*, **61**, 49–57.

Huikuri, H.V., Jokinen, V., Syvanne, M *et al.* (1999a) Heart rate variability and progression of coronary atherosclerosis. *Arteriosclerosis Thrombosis and Vascular Biology*, **19**, 1979–1985.

Huikuri, H.V., Makikallio, T., Airaksinen, J. *et al.* (1998) Power-law relationship of heart rate variability as a predictor of mortality in the elderly. *Circulation*, **97**, 2031–2036.

Huikuri, H.V., Makikallio, T., Airaksinen, J., Mitrani, R., Castellanos, A. & Myerburg, R (1999b) Measurement of heart rate variability: a clinical tool or a research toy? *Journal of the American College of Cardiology*, **34**, 1878–1883.

Huikuri, H.V., Pikkujamsa, S.M., Airaksinen, K.E. *et al.* (1996) Sex-related differences in autonomic modulation of heart rate in middle-aged subjects. *Circulation*, **94**, 122–125.

Jensen-Urstad, K. Storck, N., Bouvier, F., Ericson, M., Lindblad, L.E. & Jensen-Urstad, M. (1997) Heart rate variability in healthy subjects is related to age and gender. *Acta Physiologica Scandinavica*, **160**, 235–241.

Kageyama, T., Nishikido, N., Hona, Y *et al.*(1997) Effects of obesity, current smoking status, and alcohol consumption on heart rate variability in male white-collar workers. *International Archives of Occupational and Environmental Health*, **69**, 447–454.

Kageyama, T., Nishikido, N., Kobayashi, T., Kurokawa, Y., Kaneko, T. & Kabuto, M. (1998) Long commuting time, extensive overtime, and sympathodominant state assessed in terms of short-term heart rate variability among male white-collar workers in the Tokyo megalopolis. *Industrial Health*, **36**, 209–217.

Kageyama, T., Nishikido, N., Kobayashi, T., Kurokawa, Y., Kaneko, T. & Kabuto, M. (1998) Self-reported sleep quality, job stress, and daytime autonomic activities assessed in terms of short-term heart rate variability among male white-collar workers. *Industrial Health*, **36**, 263–272.

Kamada, T., Miyake, S., Kumashiro, M., Monou, H. & Inoue, K. (1992) Power spectral analysis of heart rate variability in Type As and Type Bs during mental workload. *Psychosomatic Medicine*, **54**, 462–470.

Kawachi, I., Sparrow, D., Vokanas, P.S. & Weiss, S.T. (1995) Decreased heart rate variability in men with phobic anxiety (data from the Normative Aging Study). *American Journal of Cardiology*, **75**, 882–885.

Kleiger, R.E., Miller, J.P., Bigger, J.T. & Moss, A.J. (1987). Decreased heart rate variability and its association with increased mortality after acute myocardial infarction. *American Journal of Cardiology*, **59**, 256–262.

Korkushko, O.V., Shatilo, V.B., Plachinda, Y. & Shatilo, T.V (1991) Autonomic control of cardiac chronotrophic function in man as a function of age: assessment by power spectral analysis of heart rate variability. *Journal of the Autonomic Nervous System*, **32**, 191–198.

Koskinen, P., Virolainen, J. & Kupari, M. (1994) Acute alcohol intake decreases short-term heart rate variability in healthy subjects. *Clinical Sciences*, **87**, 225–230.

Kuch, B., Hense, H.W., Sinnreich, R. *et al.* (2001) Determinants of a short-period heart rate variability in the general population. *Cardiology*, **95**, 131–138.

Kuo, T.B.J., Lin, T., Yang, C.C.H., Li, C., Chen, C. & Chou, P. (1999) Effect of aging on gender differences in neural control of heart rate. *American Journal of Physiology*, **277** (*Heart Circulation Physiology* **46**), H2233–H2239

Kupari, M., Virolainen, J., Koskinen, P. & Tikkanen, M.J (1993) Short-term heart rate variability and factor modifying the risk of coronary artery disease in a population sample. *American Journal of Cardiology*, **72**, 897–903.

Laederach-Hofmann, K., Mussgay, L., Buchel, B., Widler, P. & Ruddel, H. (2002) Patients with erythrophobia (fear of blushing) show abnormal autonomic regulation in mental stress conditions. *Psychosomatic Medicine*, **64**, 358–365.

Lampert, R., Baron, S.J., McPherson, C.A. & Lee, F.A. (2002) Heart rate variability during the week of September 11, 2001. *JAMA (Journal of the American Medical Association)*, **288**, 575.

Liao, D., Barnes, R.W., Chambless, L.E., Simpson, R.J. & Sorlie, P., Heiss, G. (1995) Age, race and sex differences in autonomic cardiac function measured by spectral analysis of heart rate variability – the ARIC study. *American Journal of Cardiology*, **76**, 906–912.

Liao, D., Cai, J., Barnes, R.W. *et al.* (1996) Association of cardiac autonomic function and the development of hypertension. The ARIC study. *American Journal of Hypertension*, **9**, 1147–1156.

Liao, D., Cai, J., Rosamond, W.D. *et al.* (1997) Cardiac autonomic function and incident coronary heart disease: a population-based case-cohort study. The ARIC Study. Atherosclerosis Risk in Communities Study. *American Journal of Epidemiology*, **145**, 696–706.

Liao, D., Sloan, R.P., Cascio, W.E. *et al.* (1998) Multiple metabolic syndrome is associated with lower heart rate variability. *Diabetes Care*, **21**, 2116–2122.

Makikallio, T.H., Huikuri, H.V., Makikallio, A. *et al.* (2001) Prediction of sudden cardiac death by fractal analysis of heart rate variability in elderly subjects. *Journal of the American College of Cardiology*, **37**, 1395–1402.

McCraty, R., Atkinson, M., Tiller, W.A., Rein, G. & Watkins, A.D. (1995) The effects of emotions on short-term power spectrum analysis of heart rate variability [published erratum appears in *American Journal of Cardiology*, **77**(4), 333 (1996)]. *American Journal of Cardiology*, **76**, 1089–1093.

McCraty, R., Atkinson, M., Tomasino, D. & Struppy, W.P. (2001) Analysis of twenty-four hour heart rate variability in patients with panic disorder. *Biological Psychology*, **56**, 131–150.

Mensink, G.B.M. & Hoffmeister, H. (1997) The relationship between resting heart rate and all-cause, cardiovascular and cancer mortality. *European Heart Journal*, **18**, 1404–1410.

Minami, J., Yoshi, M., Todoroki, M. *et al.* (2002) Effects of alcohol restriction on ambulatory blood pressure, heart rate, and heart rate variability in Japanese men. *American Journal of Hypertension*, **15**, 125–129.

Mølgaard, H., Sorensen, K.E. & Bjerregaard, P. (1991) Circadian variation and influence of risk factors on heart rate variability in healthy subjects. *American Journal of Cardiology*, **68**, 777–784.

Mølgaard, H., Hermansen, K. & Bjerregaard, P. (1994) Spectral components of short-term *RR* interval variability in healthy subjects and effects of risk factors. *European Heart Journal*, **15**, 1174–1183.

Morcet, J., Safar, M., Thomas, F., Guize, L. & Benetos, A. (1999) Associations between heart rate and other risk factors in a large French population. *Journal of Hypertension*, **17**, 1671–1676.

O'Brien, I.A., O'Hare, P. & Corral, R.J. (1986) Heart rate variability in healthy subjects: effect of age and the derivation of normal ranges for tests of autonomic function. *British Heart Journal*, **55**, 348–354.

Palatini, P., Casiglia, E., Julius, S. & Pessina, A.C. (1999) High heart rate: a risk factor for cardiovascular death in elderly men. *Archives of Internal Medicine*, **159**, 585–592.

Ramaekers, D., Ector, H., Aubert, A.E., Rubens, A. & Van de Werf, F. (1998) Heart rate variability and heart rate in healthy volunteers. Is the female autonomic nervous system cardioprotective? *European Heart Journal*, **19**, 1334–1341.

Ryan, S.M., Goldberger, A.L., Pincus, S.M., Mietus, J. & Lipsitz, L.A. (1994) Gender- and age-related differences in heart rate dynamics: are women more complex than men? *Journal of the American College of Cardiology*, **24**, 1700–1707.

Sato, N., Miyake, S., Akatsu, J. & Kumashiro, M. (1995) Power spectral analysis of heart rate variability in healthy young women during the normal menstrual cycle. *Psychosomatic Medicine*, **57**, 331–335.

Sato, N., Kamada, T., Miyake, S., Akatsu, J., Kumashiro, M. & Kume, Y. (1998) Power spectral analysis of heart rate variability in type A females during a psychomotor task. *Journal of Psychosomatic Research*, **45**, 159–169.

Shaper, A.G., Wannamethee, G., Macfarlane, P.W. & Walker, M. (1993) Heart rate, ischaemic heart disease, and sudden cardiac death in middle-aged British men. *British Heart Journal*, **70**, 49–55.

Silvetti, M.S., Drago, F. & Ragonese, P. (2001) Heart rate variability in healthy children and adolescents is partially related to age and gender. *International Journal of Cardiology*, **81**, 169–174.

Singh, J.P., Larson, M.G., Tsuji, H., Evans, J.C., O'Donnell, C.J. & Levy, D. (1998) Reduced heart rate variability and new-onset hypertension. Insights into pathogenesis of hypertension: the Framingham Heart Study. *Hypertension*, **32**, 293–297.

Sinnreich, R., Kark, J.D., Friedlander, Y., Sapoznikov, D. & Luria, M.H. (1998). Five min recordings of heart rate variability for population studies: repeatability and age–sex characteristics. *Heart*, **80**, 156–162.

Sloan, R.P., Shapiro, P.A., Bigger, J.T., Bagiell, E., Steinman, R.C. & Gorman, J.M. (1994) Cardiac autonomic control and hostility in healthy subjects. *American Journal of Cardiology*, **74**, 298–300.

Sloan, R.P., Bagiella, E., Shapiro, P.A. *et al.* (2001) Hostility, gender, and cardiac autonomic control. *Psychosomatic Medicine*, **63**, 434–440.

Smetana, P., Batchvarov, V.N., Hnatkova, K., Camm, A.J. & Malik, M. (2002) Sex differences in repolarization homogeneity and its circadian pattern. *American Journal of Physiology (Heart Circulation Physiology)* **282**, H1889–H1897.

Stein, P.K., Kleiger, R.E. & Rottman, J.N. (1997) Differing effects of age on heart rate variability in men and women. *American Journal of Cardiology*, **80**, 302–305.

Schwartz, P.J., La Rovere, M.T. & Vanoli, E. (1992) Autonomic nervous system and sudden cardiac death. Experimental basis and clinical observations for post-myocardial infarction risk stratification. *Circulation*, **85**, 177–191.

Tasaki, H., Serita, T., Irita, A. *et al.* (2000) A 15-year longitudinal follow-up study of heart rate and heart rate variability in healthy elderly persons. *Journal of Gerontology Series A Biological Sciences and Medical Sciences*, **55**, M744–M749.

Tsuji, H., Venditti, F.J., Manders, E.S. *et al.* (1994) Reduced heart rate variability and mortality risk in an elderly cohort. The Framingham Heart Study. *Circulation*, **90**, 878–883.

Tsuji, H., Larson, M.G., Ferdinand, J.V. *et al.* (1996a) Impact of reduced heart rate variability on risk for cardiac events. *Circulation*, **94**, 2850–2855.

Tsuji, H., Venditti, F.J., Manders, E.S. *et al.* (1996b) Determinants of heart rate variability. *Journal of the American College of Cardiology*, **28**, 1539–1546.

Umetani, K., Singer, D.H., McCraty, R. & Atkinson, M. (1998) Twenty-four h time domain heart rate variability and heart rate: relations to age and gender over nine decades. *Journal of the American College of Cardiology*, **31**, 593–601.

Vrijkotte, T.G.M., van Doornen, L.J.P. & de Geus, E.J.C. (2000) Effects of work stress on ambulatory blood pressure, heart rate, and heart rate variability. *Hypertension*, **35**, 880–886.

Yamasaki, Y., Kodama, M., Matsuhisa, M. *et al.* (1996) Diurnal heart rate variability in healthy subjects: effects of aging and sex difference. *American Journal of Physiology (Heart and Circulation Physiology)*, **271**, H303–H310.

Zhang, J. & Kesteloot, H. (1999) Anthropometric, lifestyle and metabolic determinants of resting heart rate. A population study. *European Heart Journal*, **20**, 103–110.

CHAPTER 12

Heart Rate Variability in Ischaemic Disease

Robert E. Kleiger and Phyllis K. Stein

Introduction

Heart rate is not fixed. In healthy individuals with normal sinus rhythm there are continuous fluctuations in heart rate. They occur secondary to exertion, mental stress, respiration, metabolic changes, thermoregulation and long-term diurnal central and endocrine cycles. The modulation of heart rate is primarily the result of alterations of autonomic tone with parasympathetic or vagal influences slowing heart rate and sympathetic stimulation increasing it.

Measurement of cardiac autonomic modulation

These changes in heart rate can be assessed by a variety of techniques, including simple measurement of cardiac cycle lengths or the differences in length between adjacent cycles (i.e. time-domain measurements), by calculating the underlying frequencies of heart rate fluctuations using autoregressive or fast Fourier techniques (i.e. frequency-domain measurements), creating histograms of various interval frequencies, (i.e. geometric methods) or by a variety of nonlinear methods (Cerutti *et al.* 1995; Kleiger 1995; Malik 1995). In addition, baroreceptor sensitivity can be assessed by plotting cycle length vs. blood pressure, usually by acutely altering blood pressure by administration of a vasodilator drug such as nitroglycerin or a vasopressor such as phenylephrine, but also by plotting the relationship of cycle length and blood pressure (La Rovere *et al.* 2001). All of these techniques have been used to study the effects of ischaemic disease on heart rate variability (HRV) and HRV indices as potential risk stratifiers following an ischaemic event (Kleiger & Stein, 2001; Rottman *et al.* 1990; Cripps *et al.* 1991).

Early studies of the association of decreased HRV and mortality post-MI

Several early studies suggested that alterations in heart rate variability were associated with increased mortality. Hinkle *et al.* (1972) in a 7-year follow-up of 301 middle-aged men found that those with decreased sinus arrhythmia, failure to slow heart rate with sighing, and relatively fixed heart rate with failure to increase their rate by 15 beats/min during exercise had a significantly increased risk of sudden death. Wolf *et al.* (1978) found that heart rate variability, measured as the variance of cycle lengths from 30 consecutive sinus beats of the admission electrocardiogram, was a predictor of in-hospital mortality in 176 patients with acute myocardial infarction (MI). However, the study was small and the decrease in HRV was found predominantly in patients with large anterior infarctions and other unfavourable features of infarction. HRV was not an independent variable predicting adverse outcomes.

In 1987 the Multicentre Post Infarction Project (MPIP) investigators reported their findings on >800 survivors of acute MI aged <70 and in normal sinus rhythm (Kleiger *et al.* 1987). An SDNN <50 ms (standard deviation of all normal-to-normal intervals recorded from a 24-h ambulatory electrocardiogram [ECG]) was associated with a 5.3 greater risk of mortality in the 31-month follow-up compared to those with an SDNN ≥ 100 ms and a 2.8 greater risk compared to those with SDNN >50 ms. Approximately 16% of the MI survivors had an SDNN of

<50 ms, but 43 of the 127 deaths (34%) during follow-up occurred in this group of patients. Thus, the sensitivity and positive predictive accuracy of SDNN < 50 was approximately one-third. Furthermore, a low HRV plus any of the following: repetitive premature ventricular contractions (PVCs), PVCs ≥ 10/h, ejection fraction < 30%, failure to perform a low-level exercise test, and heart rate >80 beats/min, created subgroups with mortalities around 50%. Low HRV was found to be the most powerful ambulatory ECG variable in predicting mortality and to be an independent predictor of mortality even after controlling for variables such as ejection fraction, Killip class, and PVC variables. Although HRV was significantly correlated with sinus cycle length and ejection fraction, the correlations were weak and did not negate the independent relationship between mortality and low HRV. Subsequently, the MPIP investigators demonstrated, using the same database, that other HR variables including frequency domain measures such as total power, ultra and very low frequency power and other time-domain variables, such as SDANN (standard deviation of 5-min averages of the normal *RR* intervals) and SDNN index were also powerful predictors of mortality (Bigger *et al.* 1992). This study was performed before much of today's standard therapy for MI, including the routine use of reperfusion techniques, ASA, beta blockers, bypass surgery, etc. Nevertheless, there is considerable evidence that even in the modern era, HRV remains predictive of outcome in survivors of acute MI.

Confirmatory studies of decreased HRV and risk of mortality post-MI

Table 12.1 lists some of the confirmatory studies performed after the MPIP study. Particularly important were the studies from St George's Hospital in London reported by Malik, Camm and their co-investigators. An initial report by Farrell *et al.* (1991b) described results in 68 survivors of myocardial infarction. In this study both baroreceptor sensitivity and HRV measured by a geo-metric technique (HRV index) predicted mortality with the former a more powerful predictor.

In subsequent clinical studies the group at St George's reported findings in a large number of patients surviving acute myocardial infarction. Odemuyiwa *et al.* (1991), reporting on 385 patients, compared the sensitivity and specificity of HRV index and ejection fraction in predicting all cause mortality, arrhythmic events and sudden death. HRV index was obtained from 24-h recordings made 7 days post infarction and left ventricular ejection fraction calculated from either angiograms or radionuclear studies. Receiver operator curves compared sensitivity and specificity for events at given sensitivities for each of the endpoints. At a sensitivity of 75%, HRV index < 30 units had a greater specificity for sudden death and arrhythmic events than a depressed ejection fraction and a marginally better specificity for prediction of total mortality. The combination of decreased HRV index and low ejection fraction increased the specificity for all 3 endpoints.

Farrell *et al.* (1991a) subsequently extended these observations to over 400 survivors of acute myocardial infarction. Other variables used in the analysis included ejection fraction, late potentials, heart rate, ventricular arrhythmias, and Killip class. On multivariate analysis the combination of impaired HRV and abnormal late potentials was the best independent combination for predicting arrhythmic events. For cardiac mortality the strongest univariate predictor of mortality was HRV index < 20 ms. Thus, diminished HRV, implying disordered autonomic function, predicted both death and arrhythmic events with greater accuracy than conventional risk variables such as ejection fraction or PVC frequency. Depressed HRV index and other abnormal risk variables identified subgroups with very high risk of adverse events, results essentially identical to the findings of MPIP.

Algra *et al.* (1993) explored the ability of HRV to predict sudden death in 6693 consecutive post-MI patients. Patients with short-term variability <25 ms (defined as the average of 1-min SDNN) had an unadjusted relative risk of sudden death of 4.1 compared to patients with short-term variability ≥40 ms. Even after adjustment for covariates the relative risk was 2.8. Also, after adjustment for covariates, patients with a minimum heart rate ≥65 beats/min had slightly more than twice the risk of sudden death of those with a minimum heart rate of <65 beats/min.

Table 12.1 Selected post-MPIP confirmatory studies of HRV as a predictor of all-cause or cardiac mortality in post-MI (POMI) patients

Source (study name)	*No. of patients (events)*	*HRV measure, when obtained*	*Follow-up*	*HRV predictors/endpoints*
Bigger *et al.* 1993b (CAPS)	$n = 331$ (30 deaths)	24-h, 1 year after enrolling in CAPS and 1 week after stopping meds	3 years	ULF, VLF, LF, HF all significant, univariate predictors all-cause mortality. After adjustment for covariates, VLF strongest predictor
La Rovere *et al.* 1998 (ATRAMI)	$n = 1284$ (44 cardiac deaths, 5 nonfatal sudden)	24-h, 15 ± 10 days POMI	21 ± 8 months	SDNN <70 ms vs. SDNN >70 ms ($R - R = 3.2$) for cardiac mortality
Odemuyiwa *et al.* 1991.	$n = 385$ (44 deaths, 14 sudden)	24-h, predischarge	151–1618 days	HRV index ≤39 sens 75%, spec 52% compared with LVEF ≤40 which had spec of 40% for all-cause mortality. HRV + LVEF better spec for sens <60%
Quintana *et al.* 1997	$n = 74$ (18 deaths 9 nonfatal MI), 24 normal controls	24-h, Mean 4 days POMI	36 ± 15 months	Ln VLF <5.99 independent predictor of all-cause mortality ($R - R = 1.9$) or mortality/nonfatal infarction ($R - R = 2.2$)
Touboul *et al.* 1997 (GREPI)	$n = 471$ (26 deaths for/1 yr FU, 39 for long term FU, 9 sudden) 45% had thrombolysis	24-h HRV, 10 days POMI	1 year and long term (median 31.4 months)	Nighttime AVGNN <750 ms ($R - R = 3.2$), daytime SDNN <100 ms ($R - R = 2.6$). Same predictors for 1 year and long-term all-cause mortality
Viashnav *et al.* 1994	$n = 226$ (19 cardiac deaths)	24-h, mean 83 h POMI	Mean 8 months	Cox regression not performed Decreased SDNN, SDANN, SDNNIDX, LF, HF, LF/HF among non-survivors, but rMSSD and pNN50 not different
Zabel *et al.* 1998	$n = 250$ (30 endpoints)	24-h HRV, stable, before discharge	Mean 32 months	SDNN significantly higher in event-free (no VT, resuscitated VF, or death)
Zuanetti *et al.* 1996 (GISSI)	$n = 567$ males treated with thrombolysis (52 deaths, 44 cardiac)	24-h at discharge (median 13 days)	1000 days	Independent predictors of all-cause mortality: NN50+ ($R - R = 3.5$), SDNN ($R - R = 3.0$), rMSSD ($R - R = 2.8$)

As noted above, many different heart rate variables have been used to risk stratify ischaemic patients. The most widely used is probably SDNN, but many other time domain, frequency domain and geometric measures have also been studied (Copie *et al.* 1996; Hohnloser *et al.* 1997; Stein & Kleiger 1999). Most investigations have utilized 24-h recording, but since there are high correlations between short- and long-term HRV variables, recording times as short as a min (Wolf *et al.* 1978) have been used. However, data suggest the superiority of longer time periods, since most studies show better predictive power for HRV indices, such as SDNN and SDANN, that include circadian variation. Recently, there has been great interest in nonlinear variables such as short-term fractal scaling exponent, power law slope, Poincaré plots, and approximate entropy (Schmidt & Morfill 1995; Mäkikallio *et al.* 1997). Some data suggest that these measures may be better in separating those MI survivors at high risk than conventional HRV measures. The index power law slope and its intercept were applied to the MPIP data and found to the a better predictor of mortality than any time- or frequency-domain HRV index (Bigger *et al.* 1996). Nonlinear techniques were also applied to prediction of mortality in the DIAMOND trial (Huikuri *et al.* 2000). Patients were recently post-MI and had a left ventricular ejection fraction (LVEF) of < 35%. On a univariate basis, standard time domain, frequency domain and geometric indices as well as nonlinear indices (short-term fractal scaling exponent $\alpha 1$, longer-term fractal scaling exponent $\alpha 2$, and power-law slope) all predicted mortality. However, after adjustment for clinical and demographic predictors, $\alpha 1$ was the most powerful predictor of both arrhythmia and nonarrhythmic deaths.

Decreased HRV predicts mortality in the post-thrombolytic era

Multiple studies of post-MI patients done subsequent to the MPIP study and the initial studies from St George's Hospital have confirmed the predictive ability of HRV for survival post-MI. Three of the most important such studies are GISSI (Zuanetti *et al.* 1996) and ATRAMI (La Rovere *et al.* 1998). Zuanetti *et al.* (1996) addressed the measurement of HRV in the era of reperfusion. HRV was measured in a subset of post-MI patients who received either streptokinase or tissue-type plasminogen activator (TPA). Five hundred and sixty-seven patients, in sinus rhythm, had 24-h ambulatory ECGs. Median time of recording was 13 days post-MI. Three time domain variables were determined: SDNN, rMSSD, and $NN50^+$ (the number of cycles with a 50 ms or more increase from the preceding cycle). The best cut-off was chosen for each variable, with low HRV groups ranging between 10% and 35% of the population. Other risk variables which were related to survival in the total GISSI population were: sex, age < or ≥ 70 years, previous MI, Killip class, signs of late left ventricular dysfunction, history of diabetes or hypertension, non-Q-MI, PVCs > 10 h, ineligibility for exercise test, beta blocker administration and heart rate were determined in the low and high HRV groups. Low HRV was associated with multiple adverse factors, including: type of MI, female sex, previous MI, signs of failure, rapid heart rate, etc., but even after controlling for these factors, low HRV remained an independent risk variable. In their study the best cut-off was found for $NN50^+$, a short-term measure that assesses parasympathetic modulation. This is in contrast to most other studies that have found longer-term measurements of HRV which include circadian rhythms to be the best predictors of survival (Stein & Kleiger 1999). Thus, the GISSI study confirmed the predictive value of HRV measurement in a reperfused MI population.

Coronary artery bypass surgery (CABG) is the reperfusion therapy of choice in many patients with myocardial ischaemia. Recently, it has become clear that CABG surgery is associated with marked reduced HRV even though post-CABG patients are, if anything at reduced risk of cardiovascular events (Stein *et al.*, 2000). Moreover, this reduction is HRV continues for many months after the surgery. Thus, decreased HRV in post-CABG patients does not have predictive value for mortality.

In ATRAMI (the Autonomic Tone and Reflexes After Myocardial Infarction Investigation) 1284 patients with acute MI occurring less than 28 days before entry had 24-h ambulatory monitoring and phenylephrine derived baroreceptor sensitivity recorded approximately 2 weeks post entry (La Rovere *et al.* 1998). Sixty-three per cent of the patients had received thrombolytic therapy. They were then followed for a mean of 21 months. There were 44 cardiac deaths and five nonfatal cardiac arrests. Both a low SDNN (<70) ms and a low baroreflex sensitivity (BRS) (<3.0) were strongly associated with an adverse outcome with relative risks 3.2 and 2.8, respectively. Although BRS and SDNN were significantly correlated, they were not surrogates for each other. Indeed, 2-year mortality associated with having both a low SDNN and low BRS was 17% vs. only 2% when neither was found. Either a low BRS or low SDNN combined with an ejection fraction (EF) < 35% was associated with an elevated risk ratio of 6.7 for low SDNN and low EF, and 8.7 for low BRS and low EF. Because patients had to survive for at least 2 weeks to be studied, this was a low risk post-MI population. As a result, the positive predictive accuracy of SDNN or BRS alone was low but improved greatly with combined with EF. BRS failed to predict adverse events in patients 65 years old or older, but SDNN was actually a better predictor in this age group compared to younger patients. Both BRS and SDNN were inversely correlated with age, female sex, peak CK and directly correlated with ejection fraction. About 15% of patients were in the lowest BRS or SDNN categories, 35% in the mid levels and 50% in the high BRS and SDNN groups. Although the low SDNN and low BRS groups had a high prevalence of adverse prognostic variables, such as low ejection fraction, high CK levels, and female sex, on multivariate analysis SDNN and BRS remained independent predictors of adverse events.

Tapanainen *et al.* (2002) reported on the results of the Nordic implantable cardioverter-defibrillator pilot study which aimed to assess the predictive power for mortality of HRV and of LVEF post-MI. Follow-up was for up to 2 years in 806 patients of whom 697 had analysable Holter recordings and 49 died. Several time- and frequency-domain variables, including SDNN, were associated with mortality, but upon multivariate analysis, the short-term fractal scaling exponent proved to be the most powerful predictor (relative risk 3.9).

Short-term HRV measurements and risk stratification

Most studies assessing HRV for post-MI risk stratification have utilized 24-h ambulatory ECG data. There is some information about shorter monitoring periods. Fei *et al.* (1996) from the St George's group reported on 700 post-MI patients. They were risk stratified 5–8 days post event with stress testing, late potential measurements, 24-h ambulatory monitoring and left ventricular ejection fraction. The follow-up period was a minimum of 1 year. The endpoint was total cardiac mortality. A short-term HRV measurement, the SDNN of the first 5-min period on the 24-h tape exhibiting sinus rhythm and no ectopics or intervals >20% differ-ent from the first *RR* interval in the sequence, was obtained on 663 of the 700 patients. Long-term HRV was measured by heart rate index, a geometrical variable reflecting long duration heart rate variability. The correlation between HRV index and 5-min SDNN was relatively weak (r = 0.51). In the 1-year follow-up, 45 patients died. Both long- and short-term HRV predicted mortality and remained independent predictors even after controlling for the other risk variables, such as ejection fraction, stress testing, and late potentials. For any sensitivity, long-term HRV had stronger positive predictive accuracy than 5-min SDNN.

Faber *et al.* (1996) extended the study to 729 patients and a 2-year follow-up looking at not only total mortality, but also at arrhythmic death, and arrhythmic death combined with nonfatal malignant ventricular arrhythmias. Again, HRV index predicted adverse outcome better than 5-min SDNN, and the two HRV variables were only modestly correlated with each other. However, a low 5-min SDNN could select a smaller population for whom 24-h analysis for risk stratification was appropriate and in whom there was similar sensitivity and positive predictive accuracy to that derived from the total population.

These results are similar to those in a study by Bigger *et al.* (1993a) from the MPIP population which found that random 5-min time- and frequency-domain HRV measurements correlated well with the same variables calculated over 24 h and also predicted outcome, but not as strongly as the 24-h measures.

Risk stratification using HRV measured long after MI

Ambulatory ECG recordings have generally been performed from 5 to 21 days post event. Bigger *et al.* (1993b) obtained 24-h ambulatory ECGs from 1-year survivors of acute myocardial infarction in the CAPS study. The CAPS population were survivors of acute MI with ≥10 PVCs/h who were then randomized to a variety of antiarrhythmic drugs or placebo. Three hundred and thirty-one patients from the CAPS population had usable 24-h ECGs obtained after drug washout and were not on antiarrhythmic drugs. They had several frequency measures determined including: ULF, LF, and VLF power, total power, the LF/HF ratio, as well as HR. They were then followed for total mortality for a mean of 788 days, with 30 deaths, slightly less than 10%, recorded. The group was predominantly male, and had a depressed mean ejection fraction of 46%. Thirty per cent had congestive heart failure. Patients were dichotomized into low and high HRV groups to maximize the mortality differences. The low HRV groups comprised 10–25% of the total, depending on the HRV variable assessed. There was a strong univariate association between mortality and depressed HRV values. Even after controlling for other adverse factors, depressed ULF and VLF remained significant predictors of mortality. The authors also applied the cut-off points derived from MPIP to this population. Although the low HRV groups using these cut-offs represented only 3–5% of the population, the strong independent association with total mortality was maintained. Thus, the authors concluded that low HRV predicts mortality, even 1-year post event.

Heart rate turbulence and risk stratification post-MI

A technique, which seems particularly promising, is the measurement of heart rate turbulence (HRT), a method developed by Schmidt and coworkers (Schmidt *et al.* 1999; Schmidt 2001). Heart rate turbulence measures the initial acceleration of heart rate following a PVC (turbulence onset) and the subsequent deceleration (turbulence slope). This technique has been applied to at least 3 large studies of post-MI survivors: MPIP, EMIAT (the European Myocardial Infarction Amiodarone Trial), and ATRAMI. In all three studies HRT was a powerful risk stratifier for subsequent adverse cardiac events. This is noteworthy because of the marked differences in the study populations. MPIP was a study of essentially unselected MI survivors under age 70 acquired before recent advances in therapy, such as reperfusion, the use of ASA, ACE inhibitors or generalized beta blocker therapy. ATRAMI looked at a low risk group of post-MI survivors treated in current fashion except for angioplasty or stenting. The EMIAT group on the other hand was a high-risk group of post-MI patients, all with markedly depressed ejection fraction. About 3300 patients in EMIAT were randomized to either amiodarone therapy or placebo. There was no difference in mortality by treatment, but the mode of death in the placebo group was predominantly sudden, and presumably arrhythmic. There were few arrhythmic deaths in the amiodarone group. In a retrospective analysis, amiodarone was significantly associated with both lower arrhythmic death and total mortality in those patients with depressed HRV. This suggests that in this post-MI, low ejection fraction, and low HRV population specific antiarrhythmic therapy could be useful, particularly implantation of an automatic implantable cardioverter defibrillator (AICD).

In both the EMIAT and MIPIP populations, the combination of abnormal turbulence onset (TO) and turbulence slope (TS) was the most powerful multivariate mortality predictor (Ghuran *et al.* 2002). In a multivariate analysis controlling for other significant risk factors, the relative hazard for combined TO and TS was 3.2, with P values <0.0002 for both studies. This combination had a higher hazard ratio than an ejection fraction <30%. Malik *et al.* (2000) retrospectively analysed 912 patients from the ATRAMI study utilizing heart rate turbulence techniques. They constructed ROC curves and in the 30–50% sensitivity range found heart rate turbulence to be the strongest univariate predictor. Combination of heart rate turbulence and with any other risk variable increased the association with mortality. At 40% sensitivity for mortality, the best positive predictive accuracies occurred when TS was combined with either ejection fraction or conventional HRV variables. Prospective studies

changes in autonomic activity (Clarke *et al.* 1976) and that patients with CHF had abnormal heart rate responses. Patients with CHF had been shown to display altered 24-h heart rate behaviour (Casolo *et al.* 1987) and chronotropic incompetence on exercise (Yamabe *et al.* 1987; Colucci *et al.* 1989). Computer processing of HRV offered the possibility of investigating these autonomically mediated abnormalities in detail, providing insight into the relationship between the failing heart and its neurohormonal environment.

Early investigators contrasted the HRV of patients with severe ventricular dysfunction with normal control subjects. In 1988 Saul *et al.* reported a study in which they compared 21 healthy adults with 25 CHF sufferers (NHYA grade III–IV), using 24-h Holter ECG recordings to generate time and frequency domain HRV indices. The CHF group displayed significantly low SDNN values and had significantly reduced power in all frequency domains. Residual frequency-domain power was preserved mainly in the very low frequency region (VLF). These findings were supported by Casolo's group (1989), who, using time-domain indices derived from 24-h ECG recordings, investigated a similar small group of patients with advanced heart failure. Their CHF patients displayed significantly higher mean heart rate and a lower hourly SDNN index (Fig. 13.4). Variability in heart rate was consistently lower throughout the study period, particularly during the night when the control group HRV was at its maximum. Having confirmed that patients with advanced CHF displayed abnormally low HRV, interest was directed to demonstrating the relation of measures of time and frequency analysis of HRV to functional heart failure class and disease status.

Several investigators examined autonomic modulation in different stages of ischaemic cardiomyopathy (Guzetti *et al.* 1995), dilated cardiomyopathy (Fei *et al.* 1996) and CHF of mixed aetiology (Montara *et al.* 1994; Szabo *et al.* 1995). Our research group (Nolan *et al.* 1992; Nolan 1996) demonstrated that time-domain HRV measurements influenced by parasympathetic activity were attenuated in 60% of patients with mild–moderate CHF and that this reduction in HRV was correlated to reduced systolic function (Fig. 13.5). Other investigators

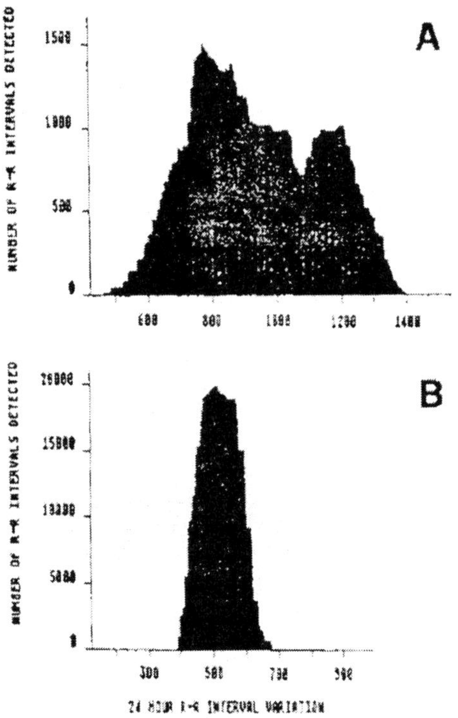

Fig. 13.4 A 24-h *RR* interval histogram in a normal individual (A) and a CHF patient (B). The standard deviation of histogram A (SDNN parameter) is considerably greater than histogram B indicating the presence of important autonomic dysfunction in the CHF patient. (Reproduced from Casolo *et al.* 1989, with permission.)

confirmed these results, demonstrating significant correlations between time-domain measurements of HRV and left ventricular dimensions (Gang Yi *et al.* 1997; Moore *et al.* 2002), left ventricular ejection fraction (Fauchier *et al.* 1997) and right heart function (Lucreziotti *et al.* 2000). Each of the clinical indices deteriorated as time-domain measures of HRV declined. Frequency-domain changes display a more intricate relationship to deteriorating cardiac function. In the early phases of disease low frequency power is exaggerated and high frequency power reduced, consistent with a shift to sympathetic dominance. As the severity of disease increases, both LF and HF power decline, leaving most of the HRV power in the VLF domain. Clearly the heightened sympathetic activity seen in patients with advanced heart failure is not captured by this type of HRV analy-

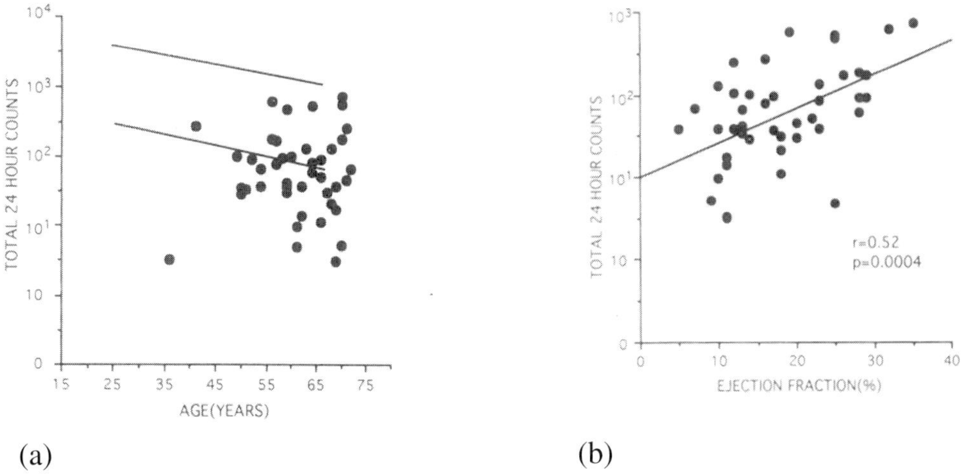

Fig. 13.5 Time-domain HRV in patients with CHF plotted against (a) age with solid lines representing 95% confidence intervals for normal subjects. 60% of the CHF patients fall below the 95% tolerance limit and thus have a significant reduction in HRV. Time-domain HRV in patients with CHF plotted against (b) ejection fraction, showing linear relationship between HRV and systolic function. (Reproduced from Nolan *et al.* 1992, with permission.)

sis. The reason for this dissociation between sympathetic drive and HRV in advanced CHF has been explored by studies that attempt to correlate spectral HRV and direct measurements of sympathetic activity.

A direct estimation of cardiac sympathetic activity can be obtained by assaying cardiac noradrenaline (NA) spillover, which is an index of sympathetic nerve firing rate and electrochemical coupling. This technique (requiring right heart catheterization and therefore unsuitable for large-scale determination of cardiac sympathetic activity) has been compared to HRV analysis. In an early study, Kingwell *et al.* (1994) investigated the relationship in 15 patients with advanced CHF. They failed to find any significant correlation between any of the HRV indices (including absolute LF spectral power) and cardiac NA release.

The lack of a direct relationship between the two methods of assessing sympathetic activity in this early study is due in part to the differing physiological processes that influence each technique. HRV reflects the sinus node reaction to sympatho-vagal balance, relying not only on the sympathetic nerve firing rates and electrochemical coupling which influence cardiac NA spillover, but also on cardiac adrenergic receptor sensitivity and postsynaptic signal transduction. The failing heart exhibits long term unopposed sympathetic sinoatrial node stimulation, impairing the responsiveness of the pacemaker cells to further sympathetic activity via down regulation and 'uncoupling' of adrenergic receptors (Fowler *et al.* 1986; Bristow *et al.* 1989). Thus as ventricular function deteriorates the cardiac pacemaker becomes less sensitive to increasing sympathetic activation and HRV is paradoxically suppressed (Cohn *et al.* 1984). This blunting of HRV has also been observed in exercise-induced sympathetic overdrive (Perini *et al.* 1990).

Tygesen *et al.* (2001) addressed some of these confounding factors in a recent study comparing NA spillover to heart variability during orthostatic stress in 15 patients suffering from mild to moderate CHF. Tygesen's group demonstrated a strong correlation between LF/HF ratio in the standing position and NA spillover ($r = 0.81$, $P = 0.0003$). They failed to demonstrate any relationship between catecholamine release and HRV indices during supine rest, consistent with the findings of Kingwell's group. Their use of a patient group with less advanced heart failure reduces the probability of selecting subjects with impaired pacemaker responsiveness, whilst the use of posturally mediated sympathetic stimulation and the LF/HF ratio diminished any potential parasympathetic contamination. These factors may explain the correlation between LF/HF ratio and NA spillover in the upright position.

Taken together, this body of data confirms that HRV is impaired in CHF, with the maximum reduction occurring in patients with severe symptoms and major ventricular dysfunction. Time-domain measurements decline in a linear fashion, while frequency domain measurements show a more complex relationship to disease severity (reflecting both autonomic and sinus node receptor dysfunction).

Various pharmaceutical agents, which have been shown to improve clinical parameters in CHF, have been investigated for their influence on HRV markers. Studies have shown a partial improvement in suppressed HRV parameters following the prescription of beta blockers (Pousset *et al.* 1992, Montara *et al.* 2000; Piccirillo *et al.* 2000; Ridha *et al.* 2002; Jansson *et al.* 1999), digoxin (Brouwer *et al.* 1995) and ACE inhibitors (Flapan *et al.* 1992; Zhang *et al.* 1995) (Fig. 13.6). This suggests that at least some of the prognostic benefit of these agents is achieved by favourable modulation of the adverse neurohumoral environment present in CHF patients.

Poincaré plots

Information on Poincaré plots in CHF is more limited. Woo *et al.* (1992) used Holter electrocardiograph recordings to retrospectively generate Poincaré plots in 24 advanced heart failure

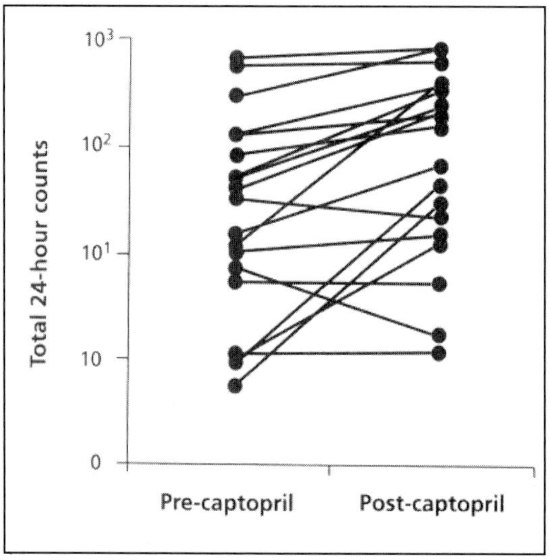

Fig. 13.6 Time-domain HRV in patients with CHF before and after the introduction of captopril, showing ACE inhibitor-mediated improvement in autonomic function. (Reproduced from Flapan *et al.* 1992, with permission.)

patients and compared the results with normal controls. The plots of the CHF patients differed markedly from the control subjects. In the control group variability decreased as heart rate rose creating a consistent 'comet' appearance. CHF patients displayed three differing patterns. One group demonstrated globally reduced variability through a marginally reduced range of heart rates producing a 'torpedo' pattern. Other patients showed a more drastic reduction in breadth of heart rate with exaggerated beat-to-beat variation producing a 'triangle' or 'fan' shaped pattern (Fig. 13.7). It was proposed that the torpedo group may represent patients whose neurohormonal state may be closer to the normal control group than the other distributions. The main limitation with this method of evaluating HRV is that it requires subjective interpretation of the plots rather than offering a straightforward quantitative measure of variability.

HRV as a prognostic indicator

HRV and mortality

Since other measures of autonomic dysfunction (such as plasma catecholamines) are related to an adverse outcome in CHF, HRV evaluation has a potential role in prognostic assessment. The ability of HRV to risk stratify CHF patients was initially evaluated in a series of small studies in patients with advanced cardiac failure. Binder *et al.* (1992) investigated the prognostic value of HRV in patients with severe and advanced CHF. Binder's group generated HRV indices using 24-h tapes and examined their ability to predict outcome in 92 patients awaiting heart transplantation. Both time and frequency domain parameters predicted cardiac death with low values of time-domain HRV being associated with a 20-fold increase in mortality risk. Montara & Tavassi (1996) examined spectral indices generated from 30 min ECG recordings in a similar patient group and observed an association between LF power, worsening clinical status and all cause mortality. It is therefore evident that in advanced cardiac failure HRV indices are univariate predictors of all cause mortality. None of these early trials subjected the HRV variables to multivariate regression to establish whether their predictive value was independent of other

Fauchier, L., Babuty, D., Cosnay, P., Autret, M.L. & Fauchier, J.P. (1997) Heart rate variability in idiopathic dilated cardiomyopathy: characteristics and prognostic value. *Journal of the American College of Cardiology*, **4**, 1009–1014.

Fei, L., Keeling, P.J., Saddoul, N. *et al.* (1996) Decreased heart rate variability in patients with congestive heart failure and chronotropic incompetence. *PACE (Pacing and Clinical Electrophysiology)*, **19**, 477–483.

Flapan, A., Nolan, J., Neilson, J. & Ewing, D. (1992) Effect of captopril on cardiac parasympathetic activity in chronic cardiac failure secondary to coronary heart disease. *American Journal of Cardiology*, **69**, 532–535.

Fowler, M.B., Laser, J.A., Hopkins, J.L. *et al.* (1986) Assessment of beta-adrenergic receptor pathway in the intact failing human heart. *Circulation*, **74**, 1290.

Guzzetti, S., Cogliati, C., Turiel, M. *et al.* (1995) Sympathetic predominance followed by functional denervation in the progression of chronic heart failure. *European Heart Journal*, **16**, 1100–1107.

Horner, S.M., Murphy, C.F., Coen, B. *et al.* (1996) Contribution to heart rate variability by mechanoelectrical feedback. Stretch of the sinus node reduces heart rate variability. *Circulation*, **94**, 1726–1767.

Huikuri, H.Y., Makaillio, T.H., Peng, C.K., Goldberger, A.L., Huize, U. & Moller, M. for the DIAMOND Study Group. (2000) Fractal correlation properties or *RR* interval dynamics and mortality in patients with depressed left ventricular function after acute myocardial infarction. *Circulation*, **101**, 47–54.

Jansson, K., Hageman, I., Ostlund, R. *et al.* (1999) The effects of metoprolol and captopril on heart rate variability in patients with idiopathic dilated cardiomyopathy. *Clinical Cardiology*, **22**, 397–402.

Jiang, W., Hathaway, W.R., McNulty, S. *et al.* (1997) Ability of heart rate variability to predict prognosis in patients with advanced congestive heart failure. *American Journal of Cardiology*, **80**, 808–811.

Kearney, M.T., Fox, K.A., Lee, A.J. *et al.* (2002) Predicting death to progressive heart failure in patients with mild to moderate chronic heart failure. *Journal of the American College of Cardiology*, **40**, 1801–1808.

Kingwell, B.A., Thompson, J.M., Kaye, D.M., McPherson, G.A., Jennings, G.L. & Esler, M.D. (1994) Heart rate spectral analysis, cardiac norepinephrine spillover and muscle sympathetic nerve activity during human sympathetic nervous activation and failure. *Circulation*, **90**, 234–240.

Lanza, G.A., Guido, V., Galeazzi, M.M. *et al.* (1998) Prognostic role of heart rate variability with a recent acute myocardial infarction. *American Journal of Cardiology*, **82**, 1323–1328.

Leimbach, W.N., Jr, Wallin, B.G., Victor, R.G. *et al.* (1986) Direct evidence from intraneural recordings for increased central sympathetic outflow in patients with heart failure. *Circulation*, **73**, 913–919.

Lubbe, W.F., Poduzuweit, T. & Opie, L. (1992) Potential arrhythmogenic role of cyclic adenosine monophosphate (AMP) and systolic calcium overload: Implications for prophylactic effects of beta blockers in myocardial infarction and proarrhythmic effects of phosphodiesterase inhibitors. *Journal of the American College of Cardiology*, **19**, 1622–1633.

Lucreziotti, S., Gavazzi, A., Scelsi, L. *et al.* (2000) Five min recordings of heart rate variability in severe chronic heart failure: correlates with right ventricular function and prognostic implications. *American Heart Journal*, **139**, 1088–1095.

Makikallio, T.H., Hoiber, S., Kober, L. *et al.* & the TRACE Investigators. (1999) Fractal analysis of heart rate dynamics in patients with depressed left ventricular function after acute myocardial infarction. *American Journal of Cardiology*, **83**, 836–839.

Mann, D.L. (1999). Mechanisms and models in heart failure: a combinatorial approach. *Circulation*, **100**, 999–1008.

Moore, R.K.G., Groves, D., Kearney, M.T. *et al.* UK HEART Study. (2002) Univariate analysis of frequency domain HRV indices as predictors of mortality in chronic heart failure; 5-year results of the UK HEART Study. *European Heart Journal*, **23** (Abstract Suppl.), 645.

Mortara, A., La Rovere, M.T., Pinna, G.D., Maestri, R., Capomolla, S. & Cobelli, F. (2000) Nonselective beta-adrenergic blocking agent carvedilol, improves arterial baroreflex gain and heart rate variability in patients with stable chronic heart failure. *Journal of the American College of Cardiology*, **36**, 1612–1618.

Mortara, A., La Rovere, M.T., Signorini, M.G. *et al.* (1994) Can power spectrum analysis of heart rate variability identify a high risk subgroup of congestive heart failure patients with excessive sympathetic activation? A pilot study before and after heart transplantation. *British Heart Journal*, **71**, 422–430.

Mortara, A. & Tavassi, L. (1996) Prognostic implications of the autonomic nervous system analysis in chronic heart failure: role of heart rate variability and baroreflex sensitivity. *Archives of Gerontology and Geriatrics*, **23**, 265–275.

Nolan, J. (1996) *Studies of a parasympathetic nervous system in chronic heart failure.* MD thesis, University of Leeds.

Nolan, J., Batin, P.D., Fox, A.A. *et al.* (1998) Prospective study of heart rate variability and mortality in chronic heart failure. *Circulation*, **98**, 1510–1516.

Nolan, J., Flapan, A.D., Capewell, S., MacDonald, T., Nielson, J.M.M. & Ewing, D.J. (1992) Decreased cardiac parasympathetic activity in chronic heart failure and its relation to left ventricular function. *British Heart Journal*, **67**, 482–486.

Nolan, J., Flapan, A.D., Goodfield, N.E. *et al.* (1996) Measurement of parasympathetic activity from 24 h ambulatory electrocardiograms and its reproducibility and sensitivity in normal subjects, patients with symptomatic myocardial ischaemia and patients with diabetes mellitus. *American Journal of Cardiology*, **77**, 154–158.

Perini, R., Orizio, C., Baselli, G., Cerutti, S. & Veicsteinas, A. (1990) The influence of exercise intensity on the power spectrum of heart rate variability. *European Journal of Applied Physiology*, **61**, 143–148.

Piccirillo, G., Luparini, R.L., Celli, V. *et al.* (2000) Effects of carvedilol on heart rate and blood pressure in subjects with chronic heart failure. *American Journal of Cardiology*, **86**, 1392–1395.

Ponikowski, P., Anker, S.D., Chua, P.D. *et al.* (1997) Depressed heart rate variability as an independent predictor of death in chronic congestive heart failure secondary to ischaemic or idiopathic dilated cardiomyopathy. *American Journal of Cardiology*, **79**, 1645–1650.

Porter, T.R., Eckberg, D.L., Fritsch, J.M. *et al.* (1990) Autonomic pathophysiology in heart failure patients: sympathetic–cholinergic interrelations. *Journal of Clinical Investigation*, **85**, 1362–1371.

Pousset, F., Copie, X., Lechat, P. *et al.* (1996) Effects of bisoprolol on heart rate variability in heart failure. *American Journal of Cardiology*, **77**, 612–617.

Pumprla, J., Howorka, K., Groves, D., Chester, M. & Nolan, J. (2002) Functional assessment of heart rate variability: physiological basis and practical applications. *International Journal of Cardiology*, **84**, 1–14.

Reid, I.A. (1992) Interactions between ANG II, sympathetic nervous system, and baroreceptor reflexes in regulation of blood pressure. *American Journal of Physiology*, **262**, E763–E778.

Ridha, M., Makikallio, T.H., Lopera, G. *et al.* (2002) Effects of carvedilol on heart rate dynamics in patients with congestive heart failure. *Annals of Noninvasive Electrocardiology*, **7**, 133–138.

Rundqvist, B., Elam, M., Bergmann-Sverrisdottir, Y. *et al.* (1997) Increased cardiac adrenergic drive precedes generalised sympathetic activation in human heart failure. *Circulation*, **95**, 169–175.

Saul, J.P., Arai, Y., Berger, R.D., Lilly, L.S., Colucci, W.S. & Cohen, R.J. (1988) Assessment of autonomic regulation in chronic congestive heart failure by heart rate spectral analysis. *American Journal of Cardiology*, **61**, 1292–1299.

Szabo, B.M., van Veldhuisen, D.J., Brouwer, J., Haaksma, J. & Lie, K.I. (1995) Relation between severity of disease and impairment of heart rate variability parameters in patients with chronic congestive heart failure secondary to coronary disease. *American Journal of Cardiology*, **76**, 713–716.

Tan, L.B., Jalil, J.E., Pick, R., Janicki, J.S. & Weber, K.T. (1991) Cardiac myocyte necrosis induced by angiotensin II. *Circulation Research*, **69**, 1185–1195.

Tygesen, H., Rundqvist, B., Waagstein, F. & Wennerbohm, B. (2001) Heart rate variability measurement correlates with cardiac noradrenaline spillover in congestive heart failure. *American Journal of Cardiology*, **87**, 1308–1311.

Wijbenga, J.A.M., Balk, H.M.M., Meij, S.H., Simoons, M.L. & Malik, M. (1998) Heart rate variability in congestive heart failure: relationship to clinical variables and prognosis. *European Heart Journal*, **19**, 1719–1724.

Woo, M.A., Stevenson, W.G., Moser, D.K. *et al.* (1992) Patterns of beat-to-beat heart rate variability in advanced heart failure. *American Heart Journal*, **123**, 704–710.

Yamabe, H., Kobayashi, K. & Takata, T. (1987) Reduced chronotropic reserve to the metabolic requirement during exercise in advanced heart failure with old myocardial infarction. *Japanese Circulation Journal*, **51**, 259–264.

Yi, G., Goldman, J.H., Keeling, P.J., Reardon, M., McKenna, W.J. & Malik, M. (1997) Heart rate variability in idiopathic dilated cardiomyopathy: relation to disease severity and prognosis. *Heart*, **77**, 108–114.

Zhang, Y., Song, Y., Zhu, J., Hu, T. & Wan, L. (1995) Effects of enalapril on heart rate variability in patients with congestive heart failure. *American Journal of Cardiology*, **76**, 1045–1048.

CHAPTER 14

Heart Rate Variability in Diabetes and Neuropathies

Ernest L. Fallen

Introduction

Table 14.1 is an abbreviated list of clinical entities for which abnormal heart rate variability (HRV) has been reported. This hodgepodge of seemingly unrelated conditions raises several questions. Do they all qualify as neuropathies? Is HRV so convenient a noninvasive measurement that, as with Pirandello's six characters, it is forever in search of clinical 'authors' to justify its easy applicability? Or, because the heart affords an accessible neuroefferent window through which many autonomic processes can be examined, may we assume that HRV is less a surrogate marker than a true measure of autonomic function? In other words can the measurements of HRV be used convincingly to study the nature, extent, prognosis and clinical course of the autonomic neuropathies? The fact that autonomic neuropathy, once clinically manifest, confers a rather poor prognosis, these questions are not without clinical relevance. The aim of this chapter is to provide a clinical perspective on the utility of HRV as a noninvasive measure of cardiac autonomic function in diabetes mellitus and selective neuropathies. The major portion of the chapter focuses on diabetic autonomic neuropathy.

Diabetic autonomic neuropathy (DAN)

General comments

Few biological systems can escape the widespread integrated control of the autonomic nervous system. It is not surprising therefore that the clinical manifestations of DAN are so ubiquitous (Spallone *et al.* 1995). Among the cardiovascular features are: persistent tachycardia, obliteration of the normal diurnal variation in both blood pressure and heart rate, postural hypotension, and silent myocardial ischaemia. Among the myriad noncardiac manifestations are reactive bronchoconstriction, gastroparesis, sudomotor dysfunction, impotence and urinary bladder dysfunction to name a few. It is even postulated that the more common diabetic complications of nephropathy, retinopathy and vasculopathy may share a neuropathic pathogenesis (Winocour *et al.* 1986; Krolewski *et al.* 1992).

Autonomic neuropathy is prevalent in up to 40% of patients with insulin-dependent diabetes (Ewing *et al.* 1985). What is worrisome is the dreadful prognosis once clinical manifestations of autonomic impairment appear (Fig. 14.1). The cumulative 5-year mortality rate from the time of clinical diagnosis ranges from 23% to 56% (Ewing *et al.* 1980; O'Brien *et al.* 1991; Spallone & Menzinger 1997). Moreover, DAN is a predictor of adverse outcome independent of renal or vascular complications (O'Brien *et al.* 1991). On a more optimistic note, irreversible structural changes vis-à-vis axonal degeneration or demyelination probably do not occur *de novo* but are preceded by functional/metabolic alterations in neurophysiological performance (Pfeifer and Schumer 1994). We may assume that it is during this so-called functional phase that reversibility of the neuropathic process is feasible. Hence, a search for noninvasive tests capable of detecting preclinical evidence of DAN are laudable despite the evidence, so far, that specific treatment to reverse the neuropathy is lacking.

Noninvasive testing

The literature is replete with different applications and formulations of HRV in the detection of DAN. Basically, there are three separate but complementary approaches:

1 the standardized bedside battery of reflexogenic tests;

2 frequency and nonlinear domains of HRV;

3 tests of arterial baroreceptor sensitivity.

Regardless of which test is used, each approach has demonstrated impairment of autonomic function in patients with clinical signs suggestive of DAN (Ewing *et al.* 1985; Pagani *et al.* 1988; Malpas & Maling 1990; Bernardi, 2000; Bellavere *et al.* 1992). The critical questions are: (a) Can any one test or a combination of approaches reliably identify pre-clinical signs of autonomic dysfunction? (b) How do they perform and compare with respect to sensitivity, specificity and predictive accuracy? (c) Can they discriminate between sympathetic and/or parasympathetic involvement? If so, does it matter? (d) How predictive are they of clinical outcome?

Table 14.1 List of clinical entities with abnormal heart rate variability

Diabetes mellitus	Alzheimer's disease
Uraemia	Cluster headaches
Alcoholism	Multiple sclerosis
Guillain–Barre syndrome	Cerebrovascular attack
Focal hyperhydrosis	Narcolepsy
Systemic sclerosis	Irritable bowel syndrome
Growth hormone deficiency	Behçet's disease
Familial amyloidosis	Lupus erythematosis
Secondary amyloidosis	Epilepsy
Sjögren's syndrome	Botulism
Muscular dystrophy	Pre-eclampsia
Parkinson's disease	Obesity
Fibromyalgia	Acute intermittent porphyria
Hyperthyroidism	Asthma
Hypothyroidism	Leprosy
Hypoxaemic chronic obstructive pulmonary disease	Functional dyspepsia
Chagas' disease	

Reflexogenic tests

The Ewing battery of tests comprises five bedside manoeuvres each requiring the active participation of the subject (Ewing *et al.* 1985). These include three tests of heart rate responses said to reflect parasympathetic activity. They are: (1) the Valsalva manoeuvre where one computes the ratio of the longest *RR* interval following the release phase to the shortest *RR* interval during the strain phase; (2) the heart rate response to orthostatic stress is measured as the ratio of the longest *RR* interval at the 30th beat to the *RR* interval of the 15th beat after standing erect from a supine position; and (3) the maximum and minimum heart rate is determined during deep breathing for 6 min. The index measurement is taken as the mean of the differences during three successive breathing cycles. The two tests of blood pressure (*BP*) responses are, more or less, examples of sympathetic activity. They are: (4) The difference in peak systolic *BP* between standing and supine states, a measure of orthostatic hypotension; and (5) The diastolic *BP* just before release of sustained handgrip for five min at 30% maximum squeeze is compared to the resting pre-grip diastolic *BP*. When applied

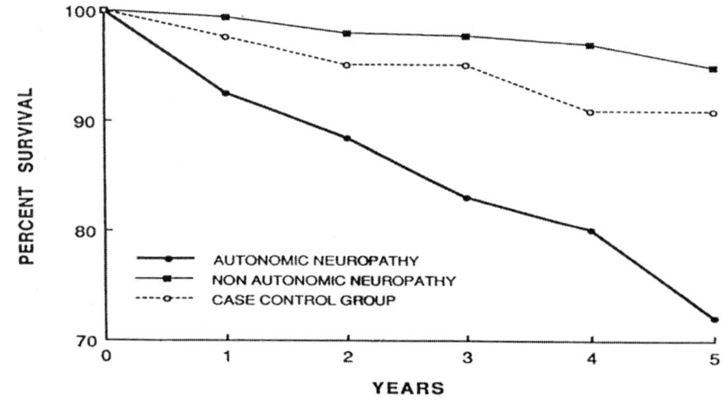

Fig. 14.1 Survival in diabetic patients with and without autonomic neuropathy. (From O'Brien *et al.* 1991, with permission.)

to diabetic patients this battery of tests has proven to be reproducible and prognostic (Ewing 1985). It has earned the distinction of being the standard against which other noninvasive tests have been validated. Among the battery's disadvantages are: reliance on patient participation, questionable inferences regarding pathophysiological mechanisms and a requirement for all five tests to be performed because individual components lack independent prognostic power. None the less, this bedside approach has been well standardized, has stood the test of time and remains useful as a determinant of both severity and prognosis. Whether it can reliably identify the early pre-clinical phases of functional (potentially reversible) autonomic neuropathy is debatable.

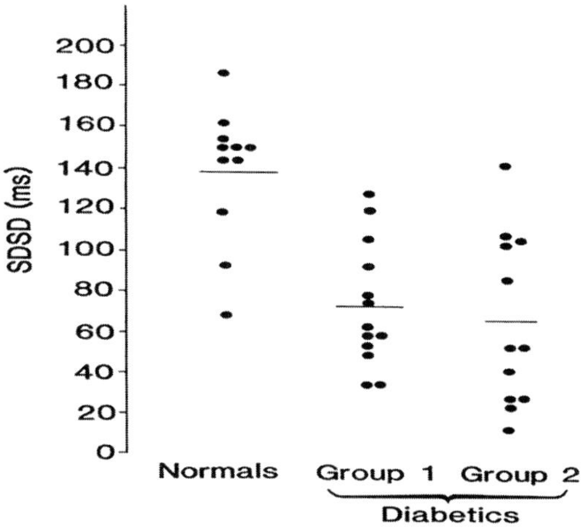

Fig. 14.2 Individual mean heart rate variability (SD) values in three groups for 24 h. Normal, nondiabetic subjects; group 1, diabetic subjects without vagal neuropathy; group 2, diabetic subjects with vagal neuropathy. Groups 1 and 2 were significantly different from normal subjects. (From Malpas & Maling 1990, with permission.)

Tests of heart rate variability

Time-domain statistics

Both descriptive (e.g. SDNN) and differencing (e.g. rMSSD, pNN50) statistics derived from 24-h successive *RR* intervals enjoy the advantages of robustness, reproducibility, proven prognostic power, applicability to ambulatory states, ability to assess diurnal variations and simplicity of use. Their major disadvantages are the temptation to ascribe pathophysiological meaning to the data and their sensitivity to cofactors such as age, gender, drugs and comorbid states.

When applied to patients with DAN, studies using time-domain HRV have consistently reported significant decreases in *RR* variability whether measured as 24-h SDNN or any of the differencing methods (Malpas & Maling 1990; Ewing 1992; Ziegler *et al.* 2001). In many studies the standardized reflexogenic tests were used as the gold standard. In other words the patients selected were already demonstrating clinical signs of autonomic dysfunction. With respect to sensitivity, Malpas & Maling (1990) measured the SDNN over 24 h in 25 insulin-dependent diabetic subjects and 11 age-matched controls. They found the SDNN to be significantly reduced in 13 of the diabetic patients whose 'vagal' indices, according to the Ewing protocol, were considered normal (Fig. 14.2). In an interesting experiment, Mølgaard *et al.* (1992) described a linear inverse correlation between HRV computed from 24-h successive *RR* intervals and urinary albumin excretion in diabetics with varying degrees of nephropathy. This lends credence to the hypothesis that HRV is less a surrogate marker than a quantifiable measure of neurocardiac regulation in DAN. Moreover, the reduced HRV (based on a differencing technique) was present in 33% of their diabetic patients deemed normal by conventional bedside tests, a clear indication of the heightened sensitivity of HRV.

These studies while intriguing are based on small sample sizes ranging from 20 to 50 patients per study. It follows that large scale prospective studies using time domain methods to identify pre-clinical cases of DAN, functional or otherwise, are sorely needed.

Power spectral analysis (PSA)

The autonomic neuropathy associated with diabetes may involve either or both limbs of the autonomic nervous system (Spallone & Menzinger 1997; Pagani 2000). Moreover, functional or structural changes need not evolve simultaneously but rather sequentially with parasympathetic impairment usually manifest before detectable sympathetic involvement. The power density spectrum of successive *RR* intervals captures the dynamics of vagal and sympathetic

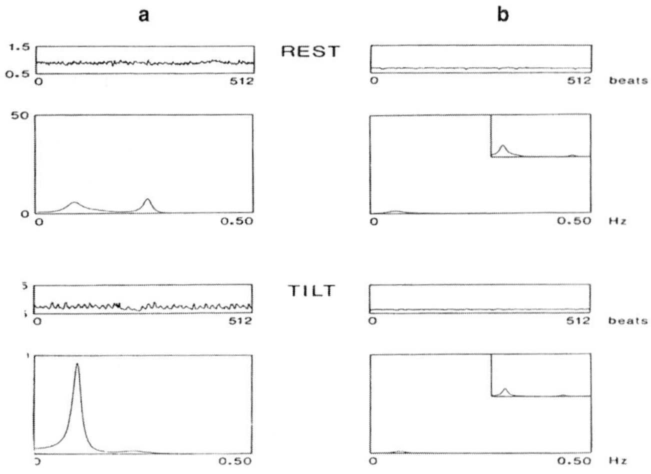

Fig. 14.3 Representative examples of *RR* variability and power spectra in a diabetic patient with no signs of autonomic neuropathy (left panels, a) and in a patient with signs of neuropathy (right panels, b). Note the increase in the low frequency component with tilt only in the patient without neuropathy. The spectra of the patient with neuropathy show very low power, magnified ×10 in the inserts.

efferent modulation of sinus node activity (Akselrod *et al.* 1981; Malliani *et al.* 1991; Kamath & Fallen1993). Its ability to differentiate between vagal and sympathetic modulation of sinus node activity makes it at least faithful in providing a measure of sympatho-vagal balance (Pagani *et al.* 1986) Its disadvantages are the requirement for steady-state recording conditions, a comparatively low power contained within the spectral bands of interest and a low signal-to-noise ratio especially under quiescent supine states in conditions such as heart failure and diabetes where overall HRV is significantly reduced. To amplify the deterministic signals some investigators study their subjects under different controlled conditions such as tilt (Pagani *et al.* 1988; Freeman *et al.* 1991). When orthostatic stress is applied to diabetic patients there is often a failure of the LF (HRV) power to increase indicating a fundamental abnormality in neuroeffector control presumably owing to a defect in arterial baroreceptor function (Fig. 14.3).

Again, as with time-domain methods, most studies using PSA have simply validated the technique against the standardized tests in patients who already exhibit some clinical manifestation of DAN (Bianchi *et al.* 1990; Freeman *et al.* 1991; Ziegler *et al.* 2001; Takase *et al.* 2002). None the less, PSA has proven useful in teasing out some interesting characteristics of the pathophysiology of DAN. In general, the LF and HF power are both depressed with a net decrease in the LF:HF ratio. In terms of early detection, Ziegler *et al.* (2001) computed the cross correlation between *HR* and *BP* spectral components and showed an abnormal variance in some diabetic patients without clinical evidence of autonomic neuropathy. Using autoregressive PSA in 53 insulin-dependent diabetic patients and 20 controls, Belavere *et al.* (1992) showed spectral analysis of HRV not only discriminated the severity of DAN based on conventional tests but demonstrated that parasympathetic and sympathetic abnormalities seem to arise simultaneously. Although these observations require validation there is little doubt that PSA provides more insight than conventional tests into the pathophysiological mechanisms that underlie the neuropathic process in diabetes.

Thus, it is now acknowledged that before any perceptible changes in standard cardiovascular tests, abnormalities in power spectral indices are already present in DAN (Pagani 2000). In other words, alterations in Ewing's battery of tests are apparent only when moderate to severe alterations in spectral parameters have already occurred. Vagal related changes seem to appear earlier than sympathetic-related PSA changes. DAN is also characterized by a flattening of the circadian pattern of LF:HF ratio in so far as the normal night-time increase in HRV is attenuated. (Spallone *et al.* 1993; Takase *et al.* 2002).

Other HRV parameters

Using cross-correlation techniques between *HR* and respiratory waveforms, Bernardi *et al.* showed significant distortion in the linkage in patients with DAN (Bernardi *et al.* 1989). Speaking of biophysical linkages in dynamical systems, Mukkamala *et al.* applied a novel approach called 'cardiovascular system identification' to characterize closed loop regulation in patients with DAN (Mukkamula *et al.* 1999). They measured beat to beat fluctuations in *HR*, *BP* and instantaneous lung volume (*ILV*). Of the four physiological coupling mechanisms they found that the autonomically coupled ones (i.e. the *HR*-baroreflex and *HR-ILV*) were inversely correlated with severity of DAN based on standard tests. Conversely, the mechanically mediated couplings (e.g. respiration-*BP*) bore no correlation with autonomic severity. The potential advantage of this approach is its quantitative ability to track the pathophysiological changes that accompany the progression of DAN.

Nonlinear methods, such as fractal dimensions and approximate entropy, may help determine the ability of a complex biological system to adapt to external stress. In this respect, patients with DAN behave similarly to aged subjects in that several nonlinear tests show reduced complexity (Chau *et al.* 1993; Ducher *et al.* 1999; Ziegler *et al.* 2001). Since nonlinear indices correlate weakly with time or frequency HRV, the alterations in fractal dimensions in DAN may shed new light on its pathophysiology.

Arterial baroreceptor sensitivity

The slope of the baroreceptor sensitivity loop is significantly reduced in diabetics even without overt signs of neuropathy (McDowell *et al.* 1994; Bernardi 2000). It is postulated therefore that arterial baroreceptor dysfunction may occur at a functional state of DAN before structural changes occur. This approach has several advantages including the ability to analyse and differentiate both cardiac and vascular responses to changes in vagoafferent drive from the carotid sinus. It is sensitive, reproducible under steady-state conditions and prognostic. The shift towards a more flattened slope in DAN suggests either reduced vagoafferent signalling or impaired central control although the reflex embodies many integrative circuits and influences that render precise discrimination difficult.

Follow-up

Prospective studies on the utility of HRV as a tracking method for patients with DAN have been sparse. Gerritson *et al.* (2001) followed 605 patients (ages 50–75 years), stratified according to glucose tolerance indices, for 9 years. No less than seven parameters of autonomic function were employed including one of Ewing's test manoeuvres, five HRV parameters and baroreceptor sensitivity. Forty-three patients died of cardiovascular causes. Of interest, the autonomic function parameters were associated with both all-cause and cardiovascular death even after adjustment were made for age, gender, glucose tolerance and antihypertensive medication. Moreover, in patients with diabetes there was double the mortality risk for those with low HRV scores. More studies like these are needed to evaluate the utility of HRV tests for screening, for prognosis and for determining response to therapeutic interventions.

Regardless of the technique used there are a host of confounders that ought to be acknowledged before applying any HRV method to a group of diabetic patients (Spallone & Menzinger 1997). These include age and gender dependency, sensitivity to respiratory variation, essential hypertension, coronary artery disease, alcohol, diet, physical exercise and a host of drugs. Comparisons between tests may have limited value since there is no gold standard for the diagnosis of DAN and individual tests may succeed in identifying different characteristics of DAN. Until such time as a bona fide gold standard test encompassing all aspects of DAN emerges it is probably wise to view the above approaches as complementary at best.

To summarize, an array of noninvasive tests are available for the detection and assessment of severity and prognosis of autonomic neuropathy in patients with diabetes. It remains to be determined if they can be relied on to detect the early, potentially reversible, preclinical or functional status of autonomic dysregulation. In this regard HRV using both time and frequency domain parameters have been shown to detect autonomic abnormalities before their identification by standard bedside reflexogenic tests. It is too early to state with certainty whether nonlinear methods will provide incremental value to the aforementioned tests. To date, no therapeutic intervention has been shown to reverse the neuropathy although the ACE inhibitor quinipril shows promise by restoring circadian HF and

LF:HF ratio in DAN patients after one year of treatment (Athyros *et al.* 1998). This may not be surprising for a class of drugs with proven benefit in diabetic patients with cardiovascular complications. The jury is still out on the effectiveness of aldose reductase inhibitors on nerve conduction in diabetes while the salutary effect of tight blood glucose control on the progression of retinopathy and nephropathy may have similar positive effects in patients with DAN. Future studies using HRV methods should begin to focus on clinical outcomes and pathophysiological correlates in the context of large scale prospective population based studies. Standardization is an issue but there already exists useful guidelines for HRV (ESC/NASPE Task Force 1996) and conventional testing (Ewing *et al.* 1985).

Other neuropathies

One would be hard pressed to ascribe a neuropathic process to each and every entity listed in Table 14.1. Just as the slope of the baroreceptor curve is exquisitely sensitive to small perturbations so is the short-term power spectral indices of HRV. Thus autonomic neuropathy should not be defined simply by evanescent changes in HRV any more than a reduced left ventricular ejection fraction be the definition of a dilated congestive cardiomyopathy. To illustrate this point, both hypothyroidism and hyperthyroidism seem to share the same directional changes in HRV, namely an elevated LF:HF ratio (Cacciatori *et al.* 2000). Are they both hyperadrenergic states? Others have gone to some lengths to refute autonomic involvement in entities such as Sjögren's syndrome (Niemela *et al.* 2000). An overdue publication of a negative study? Why the confusion? And why should all of these conditions be affecting cardiac autonomic regulation unless it is part of a widespread neuropathic phenomenon? It is important to bear in mind that HRV indices often reflect physiological changes that are evanescent and sensitive to external perturbations even under so-called steady-state conditions. Therefore it should not be inferred that a departure from normal values in age-matched populations necessarily implies an underlying neuropathy. This is important to bear in mind because established autonomic neuropathy is a serious condition carrying a poor prognosis.

Of the entities on the list (Table 14.1) at least three have earned the distinction of being associated with true neuropathy. They are (1) Chagas' disease where a distinct pathologic involvement of peripheral vagal nerve fibres is well known (Mott and Hagstrom 1965); (2) Uraemia due to chronic renal disease; and (3) Alcoholic and non-alcoholic liver cirrhosis especially in advanced stages.

Chagas' disease

Guzzetti *et al.* evaluated the power spectrum of HRV at rest, standing and following handgrip in three groups of Chagasic subjects; controls, those with ECG evidence of cardiac involvement and those with positive serology only (Guzzetti *et al.* 1991). They found that the failure to increase LF power on standing occurred in both the preclinical and clinical groups positive for Chagas' disease. While these results indicate an impairment in sympathetic response others have shown defects primarily in vagal activity (Marin-Neto *et al.* 1986).

Uraemia

Patients with chronic renal failure have a high prevalence of autonomic dysfunction. Regardless of the autonomic test used it is estimated that over 60% of chronic uraemic patients will develop some abnormality of HRV. For instance in one report there was a 40% incidence of impaired parasympathetic responses among 30 chronic uraemic patients on periodic haemodialysis and a 13% incidence of combined parasympathetic and sympathetic involvement (Vita *et al.* 1999). Galetta *et al.* confirmed the low HRV in their chronic uraemic patients. They also demonstrated that high ultrafiltration haemodialysis exacerbated the abnormal HRV indices whereas low rates of ultrafiltration restored the indices, an example of the sensitivity of HRV to the physiological perturbation of volume depletion (Galetta *et al.* 2001).

Liver cirrhosis

Autonomic dysfunction, especially along vagal nerve pathways, has been reported in patients with both alcoholic and non-alcoholic cirrhosis (Lazzeri *et al.* 1997; Rangari *et al.* 2002). The degree of impairment was prognostic of clinical outcome again attesting to the clinical utility of

HRV measurements. Rangari *et al.* found an 80% incidence of significantly reduced HRV and standardized test performances in patients with cirrhosis and a 67% incidence in those with extrahepatic portal hypertension (Rangari *et al.* 2002). They suggest that both limbs of the autonomic nervous system play a role in the neuropathy.

In summary, a number of nondiabetic conditions including chronic renal disease with uraemia, Chagas' disease and liver cirrhosis have been associated with a high incidence of autonomic dysfunction. From a pathophysiological perspective, the best that can be said is that these conditions are not uncommonly complicated by neurocardiac dysregulation involving, at times, one or both limbs of the autonomic nervous system. There is promise that therapeutic interventions such as dialysis in the case of uraemia, liver transplant in the case of advanced liver disease and tight diabetic control in the case of diabetes may be shown to retard or reverse the progression of neuropathy. The proper use of HRV methods may allow us to witness these hopeful outcomes.

References

Akselrod, S., Gordon, D., Ubel, F.A., Shannon, D.C., Barger, A.C., & Cohen, R.J. (1981) Power spectrum of heart rate fluctuation: a quantitative probe of beat to beat cardiovascular control. *Science*, **213**, 220–222.

Athyros, V.G., Didangelos, T.P., Karamitsos, D.T., Papagiorgion, A.A., Boudoulas, H. & Kontopoulos, A.G. (1998) Long term effect of converting enzyme inhibition on circadian sympathetic and parasympathetic modulation in patients with diabetic autonomic neuropathy. *Acta Cardiologica*, **53**, 201–209.

Bellavere, F., Belzani, I., De Masi, G. *et al.* (1992) Power spectral analysis of heart rate variations improves assessment of diabetic cardiac autonomic neuropathy. *Diabetes* **41**, 633–640.

Bernardi, L. (2000) Clinical evaluation of arterial baroreflex activity in diabetes. *Diabetes Nutrition and Metabolism*, **13**, 331–340.

Bernardi, L., Rossi, M., Soffiantino, F. *et al.* (1989) Cross correlation of heart rate and respiration versus deep breathing. Assessment of new test of cardiac autonomic function in diabetes. *Diabetes*, **38**, 589–596.

Bianchi, A., Bontempi, B., Cerutti, S., Gianoglio, P., Comi, G. & Natali Sora, M.G. (1990) Spectral analysis of heart rate variability signal and respiration in diabetic subjects. *Medical & Biological Engineering & Computing*, **28**, 205–211.

Cacciatori, V., Gemma, M.L., Bellavere, F. *et al.* (2000) Power spectral analysis of heart rate in hypothyroidism. *European Journal of Endocrinology* **143**, 327–333.

Chau, N.P., Chanudet, X., Bauduceau, B., Gautier, D. & Larroque, P. (1993) Fractal dimension of heart rate and blood pressure in healthy subjects and in diabetic subjects. *Blood Press* **2**, 101–107.

Ducher, M., Cerutti, C., Gustin, M. *et al.* (1999) Non-invasive exploration of cardiac autonomic neuropathy. *Diabetes Care* **22**, 388–393.

ESC/NASPE (European Society of Cardiology/North American Society of Pacing and Electrophysiology) Task Force (1996) Heart rate variability. *Circulation* **93**, 1045–1065.

Ewing, D.J. (1992) Analysis of heart rate variability and other noninvasive tests with special reference to diabetes mellitus. In: *Autonomic Failure* (eds R. Bannister & C. J. Mathias) 3rd edn, pp. 312–333. Oxford Medical, Oxford.

Ewing, D.J., Martyn, C.N., Young, R.J. & Clarke, B.F. (1985) The value of cardiovascular autonomic tests: 10 years experience in diabetes. *Diabetes Care*, **8**, 491–498.

Ewing, D.J., Campbell, I.M. & Clarke, B.F. (1980) The natural history of diabetic autonomic neuropathy. *Quarterly Journal of Medicine* **49**, 95–108.

Freeman, R., Saul, J.P., Roberts, M.S., Berger, R.D., Broadbridge, C. & Cohen, R.J. (1991) Spectral analysis of heart rate in diabetic autonomic neuropathy. *Archives of Neurology*, **48**, 185–190.

Galetta, F., Cupisti, A., Franzoni F. *et al.* (2001) Changes in heart rate variability during ultrafiltration and hemodialysis. *Blood Purification*, **19**, 395–400.

Gerritsen, J., Dekker, J.M., TenVoorde, B.J. *et al.* (2001) Impaired autonomic function is associated with increased mortality especially in subjects with diabetes, hypertension or a history of cardiovascular disease. *Diabetes Care* **24**, 1793–2001.

Guzzetti, S., Iosa, D., Pecis, M., Bonura, L., Prosdocimi, M. & Malliani, A. (1991) Impaired heart rate variability in Chagas' disease. *American Heart Journal*, **121**, 1727–1734.

Kamath, M.V. & Fallen, E.L. (1993) Power spectral analysis of heart rate variability: a noninvasive signature of cardiac autonomic function. *Critical Reviews in Biomedical Engineering* **21**, 245–311.

Krolewski, A.S., Barzilay, J., Warram, J.H., Martin, B.C., Pfeifer, M. & Rand, L.I. (1992) Risk of early onset proliferative retinopathy in IDDM is closely related to cardiovascular autonomic neuropathy. *Diabetes* **41**, 430–437.

Lazzeri, C., LaVilla, G., Laffi, G. *et al.* (1997) Autonomic regulation of heart rate and *QT* interval in nonalcoholic cirrhosis with ascites. *Digestion*, **58**, 580–586.

Malliani, A., Pagani, M., Lombardi, F. *et al.* (1991) Cardiovascular neural regulation explored in the frequency domain. *Circulation*, **84**, 482–492.

Malpas, S.C. & Maling, T.J.B. (1990) Heart rate variability and cardiac autonomic function in diabetes. *Diabetes* **39**, 1177–1181.

Marin-Neto, J.A., Marciel, B.C., Gallo, L., Junquiera, L. & Amorin, D.S. (1986) effects of parasympathetic impairment of the hemodynamic response to handgrip in Chagas' heart disease. *British Heart Journal*, **55**, 204–210.

McDowell, T.S., Chapleau, M.W., Hajduczok, G. & Abboud, F.M. (1994) Baroreflex dysfunction in diabetes mellitus. I. Selective impairment of parasympathetic control of heart rate. *American Journal of Physiology*, **266**, H235–H243.

Molgaard, H., Christensen, P.D., Sorensen, K.E., Christensen, C.K. & Mogensen, C.E. (1992) Association of 24-h cardiac parasympathetic activity and degree of nephropathy in IDDM patients. *Diabetes*, **41**, 812–817.

Mott, K.E. & Hagstrom, J.W.C. (1965) The pathologic lesions of the cardiac autonomic nervous system in chronic Chagas' myocarditis. *Circulation*, **31**, 273–286.

Mukkamala, R., Mathias, J.M., Mullen, T.J., Cohen, R.J. & Freeman, R. (1999) System identification of closed loop cardiovascular control mechanisms: diabetic autonomic neuropathy. *American Journal of Physiology*, **276**, R905–R912.

Niemela, R.K., Pikkujamsa, S.M., Hakala, M., Huikuri, H.V. & Airaksinen, K.E.J. (2000) No signs of autonomic nervous system dysfunction in primary Sjögren's syndrome evaluated by 24 hour heart rate variability. *Journal of Rheumatology*, **27**, 2605–2610.

O'Brien, J.A., McFadden, J.P. & Corrall, R.J.M. (1991) The influence of autonomic neuropathy on mortality in insulin-dependent diabetes. *Quarterly Journal of Medicine*, **79**, 495–502.

Pagani, M. (2000) Heart rate variability and autonomic diabetic neuropathy. *Diabetes Nutrition and Metabolism*, **13**, 341–346.

Pagani, M., Malfatto, G., Pierini, S. *et al.* (1988) Spectral analysis of heart rate variability in the assessment of autonomic diabetic neuropathy. *Journal of the Autonomic Nervous System*, **23**, 143–153.

Pagani, M., Lombardi, F., Guzzetti, S. *et al.* (1986) Power spectral analysis of heart rate and arterial pressure variabilities as a marker of sympatho-vagal interaction in man and conscious dogs. *Circulation Research*, **59**, 178–193.

Pfeifer, M.A. & Schumer, M.P. (1994) Cardiovascular autonomic neuropathy. *Diabetes Care*, **17**, 1545–1546.

Rangari, M., Sinha, D.M., Kapoor, D., Mohan, J.C. & Sarin, S.K. (2002) Prevalence of autonomic dysfunction in cirrhotic and non-cirrhotic portal hypertension. *Americam Journal of Gastoenterology*, **97**, 707–713.

Spallone, V. & Menzinger, G. (1997) Diagnosis of cardiovascular autonomic neuropathy in diabetes. *Diabetes*, **46** (Suppl. 2), S67–S76.

Spallone, V., Uccioli, L. & Menzinger, G. (1995) Diabetic autonomic neuropathy. *Diabetes Metabolism Reviews*, **11**, 227–257.

Spallone, V., Bernardi, L., Ricordi, L. *et al.* (1993) Relationship between the circadian rhythms of blood pressure and sympatho-vagal balance in diabetic autonomic neuropathy. *Diabetes*, **42**, 1745–1752.

Takase, B., Kitamura, H., Noritake, M. *et al.* (2002) Assessment of diabetic autonomic neuropathy using 24 h spectral analysis of heart rate variability: a comparison with the findings of the Ewing battery. *Japanese Heart Journal*, **43**, 127–135.

Vita, G., Bellinghieri, G., Trusso, A. *et al.* (1999) Uremic autonomic neuropathy studied by spectral analysis of heart rate. *Kidney International*, **56**, 232–237.

Winocour, P.H., Hanka, D. & Andersen, D.C. (1986) The relationship between autonomic neuropathy and urinary sodium and albumin excretion in insulin treated diabetics. *Diabetic Medicine*, **3**, 436–440.

Ziegler, D., Laude, D., Akila, F. & Elghozi, J.L. (2001) Time and frequency domain estimation of early diabetic cardiovascular autonomic neuropathy. *Clinics in Autonomic Research*, **11**, 369–376.

SECTION II
Baroreflex

CHAPTER 15

Physiological Background of Baroreflex

Barbara Casadei

Introduction

The main function of the arterial baroreflex is to prevent wide fluctuations of arterial blood pressure by rapidly adjusting cardiac output and peripheral vascular resistance. Baroreceptor nerve endings embedded in the carotid sinuses, aortic arch and great thoracic vessels detect the level of distension of the vessel wall (which, in physiological conditions, is mostly determined by the intravascular pressure as well as by the tone of the vessel wall itself) and send this information to the brain stem via the glossopharyngeal and vagi nerves. Integration of this afferent information in the nucleus tractus solitarii (NTS) in the dorsal medulla results in continuous fine-tuning of efferent autonomic neural activity to the cardiovascular system. These adjustments are instrumental in the short-term control of arterial blood pressure and are necessary to maintain optimal brain perfusion in the face of significant shifts in central blood volume, such as those occurring in response to physiological stimuli, e.g. postural stress, or in potential life-threatening emergencies, such as acute haemorrhage.

Several publications have reviewed this topic in detail (e.g. Eckberg and Sleight 1992; Chapleau *et al.* 1995; Lanfranchi and Somers, 2002), thus the aim of this short chapter is to update some of the well-established knowledge on the physiology of the arterial baroreceptor by focussing on recently published evidence.

The baroreflex mechanosensor

Unlike other sensory receptors, the arterial baroreceptors do not associate with specialised cells but detect mechanical deformation of the vessel wall (in response to changes in transmural pressure) by forming a vastly arborised network of mostly 'naked' unmyelinated fibres in the adventitia and media layers of the aorta and carotid arteries (Rees 1967). Extended contact of the baroreceptor nerve endings with deformable elements of the vessel wall is likely to be important for the transfer of force from the vascular wall to the sensory nerve terminals. Indeed, a close relationship between baroreceptor neurites and collagen bundles or elastic elements of the vessel wall has consistently been detected in histological studies providing some anatomical support to the large body of physiological data indicating that baroreceptors are essentially 'stretch' sensors (Fig. 15.1).

Surprisingly, however, the molecular identity of the baroreceptor mechanoelectrical transducer has remained elusive until very recently. There were findings suggesting that stretch-activated ion channels capable of generating depolarizing currents might be present in baroreceptor neurones (Hajduczok *et al.* 1994; Kraske *et al.* 1998), but, their identity remained unknown until 1998 when Drummond *et al.* (Drummond *et al.* 1998) demonstrated that the degenerin (DEG)/ENaC family of cation channels, which are responsible for touch sensation in the *C. elegans* worm, may be an important component of the baroreceptor mechanosensor. Some DEG proteins share homology with the amiloride-sensitive epithelial sodium channel (ENaC) (Snyder *et al.* 1998) suggesting that 'touch' channels in the *C. elegans* comprise subunits of a stretch gated channel related to ENaC. Further findings have indicated that the β and γ subunits of ENaC are present in cell bodies of baroreceptor neurones and that small baroreceptor nerve terminals innervating the aortic

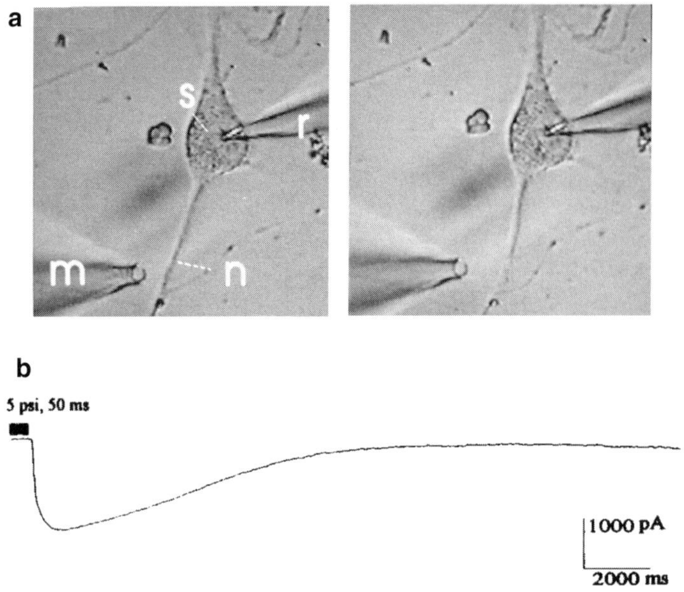

Fig. 15.1 (a) Mechanical stimulation of the neurite (n) of a cultured baroreceptor neurone by ejection of saline from a micropipette (m, see the effect on the right panel). (b) Inward current (recorded with a voltage clamp pipette, r, on the cell soma, s) that results from the mechanical stimulation of the neurite. (From Chapleau *et al.* 1995, with permission.)

arch and the carotid sinus can be stained by anti-γ ENaC antibodies, providing compelling evidence in support of the hypothesis that DEG/ENaC channels are the basic mechanotransducer in the baroreceptor nerve endings. A crucial piece of evidence supporting an important role of this class of channels in baroreceptor function is the finding that baroreceptor nerve activity can be inhibited by amiloride and its analogues, which are known to inhibit the DEG/ENaC channels (Drummond *et al.* 1998) (Fig. 15.2).

Can baroreceptors sense mechanical stimuli other than changes in transmural pressure across the vessel wall?

Evidence suggests that this may be the case since increases in blood flow stimulate carotid sinus nerve activity and decrease the pressure threshold for baroreceptor discharge in the dog isolated carotid sinus, in the absence of changes in intravascular pressure or strain (Hajduczok *et al.* 1988). These findings indicate that shear stress may be an important and previously unrecognized modulator of baroreceptor function and suggest that such flow sensitivity reflects the endothelial release of diffusible substances, of which nitric oxide (NO) might seem a plausible candidate. However, this idea is not supported by data showing that constitutive NO production has either no effect (Murakami *et al.* 1998; Fujisawa *et al.* 1999) or tonically inhibits (Minami *et al.* 1995; Liu *et al.* 1996) the gain of the baroreflex in conscious animals. These findings are consistent with data reporting that infusion of NO donors (Matsuda *et al.* 1995; Zanzinger *et al.* 1996) or stimulation of endothelial NO release (Chapleau *et al.* 1988; Matsuda *et al.* 1995) in the isolated carotid sinus inhibits baroreceptor activity in anaesthetised rats or rabbits. Similarly, in human subjects systemic infusion of the NO donor, sodium nitroprusside, in the presence of arterial pressure clamp had no effect on the cardiac-vagal limb of the baroreflex, but caused a substantial reduction in the low-frequency oscillations of arterial blood pressure, consistent with a decreased baroreflex/sympathetic control of peripheral resistance (Hogan *et al.* 1999b).

Recent findings highlighting the importance of non-endothelial NOS may help shed some light on the role of NO in baroreceptor function. The presence of a neuronal isoform of NO synthase (nNOS) in afferent baroreceptor fibres from the carotid sinus (Hohler *et al.* 1994; Tanaka and Chiba 1994) suggests that NO may be involved in the regulation of baroreceptor activity. However, some evidence in support of this hypothesis has only recently come forward as NO has been shown to inhibit both TTX-sensitive and insensitive sodium currents in autonomic

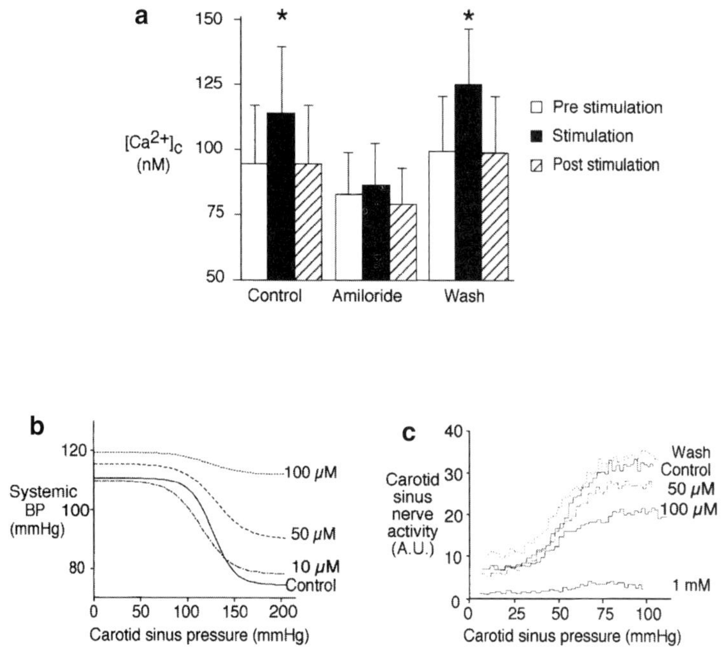

Fig. 15.2 Effect of amiloride on baroreceptor function *in vitro* and *in vivo*. (a) Effect of amiloride on mechanically activated Ca^{2+} transients in cultured baroreceptor neurones. The bars show the average per cent increase in $[Ca^{2+}]_c$ in cultured baroreceptor neurones before, immediately following, and 30 s after mechanical stimulation with a brief puff with buffer solution (as shown in Fig. 15.1). Responses were recorded under control conditions, in the presence of 100 nM amiloride, and after amiloride washout. $^*P < 0.05$ vs. prestimulation. (From Drummond *et al.* 1998, with permission.) (b) Effect of a range of concentrations of benzamil, an amiloride analogue, on carotid baroreflex control of systemic blood pressure (BP). Reflex changes in blood pressure were measured in response to a ramp increase in carotid sinus pressure. Benzamil decreased the slope of the response (mmHg systemic BP/mmHg carotid sinus pressure) in a dose-dependent fashion. (c) Effect of benzamil on carotid baroreceptor discharge. Carotid sinus nerve activity (in arbitrary units) was measured in one rabbit in response to a ramp increase in carotid sinus pressure in the presence of intraluminal benzamil. Benzamil reversibly blunted baroreceptor activation.

sensory neurones via a cyclic GMP-independent mechanism involving nitrosylation of cysteine residues within the sodium channel protein (Li *et al.* 1998; Bielefeldt *et al.* 1999). On the basis of these data, Li *et al.* (1998) postulated that the increase in intracellular calcium observed in response to mechanical stimuli in baroreceptor neurones (Sharma *et al.* 1995; Sullivan *et al.* 1997) might enhance nNOS-derived production of NO, which in turn would inhibit voltage-sensitive sodium channels and action potential discharge of baroreceptor neurones in an autocrine negative feedback fashion.

Taken together, these data suggest that endothelial-dependent factors and neuronal NO release may exert opposite effects upon baroreceptor discharge. The flow and endothelial-dependent facilitation of baroreceptor discharge may be lost in pathological states characterized by endothelial dysfunction and increased oxygen-derived free radical formation (Li *et al.* 1996; Angell-James 1974), contributing to the reduction in baroreflex sensitivity that has consistently been found in these conditions. Whether upregulation of nNOS expression in afferent nerves contributes to the impaired arterial baroreflex observed after myocardial infarction (see Takimoto *et al.* 2002; Vaziri *et al.* 2000) remains to be investigated.

Central regulation of baroreflex responses

Afferent information from arterial baroreceptors is relayed to the nucleus tractus solitarii (NTS) in the brain stem, where it is processed and integrated (reviewed by Blessing 1997). In recent years, it has become apparent that locally released NO plays an important role in the integration of the autonomic control of the cardiovascular system in the NTS. Both NTS neurones and afferent terminals within the NTS contain nNOS (Vincent & Kimura 1992; Tagawa *et al.* 1994; Ruggiero *et al.* 1996) and evidence suggests that NO and excitatory amino acids stimulate each other's release within the NTS (Lo *et al.* 1996). Furthermore, NO has been shown to increase neuronal activity in the NTS in a cyclic GMP-dependent fashion (Tagawa *et al.* 1994; Ma *et al.* 1995), suggesting that constitutive NO release in the NTS may potentiate the reflex autonomic control of cardiovascular functions. However, the effect of NTS NO production on the sensitivity of the arterial baroreflex is unclear and may vary depending on the preparation (anaesthetised vs. conscious), the type of neurones targeted by NO (inhibitory vs. excitatory), the NOS isoform involved (e.g. eNOS vs. nNOS), and the effect studied (i.e. the baroreflex control of heart rate vs. blood pressure).

Recent investigations have demonstrated that the integrity of eNOS is critical to the inhibition of the baroreceptor–heart rate reflex brought about by the injection of angiotensin II in the NTS in a rat heart–brain stem preparation (Paton *et al.* 2001; Wong *et al.* 2002; Waki *et al.* 2003) (Fig. 15.3a), suggesting that eNOS-derived NO may have an inhibitory effect on the baroreceptor–cardiac reflex. Other studies in conscious chronically instrumented rats showed that the

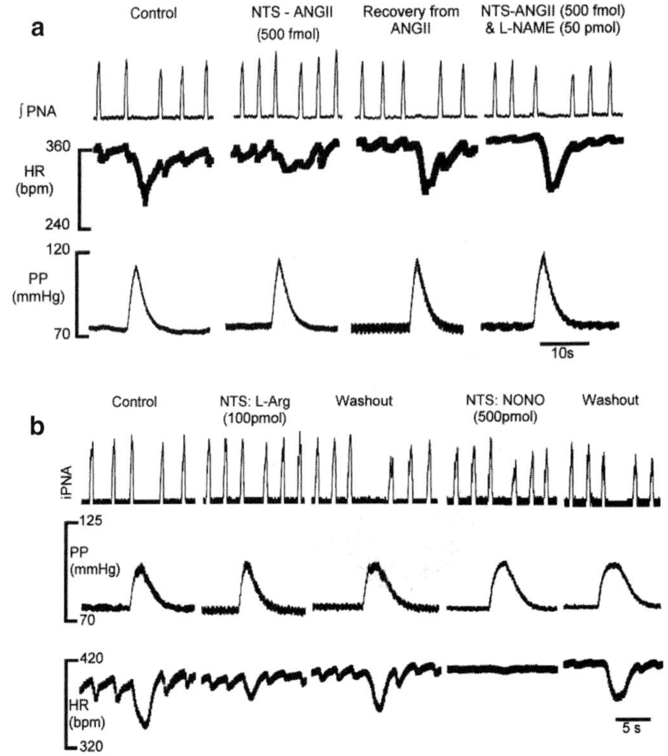

Fig. 15.3 (a) Raw data showing bilateral NTS microinjection of angiotensin II (ANG II) into the NTS attenuated the reflex cardiac and phrenic nerve responses. This effect of ANGII was prevented by a prior microinjection of a NOS inhibitor (L-NAME). (b) Nitric oxide derived from either a precursor (L-arginine, L-Arg) or a donor (diethylamine nonoate, NONO) reduce both baroreceptor reflex-induced cardiac and phrenic nerve activity responses. The baroreceptor reflex was stimulated by increases in perfusion pressure. Note the reduction in respiratory sinus arrhythmia, which may represent a reduced excitatory drive from the NTS to cardiac vagal motoneurones or possible spread of injectate to cardiac vagal motoneurones in the dorsal vagal nucleus. HR, heart rate in beats/min; iPNA, integrated phrenic nerve activity; PP, perfusion pressure. (Adapted from Paton *et al.* 2001, with permission.)

sensitivity of baroreceptor–heart rate reflex was unchanged after inhibition of constitutive NO production in the NTS (Pontieri *et al.* 1998). Similarly, both NOS inhibition and application of NO donors in the NTS had no effect on the baroreflex control of renal sympathetic activity in anaesthetised cats (Zanzinger *et al.* 1995) but suppressed the heart rate reflex response to an increase in perfusion pressure in rat heart–brain stem preparations (Fig. 15.3b) (Paton *et al.* 2001).

How does the baroreflex mediate rapid adjustments in arterial blood pressure?

Once arterial blood pressure increases above the threshold for activation of the arterial baroreceptors (which fluctuates with the prevailing arterial pressures), receptor firing begins abruptly. The reflex bradycardia that follows with almost no time lag, results from an increase in vagal efferent activity, whereas vasodilatation develops with a delay of a few seconds through a reduction in sympathetic vasoconstrictor tone (Borst & Karemaker 1983). Whereas the reduction in α-adrenergic-mediated vasoconstriction seems to be the most important factor in determining the baroreflex control of blood pressure in man, some evidence suggests that the very early hypotensive effect following baroreceptor stimulation may be owing to a vagally-mediated reflex reduction in cardiac output, resulting from an inhibitory action of the vagus nerve on both sinoatrial node activity and left ventricular contractility.

Whether the vagus exerts a direct negative inotropic action on the left ventricle of mammals has long been a matter of debate (reviewed by Casadei 2001). In humans, there is evidence for an efferent parasympathetic innervation of the left myocardium (Kent *et al.* 1974) and for the presence of muscarinic M_2 receptors (Deighton *et al.* 1990). However, evidence in support of vagal control of ventricular function is not clear-cut.

Some studies have shown that the increase in vagal firing during expiration may exert a negative inotropic effect (Karlocai *et al.* 1998). Similarly muscarinic receptor stimulation in healthy subjects antagonizes the positive inotropic effect of isoproterenol (Von Scheidt *et al.* 1992). However, muscarinic receptor inhibition by atropine seems to have no effect on basal and isoproterenol-stimulated left ventricular contractility, suggesting that cardiac vagal 'tone' does not significantly control basal and beta adrenergic myocardial inotropy.

These issues have recently been revisited by Lewis *et al.* (2001) who have shown that electrical stimulation of the left thoracic vagus nerve in patients undergoing cardiac surgery produces a rapid 40% reduction in left ventricular inotropy. This effect was only partially attenuated by selective β_1-adrenergic receptor blockade, suggesting that stimulation of vagal discharge exerts a significant negative inotropic effect in humans both directly and by antagonising the effect of sympathetic adrenergic activity.

Pulsed aortic Doppler velocimetry has proved a useful tool for assessing beat-by-beat changes in stroke volume noninvasively in humans. By using this technique, it has been possible to show that activation of the arterial baroreflex causes a reduction in cardiac output through a rapid and simultaneous effect on both stroke volume and heart rate (Casadei *et al.* 1992). Baroreflex activation by the phenylephrine bolus technique is immediately followed by a fall in cardiac output that seems to be mediated by the vagus via the muscarinic cholinergic receptors since it is virtually abolished by atropine. Furthermore, the largest reduction in stroke volume was observed in subjects with high baroreflex sensitivity where the pressor response was small compared with that observed in the group with low sensitivity (Fig. 15.4). This observation and the results obtained after muscarinic receptor blockade suggest that the fall in stroke volume in response to phenylephrine cannot be entirely attributed to the increase in arterial blood pressure and left ventricular afterload that follows α-adrenergic receptor stimulation.

Further evidence in support of this hypothesis was obtained by stimulating carotid baroreceptors with neck suction. Short bursts of negative pressure (−40 mmHg for 6 s) applied to the anterior neck of subjects with a dual-chamber pacemaker inserted for idiopathic atrioventricular block caused a similar reduction in cardiac output and in mean blood pressure when the subjects were in sinus rhythm and when heart rate was kept constant by overdrive atrial pacing. A significant reduction of stroke volume,

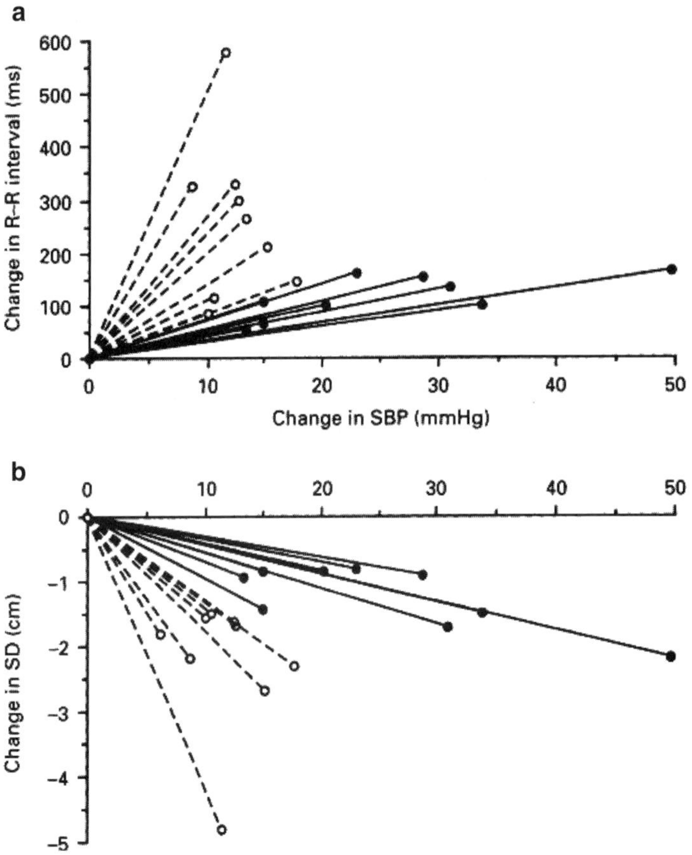

Fig. 15.4 Individual regression lines between changes in *RR* interval (a) and in the Doppler-derived index of stroke volume (stroke distance, SD) (b) in response to the rise in systolic arterial blood pressure (SBP) induced by a bolus injection of phenylephrine. Subjects are divided arbitrarily into a group with higher baroreflex sensitivity (dotted lines) and a group with lower baroreflex sensitivity (solid lines). Note that the group with higher baroreflex sensitivity showed the greatest fall in stroke distance despite a smaller rise in systolic blood pressure. (From Casadei *et al.* 1992, with permission.)

however, was only evident when the reflex lengthening of the pulse interval was prevented by pacing (Casadei *et al.* 1991; Casadei, 2001). All reflex changes in heart rate, stroke volume, and mean blood pressure were abolished after muscarinic receptor blockade with atropine.

These findings indicate that the rapid reduction in stroke volume that follows the activation of the arterial baroreflex is mediated by the vagus and that this effect is functionally important since it contributes to the fast adjustment in arterial blood pressure mediated by the arterial baroreflex.

Does the arterial baroreflex contribute to the set level of arterial blood pressure in mammals?

Experimental findings suggest that this is unlikely as persistence of the stimulus (e.g. a sustained elevation in arterial blood pressure) is not associated with sustained baroreceptors firing. On the contrary, the baroreceptor response tends to decay progressively, reaching 50% of the initial response after only 0.1 s (Landgreen 1952). The same occurs after a sudden reduction in arterial blood pressure leading to a reduction in the firing of the baroreceptor and an efferent autonomic response characterized by increased sympathetic efferent activity and withdrawal of cardiac vagal activity.

The mechanism responsible for non-sustained baroreflex responses in the presence of a sustained stimulus is not clear and likely to be a composite of different adaptations occurring at the level of the baroreceptors, within the central nervous system and possibly at the level of the sinus node, where it is known that the rate response to vagal stimulation 'fades' with time (Boyett & Roberts 1987). The adaptation of the baroreceptors to a sustained stimulus is a phenomenon termed 'resetting'. In other words, if an elevation in arterial blood pressure were maintained, the initial increase in baroreceptor firing,

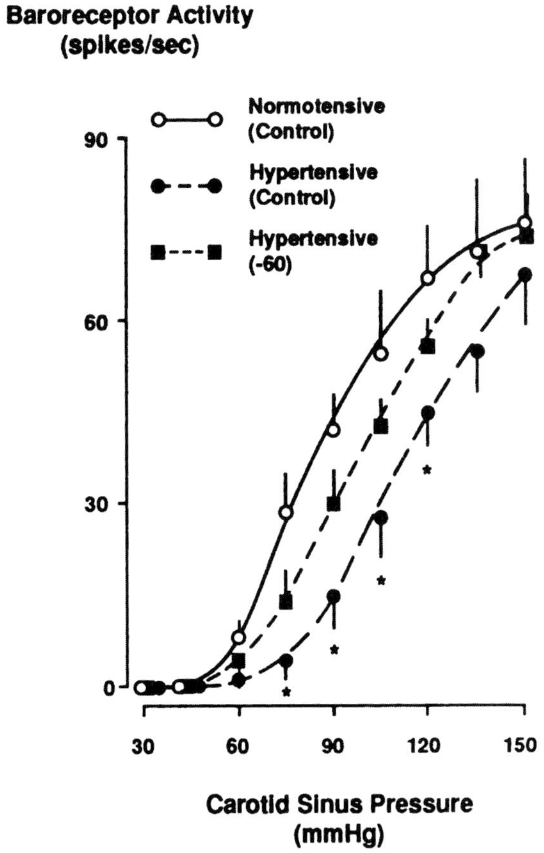

Fig. 15.5 Line graphs showing that resetting of the pressure–activity curve of baroreceptors in chronically hypertensive rabbits can be rapidly reversed towards normal. This is achieved by exposing the isolated carotid sinus of the hypertensive animal to a holding pressure that is lower than the 'usual' pressure by 10–15 min. These findings suggest that resetting of the arterial baroreflex occurs rapidly and that arterial structural changes in hypertension are not the main mechanism responsible for it. (From Xie *et al.* 1991, with permission.)

resulting in bradycardia and decreased sympathetic activity, would progressively decrease and return to normal (i.e. reach the new 'set point' from which the baroreflex would respond as usual to acute changes in pressure) (Fig. 15.5). This finding suggests that the baroreflex is unlikely to be an important determinant of the level of blood pressure and the clinical presentation of 'baroreflex failure' in humans is consistent with this idea. Indeed, this rare syndrome is mostly characterized by wide fluctuations in blood pressure level, comprising severe pressure surges in response to stimuli that elicit an increase in sympathetic outflow (e.g. mental or physical stress) as well as hypotension when sympathetic outflow is diminished (e.g. during sleep) (Jordan *et al.* 1997; Ketch *et al.* 2002) rather that by sustained hypertension (Fig. 15.6).

Methodological considerations

The methods that are most commonly used to test the sensitivity of the arterial baroreflex in humans involve the use of drugs that would alter systemic arterial blood pressure and hence the degree of baroreceptor activity, without allegedly having any direct effect on heart rate, autonomic responses or baroreceptor transmission (reviews by Casadei & Paterson, 2000; Parati *et al.* 2000). After injecting the vasoactive drug of choice, baroreflex sensitivity is evaluated as the slope of the relationship between changes in pulse interval and the increase or decrease in systolic arterial pressure elicited by the drug. This method, therefore, only assesses the autonomic responsiveness of the sinoatrial node to reflex changes in autonomic nerve activity (mostly vagal), making the assumption that the vascular/sympathetic limb of the reflex would show a similar response. This assumption, however, cannot be extrapolated to all situations. For instance, during moderate dynamic exercise (when sympathetic activity is increased but cardiac vagal activity is withdrawn) baroreflex-mediated control of arterial pressure and muscle sympathetic nerve activity is maintained whereas heart rate responses may be suppressed (e.g. Staessen *et al.* 1987; Papelier *et al.* 1994; Fadel *et al.* 2001). In addition, as our knowledge of the mechanism of action of vasoactive drugs increases, it is becoming increasingly difficult to find an agent that would change arterial blood pressure without affecting heart rate, baroreflex transmission or the activity of autonomic nervous system directly (reviewed by Casadei & Paterson, 2000).

By 1969 it had already become apparent that angiotensin (the pressor agent initially employed to test baroreflex sensitivity) could have 'direct' effects on both the vasomotor centres and the heart, thus phenylephrine has since been the drug of choice for testing the arterial baroreflex (Bristow *et al.* 1969; Smyth *et al.* 1969). Yet,

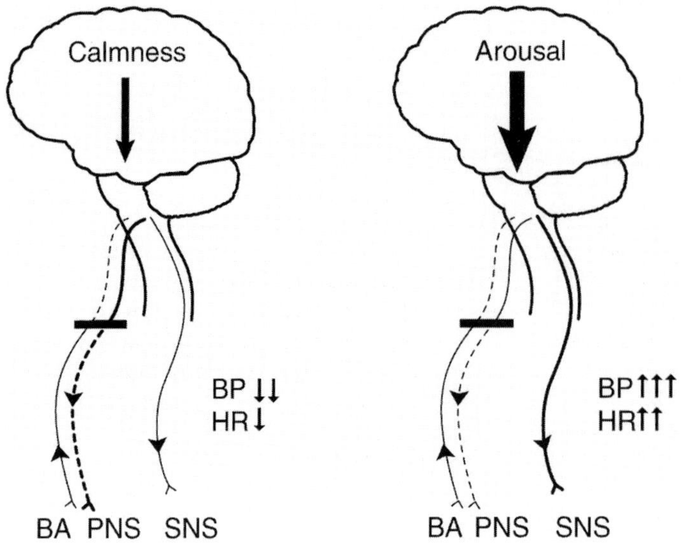

Fig. 15.6 In baroreflex failure, baroreceptor afferents (BA) and often vagal efferent fibres (PNS) are damaged. This results in paroxysms of arterial hypertension, tachycardia, flushing and headache in response to stimuli that elicit an increase in sympathetic outflow (SNS) and hypotension when sympathetic outflow is diminished. In some patients with preserved vagal efferent activity, malignant vagotonia and asystole can occur during sleep. (From Jordan *et al.* 1997, with permission.)

phenylephrine can also interfere with the assessment of baroreflex sensitivity by enhancing baroreceptor stimulation through an increase in smooth muscle tone in the carotid arteries (Peveler *et al.* 1983) and by exerting a small direct positive chronotropic effect (Williamson *et al.* 1994; Casadei *et al.* 1996; El-Omar *et al.* 2000).

Similar problems may occur when NO donors are used to lower arterial blood pressure and deactivate the arterial baroreflex. As I have mentioned earlier, it is now known that NO can modulate baroreflex responses by directly altering the firing rate and pressure threshold of arterial baroreceptors as well as affecting the integration of baroreflex afferent information in the NTS. Furthermore, recent *in vitro* and *in vivo* experiments suggest that NO could depress the sinoatrial response to a fall in arterial blood pressure (i.e. to baroreceptor deactivation) by inhibiting cardiac sympathetic neurotransmission (Schwarz *et al.* 1995; Elvan *et al.* 1997; Choate & Paterson 1999; Mohan *et al.* 2000) and by interfering with the beta-adrenergic intracellular signalling pathway (reviewed by Balligand 1999).

A further complication is that NO donors have a concentration-dependent, biphasic effect on 'intrinsic' pacemaker activity *in vitro* and *in vivo*; e.g. nano- to micromolar concentrations of NO donors gradually increase rate whereas higher concentrations (mM) decrease it (Musialek *et al.* 1997; Hogan *et al.* 1999a, b).

Further investigations have shown that the positive chronotropic response to NO donors is due to the activation of a novel intracellular pathway involving NO, cGMP and the stimulation of the hyperpolarisation activated current, I_f (Musialek *et al.* 1997, 2000). *In vivo*, however, the direct positive chronotropic effect of NO donors develops more slowly than the baroreflex-mediated increase in heart rate (Hogan *et al.* 1999b), implying that the direct effect of NO donors on heart rate is unlikely to affect the assessment of baroreflex sensitivity, unless NO donors are infused over minutes rather than injected as a bolus.

In summary, research in the arterial baroreflex has taken advantage of new techniques to cover important ground both at the 'bench' and at the 'bed side' (as illustrated in the following chapters). A high baroreflex sensitivity (assessed by the baroreceptor–heart rate reflex) has become a synonym for cardiovascular 'well-being' and studies on patients with autonomic failure have stressed the importance of the baroreflex in regulating arterial blood pressure as well as controlling sympathetic and vagal outflow to the vasculature and the heart. Indeed, in spite of the many mechanisms that nature has in place to stabilise arterial pressure, failure of baroreflex regulation results in a dramatic clinical syndrome.

References

Angell-James, J.E. (1974) Arterial baroreceptor activity in rabbits with experimental atherosclerosis. *Circulation Research*, **34**, 27–39.

Balligand, J.L. (1999) Regulation of cardiac beta-adrenergic response by nitric oxide. *Cardiovascular Research*, **43**, 607–620.

Bielefeldt, K., Whiteis, C.A., Chapleau, M.W. & Abboud, F.M. (1999) Nitric oxide enhances slow inactivation of voltage-dependent sodium current in rat nodose neurons. *Neuroscience Letters*, **271**, 159–162.

Blessing, W.W. (1997) Anatomy of the lower brainstem. In: *The Lower Brainstem and Bodily Homeostasis*, pp. 29–99. Oxford University Press, New York.

Borst, C. & Karemaker, J.M. (1983) Time delays in the human baroreceptor reflex. *Journal of the Autonomic Nervous System*, **9**, 399–409.

Boyett, M.R. & Roberts, A. (1987) The fade of the response to acetylcholine at the rabbit isolated sino-atrial node. *Journal of Physiology*, **393**, 171–194.

Bristow, J.D., Honour, A.J., Pickering, G.W., Sleight, P. & Smyth, H.S. (1969) Diminished baroreflex sensitivity in high blood pressure. *Circulation*, **39**, 48–54.

Casadei, B. (2001) Vagal control of myocardial contractility in humans. *Experimental Physiology*, **86**, 817–823.

Casadei, B., Meyer, T., Coats, A.J.S., Conway, J. & Sleight, P. (1991) The stroke volume reduction by baroreceptor activation in human volunteer subjects is mediated by the vagus. *Journal of Physiology*, **438**, 87P.

Casadei, B., Meyer, T.E., Coats, A.J., Conway, J. & Sleight, P. (1992) Baroreflex control of stroke volume in man: an effect mediated by the vagus. *Journal of Physiology*, **448**, 539–550.

Casadei, B., Moon, J., Caiazza, A. & Sleight, P. (1996) Is respiratory sinus arrhythmia a good index of cardiac vagal activity during exercise? *Journal of Applied Physiology*, **81**(2), 556–564.

Casadei, B. & Paterson, D.J. (2000) Should we still use nitrovasodilators to test baroreflex sensitivity? *Journal of Hypertension*, **18**(1), 3–6.

Chapleau, M.W., Cunningham, J.T., Sullivan, M.J., Wachtel, R.E. & Abboud, F.M. (1995) Structural vs. functional modulation of the arterial baroreflex. *Hypertension*, **26**, 341–347.

Chapleau, M.W., Hajduczok, G., Shasby, D.M. & Abboud, F.M. (1988) Activated endothelial cells in culture suppress baroreceptors in the carotid sinus of dog. *Hypertension*, **11**, 586–590.

Choate, J.K. & Paterson, D.J. (1999) Nitric oxide inhibits the positive chronotropic and inotropic responses to sympathetic nerve stimulation in the isolated guinea-pig atria. *Journal of the Autonomic Nervous System*, **75**, 100–108.

Deighton, N.M., Motomura, S., Borquez, D., Zerkowski, H.R., Doetsch, N. & Brodde, O.E. (1990) Muscarinic cholinoceptors in the human heart: demonstration, subclassification, and distribution. *Naunyn-Schmiedebergs Archives of Pharmacology*, **341**, 14–21.

Drummond, H., A., Price, M.P., Welsh, M.J. & Abboud, F.M. (1998) A molecular component of the arterial baroreceptor mechanotransducer. *Neuron*, **21**, 1435–1441.

Eckberg, D.L. & Sleight, P. (1992). *Human Baroreflexes in Health and Disease*. Clarendon Press, Oxford.

El-Omar, M., Kardos, A. & Casadei, B. (2000) Mechanisms of respiratory sinus arrhythmia in patients with mild heart failure. *American Journal of Physiology*, **280**, H125–H131.

Elvan, A., Rubart, M. & Zipes, D.P. (1997) NO modulates autonomic effects on sinus discharge rate and AV nodal conduction in open-chest dogs. *American Journal of Physiology*, **272**, H263–H271.

Fadel, P.J., Ogoh, S., Watenpaugh, D.E. *et al.* (2001) Carotid baroreflex regulation of sympathetic nerve activity during dynamic exercise in humans. *American Journal of Physiology*, **280**, H1383–H1390.

Fujisawa, Y., Mori, N., Yube, K., Miyanaka, H., Miyatake, A. & Abe, Y. (1999) Role of nitric oxide in regulation of renal sympathetic nerve activity during hemorrhage in conscious rats. *American Journal of Physiology*, **277**, H8–H14.

Hajduczok, G., Chapleau, M.W. & Abboud, F.M. (1988) Rheoreceptors in the carotid sinus of dog. *Proceedings of the National Acadamy of Sciences of the United States of America*, **85**, 7399–7403.

Hajduczok, G., Chapleau, M.W., Ferlic, R.J., Mao, H.Z. & Abboud, F.M. (1994) Gadolinium inhibits mechano-electrical transduction in rabbit carotid baroreceptors. Implication of stretch-activated channels. *Journal of Clinical Investigation*, **94**, 2392–2396.

Hogan, N., Casadei, B. & Paterson, D.J. (1999a) Nitric oxide donors can increase heart rate independent of autonomic activation. *Journal of Applied Physiology*, **87**(1), 97–103.

Hogan, N., Kardos, A., Paterson, D.J. & Casadei, B. (1999b) Effect of exogenous nitric oxide on baroreflex function in humans. *American Journal of Physiology*, **277**, H221–H227.

Hohler, B., Mayer, B. & Kummer, W. (1994) Nitric oxide synthase in the rat carotid body and carotid sinus. *Cell Tissue Research*, **276**, 559–564.

Jordan, J., Shannon, J.R., Black, B.K. *et al.* (1997) Malignant vagotonia due to selective baroreflex failure. *Hypertension*, **30**, 1072–1077.

Karlocai, K., Jokkel, G. & Kollai, M. (1998) Changes in left ventricular contractility with the phase of respiration. *Journal of the Autonomic Nervous System*, **73**, 86–92.

Kent, K.M., Epstein, S.E., Cooper, T. & Jacobowitz, D.M.

(1974) Cholinergic innervation of the canine and human ventricular conducting system: Anatomic and electrophysiological correlations. *Circulation*, **50**, 948–955.

Ketch, T., Biaggioni, I., Robertson, R. & Robertson, D. (2002) Four faces of baroreflex failure: Hypertensive crisis, volatile hypertension, orthostatic tachycardia, and malignant vagotonia. *Circulation*, **105**, 2518–2523.

Kraske, S., Cunningham, J.T., Hajduczok, G., Chapleau, M.W., Abboud, F.M. & Wachtel, R.E. (1998) Mechanosensitive ion channels in putative aortic barorecptor neurons. *American Journal of Physiology*, **275**, H1497–H1501.

Landgreen, S. (1952) On the excitation mechanism of the carotid baroreceptors. *Acta Physiologica Scandinavica*, **26**, 1–34.

Lanfranchi, P.A. & Somers, V.K. (2002) Arterial baroreflex function and cardiovascular variability: interactions and implications. *American Journal of Physiology*, **283**, R815–826.

Lewis, M.E., Al-Khalidi, A.H., Bonser, R.S. *et al.* (2001) Vagus nerve stimulation decreases left ventricular contractility *in vivo* in the human and pig heart. *Journal of Physiology*, **534.2**, 547–552.

Li, Z., Chapleau, M.W., Bates, J.N., Bielefeldt, K., Lee, H.C. & Abboud, F.M. (1998) Nitric oxide as an autocrine regulator of sodium currents in baroreceptor neurons. *Neuron*, **20**, 1039–1049.

Li, Z., Mao, H.Z., Abboud, F.M. & Chapleau, M.W. (1996) Oxygen-derived free radicals contribute to baroreceptor dysfunction in atherosclerotic rabbits. *Circulation Research*, **79**, 802–811.

Liu, J.L., Murakami, H. & Zucker, I.H. (1996) Effects of NO on baroreflex control of heart rate and renal nerve activity in conscious rabbits. *American Journal of Physiology*, **270**, R1361–R1370.

Lo, W.J., Liu, H.W., Lin, H.C., Ger, L.P., Tung, C.S. & Tseng, C.J. (1996) Modulatory effects of nitric oxide on baroreflex activation in the brainstem nuclei of rats. *Chinese Journal of Physiology*, **39**, 57–62.

Ma, S., Abboud, F.M. & Felder, R.B. (1995) Effects of L-arginine-derived nitric oxide synthesis on neuronal activity in nucleus tractus solitarius. *American Journal of Physiology*, **268**, R487-R491.

Matsuda, T., Bates, J.N., Lewis, S.J., Abboud, F.M. & Chapleau, M.W. (1995) Modulation of baroreceptor activity by nitric oxide and S-nitrosocysteine. *Circulation Research*, **76**, 426–433.

Minami, N., Imai, Y., Hashimoto, J. & Abe, K. (1995) The role of nitric oxide in the baroreceptor-cardiac reflex in conscious Wistar rats. *American Journal of Physiology*, **269**, H851–H855.

Mohan, R.M., Choate, J.K., Golding, S., Herring, N., Casadei, B. & Paterson, D.J. (2000) Peripheral presynaptic pathway reduces the heart rate response to sympathetic activation following exercise training: role of NO. *Cardiovascular Research*, **47**(1), 90–98.

Murakami, H., Liu, J.L., Yoneyama, H. *et al.* (1998) Blockade of neuronal nitric oxide synthase alters the baroreflex control of heart rate in the rabbit. *American Journal of Physiology*, **274**, R181–R186.

Musialek, P., Lei, M., Brown, H.F., Paterson, D.J. & Casadei, B. (1997) Nitric oxide can increase heart rate by stimulating the hyperpolarization-activated inward current, I_f. *Circulation Research*, **81**, 60–68.

Musialek, P., Rigg, L., Terrar, D.A., Paterson, D.J. & Casadei, B. (2000) Role of cGMP-inhibited phosphodiesterase and sarcoplasmic calcium in mediating the increase in basal heart rate with nitric oxide donors. *Journal of Molecular and Cellular Cardiology*, **32**, 1831–1840.

Papelier, Y., Escourrou, P., Gauthier, J.P. & Rowell, L.B. (1994) Carotid baroreflex control of blood pressure and heart rate in men during dynamic exercise. *Journal of Applied Physiology*, **77**, 502–506.

Parati, G., Di Rienzo, M. & Mancia, G. (2000) How to measure baroreflex sensitivity: from the cardiovascular laboratory to daily life. *Journal of Hypertension*, **18**, 7–19.

Paton, J.F.R., Deuchars, J., Ahmad, Z., Wong, L.-F., Murphy, D. & Kasparov, S. (2001) Adenoviral vector demonstrates that angiotensin II-induced depression of the cardiac baroreflex is mediated by endothelial nitric oxide synthase in the nucleus tractus solitarii of the rat. *Journal of Physiology*, **531.2**, 445–458.

Peveler, R.C., Bergel, D.H., Robinson, J.L. & Sleight, P. (1983) The effect of phenylephrine upon arterial pressure, carotid sinus radius and baroreflex sensitivity in the conscious greyhound. *Clinical Science*, **64**, 455–461.

Pontieri, V., Venezuela, M.K., Scavone, C. & Michelini, L.C. (1998) Role of endogenous nitric oxide in the nucleus tratus solitarii on baroreflex control of heart rate in spontaneously hypertensive rats. *Journal of Hypertension*, **16**, 1993–1999.

Rees, P.M. (1967) Observation of the fine structure and distribution of presumptive baroreceptor nerves at the carotid sinus. *Journal of Comparative Neurology*, **131**, 517–548.

Ruggiero, D.A., Mtui, E.P., Otake, K. & Anwar, M. (1996) Central and primary visceral afferents to nucleus tractus solitarii may generate nitric oxide as a membrane-permeant neuronal messenger. *Journal of Comparative Neurology*, **364**, 51–67.

Schwarz, P., Diem, R., Dun, N.J. & Forstermann, U. (1995) Endogenous and exogenous nitric oxide inhibits noradrenaline release from rat heart sympathetic nerves. *Circulation Research*, **77**, 841–848.

Sharma, R.V., Chapleau, M.W., Hajduczok, G. *et al.* (1995)

Mechanical stimulation increases intracellular calcium concentration in nodose sensory neurons. *Neuroscience*, **66**, 433–441.

Smyth, H.S., Sleight, P. & Pickering, G.W. (1969) Reflex regulation of arterial pressure during sleep in man: a quantitative method of assessing baroreflex sensitivity. *Circulation Research*, **24**, 109–121.

Snyder, P.M., Cheng, C., Prince, L.S., Rogers, J.C. & Welsh, M.J. (1998) Electrophysiological and biochemical evidence that DEG/ENaC cation channels are composed of nine subunits. *Journal of Biological Chemistry*, **273**, 681–684.

Staessen, J., Fiocchi, R., Fagard, R., Hespel, P. & Amery, A. (1987) Progressive attenuation of the carotid baroreflex control of blood pressure and heart rate during exercise. *American Heart Journal*, **114**, 765–772.

Sullivan, M.J., Sharma, R.V., Wachtel, R.E. *et al.* (1997) Non-voltage-gated Ca^{2+} influx through mechanosensitive ion channels in aortic baroreceptor neurons. *Circulation Research*, **80**, 861–867.

Tagawa, T., Imaizumi, T., Harada, S. *et al.* (1994) Nitric oxide influences neuronal activity in the nucleus tractus solitarius of rat brainstem slices. *Circulation Research*, **75**, 70–76.

Takimoto, Y., Aoyama, T., Tanaka, K., Keyamura, R., Yui, Y. & Sasayama, S. (2002) Augmented expression of neuronal nitric oxide synthase in the atria parasympathetically decreases heart rate during acute myocardial infarction in rats. *Circulation*, **105**, 490–496.

Tanaka, K. & Chiba, T. (1994) Nitric oxide synthase containing neurones in the carotid body and sinus of the guinea pig. *Microscopy Research and Technique*, **29**, 90–93.

Vaziri, N.D., Ding, Y., Sangha, D.S. & Purdy, R.E. (2000) Upregulation of NOS by simulated microgravity, potential cause of orthostatic intolerance. *Journal of Applied Physiology*, **89**, 338–344.

Vincent, S.R. & Kimura, H. (1992) Histochemical mapping of nitric oxide synthase in the brain. *Neuroscience*, **46**, 755–784.

Von Scheidt, W., Bohm, M., Stablein, A., Autenrieth, G. & Erdmann, E. (1992) Antiadrenergic effect of M-cholinoceptor stimulation on human ventricular contractility *in vivo*. *American Journal of Physiology*, **263**, H1927–H1931.

Waki, H., Kasparov, S., Wong, L.-F., Murphy, D., Shimizu, T. & Paton, J.F.R. (2003) Chronic inhibition of endothelial nitric oxide synthase activity in nucleus tractus solitarii enhances baroreceptor reflex in conscious rats. *Journal of Physiology*, **546**, 233–242.

Williamson, A.P., Seifen, E., Lindemann, J.P. & Kennedy, R.H. (1994) Alpha 1a-adrenergic receptor mediated positive chronotropic effect in right atria isolated from rats. *Canadian Journal of Physiology and Pharmacology*, **72**, 1574–1579.

Wong, L.-F., Polson, J.W., Murphy, D., Paton, J.F.R. & Kasparov, S. (2002) Genetic and pharmacological dissection of pathways involved in the angiotensin II-mediated depression of baroreflex function. *FASEB (Federation of American Societies for Experimental Biology) Journal*, **16**, 1595–1601.

Xie, P.L., Mcdowell, T.S., Chapleau, M.W., Hajduczok, G. & Abboud, F.M. (1991) Rapid baroreceptor resetting in chronic hypertension. Implications for normalization of arterial pressure. *Hypertension*, **17**, 72–79.

Zanzinger, J., Czachurski, J. & Seller, H. (1995) Effects of nitric oxide on sympathetic baroreflex transmission in the nucleus tractus solitarii and caudal ventrolateral medulla in cats. *Neuroscience Letters*, **197**, 199–202.

Zanzinger, J., Czachurski, J. & Seller, H. (1996) Lack of nitric oxide sensitivity of carotid sinus baroreceptors activated by normal blood pressure stimuli in cats. *Neuroscience Letters*, **208**, 121–124.

CHAPTER 16

Invasive Determination of Baroreflex Sensitivity

Maria Teresa La Rovere

Introduction

The possibility of using the analysis of baroreflex sensitivity (BRS) as a means to quantify sympatho-vagal modulation at the sinus node level and the critical role played by abnormalities in arterial baroreflex function in arrhythmia genesis, have made of this methodology a useful tool for diagnostic and prognostic evaluation of cardiovascular disease.

This chapter will address the pathophysiological background, the current methodology, the main clinical findings and their most relevant implications. Special attention will be given to the potential impact of the analysis of BRS on risk stratification and on the use of Implantable Cardioverter Defibrillators for primary prevention.

Pathophysiological background

From the standpoint of its physiological role, the arterial baroreceptor reflex system constitutes one of the most powerful and rapidly acting mechanisms aimed at maintaining circulatory control in response to short-term blood pressure fluctuations. Humoral factors, however, such as the renin–angiotensin system, which are mainly involved in long-term control, may also interact with the activity of baroreceptors. Arterial baroreceptors provide the central nervous system with a continuous stream of information on changes in blood pressure (which are sensed by the stretch receptors in the wall of the carotid arteries and the aorta), on the basis of which efferent autonomic neural activity is dynamically modulated. When baroreceptor afferents are activated by a rise in systemic arterial pressure, their reflex circulatory effects result from vagal stimulation and sympathetic inhibition, thus leading to bradycardia, vessel dilation, and decrease of contractility and venous return (Kirchheim 1976; Abboud & Thames 1983). Conversely, a decrease in systemic arterial pressure causes the deactivation of baroreceptors with subsequent enhancement of sympathetic activity and vagal inhibition, leading to tachycardia and an increase in vascular resistance, contractility and venous return. Figure 16.1 illustrates baroreceptor-mediated changes in efferent cardiac vagal neural traffic according to different levels of arterial pressure (Cerati & Schwartz 1991).

Many central neural structures as well as humoral, behavioural and environmental factors are also involved in the regulation of the cardiovascular system and contribute to the functioning of the baroreflex. Respiration continuously interacts with baroreflex modulation of heart rate. Inspiration decreases while expiration increases baroreceptor stimulation of vagal motoneurons and vagal efferent firing (Eckberg & Orshan 1977). In physiological conditions and with normal levels of arterial pressure, baroreceptors are constantly active and exert a continuous inhibition on sympathetic efferent activity. Studies in humans support a major role for carotid as compared to other baroreceptor areas, as shown by sinoaortic denervation which results in an increase in arterial pressure and its variability which is insufficiently buffered by other reflex mechanisms in the long-term (Smit *et al.* 2002).

Any form of cardiac damage can impair the

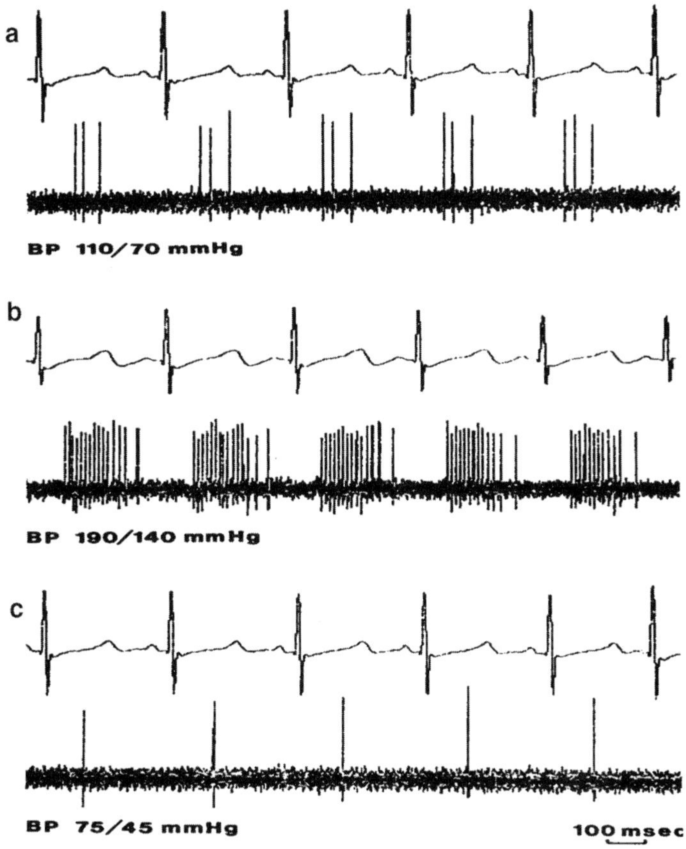

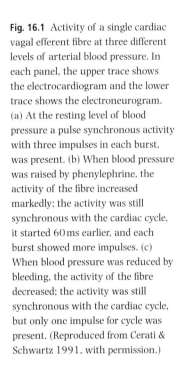

Fig. 16.1 Activity of a single cardiac vagal efferent fibre at three different levels of arterial blood pressure. In each panel, the upper trace shows the electrocardiogram and the lower trace shows the electroneurogram. (a) At the resting level of blood pressure a pulse synchronous activity with three impulses in each burst, was present. (b) When blood pressure was raised by phenylephrine, the activity of the fibre increased markedly; the activity was still synchronous with the cardiac cycle, it started 60 ms earlier, and each burst showed more impulses. (c) When blood pressure was reduced by bleeding, the activity of the fibre decreased; the activity was still synchronous with the cardiac cycle, but only one impulse for cycle was present. (Reproduced from Cerati & Schwartz 1991, with permission.)

function of baroreceptors with a reduction of inhibitory activity and imbalance of the physiological sympathetic–vagal interaction, resulting in a chronic adrenergic activation. A reduction in baroreflex control of heart rate has been reported in a number of cardiovascular disease including hypertension, coronary artery disease, myocardial infarction and heart failure (Sleight & Eckberg 1992). Sustained baroreflex-mediated increase in sympathetic activity may contribute to increased end-organ damage and to the progression of the underlying disease and a blunted baroreflex gain is predictive of cardiovascular risk in post-myocardial infarction and heart failure patients.

Baroreflex sensitivity and cardiovascular risk

An impairment in baroreflex control of cardiac function has been observed first in the post-myocardial infarction phase. The experimental data obtained from a group of dogs before and after the induction of an anterior myocardial infarction showed that in 70% of the animals the myocardial scar caused a definitive alteration in baroreflex function, while in the remaining 30% of animals there were no significant changes (Schwartz *et al.* 1988). Similarly, a group of patients with a recent myocardial infarction showed a reduction in baroreflex cardiac control when compared with normal subjects matched for age and sex (Schwartz *et al.* 1988). Although the mechanisms mediating reduced baroreflex function after myocardial infarction are unknown, it has been proposed that necrotic non-contractile myocardial segments can alter cardiac geometry and cause a mechanical distortion of sensorial fibres resulting in activation of sympathetic afferent fibres with subsequent inhibition of vagal efferent fibres and reduced responsiveness to baroreceptor-mediated blood pressure changes (Malliani *et al.* 1973; Schwartz *et al.* 1973). However, a reduced responsiveness of the sinus node as well as a central abnormality in autonomic modulation cannot be excluded. The ensuing autonomic imbalance, characterized by a decrease in vagal and/or an increase in sympathetic activity can increase cardiac electrical instability and enhance cardiac lethal arrhythmias by the interaction with other electrophysiological mechanisms such as re-entry, enhanced automaticity and triggered activity (Schwartz *et al.* 1973; Corr *et al.* 1986).

In the studies carried out in the experimental preparation cited above (Schwartz *et al.* 1988), the relationship between outcome and autonomic profile become evident. When the post-myocardial infarction dogs were submitted to a test combining physical exercise and acute myocardial ischaemia, it was found that the occurrence of ventricular fibrillation was much more frequent in the animals with an impaired baroreflex sensitivity as compared to those with a better preserved baroreflex cardiac control. This finding suggested that the ability to increase vagal activity may have a protective effect from ischaemic ventricular fibrillation, as also supported by interventions which enhance vagal activity such as direct neural stimulation, physical training and the administration of muscarinic agonists (Schwartz & Zipes 2000). There is also growing evidence that the autonomic balance is partially under genetic control (Singh *et al.* 1999; Schwartz, 2001). This would imply that alterations in tonic or reflex vagal activity might also be related to mutations on some of the genes involved in the neural control of the circulation.

Although it may be difficult to appreciate how changes in neural activity at the sinus node level might correlate with an increased electrical instability at the ventricular level, recent clinical data are well in line with this concept. Mitrani *et al.* (1998) have reported that a preserved response to phenylephrine-induced baroreflex activation was accompanied by an increase in the ventricular fibrillation threshold while the ventricular susceptibility did not change significantly in those subjects who were not able to increase vagal activity. This confirms the link between responses at the sinus node and at the ventricular level.

Methods of measurement

Arterial baroreflex function in humans is commonly assessed through various methods based on quantification of the extent of change in interbeat interval per unit change in systolic blood pressure. In standardized laboratory conditions, baroreflex modulation of heart rate can be analysed by the application of a variety of pharmacological or mechanical manipulations that cause sudden increases or decreases in arterial pressure. With these methods, owing to the need of external stimuli, mainly because of the use of drugs, the response of the cardiovascular system has been referred to as 'invasive'. More recent techniques, have allowed evaluation of baroreflex cardiovascular control without externally induced changes in arterial pressure, by the analysis of spontaneously occurring fluctuations in arterial pressure and heart rate. By contrast, this approach is defined as noninvasive and will be discussed in a different chapter.

Among the pharmacological perturbations, both vasoconstrictor and vasodilator drugs have been applied to study the reflex heart rate response to baroreceptor activation or deactivation, respectively. Vasoconstrictor drugs have been most widely used in the clinical setting. Smyth *et al.* (1969) first measured bradycardia produced in humans by an intravenous bolus of a pressor drug. The use of angiotensin as a pressor agent was subsequently replaced by the use of phenylephrine, a pure α-adrenoreceptor agonist, devoid of direct effects on cardiac contractility and the central nervous system.

The administration of the drug is performed in standardized laboratory conditions including a quiet, temperature-controlled environment, during a continuous and simultaneous recording of one lead electrocardiographic signal and beat-to-beat arterial pressure. Although noninvasive devices have been shown to overestimate blood pressure variabilities mainly in the lower frequencies bands (Pinna *et al.* 1996), noninvasive measurements during drug injection are highly correlated to the invasive ones and provide a quantification of the baroreflex gain of similar prognostic value (Pinna *et al.* 2000). Graded bolus injections of phenylephrine, beginning with 1–2 μg/kg in normal subjects, with 25–50 μg increments are administered until systolic arterial pressure increases by 20–30 mmHg. In patients with chronic heart failure up to 10 µg/kg have been safely administered (Mortara *et al.* 1997). It is commonly assumed that, given the rapidity of vagal response, the relation between pressure variation and *RR* interval is linear. Thus, systolic pressure for each beat and corresponding *RR* intervals with one-beat delay are fitted by a least-squares linear regression equation between the beginning and the end of systolic arterial pressure increase. The quantitative measure of the sensitivity of the baroreflex control of heart rate is provided by the slope of the regression line as the change in *RR* interval in ms per one millimeter mercury change in systolic pressure. The evaluation of the goodness of the linear association between systolic arterial pressure and *RR* interval is obtained by Pearson's correlation coefficient. Responses with low correlation coefficients and $P > 0.05$ are not usually considered. However, when the extent of change in *RR* interval is very limited and the sensitivity of the baroreceptor–heart rate reflex is near to zero, the correlation coefficient is obviously non-significant. In these cases, provided an adequate increase in systolic arterial pressure has been obtained, the measure is accepted independently of the correlation coefficient value. To reduce measurement variability, several administrations of phenylephrine are performed at 5- to 10-min intervals and the mean of the slopes obtained by every single test is calculated.

Figure 16.2 displays the baroreceptor-heart rate reflex in a normal subject: a steep slope is regarded as the result of the interplay between effective vagal reflexes and tonic sympathetic activity. By contrast, a flat slope may be due to abnormal vagal response or is the result of the inability of vagal reflexes to counterbalance sympathetic activation (Fig. 16.3).

With the phenylephrine method, average values of 15 ms/mmHg have been reported in normal subjects. Baroreflex dysfunction in post-myocardial infarction patients has been quantified by a mean value of 7 ms/mmHg (La Rovere *et al.* 1988a,b) and it is largely more pronounced in patients with heart failure (Mortara *et al.* 1997). In the more advanced stages of the disease values close to zero are often observed, thus describing a major derangement in reflex neural circulatory regulation. Paradoxical responses to baroreceptor stimulation, characterized by tachycardia and negative estimates of the baroreflex gain, have also been described, frequently associated with severe mitral regurgitation.

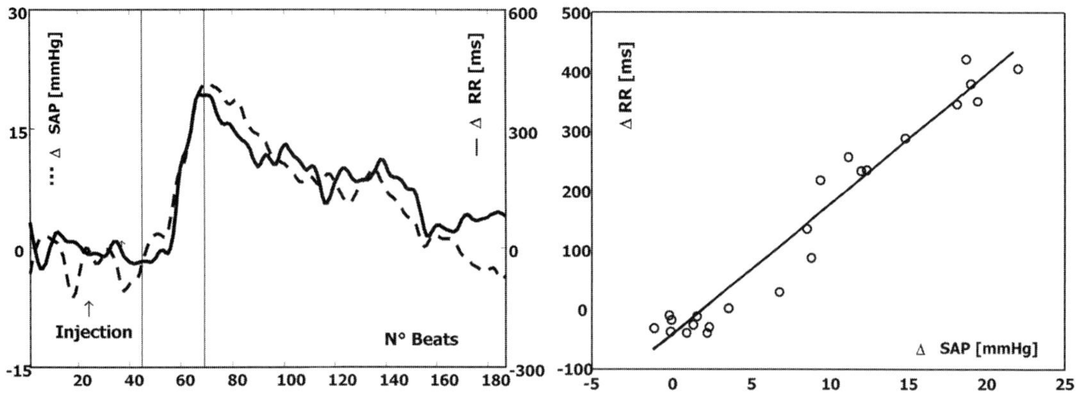

Slope = 21.8 ± 2.14 ms/mmHg r = 0.97

Fig. 16.2 Example of a normal BRS. On the left, beat-to-beat changes in systolic arterial pressure (SAP) (dotted line) and in *RR* intervals (solid line) with respect to baseline value are reported. Analysis is performed from the beginning to the end of the increase in SAP with the attendant changes in *RR* interval (points included between dotted lines). These points are used for calculation of the regression line (on the right). The increase in SAP, >20 mmHg, is associated to an increase in *RR* interval of *c.* 400 ms. The calculated slope is 21.8 ms per each mmHg increase in SAP. Such a slope identifies a baroreceptor response characterized by a prevailing increase in vagal efferent neural traffic to the sino-atrial node.

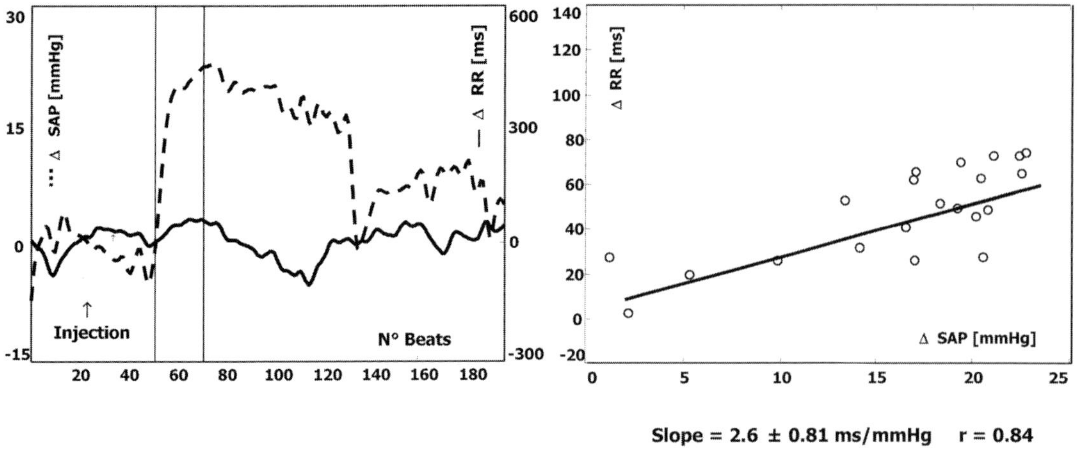

Fig. 16.3 Example of a poor BRS. Detailed description as in Fig. 16.2. The increase in SAP is accompanied by a limited change in *RR* interval and the calculated slope (lower than 3 ms/mmHg) identifies a response characterized by weak vagal reflexes or the inability of vagal reflexes to counterbalance increased sympathetic activity.

While vasoconstrictor drugs mainly explore the vagal component of the baroreceptor control of heart rate, vasodilators have been used to obtain information on the sympathetic branch of heart rate control. The injection of 100–200 μg of nitroglycerin determines an immediate and progressive fall in systolic arterial pressure of about 20 mmHg over the following 8–15 beats (Osculati *et al.* 1990). Baroreflex slopes obtained by vasodilators are lower than those obtained by increasing arterial pressure to a similar extent, suggesting that the two responses are not really mirror images (Pickering *et al.* 1972); yet it cannot be excluded that the tachycardia is produced by a direct effect on pacemaker cells (Musialek *et al.* 1997).

The lack of selectivity in the response has been claimed as one of the major limitations of the use of vasoactive drugs. Indeed, the pressure stimulus causes a simultaneous activation of multiple reflexogenic areas and the observed response is the result of multiple factors (including the stiffness of the arterial wall and transduction processes, the central integration, the sensitivity of the sinus node etc.). However, all these factors do not detract from the clinical value of baroreflex sensitivity when the test is used to obtain indirect information on the quantity of mediator (acetylcholine, noradrenaline) released at the cardiac level.

At variance with pharmacological manipulation, the mechanical manipulation provided with the neck chamber technique allows a direct activation or deactivation of carotid baroreceptors by application of measurable positive and negative pneumatic pressures to the neck region. An increase in neck chamber pressure is sensed by the baroreceptors as a decrease in arterial pressure and activates a double response that determines vagal withdrawal and sympathetic activation to the heart and arterial vessels. Conversely, a decrease in neck chamber pressure results in reflex reduction of blood pressure and heart rate. Neck suction is easier to use and better tolerated by the subjects (Eckberg *et al.* 1975). The negative pressure is applied in separate steps and ranges in magnitude from –7 to –40 mmHg. The maximal lengthening in *RR* interval observed over the three beats following the neck suction application generally represents the reflex response and the slope of the regression of *RR* interval over neck pressure is taken as the carotid baroreflex sensitivity. This method, although less invasive than drug injection, is used only in research laboratories and for particular pathophysiological purposes (Bernardi *et al.* 1995; Sleight *et al.* 1995).

Clinical applications of baroreflex study

Results from the ATRAMI (Autonomic Tone and Reflexes After Myocardial Infarction) study (La Rovere *et al.* 1998a) have defined the clinical implications of the analysis of baroreflex sensitivity in risk stratification of patients with a previous myocardial infarction. This study enrolled almost 1300 patients under 80 years of age and showed that the sympathetic–parasympathetic imbalance, expressed by a depressed baroreflex sensitivity (<3 ms/mmHg), was a significant and independent predictor of total cardiac mortality with a relative risk of 2.8 (95% CI 1.40–6.16), when compared with well-established risk factors such as depressed left ventricular function and the number of ectopic beats/h. Half of total cardiac mortality was due to sudden (presumably arrhythmic) death. The combination of a depressed left ventricular function together with a depressed baroreflex sensitivity significantly increased the predictive power of each parameter. Accordingly, the Task Force of the European Society of Cardiology has given the alteration in autonomic balance a Class I indication, level of evidence A in risk stratification for sudden cardiac death (Priori *et al.* 2001).

This observation has a particular relevance in light of the important weight that risk stratification has gained for the economical impact of medical care in the era of implantable cardioverter defibrillators (ICDs).

The problem of primary prevention of sudden cardiac death by ICD implantation is still debated (Zipes, 2001). On the basis of two large trials, the Multicentre Automatic Defibrillator Trial (MADIT) (Moss *et al.* 1996) and the Multicentre Unsustained Ventricular Tachycardia Trial (MUSST) (Buxton *et al.* 2000) 'high risk' patients were identified on the basis of a reduced left ventricular function ("40%), unsustained ventricular tachycardia at Holter monitoring and inducible ventricular tachyarrhythmias on electrophysiological study. The benefit in survival among patients meeting these criteria who also received a prophylactic ICD led to a class I indication for the implantation of the device (Priori *et al.* 2001). However, this stratification strategy could be applied to a very limited portion of patients with previous myocardial infarction (Every *et al.* 1998). On the other hand MADIT-II (Moss *et al.* 2002) criteria extended the indication for ICD implantation to all post-myocardial infarction patients with depressed left ventricular function (<30%). It is important to underscore that although this strategy could lead to an improved survival of a larger number of patients as compared to MADIT-I and MUSST (about 15% of postinfarction patients have reduced left ventricular function), it could also lead to an increase in the number of unnecessary ICDs as the positive predictive value of reduced ejection fraction in populations under optimal medical treatment is very low.

More recent data from the ATRAMI study (La Rovere *et al.* 2001) show that the analysis of BRS could provide a meaningful middle way between the 'restrictive' MADIT-I/MUSST criteria and the too 'extensive' of the MADIT-II ones. Indeed, among postinfarction patients with depressed left ventricular ejection fraction and without non sustained spontaneous ventricular tachycardia (who could be considered at low risk, following MADIT-I/MUSST) the presence or absence of an impaired baroreflex gain could identify two subgroups at significantly different two-year cardiac mortality: 18% vs 4.6% ($P = 0.01$) (Fig. 16.4). In this subset of patients, a depressed BRS carried a sensitivity of 64% and a specificity of 72%, with positive and negative predictive values of 18% and 95%, respectively. Importantly, the group of patients with reduced ejection fraction and

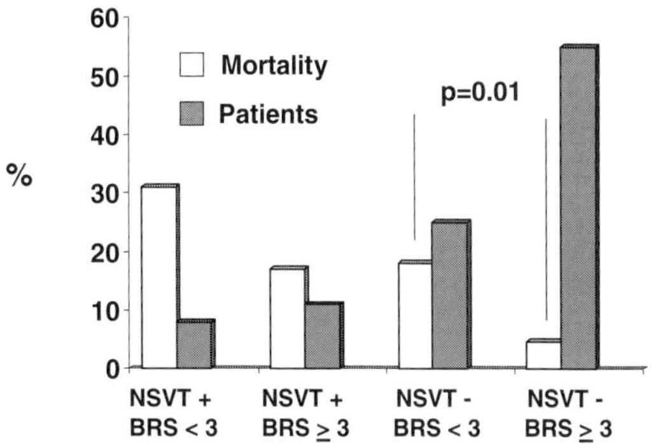

Fig. 16.4 Relation among different combinations of NSVT and BRS in patients with LVEF <35% and their relation to size of the subgroups under evaluation. Note that for patients without NSVT, presence of depressed (<3 ms/mmHg) BRS identifies a subset of patients accounting for >20% of patients with reduced LVEF (greater than entire group of patients with NSVT) with a 2-year mortality rate similar to that of patients with NSVT as a whole. A subgroup with a very low mortality rate, which accounts for >50% of patients with reduced LVEF, is identified by absence of NSVT (NSVT–) and preserved autonomic balance. (Reproduced from La Rovere *et al.* 2001, with permission.)

without nonsustained ventricular tachycardia but with a preserved autonomic balance accounts for about 50% of the patients with reduced left ventricular function. Compared with the MADIT-II strategy, this approach based on BRS analysis could significantly reduce the number of inactive defibrillators implanted. Specifically, a combined presence of a reduced left ventricular function and a depressed BRS was observed in 52 patients, 8 of whom had an arrhythmic death for a positive predictive accuracy of 15%. If the ATRAMI study population had been stratified according to the MADIT-II criteria, with 11 arrhythmic deaths out of 157 patients with reduced left ventricular function, there would have been a positive predictive accuracy of only 7%. Thus, using the MADIT-II criteria, three more lives could be saved (37%), but this would be achieved at the cost of implanting 105 more ICDs, an increase of 202%.

Conclusions

Experimental and clinical data have recognized the pathophysiological role of arterial baroreceptors in neural circulatory control and in the evolution of cardiac disease. The measurement and quantification of the effectiveness of baroreflex control supplies prognostic information in several cardiac disease, particularly in ischaemic cardiomyopathy. The 'invasive' determination of BRS seems to be particularly relevant in the stratification of patient candidates to ICD implantation, providing information which help to maximize the cost-effectiveness of the ICD.

References

Abboud, F.M. & Thames, M.D. (1983) Interaction of cardiovascular reflexes in circulatory control. In: *The Cardiovascular System* (eds J. T. Shepherd & F. M. Abboud), pp. 675–754. American Physiological Society, Bethesda, MD.

Bernardi, L., Bianchini, B., Spadacini, G. *et al.* (1995) Demonstrable cardiac reinnervation after human heart transplantation by carotid baroreflex modulation of *RR* interval. *Circulation*, **92**, 2895–2903.

Buxton, A.E., Lee, K.L., Di Carlo, L. *et al.* for the Multicenter Unsustained Tachycardia Trial Investigators (2000) Electrophysiologic testing to identify patients with coronary artery disease who are at risk for sudden death. *New England Journal of Medicine*, **342**, 1937–1945.

Cerati, D., Schwartz, P.J. (1991) Single cardiac vagal fiber activity, acute myocardial ischaemia, and risk for sudden death. *Circulation Research*, **69**, 1389–1401.

Corr, P.B., Yamada, K.A., Witkowski, F.X. (1986) Mechanisms controlling cardiac autonomic function and their relation to arrhythmogenesis. In: *The Heart and Cardiovascular System*, Vol. 2 (eds H. A. Fozzard, E. Haber, R. B. Jennings, A. N. Katz & H. E. Morgan), pp. 1343–1403. Raven Press, New York.

Eckberg, D.L., Cavanaugh, M.S., Mark, A.L. & Abboud, F.M. (1975) A simplified neck suction device for activation of carotid baroreceptors. *Journal of Laboratory Clinical Medicine*, **85**, 167–173.

Eckberg, D.L. & Orshan, C.R. (1977) Respiratory and baroreceptor reflex interactions in man. *Journal of Clinical Investigation*, **59**, 780–785.

Every, N.R., Hlatky, M.A., McDonald, K.M. *et al.* (1998) Estimating the proportion of post-myocardial infarction patients who may benefit from prophylactic implantable defibrillator placement from analysis of the CAST registry. *American Journal of Cardiology*, **82**, 683–685.

Kirchheim, H.R. (1976) Systemic arterial baroreceptor reflexes. *Physiological Review*, **56**, 100–177.

La Rovere, M.T., Bigger, J.T., Jr, Marcus, F.I. *et al.* for the ATRAMI (Autonomic Tone and Reflexes After Myocardial Infarction) Investigators (1998) Baroreflex sensitivity and heart rate variability in prediction of total cardiac mortality after myocardial infarction. *Lancet*, **351**, 478–484.

La Rovere, M.T., Pinna, G.D., Hohnloser, S.H. *et al.* (2001) Baroreflex sensitivity and heart rate variability in the identification of patients at risk for life-threatening arrhythmias. Implications for clinical trials. *Circulation*, **103**, 2072–2077.

La Rovere, M.T., Specchia, G., Mortara, A. & Schwartz, P.J. (1988) Baroreflex sensitivity, clinical correlates and cardiovascular mortality among patients with a first myocardial infarction. A prospective study. *Circulation*, **78**, 816–824.

Malliani, A., Recordati, G. & Schwartz, P.J. (1973) Nervous activity of afferent cardiac sympathetic fibres with atrial and ventricular endings. *Journal of Physiology*, **229**, 457–469.

Mitrani, R.D., Miles, W.M., Klein, L.S. *et al.* (1998) Phenylephrine increases T wave shock energy required to induce ventricular fibrillation. *Journal of Cardiovascular Electrophysiology*, **9**, 34–40.

Mortara, A., La Rovere, M.T., Pinna, G.D. *et al.* (1997) Arterial baroreflex modulation of heart rate in chronic heart failure. Clinical and hemodynamic correlates and prognostic implications. *Circulation*, **96**, 3450–3458.

Moss, A.J., Hall, W.J., Cannom, D.S. *et al.* for the Multicentre Automatic Defibrillator Implantation Trial Investigators (1996) Improved survival with an implanted defibrillator in patients with coronary disease at high risk for ventricular arrhythmia. *New England Journal of Medicine*, **335**, 1933–1940.

Moss, A.J., Zareba, W., Hall, W.J. *et al.* for the Multicentre Automatic Defibrillator Implantation Trial Investigators (2002) Prophylactic implantation of a defibrillator in patients with myocardial infarction and reduced ejection fraction. *New England Journal of Medicine*, **346**, 877–883.

Musialek, P., Lei, M., Brown, H.F., Paterson, D.J. & Casadei, B. (1997) Nitric oxide can increase heart rate by stimulating the hyperpolarization-activated inward current If. *Circulation Research*, **81**, 60–68.

Osculati, G., Grassi, G., Giannattasio, C. *et al.* (1990) Early alterations of the baroreceptor control of heart rate in patients with acute myocardial infarction. *Circulation*, **81**, 939–948.

Pickering, T.G., Gribbin, B. & Sleight, P. (1972) Comparison of the reflex heart rate response to rising and falling arterial pressure in man. *Cardiovascular Research*, **6**, 277–283.

Pinna, G.D., La Rovere, M.T., Maestri, R. *et al.* (2000) Comparison between invasive and noninvasive measurements of baroreflex sensitivity: implications for studies on risk stratification after a myocardial infarction. *European Heart Journal*, **18**, 1522–1529.

Pinna, G.D., Maestri, R. & Mortara, A. (1996) Estimation of arterial blood pressure variability by spectral analysis: comparison between Finapres and invasive measurements. *Physiological Measurement*, **17**, 147–169.

Priori, S.G., Aliot, E., Blomstrom-Lundqvist, C. *et al.* (2001) Task Force on Sudden Cardiac Death of the European Society of Cardiology. *European Heart Journal*, **22**, 1374–1450.

Schwartz, P.J., Pagani, M., Lombardi, F. *et al.* (1973) A cardiocardiac sympatho-vagal reflex in the cat. *Circulation Research*, **32**, 215–220.

Schwartz, P.J., Vanoli, E., Stramba-Badiale, M. *et al.* (1988) Autonomic mechanisms and sudden death. New insights from analysis of baroreceptor reflexes in conscious dogs with and without a myocardial infarction. *Circulation* **78**, 969–979.

Schwartz, P.J., Zaza, A., Pala, M. *et al.* (1988) Baroreflex sensitivity and its evolution during the first year after myocardial infarction. *Journal of the American College of Cardiology*, **12**, 629–636.

Schwartz, P.J. & Zipes, D.P. (2000) Autonomic modulation of cardiac arrhythmias. In: *Cardiac Electrophysiology. From Cell to Bedside* (eds D. P. Zipes & J. Jalife), 3rd edn, pp. 300–314. W. B. Saunders, Philadelphia.

Schwartz, P.J. (2001) Another role for the sympathetic nervous system in the long QT syndrome? *Journal of Cardiovascular Electrophysiology*, **12**, 500–502.

Singh, J.P., Larson, M.G., O'Donnell, C.J. *et al.* (1999) Heritability of heart rate variability. The Framingham Heart Study. *Circulation*, **99**, 2251–2254.

Sleight, P. & Eckberg, D.L. (1992) *Human Baroreflexes in Health and Disease*. Clarendon Press, Oxford.

Sleight, P., La Rovere, M.T., Mortara, A. *et al.* (1995) Physiology and pathophysiology of heart rate and blood pressure variability in humans: is power spectral analysis largely an index of baroreflex gain? *Clinical Science*, **88**, 103–109.

Smit, A.A.J., Timmers, H.J., Wieling, W. *et al.* (2002) Long-term effects of carotid sinus denervation on arterial blood pressure in humans. *Circulation*, **105**, 1329–1335.

Smyth, H.S., Sleight, P., Pickering, G.W. (1969) Reflex regulation of arterial pressure during sleep in man. A quantitative method for assessing baroreflex sensitivity. *Circulation Research*, **24**, 109–121.

Zipes, D.P. (2001) Implantable cardioverter defibrillator: a Volkswagen or a Rolls Royce. How much will we pay to save a life? *Circulation*, **103**,1372–1374.

CHAPTER 17

Noninvasive Provocations of Baroreflex Sensitivity

Josef Kautzner

Introduction

The baroreflex mechanism has been recognized as a key part of the cardiovascular regulation. Its main role is to dump variations in blood pressure. In fact, the baroreflexes originating from mechanoreceptors in the aortic arch and the carotid sinuses provide the clearest example of a negative-feedback control system (Rowell 1993). The efferent arm of the arterial baroreflex varies depending on whether blood pressure rises or falls. While the responses to a fall in blood pressure are corrected by slower responding sympathetic nervous system and directed to the resistance vessels, the reaction to a rise in blood pressure occurs fast (literally within one beat), and is executed through the vagal nerve and directed to the heart. This baroreflex control of heart rate can be quantified by baroreflex sensitivity (BRS), which represents the amount of change in heart rate attributable to changes in systolic blood pressure. Traditionally, BRS has been assessed by relating the change in heart rate to the prevailing sudden increase in blood pressure caused by intravenous injection of pure β-adrenergic agent, phenylephrine and expressed in units ofms/mmHg (Smyth *et al.* 1969). However, the need for intravenous cannulation and the use of the drug limits applicability of the technique. Therefore, the search for a simple, noninvasive method of BRS assessment is of practical interest. The aim of this chapter is to briefly review noninvasive provocations of BRS.

At present, several noninvasive alternatives to the phenylephrine method are in the process of clinical testing including: (1) the Valsalva manoeuvre; (2) spontaneous variations of the blood pressure and the *RR* intervals; (3) the neck suction method; (4) downward tilt; (5) carotid diameter variations.

The Valsalva manoeuvre

This manoeuvre represents a natural challenge for the baroreceptors and therefore, seems to be the most physiological surrogate for the phenylephrine method of BRS assessment (Palmero *et al.* 1981; S. A. Smith *et al.* 1987). While changes in systolic blood pressure that take place in phases I and III of the manoeuvre are mainly mechanical in origin, perturbations caused in phases II and IV do predominantly reflect the activity of both sympathetic and parasympathetic limbs of the autonomic nervous system (M. L. Smith *et al.* 1996). Regarding the use for the purpose of BRS assessment, it is the analysis of systolic blood pressure and heart rate during phase IV of the manoeuvre that is commonly used (Fig. 17.1). The advantages of this approach comprise the physiological nature of the stimulus, absence of significant side effects, relative simplicity and low cost. There is only one generally accepted contraindication to Valsalva manoeuvre – severe proliferative diabetic retinopathy.

Technically, both a single ECG lead plus a continuous noninvasive blood pressure signal from the finger (Finapres or Finometer) are recorded in a digital format. Tachograms of instantaneous *RR* intervals and corresponding blood pressure values are edited, and the period of interest is selected during phase IV to calculate BRS using linear regression. It could be the whole phase IV

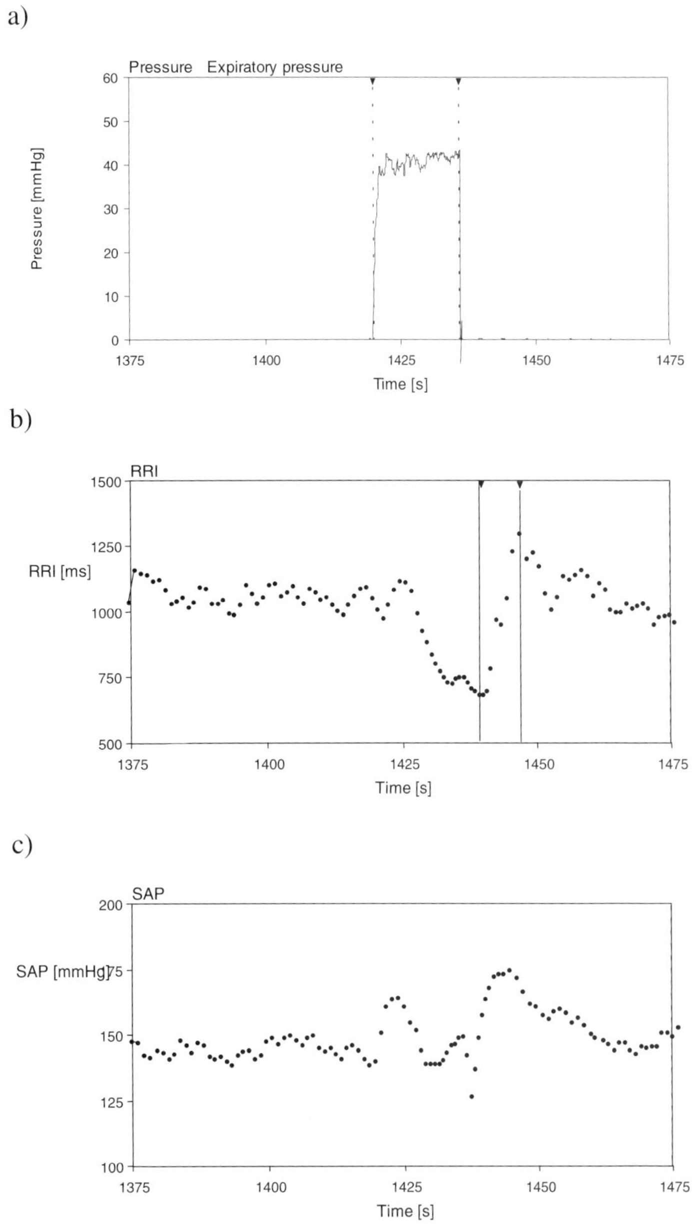

Fig. 17.1 Graphic depiction of the Valsalva manoeuvre in a normal subject: a) the subject blows into a pressure manometer to keep 40 mmHg pressure for 15 s (dotted lines), b) the course of duration of *RR* intervals (RRI) in response to changes in c) systolic blood pressure. Two lines in panel b) mark an increase in RRI during phase IV of the manoeuvre.

incorporating the increase in systolic blood pressure or just the so-called overshoot part that corresponds with a period when systolic blood pressure increases above the pretest value. In our previous study in subjects without organic heart disease we showed that this analysis could be further simplified by using the so-called BRS index, that is the ratio between the differences between the maximum and minimum *RR* interval and the differences between the maximum and minimum systolic blood pressure. Comparing this index with BRS value obtained by linear regression technique, we demonstrated that both techniques give reproducible results, provided an appropriate resting period between tests is left (5 min). Despite a good correlation between these two techniques, systematic overestimation of the BRS index was noticed (Kautzner *et al.* 1996). No comprehensive data about the performance of this index in a population of patients with heart disease are available yet.

Regarding the linear regression technique,

several studies have shown that the baroreflex slopes obtained by the phenylephrine method and by the Valsalva manoeuvre correlate to each other. However, most of these studies were performed in normal subjects and/or in patients with arterial hypertension and thus, their relevance to population of patients at risk of sudden death is less known. In addition, it is difficult to compare the findings of individual studies due to methodological differences. Some authors used the whole phase IV of the Valsalva manoeuvre to calculate the BRS while the others limited an analysis window to the overshoot part only. Not surprisingly, the correlation coefficients describing the relationship between these techniques varied accordingly from 0.27 to 0.91 (Palmero *et al.* 1981; Goldstein *et al.* 1982; S. A. Smith *et al.* 1987). In addition, the correlation analysis is not the best method to evaluate the agreement between any two different techniques of measurement. In this respect, Raczak *et al.* (2001) studied 104 postinfarction patients using both the phenylephrine method and the Valsalva manoeuvre-based method. They found that clinical utility of the Valsalva manoeuvre is hampered by a large number of non-measurable cases. Specifically, they revealed that BRS could not be computed using phase IV of the Valsalva manoeuvre or its overshoot part in 26% and in 39% of patients, respectively. This was the case especially among patients with LV ejection fraction <40% and in subjects who had significantly lower values of BRS using the phenylephrine method. Although the measurements obtained by the Valsalva manoeuvre were well correlated with those obtained by the phenylephrine method, the large limits of agreement do not indicate that both methods could be used interchangeably. Therefore, it remains that the Valsalva method could be used as a simple screening test in about two thirds of postinfarction population. Prospective studies, especially in a population of subjects with low LV ejection fraction are needed.

The Valsalva manoeuvre was used to evaluate the relationship between BRS and clinical severity of heart failure in a mixed population of patients (32 with dilated cardiomyopathy and 26 with coronary artery disease) (Rostagno *et al.* 1999). A decrease in BRS was already demonstrable in NYHA class I, while it was more profound in NYHA class II and III. The prognostic significance of the Valsalva-based BRS was evaluated in patients with mid-to-moderate heart failure by Rostagno *et al.* (Rostagno *et al.* 2000). Of the 52 patients who entered the study 15 died of cardiac cause at the end of long-term follow-up (mean 26 months) and five underwent heart transplant. While NYHA class, LV ejection fraction or end-diastolic diameters were significantly associated with event-free survival, BRS was not. Therefore, it seems to be of limited prognostic value.

Spontaneous variations of the blood pressure and the *RR* intervals

Other noninvasive methods to assess BRS employ measurements of arterial blood pressure and the joint analysis of spontaneous coherent changes in both systolic arterial pressure and heart rate (De Boer *et al.* 1987; Robbe *et al.* 1987). There are principally two different techniques for analysis of the relationship between spontaneous fluctuations in blood pressure and in the *RR* interval available: (a) the sequence technique that evaluates BRS in a time-domain; (b) the frequency-domain methods. As the latter techniques will be discussed in detail in a separate chapter, these will be mentioned only briefly here.

The sequence method

This technique analyses time series of *RR* interval and systolic blood pressure to identify sequences in which both *RR* and blood pressure increase or decrease concurrently over three and more beats (di Rienzo *et al.* 1985; Parati *et al.* 1994). The linear correlation between *RR* and systolic blood pressure is then computed for each sequence. A minimum change of 1 mmHg for systolic blood pressure and 4–6 ms for *RR* interval are required. The regression slope is calculated in those sequences with correlation coefficient above 0.8. Subsequently, the average value of the individual slopes over the 5-min episode is taken as a measure of BRS. The results are the same when comparing systolic blood pressure rises and falls.

The sequence technique has been compared in individual subjects with the phenylephrine method (Parati *et al.* 1994; Pitzalis *et al.* 1998). In most cases, high correlation coefficients between estimates of BRS obtained with the two techniques were found. However, as discussed above with the Valsalva manoeuvre technique, the absolute figures of BRS quantified by the two techniques were not identical. The explanation seems to be that both of them assess baroreflex influences on sinus node in a different way (Blaber *et al.* 1995; Parlow *et al.* 1995). It may reflect the fact that vasoactive drugs induce changes in mechanical properties of the arterial wall containing baroreceptors, which may result in a stronger and less physiological stimulus at any given change in blood pressure (di Rienzo *et al.* 1985; Pitzalis *et al.* 1998). In addition, vasoactive drug-induced blood pressure changes are usually relatively large resulting in BRS assessment over a larger segment of stimulus–response curve that is not limited solely to its linear portion. This may result in lower BRS values. On the other hand, the sequence method analyses only a part of the linear portion of the stimulus–response curve. Therefore, both methods should be regarded rather as complementary approaches to assess baroreflex function. It is not surprising then, that the best agreement between the sequence and the vasoactive drugs could be obtained by comparing the spontaneous BRS with the slope computed after administration of both phenylephrine and nitroglycerine (Parlow *et al.* 1995).

From a methodological point of view, the sequence method may be further simplified by analysing the blood pressure signal only, provided the sampling frequency of the signal is sufficiently high and the waveform undergoes a parabolic interpolation of its peak (Parati *et al.* 1990; Davies *et al.* 2002). The use of continuous blood pressure monitoring may allow noninvasive assessment of BRS in ambulatory conditions (Omboni *et al.* 1993). On the other hand, there are some suggestions to use only analysis of *RR* intervals without blood pressure measurement. The background for this reflects the fact that breathing at 0.1 Hz provides a standardized blood pressure stimulus and concentrates spectral power of heart rate at one frequency. In a study including 55 patients with chronic heart failure and 20 healthy controls, oscillations in blood pressure and *RR* interval over a 5-min period of controlled breathing were measured (Davies *et al.* 2002). Although the size of oscillations in blood pressure was not different in both groups, significant difference was found in the amplitude of *RR* interval oscillations (77 ms vs 31 ms, $P < 0.0001$) and the amplitude of the *RR* interval oscillations correlated strongly with BRS ($r = 0.81$, $P < 0.0001$). However, potential clinical utility of these simplified measurements remains unknown.

Frequency-domain techniques

These techniques use spectral analyses of nonrandom oscillations of *RR* intervals and systolic blood pressure in specific frequency bands. Technically, the method is based on analysis of short segments of both recordings, ranging from 128 to 1024 beats (De Boer *et al.* 1987; Robbe *et al.* 1987). Both signals in such segments then undergo either fast Fourier transform or autoregressive analysis. If frequency of linearly coherent oscillation of *RR* and blood pressure is detected in the range of 0–0.5 Hz, the modulus of the transfer function between these oscillations expresses BRS. Initially, as described by Robbe *et al.* (Robbe *et al.* 1987), fluctuations in low frequency band (around 0.1 Hz) were used for the analysis. More recently, estimates of BRS have been calculated both in low and high (between 0.15–0.40 Hz) frequency bands as the square root of the ratio of the spectral powers of *RR* intervals and systolic blood pressure powers in the frequency region where they are most often coherent (Fig. 17.2) (Pagani *et al.* 1988). Frequently, the mean of both bands is used as a measure of the global gain and referred to as the α-coefficient.

Few studies have demonstrated a close correlation between α-coefficient and the phenylephrine BRS estimates in small groups of normal or hypertensive subjects (Robbe *et al.* 1987; Pagani *et al.* 1988; Parlow *et al.* 1995; Watkins *et al.* 1996). More recently, studies have been published that used the more appropriate method for agreement assessment. Although there was moderate linear association, a lack of agreement between the two techniques was revealed. The limits of agreement were around (5 ms/mmHg for normotensive or hypertensive subjects, and even more in postinfarction population (13 ms/mmHg and more)) (James *et al.*

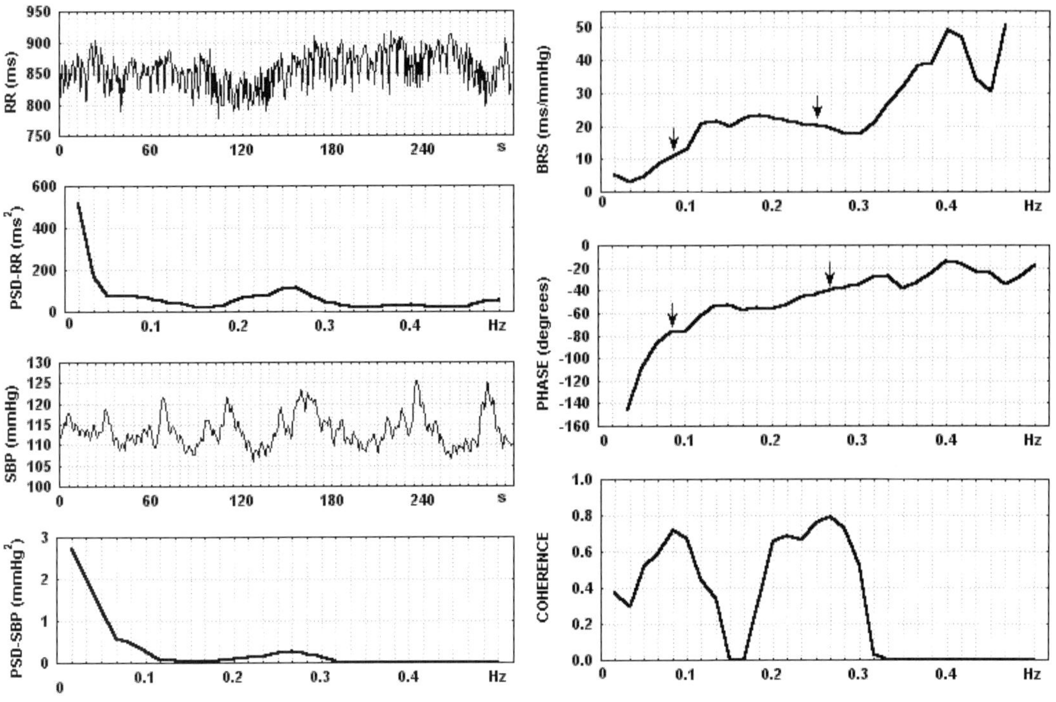
RR (ms)
950
900
850
800
750
0 60 120 180 240 s
PSD-RR (ms^2)
600
400
200
0
0 0.1 0.2 0.3 0.4 Hz
SBP (mmHg)
130
125
120
115
110
105
100
0 60 120 180 240 s
PSD-SBP (mmHg^2)
3
2
1
0
0 0.1 0.2 0.3 0.4 Hz
BRS (ms/mmHg)
50
40
30
20
10
0
0 0.1 0.2 0.3 0.4 Hz
PHASE (degrees)
0
-20
-40
-60
-80
-100
-120
-140
-160
0 0.1 0.2 0.3 0.4 Hz
COHERENCE
1.0
0.8
0.6
0.4
0.2
0.0
0 0.1 0.2 0.3 0.4 Hz

a)

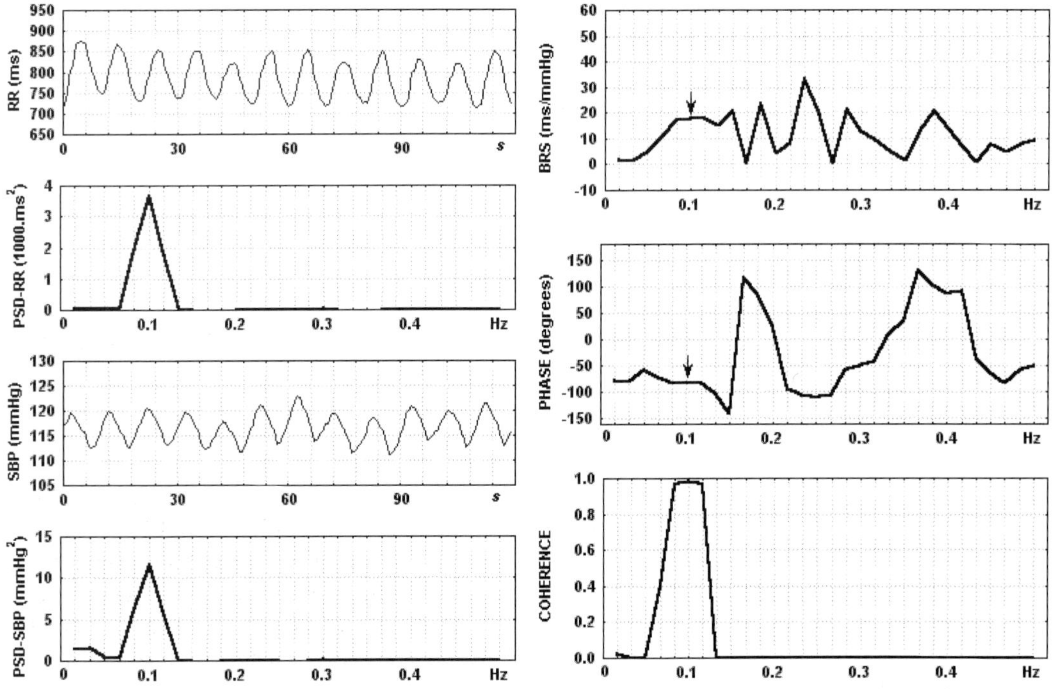
RR (ms)
950
900
850
800
750
700
650
0 30 60 90 s
PSD-RR (1000.ms^2)
4
3
2
1
0
0 0.1 0.2 0.3 0.4 Hz
SBP (mmHg)
130
125
120
115
110
105
0 30 60 90 s
PSD-SBP (mmHg^2)
15
10
5
0
0 0.1 0.2 0.3 0.4 Hz
BRS (ms/mmHg)
60
50
40
30
20
10
0
-10
0 0.1 0.2 0.3 0.4 Hz
PHASE (degrees)
150
100
50
0
-50
-100
-150
0 0.1 0.2 0.3 0.4 Hz
COHERENCE
1.0
0.8
0.6
0.4
0.2
0.0
0 0.1 0.2 0.3 0.4 Hz

b)

1998; Maestri *et al.* 1998; Pitzalis *et al.* 1988). Similarly, these two methods were compared in a group of 31 patients with congestive heart failure (Davies *et al.* 1999).

Others demonstrated reasonable reproducibility of different noninvasive indices of BRS in healthy controls, with coefficient of variation ranging from 25 to 29% (Lord *et al.* 1998). Comparing these indices with the phenylephrine method showed overestimation of the values [bias of low-frequency component of the spectral method 1.17 (0.38–3.6) and that of the Valsalva method 1.13 (0.19–6.7)]. Interestingly, the spectral analysis had the least failure as compared with the phenylephrine method.

The explanation for the above discrepancies between the spectral techniques and the phenylephrine method reflect different nature of the stimulus (i.e. input). Phenylephrine provides a strong stimulus and the derived value of BRS appear to represent the net autonomic output to the heart. In addition, it produces other effects such as direct activation of cardiac parasympathetic nerves, stimulation of vascular α_1 receptors and/or changes in venous compliance (Goldstein *et al.* 1982; Pardini *et al.* 1991). On the contrary, spontaneous oscillation of systolic blood pressure and *RR* intervals seems to be a result of multiple reflexes from the cardiovascular system.

The sequence technique has the advantage of detecting minute-to-minute variability in BRS as it requires only a few seconds of recording for analysis. It also seems to be a more comprehensive index of BRS as it focuses on changes in blood pressure and *RR* interval that may have wider frequency content. Finally, the sequence method allows separate evaluation of BRS during baroreceptor activation or deactivation (Parati *et al.* 1997). Despite some differences between both techniques, both provide similar results when averaged over a time window lasting several minutes (di Rienzo *et al.* 1997a).

Downward tilting

Recently, a technique has been described that evalu-ates BRS during downward tilting from upright back to the supine position (Takahashi *et al.* 1999). Briefly, the method requires passive head-up tilt up to 70° and controlled breathing at 15 breaths/min, with subsequent rapid return to the supine position. BRS measured by the downward tilting was calculated as the slope of the linear regression line relating systolic blood pressure changes to *RR* interval changes. Regression lines with >12 data points and *r* coefficent >0.8 are then selected for analysis. This method provided values that correlated significantly with the phenylephrine method in a group of healthy controls ($r = 0.79$, $P = 0.0003$). However, more experience with the method is needed.

The neck suction

The neck chamber device consists of a box sealed around the neck of the subject that is connected to a suction apparatus. The negative air pressure applied to the chamber results in graded reductions in carotid transmural pressure. However, only carotid baroreceptor function is evaluated, being counterbalanced by the aortic baroreflex. In addition, pressure changes are not fully transmitted through the neck tissues to the carotid baroreceptors and a correction factor is needed. The use of the method is rather cumbersome and requires training of the subject under investigation. Therefore, a simplified variable-pressure paired neck chamber was developed and tested (Raine & Cable 1999). No information is available on clinical utility of this approach.

Fig. 17.2 Examples of *RR* tachograms, corresponding spectra of *RR* intervals (PSD *RR*) together with recording of fluctuations in systolic blood pressure (SBP) and corresponding spectrum of SBP in a healthy volunteer: a) during spontaneous breathing, b) during metronome-controlled ventilation (6 breaths/min – i.e. 0.1 Hz). Right panels show gain (i.e. BRS value), phase and coherence over the whole spectral range. Note remarkable difference between both breathing patterns with shift in spectral power towards 0.1 Hz during controlled ventilation. Arrows in panel a) mark 2 regions with maximum coherence where BRS value is read. In panel b), the arrow indicates the value of BRS taken at 0.1 Hz.

Carotid diameter variations

The stretch-sensitive baroreceptors, which are located in the wall of the bulbus of the internal carotid arteries and in the wall of the aortic arch, are not only sensitive to absolute changes in arterial pressure but also to the rate of pressure change. Therefore, both absolute distension and the rate of cyclic change in distension of the arterial wall influence baroreceptor activity. A noninvasive ultrasound technique has recently been developed that enables determination of end-diastolic diameter and distension over s long time period (Kornet *et al.* 2002). In a group of 10 young subjects, variability in distension rate of the common carotid artery, i.e. increase in diameter during the cardiac cycle per systolic time interval, was a more accurate predictor of *RR* interval variability as compared with variability in systolic arterial finger pressure, conventionally used to evaluate BRS. In addition, the reduced BRS was observed in the elderly in spite of the elimination of the influence of the stiffness of the vessel wall. It remains to be confirmed that variations in signals derived from carotid artery diameter is superior to conventional assessment of signals obtained from peripheral arterial finger pressure.

Conclusion

At present, there is a wide spectrum of noninvasive methods for assessment of BRS available. Some of them are ready to be tested in larger scale trials whether other need to be further evaluated in smaller, well-defined patient populations. In addition, techniques for spontaneous BRS analysis have provided us with valuable data on mechanism of cardiovascular regulation. Recent observation on the correlation of spontaneous BRS with multiple cardiovascular risk factors even suggests that this measure might even constitute a comprehensive marker of the cardiovascular risk status (Lantelme *et al.* 2002).

References

Blaber, A.P., Yamamoto, Y. & Hughson, R.L. (1995) Methodology of spontaneous baroreflex relationship assessed by surrogate data analysis. *American Journal of Physiology*, **268**, H1682–H1687.

Davies, L.C., Colhoun, H., Coats, A.J. *et al.* (2002) A noninvasive measure of baroreflex sensitivity without blood pressure measurement. *American Heart Journal*, **143**, 441–447.

Davies, L.C., Francis, D., Jurak, P. *et al.* (1999) Reproducibility of methods for assessing baroreflex sensitivity in normal controls and in patients with chronic heart failure. *Clinical Science*, **97**, 515–522.

De Boer, R.W., Karemaker, J.M. & Strackee, J. (1987) Hemodynamic fluctuations and baroreflex sensitivity in humans: a beat-to-beat model. *American Journal of Physiology*, **253**, H680–H689.

Goldstein, D.S., Horwitz, D. & Keiser, H.R. (1982) Comparison of techniques for measuring baroreflex sensitivity in man. *Circulation*, **66**, 432–439.

James, M.A., Panerai, R.B. & Potter, J.F. (1998) Applicability of new techniques in the assessment of arterial baroreflex sensitivity in the elderly: a comparison with established pharmacological methods. *Clin. Sci.* **94**, 245–253.

Kautzner, J., Hartikainen, J.E., Camm, A.J. *et al.* (1996) Arterial baroreflex sensitivity assessed from phase IV of the Valsalva manoeuver. *American Journal of Cardiology*, **78**, 575–579.

Kornet, L., Hoeks, A.P., Janssen, B.J., Willigers, J.M. & Reneman, R.S. (2002) Carotid diameter variations as a noninvasive tool to examine cardiac baroreceptor sensitivity. *Journal of Hypertension*, **20**, 1165–1173

Lantelme, P., Khettab, F., Custaud, M.A. *et al.* (2002) Spontaneous baroreflex sensitivity: toward an ideal index of cardiovascular risk in hypertension? *Journal of Hypertension*, **20**, 935–944.

Lord, S.W., Clayton, R.H., Hall, M.C. *et al.* (1998) Reproducibility of three different methods of measuring baroreflex sensitivity in normal subjects [see comments]. *Clinical Science*, **95**, 575–581.

Maestri, R., Pinna, G.D., Mortara, A. *et al.* (1998) Assessing baroreflex sensitivity in post-myocardial infarction patients: comparison of spectral and phenylephrine techniques. *Journal of the American College of Cardiology*, **31**, 344–351.

Omboni, S., Parati, G., Frattola, A. *et al.* (1993) Spectral and sequence analysis of finger blood pressure variability. Comparison with analysis of intra-arterial recordings. *Hypertension*, **22**, 26–33.

Pagani, M., Somers, V., Furlan, R. *et al.* (1988) Changes in autonomic regulation induced by physical training in mild hypertension. *Hypertension*, **12**, 600–610.

Palmero, H.A., Caeiro, T.F., Iosa, D.J. *et al.* (1981) Baroreceptor reflex sensitivity index derived from Phase 4 of the Valsalva manoeuver. *Hypertension*, **3**, 134–137.

Parati, G., Castiglioni, P., di Rienzo, M. *et al.* (1990) Sequential spectral analysis of 24-h blood pressure and pulse interval in humans. *Hypertension*, **16**, 414–421.

Parati, G., Mutti, E., Frattola, A. *et al.* (1994) Beta-adrenergic blocking treatment and 24-h baroreflex sensitivity in essential hypertensive patients. *Hypertension*, **23**, 992–996.

Parati, G., di Rienzo, M., Bonsignore, M.R. *et al.* (1997) Autonomic cardiac regulation in obstructive sleep apnea syndrome: evidence from spontaneous baroreflex analysis during sleep. *Journal of Hypertension*, **15**, 1621–1626.

Pardini, B.J., Lund, D.D. & Schmid, P.G. (1991) Contrasting preganglionic and postganglionic effects of phenylephrine on parasympathetic control of heart rate. *American Journal of Physiology*, **260**, H118–122.

Parlow. J., Viale, J.P., Annat, G. *et al.* (1995) Spontaneous cardiac baroreflex in humans. Comparison with drug-induced responses. *Hypertension*, **25**, 1058–1068.

Pitzalis, M.V., Mastropasqua, F., Passantino, A. *et al.* (1998) Comparison between noninvasive indices of baroreceptor sensitivity and the phenylephrine method in post-myocardial infarction patients. *Circulation*, **97**, 1362–1367.

Raczak, G., la Rovere, M.T., Pinna, G.D. *et al.* (2001) Assessment of baroreflex sensitivity in patients with preserved and impaired left ventricular function by means of the Valsalva manoeuvre and the phenylephrine test. *Clinical Science*, **100**, 33–41.

Raine, N.M. & Cable, N.T. (1999) A simplified paired neck chamber for the demonstration of baroreflex blood pressure regulation. *American Journal of Physiology*, **277**, S60–S66.

di Rienzo, M. Bertinieri, G., Mancia, G. & Pedotti, A. (1985) A new method for evaluating the baroreflex role by a joint pattern analysis of pulse interval and systolic blood pressure series. *Medical & Biological Engineering & Computing*, **23**, 313–314.

di Rienzo, M., Castiglioni, P., Mancia, G. *et al.* (1997a) Critical appraisal of indices for the assessment of baroreflex sensitivity. *Methods of Information in Medicine*, **36**, 246–249.

di Rienzo, M., Parati, G., Mancia, G. *et al.* (1997b) Investigating baroreflex control of circulation using signal processing techniques. *IEEE Engineering in Medicine & Biology Magazine*, **16**, 86–95.

Robbe, H.W., Mulder, L.J., Ruddel, H. *et al.* (1987) Assessment of baroreceptor reflex sensitivity by means of spectral analysis. *Hypertension*, **10**, 538–543.

Rostagno, C., Felici, M., Caciolli, S. *et al.* (1999) Decreased baroreflex sensitivity assessed from phase IV of Valsalva manoeuver in mild congestive heart failure. *Angiology*, **50**, 655–664.

Rostagno, C., Galanti, G., Felici, M.,*et al.* (2000) Prognostic value of baroreflex sensitivity assessed by phase IV of Valsalva manoeuvre in patients with mild-to-moderate heart failure. *European Journal of Heart Failure*, **2**, 41–45.

Rowell, L.B. (1993) Reflex control during orthostasis. In: *Human Cardiovascular Control* (ed. L. B. Rowell), pp. 37–77. Oxford University Press, New York.

Smith, M.L., Beightol, L.A., Fritsch-Yelle, J.M. *et al.* (1996) Valsalva's manoeuver revisited: a quantitative method yielding insights into human autonomic control. *American Journal of Physiology*, **271**, 1240–1249.

Smith, S.A., Stallard, T.J., Salih, M.M. *et al.* (1987) Can sinoaortic baroreceptor heart rate reflex sensitivity be determined from phase IV of the Valsalva manoeuvre? *Cardiovascular Research*, **21**, 422–427.

Smyth, H.S., Sleight, P. & Pickering, G.W. (1969) Reflex regulation of arterial pressure during sleep in man: a quantitative method of assessing baroreflex sensitivity. *Circulation Research*, **24**, 109–121.

Takahashi, N., Nakagawa, M., Saikawa, T. *et al.* (1999) Noninvasive assessment of the cardiac baroreflex: response to downward tilting and comparison with the phenylephrine method. *Journal of the American College of Cardiology*, **34**, 211–215.

Watkins, L.L., Grossman, P. & Sherwood, A. (1996) Noninvasive assessment of baroreflex control in borderline hypertension. Comparison with the phenylephrine method. *Hypertension*, **28**, 238–243.

CHAPTER 18

Analysis of the Interactions Between Heart Rate and Blood Pressure Variabilities

Sergio Cerutti, Guiseppe Baselli, Anna M. Bianchi, Luca T. Mainardi and Alberto Porta

Introduction

The contemporaneous analysis of *RR* interval (or equivalently heart rate) and of arterial pressure (*AP*) short-term variabilities yields information far beyond the separate analysis of both variability signals (Akselrod *et al.* 1985; De Boer *et al.* 1985; Baselli *et al.* 1986). The reason is in the physiological interactions which govern the temporal relationships of the two variables. Conversely, the difficulty and multiplicity of approaches is related to the interpretation of underlying mechanisms considered (Koepchen 1984; Baselli *et al.* 1995, 2002b).

Observing the two variability signals over a period of few minutes (few hundreds of beats), it is usually noted the presence in both of them of fast fluctuations synchronous with respiration representing a high frequency (HF) spectral component (0.25–0.3 Hz in humans at rest) and slower waves at low frequency (LF, around 0.1 Hz in humans). Both fluctuations are largely irregular and are also blurred by even slower changes which contribute to a very low frequency component (VLF, below 0.03 Hz) not characterized by a defined spectral peak; analyses over long periods, up to 24 h, reveal the $1/f$ nature of the slow fluctuations (Kobayashi & Musha 1982).

The challenge is in trying to disentangle quantitative information from this superposition of irregularly cyclical changes and connect it to the reflex responses studied in physiological experiments or in invasive clinical tests. The latter ones address transient responses with clear input–output relationships; in contrast, spontaneous variability is the result of closed loop interactions (Akselrod *et al.* 1985; Baselli *et al.* 1988) and distributed driving effects (Baselli *et al.* 2002b).

RR and *AP* are in a closed loop formed by the feed-forward mechanical effects of *RR* changes on *AP* and by the neural feedbacks elicited by baroreflex mechanisms. The former branch of the loop is intrinsically twofold: (1) an increase of *RR* duration augments diastolic runoff and decreases the diastolic value at the end of the heart period; (2) the same *RR* change can, in contrast, increase the left ventricular filling and consequently next pulse pressure. The resulting systolic *AP* (*SAP*) is thus the sum of the two effects, most often with a prevalence of the former negative term.

The recognition of this almost immediate mechanical action is complicated by dynamics lasting several beats because the *AP* change following a *RR* change perturbs the vascular side of the system and its control mechanisms. A first-order effect is simply related to the inertia of the arterial windkessel, that displays a time constant longer than a single cardiac cycle. Also, the activation of *AP* control mechanisms, mainly the baroreflex modulation of peripheral resistances, prolongs the tail of any perturbation. These effects are lumped into an *AP–AP* loop in parametric models.

The feedback side of the loop, attains to the *RR* changes elicited by arterial baroreflex mechanisms in response to *AP* changes. Mainly negative feedback responses are activated by the baroreceptors in the aortic arch and carotid sinuses; however, this reflex is integrated with and modulated by the activation of diffused receptors and sympathetic afferences, as those experimentally revealed in the abdominal aorta (Malliani *et al.* 1986). Reflex *RR* changes are usually related to *SAP* changes both in classical invasive tests and also in the analysis methods and models of the spontaneous variability considered in this chapter; therefore, in the following the beat-by-beat series of only *SAP* values is referred to.

The efferent pathways to the sinus node are composed by the opposite action of both vagal (accelerating) and sympathetic (decelerating) fibres; however, vagal modulation is thought to explain a larger part of the *RR* variability amplitude as this is dramatically reduced in conditions of vagal inhibition and tachycardia. A cholinergic response to vagal activation is started in a very short-term and is able to prolong the very same *RR* interval in which it takes place with a rapidly decaying effect over the next beats. In contrast, a sluggish response of β-adrenergic receptors to sympathetic activation is usually described as a low pass filter with a cut frequency slightly above 0.1 Hz, thus justifying a relative insensitivity of sympathetic modulation to HF.

Once the closed loop interaction is acknowledged, the problem of recognizing the inputs by which the loop is perturbed becomes of primary importance in order to disentangle the feed-forward and feed-back branches of the loop. Indeed, in presence of a drive univocally concentrated on *SAP*, the *RR*/*SAP* relationships would be completely determined by the baroreceptive feedback while the opposite condition would reveal the sole feed-forward pathway. In fact, a mixed situation is usually found. Respiratory activity is one of the most relevant disturbances inducing cardiovascular variability. It enters on *SAP* through changes in stroke volume and also on *RR* through cardiopulmonary reflexes. In addition, a disturbance of the baroreceptors (via a dependence of aortic transmural pressure on thoracic pressure) elicits both reflexes affecting *SAP* and the *RR*. Vasomotor activity can introduce disturbances on *SAP* while central drives may affect both the vascular side and the heart side of the loop.

In the following section various methods for the analysis of *RR*/*SAP* interactions will be revisited having in mind the simple statements recalled above, which can help in choosing time to time the most appropriate approach and also indicate the physiological components contributing to the quantities extracted.

Frequency-domain approaches

A joint analysis in the frequency domain addresses cross-spectral features in addition to the spectral features provided by a separate analysis. The latter ones are described by the spectra $S_{rr}(f)$ and $S_{sap}(f)$ of *RR* and *SAP* respectively, which are real functions of the frequency f and express the power spectral density in [s^2/Hz] and [$mmHg^2$/Hz] respectively.

The cross spectrum $C(f) = |C(f)| \exp(j\varphi(f))$ is a complex function. The cross-spectral amplitude, $|C(f)|$ in [s mmHg/Hz], depends on the power exchanged in each bandwidth. This can be better appreciated by introducing the squared coherence function $K^2(f)$, which at each frequency is an index between 0 and 1 of the amount of squared correlation: the relationship $|C(f)|^2 = K(f)^2 \; S_{rr}(f) \; S_{sap}(f)$ indicates that the squared modulus is the product of both spectral densities cleaned off the contribution of uncorrelated effects (noise or other interactions). As shown in Fig. 18.1, high squared coherence values, above 0.5, are commonly found in both LF and HF bands (De Boer *et al.* 1985).

The phase spectrum $\varphi(f)$, indicates the phase relationships in the range −≠ to +≠ rad or −180° to 180°. Adopting the convention of positive phases for a leading *RR*, negative phases are often found. Unfortunately, these are not easily put in relation with a single branch of the closed loop interaction as they are in accordance both with a *SAP* maximum leading an *RR* maximum (reflex bradycardia) and with an *RR* maximum leading a *SAP* minimum (mechanical negative effect).

Indeed spectral and cross-spectral features derive from all interactions and inputs of *RR* and *SAP*. However, in some conditions and bands, changes in amplitude relationships were shown to parallel changes in baroreceptive gain, thus providing useful clinical indexes, though with consistent biases. These approaches assume that, at LF or both at LF and HF, variability is mainly driven by *SAP*; consequently, sinus arrhythmia is largely a consequence of baroreceptive response. If this simplified hypothesis is modelled as a closed loop in which all inputs are directed pri-

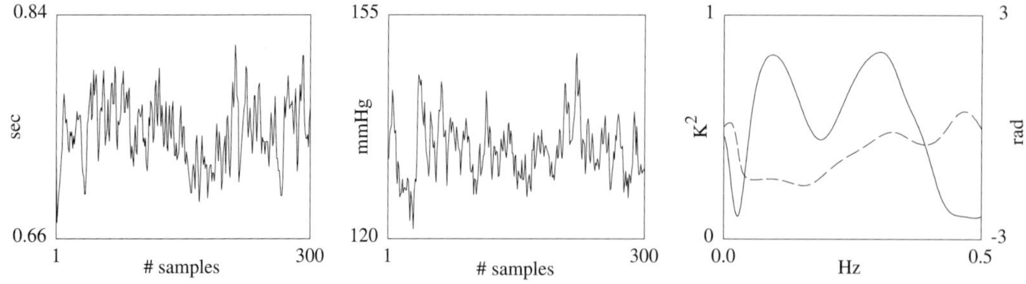

Fig. 18.1 Example of *RR* interval (left panel) and systolic arterial pressure (*SAP*) series (middle panel) in a healthy human subject at rest. The squared coherence (solid line) and phase (dashed line) derived via bivariate autoregressive analysis are shown in the right panel. Coherence exhibits two clear peaks (at low and high frequencies). Phase is negative at low frequency (*RR* interval lags behind *SAP* series) and about zero at high frequency.

marily on *SAP*, then an estimate of the feedback branch transfer function is given by the square root of the spectral ratio, $(S_{rr}(f)/S_{sap}(f))^{1/2}$. If it is assumed an open loop effect of *SAP* over an *RR* blurred with noise, then the classical open loop transfer function estimate is applied, $C(f)/S_{sap}(f)$. It is easily shown that the latter index (based on the cross-spectrum) is equal to the former one (based on the spectral ratio) times $K(f)$, with a minimum difference whenever coherence is high (Baselli *et al.* 1995).

These functions are usually averaged over a bandwidth of interest (or, almost equivalently, are based on spectral components centred on a specific frequency) thus obtaining gain indexes with the dimension of [s/mmHg] (the unit of ms/mmHg is classically employed). The spectral ratio has been used both in the HF and LF band, while the cross-spectral method was originally proposed for the LF band assuming a vasomotor origin of these oscillations (Robbe *et al.* 1987). Nonetheless, attempts to estimate the whole transfer function shape have been carried out in presence of broad band inputs, e.g. introduced by a randomly paced respiration (Saul *et al.* 1996)

Parametric models

The irregular features of spontaneous cardiovascular variabilities, which confound the search for precise patterns and oscillations, are on the contrary exploited by the identification methods of parametric models. An unexpected change due to whatever input represents the *innovation* of the process which permit to disentangle the elements of the described interactions.

A general purpose approach, is provided by a bivariate autoregressive (AR) model:

$$sap(i) = \sum_{k=1}^{p} h_{sap-sap,k} \cdot sap(i-k) + \sum_{k=1}^{p} h_{sap-rr,k} \cdot rr(i-k) + w_{sap}(i), \quad (1)$$

$$rr(i) = \sum_{k=1}^{p} h_{rr-rr,k} \cdot rr(i-k) + \sum_{k=0}^{p} h_{rr-sap,k} \cdot sap(i-k) + w_{rr}(i), \quad (2)$$

where $h_{sap\text{-}sap,k}$ represents the linear regression parameter of a *SAP* value at beat (*i*) over the value preceding by (*k*) beats; $h_{sap\text{-}rr,k}$ is the regression parameter of the *RR* interval preceding by (*k*) beats, and so on. The parameters are easily identified from *SAP* and *RR* series via the least squares. Akaike's information criterion or similar figures of merit are applied to optimise the model order. The residuals (alias input noises) w_{sap} and w_{rr} must be tested to be white and uncorrelated, otherwise the model order *p* has to be increased. Their variance matrix $\boldsymbol{W} = \mathbf{Var}\ |w_{sap}\ w_{rr}|$ should result to be diagonal in accordance with the presence of an immediate relationship inserted in the *RR*/*SAP* loop; i.e. parameter $h_{rr\text{-}sap,0}$ describing baroreceptive responses faster than one beat. This is the configuration (canonical form) that best fits the physiological problem; however, the canonical form with no immediate effect and a non-diagonal $\boldsymbol{W}$ finds a general-purpose application, when causal effects are not directly addressed (see next paragraph).

The bivariate AR is formed by two ARX (AR

with eXogenous input) single output models: eqn 1, *SAP* determined by *SAP* past values (AR part) and *RR* past values (X part); eqn 2, *RR* determined by past *RR* and *SAP* values. So, (if the hypothesis of uncorrelated residuals is verified) the former relationships disentangle the mechanical feed-forward effects, while the latter provides an estimate of the baroreceptive feedback dynamics and gain.

Spectral and cross-spectral analysis is obtained as a by-product of parametric identification:

$$\boldsymbol{S}(f)=\begin{vmatrix} S_{sap}(f) & C(f) \\ C(f) & S_{rr}(f) \end{vmatrix}=\left|\boldsymbol{H}(z)\boldsymbol{W}\,\boldsymbol{H}(z)^{\mathrm{H}}\right|_{z=e^{j2\pi f}}, \quad (3)$$

where $\boldsymbol{H}(z)$ is the transfer function matrix from the input noises to the signals ($\boldsymbol{H}(z)^{\mathrm{H}}$ is its hermitian, z^{-1} is the one-lag operator),

$$\boldsymbol{H}(z)=\begin{vmatrix} 1-\sum_k h_{sap-sap,k}\cdot z^{-k} & -\sum_k h_{sap-rr,k}\cdot z^{-k} \\ -\sum_k h_{rr-sap,k}\cdot z^{-k} & 1-\sum_k h_{rr-rr,k}\cdot z^{-k} \end{vmatrix}^{-1}. \quad (4)$$

The bivariate AR model is appealing for many reasons: it is of general use, easily identifiable, easily extended to time variant applications (see next paragraph). However, it suffers several simplifications in relation to the complex interactions introduced above: (1) all oscillation sources are lumped into the loop described by the bivariate auto-regression (technically, in the poles of the bivariate AR model determinant), even those clearly external to the *SAP/RR* interactions such as respiratory frequency or vasomotor waves; (2) correlations between *SAP* and *RR* owing to inputs (e.g. respiration) acting independently on them is attributed again to the AR interactions. As a result all reflexes impinging on *RR* variability are put together in this type of estimate and generically classified as baroreflex.

More complex though identifiable structures have been proposed. The need to overcome the former limitation requires to introduce an autoregression over the residuals *before* they are fed to the *SAP/RR* interaction; thus, coloured residuals are considered (u_{sap} and u_{rr} for *SAP* and *RR* respectively), which are allowed to convey oscillations described by their own AR poles (in parametric models a spectral peak corresponding to an oscillation is described by a pair of complex conjugate poles). This leads to ARXAR (alias dynamic adjustment) family of models, where the trailing AR refers to the residuals. The latter drawback is considerably limited if it is possible to utilise a respiration signal (thoracic movements, volume, flow etc.); this adds not only information about respiratory interactions but also permits a better assessment of the real *SAP/RR* interactions. A common exogenous input is added to the joint *SAP/RR* process and becomes a second exogenous input to each branch of the closed loop model:

$$sap(i)=\sum_{k=1}^{p}h_{sap-sap,k}\cdot sap(i-k)+h_{sap-rr,1}\cdot rr(i-1)$$
$$+\sum_{k=0}^{p}h_{sap-resp,k}\cdot resp(i-k)+u_{sap}(i), \quad (5)$$

$$u_{sap}(i)=\sum_{k=1}^{p}h_{usap-usap,k}\cdot u_{sap}(i-k)+w_{sap}(i), \quad (6)$$

$$rr(i)=\sum_{k=0}^{p}h_{rr-sap,k}\cdot sap(i-k)$$
$$+\sum_{k=0}^{p}h_{rr-resp,k}\cdot resp(i-k)+u_{rr}(i), \quad (7)$$

$$u_{rr}(i)=\sum_{k=1}^{p}h_{urr-urr,k}\cdot u_{rr}(i-k)+w_{rr}(i). \quad (8)$$

It can be noted that the *SAP* prediction model (eqns. 5 and 6) develops a full ARXXAR structure: AR recursion of *SAP* (vascular control mechanisms); *RR* seen as eXogenous input to this branch of the closed loop (mechanical effects); respiration (resp) as true eXogenous input (vascular effects of breathing); the AR coloured residual u_{sap} (possible vascular oscillations).

The symmetric branch for *RR* prediction (eqns. 7 and 8) has a simpler XXAR structure: *SAP* seen as eXogenous input to *RR* (baroreflex); eXogenous input of respiration (non-baroreflex respiratory sinus arrhythmia); u_{RR} coloured residual (other rhythms modulating the sinus node). No recursion on *RR* is considered in eqn. 7; however, recently (Porta *et al.* 2003) the addition of a limited first order recursion on *RR* has been explored, which describes the intrinsic memory of the sinus node lumping the effects of the fast cholinergic and slow adrenergic washouts.

The identification of eqns. 5–8, plus an identification of *resp*(i) as AR process, provides a spectral decomposition of both *sap*(i) and *rr*(i) into partial spectra due to $u_{sap}(i)$, $u_{rr}(i)$, and *resp*(i) respectively. In fact, provided that the residuals

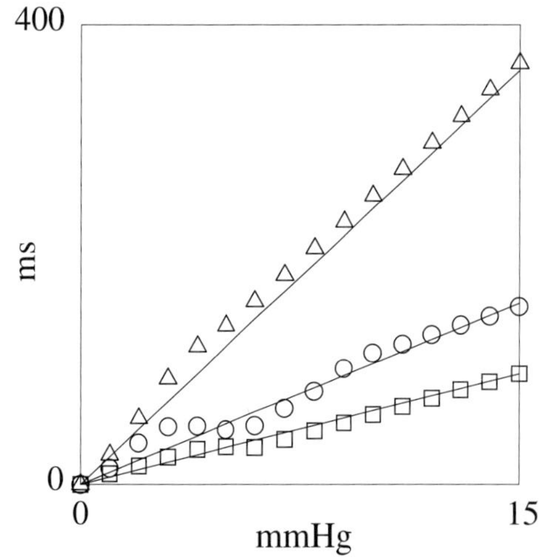

Fig. 18.2 Responses of the *RR/SAP* block to a unitary ramp simulating a pressure rise in open loop X, XAR and XXAR models (triangles, circles and squares respectively). The coefficients of *RR/SAP* blocks are identified from series derived from a dog at control. Also the linear fitting is reported, the slope of which is taken as a measure of the baroreflex gain (24, 10.5 and 6.4 ms/mmHg in X, XAR and XXAR, respectively).

(including the residual of respiration model) are uncorrelated, partial spectra are obtained as the squared modulus of the transfer function from the residual to the signal scaled by the residual variance (see Baselli *et al.* 1995 for details).

The XXAR model of *RR* prediction from *SAP* and respiration was validated on human data in its capability to selectively address the arterial baroreceptive response disentangled by cardiopulmonary reflexes (Lucini *et al.* 2000), thus addressing the main control mechanisms originating from high pressure and low pressure areas. The degradation in performance when respiration is not available (XAR structure) and also when no coloured residual is considered (X structure) was analysed in detail (Porta *et al.* 2000a); the example of Fig. 18.2, shows the increased bias of baroreceptive gain estimate passing from the complete to the simplified models due to *RR* variability components not disentangled from the true arterial baroreflex.

When only the baroreflex mechanisms are addressed, the identification of the feed-forward parameters (eqn. 1 for the bivariate AR or eqn 5 for the ARXAR) can be omitted acting as if the interactions relevant to *RR* modulation (eqn 2 for the bivariate AR or eqn 7 for the ARXAR) were in an open loop (Nollo *et al.* 2001; Baselli *et al.* 2002b). Identification results are similar to those of a full identification, as none of the constraints relevant to the direction of causal interactions is relaxed; simply, it is not possible to verify the whiteness and uncorrelation of both the residuals; therefore a correct model order should have already been determined by a previous study considering the whole model.

Time–frequency analyses

Many pathological and physiological phenomena are characterized by time-variant *RR/SAP* relationships: cardiac ischaemic episodes, effects of drug infusion, stress responses, syncope; so, it is required to assess the dynamical changes occurring in spectral parameters (Keselbrener & Akselrod 1996; Akay 1998; Akselrod *et al.* 2001) as well as in coherence, in baroreflex and mechanical gains, and in phase relationships (Bianchi *et al.* 1993; Novak *et al.* 1993; Pola *et al.* 1996; Mainardi *et al.* 2002).

The bivariate model structure presented in relation (1) and (2) can be recursively estimated according to the following relations:

$$
\begin{aligned}
&\Theta(i)=\Theta(i-1)+\boldsymbol{C}(i)\varepsilon^{T}(i)\\
&\boldsymbol{C}(i)=\boldsymbol{P}(i)\Theta(i)\\
&\varepsilon^{T}(i)=\boldsymbol{Y}^{T}(i)-\Phi^{T}(i)\Theta(i-1)\\
&\boldsymbol{P}(i)=\frac{1}{\mu}\left\{\boldsymbol{P}(i-1)-\frac{\boldsymbol{P}(i-1)\Phi(i)\Phi^{T}(i)\boldsymbol{P}(i-1)}{\mu+\Phi^{T}(i)\boldsymbol{P}(i-1)\Phi(i)}\right\}
\end{aligned}
\tag{9}
$$

where $\boldsymbol{Y}(i)=|sap(i)\ \ rr(i)|^{T}$ and where

$$
\Theta(i)=\left|\begin{matrix} h_{sap-sap,1}(i) & h_{sap+rr,1}(i) & \cdots \\ h_{rr-sap,1}(i) & h_{rr-rr,1}(i) & \cdots \end{matrix}\right.
\left.\begin{matrix} \cdots & h_{sap-sap,p}(i) & h_{sap-rr,p}(i) \\ \cdots & h_{rr-sap,p}(i) & h_{rr-rr,p}(i) \end{matrix}\right|^{T}
\tag{10}
$$

is a [2p × 2] matrix containing the model parameters h (note that the canonical form with no immediate effect is here considered), $\boldsymbol{P}(i)$[2p × 2p], is the inverse of the p-th order cross-correlation matrix of the two signals; the observation matrix $\Phi(i)$[2p × 1] contains the last p samples of the signals. Figure 18.3 shows the block diagram of the recursive estimation procedure.

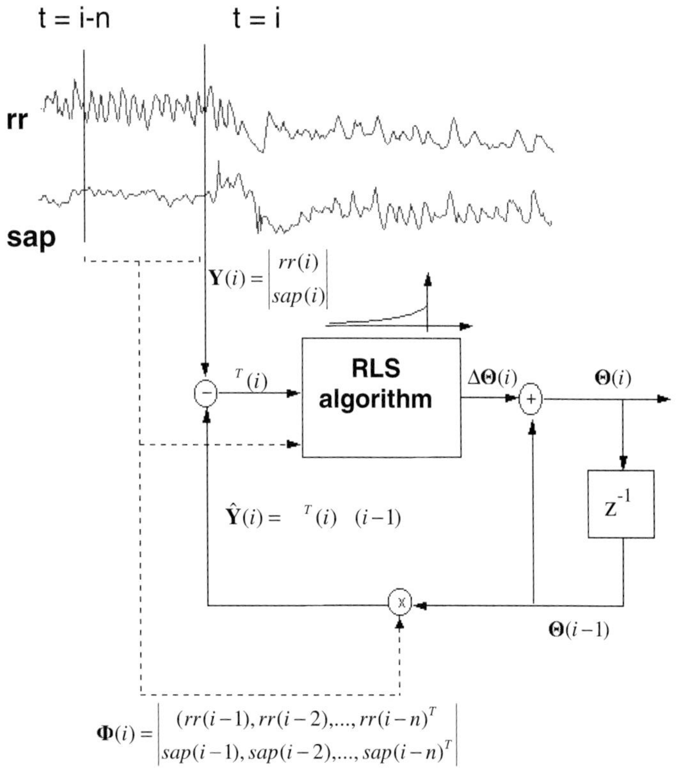

Fig. 18.3 Block diagram of the bivariate recursive identification procedure. The vector of the actual model parameters Θ(*i*) is obtained by adding an innovation term ΔΘ(*i*) to the parameters evaluated at the previous step, Θ(*i*-1). The innovation is calculated by properly weighing the prediction error $\varepsilon(i) = \mathbf{Y}(i) - \Phi^T(i)\Theta(i-1)$ where $\Phi^T(i)$ is the observation matrix containing data from time $t = i$, backward to time $t = i - p$ (p is the model order). In the example shown in the figure, the signals are *rr* and *sap*.

At time (*i*), the model parameters are updated by summing an innovation term calculated by weighing the prediction error vector ε(*i*) by a proper gain **C**(*i*)[2p×1], which is also updated sample by sample. The forgetting factor μ performs an exponential decay on the previous error terms and makes the model able to track non-stationarities in the signals (Soderstrom and Stoica 1989; Bittanti *et al.* 1994a; Bittanti *et al.* 1994b).

AR parameters in Θ(*i*), permit to update a joint spectral estimate at each time sample (*i*) (see eqns 3 and 4 with time variant parameters) thus obtaining a time-frequency description **S**(*i*, *f*). In the following example the description and the application are limited to the bivariate case, and is employed for describing the interrelationships between *RR* and *SAP* series during an episode of vaso-vagal syncope.

Syncope events are episodes of sudden loss of consciousness and fainting and may be artificially induced in inclined subjects by prolonged passive tilting, probably due to an alteration in autonomic control leading to an abnormal vasovagal reflex. Figure 18.4 shows the *RR* (a) and *SAP* (b) series during a tilting manoeuvre (T), that led to a syncope (S). In correspondence of the syncope a failure in the cardiovascular control is clearly testified by the dramatic drop of *SAP*, associated with an increased bradycardia. A time-variant analysis (Novak *et al.* 1995; Mainardi *et al.* 1997; Furlan *et al.* 1998) permits to assess transient modifications in the *SAP*/*RR* before the beginning of the episode. Panel (c) shows the contour plot of the time variant squared coherence $K^2(i,f) = |C(i,f)|^2/S_{rr}(i,f)\,S_{sap}(i,f)$ function obtained from the time-variant cross-spectral analysis: before the onset of the syncope the coherence between the signals decreases testifying a diminished loop regulation. A detail of the time course of spectral and derived parameters is shown in Fig. 18.5. In particular in Fig. 18.5(b) the $K^2(i,f)$ function, evaluated in the LF band, is characterized by a notch before the syncope, in correspondence of which the spectral baroreceptive gain at LF (Fig. 18.5c) assumes a lower value that is maintained up to the syncope.

The results described in Mainardi *et al.* (1997)

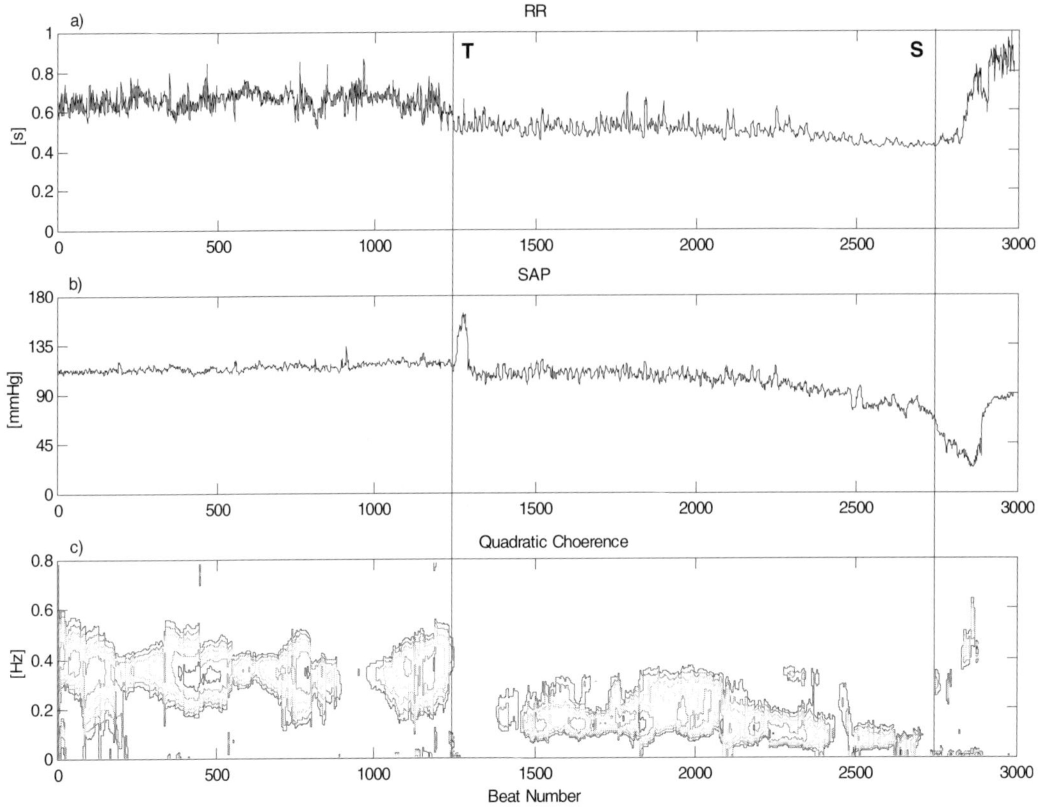

Fig. 18.4 Example of variability signal obtained during a syncope event induced by a tilting manoeuvre. *rr* is shown in (a), while *sap* is shown in (b); (c) represents the contour plot of the squared coherence function evaluated through a bivariate time-variant model: the time is on the horizontal axis, the frequency is on the vertical one, while the coherence values are represented as isocontour maps. The T marks the time instant in which the subject passed from rest to tilt position, while S marks the beginning of the syncope. During the resting condition the signals are characterized by high values of coherence in the HF frequency range. After tilting the coherence becomes high in the LF frequency range, but in the time interval before the beginning of the syncope, the coherence between signals is strongly decreased and goes below the significant level.

put into evidence that the withdrawal of sympathetic drive on pressure precedes the vagal reflex on heart. The coherence index confirms a lowered interaction in the regulation of heart and vessels. This is also confirmed by the decrease in $\alpha_{LF}(i) = (S_{rr}(i,\text{LF})/S_{sap}(i,\text{LF}))^{1/2}$ that is another index of the separation between cardiac and vascular control.

Other authors (Novak *et al.* 1995) evidenced a decrease in the VLF component in the range 0.02–0.05 Hz and gave the interpretation of an early sign of central inhibitory vasodepressor reflex, resulting in an inhibition of the baroreflex through negative feedback loops, in accordance with a decreased sympathetic discharge recorded on microneurography.

Nonlinear analysis

Coherence function is widely utilized to evaluate the degree of correlation between two signals as a function of frequency. It ranges from 0 (null correlation) to 1 (perfect correlation). Unfortunately, this tool has some drawbacks when nonlinear interactions between signals are present. For example, if the two signals are 1:2 locked (perfect coupling), their power spectra exhibit dominant peaks at different frequencies (i.e. f^* and $f^*/2$ respectively) and the coherence function may be close to zero at those frequencies. In order to overcome this limitation measures of information exchange are proposed (Hoyer *et al.* 1998; Palus *et al.* 1998; Schafer *et al.* 1998;

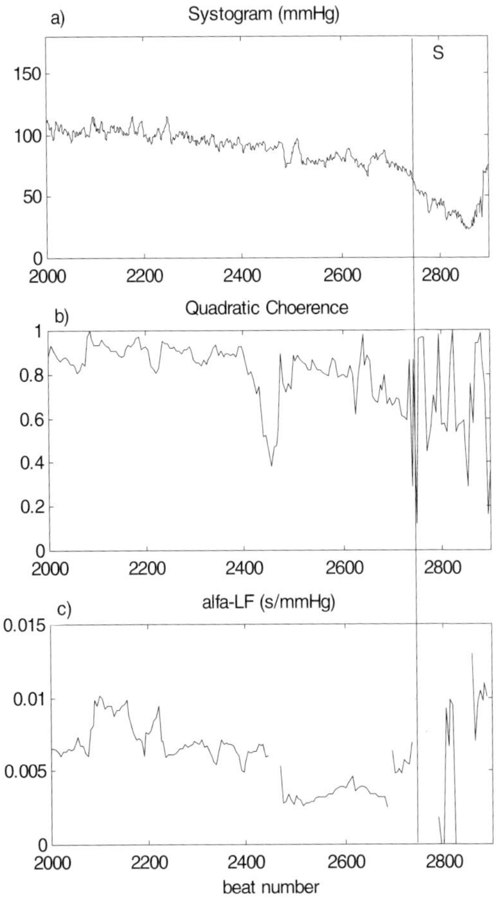

Fig. 18.5 Detail of analyses shown in Fig. 18.4 corresponding to the syncope event: (a) *sap* series; (b) maximum value of the squared coherence function in the LF band; (c) baroreceptive alfa gain in LF band. The signal and the parameters are plotted after the tilting manoeuvre, up to the syncope. After beat *n*. 2400 we can see a decrease in the coherence function, which was very close to 1 in the preceding time interval. At the same time the alfa gain is abruptly reduced.

Porta *et al.* 1999; Baselli *et al.* 2002a). Indexes of information exchange such as cross-conditional entropy and mutual information are based on the probability distribution of patterns involving both signals. The assessment of specific *RR/SAP* patterns, e.g. sequences of contemporaneous pressure rise and cardiac deceleration connected with baroreflex responses (Bertinieri *et al.* 1985), has a long tradition in the time domain analysis of variability. An information domain analysis, rather than searching for an a-priori defined type of sequence, addresses the presence of *any* repetitive pattern. As an example here we consider the measure of synchronization proposed by Porta *et al.* (1999). It is based on the evaluation of the normalized cross-conditional entropy (Fig. 18.6). Given the pair of signals $rr(i)$ and $sap(i)$, the cross-conditional entropy $NCCE_{rr/sap}$ evaluates the amount of information carried by the current sample of *RR*, $rr(i)$, when a pattern of (L-1) samples of *SAP* (i.e. $sap_{L-1}(i) = |sap(i) \ldots sap(i-L+2)|$) is known. Similarly also $NCCE_{sap/rr}$ can be calculated, thus evaluating the information exchange in the reverse causal direction. $NCCE_{rr/sap}$ and $NCCE_{sap/rr}$ are used to derive indexes of synchronization fixing the causal direction of the influences ($\chi_{rr/sap}$ and $\chi_{sap/rr}$) and the index $\chi_{rr,sap} = \max(\chi_{rr/sap}, \chi_{sap/rr})$ is proposed as a global index of synchronization beyond causality (Porta *et al.* 1999). Special care should be paid in estimating these indexes when short segments of data are considered and corrective terms are necessary to avoid the consequent underestimate of the cross-conditional entropy. Three main advantages are provided by this approach: (1) the extraction of indexes taking into account both linear and nonlinear interactions (i.e. $\chi_{rr,sap}$, $\chi_{rr/sap}$ and $\chi_{sap/rr}$); (2) the calculation, in addition to a global index of synchronization ($\chi_{rr,sap}$), of indexes strictly related to specific causal direction ($\chi_{rr/sap}$ and $\chi_{sap/rr}$); (3) the detection of nonlinear interactions via a surrogate data approach (Palus 1997). These indexes have allowed us to find out that the global index of synchronization between *sap* and *rr* increased during tilt (Porta *et al.*, 2000b), the nonlinear interactions between *sap* and *rr* gained importance after myocardial infarction and the information exchange along the baroreflex path decreased while that along the mechanical path increased in old healthy subjects (Nollo *et al.* 2002).

Conclusion

A variety of approaches can be applied to the analysis of the interactions between *RR* and *AP* variabilities, in accordance with the high complexity of the underlying physiological mechanisms, the different pathophysiological conditions and the specific clinical purposes. In this chapter an effort has been devoted in proposing the basic elements of different methods and

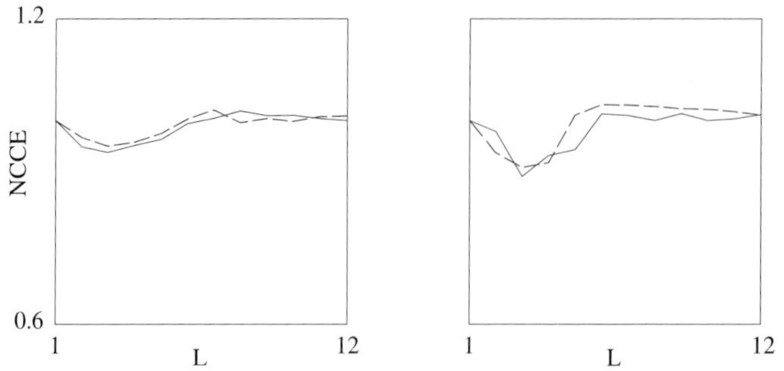

Fig. 18.6 Normalized cross-conditional entropy (NCCE) from *sap* to *rr* (dashed line) and from *rr* to *sap* (solid line) in a healthy human subject at rest (left panel) and during 90° head-up tilt (right panel). The synchronization indexes $\chi_{rr/sap}$ and $\chi_{sap/rr}$ are equal to 5.1 and 6.2 at rest while they are 9.2 and 10.9 during tilt. The indexes are similar along opposite causal directions (this is not true after recent myocardial infarction). The global index of synchronization $\chi_{rr,sap}$ is obtained as $\max(\chi_{rr/sap}, \chi_{sap/rr})$. During tilt, *rr* and *sap* series are more coupled.

in disclosing their potentials and limits having in mind the related modelling of physiological interactions. In this perspective, the availability of many algorithms for data processing and feature extraction can be fully exploited in order to gain flexibility and insight depth.

References

Akay, M. (1998) *Time Frequency and Wavelets in Biomedical Signal Processing*. IEEE Press, New York.

Akselrod, S., Barak, Y., Ben-Dov, Y., Keselbrener, L. & Baharav A. (2001) Estimation of autonomic response based on individually determined time axis. *Autonomic Neuroscience Basic & Clinical*, **90**, 13–23.

Akselrod, S., Gordon, D., Madwed, J. B., Snidman, N. C., Shannon, D. C. & Cohen, R. J. (1985) Hemodynamic regulation: investigation by spectral analysis. *American Journal of Physiology*, **249** (4 Pt 2), H867–H875.

Baselli, G., Cerutti, S., Civardi, S. *et al.* (1986) Spectral and cross-spectral analysis of heart rate and arterial blood pressure variability signals. *Computers and Biomedical Research*, **19** (6), 520–534.

Baselli, G., Cerutti, S., Civardi, S., Malliani, A. & Pagani, M. (1988) Cardiovascular variability signals: towards the identification of a closed-loop model of the neural control mechanisms. *IEEE (Institute of Electrical and Electronic Engineers) Transactions on Biomedical Engineering*, **35** (12), 1033–1046.

Baselli, G., Porta, A. & Ferrari G. (1995) Models for the analysis of cardiovascular variability signals. In: *Heart Rate Variability* (eds M. Malik & A. J. Camm), pp. 135–145. Futura Publishing, Armonk, NY.

Baselli, G., Cerutti, S., Porta, A. & Signorini, M. G. (2002a) Short and long term nonlinear analysis of *RR* variability series. *Medical Engineering & Physics*, **24**, 21–32.

Baselli, G., Caiani, E, Porta, A., Montano, N., Signorini, M. G. & Cerutti, S. (2002b) Biomedical signal processing and modelling in cardiovascular system. *Critical Reviews in Biomedical Engineering*, **30**, 57–87

Bertinieri, G., di Rienzo, M., Cavallazzi, A., Ferrari, A. U., Pedotti, A. & Mancia, G. (1985) A new approach to analysis of the arterial baroreflex. *Journal of Hypertension*, **3**, S79-S81.

Bianchi, A. M., Mainardi, L., Petrucci, E., Signorini, M. G., Mainardi, M. & Cerutti, S. (1993) Time-variant power spectrum analysis for the detection of transient episodes in HRV signal. *IEEE (Institute of Electrical and Electronic Engineers) Transactions on Biomedical Engineering*, **40** (2) 136–144

Bittanti, S. & Campi, M (1994a) Least squares identification of autoregressive models with time-varying parameters. In: *Decision and Control, Proceedings of the 33rd IEEE Conference*, Vol. 4, pp. 3610–3611.

Bittanti, S. & Campi, M. (1994b) Bounded error identification of time-varying parameters by RLS techniques. *IEEE (Institute of Electrical and Electronic Engineers) Transactions on Automatic Control*, **39** (5), 1106–1110.

De Boer, R. W., Karemaker, J. M. & Strackee, J. (1985) Relationships between short-term blood-pressure fluctuations and heart-rate variability in resting subjects (parts I and II). *Medical & Biological Engineering & Computing*, **23** (4), 352–364.

Furlan, R., Piazza, S., Dell Orto, S. *et al.* (1998) Cardiac autonomic patterns preceding occasional vasovagal reactions in healthy humans. *Circulation*, **98** (17), 1756–1761.

Hoyer, D., Bauer, R., Walter, B. & Zwiener, U. (1998) Estimation of nonlinear couplings on the basis of complexity and predictability: a new method applied to cardiorespiratory coordination. *IEEE (Institute of Electrical and Electronic Engineers) Transactions on Biomedical Engineering*, **45**, 545–552.

Keselbrener, L. & Akselrod, S. (1996) Selective discrete Fourier transform algorithm for time–frequency analysis: method and application on simulated and cardiovascular signals. *IEEE (Institute of Electrical and Electronic Engineers) Transactions on Biomedical Engineering*, **43** (8), 789–802.

Kobayashi, M. & Musha, T. (1982) 1/*f* fluctuation of heartbeat period. *IEEE (Institute of Electrical and Electronic Engineers) Transactions on Biomedical Engineering*, **29**, 456–457.

Koepchen, H. P. (1984) History of studies and concepts of blood pressure waves. In: *Mechanisms of blood pressure waves* (eds K. Miyakawa, H. P. Koepchen & C. Polosa), pp. 3–27. Springer-Verlag, New York.

Lepicovska, V., Novak, P. & Nadeau, R. (1992) Time–frequency dynamics in neurally mediated syncope. *Clinical Autonomic Research*, **2** (5), 317–326.

Lucini, D., Porta, A., Milani, O., Baselli, G. & Pagani, M. (2000) Assessment of arterial and cardiopulmonary baroreflex gains from simultaneous recordings of spontaneous cardiovascular and respiratory variability. *Journal of Hypertension*, **18** (3), 281–286.

Mainardi, L. T., Bianchi, A. M., Furlan, R. *et al.* (1997) Multivariate time-variant identification of cardiovascular variability signals: a beat-to-beat spectral parameter estimation in vasovagal syncope. *IEEE (Institute of Electrical and Electronic Engineers) Transactions on Biomedical Engineering*, **44** (10), 978–989.

Mainardi, L. T., Bianchi, A. M. & Cerutti, S. (2002) Time–frequency and time-varying analysis for assessing the dynamic responses of cardiovascular control. *Critical Reviews in Biomedical Engineering*, **30**, 175–217

Malliani, A., Pagani, M. & Lombardi, F. (1986) Positive feedback reflexes. In: *Handbook of Hypertension* (eds A. Zanchetti & R. C. Tarazzi), pp. 69–81. Elsevier, New York.

Nollo, G., Faes, L., Porta, A. *et al.* (2002) Evidence of unbalanced regulatory mechanism of heart rate and systolic pressure after acute myocardial infarction. *American Journal of Physiology (Heart Circulation, Physiology)*, **283**, H1200–H1207.

Nollo, G., Porta, A., Faes, L., Del Greco, M., Disertori, M. & Ravelli, F. (2001) Causal linear parametric model for baroreflex gain assessment in patients with recent myocardial infarction. *American Journal of Physiology (Heart Circulation, Physiology)*, **280**, H1830–H18399.

Novak, P. & Novak, V. (1993) Time/frequency mapping of the heart rate, blood pressure and respiratory signals. *Medical & Biological Engineering & Computing*, **31** (2), 103–110.

Novak, V., Novak, P., Kus, T. & Nadeau, R. (1995) Slow cardiovascular rhythms in tilt and syncope. *Journal of Clinical Neurophysiology*, **12** (1), 64–71.

Palus, M. (1997) Detecting phase synchronization in noisy systems. *Physics Letters A*, **235**, 341–351.

Pola, S., Macerata, A., Emdin, M. & Marchesi, C. (1996) Estimation of the power spectral density in nonstationary cardiovascular time series: assessing the role of the time–frequency representations. *IEEE (Institute of Electrical and Electronic Engineers) Transactions on Biomedical Engineering*, **43**, 46–59.

Porta, A., Baselli, G., Lombardi F., Montano, N., Malliani A. & Cerutti S. (1999) Conditional entropy approach for the evaluation of the coupling strength. *Biological Cybernetics*, **81**, 119–129.

Porta, A., Baselli, G., Rimoldi, O., Malliani, A. & Pagani, M. (2000a) Assessing baroreflex gain from spontaneous variability in conscious dogs: role of causality and respiration. *American Journal of Physiology (Heart Circulation Physiology)*, **279** (5), H2558–H2567.

Porta, A., Guzzetti, S., Montano, N. *et al.* (2000b) Information domain analysis of cardiovascular variability signals: evaluation of regularity, synchronization and co-ordination. *Medical & Biological Engineering & Computing*, **38**, 180–188.

Porta, A., Montano, N., Pagani, M. *et al.* (2003) Noninvasive model-based estimation of the sinus node dynamic properties from spontaneous cardiovascular variability series. *Medical & Biological Engineering & Computing*, **41**, 52–61.

Robbe, H. W., Mulder, L. J., Ruddel, H., Langewitz, W. A., Veldman, J. B. & Mulder, G. (1987) Assessment of baroreceptor reflex sensitivity by means of spectral analysis. *Hypertension*, **10** (5), 538–543.

Saul, J. P. (1996) Transfer function analysis of cardiorespiratory variability to assess autonomic regulation. *Clinical Science*, **91** (Suppl.), 101.

Schafer, C., Rosemblum, M. G., Kurths, J. & Abel, H. H. (1998) Heartbeat synchronised with ventilation. *Nature (London)*, **392**, 239–240.

Soderstrom, T. & Stoica, P. (1989) *System Identification*. Prentice-Hall, Englewood Cliffs, NJ.

CHAPTER 19

Arterial Baroreflexes in Ischaemic Heart Disease, and Their Role in Sudden Cardiac Death

Dwain L. Eckberg

Introduction

Arterial baroreflex mechanisms are impaired in patients with coronary artery disease. Evidence for this came first from cross-sectional surveys of coronary patients and healthy volunteers. Subsequently, a wealth of studies conducted in animals and patients documented the fluidity of baroreflex responses during and after myocardial ischaemia, mapped out the time course of restoration of baroflex function after acute myocardial infarction, and related baroflex gain to the severity of the cardiac dysfunction and the prognosis of patients. This chapter begins with a history of baroflex research in coronary patients (including those with myocardial infarctions and varying degrees of left ventricular dysfunction), and ends with a discussion of some practical consequences of impairment of arterial baroflex mechanisms.

History

Although the technique of stimulating carotid baroreceptors with neck suction was described in 1957 (Ernsting & Parry 1957), quantitative study of human baroreflex responses did not gain wide acceptance until 1969, when Smyth, Sleight and Pickering correlated *RR* interval lengthening with systolic pressure elevations, after bolus injections of pressor agents (Smyth *et al.* 1969). The Oxford group initially focused on hypertensive patients, and did not use their new technique to study patients with organic heart diseases. However, in 1971, Eckberg, Drabinsky and Braunwald used the Oxford method to evaluate a disparate group of patients with heart disease, and reported that cardiac patients have subnormal vagal baroreflex gain (Eckberg *et al.* 1971). The results of this effort prefigured several themes that emerged in subsequent studies of baroreflex function in coronary artery disease patients.

First, cardiac patients have subnormal vagal baroreflex gain; the average gain in patients was only 23% of the average gain in aged-matched healthy subjects (16.0 vs 3.7 ms mmHg^{-1}). In fact, two of 22 patients had negative values – heart rate speeding during pressure elevations. It is likely that these patients could not marshal baroreflex responses to increase their vagal-cardiac nerve activity, and experienced cardioacceleration because of the weak β-adrenergic agonist property of phenylephrine (White *et al.* 1973). Figure 19.1 shows *RR* interval prolongation after bolus injections of phenylephrine, in a healthy subject and a patient with cardiomyopathy.

Second, vagal baroreflex impairment was unrelated to the severity of cardiac symptoms; six symptom-free patients (New York Heart Association Functional Class I) had an average vagal baroreflex gain of only 4.0 ms mmHg^{-1}. Third, cardiac patients also had subnormal cardioacceleration, when large dose atropine was given after β-adrenergic blockade. Average responses of all subjects to propranolol and atropine are shown in Fig. 19.2. These findings confirmed results published earlier by Jose & Taylor (1969) and indicated that cardiac patients with subnor-

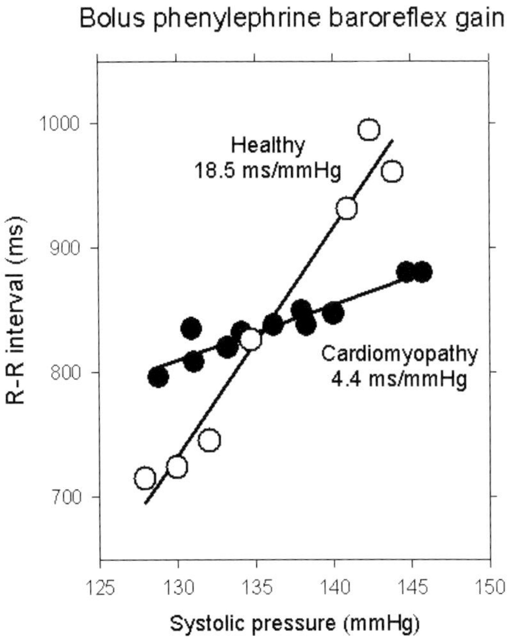

Fig. 19.1 *RR* interval and systolic pressure responses to bolus injections of phenylephrine in a healthy subject and in a patient with cardiomyopathy. The slopes were calculated with least squares linear regression. (Adapted from Eckberg *et al.* 1971, with permission.)

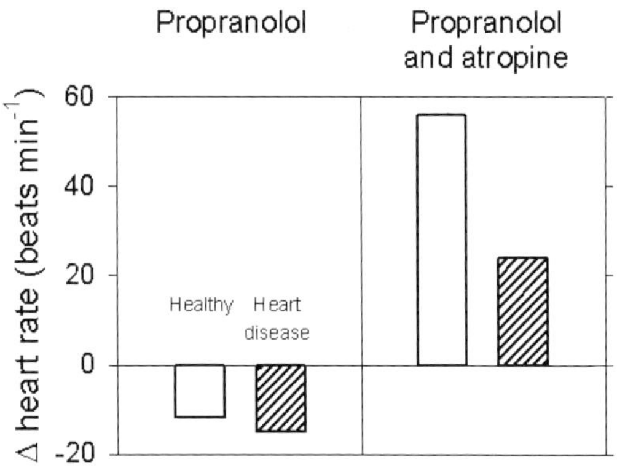

Fig. 19.2 Changes of heart rate after intravenous propranolol, 0.2 mg kg^{-1}, and propranolol and atropine, 0.04 mg kg^{-1}. Heart rate slowing after propranolol was comparable in healthy subjects (n = 13) and cardiac patients (n = 9). Heart rate speeding after addition of atropine was significantly greater in healthy subjects than in patients with heart diseases. (Adapted from Eckberg *et al.* 1971, with permission.)

mal acute increases of vagal-cardiac nerve activity during abrupt arterial pressure elevations, also have subnormal *tonic* levels of vagal-cardiac nerve activity.

Baroreflex function and heart disease

Animal and human studies indicate that acute myocardial ischaemia impairs both vagal and sympathetic responses to baroreflex challenges. Trimarco and coworkers studied the effects of left circumflex coronary artery occlusion on baroreflex responses to phenylephrine and nitroprusside injections in anaesthetized dogs (Trimarco *et al.* 1987). They reported that acute inferior ischaemia reduces both heart rate decreases and increases during arterial pressure elevations and reductions. Importantly, ischaemia also reduces changes of hindlimb vascular resistance provoked by changes of arterial pressure. Therefore, acute myocardial ischaemia impairs arterial baroreflex modulation of both *vagal* and *sympathetic* neural outflows.

In most studies of patients with coronary artery disease, only vagal baroreflex responses are evaluated. It is likely, but not conclusively proven, that in such patients, vagal baroreflex impairment provides inferential evidence for *sympathetic* baroreflex impairment. One study by Hartikainen and coworkers supports this possibility (Hartikainen *et al.* 1995). Hartikainen measured an index of sympathetic nerve activity, plasma noradrenaline concentrations (Wallin *et al.* 1981), and vagal baroreflex gain serially, in 37 patients after their first myocardial infarctions. The changes that occurred between measurements made early after infarction, and three months later, in 31 of these patients, are shown in Fig. 19.3. There was a loose, but statistically-significant trend in vagal and sympathetic changes. Patients whose plasma noradrenaline levels declined during recovery from infarction (extreme left) tended to have increases of vagal baroreflex gain. Conversely, patients whose plasma noradrenaline levels increased (extreme right) tended to have decreases of vagal baroreflex gain.

Patients are more complex than healthy dogs, and closely-controlled animal experiments cannot be conducted in humans. However, Airaksinen *et al.* (1998) obtained results that were concordant with those obtained in dog

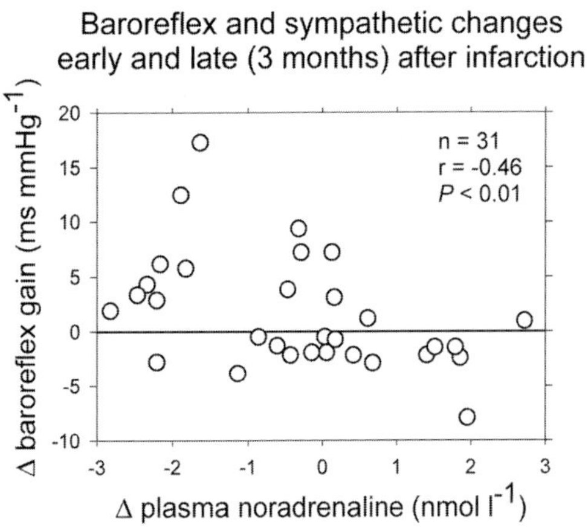

Fig. 19.3 Changes of antecubital vein plasma noradrenaline and vagal baroreflex gain (see Fig. 19.1) measured early after a first infarction and three months later. Results in inset are from least squares linear regression analysis. (Adapted from Hartikainen *et al.* 1995, with permission.)

experiments (Trimarco *et al.* 1987), during percutaneous coronary angioplasty, in patients with single vessel coronary artery disease and no history of myocardial infarction. During coronary occlusion, baroreflex gain declines significantly. In some patients, the close relation between *RR* interval prolongation and systolic pressure elevation after phenylephrine injections that is present before coronary artery occlusion is lost during coronary occlusion. This finding suggests that acute myocardial ischaemia fundamentally disrupts human vagal baroreflex mechanisms. Airaksinen also reported that phenylephrine injections provoke less systolic pressure elevation during than before myocardial ischaemia. One interpretation of this latter result is that during ischaemia, increases of afferent input from myocardial receptors provoke powerful withdrawal of sympathetic vasoconstrictor activity, which overrides the direct vasoconstrictor actions of phenylephrine (Halliwill *et al.* 1993).

Why is baroreflex function deranged in coronary artery disease patients?

There are at least three potential explanations for the baroreflex impairment that is found in patients with myocardial ischaemia. That said, it must be recognized that any division of the manifold possibilities that exist into a discrete manageable number is artificial, and likely does not represent pathophysiological facts as thy exist.

Afferent inputs

Patients with coronary artery disease must have profoundly altered firing of *myocardial receptors*, and therefore, profoundly altered sensory inputs to the central nervous system. It is improper to lump the wide variety of sensory receptors located in the atria, ventricles, great veins and arteries, and lungs into a single category, 'cardiopulmonary receptors', and then regard this disparate group of neurones as a class that subserves one physiological function (Hainsworth 1991). That said, however, it is clear that the heart provides important sensory information which modulates autonomic neural outflow.

Halliwill and coworkers studied interrelations between cardiac receptors and arterial baroreceptors in anaesthetized dogs, by determining the contributions from each group to haemodynamic adjustments to abrupt hypotension provoked by rapid right ventricular pacing [used to simulate ventricular tachycardia (Halliwill *et al.* 1993)]. His study showed that ventricular pacing presents the central nervous system with conflicting information: rapid pacing provokes increases of left atrial pressure (and presumably, increases of firing of cardiac receptors), and decreases of arterial pressure (and presumably, decreases of firing of arterial baroreceptors). In otherwise healthy, intact dogs, this combination leads to *inhibition* of renal sympathetic nerve activity. Therefore, in this model, cardiac receptors are prepotent, and override arterial baroreceptor responses to hypotension. However, after vagal cardiac (and pulmonary) receptors are denervated, ventricular tachycardia augments renal sympathetic nerve activity.

The results from Halliwill's dog experiment are different from results obtained from patients. Smith *et al.* reported that in intact patients with cardiac diseases, rapid ventricular pacing leads to increases of muscle sympathetic nerve activity (Smith *et al.* 1991). Smith subsequently revisited this pathophysiology in dogs with or without healed anteroapical left ventricular infarctions

(Smith *et al.* 1996). Dogs with infarctions behaved as patients did – arterial hypotension was met by increased renal sympathetic nerve activity. However, dogs without infarctions behaved as the healthy dogs reported earlier by Halliwill *et al.* (1993) – increases of pulmonary capillary wedge pressure were met by decreases of renal sympathetic nerve activity. These results suggest that patients with cardiac diseases have deranged inputs from cardiac receptors, and therefore, their responses to hypotension during rapid ventricular pacing are driven by arterial baroreceptors.

Sensory inputs from cardiac receptors may be altered by a variety of mechanisms in patients with ischaemic heart disease. First, ischaemia may alter firing of receptors whose afferent axons travel with both sympathetic (Schwartz *et al.* 1973) and vagal efferent nerves (Felder & Thames 1979), and modulate arterial baroreflex responses. As mentioned, Trimarco *et al.* (1987) showed that circumflex coronary artery occlusion impairs both sympathetic and vagal baroreflex responses. In his study, baroreflex impairment did not occur during coronary artery occlusion after application of lidocaine to the left ventricular epicardium; therefore, the acute autonomic neural changes provoked by ischaemia that he recorded are mediated by altered firing of receptors located near the epicardial surface of the left ventricle. Altered cardiac receptor firing could result from neuronal changes provoked by ischaemia, or from altered firing of uninvolved sensory receptors, located near hypocontractile ischaemia or infarcted ventricular myocardium.

Second, infarction may destroy cardiac receptors, which, in consequence, cannot fire at all (Stanton *et al.* 1989). In dogs (Schwartz 1986) and patients (Mortara *et al.* 1996) with healed infarctions, the largest reductions of baroreflex gain may be associated with the largest infarctions.

Arterial pressure profile

Any change of left ventricular contraction, whether mediated by acute ischaemia, or death of myocardial cells, must lead to altered left ventricular contraction patterns, and thereby to altered arterial pressure profiles (Eckberg & Sleight 1992). However, there are at least two problems that arise with attempts to quantitate these inevitable changes of baroreceptive artery pulsations. First, in nearly all human studies, physical parameters or arterial pulsations are not measured; rather arterial pressures are used as surrogates for arterial pulsations. This leads to the second problem, arterial pressures reflect not only changes mediated by differences of arterial pulsation, but also, baroreflex *responses* to those changes. For example, systolic and diastolic pressures may *increase* during passive upright tilt, notwithstanding certain reductions of baroreceptive artery dimensions (Morillo *et al.* 1997), or arterial pressure may remain constant, notwithstanding sequestration of blood in the lower body during mild lower body suction (Taylor *et al.* 1995). In these circumstances, measurements of arterial pressure give no indication of the profound changes of baroreceptive artery dimensions that have occurred.

Arterial baroreceptors

Impaired arterial baroreflex function in coronary artery disease patients may occur because of intrinsic disease in baroreceptive arteries. Some evidence supports this possibility. Clearly, in older healthy subjects (Kaushal & Taylor 2002) and in patients with coronary artery disease (Tomiyama *et al.* 1996), baroreflex gain (and reduced heart rate variability) can be ascribed importantly to reduced distensibility of baroreceptive arteries. However, this factor is unlikely to explain all of the reduced baroreflex gain found in cardiac patients. Heart failure patients who receive orthotopic heart transplants, experience major improvement of baroreflex gain (Ellenbogen *et al.* 1989). Therefore, physical changes in baroreceptive arteries associated with atherosclerosis may not be sufficient to explain baroreflex impairment in cardiac patients.

The methods available for studying cardiac patients are limited, and withal, crude. Afferent inputs from cardiac receptors cannot be measured. Measurements of left ventricular ejection fraction provide extremely limited information regarding myocardial cell deformation or the influence of metabolic changes on myocardial cell function. Measurements of arterial pressure provide extremely limited information on baroreceptor deformation, and may not even indicate that major changes of pulsatile baroreceptor stimulation have occurred. The above discussion catalogues some possible mechanisms likely to be involved in the derangements of arterial baroreflex function seen in patients with coronary artery occlusion. This list is not inclusive; moreover, it is likely that *all* of the above mechanisms contribute to baroreflex derangements in patients, to greater or lesser degrees.

Practical consequences of baroreflex malfunction

There are several central questions that should be asked regarding baroreflex mechanisms in ischaemic heart disease: Does baroreflex impairment represent a *marker* for the extensiveness of cardiac disease, or for the degree of autonomic impairment? Does baroreflex impairment have practical consequences? Could it be that baroreflex mechanisms importantly orchestrate responses to acute haemodynamic insults, and thereby, determine their outcomes? Some answers to these questions have come from prospective research based on the dog model of sudden cardiac death developed by Billman, Schwartz & Stone (1982): intense treadmill exercise (which physiologically augments sympathetic stimulation and withdraws vagal restraint) in animals with healed anterior myocardial infarctions, and superimposed acute inferior ischaemia (balloon occlusion of the left circumflex coronary artery). Some of these exercising dogs develop ventricular tachycardia, which degenerates into ventricular fibrillation ('susceptible'), and others tolerate exercise plus ischaemia and do not develop ventricular dysrhythmias ('resistant'). In this model, circumflex coronary artery occlusion is maintained after cessation of exercise into the recovery period, and it is at this time that ventricular fibrillation is most likely to occur (Schwartz *et al.* 1984). [In humans, sudden death also may occur after, rather than during exercise (Albert *et al.* 2000).] The physiologically-relevant dog model of sudden death has yielded important insights into baroreflex mechanisms in ischaemic heart disease.

1 Myocardial infarction reduces vagal baroreflex gain. In dogs studied before and after anterior infarctions, baroreflex gain declines by at least 3 ms mmHg^{-1} in 73% (Schwartz *et al.* 1988). (Baroreflex impairment does not develop in sham-operated dogs, and therefore, is secondary to infarction.)

2 Reductions of baroreflex gain correlate with the occurrence of sudden death: dogs with baroreflex gains >15 ms mmHg^{-1} have a 20% likelihood of ventricular fibrillation during exercise plus ischaemia, and dogs with baroreflex gains <9 ms mmHg^{-1} have a 91% risk of ventricular fibrillation.

3 The occurrence of sudden death is not a simple function of infarct size (Schwartz *et al.* 1984), and heart rate before exercise, an index of the degree of haemodynamic compensation (Schwartz *et al.* 1988), are comparable in susceptible and resistant dogs.

4 Baroreflex impairment correlates with heart rate responses. Notwithstanding exercise-induced tachycardia, resistant dogs experience heart rate *slowing* when ischaemia is added, and susceptible dogs experience further heart rate *speeding*.

5 The physiological importance of baroreflex responsiveness is underscored by baroreflex function before infarctions occur: low baroreflex gain before infarctions predicts susceptibility to sudden death after infarctions during exercise plus ischaemia (Schwartz *et al.* 1988).

6 Susceptible dogs have lower heart rate variability than resistant dogs at rest (Hull *et al.* 1990), and greater reductions of an indirect index of vagal-cardiac nerve activity, i.e. high-frequency *RR* interval variability (Eckberg 1983), during exercise plus ischaemia than resistant dogs. They also have less speeding of the heart rate after parasympathetic blockade with atropine (Billman & Hoskins 1989).

7 Heart rate showing during exercise plus ischaemia in resistant dogs likely reflects increases of vagal-cardiac nerve activity. Cholinergic blockade with atropine may convert resistant dogs into susceptible dogs (De Ferrari *et al.* 1991). [In a different model of sudden death, anaesthetized cats with acute anterior ischaemia, single-fibre vagal-cardiac nerve activity increases in cats that do not develop ventricular fibrillation, and does not change in cats that develop ventricular fibrillation (Cerati & Schwartz 1991).]

8 Improvement of vagal baroreflex gain and heart rate variability following exercise training moves dogs from susceptible to resistant categories (Hull *et al.* 1994).

The dog model seems to be extremely relevant to patients who are at risk of experiencing sudden cardiac death. In patients followed after their first myocardial infarctions, both low vagal baroreflex gain (La Rovere *et al.* 1998) and low heart rate variability (Kleiger *et al.* 1987; La Rovere *et al.* 1998) are associated with augmented risk of death. Moreover, the high risk associated with low baroreflex gain or heart rate variability, exists independent of myocardial function, as reflected by left ventricular ejection fraction. In patients, ventricular tachycardias whose QRS complexes are similar to those of the premature ventricular beats that trigger them, is preceded by reductions of very low- and low-frequency *RR* interval fluctuations (Anderson *et al.* 1999). Since virtually all heart rate variability is abolished by high-dose atropine (Taylor *et al.* 1998), reductions of very low- and low-frequency likely reflect reductions of vagal-cardiac nerve activity. Moreover, heart rate variability also declines before spontaneous ventricular tachycardia in patients treated with β-adrenergic blocking drugs (Pruvot *et al.* 2000), an observation that strongly implicates vagal withdrawal. Finally, pharmacological interventions that increase vagal-cardiac nerve activity, including β-adrenergic (Eckberg *et al.* 1976) and angiotensin converting enzyme (Anderson *et al.* 1999) blockade, and exercise training, reduce the incidence of sudden cardiac death in patients (Chadda *et al.* 1986; SOLVD Investigators 1991).

The dog experiments described above establish the likelihood that depression of vagal baroreflex function is not simply an epiphenomenon that appears after infarction, but rather, a factor that has functional importance. The question, Why should vagal baroreflex function determine life or death? merits close consideration. I conclude this chapter by making a case (intending to be provocative) that in many patients, under extraordinary circumstances which may come together uniquely in a patient's life, the quality of arterial baroreflex responses spells the difference between life and death.

In patients who die wearing Holter monitors, most sudden deaths result from ventricular tachycardia that degenerates into ventricular fibrillation (Bayes de Luna *et al.* 1989). In patients monitored in the hospital after they have been resuscitated from sudden death, a variety of rhythms, including supraventricular tachycardias, may precipitate ventricular fibrillation (Bardy & Olson 1990). In both circumstances, death is presaged by major haemodynamic perturbations.

During very rapid ventricular rhythms, systolic and diastolic pressure fall precipitously, in proportion to the extent of pre-existing myocardial disease (Steinbach *et al.* 1994). Tachycardia increases myocardial infarction oxygen needs, but at the same time reduces myocardial oxygen delivery by shortening the time available for coronary perfusion during diastole, and reducing diastolic pressure. Therefore, a critical issue during tachycardia is, How rapidly is arterial pressure restored towards normal levels? This question is important because restoration of *systemic arterial* pressure signifies restoration of *coronary artery* perfusion pressure, and thereby augmentation of myocardial oxygen delivery. Figure 19.4 illustrates average systolic pressure and muscle sympathetic nerve responses of eight patients to ventricular tachycardia, as simulated by right ventricular pacing at three rates: 100, 120 and 150 beats min^{-1} (Smith *et al.* 1991).

These systolic pressure measurements illustrate several features of human responses to tachydysrhythmias. First, systolic pressure declines precipitously at the beginning of tachycardia. Since all of the patients studied had myocardial disease, no conclusions can be drawn regarding the contribution of impaired left ventricular function to the fall of pressure. Second, as expected, the faster the ventricular rate, the greater the reduction of systolic pressure. Third, systolic pressure neither continued to fall, nor remained at the same low level – systolic pressure *rose*, notwithstanding persistence of tachycardia at constant rates. Therefore, during tachycardia, coronary perfusion pressure increases, and with it, myocardial oxygen delivery. The importance of these haemodynamic responses is illustrated by cases of supraventricular tachycardia: recovery of blood pressure may terminate the dysrhythmia, an effect that is vagally mediated, because it does not occur after cholinergic blockade (Waxman *et al.* 1982).

Why does systolic pressure increase during

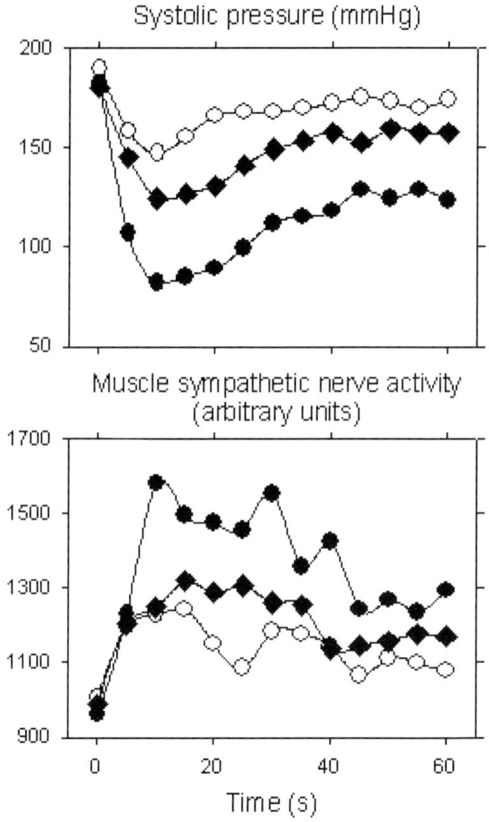

Fig. 19.4 Average changes of systolic pressure and muscle sympathetic nerve activity with right ventricular pacing at 100 (open circles), 120 (diamonds), and 150 (closed circles) beats min^{-1} from eight patients. (Adapted Smith *et al.* 1991, with permission.)

tachycardia? The obvious answer is that hypotension is reversed in a major way by augmentation of muscle sympathetic nerve activity, as shown in the lower panel of Fig. 19.4. Sympathetic firing increases abruptly, in rough proportion to the degree of hypotension. It is reasonable to assume that arterial pressure increases because of this increase of sympathetic nerve activity. Further, it is reasonable to assume that sympathetic nerve activity increases because of the intervention of arterial baroreflex mechanisms. The validity of these assumptions cannot be tested in humans, but can be tested in experimental animals. In this connection, a dog study of Smith *et al.* (1996) is informative. Dogs with anteroapical infarctions, whose afferent cardiac receptor activity was presumably deranged, restored arterial pressure more rapidly than dogs without infarctions. [It is likely that the presence of the infarctions resolved the *conflict* that exists between cardiac receptors and arterial baroreceptors – see above – by minimizing sympathoinhibition secondary to the increased activity of cardiac receptors (Halliwill *et al.* 1993).] Smith also showed that the return of arterial pressure during tachycardia is mediated by arterial baroreceptors: arterial pressure during tachycardia remains low after arterial baroreceptor denervation.

Smith and coworkers modelled factors responsible for restoration of systolic pressure during ventricular tachycardia in patients (Smith *et al.* 1991). They reported that the most important factor is the tachycardia rate; extremely rapid ventricular rates lead to critically shortened diastolic filling periods (Steinbach *et al.* 1994), impaired diastolic left ventricular relaxation (Saksena *et al.* 1984), and greater arterial pressure reductions. Even robust sympathetic responses to ventricular tachycardia cannot restore arterial pressure to normal if there is insufficient time for diastolic ventricular filling to occur. Smith identified two other factors that improved his model: ejection fraction and sympathetic baroreflex gain (the intensity of the sympathetic nerve augmentation that occurred in response to hypotension at the beginning of tachycardia). [A subsequent study showed that rapid return of arterial pressure during tachycardia is associated with higher vagal, as well as sympathetic baroreflex gain (Hamdan *et al.* 1999).] Other factors include loss of synchrony between atria and ventricles (Steinbach *et al.* 1994), and ischaemia itself [the faster the tachycardia, the greater the ischaemia in coronary artery disease patients (van Boven *et al.* 1995)].

The above considerations establish the importance of adequate baroreflex responses to ventricular tachycardia. The great majority of ventricular tachycardia episodes terminate spontaneously, no doubt aided by adequate baroreflex responses. Several pieces of evidence suggest that patients who fail to mount adequate baroreflex responses to ventricular tachycardia fare poorly. Landolina and coworkers divided 24 patients with sustained monomorphic ventricular tachycardia and healed myocardial infarctions into two groups: those who tolerated ventricular tachycardia well, and those who did not tolerate ventricular tachycardia well, and developed faintness, syncope, or hypotension (Landolina *et al.* 1997). Patients in two groups were comparable in terms of their average ages, left ventricular function, and ventricular tachycardia rate, but different in terms of their vagal baroreflex gain. Ventricular tachycardia was tolerated well in patients with higher vagal baroreflex gain, and poorly in patients with lower baroreflex gain [average values: 7.1 in patients who tolerated ventricular tachycardia, and 3.4 $ms\,mmHg^{-1}$ in patients who did not tolerate ventricular tachycardia ($P = 0.003$)].

Huikuri and colleagues studied patient responses to induced ventricular tachycardia, and used the atrial rate, recorded with a right atrial electrode as an indirect indicator of changes of efferent autonomic nerve traffic to the sinoatrial node (Huikuri *et al.* 1989). Their study yielded several important insights. First, across all patients, ventricular tachycardia is associated with an increase of the atrial rate. Since this speeding occurs after, as well as before β-adrenergic blockade, it likely reflects withdrawal of vagal restraint. Some patients tolerate ventricular tachycardia well, and do not require emergent termination with electrical countershock. Other patients are unstable (they lapse into unconsciousness), and require emergent countershock. Atrial rates in the two groups of patients diverged during the tachycardia. Patients who tolerate ventricular tachycardia well maintain and even increase the frequency of their accelerated atrial rates, and patients who do not tolerate ventricular tachycardia experience an abrupt slowing of their atrial rates. I suspect that the two groups had different autonomic reactions to hypotension (beat-by-beat arterial pressures were not recorded). Patients who tolerated ventricular tachycardia well had adequate baroreflex responses and maintained arterial pressure at acceptable levels. Patients who did not tolerate ventricular tachycardia well had impaired baroreflex responses, were not able to maintain arterial pressure, and as a result of falling pressures, developed full-blown vasovagal reactions. The development of vasovagal physiology during ventricular tachycardia presents an extremely serious problem because sympathetic firing stops, and arterial pressure, already reduced by ventricular tachycardia, falls further (Morillo *et al.* 1997).

Conclusions

Acute myocardial ischaemia and myocardial infarction impair vagal and sympathetic arterial baroreflex mechanisms. It is likely that several mechanisms contribute to arterial baroreflex impairment in patients with coronary artery disease. A partial list includes changing autonomic sensory inputs form cardiac receptors; altered arterial pulse profiles secondary to disordered left ventricular contraction; and intrinsic disease of baroreceptive arteries, secondary to generalized atherosclerosis. Baroreflex impairment has major adverse prognostic implications, and adds to cardiovascular risk, independent of coexisting left ventricular impairment. I make the argument that baroreflex impairment is not simply a marker for the extensiveness of disease, but reflects a serious inability of patients to respond to haemodynamic challenges, including especially, those presented by ventricular tachycardia. Adequate baroreflex responses to ventricular tachycardia restore arterial pressure towards normal, and increase vagus nerve traffic to the myocardium. Increased vagus traffic prolongs ventricular refractoriness (Ellenbogen *et al.* 1990), opposes the pernicious influence of increased sympathetic stimulation (Taylor *et al.* 2001), and reduces vulnerability of the ventricle to the occurrence of the ventricular fibrillation (Kolman *et al.* 1975).

References

Airaksinen, K.E.J., Tahvanainen, K.U.O., Eckberg, D.L., Niemelä, M., Yitalo, A. & Huikuri, H.V. (1998) Arterial baroreflex impairment in patients during acute coronary occlusion. *Journal of the American College of Cardiology*, **32**, 1641–1647.

Albert, C.M., Mittleman, M.A., Chae, C.U., Lee, L.-M., Hennekens, C.H. & Manson, J.E. (2000) Triggering of sudden death from cardiac causes by vigorous exertion. *New England Journal of Medicine*, **343**, 1355–1361.

Anderson, K.P., Shusterman, V., Aysin, B., Weiss, R., Brode, S. & Gottipaty, V. and ESVEM Investigators (1999) Distinctive *RR* dynamics preceding two modes of onset of spontaneous sustained ventricular tachycardia. *Journal of Cardiovascular Electrophysiology*, **10**, 897–904.

Bardy, G.H. & Olson, W.H. (1990) Clinical characteristics of spontaneous-onset sustained ventricular tachycardia and ventricular fibrillation in survivors of cardiac arrest. In: *Cardiac Electrophysiology. From Cell to Bedside* (eds D. P. Zipes & J. Jalife), pp 778–790. W.B. Saunders, Philadelphia.

Bayes de Luna, A., Coumel, P. & Leclercq, J.F. (1989) Ambulatory sudden cardiac death: mechanisms of production of fatal arrhythmia on the basis of data from 157 cases. *American Heart Journal*, **117**, 151–159.

Billman, G.E. & Hoskins, R.S. (1989) Time-series analysis of heart rate variability during submaximal exercise. Evidence for reduced cardiac vagal tone in animals susceptible to ventricular fibrillation. *Circulation*, **80**, 146–157.

Billman, G.E, Schwartz, P.J. & Stone, H.L. (1982) Baroreceptor reflex control of heart rate: a predictor of sudden cardiac death. *Circulation*, **66**, 874–880.

van Boven, A.J., Jukema, J.W., Crijns, H.J.G.M. & Lie, K.I. (1995) Heart rate variability profiles in symptomatic coronary artery disease and preserved left ventricular function: relation to ventricular tachycardia and transient myocardial ischemia. *American Heart Journal*, **130**, 1020–1025.

Cerati, D. & Schwartz, P.J. (1991) Single cardiac vagal fiber activity, acute myocardial ischemia, and risk for sudden death. *Circulation Research*, **69**, 1389–1401.

Chadda, K., Goldstein, S., Byington, R. & Curb, J.D. (1986) Effect of propranolol after acute myocardial infarction in patients with congestive heart failure. *Circulation*, **73**, 503–510.

De Ferrari, G.M., Vanoli, E., Stramba-Badiale, M., Hull, S.S., Jr, Foreman, R.D. & Schwartz, P.J. (1991) Vagal reflexes and survival during acute myocardial ischemia in conscious dogs with healed myocardial infarction. *American Journal of Physiology*, **261**, H63–H69.

Eckberg, D.L. (1983) Human sinus arrhythmia as an index of vagal cardiac outflow. *Journal of Applied Physiology*, **54**, 961–966.

Eckberg, D.L., Abboud, F.M. & Mark, A.L. (1976) Modulation of carotid baroreflex responsiveness in man: effects of posture and propranolol. *Journal of Applied Physiology*, **41**, 383–387.

Eckberg, D.L., Drabinsky, M. & Braunwald, E. (1971) Defective cardiac parasympathetic control in patients with heart disease. *New England Journal of Medicine*, **285**, 877–883.

Eckberg, D.L. & Sleight, P. (1992) *Human Baroreflexes in Health and Disease*. Clarendon Press, Oxford.

Ellenbogen, K.A., Mohanty, P.K., Szentpetery, S. & Thames, M.D. (1989) Arterial baroreflex abnormalities in heart failure. Reversal after orthotopic cardiac transplantation. *Circulation*, **79**, 51–58,

Ellenbogen, K.A., Smith, M.L. & Eckberg, D.L. (1990) Increased vagal cardiac nerve traffic prolongs ventricular refractoriness in patients undergoing electrophysiology testing. *American Journal of Cardiology*, **65**, 1345–1350.

Ernsting, J. & Parry, D.J. (1957) Some observations on the effects of stimulating the stretch receptors in the carotid artery of man. *Journal of Physiology*, **137**, 45P–46P.

Felder, R.B. & Thames, M.D. (1979) Interaction between cardiac receptors and sinoaortic baroreceptors in the control of efferent cardiac sympathetic nerve activity during myocardial ischemia in dogs. *Circulation Research*, **45**, 728–736.

Hainsworth, R. (1991) Reflexes from the heart. *Physiological Reviews*, **71**, 617–658.

Halliwill, J.R., Minisi, A.J., Smith, M.L. & Eckberg, D.L. (1993) Renal sympathetic responses to conflicting baroreceptor inputs: rapid ventricular pacing in dogs. *Journal of Physiology*, **471**, 365–378.

Hamdan, M., Joglar, J.A., Page, R.L *et al.* (1999) Baroreflex gain predicts blood pressure recovery during simulated ventricular tachycardia in humans. *Circulation*, **100**, 381–386.

Hartikainen, J., Fyhrquist, F., Tahvanainen, K., Lansimies, E. & Pyörälä, K. (1995) Baroreflex sensitivity and neurohormonal activation in patients with acute myocardial infarction. *British Heart Journal*, **74**, 21–26.

Huikuri, H.V., Zaman, L., Castellanos, A. *et al.* (1989) Changes in spontaneous sinus node rate as an estimate of cardiac autonomic tone during stable and unstable ventricular tachycardia. *Journal of the American College of Cardiology*, **13**, 646–652.

Hull, S.S., Jr, Evans, A.R., Vanoli, E. *et al.* (1990) Heart rate variability before and after myocardial infarction in conscious dogs at high and low risk of sudden death. *Journal of the American College of Cardiology*, **16**, 978–985.

Hull, S.S., Jr, Vanoli, E., Adamson, P.B., Verrier, R.L., Foreman, R.D. & Schwartz, P.J. (1994) Exercise training confers anticipatory protection from sudden death during acute myocardial ischemia. *Circulation*, **89**, 548–552.

Jose, A.D. & Taylor, R.R. (1969) Autonomic blockade by propranolol and atropine to study intrinsic myocardial function in man. *Journal of Clinical Investigation*, **48**, 2019–2031.

Kaushal, P. & Taylor, J.A. (2002) Inter-relations among declines in arterial distensibility, baroreflex function and respiratory sinus arrhythmia. *Journal of the American College of Cardiology*, **39**, 1524–1530.

Kleiger, R.E., Miller, J.P., Bigger, J.T., Jr, Moss, A.J. & Multicenter Post-Infarction Research Group (1987) Decreased heart rate variability and its association with increased mortality after acute myocardial infarction. *American Journal of Cardiology*, **59**, 256–262.

Kolman, B.S., Verrier, R.L. & Lown, B. (1975) The effect of vagus nerve stimulation upon vulnerability of the canine ventricle. Role of sympathetic–parasympathetic interactions. *Circulation*, **52**, 578–585.

La Rovere, M.T., Bigger, J.T., Jr, Marcus, F.I., Mortara, A. & Schwartz, P.J. (1998) Baroreflex sensitivity and heart-rate variability in prediction of total cardiac mortality after myocardial infarction. *Lancet*, **351**, 478–484.

Landolina, M., Mantica, M., Pessano, P. *et al.* (1997) Impaired baroreflex sensitivity is correlated with hemodynamic deterioration of sustained ventricular tachycardia. *Journal of the American College of Cardiology*, **29**, 568–575.

Morillo, C.A., Eckberg, D.L., Ellenbogen, K.A. *et al.* (1997) Vagal and sympathetic mechanisms in patients with orthostatic vasovagal syncope. *Circulation*, **96**, 2509–2513.

Mortara, A., Specchia, G., LaRovere, M.T., Bigger, J.T., Jr, Marcus, F.I. & Camm, A.J. (1996) Patency of infarct-related artery: effect of restoration of anterograde flow on vagal reflexes. *Circulation*, **93**, 1114–1122.

Pruvot, E., Thonet, G., Vesin, J.-M. *et al.* (2000) Heart rate dynamics at the onset of ventricular tachyarrhythmias as retrieved from implantable cardioverter-defibrillators in patients with coronary artery disease. *Circulation*, **101**, 2398–2404.

Saksena, S., Ciccone, J.M., Craelius, W., Pantopoulos, D., Rothbart, S.T. & Werres, R. (1984) Studies on left ventricular function during sustained ventricular tachycardia. *Journal of the American College of Cardiology*, **4**, 501–508.

Schwartz, P.J. (1986) An experimental approach to the problem of postinfarction angina and sudden cardiac death. *European Heart Journal*, **7** (Suppl. C), 7–17.

Schwartz, P.J., Billman, G.E. & Stone, H.L. (1984) Autonomic mechanisms in ventricular fibrillation induced by myocardial ischemia during exercise in dogs with healed myocardial infarction. An experimental preparation for sudden cardiac death. *Circulation*, **69**, 790–800.

Schwartz, P.J., Pagani, M., Lombardi, F., Malliani, A. & Brown, A.M. (1973) A cardiocardiac sympatho vagal reflex in the cat. *Circulation Research*, **32**, 215–220.

Schwartz, P.J., Vanoli, E., Stramba-Badiale, M., De Ferrari, G.M., Billman, G.E. & Foreman, R.D. (1988) Autonomic mechanisms and sudden death. New insights from analysis of baroreceptor reflexes in conscious dogs with and without a myocardial infarction. *Circulation*, **78**, 969–979.

Smith, M.L., Ellenbogen, K.A., Beightol, L.A. & Eckberg, D.L. (1991) Sympathetic neural responses to induced ventricular tachycardia. *Journal of the American College of Cardiology*, **18**, 1015–1024.

Smith, M.L., Kinugawa, T. & Dibner-Dunlap, M.E. (1996) Reflex control of sympathetic activity during ventricular tachycardia in dogs. Primary role of arterial baroreceptors. *Circulation*, **93**, 1033–1042.

Smyth, H.S., Sleight, P. & Pickering, G.W. (1969) Reflex regulation of arterial pressure during sleep in man. A quantitative method of assessing baroreflex sensitivity. *Circulation Research*, **24**, 109–121.

SOLVD Investigators (1991) Effect of enalapril on survival in patients with reduced left ventricular ejection fractions and congestive heart failure. *New England Journal of Medicine*, **325**, 293–302.

Stanton, M.S., Tuli, M.M., Radtke, N.L. *et al.* (1989) Regional sympathetic denervation after myocardial infarction in humans detected noninvasively using I-123-metaiodobenzylguanidine. *Journal of the American College of Cardiology*, **14**, 1519–1526.

Steinbach, K.K., Merl, O., Frohner, K. *et al.* (1994) Hemodynamics during ventricular tachyarrhythmias. *American Heart Journal*, **127**, 1102–1106.

Taylor, J.A., Carr, D.L., Myers, C.W. & Eckberg, D.L. (1998) Mechanisms underlying very-low-frequency *R–R*-interval oscillations in humans. *Circulation*, **98**, 547–555.

Taylor, J.A., Halliwill, J.R., Brown, T.E., Hayano, J. & Eckberg, D.L. (1995) 'Non-hypotensive' hypovolaemia reduces ascending aortic dimensions in humans. *Journal of Physiology*, **483**, 289–298.

Taylor, J.A., Myers, C.W., Halliwill, J.R., Seidel, H. & Eckberg, D.L. (2001) Sympathetic restraint of respiratory sinus arrhythmia: implications for assessment of vagal-cardiac tone in humans. *American Journal of Physiology*, **280**, H2808–H2814.

Tomiyama, H., Kihara, Y., Nishikawa, E. *et al.* (1996) An impaired carotid sinus distensibility and baroreceptor sensitivity alter autonomic activity in patients with effort angina associated with significant coronary artery disease. *American Journal of Cardiology*, **78**, 225–227.

Trimarco, B., Ricciardelli, B., Cuocolo, A. *et al.* (1987) Effects of coronary occlusion on arterial baroreflex control of heart rate and vascular resistance. *American Journal of Physiology*, **252**, H749–H759.

Wallin, B.G., Sundlöf, G., Eriksson, B.-M., Dominiak, P., Grobecker, H. & Lindblad, L.E. (1981) Plasma noradrenaline correlates to sympathetic muscle nerve activity in normotensive man. *Acta Physiologica Scandinavica*, **111**, 69–73.

Waxman, M.B., Sharma, A.D., Cameron, D.A., Huerta, F. & Wald, R.W. (1982) Reflex mechanisms responsible for early spontaneous termination of paroxysmal supraventricular tachycardia. *American Journal of Cardiology*, **49**, 259–272.

White, C.W., Eckberg, D.L. & Inasaka, T. (1973) Direct effects of methoxamine and phenylephrine on sinus mode function. *American Journal of Cardiology*, **31**, 164 (abstract).

CHAPTER 20

Heart Rate Turbulence on Holter

Raphael Schneider, Petra Barthel and Mari Watanabe

Introduction

The goal of this chapter is to describe in detail the quantification of heart rate turbulence (HRT) in Holter recordings. The source code for HRT calculation described here can be downloaded at the website www.h-r-t.org.

For the analyses and figures in this chapter, we used Holter data from a subset of 428 patients from the ISAR-HRT postinfarction study (Barthel *et al.*, 2003), if not stated otherwise. All patients presented with sinus rhythm and had frequent (>30 per 24 h) ventricular premature complexes (VPC) with a normal HRT pattern.

Background

The term heart rate turbulence (HRT) was coined to describe the short-term fluctuation in sinus cycle length that follows a ventricular premature complex (VPC) (Schmidt *et al.* 1999). In normal subjects, sinus rate accelerates then decelerates back to baseline following a VPC (Fig. 20.1a). The precise mechanism underlying normal heart rate turbulence is unknown, but it is likely that the sudden drop in blood pressure with the VPC results in vagal withdrawal and sympathetic recruitment, both of which accelerate sinus rate, while the ensuing compensatory pause and subsequent increase in blood pressure induce vagal recruitment and sympathetic withdrawal, both of which would decelerate sinus rate (Schmidt *et al.* 1999; Bauer *et al.* 2001a, b).

The clinical significance of HRT lies in its ability to predict mortality and sudden cardiac death following myocardial infarction (Schmidt *et al.* 1999; Ghuran *et al.* 2002). In patients at risk for subsequent death, HRT is blunted or entirely missing (Fig. 20.1b).

Assessment of HRT

Turbulence onset

The initial acceleration of sinus rhythm is quantified by turbulence onset (TO), which is the relative change of *RR* intervals immediately after compared with immediately before a VPC. TO is calculated using the following equation:

$$\text{TO}[\%] = \frac{(RR_1 + RR_2) - (RR_{-2} + RR_{-1})}{(RR_{-2} + RR_{-1})} \times 100$$

where RR_{-2} and RR_{-1} are the two *RR* intervals immediately preceding the VPC and RR_1 and RR_2, the two *RR* intervals immediately following the compensatory pause (Fig. 20.2). The calculations were performed for each single VPC and then averaged over the entire Holter recording to obtain the value characterizing the patient. Positive values of TO signify sinus rhythm deceleration after a VPC, and negative values signify sinus rhythm acceleration after a VPC.

Turbulence slope

The deceleration phase of sinus rhythm is quantified by turbulence slope (TS). TS is assessed in the average HRT tachogram as the slope of the steepest regression line observed over any sequence of five consecutive *RR* intervals (Figure 2). The beginning of this sequence is usually found within the first 10 intervals (Fig. 20.3). Thus, for the calculation of TS, it is sufficient to use only the first 15 *RR* intervals after the VPC.

Normal values

TO values <0 and TS values >2.5 ms/*RR* interval are considered normal in post-myocardial infarction (MI) patients. TO and TS can be used

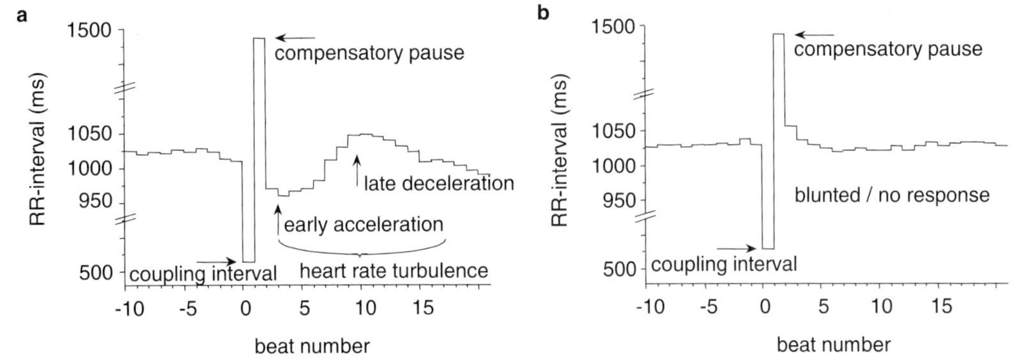

Fig. 20.1 Examples of heart rate turbulence patterns in two postinfarction patients. (a) Typical acceleration–deceleration sequence of *RR* intervals after coupling interval and compensatory pause of a VPC recorded in a 64-year-old woman with anterior myocardial infarction who survived during follow-up. (b) Almost random pattern recorded in a 77-year-old man with inferior myocardial infarction who died 7 months after the index infarction.

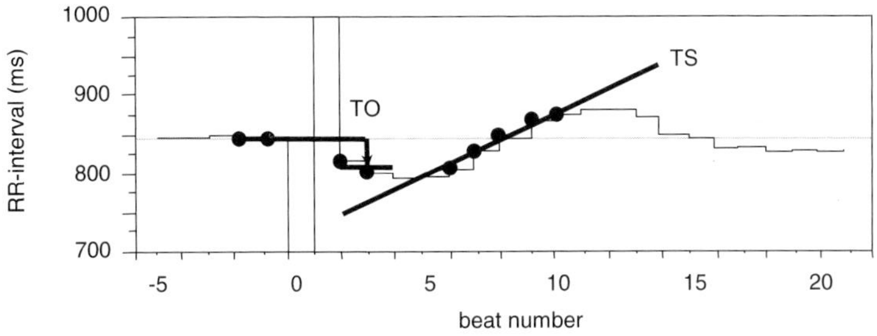

Fig. 20.2 Calculation of the heart rate turbulence parameters turbulence onset (TO) and turbulence slope (TS). TO is the relative change of heart rate before and after the VPC. TS is the slope of the steepest regression line over any sequence of five subsequent sinus-rhythm *RR* intervals within the first 15 *RR* intervals after the VPC.

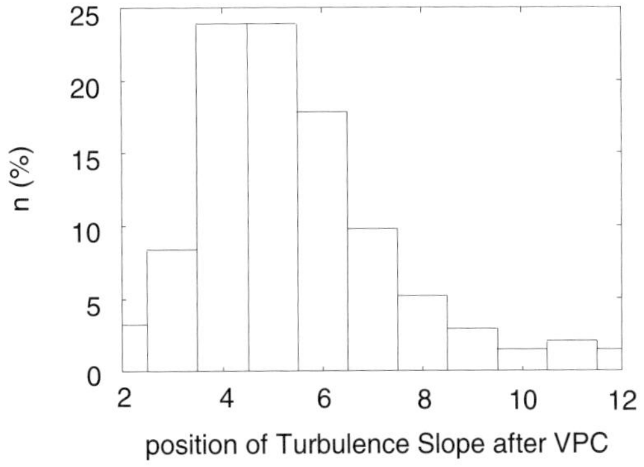

Fig. 20.3 Distribution (%) of the positions of turbulence slope. The position is the beginning of the *RR* interval sequence used for the calculation of TS (i.e. if the *RR* interval sequence RR5–RR9 is used for TS, the position of TS is 5). For the majority (>90%) of the Holter recordings, the position of TS lies within the first 10 *RR* intervals.

both as separate variables, and in combination. For the combination, we recommend the use of three categories: HRT0, TO & TS normal; HRT1, TO or TS abnormal; and HRT2, TO & TS abnormal.

Filtering

Sinus intervals

Sinus rhythm is required for measurement of HRT; assessment of HRT does not make sense in presence of atrial fibrillation or during pacing. To exclude sections of misclassified rhythm, we recommend excluding *RR* interval sequences containing exceptionally long or short intervals (<300 ms, >2000 ms) and large changes in *RR* intervals, namely those with >200 ms difference to the preceding sinus interval or >20% differ-

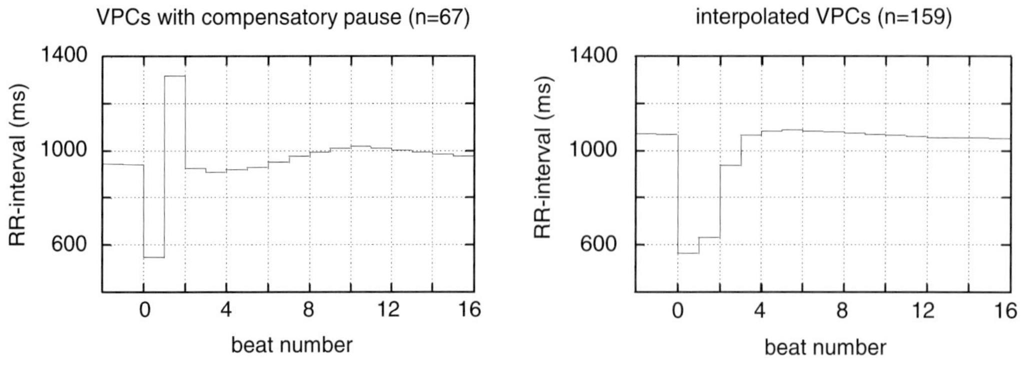

Fig. 20.4 Tachograms from a patient showing VPCs with (left) and without (right) compensatory pauses. Only the former induce the typical HRT pattern.

ence to the reference interval (defined as the mean of the five last sinus intervals before the VPC).

VPC-related intervals

The postextrasystolic drop in arterial pressure during the compensatory pause is the main trigger of HRT. Accordingly, interpolated VPCs without compensatory pauses do not set off a typical HRT response (Fig. 20.4) and can artificially reduce the TS measurement. We therefore exclude VPC sequences containing coupling intervals >80% and postextrasystolic pauses <120% of the reference interval (defined as mean of the five last sinus intervals before the VPC).

Number of VPC sequences required for HRT calculation

To a certain extent, HRT is masked by heart rate fluctuations of non-VPC related origin. As a result, the HRT response varies from one VPC to the next. Figure 20.5 shows HRT tachograms of a patient with frequent VPCs, in whom several HRT tachograms were calculated on the basis of averaging different numbers of VPCs. With increasing numbers of VPC sequences, the HRT pattern becomes more distinct. And indeed, restriction of HRT assessment to patients with a minimum number of VPCs, e.g. ≥5 in 24 h, increases the positive predictive value. However, this increase is slight, and is achieved at the cost of decreasing values for relative risk and sensitivity. Therefore, we

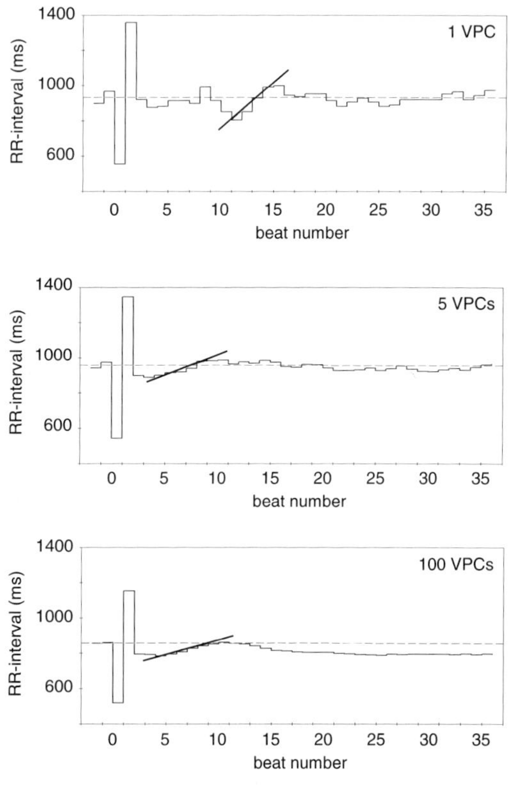

Fig. 20.5 Effect of averaging HRT tachograms. Top panel: HRT tachogram based on one VPC sequence; no clear HRT; 'noisy' sinus-rhythm. Middle panel: HRT tachogram based on 5 VPC sequences; HRT is more distinct. Bottom panel: HRT tachogram based on 100 VPC sequences; clear HRT reaction; factors other than HRT are removed by the averaging process.

recommend calculating HRT in all patients presenting with ≥1 VPC(s).

Novel HRT measures

In addition to TO and TS, there are various HRT parameters that have been proposed and studied. The relationship between HRT and HR can be quantified by a parameter termed *turbulence dynamics* (Bauer *et al.*, 2002). In a retrospective study, linear regression showed correlations between HRT parameters and HR (all $P < 0.0001$), both for survivors and non-survivors. In survivors, turbulence dynamics was significantly greater than in non-survivors.

Turbulence frequency decrease is a parameter that measures HRT in the frequency domain (Schneider *et al.* 1999). This parameter is obtained by fitting a sine wave equation to the post-compensatory pause *RR* values with a frequency term that decreases over time. It seems to contain mortality information independent of the time domain parameters TO and TS.

Turbulence timing is a parameter that notes the first beat number of the 5 *RR* interval sequence where TS is found (where the slope of *RR* change is maximum) (Watanabe & Josephson 2000; Watanabe *et al.* 2002). Turbulence timing is dependent on HR, and the relationship indicates that the sinus deceleration phase of HRT is earlier at slow heart rates.

Turbulence jump is a parameter which quantifies the maximum difference between adjacent *RR* intervals (Berkowitsch *et al.* 2001). It was found to predict recurrence of ventricular tachycardia and fibrillation in patients with dilated cardiomyopathy.

Correlation coefficient of TS is the correlation coefficient of the regression line fitted to the 5 *RR* intervals giving the maximum slope (i.e. where TS is defined) (Schmidt *et al.* 2001). It is an independent predictor of mortality in postinfarction patients, but its risk ratio is lower than that for TO or TS.

Further studies are needed to see if any of these parameters provide significantly superior risk stratification to TO and TS, given that TO and TS are simpler to measure than some of these parameters, and can be measured in short records.

References

Barthel, P., Schneider, R., Bauer, A. *et al.* (2003) Risk stratification after acute myocardial infarction by heart rate turbulence. *Circulation*, **108** (10), 1221–1226.

Bauer, A., Barthel, P., Schneider, R., Malik, M. & Schmidt, G. (2001a) Impact of coupling interval on heart rate turbulence. *European Heart Journal*, **22** (Suppl.), 438.

Bauer, A., Barthel, P., Schneider, R. & Schmidt, G. (2001b) Dynamics of heart rate turbulence. *Circulation*, **104** (Suppl. II), 339.

Bauer, A., Barthel, P., Schneider, R. and Schmidt, G. (2002) Dynamics of heart rate turbulence predicts mortality after acute myocardial infarction. *Circulation*, **106** (Suppl. II), 373.

Berkowitsch, A., Guettler, N., Neumann, T. *et al.* (2001) Turbulence jump – a new descriptor of heart-rate turbulence after paced premature ventricular beats. A study in dilated cardiomyopathy patients. *European Heart Journal*, 22 (Suppl.), 547.

Ghuran, A., Reid, F., La Rovere, M.T. *et al.* (2002) Heart rate turbulence-based predictors of fatal and nonfatal cardiac arrest (the Autonomic Tone and Reflexes After Myocardial Infarction substudy). *American Journal of Cardiology*, **89** (2), 184–190.

Schmidt, G., Malik, M., Barthel, P. *et al.* (1999) Heart-rate turbulence after ventricular premature beats as a predictor of mortality after acute myocardial infarction. *Lancet*, **353** (9162), 1390–1396.

Schmidt, G., Schneider, R. & Barthel, P. (2001) Correlation coefficient of the heart rate turbulence slope: new risk stratifier in postinfarction patients. *European Heart Journal*, **22** (Suppl.), 72.

Schneider, R., Röck, A., Barthel, P., Malik, M., Camm, A. J. & Schmidt, G. (1999) Heart rate turbulence: rate of frequency decrease predicts mortality in chronic heart disease patients. *PACE (Pacing and Clinical Electrophysiology)*, **22** (Part II), 879.

Watanabe, M. & Josephson, M. E. (2000) Heart rate turbulence in the spontaneous ventricular tachyarrhythmia database. *PACE (Pacing and Clinical Electrophysiology)*, **23** (Part II), 686.

Watanabe, M. A., Marine, J. E., Sheldon, R. & Josephson, M. E. (2002) Effects of ventricular premature stimulus coupling interval on blood pressure and heart rate turbulence *Circulation*, **106** (3), 325–330.

CHAPTER 21

Heart Rate Turbulence in Pacing Studies

Dan Wichterle and Marek Malik

Introduction

Following the first description of heart rate turbulence (HRT) (Schmidt *et al.* 1999), analyses of Holter recordings from other large trials in postinfarction populations confirmed risk-prediction power of HRT quantifiers (Makikallio *et al.* 2000; Barthel *et al.* 2001; Batchvarov *et al.* 2001; Huikuri *et al.* 2001; Ghuran *et al.* 2002). Considerable effort has been made to define pathophysiological background of HRT since only proper understanding of the underlying mechanisms may offer an explanation of why is HRT such a potent postinfarction risk stratifier.

While Holter-based studies provided some preliminary hypotheses about the mechanisms of HRT, specific electrophysiological studies in smaller populations offer a more direct insight into the pathophysiology of HRT. Consequently, this text focuses on the description of pacing studies and of their contribution to the HRT research.

In HRT pacing studies, two approaches have been used to induce ectopic beats. Extrastimuli were delivered from right ventricular apex (or high right atrium) during invasive electrophysiological examinations (Roach *et al.* 2000; Guettler *et al.* 2001; Marine *et al.* 2002; Watanabe *et al.* 2002; Lin *et al.* 2002; Savelieva *et al.* 2003; Wichterle *et al.* 2003). Alternatively, extrastimuli were noninvasively provoked via an implanted device (Berkowitsch *et al.* 2000; Berkowitsch *et al.* 2001). Although artificially induced ectopic beats might differ from the spontaneous premature depolarizations, programmed stimulation during sinus rhythm enables to collect sufficient number of isolated monomorphic ectopic beats with pre-specified coupling interval within a short period of time. Consequently, HRT-related investigations do not need to be limited to patients with frequent spontaneous ectopic activity.

Pacing protocols are essential in studies investigating HRT during pharmacological autonomic intervention, especially since vagal blockade effectively abolishes the presence of spontaneous ectopic beats. Compared to Holter recordings, pacing studies also benefit from a 'random' delivery of extrastimuli with respect to instant heart rate. Indeed, heart rate variability might significantly interfere with the assessment of HRT quantifiers, particularly if a relation exists between instant autonomic modulation and occurrence of spontaneous ectopic beats. Compared to Holter studies, recordings obtained during electrophysiological study are usually also of better quality with higher sampling frequency and better signal-to-noise ratio. When available, intracardiac electrograms are useful during visual scanning and editing that can be performed to higher procedural standard than in Holter recording.

HRT and autonomic blockades

It has been hypothesized from the very beginning that HRT is triggered by the transient loss of vagal activity in response to the missed baroreflex afferent input due to haemodynamically inefficient ventricular contraction, which is responsible for the early acceleration of heart rate. Sympathetically mediated overshoot of arterial pressure subsequently causes deceleration of heart rate through a vagal activation (Malik *et al.* 1999).

Therefore, a logical step is to establish the vagal involvement in HRT. The effect of vagal blockade on HRT indices was studied 12 middle-aged patients without structural heart diseases (Guettler *et al.* 2001). Ten ventricular premature extrastimuli were applied during sinus rhythm before and after 0.04 mg/kg atropine administered intravenously. Blood pressure dynamics did not change significantly after vagal blockade. In contrast, atropine abolished heart rate response after ventricular premature complexes (VPCs), so that HRT quantifiers, Turbulence Onset (TO) and Turbulence Slope (TS), became near zero. This observation was later confirmed by Marine *et al.* (2002). In their pacing study, at least five isolated extrastimuli with 60% prematurity were delivered from right ventricular apex during electrophysiological study in heterogeneous population of 12 patients with cardiac diseases. After intravenous administration of atropine (1 mg), TS consistently decreased from 11.5 ± 6.4 to 1.2. ± 0.5 ms/*RR*, $P = 0.0002$, and TO changed from −1.4 ± 2.2 to 1.0 ± 1.1%, $P = 0.0012$ (Figs 21.1 and 21.2). It was concluded that preserved vagal influence on sinus node is an essential condition for normal HRT.

In another pacing study by Lin *et al.* (2002), not only vagal blockade, but also sympathetic and combined autonomic blockade was investigated. The study was performed in 16 middle-aged patients (10 males) without structural heart disease referred for invasive electrophysiological study due to paroxysmal AV (or AV nodal) re-entrant tachycardia. Isolated right ventricular apex extrastimuli were delivered with initial coupling interval of 60% which was decremented in 2% steps until a total of 10 VPCs induced. TS was 5.2 ± 4.0 ms/*RR* and TO was −0.45 ± 0.94% at baseline. While there

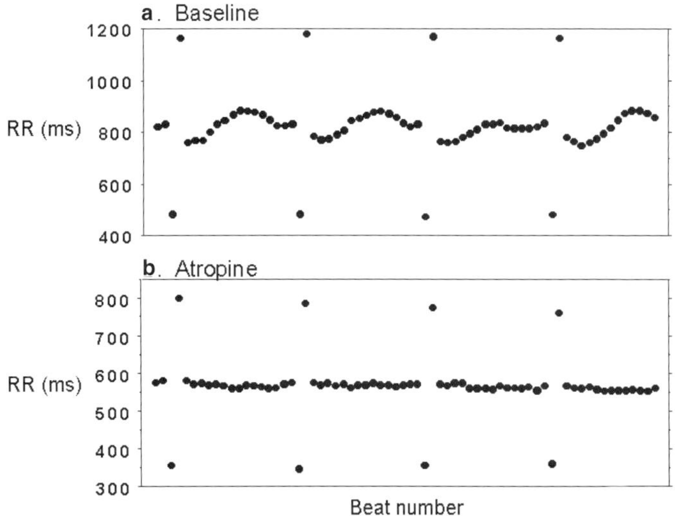

Fig. 21.1 Modulations of *RR* sensing intervals following isolated ventricular extrastimuli with 60% prematurity at baseline (a) and after atropine administration (b). (Reproduced from Marine *et al.* 2002, with permission.)

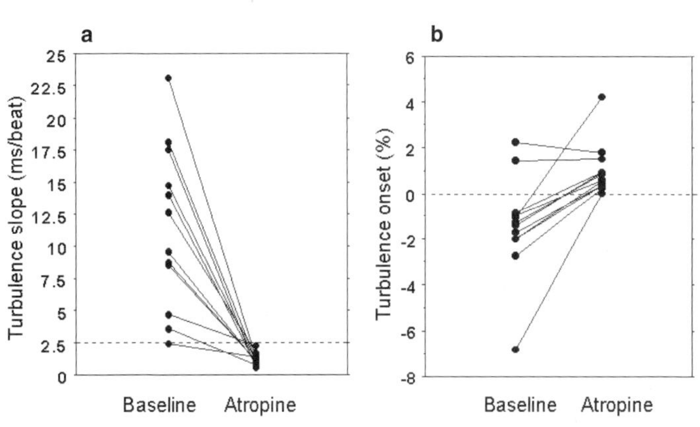

Fig. 21.2 Values of Turbulence Slope and Turbulence Onset measured in the pacing study by Marine *et al.* at baseline and after atropine administration. Dashed lines: normal limits of TS > 2.5 ms/RR and TO < 0% (Reproduced from Marine *et al.* 2002, with permission.)

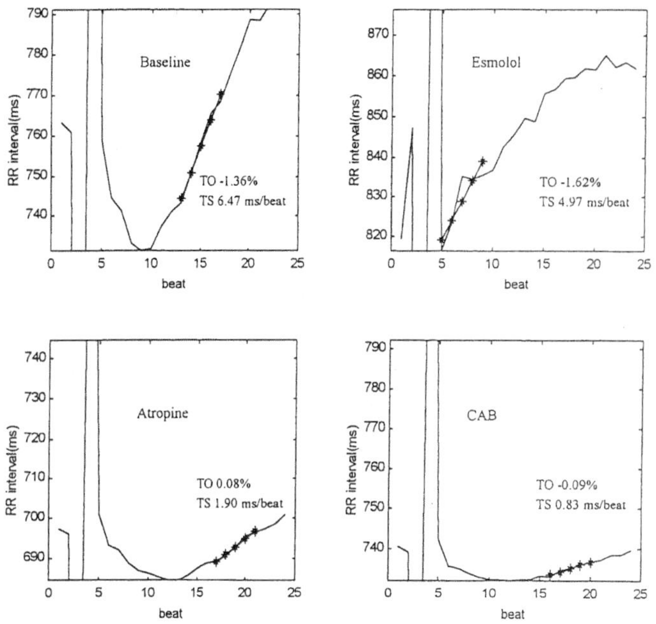

Fig. 21.3 Patterns of *RR* interval dynamics triggered by isolated ventricular extrastimuli at baseline, after beta-blockade with esmolol, after vagal blockade with atropine, and after combined autonomic blockade (CAB). (Reproduced from Lin *et al.* 2002, with permission.)

was significant attenuation of HRT after vagal blockade with atropine (TS: 0.71 ± 0.50 ms/*RR*, $P < 0.01$; TO: 0.32 ± 0.35%, $P < 0.01$), no significant change was observed after beta-blockade with esmolol (TS: 4.5 ± 3.3 ms/*RR*; TO: −0.62 ± 1.33%). Not surprisingly, HRT after combined autonomic blockade did not differ significantly from that after vagal blockade, because vagal blockade alone almost completely abolished HRT (Fig. 21.3). Although the effect of beta-blockade was not discussed and blood pressure dynamics after sympathetic blockade was not presented, the explanation seems to be simple. First of all, administration of beta-blocker does not provide the complete sympathetic blockade. Beta-blockade influences more the modulation of sinus node discharge than the modulation of peripheral vascular resistance. As a result, sympathetically mediated overshoot of systolic blood pressure in the late phase of HRT is not significantly affected, and consequently, late deceleration of heart rate due to preserved vagal response is unchanged compared to baseline. Moreover, HRT has dominant frequency component of ~0.1 Hz. At this frequency, sympathetic modulation of heart rate has rather anti-oscillatory role (De Boer *et al.* 1987), so that beta-blockade may even enhance heart rate response to the ectopic contraction.

HRT and baroreflex sensitivity

Already a retrospective analysis of the ATRAMI study suggested the importance of baroreflex as an underlying mechanism of HRT (Ghuran *et al.* 2000). Both TO and TS correlated mildly but significantly with baroreflex sensitivity (BRS) assessed by the phenylephrine method ($r = -0.34$ and $r = 0.44$, both $P < 0.001$, respectively).

A seminal pacing study that directly addressed the relationship of baroreflex and HRT was performed by Roach *et al.* (2000). They investigated heart rate and blood pressure response to single ventricular extrastimuli in 15 patients undergoing electrophysiological examination. Transient hypertension that reached peak at beat 7 after the extrastimulus was followed by transient bradycardia peaking at beat 8. This pattern was fully compatible with baroreflex action and BRS of 10.4 ms/mmHg was estimated from this dynamics.

Davies *et al.* (2001) studied HRT and BRS in 45 patients with congestive heart failure and spontaneous VPCs. It was shown that both TS and turbulence-derived BRS correlated markedly with spectral measure of BRS (autoregressive method, α-index) giving correlation coefficients $r = 0.70$ and $r = 0.67$ (both $P < 0.00001$), respectively. This correspondence was attributable to surprisingly uniform turbulence of systolic blood pressure. The conclusion was offered that heart rate slope rather than blood pressure slope after VPB conveys the information relevant to BRS. Comparable results were reported in pacing study of Lin *et al.* (2002). Both TS and TO significantly correlated with spontaneous BRS assessed by the sequence method ($r = 0.78$, $P = 0.001$ and $r = -0.61$, $P = 0.01$, respectively) and by spectral method ($r = 0.49$, $P = 0.05$ and $r = -0.69$, $P = 0.003$, respectively).

HRT and prematurity of ectopic complexes

Another evidence of baroreflex involvement in HRT has been derived from the analysis of Holter recordings in the EMIAT trial (Schmidt *et al.* 2000; Bauer *et al.* 2001), where both TO and TS depended on the coupling interval of the preceding VPC. This observation was compatible with a greater baroreflex response to a more premature (and less haemodynamically efficient) ventricular contractions.

The effects of VPC coupling interval on HRT was directly addressed in two pacing studies (Watanabe *et al.* 2002; Savelieva *et al.* 2003) with rather conflicting results.

In the study by Watanabe *et al.* (2002), a total of 28 patients (21 men, 12 with a history of previous MI, aged 60 ± 18 years) were examined for documented or suspected arrhythmias (16 ventricular, 12 supraventricular). Extrastimuli were delivered from the right ventricular apex after every 20th beat during sinus rhythm. The first extrastimulus was induced with a prematurity of 100 ms and subsequent coupling intervals were decremented by 20–30 ms until refractoriness was reached. Relationship of HRT indices and coupling intervals (CI) analysed by linear regression in individual patients were not conclusive. Having in mind the pathophysiological background of HRT, the correlation between TS and CI should be negative and correlation between TO and CI should be positive. However, the inverse relationship was frequently found in this study (Fig. 21.4). Irrespective of statistical significance of correlation coefficients, 10 patients had a positive correlation between TS and CI and 14 patients had a negative correlation between TO and CI. Regressions between TS and CI had a negative slope significantly different from zero only in three patients. Moreover, in three patients, who had non-zero regression slope regression between TO and CI, the correlation was negative. When regression analysis was performed on pooled patient data using normalized coupling interval, no significant relationship between HRT indices and CI was found.

The study by Savelieva *et al.* (2003) investigated 40 patients (34 men, aged 54 ± 16 years) referred for electrophysiological evaluation. Twenty of them had a coronary artery disease, 12 patients had a structurally normal heart and idiopathic VT, and the remaining eight patients presented with other underlying cardiac pathology. The stimulation protocol consisted of three series of single extrastimuli delivered from right ventricular apex every 20 s with a coupling interval ranging from 750 to 400 ms at a 50-ms steps. There were significant correlations between normalized coupling interval and TO and TS ($r = 0.30$, $P < 0.0001$ and $r = -0.22$, $P < 0.0001$, respectively) assessed on pooled patient data. In

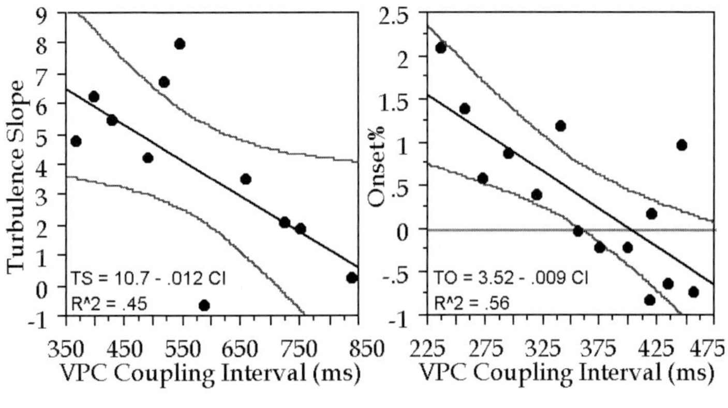

Fig. 21.4 Relationship between Turbulence Slope and Turbulence Onset and the coupling interval (CI) of ventricular extrastimuli. Left panel shows 'proper' negative correlation between Turbulance Slope and CI. Right panel shows inverse relationship between Turbulence Onset and CI which is not in agreement with pathophysiological background of HRT. (Reproduced from Watanabe *et al.* 2002, with permission.)

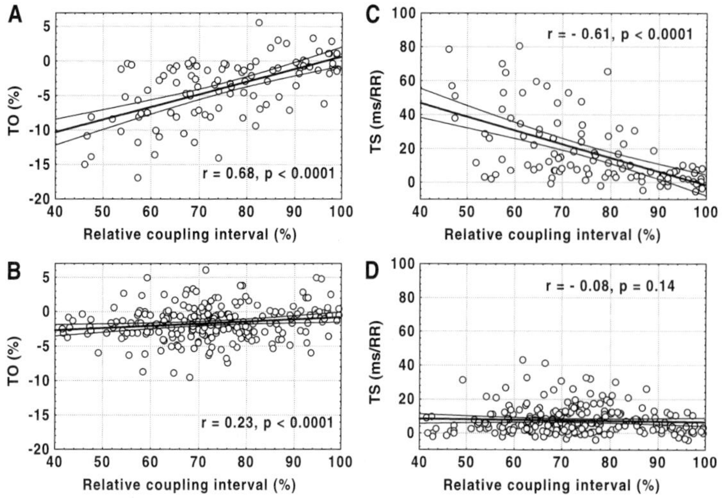

Fig. 21.5 Relationship between Turbulence Onset (TO) and Turbulence Slope (TS) and relative coupling interval in cardiac patients with preserved left ventricular function (ejection fraction > 40%; top panels) and in patients with left ventricular dysfunction (ejection fraction ≤40%; bottom panels). (Redrawn from Savelieva *et al.* 2003, with permission.)

patients with preserved left ventricular (LV) function (ejection fraction > 40%, n = 13), the relationship was even stronger (r = 0.68, P < 0.0001 and r = –0.61, P < 0.0001), while in patients with LV dysfunction (ejection fraction ″ 0.40, n = 27), a weak correlation was observed only for TO (r = 0.23, P < 0.0001) and not for TS (r = –0.08, P = 0.14) (Fig. 21.5). The lack of correlation between HRT indices and CI in patients with LV dysfunction might be explained by a notably depressed BRS in these patients. Consequently, HRT is significantly attenuated not only after VPCs with a long CI but also after VPCs with a short CI despite their greater haemodynamic impact.

At least one methodological issue might be responsible for the difference between both studies. While in the study by Watanabe *et al.*, there were no limits for turbulence timing (i.e. the first *RR* interval of five *RR* intervals sequence giving the maximum regression slope for the quantification of TS), the turbulence timing was fixed between the third and fifth sinus *RR* interval after VPC in the study by Savelieva *et al.* (2003). When TS is assessed for individual VPCs, its value tends to be falsely overestimated due to the freedom of turbulence timing which allows non-HRT variability (e.g. respiratory arrhythmia) to interfere with the calculation of TS. Of course, this bias does not apply to the assessment of TO.

Hence, the study by Savelieva *et al.* (2003) conforms more to the presumed pathophysiology of HRT. Also, another Holter study in 10 healthy subjects (Indik *et al.* 2002) confirmed the negative correlation between TS and CI. Whether the adjustment of TS for corresponding CI might improve the predictive power of TS in postinfarction patients remains to be established.

HRT and left ventricular function

The analysis of Holter data from the EMIAT trial showed that TO and TS are significantly influenced by left ventricular ejection fraction (Yap *et al.* 2001). The direct comparison of patients with congestive heart failure (34 DCM, 16 CAD post MI) and controls revealed that HRT indices were significantly depressed in patients with CHF compared to healthy controls. TS was 3.7 ± 1.7 and 16.4 ± 5.3 ms/*RR*, and TO was –1.1 ± 1.9% and –3.6 ± 1.7%, respectively (Koyama *et al.* 2002). On the other hand, it was also shown that even in the case of preserved LV function, the presence of organic heart disease affected HRT indices to a similar extent (Sestito *et al.* 2002). TS was 2.8 ± 1.9 and 10.8 ± 7.4 ms/*RR* (P = 0.0001) and TO was –0.20 ± 1.7 and –0.67 ± 2.2% (P = 0.00001) in CAD patients and controls, respectively

Recent re-analysis of the pacing study of Savelieva *et al.* (2003) provided similar information about relationship of HRT and LV function. When HRT indices were assessed using averaged post-VPC profiles of *RR* intervals (instead of analysis of individual VPC episodes), and when at least 3 VPC episodes with CI < 90% were required for the valid analysis, there was a significant difference between patients with abnormal and normal LV function. TS was 6.1 ± 4.0 and 17.9 ± 20.4 ms/*RR* ($P = 0.014$), and TO was −1.3 ± 1.8% and −4.3 ± 3.4% ($P = 0.004$), respectively. The differences were independent of age and mean heart rate (TS: $P = 0.013$; TO: $P = 0.045$; ANCOVA).

HRT assessed using an implanted device

The induction of extrastimuli via the implanted device is a promising tool for the noninvasive investigation of HRT. Two studies were reported so far (Berkowitsch *et al.* 2000, 2001). The first of them found a significant association between abnormal TS and an incidence of ventricular tachyarrhythmias in 44 ICD patients with LV dysfunction of mixed ischaemic and nonischaemic origin. The later study investigated HRT in 33 ICD patients with dilated cardiomyopathy. New risk predictor, turbulence jump (TJ), was defined as a maximal proportional difference between two *RR* intervals within 10 *RR* intervals after VPC. While TS had no predictive value, TJ dichotomized at 42.5% (median value) provided specificity of 81% and sensitivity of 85% for the prediction of VT/VF. However, these studies should be interpreted with caution, as they investigated a small number of patients, used retrospectively defined predictors and the used cut-off values were not independently validated.

HRT after atrial premature complexes

In the study by Savelieva *et al.* (2003) that was already mentioned in detail, the identical stimulation protocol was performed with extrastimuli delivered from the high right atrium instead of right ventricular apex. Dynamics of heart rate after atrial premature complexes (APCs) was different from that after VPCs (Fig. 21.6). There was an abrupt deceleration of heart rate immediately after APC that decayed in time and was followed by a second transitory heart rate deceleration. It is plausible to speculate that the abrupt deceleration is due to temporary suppression of sinus node automaticity by the direct effect of atrial stimulation (Heddle *et al.* 1985), which masks (and on average overwhelms) the autonomic component of early acceleration phase of HRT. The late deceleration has the same mechanism as that after VPC.

When HRT was quantified identically after APCs and VPCs, in pairwise comparison, TO was −2.1 ± 2.8 and 1.4 ± 2.4% ($P < 0.0001$), and TS was 9.2 ± 12.5 and 3.4 ± 2.5 ms/*RR* ($P = 0.017$) after VPCs and APCs, respectively. The difference in TO is obviously caused by different mechanisms of early change of heart rate after VPCs or APCs, while significantly attenuated TS after APCs can be explained by a weaker haemodynamic impact of APCs in comparison to VPCs. Not only significant correlation between TO and TS after VPCs ($r = -0.80$, $P < 0.0001$) and APCs ($r = -0.54$, $P = 0.005$), but also significant correlation between TO after VPCs and APCs ($r =$

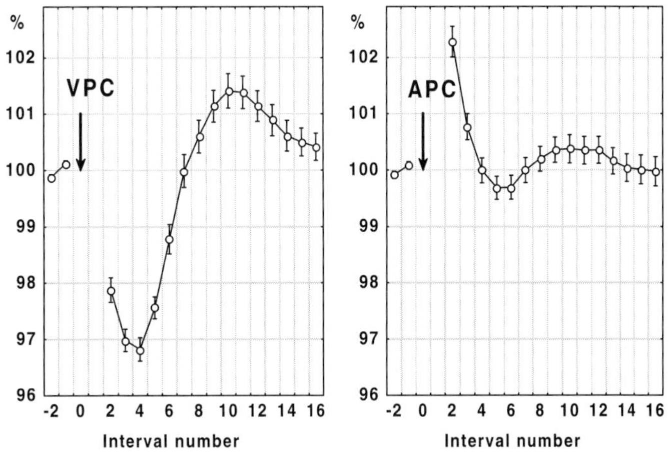

Fig. 21.6 Relative changes in *RR* intervals as percentages of pre-extrasystolic values (vertical axis) after ventricular premature complex (left panel) and after atrial premature complex (right panel). The horizontal axes indicate the *RR* interval order number relative to the ventricular or atrial premature complex.

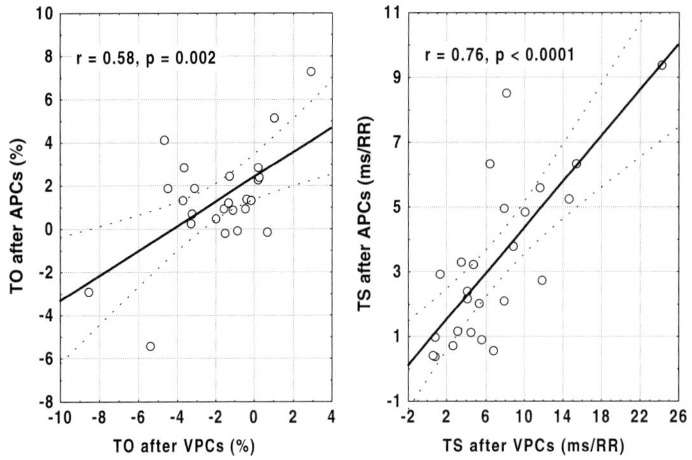

Fig. 21.7 Relationship between Turbulence Onset (TO) and Turbulence Slope (TS) after ventricular premature complexes (VPCs) and after atrial premature complexes (APCs).

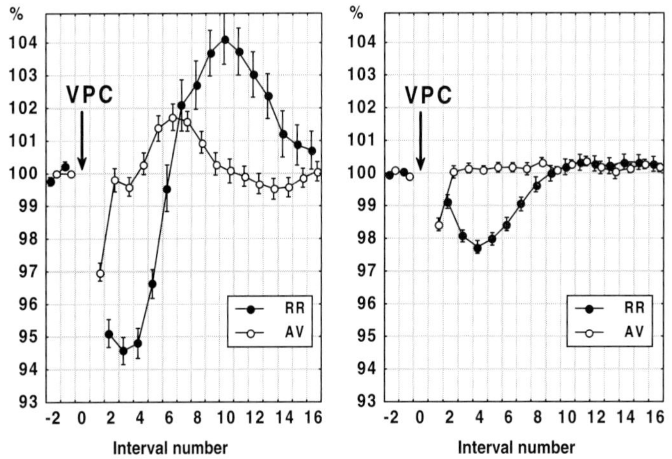

Fig. 21.8 Relative changes in *RR* intervals and in atrioventricular conduction intervals (*AV*) following a single ventricular premature complex (VPC) in patients with preserved left ventricular function (left panel) and in patients with left ventricular dysfunction (right panel). The vertical axis shows the relative change of the intervals compared to the average of two intervals before the VPC. The horizontal axis shows the order number of the *RR* intervals relative to the VPC. (Redrawn from Wichterle *et al.* 2003, with permission.)

0.58, $P = 0.002$) and TS after VPCs and APCs ($r = 0.76$, $P < 0.0001$) was observed (Fig. 21.7). This finding is of considerable practical importance as it offers an opportunity of assessing HRT (and thus cardiovascular risk) even in patients without ventricular ectopy. There is only one published Holter study to date (Indik *et al.* 2002) also showing that HRT is present after APCs and that TS is attenuated after an APCs compared to that after VPCs.

Other ECG phenomena associated with HRT

The biphasic profile of *AV* intervals consisting of early shortening and later prolongation of *AV* intervals after a single VPC was observed in a pacing study (Wichterle *et al.* 2003) (Fig. 21.8). This phenomenon was fully expressed only in patients with normal LV function. The major observation was that AV interval dynamics significantly precedes the change of *RR* intervals, which is in conflict with near to zero phase of transfer function between *RR* and *AV* intervals in previous studies (Leffler *et al.* 1994; Chen *et al.* 1999). Again, the early dynamics of *AV* intervals after a VPC may be more influenced by purely electrophysiological mechanisms rather than by a vagal withdrawal. However, in the late HRT phase, where nonautonomic effects are less likely to occur, the temporal dissociation between *RR* and *AV* interval response was even more pronounced and no plausible explanation was found. In absolute values, the response of AV conduction to a VPB was approximately 25-times and 15-times weaker in the early and late

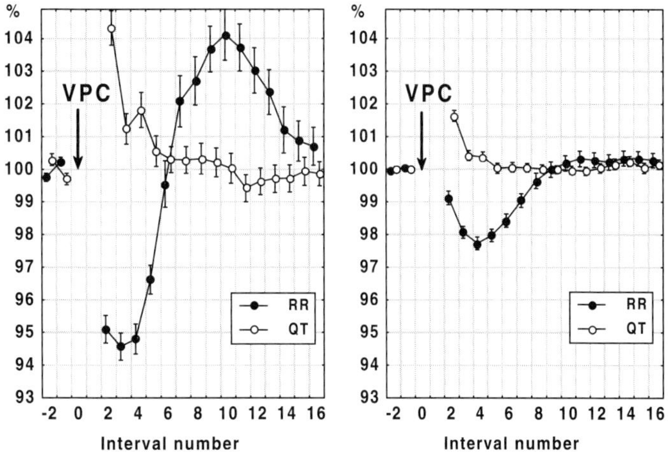

Fig. 21.9 The dynamics of *RR* intervals and of *QT* intervals (*QT*) following a single ventricular premature complex (VPC) in patients with preserved left ventricular function (left panel) and in patients with left ventricular dysfunction (right panel). The vertical axis shows the relative change of the intervals compared to the average duration of the two intervals before the VPC, the horizontal axis shows the order number of the interval relative to the VPC.

phases, respectively, than that of *RR* intervals. Therefore, the dynamics of AV delay has a little impact on accuracy of HRT assessment using the surface ECG. This is in agreement with the findings of the study by Marine *et al.* (2002) that indicated that almost all post-VPC variation in VV intervals is due to a corresponding variation in *AA* and not in *AH* and *HV* intervals.

Recently (unpublished data) we investigated the dynamics of ventricular repolarization associated with HRT. The study population and pacing protocol has been already described (Savelieva *et al.* 2003). *QT* intervals were analysed by automated procedure that utilised the area method for the detection of the end of T wave. Specifically, *QT*end was defined as a point at which 95% of total integral of the first derivative of T wave was accumulated. The calculation was performed separately in all standard surface leads and *QT* intervals from 6 leads with the most prominent T wave morphology were averaged. *QT* interval dynamics after VPCs was characterized by an abrupt prolongation immediately after VPC suggesting non-neural mechanism and by a slow return to baseline values (Fig. 21.9). There was not any dynamics in *QT* interval corresponding to vagal activation in late phase of HRT. On average, the early prolongation (*QT*onset) by 2.1 ± 2.9% was observed. It was more prominent in patients with preserved and impaired LV function (4.1 ± 4.5 and 1.3 ± 1.5%, $P = 0.013$, respectively). At present, there is only one similar Holter study (Szydlo *et al.* 2002) with rather conflicting results. It investigated post-VPCs dynamics of *QT* intervals in 59 patients with either benign ventricular arrhythmia or with history of VT/VF. A more positive *QT*onset was found in high-risk patients (4.6 ± 14 vs. −0.23 ± 11%).

References

Barthel, P., Ulm, K., Schneider, R. *et al.* (2001). Role of risk stratifiers in postinfarction patients with acute PTCA/stenting (abstract). *Journal of the American College of Cardiology*, **37** (2 Suppl. A), 134A–135A.

Batchvarov, V., Hnatkova, K., Poloniecki, J., Ghuran, A., Camm, A.J. & Malik, M. (2001) Distinction between risk for early and for late cardiac mortality following myocardial infarction (abstract). *European Heart Journal*, **22** (Suppl.), 72.

Bauer, A., Barthel, P., Schneider, R., Malik, M. & Schmidt, G. (2001) Impact of coupling interval on heart rate turbulence (abstract). *European Heart Journal*, **22** (Suppl.), 438.

Berkowitsch, A., Guettler, N., Schulte, B. *et al.* (2000) Heart-rate turbulence slope after paced premature ventricular beats as a predictor for the recurrence of ventricular tachyarrhythmias: A study in defibrillator patients (abstract). *Circulation*, **102** (18 Suppl. II), II-525.

Berkowitsch, A., Guettler, N., Neumann, T. *et al.* (2001) Turbulence jump – a new descriptor of heart-rate turbulence after paced premature ventricular beats. A study in dilated cardiomyopathy patients (abstract). *European Heart Journal*, **22** (Suppl.), 547.

Chen, S.L., Kawada, T., Inagaki, M. *et al.* (1999) Dynamic counterbalance between direct and indirect vagal controls of atrioventricular conduction in cats. *American Journal of Physiology*, **277**, H2129–H2135.

Davies, L.C., Francis, D.P., Ponikowski, P., Piepoli, M.F. & Coats, A.J. (2001) Relation of heart rate and blood pressure turbulence following premature ventricular complexes to baroreflex sensitivity in chronic congestive heart failure. *American Journal of Cardiology*, **87**, 737–742.

DeBoer, R.W., Karemaker, J.M. & Strackee, J. (1987) Hemodynamic fluctuations and baroreflex sensitivity in humans: a beat-to-beat model. *American Journal of Physiology*, **253**, H680–H689.

Ghuran, A., Schmidt, G., La Rovere, M.T *et al.* (2000) Pathophysiological correlate of heart rate turbulence and baroreceptor reflex sensitivity from the ATRAMI study. *European Heart Journal*, **21** (Suppl.), 333 (abstract).

Ghuran, A., Reid, F., La Rovere, M.T. *et al.* (2002) Heart rate turbulence-based predictors of fatal and nonfatal cardiac arrest (The Autonomic Tone and Reflexes After Myocardial Infarction substudy). *American Journal of Cardiology*, **89**,184–190.

Guettler, N., Vukajlovic, D., Berkowitsch, A. *et al.* (2001) Effect of vagus blockade with atropine on heart-rate turbulence (abstract). *PACE (Pacing and Clinical Electrophysiology)*, **24** (4 Part II), 625.

Heddle, W.F., Jones, M.E. & Tonkin, A.M. (1985) Sinus node sequences after atrial stimulation: similarities of effects of different methods. *British Heart Journal*, **54**, 568–576.

Huikuri, H.V., Lindgren, K., Tapanainen, J. *et al.* (2001) Prognostic power of traditional and new heart rate variability indices in patients with optimized therapy after myocardial infarction. Results of a prospective study [abstract]. *Circulation*, **104** (17 Suppl. II), II-637.

Indik, J.H., Ott, P. & Marcus, F.I. (2002) Heart rate turbulence and fractal scaling coefficient in response to premature atrial and ventricular complexes and relationship to the degree of prematurity (abstract). *Journal of the American College of Cardiology*, **39** (5 Suppl. A), 97A.

Koyama, J., Toda, S., Kon-No, Y. *et al.* (2002) Evaluation of heart-rate turbulence as a new prognostic marker in patients with chronic heart failure (abstract). *PACE (Pacing and Clinical Electrophysiology)*, **25** (4 Part II), 608.

Leffler, C.T., Saul, J.P. & Cohen, R.J. (1994) Rate-related and autonomic effects on atrioventricular conduction assessed through beat-to-beat PR interval and cycle length variability. *Journal of Cardiovascular Electrophysiology*, **5**, 2–15.

Lin, L.Y., Lai, L.P., Lin, J.L. *et al.* (2002) Tight mechanism correlation between heart rate turbulence and baroreflex sensitivity: sequential autonomic blockade analysis. *Journal of Cardiovascular Electrophysiology*, **13**, 427–431.

Makikallio, T.H., Hintze, U., Huikuri, H.V. *et al.* (2000) Comparison of post-ectopic turbulence analysis, fractal analysis and traditional heart rate variability analysis as predictors of mortality in patients with a recent and remote myocardial infarction (abstract). *Journal of the American College of Cardiology*, **35** (2 Suppl. A), 107A.

Malik, M., Wichterle, D. & Schmidt, G. (1999) Heart-rate turbulence. *Giornale Italiano di Cardiologia*, **29** (Suppl. 5), 65–69.

Marine, J.E., Watanabe, M.A., Smith, T.W. & Monahan, K.M. (2002) Effect of atropine on heart rate turbulence. *American Journal of Cardiology*, **89**, 767–769.

Roach, D., Koshman, M.L. & Sheldon, R. (2000) Turbulence: a focal, inducible, source of heart period variability associated with induced, transient hypertension (abstract). *PACE (Pacing and Clinical Electrophysiology)*, **23** (4 Part II), 709.

Savelieva, I., Wichterle, D., Haries, M., Meara, M., Camm, A.J. & Malik, M. (2003) Heart rate turbulence after atrial and ventricular premature beats: relation to left ventricular function and coupling intervals. *PACE (Pacing and Clinical Electrophysiology)*, **26**, 401–405.

Schmidt, G., Malik, M., Barthel, P. *et al.* (1999) Heart-rate turbulence after ventricular premature beats as a predictor of mortality after acute myocardial infarction. *Lancet*, **353**,1390–1396.

Schmidt, G., Bauer, A., Schneider, R. *et al.* (2000) Heart rate turbulence: impact of coupling interval and preceding sinus interval (abstract). *European Heart Journal*, **21** (Suppl.), 552.

Sestito, A., Valsecchi, S., De Filippis, M., Bencardino, G., Bellocci, F. & Lanza, G.A. (2002) Differences in heart rate turbulence between patients with coronary artery disease and patients with complex ventricular arrhythmias but structurally normal heart [abstract]. *Journal of the American College of Cardiology*, **39** (5 Suppl. A), 97A.

Szydlo, K. Trusz-Gluza, M., Orszulak, W., Wita, K. & Urbanczyk, D. (2002) HR- and *QT*-turbulence in patients with ventricular arrhythmias [abstract]. *Europace*, **3** (Suppl.), A42.

Watanabe, M.A., Marine, J.E., Sheldon, R. & Josephson, M.E. (2002) Effects of ventricular premature stimulus coupling interval on blood pressure and heart rate turbulence. *Circulation*, **106**, 325–330.

Wichterle, D., Savelieva, I., Meara, M., Camm, A.J. & Malik, M. (2003) Paradoxical autonomic modulation of atrioventricular nodal conduction during heart rate turbulence. *PACE (Pacing and Clinical Electrophysiology)*, **26**, 440–443.

Yap, Y.G., Camm, A.J., Schmidt, G. & Malik, M. (2001) Heart rate turbulence is influenced by heart rate, age, LVEF, NYHA class, diabetes, drugs and frequency of ventricular extopics in patients after acute myocardial infarction – EMIAT substudy [abstract]. *Journal of the American College of Cardiology*, **37** (2 Suppl. A), 133A.

CHAPTER 22

Physiological Hypotheses on Heart Rate Turbulence

Andreas Voss, Vico Baier, Alexander Schirdewan and Uwe Leder

Introduction

Since the description of an early acceleration and late deceleration in heart rate following ventricular premature beats, called heart rate turbulence (HRT) (Schmidt *et al.* 1999), considerable progress has been made in the understanding of physiological mechanisms underlying this regulatory process. The response to an endogenous disturbance of the heart rate–blood pressure sequence provides unique insights into regulation phenomena. In contrast to alternative methods that use exogenous stimuli as the baroreflex stimulation with phenylephrine the HRT method enables a quantification and characterization of blood pressure regulation mechanisms caused by intrinsic triggers.

Discovering the pathophysiological mechanisms involved in HRT offers not only an explanation of why this method is particularly suitable for risk stratification after myocardial infarction but also gives new insights into different consequences of arrhythmias on cardiac mortality.

In previous studies several mechanisms that might have influence on HRT have been discussed. At the early beginning it was assumed that it is caused by ventriculophasic sinus arrhythmia (Döhlemann *et al.* 1979), whereas presently available data support only hypotheses of mechanisms mediated by the autonomic reflex arch (Wichterle *et al.* 2002). Beside the loss of baroreflex sensitivity in heart failure patients due to a shifted sympatho-vagal balance, the influences of postextrasystolic potentiation, pulsus alternans, baseline heart rate, coupling interval, and compensatory pause were investigated in several studies. The schematic representation of these interdependencies is summarized in Fig. 22.1.

Influence of the autonomic nervous system

An early acceleration in heart rate after ventricular premature beats (VPBs) was described first in 1979 by Döhlemann *et al.* They attributed this observation to ventriculophasic sinus arrhythmia. This phenomenon is predominantly described in patients with various degrees of atrioventricular blockade, where *PP* intervals containing a QRS complex being slightly shorter than *PP* intervals without a QRS complex. Although ventriculophasic sinus arrhythmia was primarily discussed as a possible mechanism affecting HRT (Schmidt *et al.* 1999), it is preferred not to attribute a substantial role to this mechanism in HRT (Wichterle *et al.* 2002).

Several studies support the theory that HRT is vagally mediated (Lin *et al.* 2002). A transient loss of vagal efferent activity is caused by lowering of baroreflex afferent input during haemodynamically inefficient contractions by the VPB (Schmidt 2001).

This was initially assumed using a physiological model involving excitation generation in the heart, haemodynamic situation in the aorta, and baroreceptor feedback mechanisms (Mrowka *et al.* 2000). In case of intact baroreflex sensitivity the model produced HRT patterns similar to those of low risk patients, whereas after reducing baroreflex sensitivity the pattern was comparable to those of high-risk patients.

In the retrospective analysis of the ATRAMI (Autonomic Tone and Reflexes After Myocardial

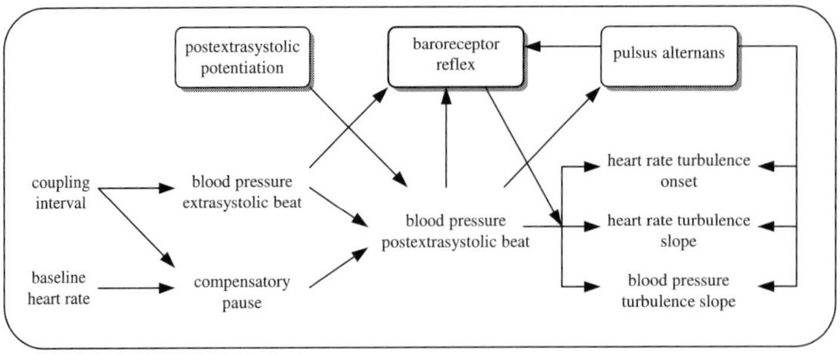

Fig. 22.1 Schematic representation of the different mechanisms influencing heart rate and blood pressure turbulence. The baroreceptor reflex represents the main mechanism of postextrasystolic regulation. Postextrasystolic potentiation and pulsus alternans might superimpose the vagally mediated baroreceptor response particularly in patients with compromised left ventricular function.

Table 22.1 Correlations of spontaneous baroreflex sensitivity (b_BRS, t_BRS) with turbulence derived BRS as well as heart rate turbulence slope (HRTS) and blood pressure turbulence slope (BPTS). Note the lack of correlation of BPTS with spontaneous BRS

		turb_BRS	*HRTS*	*BPTS*
Healthy subjects	b_BRS	0.97**	0.86**	NS
	t_BRS	0.85**	0.78**	NS
Heart failure patients	b_BRS	0.76**	0.73**	NS
	t_BRS	0.64**	0.56**	NS

** $P < 0.001$; NS, not significant.

Infarction – Ghuran *et al.* 2002) study, turbulence onset and turbulence slope moderately but significantly correlated with baroreflex sensitivity assessed by using the phenylephrine method ($r = -0.34$ and 0.44, $P < 0.001$).

Both, the aforementioned study and the analysis of 1486 patients after myocardial infarction with a left ventricular ejection fraction below 40% (EMIAT – European Myocardial Infarct Amiodarone Trial, Yap *et al.* 2000) revealed significant correlations of turbulence slope with the heart rate variability parameter sdNN ($r \sim 0.4$, $P < 0.0001$). Reduced variability, which is associated with impaired vagal or increased sympathetic activity, causes decreased turbulence slope values.

Turbulence derived baroreflex sensitivity calculated from the ratio of heart rate and blood pressure (*BP*) turbulence slope in 45 patients with chronic heart failure was significantly correlated ($r = 0.67$; $P < 0.0001$) with the spontaneous baroreflex sensitivity (alpha-index method – Davies *et al.* 2001). This relation was attributed to the correlation of heart rate turbulence slope and baroreflex sensitivity ($r = 0.70$; $P < 0.0001$), whereas *BP* turbulence slope did not correlate with baroreflex sensitivity ($r = 0.10$; $P = n.s.$).

We recently demonstrated these dependencies in healthy subjects (Voss *et al.* 2002a,b), where spontaneous baroreflex sensitivity was also highly correlated ($r \sim 0.9$) with turbulence derived baroreflex sensitivity and heart rate turbulence slope ($r \sim 0.8$) but not with *BP* turbulence slope ($r < 0.1$, Table 22.1).

During atropine-induced vagal blockade the turbulence slope significantly ($P = 0.0002$) decreased and turbulence onset increased significantly ($P = 0.0012$, Marine *et al.* 2002) in patients without structural heart disease. The influence of vagal activity was tested during programmed ventricular pacing with systematically introduced VPBs in 16 patients with structural heart diseases (Lin *et al.* 2002). Turbulence parameters were calculated at baseline and after sequential sympathetic (esmolol), parasympathetic (atropine) and combined (esmolol and atropine) autonomic blockade. The turbulence slope ($P < 0.01$) and the turbulence onset ($P < 0.05$) were significantly affected by vagal and combined autonomic blockade; however, there was no response to sympathetic blockade.

Furthermore, it was found that HRT is mediated by beat-to-beat changes in sinoatrial rate, because there is a relatively small effect of the VPB on subsequent atrio-His and His-ventricle intervals (atrioventricular conduction). Thus, preserved vagal influence on the sinus node is a stringent condition for normal HRT (Marine *et al.* 2002).

Coupling interval and compensatory pause

In normal subjects a negative correlation ($r = -0.4$; $P < 0.001$) between heart rate turbulence slope and the coupling interval of the VPB was reported (Indik *et al.* 2002). In the placebo arm of EMIAT ($n = 428$) strong interdependencies of heart rate and turbulence parameters were found. The influence of the coupling interval on HRT increased with decreasing heart rate. The lower the heart rate and the shorter the coupling interval the more pronounced became HRT (Bauer 2000). Watanabe *et al.* (2002) investigated the effects of ventricular premature stimulus coupling intervals and compensatory pause on *BP* and HRT. No correlation was found between the coupling interval and turbulence parameters. The positive correlation between turbulence slope and compensatory pause was abolished after normalizing the compensatory pause to the *RR* interval before the VPB, because patients with high heart rates have low turbulence slope and vice versa. Therefore, baseline heart rate did affect turbulence parameters rather than prematurity of the VPB.

Watanabe *et al.* (2002) also investigated the relationship between the VPB coupling and arterial *BP*. Systolic *BP* of VPBs was steeply related to the coupling interval, but remained constant after compensatory pause independent from the duration of the compensatory pause. Diastolic *BP* was found to be inversely related to both, coupling interval and compensatory pause. Consequently, pulse pressure (systolic *BP* minus diastolic *BP*) was steeply related to VPB coupling interval and moderately related to compensatory pause. Therefore, the independence of systolic *BP* from compensatory pause duration or the nonlinear characteristics of the baroreflex was hypothesized to be responsible for the poor correlation between coupling interval and turbulence parameters.

Postextrasystolic regulation

The blood pressure during VPBs differs from pressure set point of the baroreceptor reflex for at least one beat. The ejection of low stroke volume by the extrasystolic beat into the aorta induces lower extrasystolic pulse wave amplitude and lowered diastolic *BP* because of the compensatory pause and a reduced filling of the arterial vascular compartment. This results in a reduced distension of arterial (aortic, carotid) pressoreceptors (Voss *et al.* 2002a). It decreases tonic vagal nerve activity and its inhibitory influence on the heart (Guzik & Schmidt 2002). Vagal response to changes in *BP* starts as fast as within 500–600 ms (Borst & Karemaker 1983). This fast activation of the baroreflex enables a heart rate response to changes in *BP* on a beat-to-beat basis. The degree of activation of the pressoreceptors depends on the speed of the arterial *BP* increase, on the *BP* amplitude, and on the mean arterial *BP* (Greger & Windhorst 1996).

In patients with preserved left ventricular function as well as in healthy subjects the first postextrasystolic beat produces significantly reduced systolic *BP* and the haemodynamic deficit caused by the VPB will not become compensated (Wichterle *et al.* 2002; Voss *et al.* 2002a; Fig. 22.2). This drop in *BP* continues for the first few postextrasystolic beats. The transient loss of vagal nerve activity causes an immediate increase in heart rate and, therefore, was believed to be the cause of the early phase of acceleration of the heart rate after a VPB (Malik *et al.* 1999).

About two beats after the VPB the *BP* increases (Voss *et al.* 2002a). Heart rate is higher as long as the *BP* reaches its preextrasystolic level about four beats after the VPB (Fig. 22.2). The phase of deceleration in heart rate is preceded by this increase in *BP* and is the consequence of a baroreflex response to an increase in vagal nerve

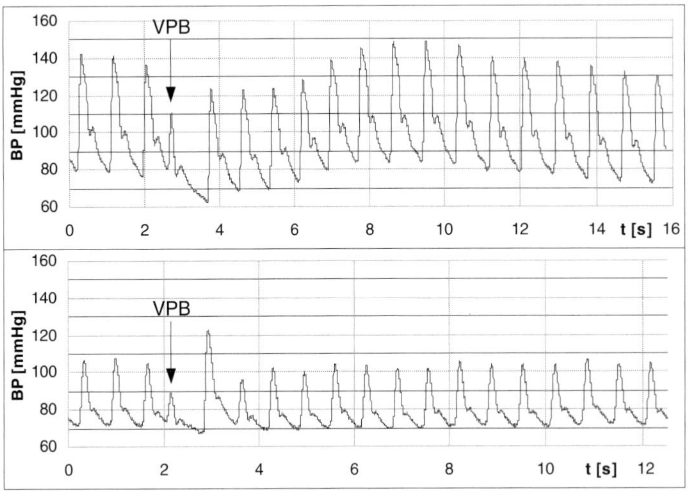

Fig. 22.2 Blood pressure (*BP*) response to a ventricular premature beat (VPB, arrow) in a healthy subject (top) and a patient with idiopathic dilated cardiomyopathy (bottom). *BP* traces were recorded noninvasively. Note the different increase in postextrasystolic *BP* amplitudes compared with preextrasystolic *BP* amplitudes.

activity (Guzik & Schmidt 2002) caused by an increased distension of pressoreceptors.

These findings let us suggest that heart rate turbulence slope reflects the instantaneous regulation by the baroreflex, whereas *BP* turbulence slope reflects the compensation of the haemodynamic deficit by a superimposition of an increase in heart rate and in peripheral vascular resistance. This might explain the poor correlation between *BP* turbulence slope and spontaneous baroreflex sensitivity.

Postextrasystolic potentiation and pulsus alternans

Supposing that the premature beat is followed by a compensatory pause, postextrasystolic potentia-tion appears (Hamby *et al.* 1975; Yamazoe 1987; Cooper 1993). Postextrasystolic potentiation is a phenomenon of augmented contractility following VPBs that is independent of ventricular loading and represents a distinct property of the myocardium (Cooper 1993). Despite a number of studies investigating the cause of postextrasystolic potentiation, the underlying mechanisms are not fully understood. Available experimental data relate this phenomenon to three main mechanisms: First, the increase in activator calcium due to augmented intracellular stores; second, an enhanced ability of the sarcoplasmatic reticulum to release calcium; and third, greater transsarcolemmal movement of calcium (Scognamiglio *et al.* 1998).

Several studies reported increased postextrasystolic potentiation in patients with idiopathic dilated cardiomyopathy (IDC) (Welch *et al.* 1989) compared with normal ventricles. In these IDC patients a postextrasystolic *BP* amplitude is twice as high as the normal ventricular systole. The degree of potentiation in *BP* obviously depends on the left ventricular end-diastolic diameter and left ventricular ejection fraction (Voss *et al.* 2002a).

Patients with compromised left ventricular function have sudden increase in systolic and diastolic *BP* of the first postextrasystolic beat caused by augmented myocardial contractility, increased stroke volume, and increased outflow velocity due to postextrasystolic potentiation. Augmented *BP* amplitude of the postextrasystolic beat overcompensates low preceding diastolic *BP* and, therefore, changes the baroreceptor response initiated by the VPB.

Furthermore, postextrasystolic potentiation triggers pulsus alternans in patients with compromised left ventricular function (Davies *et al.* 2001; Voss *et al.* 2002a,b). Pulsus alternans is a phenomenon known for a long time in the severely failing heart (Traube 1872; Schaefer *et al.* 1988) as it is for electrical alternans (Surawicz & Fisch 2002). These phenomena become obvious at macroscopic level in end-stages of heart failure. Pulsus alternans results from alternations of end-diastolic volume, probably related to Frank Starling mechanism or to an alternating contractility of the ventricle (Hada *et al.* 1982) caused by an increased avail-

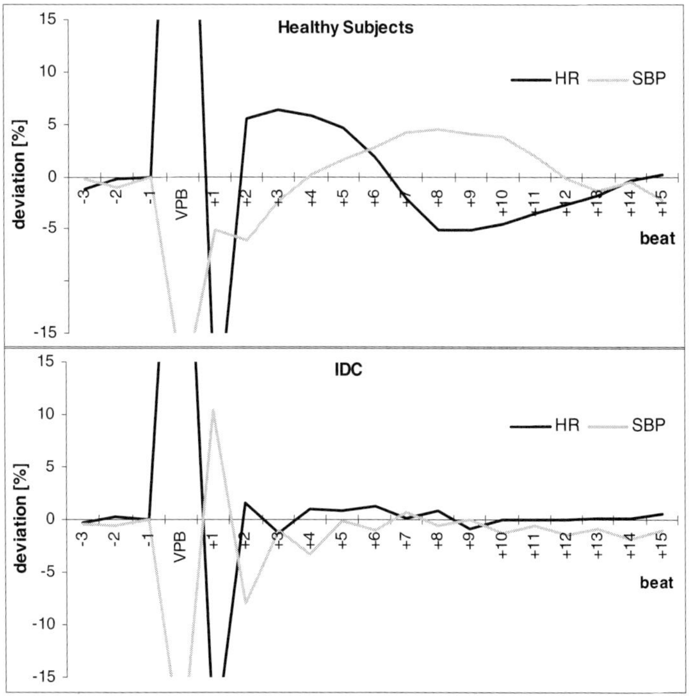

Fig. 22.3 Postextrasystolic regulation of heart rate (HR) and systolic *BP* (SBP) in 13 healthy subjects (top) and in 12 patients with idiopathic dilated cardiomyopathy (IDC). In healthy subjects a typical baroreflex response is apparent, whereas in IDC patients, the baroreflex response is superimposed by the response to postextrasystolic regulation and pulsus alternans. Group mean values are plotted as relative deviation from the reference, which is the last sinus beat preceding the ventricular premature beat (VPB).

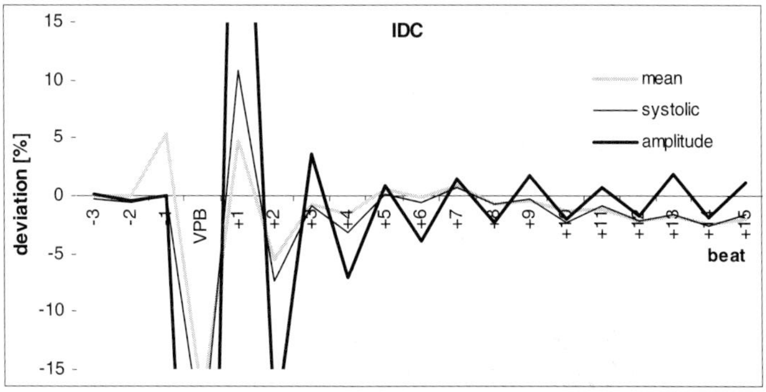

Fig. 22.4 Postextrasystolic regulation of mean *BP*, systolic *BP* and *BP* amplitude in patients with idiopathic dilated cardiomyopathy. Pulsus alternans is triggered by postextrasystolic potentiation. Otherwise the alternating amplitude would be smoothed by the averaging procedure as during the last beats preceeding the ventricular premature beat. Group mean values are plotted as relative deviation from the reference, which is the last sinus beat preceding the ventricular premature beat (VPB) for systolic *BP* and *BP* amplitude values. The reference for mean *BP* is beat$_{-2}$.

ability of intracellular calcium (Suko *et al.* 1970). Carlson & Rapaport (1984) interpreted postextrasystolic and sustained pulsus alternans as an inevitable consequence of alterations in heart rate and the relationship between ejection and diastolic filling.

The postextrasystolic *BP* regulation pattern in patients with impaired left ventricular function (IDC) is shown in Fig. 22.3. In the majority of these patients we observed pulsus alternans during long periods of sinus rhythm (Leder *et al.* 2002). Postextrasystolic pulsus alternans (amplitude alternans, Fig. 22.4) is triggered by the premature beat and postextrasystolic potentiation.

There is an interrelation of the different regulation phenomena. It is known that heart failure patients with postextrasystolic pulsus alternans have a significant lower heart rate turbulence slope and baroreflex sensitivity (turbulence derived), and lower ejection fraction than those without postextrasystolic pulsus alternans (Davies *et al.* 2001).

The increased vagal nerve activity due to postextrasystolic potentiation and furthermore the occurrence of postextrasystolic pulsus alternans significantly influence the early acceleration phase and prevent late deceleration phase in heart rate particularly in IDC patients. In this case both, the extrasystolic and postextrasystolic *BP* determine the regulation patterns following a VPB and HRT could not be observed (Voss *et al.* 2002a,b).

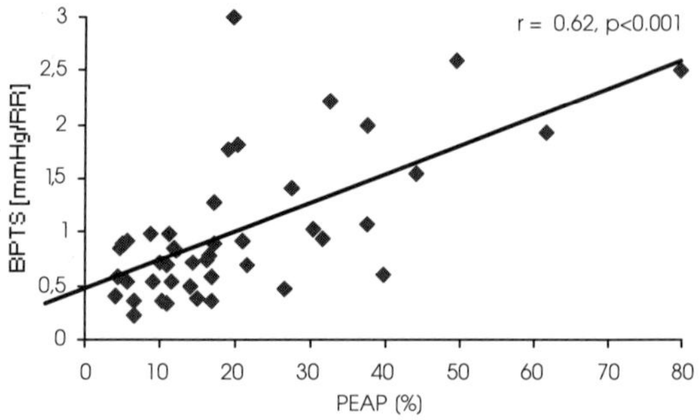

Fig. 22.5 Correlation between postextrasystolic potentiation of the blood pressure amplitude (PEAP) and blood pressure turbulence slope (BPTS) in 44 patients with heart failure.

Blood pressure turbulence slope, postextrasystolic potentiation and pulsus alternans

The reviewed literature does not fully explain the influence of postextrasystolic potentiation and pulsus alternans on *BP* turbulence slope. Therefore, in the following chapter we present new data from a recent study in 44 patients with heart failure.

We recorded ECG and noninvasive finger arterial *BP* (Portapres®) simultaneously for 30 min under standardized resting conditions. The overall number of VPBs was 413 ranging from 1 to 55 episodes in the individual patient. From these episodes we calculated heart rate turbulence onset HRTO, heart rate turbulence slope HRTS (Schmidt *et al.* 1999), slope of the mean *BP* (BPTS) (Davies *et al.* 2001; Voss *et al.* 2002a), and the ratio of post- and pre-extrasystolic *BP* amplitudes (PEAP) (Voss *et al.* 2002a). Turbulence-derived baroreflex sensitivity (turb_BRS – Davies *et al.* 2001) was determined as the ratio of HRTS and BPTS. Further on, we calculated spontaneous baroreflex sensitivity based on the sequence method (Bertinieri *et al.* 1985) for bradycardic (b_BRS, increasing *BP* with subsequent increasing sinus cycle length) and tachycardic (t_BRS, decreasing *BP* with subsequent decreasing sinus cycle length) sequences. If postextrasystolic pulsus alternans occurred, the magnitude of this alternans (MAL) was quantified by the maximum mean value of four consecutive amplitude differences (five beats) within the second to 20th postextrasystolic beats.

Spontaneous baroreflex sensitivity and the turbulence derived baroreflex sensitivity were significantly correlated ($r = 0.7$, $P < 0.001$, Table 22.1). This can be attributed to the correlation of spontaneous baroreflex sensitivity with heart rate turbulence slope rather than with *BP* turbulence slope (Table 22.1), which is in accordance with Davies *et al.* (2001).

The influence of the postextrasystolic *BP* amplitude on *BP* turbulence slope depends on the degree of potentiation, because PEAP was significantly correlated ($r = 0.62$, $P < 0.001$) with BPTS (Fig. 22.5).

19 patients developed postextrasystolic pulsus alternans. These patients had significant lower left ventricular ejection fraction (EF: 45 ± 18% vs. 59 ± 15%, $P < 0.01$), a more pronounced postextrasystolic potentiation (PEAP: 26 ± 18% vs. 14 ± 12%, $P < 0.01$) and an increased *BP* turbulence slope (BPTS: 1.30 ± 0.77 mmHg/*RR* vs. 0.74 ± 0.41 mmHg/*RR*, $P < 0.01$) than patients without pulsus alternans. Alternans magnitude and *BP* turbulence slope (that are both assessed over five consecutive beats) were significantly correlated ($r = 0.63$, $P < 0.001$, Fig. 22.6).

These results further confirm the influence of postextrasystolic potentiation and pulsus alternans on *BP* regulation following a VPB.

Summary

Heart rate turbulence is vagally dependent because of a transient loss of vagal efferent activ-

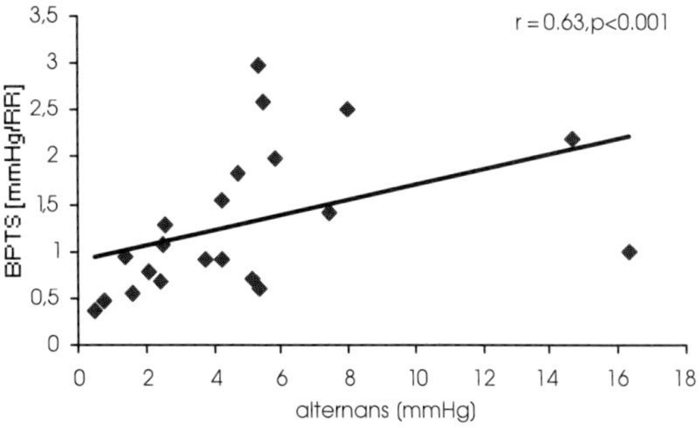

Fig. 22.6 Correlation between magnitude of postextrasystolic pulsus alternans (MAL) and blood pressure turbulence slope (BPTS) in 19 patients with heart failure.

ity. This is caused by a lowered baroreflex afferent input due to the haemodynamical inefficient contraction of the ventricular premature beat. Correlation between baroreflex sensitivity obtained with spontaneous methods and obtained with turbulence method arises from the correlation of the baroreflex sensitivity with heart rate turbulence slope rather than *BP* turbulence slope.

In patients with compromised left ventricular function the baroreflex regulation might be superimposed by the phenomena of postextrasystolic potentiation and pulsus alternans, which influence heart rate and *BP* regulation. The increased *BP* caused by postextrasystolic potentiation and the resulting increase in vagal activity significantly influence the early acceleration phase and might prevent late deceleration phase in heart rate. Therefore, the response to ventricular premature beats is both, a consequence of ventricular contractility and baroreflex activity.

References

Bauer, A. (2000) *Einfluß von Kopplungsintervall und Herzfrequenz auf die heart rate turbulence [Impact of coupling interval and heart rate on heart rate turbulence]*. PhD thesis, Technische Universität München.

Bertinieri, G., di Rienzo, M., Cavallazzi, A., Ferrari, A.U., Pedotti, A. & Mancia, G. (1985) A new approach to analysis of the arterial baroreflex. *Journal of Hypertension*, **3** (Suppl. 3), 79–81.

Borst, C. & Karemaker, J.M. (1983) Time delays in the human baroreceptor reflex. *Journal of the Autonomic Nervous System*, **9**, 399–409.

Carlson, C.J. & Rapaport, E. (1984) Postextrasystolic pulsus alternans and heart rate. *American Journal of Physiology*, **246**, 245–249.

Cooper, M.W. (1993) Postextrasystolic potentiation. Do we really know what it means and how to use it? *Circulation*, **88**, 2962–2971.

Davies, L.C., Francis, D.P., Ponikowski, P., Piepoli, M.F. & Coats, A.J. (2001) Relation of heart rate and blood pressure turbulence following premature ventricular complexes to baroreflex sensitivity in chronic congestive heart failure. *American Journal of Cardiology*, **87**, 737–742.

Döhlemann, C., Murawski, P., Theissen, K., Haider, M., Förster, C. & Pöppl, S.J. (1979) Ventriculophasische Sinusarrhythmie bei ventrikulärer Extrasystolie. [Ventricular premature systoles causing ventriculophasic sinus arrhythmia.] *Zeitschrift für Kardiologie*, **68**, 557–565.

Ghuran, A., Reid, F., La Rovere, M.T. *et al.* for the ATRAMI Investigators (2002) Heart rate turbulence-based predictors of fatal and nonfatal cardiac arrest (The Autonomic Tone and Reflexes After Myocardial Infarction substudy). *American Journal of Cardiology*, **89**, 184–190.

Greger, R. & Windhorst, U. (eds) (1996) *Comprehensive Human Physiology – From Cellular Mechanisms to Integration*. Springer, Berlin.

Guzik, P. & Schmidt, G. (2002) A phenomenon of heart-rate turbulence, its evaluation, and prognostic value. *Cardiac Electrophysiology Review*, **6**, 256–261.

Hada, Y., Wolfe, C. & Craige, E. (1982) Pulsus alternans determined by biventricular simultaneous systolic time intervals. *Circulation*, **65**, 617–626.

Hamby, R.I., Aintablian, A., Wisoff, G. & Hartstein, M.L. (1975) Response of the left ventricle in coronary artery disease to postextrasystolic potentiation. *Circulation*, **51**, 428–435.

Indik, J.H., Ott, P. & Marcus, F.I. (2002) Heart rate turbulence and fractal scaling coefficient in response to premature atrial and ventricular complexes and relationship to the degree of prematurity. *Journal of the American College of Cardiology*, **39** (Suppl. 1), 97–98.

Leder, U., Pohl, H.P., Baier, V. *et al.* (2002) Alternans of blood pressure and heart rate in dilated cardiomyopathy. *Pacing and Clinical Electrophysiology*, **25**, 1307–1314.

Lin, L.-Y., Lai, L.-P., Lin, J.-L. *et al.* (2002) Tight mechanism correlation between heart rate turbulence and baroreflex sensitivity: sequential autonomic blockade analysis. *Journal of Cardiovascular Electrophysiology*, **13**, 427–431.

Malik, M., Wichterle, D. & Schmidt, G. (1999) Heart-rate turbulence. *Giornale Italiano Cardiologia*, **29** (Suppl. 5), 65–69.

Marine, J.E., Watanabe, M.A., Smith, T.W. & Monahan,

K.M. (2002) Effect of atropine on heart rate turbulence. *American Journal of Cardiology*, **89**, 767–769.

Mrowka, R., Persson, P.B., Theres, H. & Patzak, A. (2000) Blunted arterial baroreflex causes 'pathological' heart rate turbulence. *American Journal of Physiology (Regulatory, Integrative and Comparative Physiology)* **279**, 1171–1175.

Schaefer, S., Malloy, C.R., Schmitz, J.M. & Dehmer, G.J. (1988) Clinical and hemodynamic characteristics of patients with inducible pulsus alternans. *American Heart Journal*, **115**, 1251–1257.

Schmidt, G., Malik, M., Barthel, P. *et al.* (1999) Heart-rate turbulence after ventricular premature beats as a predictor of mortality after acute myocardial infarction. *Lancet*, **353**, 1390–1396.

Schmidt, G. (2001) Heart rate turbulence. In: *Risk of Arrhythmia and Sudden Death* (ed. M. Malik), pp. 242–248. BMJ Books, London.

Scognamiglio, R., Marin, M., Miorelli, M., Palisi, M., Fasoli, G. & Dalla Volta, S. (1998) Postextrasystolic potentiation echocardiography in predicting reversible myocardial dysfunction by surgical coronary revascularization. *American Journal of Cardiology*, **81**, 36–40.

Suko, J., Ueba, Y. & Chidsey, C.A. (1970) Intracellular calcium and myocardial contractility. II. Effects of postextrasystolic potentiation in the isolated rabbit heart. *Circulation, Research*, **27**, 227–234.

Surawicz, B. & Fisch, C. (2002) Cardiac alternans: diverse mechanisms and clinical manifestations. *Journal of the American College of Cardiology*, **20**, 483–499.

Traube L. (1872) Ein Fall von Pulsus bigeminus nebst Bemerkungen über die Leberschwellungen bei Klappenfehlern und über akute Leberatrophie. *Berliner Klinische Wochenschrift*, **9**, 185–188.

Voss, A., Baier, V., Schumann, A. *et al.* (2002) Postextrasystolic regulation patterns of blood pressure and heart rate in patients with idiopathic dilated cardiomyopathy. *Journal of Physiology*, **538**, 271–8.

Voss, A., Baier, V., Hopfe, J., Schirdewan, A. & Leder, U. (2002) Heart rate and blood pressure turbulence – marker of the baroreflex sensitivity or consequence of postextrasystolic potentiation and pulsus alternans? *American Journal of Cardiology*, **89**, 110–111.

Watanabe, M.A., Marine, J.E., Sheldon, R. & Josephson, M.E. (2002) Effects of ventricular premature stimulus coupling interval on blood pressure and heart rate turbulence. *Circulation*, **106**, 325–330.

Welch, W.J., Smith, M.L., Rea, R.F., Bauernfeind, R.A. & Eckberg, D.L. (1989) Enhancement of sympathetic nerve activity by single premature ventricular beats in humans. *Journal of the American College of Cardiology*, **13**, 69–75.

Wichterle, D., Melenovsky, V. & Malik, M. (2002) Mechanisms involved in heart rate turbulence. *Cardiac Electrophysiology Review*, **6**, 262–266.

Yamazoe M. (1987) Response of the left ventricle in idiopathic dilated cardiomyopathy to postextrasystolic potentiation. *American Heart Journal*, **113**, 1449–1456.

Yap, Y.G., Camm, A.J., Schmidt, G. & Malik, M. (2000) Heart rate turbulence is influenced by sympatho-vagal balance in patients after myocardial infarction – EMIAT substudy. *European Journal of Heart Failure*, **2** (Suppl. 1), 51.

CHAPTER 23

Heart Rate Turbulence in Ischaemic Heart Disease

Axel Bauer and Georg Schmidt

Introduction

Sudden cardiac death (SCD) is the main cause of death among patients with ischaemic heart disease (Huikuri *et al.* 2001). There is clinical evidence that in patients with ischaemic heart disease who are at high risk, mortality can be substantially reduced by prophylactic implantation of an internal cardioverter defibrillator (ICD) (Moss *et al.* 1996; Buxton *et al.* 1999; Moss *et al.* 2002). However, only a small proportion of patients prone to death fulfil the inclusion criteria used in the primary prevention trials. Aim of modern risk stratification strategies is therefore to substantially enlarge the number of patients who might benefit from prophylactic ICD therapy.

It is widely accepted that reduced left ventricular ejection fraction (LVEF) is the single most important risk factor for overall mortality and SCD in patients with ischaemic heart disease (Priori *et al.* 2001). In the last decades markers of autonomic dysfunction became increasingly important and it could be shown that markers like SDNN, mean heart rate and baroreflex sensitivity significantly improve risk assessment based on LVEF (La Rovere *et al.* 1998).

Heart rate turbulence (HRT) is a novel and promising risk predictor quantifying the autonomic reflex response of heart rate to single VPC (Schmidt *et al.* 1999).

Clinical value of heart rate turbulence

HRT has been developed in an open training sample containing 100 patients with ischaemic heart disease. In this patient group, the mathematical algorithm for the calculation of HRT was defined and optimized. The exact formulae are described elsewhere (Chapter 21) (Schmidt *et al.* 1999; Malik *et al.* 1999a,b). Briefly, HRT is quantified by turbulence onset (TO) and turbulence slope (TS). TO quantifies the initial postextrasystolic acceleration of heart rate, TS quantifies the subsequent deceleration of heart rate. Within the training sample, the cut-off values for TO and TS have been determined. These cut-off values have been used for all further analyses. They were 0% for TO and 2.5ms/*RR* interval (RRI) for TS. Accordingly, abnormal HRT is characterized by a TO $\geq$0% and a TS $\leq$2.5ms/RRI.

The clinical value of HRT as risk predictor after acute myocardial infarction has been validated in three large post-myocardial infarction trials, namely the population of the Multicentre Post-Infarction Program (MPIP) (Multicentre Postinfarctions Research Group 1983), the placebo arm of the European Myocardial Infarction Amiodarone Trial (EMIAT) (Julian *et al.* 1997) and the Autonomic Tone and Reflexes after Acute Myocardial Infarction trial (ATRAMI) (La Rovere *et al.* 1998). All studies have been finished before the phenomenon of HRT has been discovered. However, the statistical analyses of HRT were performed in a blinded fashion by an independent centre (Schmidt *et al.* 1999; Ghuran *et al.* 2002).

The study characteristics, the clinical variables and the treatment of the study populations can be taken from Table 23.1. MPIP was a postinfarction study of the pre-lysis era with a comparable high overall mortality. EMIAT was a postinfarction study of the lysis era restricted to patients with reduced LVEF. ATRAMI was a postinfarction study of the lysis era with comparable low mortality. In MPIP and EMIAT, the pre-

Table 23.1 MPIP, EMIAT and ATRAMI: study characteristics, clinical variables and therapy. AMI: acute myocardial infarction; LVEF: left ventricle ejection fraction; VPC: ventricular premature complexes

	MPIP (n = 577)	*EMIAT (Placebo)* (n = 614)	*ATRAMI* (n = 981)
Inclusion criteria	AMI	AMI & LVEF (40%)	AMI
Primary endpoint	Total mortality	Total mortality	Cardiac mortality
	13% (75/577)	14% (87/614)	4% (40/981)
Follow-up (months)	22	21	20
Age (years)	57 (9)	61 (9)	57 (10)
Women (%)	22	15	13
Previous infarction (%)	26	26	7
VPC/h	16 (49)	48 (186)	14 (61)
LVEF (%)	45 (15)	30 (9)	49 (12)
Thrombolysis (%)	0	60	63

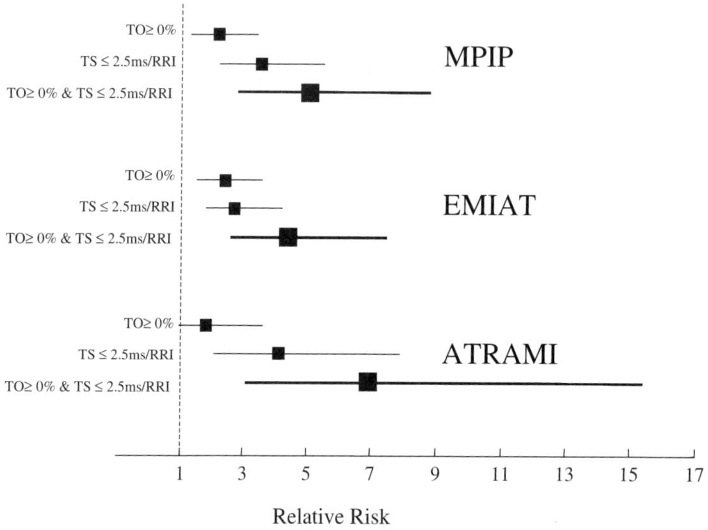

Fig. 23.1 Relative risks of total mortality (MPIP & EMIAT)/ cardiac mortality (ATRAMI) for turbulence onset (TO), turbulence slope (TS) and combined use of TO and TS in the study populations of MPIP, EMIAT (placebo) and ATRAMI, respectively.

defined primary endpoint was total mortality. In ATRAMI, the primary endpoint was total cardiac mortality, a composed endpoint of fatal and non-fatal cardiac arrest. In all three studies, mean follow-up was about 2 years.

In all studies, HRT was significantly associated with the primary endpoint. TO and TS were used both as separate variables and as combined variables. In the latter case three HRT categories were formed: 0 = TO and TS normal, 1 = TO or TS abnormal, 2 = TO and TS abnormal. Highest relative risks were achieved for HRT category 2 (Fig. 23.1). In MPIP, EMIAT and ATRAMI, the relative risks were 5.0 (2.8–8.8), 4.4 (2.6–7.5) and 6.9 (3.1–5.5), respectively.

Table 23.2 shows the results of the multivariate analyses in the MPIP, EMIAT and ATRAMI populations, respectively. The analyses included the most commonly accepted conventional risk variables: age, history of previous myocardial infarction (only MPIP and EMIAT), mean *RR* interval, heart rate variability (HRV index used in MPIP and EMIAT, SDNN used in ATRAMI), arrhythmia on Holter (VPC/h (10 and/or presence of nonsustained ventricular tachycardia used in MPIP and EMIAT, VPC/h (10 used in ATRAMI), baroreflex sensitivity (only available in ATRAMI), LVEF and HRT. All variables were dichotomized at previously established cut-off points (Table 23.2).

In all three populations, HRT category 2 and LVEF were the most important independent risk predictors with HRT being even stronger than LVEF. The relative risks of an abnormal HRT were 3.2 (1.7–6.0), 3.2 (1.8–5.6) and 4.1 (1.7–9.8) in MPIP, EMIAT and ATRAMI, respectively. In MPIP

Table 23.2 MPIP, EMIAT and ATRAMI: multivariate analyses. Same abbreviations as in Table 23.1 and in Fig. 23.1

	MPIP (n = 577)	*EMIAT (placebo)* (n = 614)	*ATRAMI* (n = 981)
Age (65 years)	–	–	–
Previous infarction	–	1.8 (1.2–2.7)	Not included
Mean *R* – *R* interval (800 ms)	–	1.8 (1.1–2.9)	–
Heart rate variability*	–	–	–
Arrhythmia†	–	–	–
Baroreflex sensitivity <3 ms/mmHg	Not available	Not available	–
LVEF‡	2.9 (1.8–4.9)	1.7 (1.1–2.7)	3.5 (1.8–7.1)
Heart rate turbulence (TO (0%) and TS (2.5 ms/RRI)	3.2 (1.7–6.0)	3.2 (1.8–5.6)	4.1 (1.7–9.8)

* HRV index (20 units (MPIP & EMIAT), SDNN <70 ms (ATRAMI).
† VPC/h (10 and/or non-sustained VT (MPIP & EMIAT), VPC/h (10 (ATRAMI).
‡ LVEF <30% (MPIP & EMIAT), LVEF (35% (ATRAMI).

and ATRAMI, LVEF and HRT were the only two independent predictors of mortality. In EMIAT, also history of previous myocardial infarction and mean *RR* interval provided independent prognostic information in addition to LVEF and HRT.

Conclusion

In postinfarction patients, HRT is a strong and independent risk predictor of total mortality and cardiac mortality, respectively. HRT is superior to other ECG based risk predictors and contributes substantially to LVEF as the single most important risk predictor in patients with ischaemic heart disease.

References

Buxton, A.E., Lee, K.L., Fisher, J.D. *et al.* (1999) A randomized study of the prevention of sudden death in patients with coronary artery disease. Multicentre Unsustained Tachycardia Trial Investigators. *New England Journal of Medicine*, **341**, 1882–1890.

Ghuran, A., Reid, F., La Rovere, M.T. *et al.* (2002) Heart rate turbulence-based predictors of fatal and nonfatal cardiac arrest (The Autonomic Tone and Reflexes After Myocardial Infarction substudy). *American Journal of Cardiology*, **89**, 184–190.

Huikuri, H.V., Castellanos, A. & Myerburg, R.J. (2001) Sudden death due to cardiac arrhythmias. *New England Journal of Medicine*, **345**, 1473–1482.

Julian, D.G., Camm, A.J., Frangin, G. *et al.* (1997) Randomised trial of effect of amiodarone on mortality in patients with left-ventricular dysfunction after recent myocardial infarction: EMIAT. European Myocardial Infarct Amiodarone Trial Investigators. *Lancet*, **349**, 667–674.

La Rovere, M.T., Bigger, J.T., Jr, Marcus, F.I. *et al.* (1998) Baroreflex sensitivity and heart-rate variability in prediction of total cardiac mortality after myocardial infarction. ATRAMI (Autonomic Tone and Reflexes After Myocardial Infarction) Investigators [see comments]. *Lancet*, **351**, 478–484.

Malik, M., Schmidt, G., Barthel, P. *et al.* (1999) Heart rate turbulence is a postinfarction mortality predictor which is independent of and additive to other recognized risk factors. *PACE (Pacing and Clinical Electrophysiology)*, **22**, 741.

Malik, M., Wichterle, D. & Schmidt, G. (1999) Heart-rate turbulence. *Giornale Italiano Cardiologia*, **29**, 65–69.

Moss, A.J., Hall, W.J., Cannom, D.S. *et al.* (1996) Improved survival with an implanted defibrillator in patients with coronary disease at high risk for ventricular arrhythmia. Multicentre Automatic Defibrillator Implantation Trial Investigators [see comments]. *New England Journal of Medicine*, **335**, 1933–1940.

Moss, A.J., Zareba, W., Hall, W.J. *et al.* (2002) Prophylactic implantation of a defibrillator in patients with myocardial infarction and reduced ejection fraction. *New England Journal of Medicine*, **346**, 877–883.

Multicentre Postinfarctions Research Group. (1983) Risk stratification and survival after myocardial infarction. *New England Journal of Medicine*, **309**, 331–336.

Priori, S.G., Aliot, E., Blomstrom-Lundqvist, C. *et al.* (2001) Task Force on Sudden Cardiac Death of the European Society of Cardiology. *European Heart Journal*, **22**, 1374–1450.

Schmidt, G., Malik, M., Barthel, P. *et al.* (1999) Heart-rate turbulence after ventricular premature beats as a predictor of mortality after acute myocardial infarction. *Lancet*, **353**, 1390–1396.

SECTION III
Ischaemic Patterns

CHAPTER 24

Electrocardiographic Background

Marian Vandyck-Acquah and Paul Schweitzer

Introduction

The 12-lead electrocardiogram (ECG) is a simple and reliable diagnostic tool in patients with suspected acute coronary syndromes (ACS). It is helpful in differentiation between various types of ACS, the timing of event and the localization of coronary artery occlusion. It is also useful in risk stratification. The purpose of this chapter is to review the electrocardiographic background of myocardial ischaemia.

Basic electrophysiology

At rest there is a negative intracellular electric potential. Stimulation of the myocardial cell creates an action potential (AP) representing depolarization and repolarization of the myocardial cell. During depolarization, positively charged ions cross the cell membrane into the cell, while during repolarization they are pumped out. A wave of depolarization spreads throughout all myocardial cells and the first cells to depolarize, begin a sequence of repolarization. The ECG summation in a single cell is depicted in Fig. 24.1 showing the opposite directions of the waves in time. However, in the whole myocardium the situation is more complex. The duration of the AP differs across the ventricular wall. The APs are longest near the endocardium, shortest near the epicardium and intermediate at mid wall sites. This difference, explains why repolarization is completed in the epicardium before the endocardium which translates into transmural gradient. During depolarization, a surface epicardial unipolar electrode records the intracellular current flow from positive to negative (endocardium to epicardium) and during repolarization from less recovered endocardium to fully recovered epicardium, hence the QRS complex and T waves are concordant and upright (Fig. 24.2).

Electrophysiology of the ischaemic myocardium

Before discussing the ECG manifestations of myocardial ischaemia, it is important to review the sequence of events following acute occlusion of a coronary artery. Figure 24.3 illustrates that mechanical wall motion abnormalities develop about 19 s after balloon inflation followed immediately by ST segment shifts and 10 s later by angina. Filling pressures also rise before the ECG changes occur.

Myocardial ischaemia markedly influences the electrophysiological properties of the myocardial cell. Ischaemia lowers the resting membrane potentials to less negative values (−60 to −65 mV) owing to a rise in extracellular potassium, which depolarizes the cell. There is also a reduction in rate of rise of phase 0 (reduction of number of sodium channels opened), and the amplitude and duration of the AP are decreased.

The electrocardiographic effect of myocardial ischaemia is the 'injury current' which results from partial depolarizations and shortened APs generating potential gradients between the ischaemic and neighbouring normal cells. These electrophysiological abnormalities produce diastolic as well as systolic injury currents (Fig. 24.4) and manifest as deviations in the ST–T segments on the surface ECG.

When ischaemia is transmural the ST vector is shifted in the direction of the epicardial layers producing ST segment elevations and tall T waves over the ischaemic zone because the early

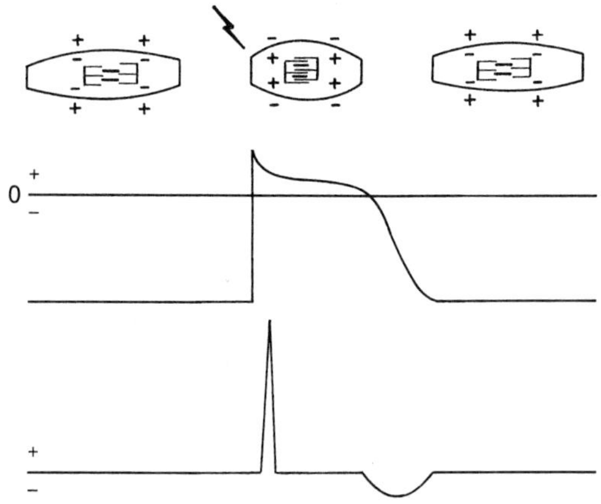

Fig. 24.1 ECG as a summation of electrical signals in a single cell. Onset of depolarization gives a high frequency waveform and repolarization is represented by a lower frequency waveform opposite to depolarization. (Modified from Marriott's *Practical Electrocardiography*, 10th edn, 2001, with permission from Lippincott Williams & Wilkins.)

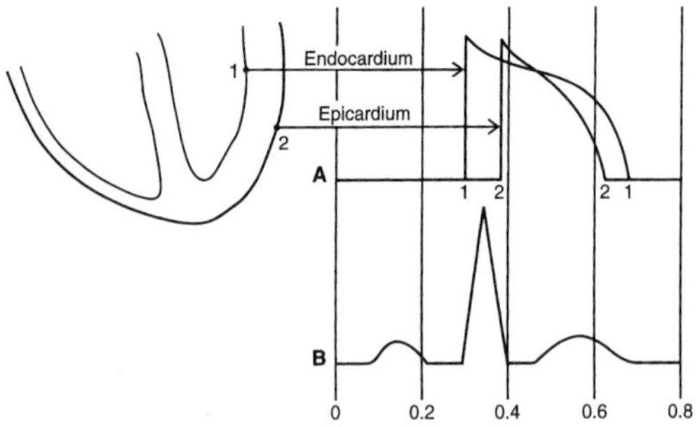

Fig. 24.2 Transmural variation in action potentials. Recordings from left-ventricular myocardial cell on: (A) the endocardial (1) and epicardial surface (2), and (B) the long-axis body surface ECG waveforms. Numbers correspond to time (s) for sequential electrical events. (Modified from Marriott's *Practical Electrocardiography*, 10th edn, 2001, with permission from Lippincott Williams & Wilkins.)

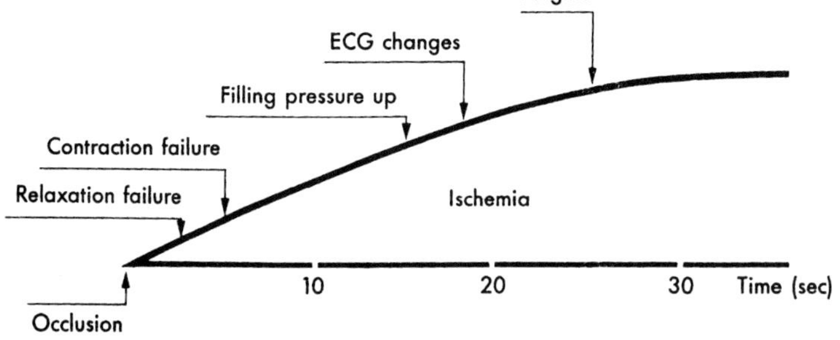

Fig. 24.3 Sequence of mechanical, electrocardiographic and clinical events after acute balloon occlusion of a coronary artery. ECG changes follow mechanical dysfunction but precedes pain. (Reproduced from *Electrocardiography, A Physiological Approach*, Chapter 15: fig. 3, Mosby-Year Book, 1993, David Mirvis, with permission from Elsevier Science.)

repolarization (phase 2 and 3) makes the ischaemic cells more negative than normal cells and intracellular current flows from normal to ischaemic cells (positive to negative).

When ischaemia is confined to the subendocardium, the ST vector shifts typically in the opposite direction towards the inner ventricular layer and the cavity (away from the epicardium, towards endocardium more recovered and negative) showing ST depression in leads overlying ischaemic zones. See Fig. 24.5.

ECG changes during myocardial ischaemia

Myocardial ischaemia influences the QRS complex, the ST segment and the T waves. The main determinants of ECG changes are the duration and degree of ischaemia. Increased demand for myocardial blood flow or decreased supply causes ST segment depression and T wave changes. The subendocardial layer is most susceptible to ischaemia, being most distant from

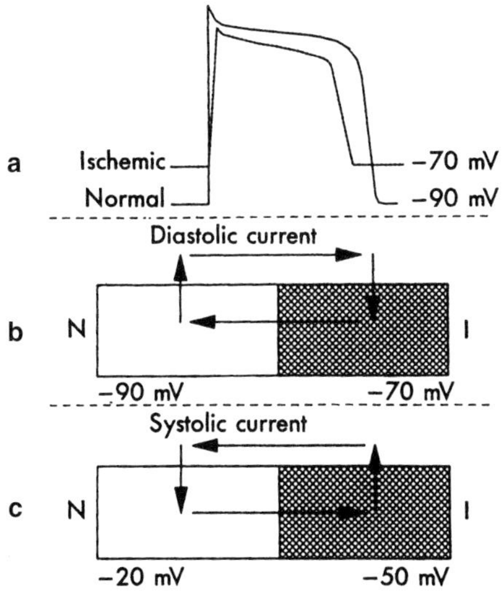

Fig. 24.4 The effects of ischaemia on action potential and resting potential. (a)The ischaemic cell has a less negative resting potential and a shorter action potential, resulting in potential gradients between normal and ischaemic cells producing diastolic (b) and systolic (c) injury currents. Arrows indicate direction of flow of intracellular and extracellular current. In (b) intracellular positive current flows from ischaemic to normal cells and in (c) during systole intracellular current flow is from normal to ischaemic cells. (Reproduced from *Electrocardiography, A Physiological Approach*, Chapter 15: fig. 7, Mosby-Year Book, 1993, David Mirvis, with permission from Elsevier Science.)

the source of blood supply. Complete cessation of flow causes ST elevation and Q wave changes as a result of depolarization abnormalities.

ST segment changes

The normal ST segment is at the TP/PR baseline. During subendocardial myocardial ischaemia there is ST segment depression that is either horizontal or downsloping. This is best illustrated during exercise (Fig. 24.6).

Sudden complete occlusion of a coronary artery causes epicardial injury which could be reversed once flow is immediately re-established and no infarction occurs. Acute ST segment elevation occurs sometimes without QRS changes, and may signify the early phase of an infarct, transient angina, or ischaemia resulting from acute coronary vasospasm.

In acute transmural myocardial injury, J point and ST segment elevation occurs. Its presence in two or more limbs or left precordial leads of 0.1 mV, or 0.2 mV in the right precordial leads are generally considered diagnostic of acute transmural infarction. (Fig. 24.7). Lesser deviations in the opposite direction often accompany ST segment elevation in larger infarcts especially during the early phase (Fig. 24.8). The significance of these is controversial and in patients with single vessel occlusions, these changes are most probably the result of reciprocal electrical alterations in opposite leads (Norrell *et al.* 1989). Others have suggested that these represent changes owing to increased metabolic demand

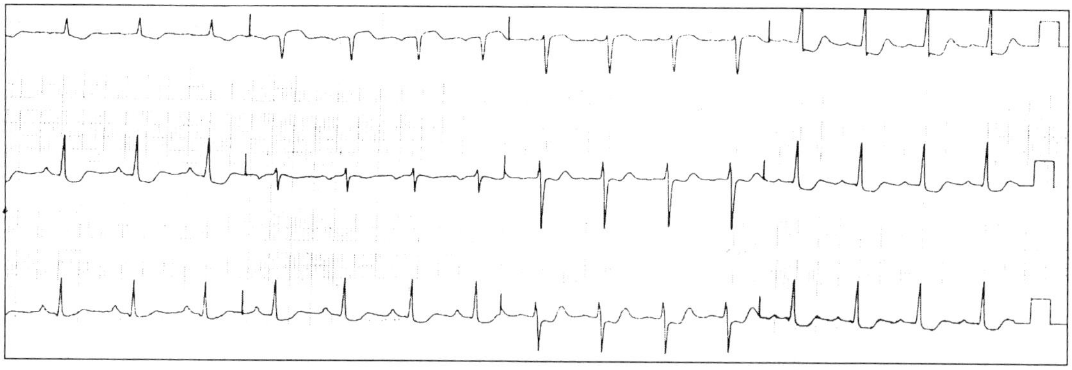

Fig. 24.5 ECG showing diffuse subendocardial ischaemia, with ST segment depression in most leads and ST segment elevation in aVR in a patient with left main disease.

or remote ischaemia, in an area dependent on collaterals (Lew *et al.* 1987).

T wave changes

A variety of T wave abnormalities are seen when ischaemia is limited to the subendocardial layer, or is transmural with or without injury or infarction. Ischaemic T waves are deep symmetrical and inverted below the isoelectric line (Fig. 24.9).

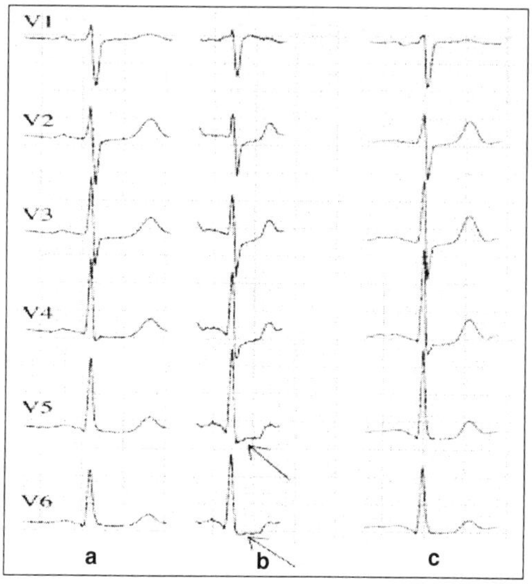

Fig. 24.6 ECG showing six precordial leads (a) at rest (b) during exercise, and (c) after 5 min of rest. ST segment depression is upsloping in V2 and V3 and horizontal in V5 and V6. (Reproduced from Marriott's *Practical Electrocardiography*, 10th edn, 2001, with permission from Lippincott Williams & Wilkins.)

This occurs owing to the earlier repolarization of the ischaemic subendocardium resulting in a change in the direction of the mean electrical vector.

With transmural ischaemia, the T wave axis shifts in the opposite direction towards the region of epicardial involvement, and is often the earliest sign of myocardial infarction. These T waves are tall, upright, symmetrical or asymmetrical, peaked or blunted, often with a prolonged *QT* interval, commonly seen in the anterior precordial leads. (Fig.24.10). T wave changes are less sensitive and specific in determining the presence of ischaemia, but may help localize ischaemia to specific regions. Inferior T wave inversion with abnormally tall T waves in the anterior leads may signify inferior–posterior ischaemia.

In some patients with coronary artery disease and inverted T waves, return to a normal upright position may occur with ischaemia. This pseudonormalization is probably the result of opposing forces in the acutely ischaemic area (Nobel *et al.* 1976).

QRS changes

With acute high grade ischaemia (minutes after balloon occlusion of a coronary artery), there is a primary deviation of the QRS complex towards the area of epicardial injury. The amplitude of this deviation may exceed that of the ST segment, and QRS may be prolonged. This deviation could be explained by ischaemia-induced delay in myocardial electrical activation, causing the epicardial layer to be depolarized later

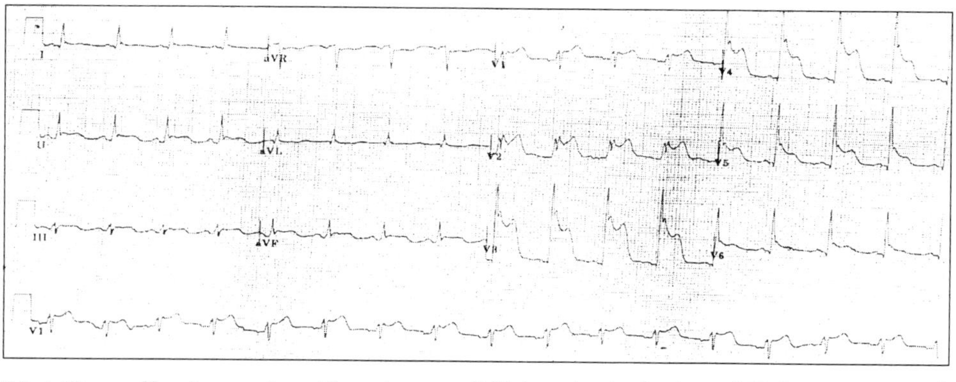

Fig. 24.7 A 48-year-old male presenting with acute myocardial injury, showing J point and ST elevation in precordial and inferior leads, after acute mid LAD occlusion. Coronary angiogram revealed, 100% mid LAD and 90% proximal RCA occlusions.

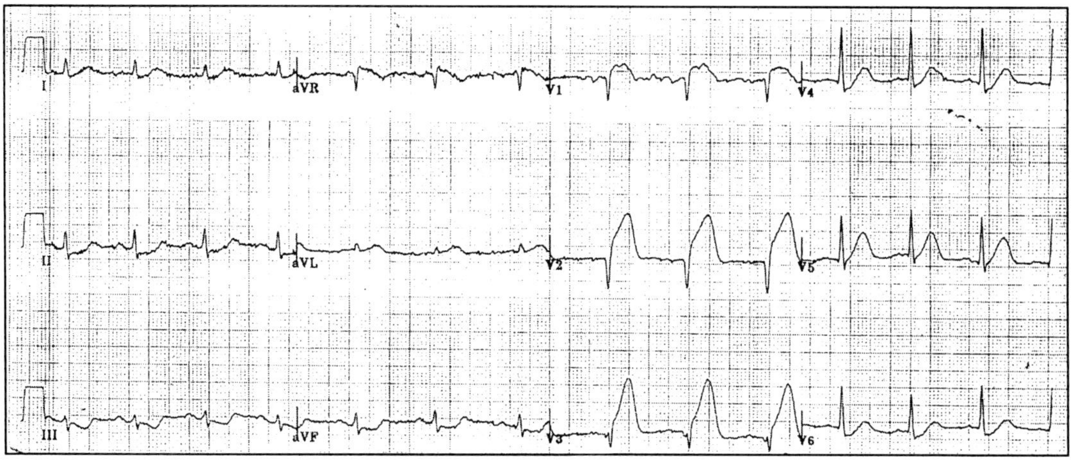

Fig. 24.8 Acute extensive anterolateral infarction with reciprocal ST segment depression in II, III and aVF in a patient with ostial LAD occlusion.

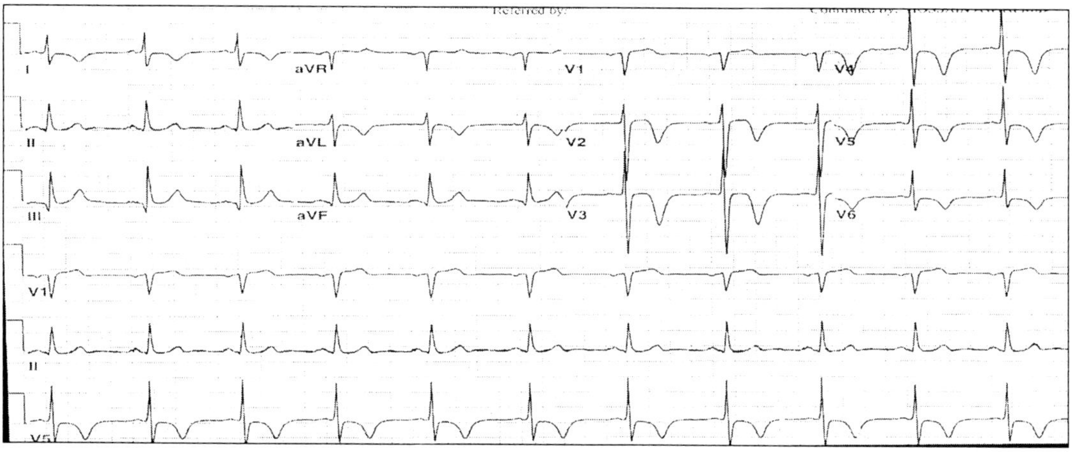

Fig. 24.9 Patient with acute coronary syndrome. Coronary angiogram revealed 90% mid LAD occlusion with distal embolization.

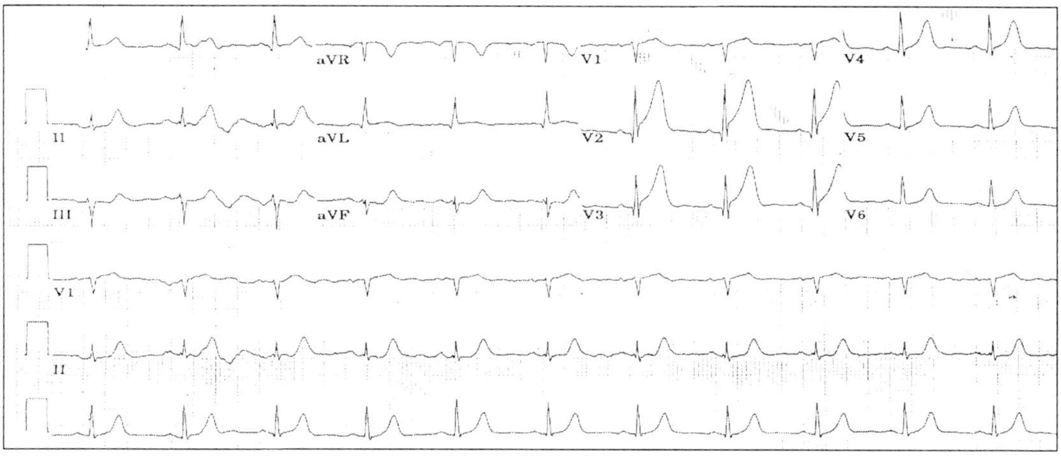

Fig. 24.10 Hyperacute T waves in 73-year-old male presenting with 2 h of substernal chest pain. In a patient with 100% proximal LAD occlusion.

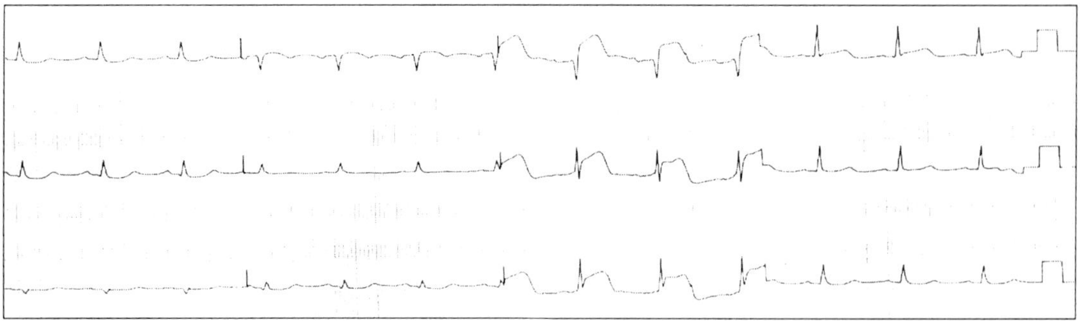

Fig. 24.11 Shows acute phase of anterior wall MI with deviation of QRS complex, especially S wave, 0.04 mV above the PR segment baseline in lead V3.

Table 24.1 Localization of infarct based on ECG Q wave pattern

Q wave pattern	*Location of infarct*
QS in V1, V2, V3, and sometimes, V4	Anteroseptal
rS in V1 with Q in one or more of V2 to V4	Anterior
Q in V4 or V5 through V6, I, and aVL	Anterior lateral
QS in all precordial, with or without I and aVL	Extensive anterior
Q in I and aVL	High lateral or lateral
Q in II, III and aVF (especially)	Inferior
Q in II, III and aVF plus abnormal Q in V5 and V6	Inferior lateral
Initial r in V1 and V2 > 0.04 s r/S > 1	True posterior
Q in II, II, aVF plus tall r in V1 0.04 s r/S > 1	Inferior posterior
Criteria for true posterior plus abnormal Q in I and aVL and or V5 and V6	Posterior lateral.

generating an 'injury current' towards the infarcted area (Figs 24.7 & 24.11). After necrosis occurs, the zone of necrosis becomes electrically silent and the resultant electrical forces during depolarization points away from the infarcted area leading to a negative QRS deflection, with a prolonged duration or loss of R wave amplitude. Any Q wave with a duration >0.04 s and amplitude >25% of the following R wave, is considered abnormal. Any Q in V1–V3 is considered abnormal (Wagner *et al.* 1982). Note that leads III and aVR have wide deep Q waves in normal subjects. In some cases diminution of R waves is considered evidence of transmural infarction (Hindman *et al.* 1985). A posterior infarct is represented by a positive and not a negative deviation of the QRS complex, leading to increased R wave amplitude in V1 and V2.

For localization of myocardial infarction based on QRS pattern, see Table 24.1.

Evolution of the ECG in ST segment elevation acute myocardial infarction

1 Hyperacute phase: tall-peaked T waves, seen within minutes to hours of onset of chest pain are often transient and easily missed.

2 Acute phase: ST segment elevation with increase in amplitude of the QRS complex and upright T waves. These are often accompanied by reciprocal ST depressions. The duration of ST elevation may last from hours to days and occasionally weeks. Mills *et al.* (1975) found that ST segment elevation resolved in 40% of anterior wall AMIs vs. 90% in inferior MIs by 2 weeks. The possibility of ventricular aneurysm or persisting wall motion abnormalities, should be considered when ST segment elevation persists.

3 Abnormal Q waves: pathologic Q waves could be seen as early as 2 h after the pain and are fully developed within 9 h, as the electrical activity deviates away from the infarcted area. In most patients they persist indefinitely, but in *c*. 6–20% (Nagase *et al.* 1998) they may regress to normal or nondiagnostic patterns by 1–2 years, especially with smaller infarcts, as recanalization occurs and regional wall motion improves.

4 Decrease in ST segment and beginning of T wave inversion: within 12 h there is a rapid decline in elevation and then, a more gradual decline as the infarct evolves. The T waves begin to invert even before normalization of the ST segment. Typically the terminal portions of T waves are the first to become inverted followed by the middle and then the initial parts. These T waves are often associated with *QT* prolongation. They may resolve in days or weeks or persist indefinitely. Spontaneous normalization of negative T waves often reflects improvement of wall motion (Nagase *et al.* 2001).

Chronic T wave inversion does not mean chronic ischaemia but rather represents the alteration in electrical recovery as a result of infarction-induced changes in electrical activation. Evolutionary changes may be accelerated with thrombolytic therapy or primary angioplasty (Fig. 24.12a–c)

Localization of infarct-related artery

The 12-lead ECG is better at the identification of the infarct-related artery in patients with ST segment elevation than non-ST segment elevation AMI. In addition the ECG is more helpful in patients with their first myocardial infarction, and in those with single vessel disease.

Left anterior descending artery

The correlation between left anterior descending artery (LAD) occlusion and the ECG is very good. The 12-lead ECG has been shown to confirm the diagnosis of anterior wall MI in 90% and 83% of patients with total and subtotal LAD occlusion, respectively (Blanke *et al.*1984). The best lead for detection of LAD occlusion is V2 followed by V1and V3. The site within the LAD can further be determined as being proximal (pre-first diagonal or first septal), if there is inferior ST segment depression (Lew *et al.* 1987), or if there is ST elevation (>1 mm) in aVL (Birnbaum *et al.* 1993). The incidence of ST elevation in aVL >1.0 mm and ST depression in the inferior leads varies between 66–81% and 58–90%, respectively (Birnbaum 1994; Engelen *et al.* 1999). Occlusion before the first septal may also cause ST segment elevation in aVR or in VI >2.5 mm (Engelen *et al.* 1999), complete right bundle branch block, and ST depression in lead V5 (Figs 24.13 & 24.14). Mid and distal LAD occlusion usually presents with elevation limited to precordial leads, depression in aVL and isoelectric or elevated inferior ST segment (Fig. 24.15). There is some controversy about the cause of the ST depression in the inferior leads. Some studies suggest that there could be accompanying inferior ischaemia while more recent studies indicate that inferior ST segment depression is more probably the result of reciprocal changes in proximal LAD occlusion. Tombstoning of the ST segment (Guo *et al.* 2000), described as absent or short initial R wave (0.04s), convex merging ST–T wave with the descending limb of R wave has been also shown to be present in 83% of anterior MIs and 92% of proximal LAD occlusions (Fig. 24.16).

Combined ST segment elevation in anterior and inferior leads is a pattern recognized (Sapin 1992; Tamura 1995; Sasaki 2001) in mid LAD occlusions, when the LAD 'wraps around' the apex, usually causing smaller infarcts with better prognosis. Rarely, however, this could mean proximal RCA occlusion with right ventricular involvement or chronic LAD disease with recent RCA occlusion suggesting that the anterior wall became ischaemic owing to loss of collaterals from the RCA (Ilia *et al.* 1990).

ST elevation in lead V1 is worth mentioning since it could represent anteroseptal AMI with occlusion before the first septal. However the degree of ST segment elevation is determined by the blood supply of the intraventricular septum from the first septal perforator and/or from the conus artery. If the conus artery is large, the ST remains isoelectric, but if it is small there is more ST elevation in V1 than in V2 (Ben-Gal *et al.* 1997).

Right coronary artery

The RCA supplies the right ventricle, inferior and posterior septal walls of the left ventricle. The 12-lead ECG can diagnose inferior wall MI in

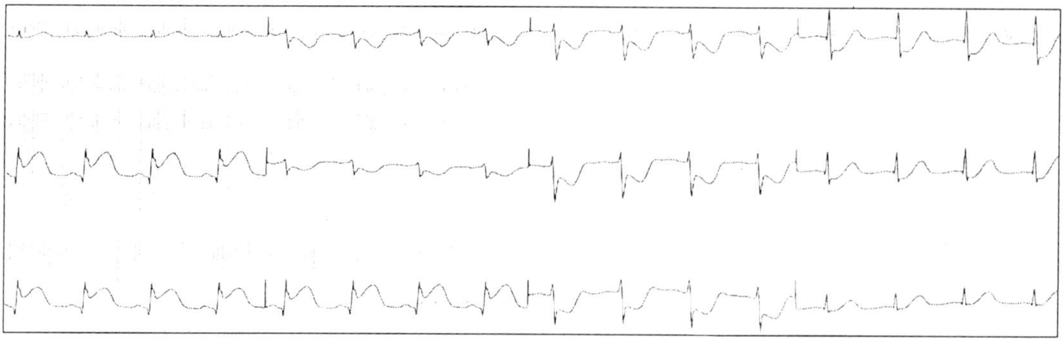

a

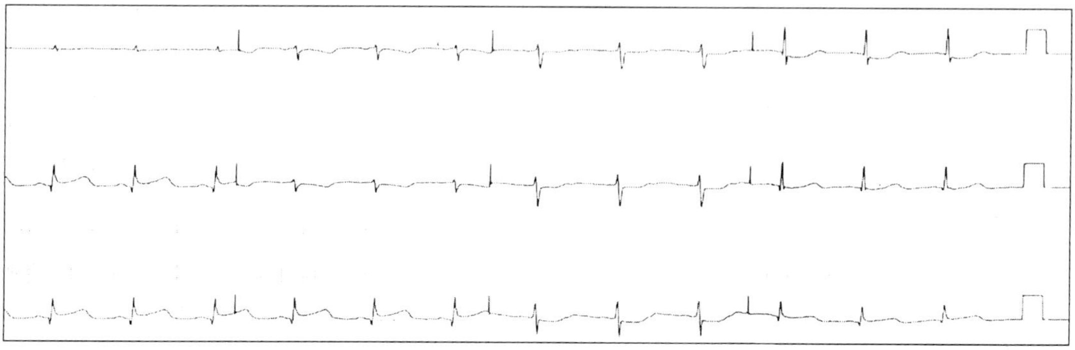

b

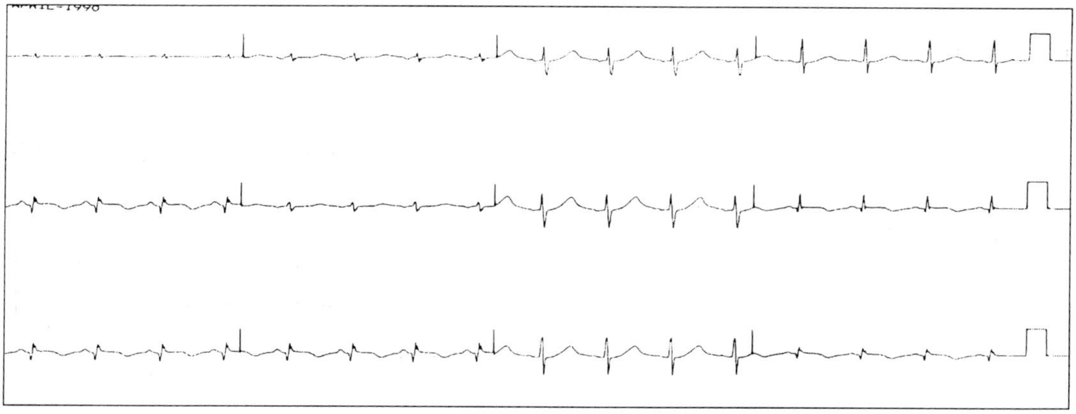

c

Fig. 24.12 Evolutionary changes in a inferior–posterior AMI: (a) at presentation; (b) after thrombolysis; (c) 24 h later. Note the increase in R wave amplitude, and upright T waves in right precordial leads.

70–90% of cases. In 60% of these the proximal or mid RCA is involved and the remainder involve the distal RCA, the posterior descending artery or the right posterolateral branch. The best criterion for proximal RCA involvement is ST elevation in V4R or V3R (signifying acute right ventricular injury), which is a transient feature in 50% of patients, normalizing in about 10 h (Fig. 24.18). Proximal RCA occlusion also causes ST segment elevation in the right precordial leads, maximally in V1 (when the right ventricle is involved,) occasionally in V1–V3 and rarely in V4 and V5 confusing it with anteroseptal MI. In addition, second and third degree AV block can

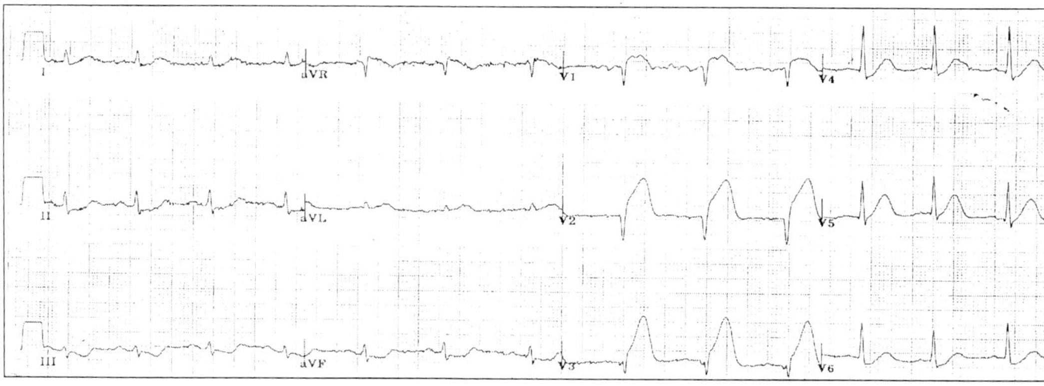

Fig. 24.13 ECG of a patient with anterior AMI due to proximal LAD occlusion.

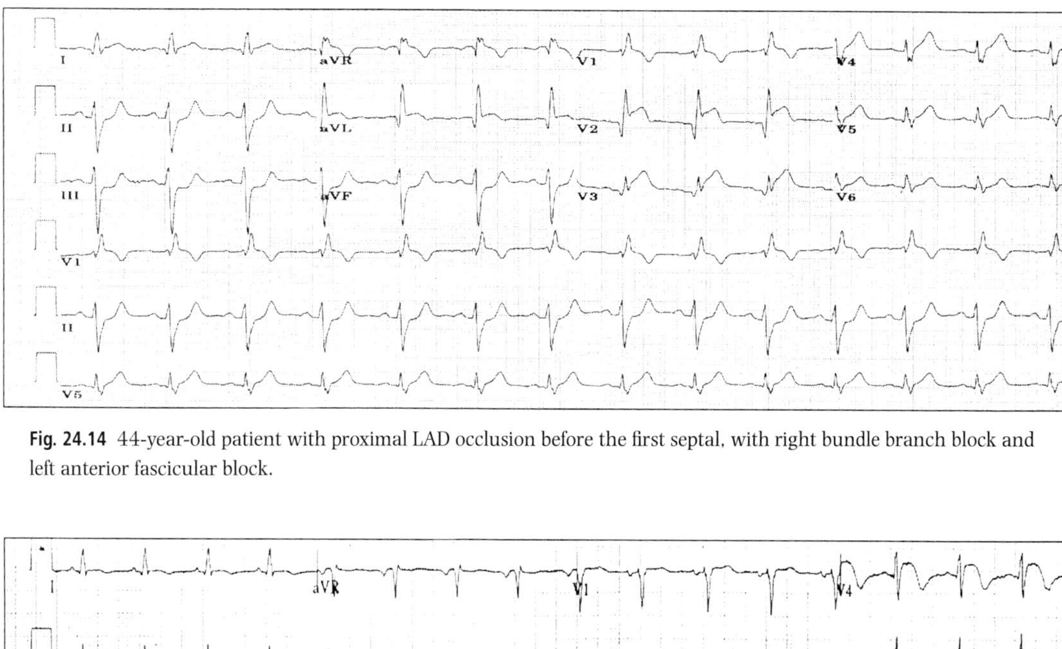

Fig. 24.14 44-year-old patient with proximal LAD occlusion before the first septal, with right bundle branch block and left anterior fascicular block.

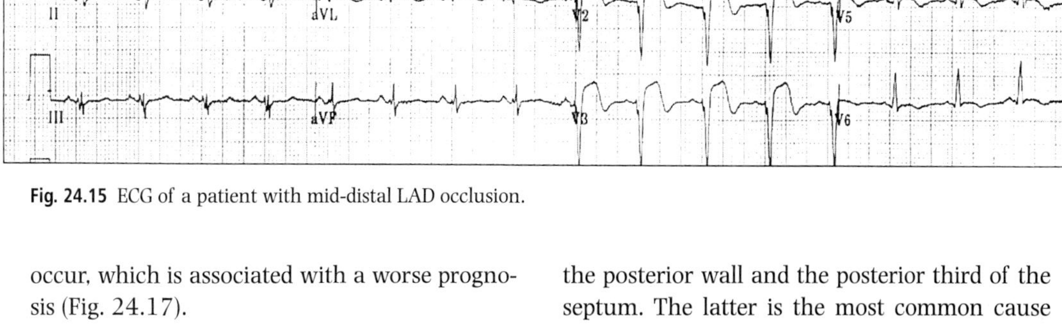

Fig. 24.15 ECG of a patient with mid-distal LAD occlusion.

occur, which is associated with a worse prognosis (Fig. 24.17).

Right precordial ST segment depression (Fig. 24.18) (Peterson *et al.* 1996) is also of interest in RCA occlusions and inferior wall infarcts signifying: (1) reciprocal changes; (2) anterior wall ischaemia or (3) extensive myocardial necrosis of the posterior wall and the posterior third of the septum. The latter is the most common cause and has been suggested as a marker of worse prognosis. These findings may mask the presence of proximal RCA involvement. Left precordial (V4–V6) ST depression has been shown to be present in patients with a higher incidence of

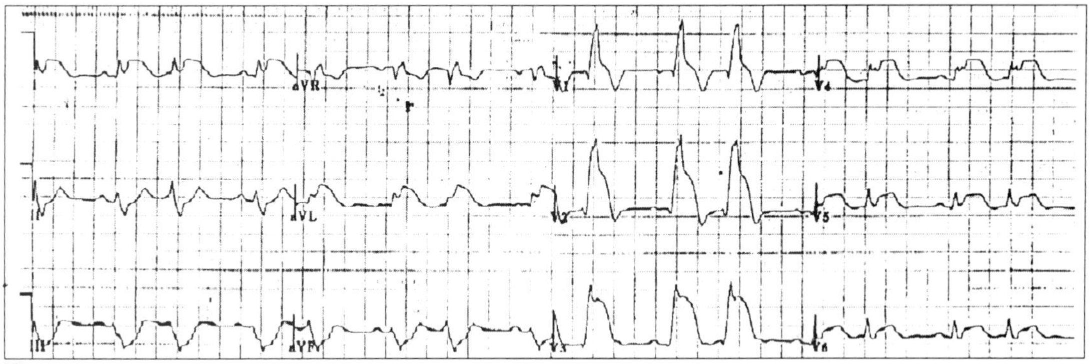

Fig. 24.16 ECG of a patient with tombstoning ST segment elevation. Coronary angiogram revealed 100% ostial LAD occlusion.

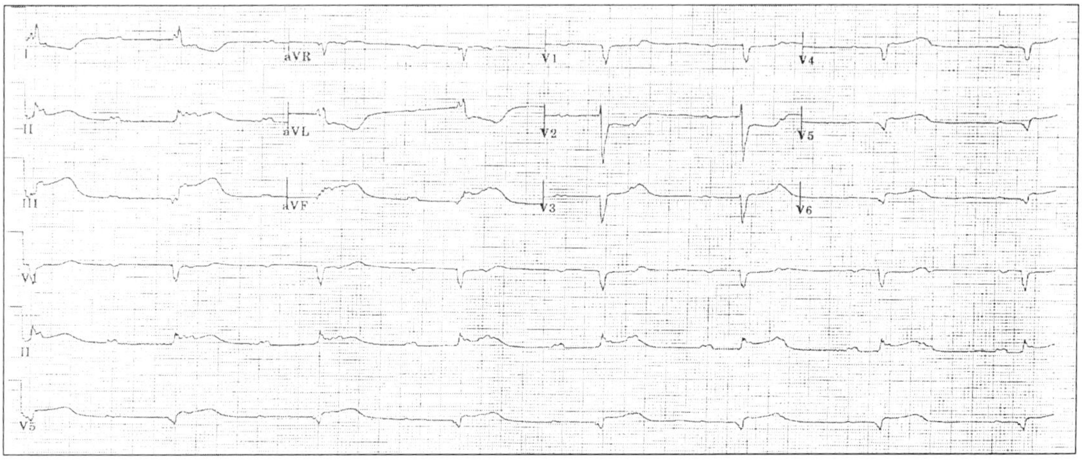

Fig. 24.17 ECG of patient with inferior AMI with right ventricular involvement and complete AV block. Note ST elevation in II, III, aVF, V4R–V6R with ST depressions in I and AVL. Coronary angiogram revealed 100% proximal RCA occlusion.

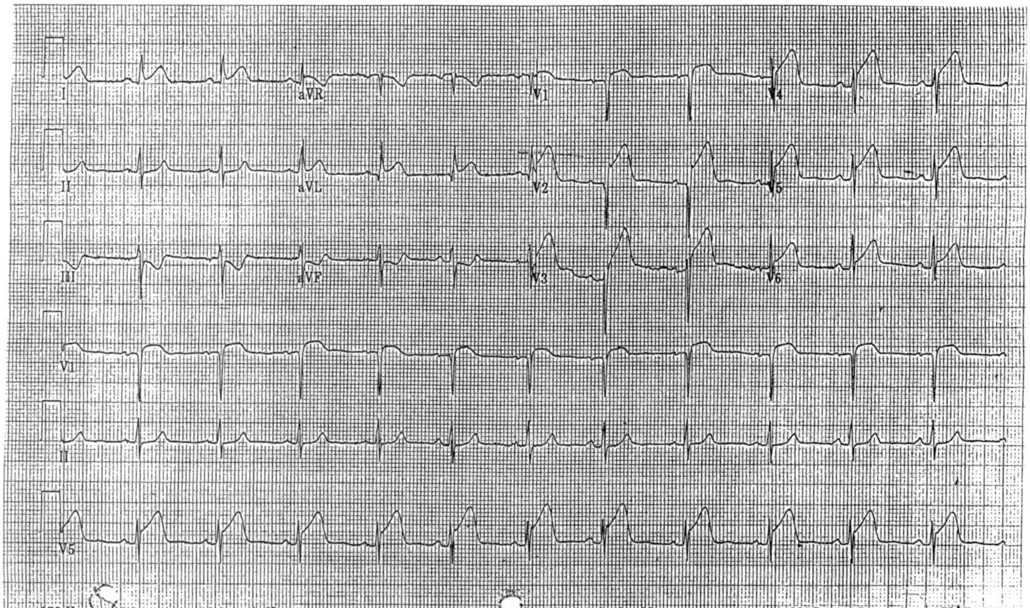

Fig. 24.18 Inferior wall MI with anterior precordial ST segment depression, in a patient with extensive inferior–posterior AMI and mid RCA occlusion.

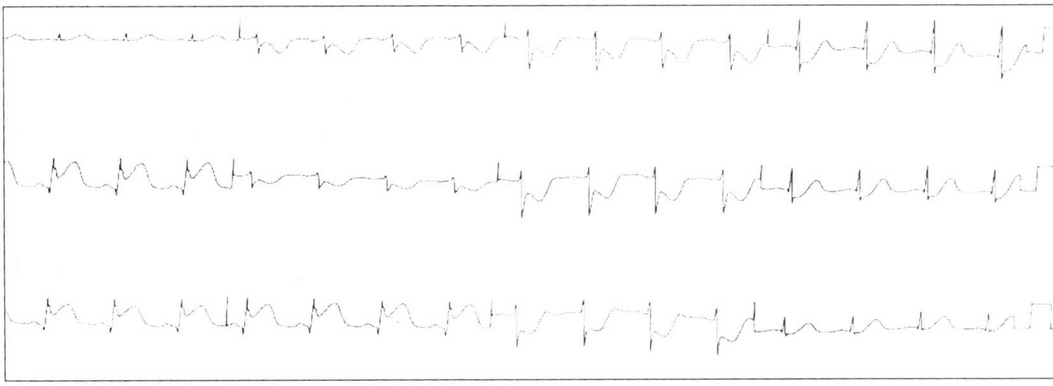

Fig. 24.19 Inferior wall AMI in a 46-year-old patient with proximal dissection of aorta involving the ostium of RCA. Note ST segment elevation in right and left precordial leads.

multivessel disease, lower ejection fraction, and increased long-term mortality (Birnbaum *et al.* 1999).

Left circumflex artery

This vessel supplies the posterior, the posterior–lateral and also the inferior wall in a left-dominant system. Occlusion presents as ST-elevation inferior AMI in a small percentage of patients, and the diagnostic accuracy of the 12-lead ECG is very low. ST-elevation in V6 and ST depression in V2 were identified as useful features in a study conducted by Blanke *et al.* (1984).

In patients presenting with inferior wall AMI, certain features on the surface ECG differentiate RCA from LCX involvement (Fig. 24.20):

1 the presence of ST segment elevation in II which is equal or greater than that in III, i.e. II/III > 1 is a strong predictor of LCX occlusion;

2 the ratio of ST depression in V3 to ST segment elevation in III; V3/III ratio >1.2 had a sensitivity and specificity for LCX of 84% and 95%, respectively;

3 when the above ratio is <0.5 sensitivity and specificity for proximal right occlusion is 91% and 91% (Herz *et al.* 1997; Kosude *et al.* 1998; Chia *et al.* 2000).

Posterior wall myocardial infarcts and leads V7–V9

Isolated posterior AMI is seen in LCX occlusion and is characterized as follows: (1) tall R waves V1 and V2 (0.04 s); (2) horizontal ST depression in leads V1–V4 with positive T waves: contrast with convex downward ST depression in anterior ischaemia with negative T waves (Fig. 24.21a, b).

Posterior leads V7–V9 (Zalensky *et al.* 1997; Matetsky *et al.* 1999; Wung *et al.* 2001) can improve the diagnostic yield of the ECG. ST segment elevation ≥1 mm is considered abnormal, and diagnostic of posterior wall AMI. Several small studies have shown that the IRA is invariably the LCX or one of its marginal branches. ST segment elevation in V7–V9, accompanying anterior precordial ST depression is helpful in distinguishing anterior wall ischaemia from posterior AMI.

Lateral wall myocardial ischaemia

ST elevation in leads I and AVL is often referred to as a high lateral infarct and involves either the first diagonal branch of the LAD or the LCX or one of its marginal branches. In diagonal occlusions (Fig. 24.22), there is often ST elevations in V2 with isoelectric ST segment in the left precordial leads while in marginal infarcts there would be ST depression in V2 with or without elevation in V6.

Left main coronary artery occlusion

ST segment elevation in lead aVR greater than in V1 has been suggested as a useful tool in recognizing acute left main (LCMA) obstruction. Yamaji *et al.* (2001) compared 16 patients with

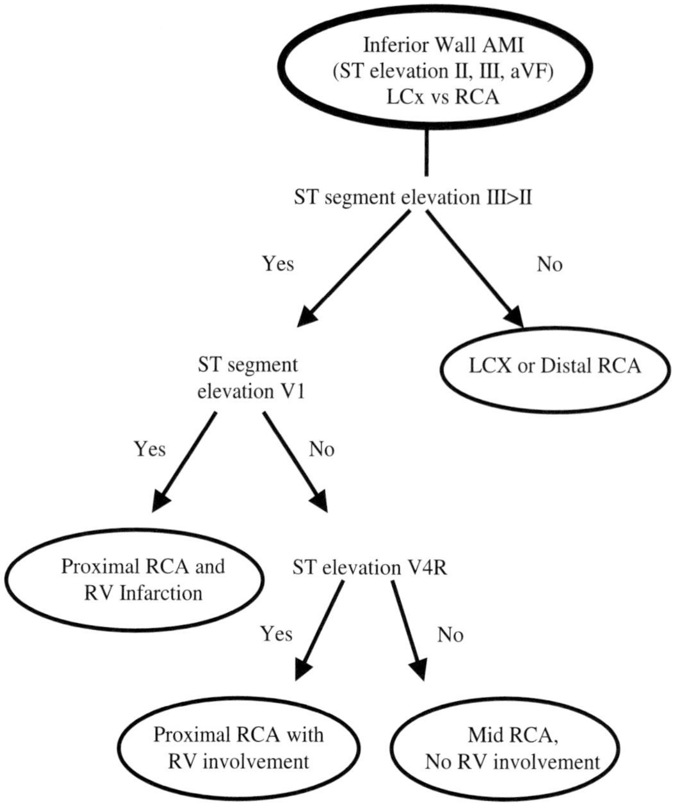

Fig. 24.20 Algorithm for determination of site of occlusion in inferior wall myocardial infarction

LCMA obstruction to 46 with LAD and 24 RCA obstructions, and found that this feature distinguished the LCMA group from the LAD group with a sensitivity of 81%, a specificity of 80% and an accuracy of 81%.

The proposed explanation was that the obstruction caused transmural ischaemia of the basal part of the septum thus less elevation in V1 was the result of electrical forces induced by posterior wall ischaemia counter balancing the effect of ischaemia in the anterior wall. This finding however has been seen in patients with triple vessel disease, and acute right ventricular overload as in pulmonary embolism (Figs 24.23 & 24.24).

Segment elevation acute myocardial infarction

The term non-ST elevation myocardial infarction (Non STEMI) has replaced the non-Q wave myocardial infarction. The ECG changes in Non STEMI ranges from normal, nonspecific ST–T wave changes to T wave inversion and ST segment depression. The diagnosis of Non STEMI usually requires elevation of troponins or creatinine kinase. Some of the pathophysiological mechanisms proposed are that smaller vessels may be involved and that there is obstruction of flow to an area supplied by collateral vessels. When a single culprit is identified (which occurs in <50% of cases) it is often incompletely occluded (Liebson & Klein 1997). However in the analysis of 350 patients in the VANQUISH trial, early angiography showed that the majority had either no identifiable culprit or multiple apparent culprits (Kerensky *et al.* 2002).

Normal or nondiagnostic ECG usually signifies a small area at risk, branch vessel ischaemia or LCX occlusion (Caceras 1995; Kontos 2001). Occasionally it might signify delayed evolution of the ST–T and Q waves. These patients have been shown to have a 1 year mortality of 8.2% and a generally good prognosis, except those with delayed evolution whose outcome depends on infarct size (Canon *et al.* 1997).

Isolated T wave abnormalities occur in 20–30% of non-ST elevation acute coronary

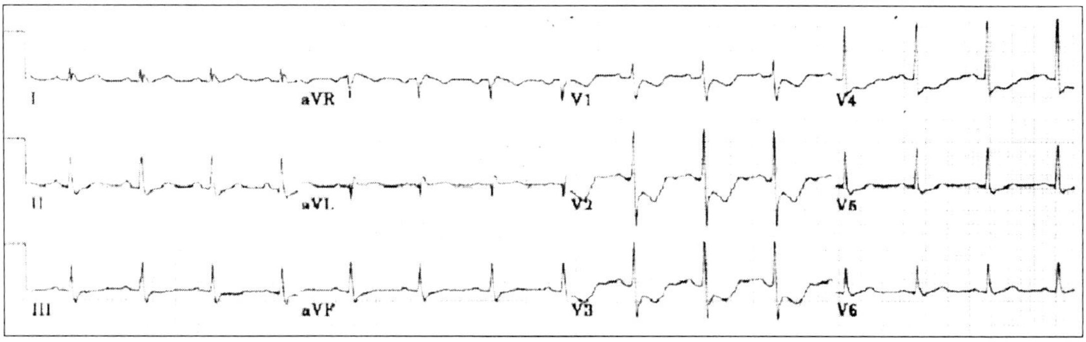

a

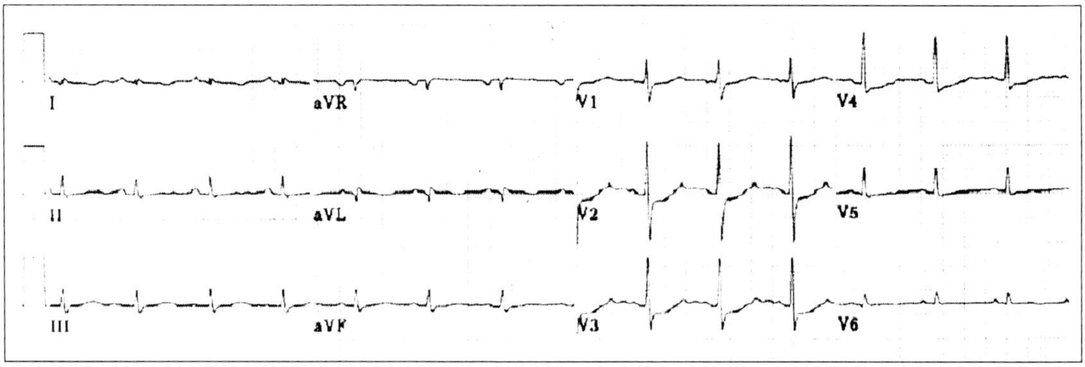

b

Fig. 24.21 (a) and (b) True posterior wall AMI. Note ST segment depression and T wave inversions in V1–V4, and prominent r in V2 and V3. ECG the next day shows less ST segment depression, with further increase in the amplitude of the R waves in V2 and V3 with positive T waves. Coronary angiogram revealed total occlusion of proximal LCX artery.

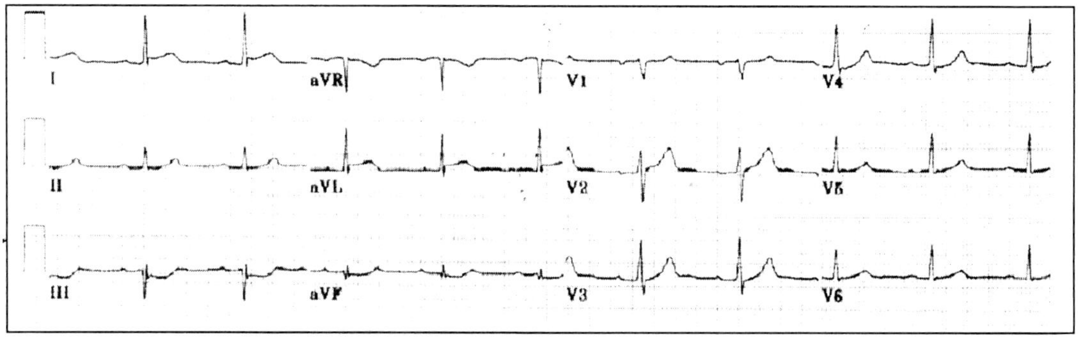

Fig. 24.22 ECG of lateral wall AMI. showing ST segment is elevation in leads I and aVL and less prominent in V2, with ST segment depression in III and aVF, because of obstruction of the first diagonal branch.

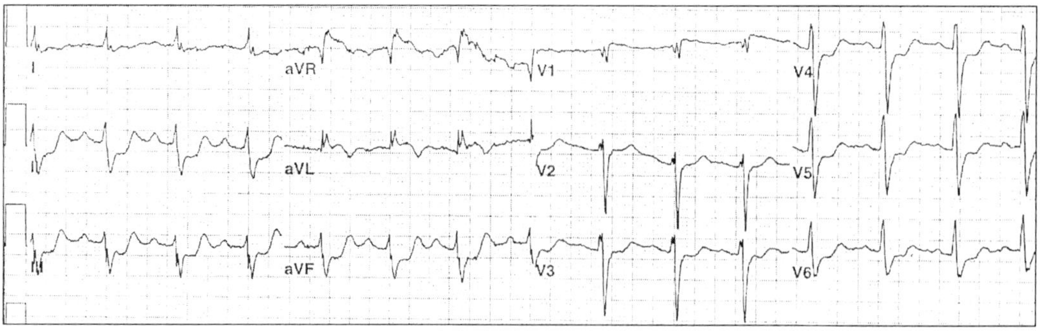

Fig. 24.23 Acute left main coronary artery occlusion.

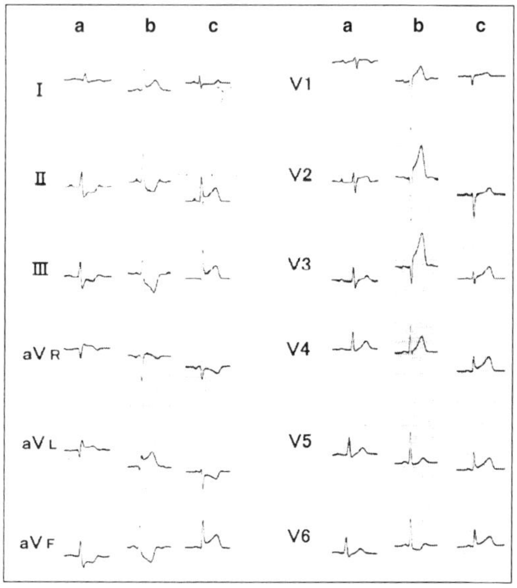

Fig. 24.24 ECG changes in patients with (a) LMCA, (b) LAD, (c) RCA occlusion. (Reproduced from the American College of Cardiology Foundation *Journal of the American College of Cardiology*, (2001), **38** (5), 1348–1354, with permission.)

syndromes and are highly predictive of future cardiac events. Event rates are lower than in ST segment depression at about 6.8%, except when present in five or more leads (Holmvang *et al.* 1999).

The incidence of ST depression varies from 12.4% to 46% and is associated with the highest incidence of death, re-infarction and recurrent ischaemia (Cannon 1997; Holmvang 1999; Savonitto 1999). The one year mortality or AMI rate in patients with 0.5 mm, 1 mm, >2 mm ST depressions were 12%, 15%, and 41%, respectively (Hyde *et al.* 1999).

Initial ST segment elevation without development of frank Q waves (with or without reperfusion) was seen in about 21.3% of the patients studied by the GUSTO-1 investigators (Barbagelata *et al.* 1997). These patients have been shown to have lower total CK rise compared to Q wave infarcts, preserved left ventricular function but more residual ischaemia on radionuclide imaging (Huey *et al.* 1987).

The direction of ST shift in the initial ECG is a poor predictor of the development of Q waves. Inverted T waves may evolve in leads with ST segment elevation or depression and are often deep. Newly developed and persistent marked ST depression with deep T wave inversion is highly suggestive of infarction.

References

Anton, P.M., Engelen, D.J.M. *et al.* (2001) Lead aVR, a mostly ignored but very valuable lead in clinical electrocardiography. *Journal of the American College of Cardiology*, **38**, 1355–1356.

Arbane, M. & Goy, J.J. (2000) Prediction of the site of total occlusion in the left anterior descending artery using admission electrocardiogram in anterior wall acute myocardial infarction. *American Journal of Cardiology*, **85**, 487.

Barbagelata, A., Califf, R.M., Sgasbossa, E.B. *et al.* (1997) Thrombolysis and Q wave vs. non-Q wave first acute myocardial infarction: a GUSTO-1 substudy. Global Utilization of Streptokinase and Tissue Plasminogen Activator for Occluded Arteries Investigators. *Journal of the American College of Cardiology*, **29**, 770.

Barrabes, J.A., Moure, C. *et al.* (2000) Prognostic significance of ST segment depression in lateral leads I, aVL, V5, and V6 on the admission electrocardiogram in patients with first acute myocardial infarction without

ST segment elevation. *Journal of the American College of Cardiology*, **35**, 1813.

Ben-Gal, T., Sclarovsky, S., Herz, I. *et al.* (1997). Importance of conal artery in patients with acute anterior wall myocardial infarction: electrocardiographic and angiographic correlation. *Journal of the American College of Cardiology*, **29**, 506–511

Birnbaum, Y., Sclarovsky, S., Solodky, A. *et al.* (1993). Prediction of the level of anterior descending coronary artery obstruction during anterior wall acute myocardial infarction by the admission EKG. *American Journal of Cardiology*, **72**, 823–826

Birnbaum, Y., Herz, I., Solodky, A. *et al.* (1994) Can we differentiate by admission electrocardiogram between anterior descending artery occlusion proximal to the origin of the first septal branch or a post septal occlusion? *American Journal of Noninvasive Cardiology*, **8**, 115–119.

Birnbaum, Y., Wagner, G.S., Barbash, G.I. *et al.* (1999) Correlation of angiographic findings in right (V1 toV3) vs. left (V4 to V6) precordial ST segment depressions in inferior wall acute myocardial infarction. *American Journal of Cardiology*, **83**, 143–148.

Birnbaum, Y., Hasdai D., Sclarovsky, S. *et al.* (1996) Acute myocardial infarction entailing ST segment elevation in lead aVL, electrocardiographic differentiation among occlusion of the left anterior descending, first diagonal, and first obtuse marginal coronary arteries. *American Heart Journal*, **131**, 38–42

Blanke, H., Cohen, M., Schlueter, G.U. *et al.* (1984). Electrocardiographic and coronary angiographic correlations during acute myocardial infarction. *American Journal of Cardiology*, **54**, 249–255

Caceres, L., Cookie, D., Zalenski, R. *et al.* (1995) Myocardial infarction with an initially normal electrocardiogram – angiographic findings. *Clinical Cardiology*, **18**, 563–568.

Casas, R.E., Marriott, H.J.L., Glancy, D.L. (1997) Value of leads V7–V9 in diagnosing posterior wall myocardial infarction and other causes of tall R wave in V1–V2. *American Journal of Cardiology*, **80**, 508.

Cannon, C.P., McCabe, C.H., Stone, P.H. *et al.* (1997) The electrocardigram predicts one year outcome of patients with unstable angina and non-Q wave myocardial infarction: results of TIMI III registry ECG ancillary study. *Journal of the American College of Cardiology*, **30**, 133–140.

Chia, B.L., Yip, J.W., Tan, H.C. & Lim, Y.T. (2000) Usefulness of ST elevation II/III ratio and ST deviation in Lead I for identifying the culprit artery in inferior wall acute myocardial infarction. *American Journal of Cardiology*, **86**, 341–3432.

Engelen, D.J., Gorgels, A.P., Cheriex, E.C. *et al.*(1999) Value of the electrocardiogram in localizing occlusion in the left anterior descending artery in acute anterior wall infarction. *Journal of the American College of Cardiology*, **34**, 389–395.

Goldberger, A.l. (1999) *Clinical Electrocardiography. A Simplified Approach*, 6th edn. Mosby, St Louis, MO.

Guey, B.L., Bellar, G.A., Kaiser, D.L. *et al.* (1988) A comprehensive analysis of myocardial infarction due to left circumflex artery occlusion: comparison with infarction due to right coronary and left anterior descending artery occlusion. *Journal of the American College of Cardiology*, **4**, 660–666.

Guo, X.H., Yap, Y.G., Chen, L.J. *et al.* (2000) Correlation of coronary angiography with 'Tombstoning' electrocardiographic pattern in patients after acute myocardial infarction. *Clinical Cardiology*, **23**, 347–352.

Haines, D.E., Raabe, D.S., Gundel, W.D. *et al.* (1983) Anatomic and prognostic significance of new T wave inversion in unstable angina. *American Journal of Cardiology*, **52**, 14.

Herz, I., Assali, A.R., Adler, Y. *et al.* (1997) New electrocardiographic criteria for predicting either right or left circumflex artery as the culprit coronary artery in inferior wall acute myocardial infarction. *American Journal of Cardiology*, **82**, 1318–1322.

Hindman, N.B., Schocken, D.D., Widmann, M. *et al.* (1985) Evaluation of a QRS scoring system for estimating myocardial infarct size. V. Specificity and method of application of the complete system. *American Journal of Cardiology*, **55**, 1485–1490.

Holmvang, L., Luscher, M.S., Clemmensen, P. *et al.* (1998). Very early risk stratification using combined ECG and biochemical assessment in patients with unstable coronary artery disease. A Thrombin Inhibition in Myocardial Ischaemia (TRIM) substudy. *Circulation*, **98**, 2004–2009.

Holmvang, L., Clemmensen, P., Wagner, G. *et al.* (1999). Admission standard electrocardiogram for early risk stratification in patients with unstable coronary artery disease not eligible for acute revascularization therapy, A TRIM substudy. *American Heart Journal*, **137**, 24–33.

Hyde, T.A., French, J.K., Wong, C.K. *et al.* (1999) Four year survival of patients with acute coronary syndrome without ST segment elevation and prognostic significance of 0.5 mm ST depression., **84**, 379–385.

Ilia, R., Goldfarb, B. & Ovsyshcher, I.A. (1990) Concomitant ST elevation in inferior and anterior leads in acute myocardial infarction. Clinical and anatomical significance. *Journal of Electrocardiology*, **23** 199–205.

Kerensky, R.A., Wade, M. *et al.* (2002) Revisiting the culprit lesion in non-Q wave myocaridial infarction, results from the VANQUISH trial angiographic core laboratory. *Journal of the American College of Cardiology*, 1456–1467.

Kontos, M.C., Kurdzeil, K.A., Ornato, J.P. *et al.* (2001). A nonischaemic electrocardiogram does not always predict a small myocardial infarction, Results with acute myocardial perfusion imaging. *American Heart Journal*, **141**, 360–366.

Kosude, M., Kimura, K., Ishikawa, T. *et al.* (1998) New electrocardiographic criteria for predicting the site of coronary artery occlusion in inferior wall acute myocardial infarction. *American Journal of Cardiology*, **82**, 1318–1322.

Liebson, P.R. & Klein, L.W. (1997) The non-Q wave myocardial infarction revisited, 10 years later. *Progress in Cardiovascular Diseases*, **39**, 399.

Lew, A.S., Hod, H., Cerek, B. *et al.* (1987). Inferior ST segment changes during acute anterior myocardial infarction: a marker of the presence or absence of concomitant inferior wall ischaemia. *Journal of the American College of Cardiology*, **10**, 519–526.

Matetzky, S., Freimark, D., Feinberg, M.S. *et al.* (1999). Acute myocardial infarction with isolated ST segment elevation in posterior chest leads V7–9. 'Hidden' ST segment elevation revealing acute posterior infarction. *Journal of the American College of Cardiology*, **34**, 748–753.

Mills, R.M., Young, E., Gorlin, R. *et al.* (1975) Natural history of ST segment elevation after acute myocardial infarction. *American Journal of Cardiology*, **35**, 609.

Mirvis, D.M. (1993) *Electrocardiography, a Physiological Approach*. Mosby-Year Book, St Louis, MO.

Mukharji, J., Murray, S., Lewis, S.E. *et al.* (1984) Is anterior ST depression with acute transmural inferior infarction due to posterior infarction? A vectorcardiographic and scintigraphic study. *Journal of the American College of Cardiology*, **4**, 28.

Nagase, K., Tamura, A., Mikuriya, Y. *et al.* (1998) Significance of Q wave regression after anterior wall acute myocardial infarction. *European Heart Journal*, 19, 742.

Nagase, K., Tamura, A., Mikuriya, Y. *et al.* (2001) Spontaneous normalization of negative T waves in infarct-related leads reflects improvement in left ventricular wall motion even in patients with persistent abnormal Q waves after anterior wall acute myocardial infarction. *Cardiology*, **96** (2), 94–96.

Nobel, R.J., Rothbaum, D.A., Knooebel, S.B. *et al.* (1976). Normalization of abnormal T waves in ischaemia. *Archives of Internal Medicine*, **136**, 391.

Norell, M.S., Lyons, J.P., Gardener, J.E. *et al.* (1989) Significance of 'reciprocal' ST segment depression: left ventriculographic observations during left anterior descending coronary angioplasty. *Journal of the American College of Cardiology*, **13**, 1270.

Peterson, E.D., Hathaway, W.R., Zabel, K.M. *et al.* (1996) Prognostic significance of precordial ST segment depression during inferior myocardial infarction in the thrombolytic era: results in 16521 patients. *Journal of the American College of Cardiology*, **28**, 305–312.

Sasaki, K., Yotsukura, M., Sakata, K. *et al.* (2001) Relation of ST segment changes in inferior leads during anterior wall acute myocardial infarction to length and occlusion site of the left anterior descending coronary artery. *American Journal of Cardiology*, **87**, 1340–1345.

Savonitto, S., Ardissino, D., Granger, C.B *et al.* (1999) Prognostic value of the admission electrocardiogram in acute coronary syndrome. *JAMA (Journal of the American Medical Association)*, **281**, 707–713.

Sapin, P.,M., Musselman, D.R., Dehmar, G.J. *et al.* (1992) Implications of inferior ST segment elevation accompanying anterior wall acute myocardial infarction for angiographic morphology of the left anterior descending coronary artery morphology and site occlusion. *American Journal of Cardiology*, **69**, 860–865.

Schweitzer, P. (1990) The electrocardiographic diagnosis of acute myocardial infarction in the thrombolytic era. *American Heart Journal*, **119**, 642–654.

Shah, P.K., Pichler, M., Bergman, D.S. *et al.* (1980) Noninvasive identification of a high risk subset of patients with acute inferior myocardial infarction. *American Journal of Cardiology*, **46**, 915–921.

Tamura, A., Kataoka, H., Nagase, K. *et al.* (1995) Clinical significance of inferior ST elevation during acute anterior myocardial infarction. *British Heart Journal*, **74**, 611–614.

Wagner, G.S., Freye, C.J., Palmeri, S.T. *et al.* (1982) Evaluation of a QRS scoring system for estimating myocardial infarct size. Specificity and observer agreement. *Circulation*, **65**, 345.

Wung, S.F. & Drew, B.J. (2001) New electrocardiographic criteria for posterior wall acute myocardial ischaemia validated by a percutaneous transluminal coronary angioplasty model of acute myocardial infarction. *American Journal of Cardiology*, **87**, 970–974.

Yamaji, H. *et al.* (2001) Prediction of acute left main coronary artery obstruction by 12-lead electrocardiography. *Journal of the American College of Cardiology*, **38**, 1348–1354.

Zalenski, R.J., Rydman, R.J., Sloan, E.P. *et al.* (1997) Value of posterior and right ventricular leads in comparison to the standard 12-lead electrocardiogram in evaluation of ST segment elevation in suspected acute myocardial infarction. *American Journal of Cardiology*, **79**, 1579–1585.

Zehender, M., Kasper, W., Kauder, E. *et al.* (1993) Right ventricular infarction as a independent predictor of prognosis after acute inferior myocardial infarction. *New England Journal of Medicine*, **328**, 981.

CHAPTER 25

Dynamics of Silent Ischaemia

Shlomo Stern

Introduction

For many years, the ST segment of the ECG was the only laboratory marker of myocardial ischaemia (Feil & Siegel 1929) and now, nearly a century later, is still its best and most easily available sign. In an Annotation in the *American Heart Journal* (Stern & Tzivoni 1976) we wrote '. . . in our experience patients with ischaemic heart disease show extremely wide variations in this (the ST) segment during normal everyday activities, at rest, or even during sleep, and very often without any accompanying chest pains'. Moreover 'there are evidently stimuli other than exercise which can provoke ST–T changes which are sometimes even more drastic than those appearing during physical effort'. We stressed in this communication, as its title tells, 'the dynamic nature of the ST–T segment in ischaemic heart disease'. In its time, this concept was somewhat new and it needed time to establish that ischaemia of the myocardium and its electrocardiographic expression, the ST–T segment, can undergo dramatic alterations without any apparent trigger and in certain individuals an adequate supply of oxygen to the heart at one moment may become inadequate a few seconds or minutes later. In other words, an imbalance between oxygen availability on the one hand and the maintenance of a steady metabolic turnover, as ischaemia is now defined (Poole-Wilson 2002) may appear abruptly and disappear subsequently.

In the following an attempt will be made to show the accuracy of this notion about ischaemia and to demonstrate the fluctuations and the dynamicity in the myocardial flow/demand ratio in persons with diseased coronary arteries. Furthermore, we will discuss the role of pain, its importance and its frequency during ischaemia of the myocardium and possible mechanisms involved with silent ischaemia (SI).

The dynamic nature of ischaemia during everyday activities

Only the technological advance producing the ability to continuously monitor the ECG during everyday activities, the method known today as 'Holter recording', enabled us to demonstrate that ischaemic episodes are not always accompanied by anginal pain, and that, the so-called 'silent' ischaemic attacks are even more frequent in patients with coronary artery disease, than are the painful ones.

These 'come and go' ischaemic episodes are easily understood if they are subsequent to a sudden or even a gradual increase in the subject's physical activity. It took several more years to realize the role of mental stress in eliciting such transient ischaemic events and today it is generally accepted that the psychological trigger is most important in the genesis of transient myocardial ischaemia. Moreover, mental stress-induced ischaemia is even more often silent than the exercise-induced one. In the PIMI study, Sheps *et al.* (2002) demonstrated that mental stress-induced new or worsened wall-motion abnormalities, using the simple speech test, even predicted subsequent death in patients with coronary artery disease. In an earlier publication this group demonstrated that mental stress usually produces higher epinephrine responses than exercise does (Goldberg *et al.* 1996) and also reported (Stone *et al.* 1999) that transient ST depression induced by mental or exercise stress testing is more predictive of ST segment depression during routine daily activities than other laboratory-based ischaemic markers.

Physical stress-provoked ischaemia

It is an ancient observation, originating with Heberden himself, that chest pain, starting during a period of increased physical activity such as walking up-hill, sexual activity or other, is typical for 'angina pectoris'. Paul Wood in the early 1950s called attention during a lecture to the interesting point that during a Master two-step test, pain is not needed for a test to be positive and ST depression, even without any symptoms, is sufficient for the diagnosis. Several decades later, nobody raised an eyebrow, when both the nuclear and the echo experts confirmed ischaemia, if a thallium scan showed a reversible perfusion defect or a stress echo demonstrated wall-motion abnormality, even if the examinee felt no symptoms during the ischaemic period. Interestingly, this is true both for a physical stress or a dipyridamole perfusion scan and for a physical stress or a dobutamine echo, even when the pathophysiological mechanisms of inducing the ischaemia are obviously different.

In a relatively large asymptomatic population Rywik *et al.* (2002) found that not only the classic ischaemic ST segment response to exercise predicted future coronary events, but also an intensification of a minor pre-excercise ST depression to levels ≥ 1 mm carried an increased risk. A poor outcome for middle-aged, apparently healthy individuals with no prior coronary artery disease, but with SI on treadmill testing was demonstrated by Laukkanen *et al.* (2001) predominantly in subjects with one of the three major coronary risk factors. In this study even the SI detected during the post-exercise recovery phase was associated with an adverse clinical outcome, emphasizing the importance of the recovery ECG. A possible explanation for the grave consequences of repeated ischaemia can be found in the important observations of Schaper (1988) who demonstrated depletion of energy stores, cell death and other processes which can lead to myocardial dysfunction over time. Therefore it is recommended that even healthy subjects who have ≥2 coronary risk factors should be screened with exercise stress testing (Deedwania 2001).

That pain itself – during transient perfusion abnormalities on thallium or during contraction abnormalities on echo – has no prognostic significance, was demonstrated by earlier investigators, and has been confirmed again and again. Recently, Elhendy *et al.* (2002) pointed out that the absence of angina in patients with reversible perfusion abnormalities during dobutamine stress 99-m technetium sestamibi SPECT should not be interpreted as a predictor of a benign outcome. Regional dysfunction on stress echo, irrespective of pain, was found to be a good predictor of significant coronary artery disease while the ST depression during the test was indicative of systemic endothelial dysfunction in these patients (Palinkas *et al.* 2002).

Silent ischaemia and related conditions

The disease most frequently associated with SI is diabetes and the high prevalence of painless ischaemia in diabetics has been stressed by Nesto *et al.* (1988). In such patients exercise testing showed a low sensitivity (50%) but higher specificity (83%) for future events. Recently, Rutter *et al.* (2002) demonstrated that in type 2 diabetics microalbuminuria was a predictor of future coronary events in asymptomatic individuals, although SI on treadmill testing showed an even higher sensitivity and positive predictive value and was independent of the presence of microalbuminuria.

Hypertension is another condition which may facilitate the development of SI and asymptomatic ST depression on 24-h ambulatory ECG was found to be a rather common event among patients with mild and moderate arterial hypertension (Florczak *et al.* 2002). For these patients stress echo, specially when using dobutamine, yields the best diagnostic accuracy, as this agent increases myocardial oxygen consumption by sympathetic stimulation which in turn increases heart rate and contractility, metabolic stimulation and increases ATP breakdown. This is in contrast to the mainly 'steal' effect of dipyridamole which causes ischaemia in the presence of critical epicardial coronary disease only (Fragasso *et al.* 1999).

High proportions of patients with a history of

congestive heart failure also show lack of pain during the acute presentation of myocardial infarction. It is generally accepted that older patients are less likely to present with chest pain during acute coronary events and so are women, even after correction for age. It should be added that these subgroups of patients with 'silent' myocardial infarction were found to have a poorer prognosis than the ones with chest pain (Dorsch *et al.* 2001).

The circadian nature of ischaemic events

A characteristic circadian pattern of ischaemic episodes was demonstrated in earlier investigations, with a peak incidence in the early morning hours, coinciding with a rise in heart rate and plasma catecholamines (Mulcahy *et al.*). This morning peak could be explained by circadian variations in platelet activity, and also there is a morning trough in fibrinolytic activity. This peak is similar to the peak observed for myocardial infarction and sudden cardiac death (Muller *et al.* 1985). This observation was confirmed recently by the CAPE (Circadian Anti-ischaemia Program in Europe) study, which used 72-h Holter and exercise testing for identifying ambulatory and exercise ischaemia, respectively (Deanfield *et al.* 2002). Although the pathophysiology of exercise-induced and transient Holter-detected ischaemia is likely to differ, in this trial the use of these two objective measurements proved consistently the efficacy of the drug regimen used, both for angina and for ischaemia.

Circadian blood pressure changes can influence the occurrence of ischaemic episodes at night in hypertensive patient with coronary artery disease, as demonstrated by Pierdomenico *et al.* (1998), as nocturnal ischaemia was found to be more frequent in patients without the usual night-time fall in blood pressure. Similar observations of a preceding systolic blood pressure rise and an increased heart rate led Quyyumi (1998) to suggest that an important and perhaps predominant trigger for myocardial ischaemia and for its distribution, is a change in myocardial oxygen demand. This increase in demand, in combination with alterations in coronary vasoconstrictor tone and the degree of compromise of blood delivery to the myocardium and variations in the ischaemic threshold (Benhorin *et al.* 1993), is responsible for the observed variability in ischaemic episodes, whether silent or accompanied by pain.

Silent infarction of the right ventricle (RV)

The clinical observation that transmural infarction of the RV is frequently silent, is not new, but is gaining importance as our ability to diagnose this condition is increasing. The lack of pain is now attributed to the fact that only about 25% of the patients with RV infarctions develop clinically evident hemodynamic manifestations (Shah *et al.* 1985). Still, caution is needed, as even this clinically silent patient may subsequently develop hypotension and mechanical complications, following septal rupture or functional tricuspid regurgitation, due to tricuspidal annular dilatation. The pathophysiology and management of the mostly silent RV infarction was recently excellently reviewed by Goldstein (2002), who called our attention to this frequently asymptomatic but not at all harmless condition.

Studies explaining the lack of pain during myocardial ischaemia

Several theories have been suggested to explain the mechanism involved in the phenomenon of SI. Individual differences in pain threshold were entertained as a possible mechanism and indeed, hyposensitivity and/or high threshold were documented in 'silent' patients, as compared with symptomatic ones (Glazier *et al.* 1986). Others supposed an insufficient generation of adenosine (Crea *et al.* 1990) or a higher rate of production of endogenous opiates in these patients (Droste 1990; Falcone *et al.* 1993) although none of these mechanisms have convincingly been demonstrated yet.

An intriguing new mechanism was put forward recently by Mazzone *et al.* (2001), who showed that the significant increase of anti-inflammatory cytokines together with the decrease of leucocyte adhesion molecule expression might identify one of the mechanisms explaining SI. In these silent patients it might be possible that the Th2 (anti-inflammatory) activation will induce higher production of anti-inflammatory cytokines together with endogenous opioid production and higher expression of peripheral benzodiazepine receptors; the result may be the reduced pain perception of these patients. Only further studies will be able to clarify the effects of these cytokines on the atherosclerotic process itself and on clinical progression of the disease and on its prognosis. Even now, however, it seems to be proven that immune system and inflammatory system activation may be crucial for developing anginal symptoms, while reduced Cd11b receptor expression and higher concentration of anti-inflammatory cytokines result in 'silent ischaemia'.

Will this new mechanism, possibly acting in tandem with the previously proposed ones, satisfactorily answer the question why one person does and the other does not feel ischaemic pain? And even more puzzling, why the same person on the same day under apparently similar conditions, during one episode does and during another doesn't have pain? These riddles still await their solution.

References

Benhorin, J., Banai, S., Moriel, M. *et al.* (1993) Circadian variation in ischaemic threshold and their relation to the occurrence of ischaemic episodes. *Circulation*, **87**, 808–814.

Crea, F., Pupita, G., Galassi AR. *et al.* (1990) Role of adenosine in pathogenesis of anginal pain. *Circulation*, **81**, 164–172.

Deanfield, J.E., Detry, J.M., Sellier, P. *et al.* (2002) Medical treatment of myocardial ischaemia in coronary artery disease: effect of drug regime and irregular dosing in the CAPE II trial. *Journal of the American College of Cardiology*, **40**, 917–925.

Deedwania, P.C. (2001) Silent ischaemia predicts poor outcome in high-risk healthy men. *Journal of the American College of Cardiology*, **38**, 80–83.

Dorsch, M.F., Lawrance, R.A., Sapsford, R.J. *et al.* (2001) Poor prognosis of patients presenting with symptomatic myocardial infarction but without chest pain. *Heart*, **86**, 494–498.

Droste, C. (1990) Influence of opiate system in pain transmission during angina pectoris. *Zeitschrift für Kardiologie*, **79S**, 31–33.

Elhendy, A., van Domburg, R.T. & Schinkel, A. (2002) Prognostic significance of silent ischaemia assessed by dobutamine stress 99-m technetium sestamibi SPECT imaging. *Circulation*, **106** (Suppl.), II-618.

Falcone, C., Guasti, L. Ochan, M. *et al.* (1993) Beta-endorphins during coronary angioplasty in patients with silent or symptomatic myocardial ischaemia. *Journal of the American College of Cardiology*, **22**, 1614–1620.

Feil, H. & Siegel, M. (1929) Electrocardiographic changes during attacks of angina pectoris. *American Journal of Medical Science*, **177**, 223–242.

Florczak, E., Makowiecka-Ciesla, M., Baranowski, R. *et al.* (2002) Asymptomatic ST segment depression in patients with primary hypertension. *Folia Cardiologica*, **9**, 319–327.

Fragasso, G., Lu, C., Dabrowski, P. *et al.* (1999) Comparison of stress/rest myocardial perfusion tomography, dipyridamole and dobutamine stress echocardiography for the detection of coronary disease in hypertensive patients with chest pain and positive exercise test. *Journal of the American College of Cardiology*, **34**, 441–447.

Glazier, JJ., Chierchia, S., Brown, MJ. *et al.* (1986) The importance of generalized defective perception of painful stimuli as a cause of silent myocardial ischaemia in chronic stable angina pectoris. *American Journal of Cardiology*, **58**, 667–672.

Goldberg, A.D, Becker, L.C., Bonsall, R. *et al.* (1996) Ischaemic, hemodynamic, and neurohormonal responses to mental and exercise stress: experience from the Psychophysiological Investigations of Myocardial Ischaemia Study (PIMI). *Circulation*, **94**, 2402–2409.

Goldstein, J.A. (2002) Pathophysiology and management of right heart ischaemia. *Journal of the American College of Cardiology*, **40**, 841–853.

Laukkanen, J.A., Kurl, S., Lakka, A. *et al.* (2001) Exercise-induced silent myocardial ischaemia and coronary morbidity and mortality in middle-aged men. *Journal of the American College of Cardiology*, **38**, 72–79.

Mazzone, A., Cusa, C., Mazzucchelli, I. *et al.* (2001) Increased production of inflammatory cytokines in patients with silent myocardial ischaemia. *Journal of the American College of Cardiology*, **38**, 1895–1901.

Mulcahy, D., Keegan, J., Cunningham, D. *et al.* (1988) Circadian variation of total ischaemic burden and its alteration with anti-anginal agents. *Lancet*, **2**, 755–759.

Muller, J.E., Stone, P.H., Turi, Z.G. *et al.* (1985) Circadian variation in the frequency of onset of acute myocardial infarction. *New England Journal of Medicine*, **313**, 1315–1322.

Nesto, R.W., Phillips, R.T., Kett, K.G. *et al.* (1988) Angina and exertional myocardial ischaemia in diabetic and nondiabetic patients: assessment by exercise thallium scintigraphy. *Annals of Internal Medicine* **108**, 170–175.

Palinkas, A., Toth, E., Amyot, R. *et al.* (2002) The value of ECG and echocardiography during stress testing for identifying systemic endothelial dysfunction and epicardial artery stenosis. *European Heart Journal*, **23**, 1587–1595.

Pierdomenico, S.D., Bucci, A., Costantini, F. *et al.* (1998) Circadian blood pressure changes and myocardial ischaemia in hypertensive patients with coronary artery disease. *Journal of the American College of Cardiology*, **31**, 1627–1634.

Poole-Wilson, P.A. (2002) Who are the enemies? Lack of oxygen. *European Heart Journal Supplements* **4**, G15–G19.

Quyyumi, A.A. (1998) Circadian variation in myocardial ischaemia: pathophysiological mechanims. In: *Silent Myocardial Ischaemia* (eds S. Stern), pp. 159–173. Martin Dunitz, London.

Rutter, M.K., Wahid, S.T., McComb, J.M. *et al.* (2002) Significance of silent ischaemia and microalbuminuria in predicting coronary events in asymptomatic patients with type 2 diabetes. *Journal of the American College of Cardiology*, **40**, 56–61.

Rywik, T.M., O'Connor, F.C., Gittings, N.S. *et al.* (2002) Role of nondiagnostic exercise-induced ST segment abnormalities in predicting future coronary events in asymptomatic volunteers. *Circulation*, **106**, 2787–2792.

Schaper, J. (1988) Effects of multiple ischemic events on human myocardium: an ultrastructural study. *European Heart Journal*, **9** (Suppl. A), 141–149.

Shah, P.K., Maddahi, J., Berman, D.S. *et al.* (1985) Scintigraphically detected predominant right ventricular dysfunction in acute myocardial infarction: clinical and hemodynamic correlates and implications for therapy and prognosis. *Journal of the American College of Cardiology*, **6**, 1264–1272.

Sheps, D.S., McMahon, R.P., Becker, L. *et al.* (2002) Mental stress-induced ischaemia and all-cause mortality in patients with coronary artery disease. *Circulation*, **105**, 1780–1784.

Stern, S. & Tzivoni, D. (1976) The dynamic nature of the ST–T segment in ischaemic heart disease. *American Heart Journal*, **91**, 820–822.

Stone, P.H., Krantz, D.S., McMahon, R.P. *et al.* (1999) Relationship among mental stress-induced ischaemia and ischaemia during daily life and during exercise: the psychophysiological investigations of myocardial ischaemia (PIMI) study. *Journal of the American College of Cardiology*, **33**, 1476–1484.

CHAPTER 26

Dynamics of ST Segment in Ischaemic Heart Disease

Divaka Perera, Sundip J. Patel and Simon R. Redwood

Introduction

The ST segment lies between the end of the QRS complex and the beginning of the T wave on a surface electrocardiogram (ECG) and represents the interval between ventricular depolarization and repolarization. Under normal circumstances, there are virtually no electrical fluxes in the myocardium during this phase and the ST segment is undisplaced from the isoelectric baseline. Alteration of the electrophysiological properties of the myocardium can cause changes in duration of the *ST* interval, which is an important component of the *QT* interval, or deflection of the ST segment away from the baseline. Ischaemia triggers a series of cellular changes in the myocyte, which give rise to electrical heterogeneity between ischaemic and normal myocardium. The resultant electrical fluxes between these regions are manifest as deviation of the ST segment, which is the earliest and most consistent ECG abnormality during ischaemia. The pattern of ST deviation depends on the nature of the ischaemic process (including time-course, transmural extent and anatomical region) and is modified by pre-existing structural and functional abnormalities such as conduction system defects.

Electrophysiological basis of ST segment changes

Within minutes of acute coronary occlusion, the resting membrane potential depolarizes and can decrease by 20–25 mV during the first 10–15 min of ischaemia. This is accompanied by a decrease in the amplitude and upstroke velocity of phase 0 of the action potential. There is concomitant pathological early repolarization, resulting in abbreviation of the plateau (phase 2) and shortening of the action potential duration (Downar, Janse & Durrer 1977) (Fig. 26.1). The action potential changes are paralleled by a marked rise in extracellular potassium concentration ($[K^+]_o$) from approximately 4 mmol/L to a plateau of 10–15 mmol/L after 10 min (Kleber 1983). The rise in $[K^+]_o$ represents an imbalance between K^+ influx via the Na^+-K^+ pump and K^+ efflux, but the latter is likely to be the predominant effect as the Na^+-K^+ pump has been shown to function during the first 10–15 min of ischaemia. Whilst several mechanisms have been proposed for this increased K^+ efflux, the most important seems to be activation of the ATP-sensitive K^+ channel (K^+_{ATP}) (Wilde *et al.* 1990). This is a ligand-gated, voltage-insensitive channel which is highly selective for K^+ and is present in high density in the cardiac sarcolemma. The channel is inhibited by intracellular ATP and remains closed under normal conditions. Intracellular [ATP] is reduced in conditions such as ischaemia or hypoxia, which results in K^+_{ATP} opening and increased K^+ efflux. Pharmacological activation of K^+_{ATP} channels has been shown to produce ECG changes which closely resemble those of ischaemia (Kubota *et al.* 1993). Conversely, transgenic homozygous knockout mice (who lack the gene which encodes a subunit of K^+_{ATP} channels) do not develop ST elevation on ligation of the LAD artery, despite undergoing a similar degree of infarction as wild-type mice (Li *et al.* 2000).

The action potential changes described above give rise to voltage gradients between healthy and ischaemic myocardium. Flow of current between these regions is represented by deflections in the surface and epicardial ECG. These are known as 'currents of injury' by analogy with the changes observed in frog myocardium that has been subjected to mechanical injury (Burdon-Sanderson & Page 1879). Systolic as well as diastolic currents of injury are thought to occur, although the relative contribution of each to changes on surface ECG remains controversial. During phase 4 of the action potential (i.e. electrical diastole or TQ segment of ECG), the membrane potential of ischaemic cells is relatively depolarized compared to healthy tissue. The extracellular space is more negatively charged in ischaemic zones than in adjacent healthy areas and as such, the current of injury in diastole is from ischaemic to healthy myocardium. This results in TQ depression but, as ECG recorders use AC coupled amplifiers which compensate for baseline shift, there is *apparent* ST elevation on the surface ECG. In systole, the decrease in action potential amplitude and duration causes ischaemic myocardium to remain relatively repolarized, i.e. the extracellular space in ischaemic regions remains more positive than normal tissue. Therefore, current of injury is directed towards the ischaemic zone in systole and is represented by *true* ST elevation in surface ECG leads overlying these areas (Kleber *et al.* 1978).

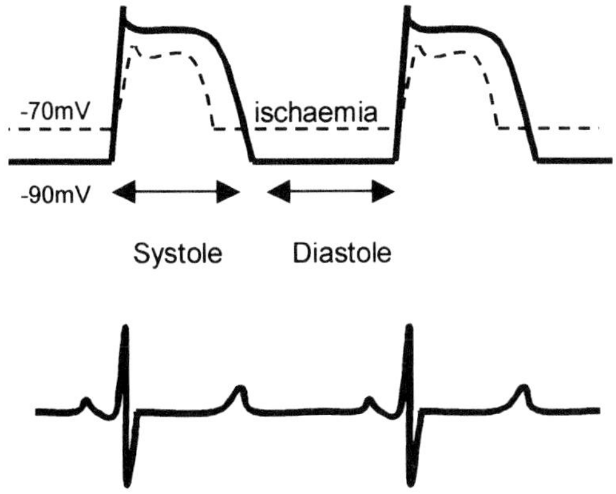

Fig. 26.1 Action potential changes during ischaemia. The resting membrane potential depolarizes rapidly when ischaemic. The action potential amplitude and duration are also decreased owing to diminished amplitude and velocity of phase 0 and early repolarization.

The direction of ST segment deviation on the surface ECG depends on the orientation of the overall ST vector (which is comprised of true systolic current and compensated diastolic current) in relation to the tissue immediately underlying the ECG electrode, i.e. the epicardium. In transmural ischaemia, as described above, the ST vector is towards the ischaemic epicardium, resulting in ST elevation and hyperacute T waves. When ischaemia is confined to the subendocardial layers however, a voltage gradient between epicardial and endocardial layers causes the ST vector to be directed towards the ischaemic zone, i.e. away from the epicardium (Fig. 26.2). This is represented by depression of the ST segment on surface ECG. This explana-

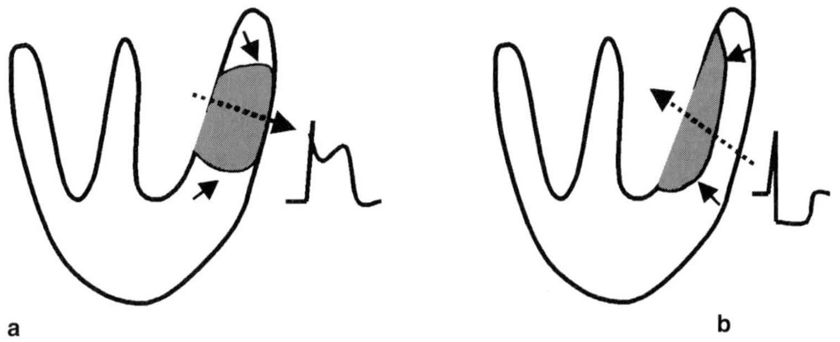

Fig. 26.2 Injury current and ST vectors. When ischaemia is transmural, current of injury flows from healthy to ischaemic myocardium and the ST vector is directed towards the epicardium, resulting in ST elevation on the ECG (a). In subendocardial ischaemia (b), the ST vector is directed away from healthy epicardium to ischaemic endocardium and is represented by ST depression.

tion, which is based on the dipole model, accounts for the nature of ST change observed during episodes of subendocardial ischaemia. Given that ST elevation has been shown to localize transmural ischaemia, the dipole model would further predict that ST depression could accurately localize regions of subendocardial ischaemia. However, this is not borne out in clinical practice and it has been shown that ST depression on surface ECG very poorly localizes ischaemia (Fuchs *et al.* 1982). One possible explanation of this discrepancy is that the major source of current flow towards the ischaemic subendocardium is the lateral border of the ischaemic zone rather than the overlying epicardium (Li *et al.* 1998). Tangential current flow away from these border zones would cause ST depression in ECG leads overlying these areas, which are adjacent to the ischaemic region (Fig. 26.2).

When ischaemia is prolonged, electrical resistance in the myocardium increases due to gap junction uncoupling. Consequently, the flow of injury current diminishes leading to a decrease in ST elevation and TQ depression at the centre of the ischaemic zone (Kleber, Janse, van Capelle & Durrer1978).

Chronic stable ischaemic heart disease

ST depression on a resting ECG can be a marker of the presence and severity of coronary disease (number of vessels involved, degree of obstruction) and impairment of left ventricular function (Mirvis *et al.* 1990). Similarly, resting ST–T changes are predictive of increased cardiovascular events and overall mortality in patients with established coronary disease (Crenshaw *et al.* 1991) as well as individuals with no prior history of ischaemic heart disease (Tervahauta *et al.* 1996). However, at least 50% of the patients with stable exertional angina and known coronary artery disease have a normal ECG at rest. When resting ECG abnormalities do occur, they tend to be nonspecific ST–T wave changes which are seen in a variety of conditions such as digoxin use or left ventricular hypertrophy. As a consequence, the resting ECG has limited sensitivity and specificity for diagnosing coronary disease. In contrast, dynamics of the ST segment during provoked ischaemia can provide valuable diagnostic and prognostic information in patients with suspected ischaemic heart disease. The two main modalities for assessing dynamic ST changes are exercise electrocardiography and ambulatory monitoring. A review of ST changes on Holter monitoring is beyond the scope of this chapter and will be covered in the section on silent ischaemia.

Exercise testing

In normal individuals, exercise causes characteristic changes in the ECG, including shortening of the *PR*, *QRS* and *QT* intervals, as well as depression of the junctional point (J point). The latter marks the onset of the ST segment and depression of the J point below the isoelectric baseline is accompanied by rapidly up-sloping ST depression. In addition to these changes, patients with coronary flow limitation develop horizontal or down-sloping ST depression (Fig. 26.3), which is the principal electrocardiographic endpoint of an exercise tolerance test (ETT). The basis of horizontal ST depression is thought to be subendocardial ischaemia of the myocardium subtended by a diseased coronary artery. Myocardial oxygen demand increases progressively during exercise and autoregulation allows increases in coronary blood flow to match this demand in healthy individuals. However, in patients with flow limiting coronary stenoses, such compensa-

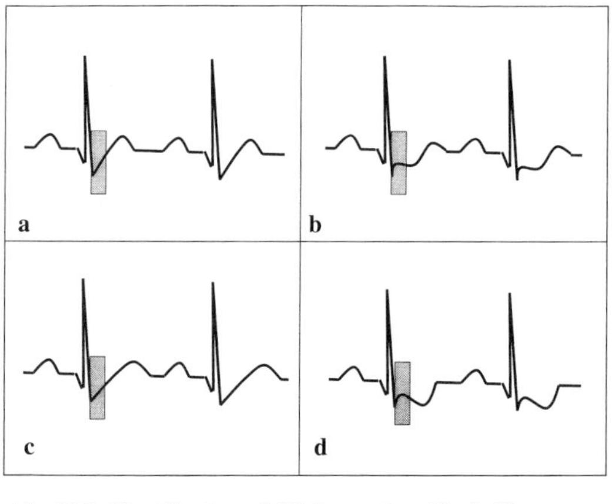

Fig. 26.3 Classification of ST depression. Shaded bar represents the 80 ms interval following the J point. (a) Up-sloping ST depression (ST80 <0.5 mm) seen in healthy subjects; (b) slow ascending ST depression (significant when ST80 >2 mm); (c) horizontal ST depression; (d) down-sloping ST depression

tion is impaired and distal coronary flow actually falls during exercise. The mismatch between myocardial oxygen demand and coronary flow results in ischaemia, which preferentially affects the endocardium owing to a concurrent drop in the endocardial:epicardial flow ratio (usually >1 but <0.5 in flow limitation (Gallagher *et al.* 1982)).

In the absence of resting Q waves, ST elevation occurs rarely (0.1–0.5%) during exercise testing (Longhurst & Kraus 1979). It is usually a manifestation of transmural ischaemia caused by vasospasm or a flow limiting coronary lesion and in contrast to ST depression, localizes ischaemia accurately and is associated with a worse prognosis. On the other hand, ST elevation occurs in leads with pre-existing Q waves in 30% of patients following anterior and 15% of patients following inferior AMI. In this context, ST elevation is often a marker of impaired ventricular function rather than residual viability in the infarcted zone (Manrique *et al.* 2001), although interpretation of this sign may depend on the degree of myocardial recovery following an infarction (Shimonagata *et al.* 1990).

The diagnostic accuracy of ETT has been extensively studied and meta-analysis of approximately 150 published reports reveals a mean (±SD) sensitivity of 67% (±16%) and specificity of 72% (±17%), using a threshold of 1mm horizontal or down-sloping ST depression measured 60–80ms following the J point (Gibbons *et al.* 2002). The predictive value of an ETT is influenced by the pre-test probability of obstructive coronary disease as well as a variety of electrocardiographic factors that affect interpretation of ST segment changes (Redwood, Borer & Epstein 1976). Conditions that cause depression of the ST segment at rest, such as left ventricular hypertrophy or digoxin use, can also produce an abnormal ST response to exercise, which reduces the specificity of exercise testing. Nevertheless, as this marker identifies a group who are more likely to have coronary disease, sensitivity is unaffected or even increased in these patients and the ETT remains a useful first line investigation. However, in the presence of LBBB, exercise-induced ST depression has no association with ischaemia and alternative tests are indicated.

While rapidly up-sloping ST depression is considered a normal response to exercise, a slower ST upslope (< 1 mV/s) can be the only finding in patients with well-defined obstructive coronary disease (Rijneke, Ascoop & Talmon 1980). However, using a slowly ascending slope as a criterion for abnormal findings would result in a greater number of false-positive results unless an increased threshold for ST depression (2 mm) is used in these cases. Computer assisted analysis of ETTs has been shown to be comparable to visual assessments and are particularly useful when combined with a clinical scoring system (Atwood *et al.* 1998). One technique that has received attention recently is adjustment of ST depression (slope and/or extent) to heart rate. It is expected that the sensitivity of ETT would be enhanced by this adjustment, which takes into account the independent association between tachycardia and ST depression. However, ST–heart rate adjustment has not been shown to improve prognostic value in symptomatic patients, although it may enhance diagnosis in asymptomatic individuals (Froelicher *et al.* 1998).

In patients with symptomatic stable coronary artery disease, the ETT is a powerful prognostic tool. Exercise-induced ST deviation provides a measure of reversible ischaemia but the strongest and most consistent prognostic marker is exercise test capacity. Combination of these variables further refines prognostic accuracy; in the CASS registry, patients who were unable to complete Stage I of the Bruce protocol and had ≥1 mm ST depression had a 5% annual mortality while mortality in those who exercised to Stage III with no ST changes was lower than 1% (Weiner *et al.* 1984). Exercise induced ST depression in this group gives a better guide to the likelihood that the patient will die than the likelihood of a nonfatal myocardial infarction (Mark *et al.* 1987), which may be explained by rupture of coronary plaques which are haemodynamically insignificant.

Unstable angina

Patients with unstable angina comprise a heterogeneous group with diverse clinical features and varying prognosis. An important aim of managing such patients is to identify those with increased risk of developing AMI or death and instituting treatment to alter these outcomes. The circumstances of presentation and severity of angina have been shown to be useful in stratifying risk within this group (Calvin *et al.* 1995) but the 12-lead ECG remains a powerful prognostic tool. In patients with ischaemic chest pain but no ST elevation on the admission ECG, the presence of ≥0.5 mm ST depression is predictive of increased mortality in the medium and long term (Cannon *et al.* 1997; Hyde *et al.* 1999).

In addition to dichotomous assessment, the extent of ST segment depression seems to allow further grading of risk in this group. Compared to patients with acute coronary syndromes and normal ECGs, the risk of death at one year is two-, four- and sixfold higher in patients with 0.5, 1 and ≥2 mm of ST depression, respectively. Involvement of distinct anatomical regions is an additional prognostic sign; patients with ≥2 mm ST depression in more than one region are 10 times more likely to die within 1 year than patients with a normal ECG (Kaul *et al.* 2001). Patients with unstable angina and ST depression have a much higher incidence of left main stem or triple vessel disease and the pathophysiology of ST changes is likely to be widespread subendocardial ischaemia. T wave abnormalities are a sensitive sign of ischaemia but are nonspecific and have limited prognostic value, particularly in the presence of concomitant ST depression. However, deep transient T-inversion (≥3 mm) is relatively specific for ischaemia.

The advent of highly sensitive markers of myocardial damage, such as cardiac troponin and C reactive protein, have allowed further stratification of risk in patients with acute coronary syndromes. However, recent studies suggest that ST depression provides prognostic information and identifies those high-risk patients who are likely to benefit from revascularization, independent of their biochemical marker status (Fig. 26.4). It seems likely that optimal risk assessment relies on a combination of clinical history, ECG changes and biochemical markers of myocardial damage such as (Diderholm *et al.* 2002a).

Myocardial infarction

The diagnosis of acute myocardial infarction (AMI) has traditionally relied on the presence of a suggestive history, specific ECG changes and detection of biochemical markers of myocardial

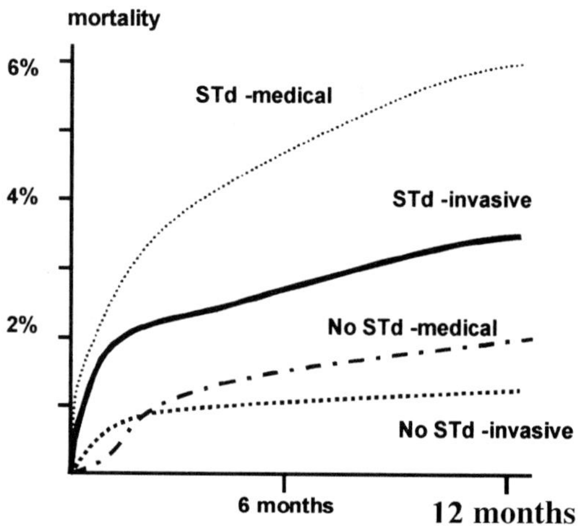

Fig. 26.4 Prognostic value of *ST* depression in acute coronary syndromes. ST depression (STd) is associated with a significantly higher mortality up to 1 year, compared to patients without STd, irrespective of treatment strategy. Invasive treatment was of benefit only in patients with STd. (Diderholm *et al.* 2002b)

damage. However, as biochemical markers frequently fail to reach diagnostic levels within 6 h, there can be considerable delays in establishing a diagnosis (Roberts & Fromm 1998). In the era of thrombolysis and acute coronary intervention, an expeditious diagnosis is often life saving and as such, the ECG has assumed an even more important role in diagnosis and management of patients with AMI.

ST elevation

Whilst Q waves are the hallmark of myocardial necrosis, ST segment elevation is the most reliable indicator of transmural ischaemia. A threshold of 1 mm ST elevation in at least one inferior or lateral lead (II, III, AVF or V5, V6, I, AVL) and 2 mm in at least one anterior lead has been shown to correctly identify 83% of patients with AMI (Menown, Mackenzie & Adgey 2000). These thresholds, which are commonly used as criteria for thrombolysis, are very specific for AMI (94%) but are not particularly sensitive (56%). A lower ST elevation threshold does improve sensitivity (to approximately 70%), although this is at the expense of specificity. The extent of ST elevation across all leads can provide a quantitative indicator of final infarct size, but the latter is strongly influenced by the time to reperfusion as well as myocardium at risk

(Christian *et al.* 1995). Multiple mechanical, anatomical and electrophysiological variables may influence this measurement and ST segment elevation as a quantitative marker of acute ischaemia should be used with caution in individual cases. Despite these limitations, the degree of ST elevation at admission is a powerful independent predictor of in hospital mortality, as well as survival for up to 10 years, even in patients treated with thrombolysis (Mauri *et al.* 2002). ST segment changes during AMI also allow noninvasive localization of the anatomic region affected and estimation of the site of occlusion of the infarct-related artery in most cases. The diagnostic ECG patterns and their predictive value are represented in Table 26.1.

Table 26.1 Electrocardiographic localization of infarct artery and affected myocardium. STe, ST elevation; STd, ST depression; sen, sensitivity; spec, specificity

	Common ECG indicators
Anterior	STe V1–V6 (max V2 or V3)
Proximal LAD	STe I, AVL; STd II, III, AVF
	STe AVR (sen 43%, spec 95%)
	Loss of lateral Q waves (sen 30%, spec 98%)
	STd V5 (sen 17%, spec 98%)
Distal LAD	<2.5 mm STe V1
	<1 mm STd II, II, AVF
High lateral	STe I, AVL
Diagonal	Concomitant precordial STe
OM	STd V2
Inferior	STe II, II, AVF
RCA	STe III > II, STd AVL
Circumflex	STd V1–V2, normal or STe AVL
Posterior	STe V7–V9 (sen 84%, spec 80%), STd V1–2
	STe II, III, AVF, V5–6, AVL (sen 57%, spec 80%)
Right ventricle	STe V1 (can mimic anterior MI with STe to V4)
	STe V4R (sen 93%, spec 93%)
Anterior plus inferior	Usually 'wrap around' LAD
	Σ STe >18 mm is 90% sensitive for LMS disease

ST depression

Although the presence of ST elevation is highly suggestive of AMI, the poor sensitivity of this sign is a major limitation. A significant proportion of cases of AMI do not present with ST elevation on ECG (Rude *et al.* 1983) but have normal or nondiagnostic ECGs, T wave inversion or isolated ST depression. Of all AMIs, 10–15% present with ST depression alone (Miller *et al.* 2001) and represent a high-risk group with poor short- and long-term prognosis (Lee *et al.* 1993). Increased mortality partly reflects the difficulty in distinguishing ischaemia from infarction but also relates to the adverse demographic profile of this group; patients with ST depression AMI tend to be older, have a history of previous myocardial infarction and have a higher incidence of triple vessel coronary disease (Lee, Cross, Rawles & Jennings1993; Mahon *et al.* 2000). The benefit of thrombolysis in these patients is controversial (Braunwald & Cannon 1996; Langer *et al.* 1996), but even amongst AMI patients who are not treated with thrombolysis on account of contra-indications, ST depression is associated with higher mortality than ST elevation or left bundle branch block (Wong *et al.* 1998). Autopsy studies have shown that the underlying basis may be widespread subendocardial ischaemia (Cook, Edwards, & Pruitt 1958) but pathophysiology is probably heterogeneous. ST depression ≥1 mm (measured 80 ms after the J point) in ≥ six leads (Menown, Mackenzie & Adgey 2000) or ≥4 mm in any lead (Lee, Cross, Rawles & Jennings 1993) are highly specific criteria for diagnosis of infarction. There is some evidence that body surface mapping may be superior to a 12-lead ECG in diagnosing infarction in these patients (Menown *et al.* 2001) but this technique is not widely available and is unlikely to influence clinical practice at present.

Reciprocal changes

ST depression can occur concurrent with ST elevation during AMI and in most cases, is associated with a poorer outcome than ST elevation alone (Savonitto *et al.* 1999). Two mechanisms have been proposed to account for this finding. The first is that ST depression is a benign electrical phenomenon, secondary or reciprocal to ST elevation and is produced by viewing an active myocardial event from the opposite perspective (some authors describe this process as 'mirroring'). This model, which is based on the dipole theory (Mirvis *et al.* 1978), suggests that every positive flux (primary ST elevation) is accompanied by an equivalent but negative flux (reciprocal ST depression) recorded at the opposite end of a theoretical sphere. Accordingly, reciprocal ST depression *always* accompanies ST elevation during AMI although its detection on the surface ECG depends on the strength and location of the lesion in relation to the position of body surface electrodes. This hypothesis has been borne out experimentally in isolated heart preparations (Wolforth *et al.* 1945) as well as animal studies (Crawford, O'Rourke & Grover 1984).

The second explanation is that ST depression, when it accompanies ST elevation, represents ischaemia at a distance. Interruption of the infarct-related artery is thought to affect a remote vascular bed supplied by a second stenosed coronary artery. Multiple mechanisms interact to produce this effect, including increased oxygen demand due to ischaemia in the infarct bed, increased left ventricular end diastolic pressure, reduced collateral flow from the infarct artery and change in compliance of the stenosed artery (Schwartz, Cohn & Bache 1983). Subendocardial hypoperfusion then causes remote ST depression, as described in an earlier section.

The commonest clinical example of concurrent ST elevation and depression is inferoposterior AMI, when the source of anterior ST depression may reflect anterior ischaemia or may merely be secondary to inferior and posterior ST elevation (Fig. 26.5). A large number of studies have demonstrated LAD lesions, anterior perfusion defects or wall motion abnormalities in such patients (supporting ischaemia at a distance) while several have not (implying reciprocal ST depression) (Mirvis 1988). Posterior infarction rather than anterior ischaemia is suggested by the presence of a tall R wave (R:S ratio >1) in addition to ST depression in leads V1 or V2, while demonstration of ST elevation in posterior leads (V7–V9) is a highly specific sign (Khaw *et al.* 1999). On balance, the evidence suggests that most patients with inferior ST elevation and anterior ST depression have inferior AMIs with extension to posterior regions, while a significant minority have true anterior ischaemia. Regardless of the mechanism, concurrent ST elevation and depression appear to reflect a greater mass of ischaemic or necrotic myocardium, whether it is inferior, posterior or anterior.

Effect of reperfusion

ST segment deflection during ischaemia is a dynamic process and resolution of these changes indicates relief of ischaemia (through reperfusion) or the onset of irreversible necrosis. Early animal studies demonstrated that myocardial reperfusion results in rapid resolution of ST elevation (Muller, Maroko & Braunwald 1975) and this finding has subsequently been borne out in humans (Clemmensen *et al.* 1990). The extent of ST resolution is strongly predictive of final infarct size, LV dysfunction and mortality, irrespective of the reperfusion strategy used (Schroder *et al.* 1994). Much of the prognostic value of ST resolution seems to relate to the ability to predict infarct artery patency. Patients with complete resolution of ST elevation following thrombolysis are 90–95% likely to have a patent infarct-related artery and the majority of these patients would have TIMI 3 flow at coronary angiography (Zeymer *et al.* 2001). However, many patients who have restoration of epicardial coronary flow fail to achieve reperfusion at the level of the coronary microcirculation and myocardium (Ito *et al.* 1992). ST resolution accurately differentiates outcome even amongst patients with normal epicardial flow (de Lemos *et al.* 2000) and is increasingly recognized as a surrogate marker of tissue-level reperfusion (Dong *et al.* 2002). The association between myocardial perfusion and ST resolution is the probable basis of its prognostic value and these observations have challenged the role of angiography as a gold standard for successful reperfusion (Shah *et al.* 2000; Roe *et al.* 2001).

A three-component definition of ST resolution is used in most fibrinolysis and percutaneous intervention trials: complete (>70% resolution of initial ST elevation), partial (30–70% resolution) and incomplete (<30% resolution). Anterior AMIs are often associated with a smaller degree of ST resolution than inferior infarcts (leading some investigators to use a threshold of 50% to define complete resolution in these cases), although greater ST resolution is associated with lower mortality in all infarcts. The optimal timing for assessment of ST resolution is unresolved; benefit has been shown with ST resolution as

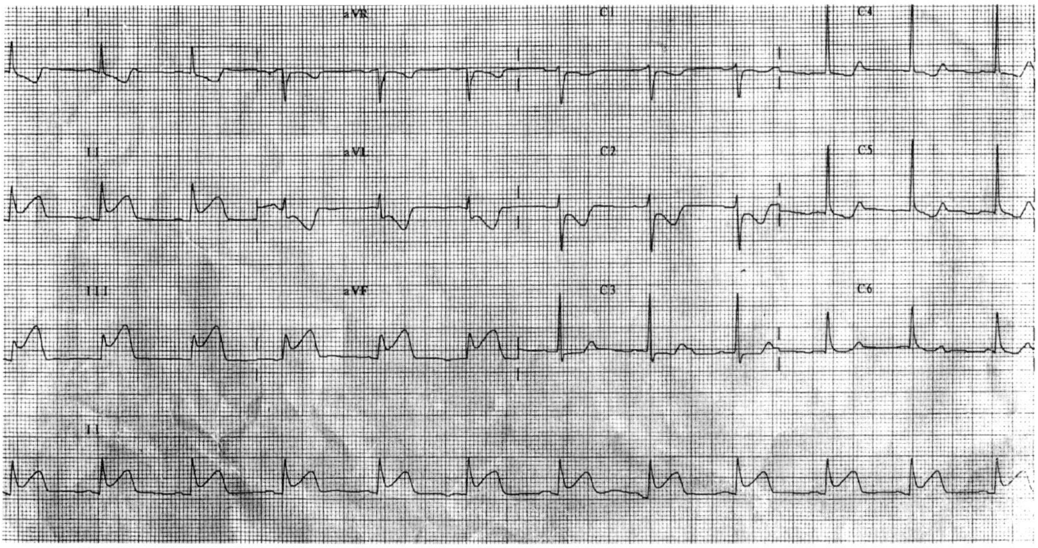

Fig. 26.5 Concomitant ST elevation and depression in AMI. ST elevation in leads II, III and AVF represent acute inferior MI. ST depression in leads I, AVL and leads V1–V5 may indicate reciprocal changes (an electrical phenomenon) or true anterior/lateral ischaemia. Angiography in this patient revealed single-vessel RCA disease, providing retrospective confirmation of secondary ST depression.

early as 60 min and up to 4 h (Schroder *et al.* 1999), while a recent study has demonstrated improved mortality benefit even when resolution occurs 24 h after fibrinolysis (Fu *et al.* 2001).

Frequency of monitoring

Continuous ST segment monitoring is superior to serial static ECGs in detecting peak ST change (Veldkamp *et al.* 1994) as well as recurrent ST elevation following initial resolution, which is associated with a poor prognosis (Langer *et al.* 1998). However, in centres where high quality ST segment monitoring facilities are unavailable, 12-lead ECGs performed 60, 90 and 180 min following thrombolysis and at least every 6 h during the subsequent 24 h should yield adequate prognostic and diagnostic information. If lead position is identical from tracing to tracing, assessing changes in a single lead showing maximal ST elevation probably provides equivalent information to multi-lead techniques which rely on summation of ST changes (Schroder *et al.* 2001).

Influence of bundle branch block

Interpretation of primary ST changes of ischaemia can be difficult when an abnormal sequence of depolarization causes altered repolarization and secondary ST–T abnormalities. Right bundle branch block seldom obscures ST changes seen during ischaemia, as the intact left bundle allows relatively normal depolarization of the septum and sites of early activation in the left ventricle (Eriksson, Gunnarsson & Dellborg 1998). However, left bundle branch block (LBBB) causes the septum to depolarize from the right and delays activation of most areas of the left ventricle, resulting in widespread secondary ST and T waves abnormalities which can mimic or mask ischaemia. In uncomplicated LBBB, the ST–T vector and QRS complex are discordant, i.e. they are oriented in opposite directions (Hurst 1997); ST elevation and tall positive T waves are frequently seen in right ventricular leads and T inversion is seen in lateral precordial leads. The appearance of concordant ST deflection ($\geq$1 mm ST elevation in V5, V6, I, AVL or ST depression in V1–3) is strongly suggestive of ischaemia. Increased discordant ST elevation ($\geq$5 mm in leads with a negative QRS) may also be due to acute ischaemia. When combined in a scoring system, these criteria are fairly specific for AMI (Sgarbossa *et al.* 1996a), although they await validation in larger groups. Changes in QRS morphology, such as the Cabrera Sign (notching of ascending limb of S wave in V3,V4), appearance of RV1 or QV6, may also aid detection of infarction in these patients (Wackers 1987).

Given the low sensitivity of these criteria, it is reasonable to treat patients with LBBB aggres-

Table 26.2 ECG discriminators of ST elevation

	Early repolarization	*Pericarditis*	*Myocardial infarction*
Location of ST elevation	Precordial leads	All leads	Leads overlying infarct
ST morphology	Concave upwards	Concave upwards	Convex upwards
Reciprocal changes	Absent	Absent	Present
ST/T ratio V6	<0.25	>0.25	N/A
PR segment	Usually depressed	Rarely depressed	Normal
QRS morphology	J point elevation (terminal QRS notch)	May be low voltage	Descending limb of QRS merges with raised ST
R waves	Normal R amplitude Abrupt transition at V2	Normal R amplitude	Loss of R amplitude
Q waves	Absent	Absent	May be present
Evolution	Temporally stable, normalizes on exercise	Evolution in 4 stages	Serial Q, ST and T changes

sively when AMI is suspected but specific ECG features are lacking or a previous ECG is unavailable (Shlipak *et al.* 1999). Right ventricular pacing causes similar diagnostic difficulty as LBBB and there is some evidence that the above criteria may be applicable (Sgarbossa *et al.* 1996b). Diagnosis of AMI can usually be made with reasonable accuracy using standard ECG criteria in patients with Wolff-Parkinson–White syndrome, although pre-excitation owing to a left accessory pathway could be misinterpreted as ST elevation in leads V2 and V3.

Nonischaemic ST elevation

Several nonischaemic conditions may be associated with ST segment elevation and some occur with sufficient frequency to warrant consideration in the differential diagnosis of AMI. A normal ECG variant which is often misdiagnosed as AMI is early repolarization. ST elevation is frequently accompanied by characteristic electrocardiographic features, which may allow differentiation of early repolarization from AMI (Table 26.2). It occurs in 1–2% of most races, is more common in younger individuals and predominantly affects males. There do not appear to be any pathological correlates to this ECG abnormality, whose natural history is benign (Mehta, Jain & Mehta 1999). Unlike in AMI, the ECG changes are non-progressive, although the ST segment and J point may normalize on exercise. Acute pericarditis is also manifest by ST elevation and may mimic acute infarction or reinfarction. ST elevation is believed to be due to epicardial injury, with consequent flow of injury current towards the affected zone (Bonnefoy *et al.* 2000). The concave upward nature of ST elevation, involvement of more than one coronary territory and other ECG discriminators (Table 26.2) are characteristic, but distinguishing from AMI can be difficult and patients with acute pericarditis are often treated with reperfusion therapy.

References

Atwood, J.E., Do, D., Froelicher, V. *et al.* (1998) Can computerization of the exercise test replace the cardiologist? *American Heart Journal*, **136** (3), 543–552.

Bonnefoy, E., Godon, P., Kirkorian, G., Fatemi, M., Chevalier, P. & Touboul, P. (2000) Serum cardiac troponin I and ST segment elevation in patients with acute pericarditis. *European Heart Journal*, **21** (10), 832–836.

Braunwald, E. & Cannon, C.P. (1996) Non-Q wave and ST segment depression myocardial infarction: is there a role for thrombolytic therapy? *Journal of the American College of Cardiology*, **27**(6), 1333–1334.

Burdon-Sanderson, J. & Page, F. (1879) On the time relation of the excitatory process in the ventricle of the heart of the frog. *Journal of Physiology*, **2**, 384–429.

Calvin, J.E., Klein, L.W., VandenBerg, B.J. *et al.* (1995) Risk stratification in unstable angina. Prospective validation of the Braunwald classification. *JAMA (Journal of the American Medical Association)*, **273** (2), 136–141.

Cannon, C.P., McCabe, C.H., Stone, P.H. *et al.* (1997) The electrocardiogram predicts one-year outcome of patients with unstable angina and non-Q wave myocardial infarction: results of the TIMI III Registry

ECG Ancillary Study. Thrombolysis in Myocardial Ischaemia. *Journal of the American College of Cardiology*, **30** (1), 133–140.

Christian, T.F., Gibbons, R.J., Clements, I.P., Berger, P.B., Selvester, R.H. & Wagner, G.S. (1995) 'Estimates of myocardium at risk and collateral flow in acute myocardial infarction using electrocardiographic indexes with comparison to radionuclide and angiographic measures. *Journal of the American College of Cardiology*, **26** (2), 388–393.

Clemmensen, P., Ohman, E.M., Sevilla, D.C., Peck, S., Wagner, N.B., Quigley, P.S., Grande, P., Lee, K.L. & Wagner, G.S. (1990) Changes in standard electrocardiographic ST segment elevation predictive of successful reperfusion in acute myocardial infarction. *American Journal of Cardiology*, **66** (20), 1407–1411.

Cook, R., Edwards, J. & Pruitt, R. (1958) Electrocardiographic changes in acute subendocardial infarction, I: large subendocardial and large nontransmural infarcts. *Circulation*, **18**, 603–612.

Crawford, M.H., O'Rourke, R.A. & Grover, F.L. (1984) Mechanism of inferior electrocardiographic ST segment depression during acute anterior myocardial infarction in a baboon model. *American Journal of Cardiology*, **54** (8), 1114–1117.

Crenshaw, J.H., Mirvis, D.M., el Zeky, F. *et al.* (1991) Interactive effects of ST–T wave abnormalities on survival of patients with coronary artery disease. *Journal of the American College of Cardiology*, **18** (2), 413–420.

Diderholm, E., Andren, B., Frostfeldt, G. *et al.* (2002a) The prognostic and therapeutic implications of increased troponin T levels and ST depression in unstable coronary artery disease: the FRISC II invasive troponin T electrocardiogram substudy. *American Heart Journal*, **143** (5), 760–767.

Diderholm, E., Andren, B., Frostfeldt, G. *et al.* (2002b) ST depression in ECG at entry indicates severe coronary lesions and large benefits of an early invasive treatment strategy in unstable coronary artery disease; the FRISC II ECG substudy. The Fast Revascularization during InStability in Coronary artery disease. *European Heart Journal*, **23** (1), 41–49.

Dong, J., Ndrepepa, G., Schmitt, C. *et al.* (2002) Early resolution of ST segment elevation correlates with myocardial salvage assessed by Tc-99m sestamibi scintigraphy in patients with acute myocardial infarction after mechanical or thrombolytic reperfusion therapy. *Circulation*, **105** (25), 2946–2949.

Downar, E., Janse, M.J. & Durrer, D. (1977) The effect of acute coronary artery occlusion on subepicardial transmembrane potentials in the intact porcine heart. *Circulation*, **56** (2), 217–224.

Eriksson, P., Gunnarsson, G. & Dellborg, M. (1998) Diagnosis of acute myocardial infarction in patients with chronic right bundle-branch block using standard 12-lead electrocardiogram compared with dynamic vector cardiography. *Cardiology*, **90** (1), 58–62.

Froelicher, V.F., Lehmann, K.G., Thomas, R. *et al.* (1998) The electrocardiographic exercise test in a population with reduced workup bias: diagnostic performance, computerized interpretation, and multivariable prediction. Veterans Affairs Cooperative Study in Health Services no. 016 (QUEXTA) Study Group. Quantitative Exercise Testing and Angiography. *Annals of Internal Medicine*, **128** (12 Pt 1), 965–974.

Fu, Y., Goodman, S., Chang, W.C., Van de, W.F., Granger, C.B. & Armstrong, P.W. (2001) Time to treatment influences the impact of ST segment resolution on one-year prognosis: insights from the assessment of the safety and efficacy of a new thrombolytic (ASSENT-2) trial. *Circulation*, **104** (22), 2653–2659.

Fuchs, R.M., Achuff, S.C., Grunwald, L., Yin, F.C. & Griffith, L.S. (1982) Electrocardiographic localization of coronary artery narrowings: studies during myocardial ischaemia and infarction in patients with one-vessel disease. *Circulation*, **66** (6), 1168–1176.

Gallagher, K.P., Osakada, G., Matsuzaki, M., Kemper, W.S. & Ross, J., Jr (1982) Myocardial blood flow and function with critical coronary stenosis in exercising dogs. *American Journal of Physiology*, **243** (5), H698–H707.

Gibbons, R.J., Balady, G.J., Timothy, B.J. *et al.* (2002) *ACC/AHA 2002 Guideline Update for Exercise Testing: A Report of the American College of Cardiology/American Heart Association Task Force on Practice Guidelines (Committee on Exercise Testing)*. American College of Cardiology Website. http://www.acc.org/clinical/guidelines/exercise/exercise_clean.pdf

Hurst, J.W. (1997) Abnormalities of the ST segment – Part I. *Clinical Cardiology*, **20** (6), 511–520.

Hyde, T.A., French, J.K., Wong, C.K., Straznicky, I.T., Whitlock, R.M. & White, H.D. (1999) Four-year survival of patients with acute coronary syndromes without ST segment elevation and prognostic significance of 0.5-mm ST segment depression. *American Journal of Cardiology*, **84** (4), 379–385.

Ito, H., Tomooka, T., Sakai, N. *et al.* (1992) Lack of myocardial perfusion immediately after successful thrombolysis. A predictor of poor recovery of left ventricular function in anterior myocardial infarction. *Circulation*, **85** (5), 1699–1705.

Kaul, P., Fu, Y., Chang, W.C. *et al.* (2001) Prognostic value of ST segment depression in acute coronary syndromes: insights from PARAGON-A applied to GUSTO-IIb. PARAGON-A and GUSTO IIb Investigators. Platelet IIb/IIIa Antagonism for the Reduction of Acute Global Organization Network. *Journal of the American College of Cardiology*, **38** (1), 64–71.

Khaw, K., Moreyra, A.E., Tannenbaum, A.K., Hosler, M.N., Brewer, T.J. & Agarwal, J.B. (1999) Improved detection of posterior myocardial wall ischaemia with the 15-lead electrocardiogram. *American Heart Journal*, **138** (5 Pt 1), 934–940.

Kleber, A.G. 1983, Resting membrane potential, extracellular potassium activity, and intracellular sodium activity during acute global ischaemia in isolated perfused guinea pig hearts. *Circulation Research*, **52** (4), 442–450.

Kleber, A.G., Janse, M.J., van Capelle, F.J. & Durrer, D. (1978) Mechanism and time course of S-T and T-Q segment changes during acute regional myocardial ischaemia in the pig heart determined by extracellular and intracellular recordings. *Circulation Research*, **42** (5), 603–613.

Kubota, I., Yamaki, M., Shibata, T., Ikeno, E., Hosoya, Y. & Tomoike, H. (1993) Role of ATP-sensitive K+ channel on ECG ST segment elevation during a bout of myocardial ischaemia. A study on epicardial mapping in dogs. *Circulation*, **88** (4 Pt 1), 1845–1851.

Langer, A., Goodman, S.G., Topol, E.J. *et al.* (1996) Late assessment of thrombolytic efficacy (LATE) study: prognosis in patients with non-Q wave myocardial infarction. (LATE Study Investigators). *Journal of the American College of Cardiology*, **27** (6), 1327–1332.

Langer, A., Krucoff, M.W., Klootwijk, P. *et al.* (1998) Prognostic significance of ST segment shift early after resolution of ST elevation in patients with myocardial infarction treated with thrombolytic therapy: the GUSTO-I *S–T* Segment Monitoring Substudy. *Journal of the American College of Cardiology*, **31** (4), 783–789.

Lee, H.S., Cross, S.J., Rawles, J.M. & Jennings, K.P. (1993) Patients with suspected myocardial infarction who present with ST depression. *Lancet*, **342** (8881), 1204–1207.

de Lemos, J.A., Antman, E.M., Giugliano, R.P. *et al.* (2000) ST segment resolution and infarct-related artery patency and flow after thrombolytic therapy. Thrombolysis in Myocardial Infarction (TIMI) 14 investigators. *American Journal of Cardiology*, **85** (3), 299–304.

Li, D., Li, C.Y., Yong, A.C. & Kilpatrick, D. (1998) Source of electrocardiographic ST changes in subendocardial ischaemia. *Circulation Research*, **82** (9), 957–970.

Li, R.A., Leppo, M., Miki, T., Seino, S. & Marban, E. (2000) Molecular basis of electrocardiographic ST segment elevation. *Circulation Research*, **87** (10), 837–839.

Longhurst, J.C. & Kraus, W.L. (1979) Exercise-induced ST elevation in patients without myocardial infarction. *Circulation*, **60** (3), 616–629.

Mahon, N.G., Codd, M.B., McKenna, C.J., O'Rorke, C., McCann, H.A. & Sugrue, D.D. (2000) Characteristics and outcomes in patients with acute myocardial infarction with ST segment depression on initial electrocardiogram. *American Heart Journal*, **139** (2 Pt 1), 311–319.

Manrique, A., Koning, R., Hitzel, A., Cribier, A. & Vera, P. (2001) Exercise-induced *ST*-elevation is related to left ventricular dysfunction but not to myocardial viability in patients with healed myocardial infarction. *European Journal of Heart Failure*, **3** (6), 709–716.

Mark, D.B., Hlatky, M.A., Harrell, F.E., Jr, Lee, K.L., Califf, R.M. & Pryor, D.B. (1987) Exercise treadmill score for predicting prognosis in coronary artery disease. *Annals of Internal Medicine*, **106** (6), 793–800.

Mauri, F., Franzosi, M.G., Maggioni, A.P., Santoro, E. & Santoro, L. (2002) Clinical value of 12-lead electrocardiography to predict the long-term prognosis of GISSI-1 patients. *Journal of the American College of Cardiology*, **39** (10), 1594–1600.

Mehta, M., Jain, A.C. & Mehta, A. (1999) Early repolarization. *Clinical Cardiology*, **22** (2), 59–65.

Menown, I.B., Allen, J., Anderson, J.M. & Adgey, A.A. (2001) ST depression only on the initial 12-lead ECG: early diagnosis of acute myocardial infarction. *European Heart Journal*, **22** (3), 218–227.

Menown, I.B., Mackenzie, G. & Adgey, A.A. (2000) Optimizing the initial 12-lead electrocardiographic diagnosis of acute myocardial infarction. *European Heart Journal*, **21** (4), 275–283.

Miller, W.L., Sgura, F.A., Kopecky, S.L. *et al.* (2001) Characteristics of presenting electrocardiograms of acute myocardial infarction from a community-based population predict short- and long-term mortality. *American Journal of Cardiology*, **87** (9), 1045–1050.

Mirvis, D.M. (1988) Physiological bases for anterior ST segment depression in patients with acute inferior wall myocardial infarction. *American Heart Journal*, **116** (5 Pt 1), 1308–1322.

Mirvis, D.M., Keller, F.W., Ideker, R.E., Zettergren, D.G. & Dowdie, R.F. (1978) Equivalent generator properties of acute ischaemic lesions in the isolated rabbit heart. *Circulation Research*, **42** (5), 676–685.

Mirvis, D.M., el Zeky, F., Vander, Z.R. *et al.* (1990) Clinical and pathophysiological correlates of ST–T wave abnormalities in coronary artery disease. *American Journal of Cardiology*, **66** (7), 699–704.

Muller, J.E., Maroko, P.R. & Braunwald, E. (1975) Evaluation of precordial electrocardiographic mapping as a means of assessing changes in myocardial ischaemic injury. *Circulation*, **52** (1), 16–27.

Redwood, D.R., Borer, J.S. & Epstein, S.E. (1976) Whither the ST segment during exercise. *Circulation*, **54** (5), 703–706.

Rijneke, R.D., Ascoop, C.A. & Talmon, J.L. (1980) Clinical significance of upsloping ST segments in exercise electrocardiography. *Circulation*, **61** (4), 671–678.

Roberts, R. & Fromm, R.E. (1998) Management of acute coronary syndromes based on risk stratification by biochemical markers: an idea whose time has come. *Circulation*, **98** (18), 1831–1833.

Roe, M.T., Ohman, E.M., Maas, A.C. *et al.* (2001) Shifting the open-artery hypothesis downstream: the quest for optimal reperfusion. *Journal of the American College of Cardiology*, **37** (1), 9–18.

Rude, R.E., Poole, W.K., Muller, J.E. *et al.* (1983) Electrocardiographic and clinical criteria for recognition of acute myocardial infarction based on analysis of 3,697 patients. *American Journal of Cardiology*, **52** (8), 936–942.

Savonitto, S., Ardissino, D., Granger, C.B. *et al.* (1999) Prognostic value of the admission electrocardiogram in acute coronary syndromes. *JAMA (Journal of the American Medical Association)*, **281** (8), 707–713.

Schroder, K., Wegscheider, K., Zeymer, U., Tebbe, U. & Schroder, R. (2001) Extent of ST segment deviation in a single electrocardiogram lead 90 min after thrombolysis as a predictor of medium-term mortality in acute myocardial infarction. *Lancet*, **358** (9292), 1479–1486.

Schroder, R., Dissmann, R., Bruggemann, T. *et al.* (1994) Extent of early ST segment elevation resolution: a simple but strong predictor of outcome in patients with acute myocardial infarction. *Journal of the American College of Cardiology*, **24** (20), 384–391.

Schroder, R., Zeymer, U., Wegscheider, K. & Neuhaus, K.L. (1999) Comparison of the predictive value of ST segment elevation resolution at 90 and 180 min after start of streptokinase in acute myocardial infarction. A substudy of the hirudin for improvement of thrombolysis (HIT)-4 study. *European Heart Journal*, **20** (21), 1563–1571.

Schwartz, J.S., Cohn, J.N. & Bache, R.J. (1983) Effects of coronary occlusion on flow in the distribution of a neighbouring stenotic coronary artery in the dog. *American Journal of Cardiology*, **52** (1), 189–195.

Sgarbossa, E.B., Pinski, S.L., Barbagelata, A. *et al.* (1996a) Electrocardiographic diagnosis of evolving acute myocardial infarction in the presence of left bundle-branch block. GUSTO-1 (Global Utilization of Streptokinase and Tissue Plasminogen Activator for Occluded Coronary Arteries) Investigators. *New England Journal of Medicine*, **334** (8), 481–487.

Sgarbossa, E.B., Pinski, S.L., Gates, K.B. & Wagner, G.S. (1996b) Early electrocardiographic diagnosis of acute myocardial infarction in the presence of ventricular paced rhythm. GUSTO-I investigators. *American Journal of Cardiology*, **77** (5), 423–424.

Shah, A., Wagner, G.S., Granger, C.B. *et al.* (2000) Prognostic implications of TIMI flow grade in the infarct-related artery compared with continuous 12-lead ST segment resolution analysis. Reexamining the 'gold standard' for myocardial reperfusion assessment. *Journal of the American College of Cardiology*, **35** (3), 666–672.

Shimonagata, T., Nishimura, T., Uehara, T., Hayashida, K., Saito, M. & Sumiyoshi, T. (1990) Exercise-induced ST segment elevation in leads over infarcted area and residual myocardial ischaemia in patients with previous myocardial infarction. *American Journal of Physiological Imaging*, **5** (3), 99–106.

Shlipak, M.G., Lyons, W.L., Go, A.S., Chou, T.M., Evans, G.T. & Browner, W.S. (1999) Should the electrocardiogram be used to guide therapy for patients with left bundle-branch block and suspected myocardial infarction? *JAMA (Journal of the American Medical Association)*, **281** (8), 714–719.

Tervahauta, M., Pekkanen, J., Punsar, S. & Nissinen, A. (1996) Resting electrocardiographic abnormalities as predictors of coronary events and total mortality among elderly men. *American Journal of Medicine*, **100** (6), 641–645.

Veldkamp, R.F., Green, C.L., Wilkins, M.L. *et al.* (1994) Comparison of continuous ST segment recovery analysis with methods using static electrocardiograms for noninvasive patency assessment during acute myocardial infarction. Thrombolysis and Angioplasty in Myocardial Infarction (TAMI) 7 Study Group. *American Journal of Cardiology*, **73** (15), 1069–1074.

Wackers, F.J. (1987) The diagnosis of myocardial infarction in the presence of left bundle branch block. *Cardiology Clinics*, **5** (3), 393–401.

Weiner, D.A., Ryan, T.J., McCabe, C.H. *et al.* (1984) Prognostic importance of a clinical profile and exercise test in medically treated patients with coronary artery disease. *Journal of the American College of Cardiology*, **3** (3), 772–779.

Wilde, A.A., Escande, D., Schumacher, C.A. *et al.* (1990) Potassium accumulation in the globally ischaemic mammalian heart. A role for the ATP-sensitive potassium channel. *Circulation Research*, **67** (4), 835–843.

Wolforth, C., Bellet, S., Livezey, M. & Murphy, F. (1945) Negative displacement of the RS-T segment in the electrocardigram and its relationship to positive displacement: an experimental study. *American Heart Journal*, **29**, 220–245.

Wong, P.S., el Gaylani, N., Griffith, K., Dixon, G., Robinson, D.R. & Norris, R.M. (1998) The clinical course of patients with acute myocardial infarction who are unsuitable for thrombolytic therapy because of the presenting electrocardiogram. UK Heart Attack Study Investigators. *Coronary Artery Disease*, **9** (11), 747–752.

Zeymer, U., Schroder, R., Tebbe, U., Molhoek, G.P., Wegscheider, K. & Neuhaus, K.L. (2001) Noninvasive detection of early infarct vessel patency by resolution of ST segment elevation in patients with thrombolysis for acute myocardial infarction; results of the angiographic substudy of the Hirudin for Improvement of Thrombolysis (HIT)-4 trial. *European Heart Journal*, **22** (9), 769–775.

CHAPTER 27

Spatial Patterns of ST Segment Shift During Myocardial Ischaemia

B. Milan Horáček and Galen S. Wagner

Introduction

Diagnostically important ST segment changes in the electrocardiograms (ECGs) of patients with acute myocardial ischaemia have been studied for over eight decades, since Pardee's seminal contribution (Pardee 1920). Among many reviews of the subject, those by Holland & Brooks (1977) and Mirvis (1988) provide description of the underlying biophysical concepts. In current clinical electrocardiography, ST segment measurements in the standard 12-lead ECG play a pivotal role in the stratification of patients with acute coronary syndromes (Ryan *et al.* 1996, 1999; Braunwald *et al.* 2000). Unfortunately, as pointed out by Braunwald & Cannon (1996), the currently used electrocardiographic criteria for such patients leave much to be desired. For instance, the recommended criterion for diagnostic ST segment changes (Ryan *et al.* 1996) – which is widely used as the indication for thrombolytic therapy – requires that two or more contiguous leads of the 12-lead ECG display an ST elevation greater than 0.1 mV. Thrombolysis is not recommended for patients with chest pain and ST depression on the 12-lead ECG, because many of these patients might have nonocclusive types of ischaemia that have not been shown to benefit from thrombolysis. In some patients, however, precordial ST depression might be the equivalent of ST elevation (Mirvis 1988) indicating an acute MI of the posterior wall, caused by the complete occlusion of the left circumflex (LCx) coronary artery, and this group of patients would be likely to benefit from thrombolysis (Braunwald & Cannon 1996).

To clarify the relationships among ST segment changes during ischaemia in various ECG leads, this chapter describes vessel-specific shifts in ST segment recorded over the entire thoracic surface during controlled regional ischaemia induced by percutaneous transluminal coronary angioplasty (PTCA). Balloon-inflation PTCA is a valuable model of supply ischaemia (Katz 1992) in humans, which occurs in response to a total interruption of blood flow through a coronary artery supplying a large region of the ventricular myocardium, e.g. due to thrombosis in patients with acute MI (Ryan *et al.* 1996) or due to coronary artery spasm in patients with 'Prinzmetal's angina' (Braunwald *et al.* 2000). Demand ischaemia (Katz 1992), occurring in a controlled fashion during exercise testing, affects the subendocardial regions of the left ventricle, and its distributions of ST segment shifts on the body surface (Kubota *et al.* 1985; Hänninen *et al.* 2001) differ from those observed during PTCA. The knowledge of ischaemia-induced spatial patterns of ST segment shifts can potentially improve and simplify the current clinical criteria for electrocardiographic recognition of acute MI and for prediction of the infarct-related artery.

Electrocardiographic mapping during myocardial ischaemia

Several studies have used body-surface potential mapping to obtain a comprehensive electrocardiographic picture of acute myocardial ischaemia; some studies dealt with the controlled

---

Supported by grants from the Canadian Institutes of Health Research and from the Heart & Stroke Foundation of Nova Scotia.

ischaemia associated with PTCA (Vondenbusch *et al.* 1985; MacLeod 1990; Spekhorst *et al.* 1990; Shenasa *et al.* 1993; Horáček *et al.* 2001), and others with the spontaneous clinical ischaemia associated with acute MI (Kornreich *et al.* 1985, 1993).

Spekhorst *et al.* (1990) recorded simultaneously 62 ECG leads during PTCA in 25 patients, for 15 dilations in the left anterior descending (LAD) artery, 7 in the right coronary artery (RCA), and 8 in the LCx artery; although these investigators were mainly interested in QRS changes induced by ischaemia, they also showed vessel-specific distributions of ST segment shifts for occlusions in each of the three main coronary arteries. MacLeod (1990) obtained simultaneously 120 ECGs during balloon-inflation PTCA, initially for 17 patients in the preliminary study and then for another group of 17 patients in the strictly controlled study that captured the evolution of ischaemia-induced ECG changes by continuous recording throughout the entire inflation–reperfusion cycle; the latter study investigated both QRS and ST changes for 18 dilations in the LAD artery, 10 dilations in the RCA, and 6 in the LCx artery. Shenasa *et al.* (1993) recorded simultaneously 63 ECG leads during PTCA in 20 patients, and investigated the thoracic patterns of ST segment changes for 10 dilations in the LAD artery, 7 dilations in the RCA, and 5 dilations in the LCx artery; they compared the ST segment maps with 12-lead ECGs and orthogonal leads, and found that their group-averaged ST distributions showed patterns specific to the occluded vessel. They also discussed the possibility of determining a set of optimal vessel-specific leads, but cautioned that one must consider both ST-amplitude shifts and optimal diagnostic discrimination when selecting such leads. To identify the optimal leads for diagnosing myocardial ischaemia associated with acute MI, Kornreich *et al.* (1993) compared body-surface potential maps of patients with an acute MI and those of normal subjects. In search of optimal leads, they used difference maps with respect to normal controls, normalized by the standard deviations, and they recommended optimal sites for the classification of patients with an acute MI. In all these studies, thoracic maps of ST segment shifts during acute ischaemia showed very similar spatial patterns that were specific to the occluded vessel: for the LAD-related ischaemia, the ST segment elevations were observed in a precordial area and posterior areas showed ST depression; for the RCA-related ischaemia, ST depression appeared on the left upper torso and the remainder of the torso showed ST elevation; and for the LCx-related ischaemia, ST depression occurred in a precordial area and ST segment elevation appeared over the back.

In a recently published study, which incorporated data previously obtained by MacLeod (1990), Horáček *et al.* (2001) recorded simultaneously 120 ECGs during balloon-inflation PTCA for 202 dilations in 91 patients with single-vessel disease. The ST amplitudes were measured during baseline and ischaemic states and the differences displayed as mean ΔST maps for three distinct groups, each including patients with regional ischaemia related to one of the three main coronary arteries (LAD = 32; RCA = 36; LCx = 23). The values of ΔST pertaining to a given lead in each patient group were expressed as mean ± standard deviation (SD), and for each mean ΔST map a corresponding discriminant (t) map was calculated by dividing the mean ΔST by the SD. In agreement with the previous findings, this study showed that there are distinct common features in the maps of body-surface potentials during the ST segment that can be identified when each of the three main coronary arteries is occluded. These features are reproducible, and they reveal the origins of the ischaemic region. The resultant changes observed during regional ischaemia caused by single-vessel occlusion are discussed below in detail for each supply vessel separately.

Acute ischaemia caused by occlusion of the LAD coronary artery

Figure 27.1(a) shows a mean spatial pattern of ST segment shifts (ΔST map) for the group of patients whose proximal LAD coronary artery was occluded by inflation of the PTCA balloon; the maximal ST elevation appears just above lead V3, and the inferior part of the map shows ST depression, which is largest in the mid-dorsal area. Figure 27.1(b) shows the corresponding discriminant map of t values associated with the mean ΔST map; this distribution indicates where

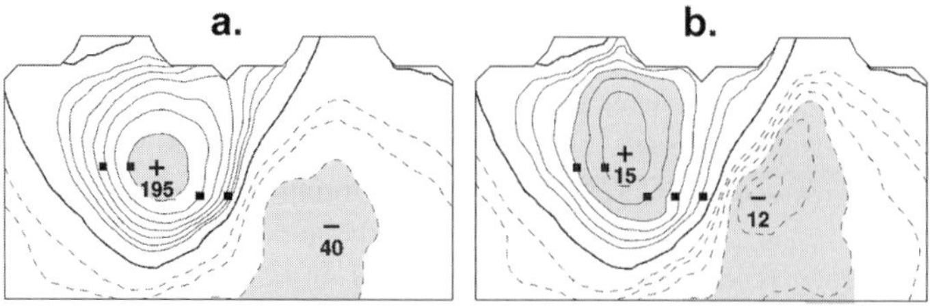

Fig. 27.1 Mean spatial patterns of ischaemia-induced ST shifts from baseline values (a) and corresponding discriminant maps of *t* values (b) for the controlled ischaemia induced by the occlusion of the LAD coronary artery in 15 patients who underwent PTCA. Maps correspond to the anterior (left half of each map) and posterior (right half) chest; sites of precordial leads V1 to V6 are marked by black squares; potential values are in microvolts (μV); contour lines progress in logarithmic steps (e.g. for the extrema at +195 and −40 μV, the contours are at +150, +100, +68, +47, ± 33, ± 22, ±15, and 0 μV); in the difference map, areas nearest to the extrema are shaded; in the discriminant map, shaded areas correspond to $|t| \geq 4.7$.

the discriminating power for distinguishing an ischaemic from a nonischaemic state lies; an oval region with high *t* values peaks more superiorly than does the ΔST map, but high *t* values extend far enough inferiorly to encompass the area of highest ΔSTs. Based on both the ΔST map and the discriminant map in Fig. 27.1, an optimal lead for detecting ischaemia related to LAD-artery occlusion would be a bipolar lead with a positive terminal connected to an electrode near precordial lead V3 and a negative terminal connected to an electrode below posterior chest lead V8. Bipolar leads are used in ambulatory monitoring (Crawford *et al.* 1999) and in exercise electrocardiography (Chaitman 2001); e.g. Krucoff *et al.* (1988) used a lead with electrodes at the V2 position and at the spinous process, and found that it sensitively detects LAD-artery-related spatial pattern of ST segment changes, for which they coined the term 'ischaemic fingerprint.'

In patients with an acute anterior MI resulting from occlusion of the LAD coronary artery, elevation of the ST segment is usually seen in the precordial leads V1–V6, and ST segment depression is sometimes observed simultaneously in the limb leads II, III, and aVF (Ferguson *et al.* 1984; Birnbaum *et al.* 1994) of the 12-lead ECG. (It should be noted that leads V1–V6 have been designated as 'precordial' because their positive terminals are connected to the positions of the 'exploring electrode' on the anterior and left lateral thorax.) This ST depression in leads II, III, and aVF has been previously considered to be a 'reciprocal change' of ST segment elevation in the precordial leads (Ferguson *et al.* 1984; Fletcher *et al.* 1993).

However, several studies have shown that the ST segment changes in body-surface ECGs seen during an acute anterior MI can be linked to the site of the occlusion of the LAD (Sapin *et al.* 1992; Birnbaum *et al.* 1993b; Tamura *et al.* 1995). Sasaki *et al.* (2001), in a study investigating the relation between LAD pathology and ST segment changes in the ECG, found that ST segment changes in limb leads II, III, and aVF during an acute anterior MI are determined by competition between changes caused by involvement of the 'high lateral wall' due to occlusion of the proximal LAD, which depress the ST segments; and involvement of the inferoapical wall due to a wrapped around LAD, which elevate the ST segments. Therefore, the minimal reduction of LV ejection fraction in the patients with inferiorly directed ST segments might simply indicate that the apical involvement due to the typical amount of 'LAD wrap around' is unopposed due to the mid to distal site of their LAD occlusion (Sadanandan *et al.* 2003). Arbane & Goy (2000) state that, in acute anterior MIs, the most important coronary anatomical determinant of the direction of ST deviation in leads II, III, and aVF seems to be the site of the LAD occlusion. For example, ST depression is not related to 'remote ischaemia', but represents the reciprocal of ST elevation in –II, –III, and –aVF in addition to the ST elevation in aVL and I (due to anterolateral extension of the infarct secondary to first-diagonal-branch ischaemia). Inferior ST depression therefore predicts a proximal LAD artery occlusion (Sapin *et al.* 1992; Birnbaum *et al.* 1993b; Tamura *et al.* 1995; Arbane & Goy 2000; Sasaki *et al.* 2001), which, in turn, is known to be associated with greater infarct size, left ventricular dysfunction, and poorer prognosis in acute MIs (Haraphongse *et al.* 1984; Willems *et al.* 1990).

Reports that correlated the admission 12-lead ECG with the angiographically determined site of LAD occlusion (Haraphongse *et al.* 1984; Sapin *et al.* 1992; Birnbaum *et al.* 1993b; Tamura *et al.* 1995; Arbane & Goy 2000; Sasaki *et al.* 2001) found that ST elevation in lead aVL and ST depression in leads II, III, and aVF were largest when the occlusion was in the proximal rather than the mid- or distal LAD artery. Birnbaum *et al.* (1993b) assessed the value of ST changes in various leads during evolving acute anterior MIs for predicting the location of the LAD coronary artery obstruction (in relation to the origin of the first diagonal branch). They showed that ST elevation in leads I and aVL and ST depression in leads II, III, and aVF indicate a culprit lesion proximal to the origin of the first diagonal branch, whereas isoelectric ST or ST elevation in the inferior leads suggests distal LAD artery occlusion. Tamura *et al.* (1995) compared ST segment measurements on admission 12-lead ECG of patients with an acute anterior MI caused by proximal or distal LAD-artery occlusion and found that ST depression in all of leads II, III, and aVF identified patients with a proximal lesion.

Willems *et al.* (1990) showed that the magnitude of the initial ST elevation as well as that of the ST depression in the admission 12-lead ECG – both summated over several leads (Bär *et al.* 1987) – are valuable for the management and assessment of thrombolytic therapy in patients with an acute MI. For LAD-artery-related acute anterior MIs, the sum of ST elevations was calculated from leads I, aVL, and V1 to V6; the absolute values of ST depressions in leads II, III, and aVF was also added. Inspection of Fig. 27.1 (also Horáček *et al.* 2001: table 3) clarifies why the summation of selected leads might be beneficial for the recognition of the LAD-artery-related ischaemia.

Clinical findings discussed in this section are all compatible with Fig. 27.1, which illustrates that in response to proximal LAD-artery occlusion, the ST segment distribution features precordial ST segment elevation, which peaks near lead V3, complemented by reciprocal changes on the inferior torso that produce ST depression in leads with their positive poles oriented inferiorly. The presence of either an isoelectric ST segment or ST segment elevation in the inferior leads suggests that an additional (inferior) ischaemic region contributes to the ST distribution; the pattern of this additional contribution resembles that caused by occlusion of the right coronary artery (Fig. 27.2, discussed later).

Acute ischaemia caused by occlusion of the RCA

Figure 27.2(a) shows that in the mean ΔST map for the group of patients whose proximal RCA was occluded by inflation of the PTCA balloon, ST elevations are on the inferior chest and ST depressions on the superior chest, including the precordial area from V1 to V6 (just as in Mirvis 1988: fig. 5B). The spatial pattern of the ST segment shifts has a vertical axis, with the maximal ST elevation occurring on the lower anterior chest. The discriminant map of *t* values associated with mean ΔSTs for RCA occlusion (Fig. 27.2b), differs notably from the ΔST map with respect to the location of the extrema; the maximal *t* value appears in the mid-dorsal region, but the more accessible umbilical and iliac crest regions feature *t* values that are almost

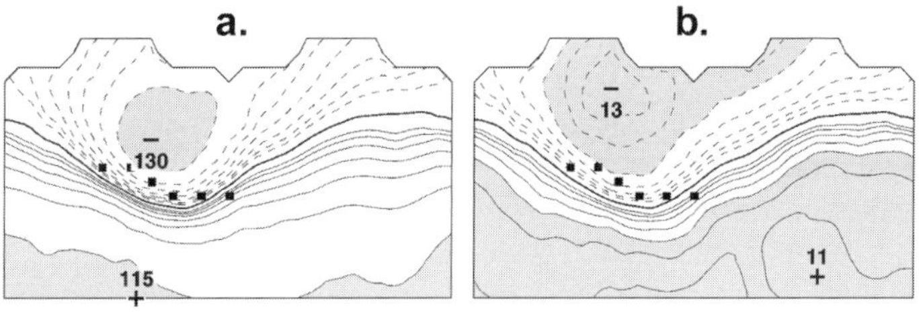

Fig. 27.2 Mean spatial patterns of ST shifts (a) and corresponding discriminant maps of *t* values (b) during controlled ischaemia induced by the occlusion of the RCA in 15 patients who underwent PTCA. For description of map display see Fig. 27.1.

as high. Based on the ΔST map and discriminant (*t*) map in Fig. 27.2, an optimal lead for detecting ischaemia related to the RCA occlusion would be a bipolar lead with a positive terminal connected to an electrode near the left iliac crest and a negative terminal connected to an electrode above precordial lead V3.

In patients with an acute inferior MI – due to occlusion of the RCA – elevation of the ST segment is typically seen in leads II, III, and aVF, and ST segment depression is often observed simultaneously in precordial leads V1–V4. Mirvis (1988) reviewed the physiological and clinical meaning of ST segment depression in the precordial leads of these patients. Such a depression may either be the result of *reciprocal* changes associated with the ST segment elevation in the inferior leads due to ischaemia of the inferior wall, or, alternatively, the primary ST segment depression reflecting ischaemia of the more laterally positioned posterior ventricular wall. Mirvis (1998) concluded that reciprocal ST segment changes *always* occur, whereas primary ST segment depression also occurs in some patients with an acute inferior MI. Numerous clinical studies dealing with patients who suffered acute inferior MI show that many patients who have ST segment depression in leads V1–V3 have multivessel coronary artery disease, and they are usually described as having a larger infarct and worse prognosis than patients without such an abnormality. Little *et al.* (1984) found that ST segment depression in V1–V3, observed in most of their patients with an acute inferior MI, resolved promptly when the occluded RCA was opened with an infusion of streptokinase; this finding supports the view that this ST segment depression is a manifestation of either the inferior infarction alone or its extension posterolaterally, and is not owing to 'anterior ischaemia at the distance', resulting from LAD-artery stenosis as has been previously suggested.

Willems *et al.* (1990) showed that, in patients with acute inferior and posterior MIs, the magnitude of the initial ST segment elevation in the admission 12-lead ECG (summed over leads II, III, aVF, I, aVL, V5, and V6) and of the ST segment depression (summed over leads V1 to V4) provide useful clinical measures. Inspection of Fig. 27.2 (and Horáček *et al.* 2001: tables 4 & 5) makes it clear why summations of ST segment elevation over leads II, III, and aVF, and of ST segment depression over V1 to V4 would be beneficial for the recognition of RCA-related ischaemia. On the other hand, the inclusion of leads I, aVL, V5, and V6 in the sum of ST segment elevations cannot be recommended on the basis of Fig. 27.2; these leads, however, can help in differentiating between acute inferior (RCA-related) and posterior (LCx-artery-related) MIs, as discussed below. With regard to lead aVL, Birnbaum *et al.* (1993a) studied a group of over one hundred patients with an acute inferior MI, some of whom had no ST segment elevation on the 12-lead ECG, and found reciprocal ST segment depression in lead aVL in all but three patients. Certainly, truly reciprocal ST depression in the more superiorly located –II, –III, and –aVF must be present.

Acute ischaemia caused by occlusion of the LCx coronary artery

Figure 27.3(a) shows the spatial pattern of mean ST segment shifts (ΔST map) for the group of patients whose LCx coronary artery was occluded by inflation of the PTCA balloon. It is evident that the ST elevations appear on the inferior chest, with the maximal elevation near posterior lead V8, and the ST depressions appear on the superior chest, including the precordial area

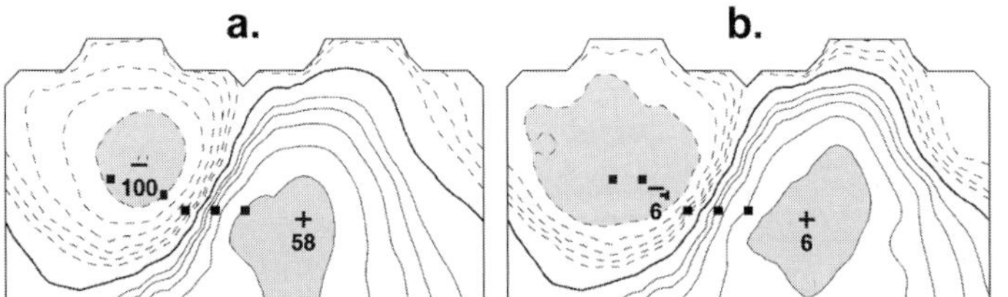

Fig. 27.3 Mean spatial patterns of ST shifts (a) and corresponding discriminant maps of *t* values (b) during controlled ischaemia induced by the occlusion of the LCx coronary artery in 15 patients who underwent PTCA. For description of map display see Fig. 27.1.

from V1 to V4. (Note that the distribution resembles that for LAD-artery occlusion, with the opposite polarity.) The discriminant map of *t* values associated with mean ΔSTs for LCx-artery occlusion is shown in Fig. 27.3b; it resembles its corresponding ΔST map with respect to the location of the extrema. Based on the ΔST map and the discriminant (*t*) map in the Fig. 27.3, an optimal lead for detecting ischaemia related to LCx-artery occlusion would be a bipolar lead with a positive terminal connected to an electrode placed below posterior lead V8, and a negative terminal connected to an electrode near precordial lead V2. This bipolar lead for detecting LCx-artery-related ischaemia is similar to that suggested for detecting LAD-artery-related ischaemia, but it has a reversed polarity. (Therefore, the same lead can be used for optimal detection of both LAD- and LCx-artery-related ischaemia; in the former case, it will record ST segment elevation and in the latter ST segment depression.) Observations based on Fig. 27.3 regarding the optimal site for detecting LCx-artery-related ischaemia agree with those of Casas *et al.* (1997), Agarwal *et al.* (1999), and Wung & Drew (2001), who noted that ST segment elevation in posterior leads V7 to V9 helps to identify LCx-artery-related ischaemia of the posterior wall.

The standard 12-lead ECG is less sensitive in detecting occlusion of the LCx coronary artery than it is in detecting one in the other arteries (Perloff 1964; Eisenstein *et al.* 1985). Huey *et al.* (1988) found that 52% of patients with an acute MI resulting from the occluded LCx artery did not have ST segment elevation in the 12-lead ECG, and Berry *et al.* (1989) reported that, despite the comparable magnitude of intracoronary ST segment elevation, LCx-artery occlusion often produces no change or only precordial ST segment depression in the 12-lead ECG. This limitation of the 12-lead system – caused by the absence of leads with their positive poles facing the posterior left-ventricular wall – hampers the diagnosis of a significant subgroup of patients with an acute MI who would benefit from the prompt initiation of reperfusion therapy (Huey *et al.* 1988; Berry *et al.* 1989). To alleviate this problem, lead systems that include the posterior chest leads have been proposed (Melendez *et al.* 1978; Agarwal 1998), and it is now becoming increasingly popular to consider that the posterior chest leads V7 through V9 can be useful in diagnosing acute posterior myocardial ischaemia and infarctions (Matetzky *et al.* 1998, 1999; Agarwal *et al.* 1999). For instance, Matetzky *et al.* (1999) studied patients who had ischaemic chest pain suggestive of an acute MI, no ST segment elevation on the standard 12-lead ECG, but isolated ST segment elevation in the posterior chest leads, and they concluded that ST segment elevation in these leads reliably identifies patients with an acute posterior MI (which in their study was confirmed by coronary angiography to be caused by LCx-artery occlusion). On the other hand, Zalenski *et al.* (1997) found in their multicentre prospective trial that the addition of posterior and right ventricular leads only modestly improved the diagnostic accuracy of the 12-lead ECG in detecting acute MIs.

Bairey *et al.* (1987) investigated whether the admission 12-lead ECG can assist in differentiating LCx-artery and RCA occlusion in patients with an acute inferior MI, and found that the presence of both ST segment elevation in two or more of leads II, III, and aVF as well as in one or more of leads aVL, V5, and V6 with an isoelectric or elevated ST segment in lead I identified LCx-artery occlusion with high diagnostic accuracy; these findings are compatible with Horáček *et al.* (2001: table 5). Shah *et al.* (1997) hypothesized that during LCx-artery occlusion, the localized precordial ST segment depression, representing the reciprocal change associated with ST segment elevation in the posterior leads V7 to V9, can be used to recognize ischaemia. However, Wung & Drew (2001) argue that, to detect ischaemia due to LCx-artery occlusion, the anterior ST segment-depression criteria are less efficacious than those using ST segment elevation in posterior leads. Inspection of Fig. 27.3 reveals that a potential difference between V8 and V2 provides the most sensitive measure of the LCx-artery-related ischaemia, by combining ST segment elevation in the posterior chest area with ST segment depression in the anterior chest area.

Langer *et al.* (1996) examined the impact of thrombolytic therapy on a subset of patients with an acute MI who took part in a trial known as the Late Assessment of Thrombolytic Efficacy (LATE) study. One of their three principal findings was that thrombolytic therapy provided a substantial benefit in the subgroup of patients presenting initially with ST segment depression in the standard 12-lead ECG. Braunwald & Cannon (1996), in their editorial comment, termed this finding 'provocative,' because 'it is surely not in concert with current practice in which thrombolytic therapy is administered to patients with a myocardial infarction with ST elevation up to 12 h after the onset of pain but not to patients with ST segment depression, irrespective of the time after the onset of chest pain.' Braunwald & Cannon pointed out that there is the possibility that, at least in some patients in the study of Langer *et al.* (1996), the ST segment depression might have represented posterior ST segment elevation caused by an occluded LCx coronary artery; thus the current concept that thrombolysis benefits only patients with ST segment elevation would be applicable even in patients with a posterior infarction, provided that the posterior leads would be considered in addition to the standard 12-lead ECG set. However, as noted by Wung & Drew (2001), it also may be necessary to readjust the threshold for a 'diagnostic' ST segment elevation.

Alternative displays of the standard 12-lead electrocardiogram

The classic display of the standard 12-lead ECG includes two segregated groups of the six limb leads (I, II, and III; and aVR, aVL, and aVF) and two integrated groups of the six precordial leads. Other methods of displaying 12-lead ECG, discussed by Pahlm-Webb *et al.* (2002), can enhance the diagnostic information that is required for making the therapeutic decisions for patients with acute coronary syndromes. Figure 27.4 presents a suggested format for the display of a '24-view ECG,' with the groups of the 12 frontal and 12 transverse leads arranged like the numbers on a clock face. The ECG tracings shown in Fig. 27.4 were recorded from a patient who had a transient occlusion of an LCx coronary artery during PTCA. Although there is no ST elevation in any of the standard 12 leads, there is ST depression in V1–V4. The appearance of ST elevation in leads –V1 to –V4 visualizes the posterior epicardial ischaemia induced by the balloon inflation; if this patient had presented with acute chest pain, use of the 24-view ECG might have facilitated true allocation to the ST-

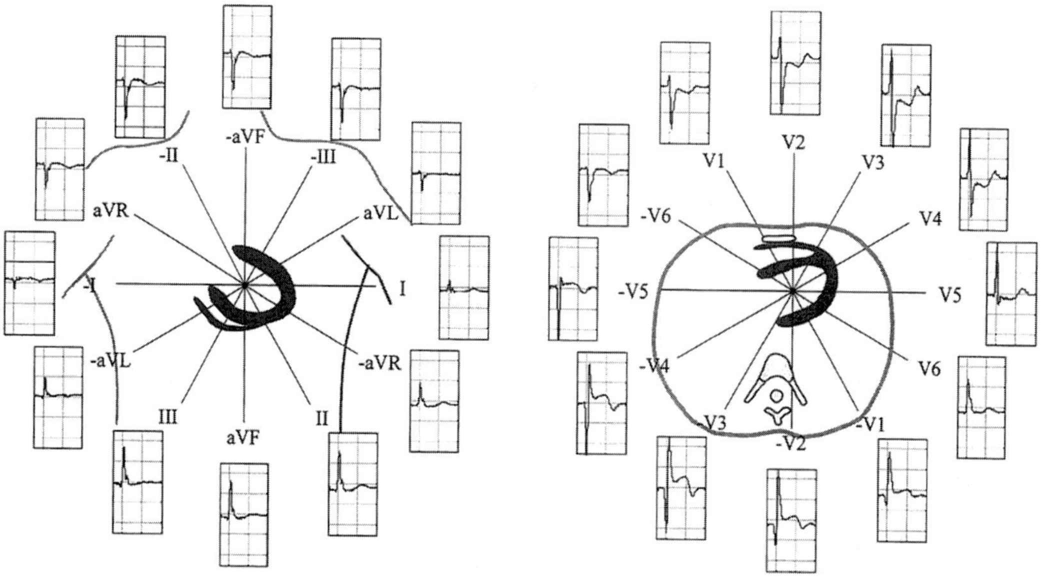

Fig. 27.4 The 24 views of the standard 12-lead electrocardiogram. The ECGs shown on this display were recorded from a patient during balloon-inflation PTCA of the LCx coronary artery; QRST complexes of simultaneously-recorded leads are arranged as numbers around a clock face for the six frontal-plane leads viewed from the front (left), and the six transverse-plane leads viewed from below (right). (Reproduced from Pahlm-Webb, 2002, with permission.)

elevation category of acute coronary syndromes, rather than false one to the non-ST-elevation category. As discussed in the previous section, some investigators have applied posterior thoracic electrodes in order to record ST elevation associated with posterior epicardial ischaemia associated with the occlusion of the LCx coronary artery. The point of this section is to demonstrate that 24-view ECG can provide waveforms that correlate with posterior leads V8 and V9 by simply inverting precordial leads V1 and V2. In acute anterior MIs, a proximal LAD artery occlusion produces inferior ST depression (Sasaki *et al.* 2001), which is accompanied by ST elevation in leads aVL (Arbane & Goy 2000), and in addition in leads –II, –III, and –aVF (Pahlm-Webb *et al.* 2002). In patients with an acute inferior MI, Birnbaum *et al.* (1993a) found in almost all patients ST segment depression in lead aVL; certainly, truly reciprocal ST depression in the more superiorly oriented leads –II, –III, and –aVF must be present.

Conclusion

The purpose of this chapter was to show both the capabilities and the limitations of the 12-lead ECG in recognizing ischaemia, and to seek alternative electrocardiographic leads, optimized for detection of ischaemia originating in different regions of the ventricular myocardium. A survey of recent clinical studies showed that the electrocardiographic manifestations of acute myocardial ischaemia observed on body-surface potential maps of ST segment shifts recorded during controlled ischaemia induced by balloon-inflation PTCA are in agreement with the ST segment measurements in admission ECGs of patients with acute myocardial infarction. Thus, based on the electrocardiographic data recorded during PTCA, leads can be judiciously chosen, which can potentially improve the clinical electrocardiographic criteria for recognizing acute myocardial infarction and for identifying the infarct-related artery. Alternatively, new ways of displaying the standard 12-lead ECG – such as the 24-view method – can be sought to enhance the diagnostic information required for making the therapeutic decisions for patients with acute coronary syndromes.

References

Agarwal, J. B. (1998) Routine use of a 15-lead electrocardiogram for patients presenting to the emergency department with chest pain. *Journal of Electrocardiology*, **31** (Suppl.), 172–177.

Agarwal, J. B., Khaw, K., Aurignac, F. & LoCurto, A. (1999) Importance of posterior chest leads in patients with suspected myocardial infarction, but nondiagnostic, routine 12-lead electrocardiogram. *American Journal of Cardiology*, **83**, 323–326.

Arbane, M. & Goy, J.-J. (2000) Prediction of the site of total occlusion of the left anterior descending coronary artery using admission electrocardiogram in anterior wall acute myocardial infarction. *American Journal of Cardiology*, **85**, 487–491.

Bairey, C. N., Shah, P. K., Lew, A. S. & Hulse, S. (1987) Electrocardiographic differentiation of occlusion of the left circumflex vs. the right coronary artery as a cause of inferior acute myocardial infarction. *American Journal of Cardiology*, **60**, 456–459.

Bär, F. W., Vermeer, F., de Zwaan, C. *et al.* (1987) Value of admission electrocardiogram in predicting outcome of thrombolytic therapy in acute myocardial infarction: a randomized trial conducted by The Netherlands Interuniversity Cardiology Institute. *American Journal of Cardiology*, **59**, 6–13.

Berry, C., Zalewski, A., Kovach, R. *et al.* (1989) Surface electrocardiogram ischaemia during coronary artery occlusion. *American Journal of Cardiology*, **63**, 21–26.

Birnbaum, Y., Sclarovsky, S., Mager, A. *et al.* (1993a) ST segment depression in aVL: a sensitive marker for acute inferior myocardial infarction. *European Heart Journal*, **14**, 4–7.

Birnbaum, Y., Sclarovsky, S., Solodky, A. *et al.* (1993b) Prediction of the level of the left anterior descending coronary artery obstruction during anterior wall acute myocardial infarction by the admission electrocardiogram. *American Journal of Cardiology*, **72**, 823–826.

Birnbaum, Y., Solodky, A., Herz, I. *et al.* (1994) Implications of inferior ST segment depression in anterior acute myocardial infarction: electrocardiographic and angiographic correlations. *American Heart Journal*, **127**, 1467–1473.

Braunwald, E. & Cannon, C. P. (1996). Non-Q wave and ST segment depression myocardial infarction: is there a role for thrombolytic therapy? *Journal of the American College of Cardiology*, **27**, 1333–1334.

Braunwald, E., Antman, E. M., Beasley, J. W. *et al.* (2000) ACC/AHA guidelines for the management of patients with unstable angina and non-ST segment elevation myocardial infarction: a report of the American College of Cardiology/American Heart Association Task Force on Practice Guidelines (Committee on Management of

Patients With Unstable Angina). *Journal of the American College of Cardiology*, **36**, 970–1062. Available at http://www.acc.org/clinical/guidelines

Casas, R. E., Marriott, H. J. L. & Glancy, D. L. (1997) Value of leads V7–V9 in diagnosing posterior wall acute myocardial infarction and other causes of tall R waves in V1–V2. *American Journal of Cardiology*, **80**, 508–509.

Chaitman, B. (2001) Exercise testing. In: *Heart Disease: A Textbook of Cardiovascular Medicine*, (eds E. Braunwald, D. P. Zipes, & P. Libby), 6th edn, pp. 129–155. W. B. Saunders, Philadelphia, PA.

Crawford, M. H., Bernstein, S. J., Deedwania, P. C. *et al.* (1999) ACC/AHA guidelines for ambulatory electrocardiography: a report of the American College of Cardiology/American Heart Association Task Force on Practice Guidelines (Committee to Revise the Guidelines for Ambulatory Electrocardiography). *Journal of the American College of Cardiology*, **34**, 912–948. Available at http://www.acc.org/clinical/guidelines

Eisenstein, I., Sanmarco, M. E., Madrid, W. L. & Selvester, R. H. (1985) Electrocardiographic and vectorcardiographic diagnosis of posterior wall myocardial infarction. *Chest* **88**, 409–416.

Ferguson, D. W., Pandian, N., Kioschos, J. M. *et al.* (1984) Angiographic evidence that reciprocal ST segment depression during acute myocardial infarction does not indicate remote ischaemia: analysis of 23 patients. *American Journal of Cardiology*, **53**, 55–62.

Fletcher, W. O., Gibbons, R. J. & Clements, I. P. (1993) The relationship of inferior ST segment depression, lateral ST elevation, and left precordial ST elevation to myocardium at risk in acute anterior myocardial infarction. *American Heart Journal*, **126**, 526–535.

Hänninen, H., Takala, P., Mäkijärvi, M. *et al.* (2001) ST segment level and slope in exercise-induced myocardial ischaemia evaluated with body surface potential mapping. *American Journal of Cardiology*, **88**, 1152–1156.

Haraphongse, M., Tanomsup, S. & Jugdutt, B. I. (1984) Inferior ST segment depression during acute anterior myocardial infarction: clinical and angiographic correlations. *Journal of the American College of Cardiology*, **4**, 467–476.

Holland, R. P. & Brooks, H. (1977) TQ–ST segment mapping: critical review and analysis of current concepts. *American Journal of Cardiology*, **4**, 110–129.

Horáček, B. M., Warren, J. W., Penney, C. J. *et al.* (2001) Optimal electrocardiographic leads for detecting acute myocardial ischaemia. *Journal of Electrocardiology*, **34** (Suppl.), 97–111.

Huey, B. L., Beller, G. A., Kaiser, D. L. & Gibson, R. S. (1988) A comprehensive analysis of myocardial infarction due to left circumflex artery occlusion: comparison with infarction due to right coronary artery and left anterior descending artery occlusion. *Circulation*, **12**, 1156–1166.

Katz, A. M. (1992) The ischaemic heart. In: *Physiology of the Heart*, 2nd edn, pp. 623–626. Raven Press, New York.

Kornreich, F., Rautaharju, P. M., Warren, J. W. *et al.* (1985) Identification of best electrocardiographic leads for diagnosing myocardial infarction by statistical analysis of body surface potential maps. *American Journal of Cardiology*, **56**, 852–856.

Kornreich, F., Montague, T. J. & Rautaharju, P. M. (1993). Body surface potential mapping of ST segment changes in acute myocardial infarction. *Circulation*, **87**, 773–782.

Krucoff, M. W., Parente, A. R., Bottner, R. K. *et al.* (1988) Stability of multilead ST segment 'fingerprints' over time after percutaneous transluminal coronary angioplasty and its usefulness in detecting reocclusion. *American Journal of Cardiology*, **61**, 1232–1237.

Kubota, I., Ikeda, K., Ohyama, T. *et al.* (1985) Body surface distributions of ST segment changes after exercise in effort angina pectoris without myocardial infarction. *American Heart Journal*, **110**, 949–955.

Langer, A., Goodman, S. G., Topol, E. J. *et al.* for the LATE study investigators (1996). Late assessment of thrombolytic efficacy (LATE) study: prognosis in patients with non-Q wave myocardial infarction. *Journal of the American College of Cardiology*, **27**, 1327–1332.

Little, W. C., Rogers, E. W. & Sodums, M. T. (1984) Mechanism of anterior ST segment depression during acute inferior myocardial infarction. *Annals of Internal Medicine* **100**, 226–229.

MacLeod, R. S. (1990) *Percutaneous transluminal coronary angioplasty as a model of cardiac ischaemia: clinical and modelling studies*. PhD thesis, Dalhousie University, Canada.

Matetzky, S., Freimark, D., Feinberg, M. S. *et al.* (1998) Significance of ST segment elevations in posterior chest leads (V7 to V9) in patients with acute inferior myocardial infarction: application to thrombolytic therapy. *Journal of the American College of Cardiology*, **31**, 506–511.

Matetzky, S., Freimark, D., Feinberg, M. S. *et al.* (1999) Acute myocardial infarction with isolated ST segment elevation in posterior chest leads $V7_{-9}$: 'hidden' ST segment elevation revealing acute posterior infarction. *Journal of the American College of Cardiology*, **34**, 748–753.

Melendez, L. J., Jones, D. T. & Salcedo, J. R. (1978) Usefulness of three additional electrocardiographic chest leads (V7, V8 and V9) in the diagnosis of acute myocardial infarction. *Canadian Medical Association Journal*, **119**, 745–748.

Mirvis, D. M. (1988) Physiological bases for anterior ST segment depression in patients with acute inferior wall myocardial infarction. *American Heart Journal*, **116**,1308–1322.

Pahlm-Webb, U., Pahlm, O., Sadanandan, S. *et al.* (2002) A new method for using the direction of ST segment deviation to localize the site of acute coronary occlusion: The 24-view standard electrocardiogram. *American Journal of Medicne*, **113**, 75–78.

Pardee, H. E. B. (1920) An electrocardiographic sign of coronary artery obstruction. *Archives of Internal Medicine*, **26**, 244–257.

Perloff, J. K. (1964) The recognition of strictly posterior myocardial infarction by conventional scalar electrocardiography. *Circulation*, **30**, 706–718.

Ryan, T. J., Anderson, J. L., Antman, E. M. *et al.* (1996) ACC/AHA guidelines for the management of patients with acute myocardial infarction: a report of the American College of Cardiology/American Heart Association Task Force on Practice Guidelines (Committee on Management of Acute Myocardial Infarction). *Journal of the American College of Cardiology*, **28**, 1328–1428. Available at http://www.acc.org/clinical/guidelines

Ryan, T. J., Antman, E. M., Brooks, N. H. *et al.* (1999) Update of ACC/AHA guidelines for the management of patients with acute myocardial infarction: a report of the American College of Cardiology/American Heart Association Task Force on Practice Guidelines (Committee on Management of Acute Myocardial Infarction). *Journal of the American College of Cardiology*, **34**, 890–911. Available at http://www.acc.org/clinical/guidelines

Sadanandan, S., Hochman, J. S., Kolodziej, A. *et al.* (2003) Clinical and angiographic characteristics of patients with combined anterior and inferior ST segment deviation on the initial electrocardiogram during acute myocardial infarction. *American Heart Journal*, (in press)

Sapin, P. M., Musselman, D. R., Dehmer, G. J. & Cascio, W. E. (1992) Implications of inferior ST segment elevation accompanying anterior wall acute myocardial infarction for the angiographic morphology of the left anterior descending coronary artery morphology and site of occlusion. *American Journal of Cardiology*, **69**, 860–865.

Sasaki, K., Yotsukura, M., Sakata, K. *et al.* (2001) Relationship of ST segment changes in inferior leads during anterior wall acute myocardial infarction to length and occlusion site of the left anterior descending coronary artery. *American Journal of Cardiology*, **87**, 1340–1345.

Shah, A., Wagner, G. S., Califf, R. M. *et al.* (1997) Comparative prognostic significance of simultaneous vs. independent resolution of ST segment depression relative to ST segment elevation during acute myocardial infarction. *Journal of the American College of Cardiology*, **30**, 1478–1483.

Shenasa, M., Hamel, D., Nasmith, J. *et al.* (1993) Body surface potential mapping of ST segment shift in patients undergoing percutaneous transluminal coronary angioplasty: correlations with the ECG and vectorcardiogram. *Journal of Electrocardiology*, **26**, 43–51.

Spekhorst, H., SippensGroenewegen, A., David, G. K. *et al.* (1990) Body surface mapping during percutaneous transluminal coronary angioplasty: QRS changes indicating regional myocardial conduction delay. *Circulation*, **81**, 840–849.

Tamura, A., Kataoka, H., Mikuriya, Y. & Nasu, M. (1995) Inferior ST segment depression as a useful marker for identifying proximal left anterior descending artery occlusion during acute anterior myocardial infarction. *European Heart Journal*, **16**, 1795–1799.

Vondenbusch, B., Silny, J., von Essen, R. *et al.* (1985) ECG-mapping during coronary dilatation: Improvement of diagnosis and therapy control. In: *Computers in Cardiology* (ed. K. L. Ripley), pp. 43–46. IEEE Computer Society Press, Washington, DC.

Willems, J. L., Willems, R. J., Willems, G. M. *et al.* for the European Cooperative Study Group for Recombinant Tissue-Type Plasminogen Activator (1990). Significance of initial ST segment elevation and depression for the management of thrombolytic therapy in acute myocardial infarction. *Circulation*, **82**, 1147–1158.

Wung, S.-F. & Drew, B. J. (2001) New electrocardiographic criteria for posterior wall acute myocardial ischaemia validated by percutaneous transluminal coronary angioplasty model of acute myocardial ischaemia. *American Journal of Cardiology*, **87**, 970–974.

Zalenski, R. J., Rydman, R. J., Sloan, E. P. *et al.* (1997) Value of posterior and right ventricular leads in comparison to the standard 12-lead electrocardiogram in evaluation of ST segment elevation in suspected acute myocardial infarction. *American Journal of Cardiology*, **79**, 1579–1585.

CHAPTER 28

ST Segment Trend Monitoring of Acute Chest Pain Patients

J. Lee Garvey

Introduction

The nature of coronary artery disease (CAD) is dynamic. While usually progressing over decades, it is manifest acutely by symptoms that evolve over minutes to hours. Our clinical tools can assist with the evaluation on this acute time frame, as well. The electrocardiogram is the instrument by which we examine the electrical function of the myocardium. We have used this tool for nearly 100 years to assist in the diagnosis of acute ischaemia. The typical 12-lead ECG collects and presents data representing about 10 s of cardiac function – a brief snap-shot of the myocardial activity. Current technology now makes possible the dynamic monitoring of such information within a time frame that is consistent with the underlying pathophysiology.

Coronary care units evolved in the 1960s as it was recognized that immediate identification of potentially lethal arrhythmias could lead to life-saving interventions. The monitors at that time could display real-time representations of a lead or two of the electrocardiogram. Technicians, and later software-based algorithms, monitored these displays in order that immediate defibrillation could be provided as rescue. With today's physiological monitors' processing speed and algorithm maturation, we can now provide surveillance for acute ischaemia on a real-time basis. Intuitively, it is preferable to intervene at an early time when ischaemia is first detected, rather than react after the development of a potentially lethal arrhythmia. The corollaries of the 'open artery hypothesis' support such a concept (French *et al.* 2002).

Chest pain evaluation is a leading reason for patient presentation to the emergency department (ED). While most of these patients will ultimately be found to have a 'non-cardiac' aetiology of their chest pain, the need for urgent interventions in acute coronary syndromes (ACS) drives the evaluation protocols for these patients (Sarko and Pollack, Jr., 1997; Graff *et al.* 1995; Gomez *et al.* 1996). According to most large studies, patients presenting to emergency departments with acute myocardial infarction have diagnostic electrocardiograms only roughly 50% of the time (Aufderheide and Brady, 1994). This unfortunately means that roughly half of the patients in the midst of an evolving infarction will have initial electrocardiograms that are not diagnostic for the condition. However, many additional patients ultimately will be found to have abnormal ECGs during their hospitalization. At some point an initially nondiagnostic ECG becomes diagnostic for ischaemia, injury, or arrhythmia. A principal goal of ST segment trend monitoring in the acute chest pain patient is to provide surveillance for these changes in the ECG reflecting ischaemia and infarction. Additionally, ST segment trend monitoring can be useful as an aid in managing patients with acute ischaemia or infarction on the ECG available at presentation.

Technical considerations

ST segment trend monitoring is the process of dynamic surveillance for cardiac ischaemia. ECGs are automatically and repetitively collected by the hardware device. The amplitude of the ST segment in each of the constituent standard 12 leads is analysed by software algorithms. The ST

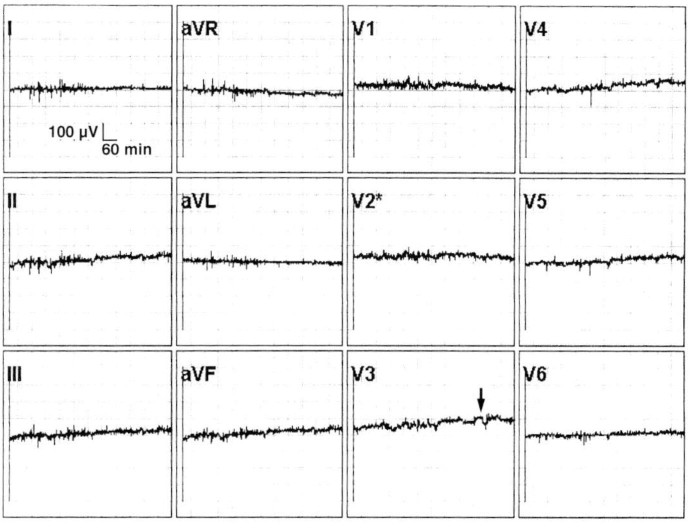

Fig. 28.1 Normal ST segment trend monitoring display from a patient being evaluated for chest pain. ST amplitudes remain unchanged over the period of monitoring. Small changes in amplitude (arrow) reflect changes in patient position.

segment amplitude is plotted over time, and displayed. Limits can be set within the device to automatically detect changes in the ST segment amplitude that suggest acute ischaemia. Monitors obtain a typical 10-s ECG as often as one or two times per min, and compare the ST amplitudes to the initial ECG. This transforms a static snapshot into a dynamic image. Figure 28.1 shows an example of normal ST segment trend monitoring in an individual who presented to the emergency department (ED) with chest pain. This graphical presentation provides a means by which the information from several hundred ECGs may be viewed at a glance. Changes from baseline may be readily visualized and predetermined alarm thresholds can provide visual and auditory alerts to caregivers when acute ischaemia is detected.

The ST amplitude is defined as the voltage difference between isoelectric level and the ST point. The isoelectric point is typically defined as a low-noise area within the *TP* interval. The ST point is defined as either the J point, or at some fixed position following the J point (e.g. J point + 60 ms). Since changes in heart rate influence *QT* interval (and resulting ST/T wave duration), some algorithms locate the ST point as the J point plus a fraction of the *RR* interval (e.g. J point + $1/12^{th}$ of the *RR* interval). If uncorrected for changes in heart rate, the ST point could otherwise creep up the ascending portion of the T wave during a tachycardia, falsely suggesting a rise in the ST segment amplitude.

As with all diagnostic tools, a balance between sensitivity and specificity dictates the usefulness of ST segment ischaemia monitoring. Typical monitor settings require a change in ST amplitude of > 100 µV in two or more contiguous leads, occurring over two or three successive recordings. This would require ECG changes to be present for only 2 or 3 min to be recognized as abnormal. Several ECGs are required in order that brief changes, such as electrical noise or suboptimal skin-electrode contact, are not classified as ischaemia. Even such thresholds will not capture all dynamic changes that actually reflect acute ischaemia. (Fig. 28.2) Note, also, that a *change* from baseline is the entity that is being evaluated. It is possible that the initial ECG, to which subsequent ECGs are compared, could have ST segment abnormalities that are not initially diagnostic (e.g. ST depression of 60 µV). Further ischaemia with additional ST depression will not violate the ST segment monitor's alarm criteria until the magnitude of the ST segment amplitude reaches 160 µV, reflecting a change of 100 µV.

While standard electrocardiographic recordings are made with the patient resting quietly in a supine position, continuous ST segment monitoring is accomplished while the patient is able to change position and move about to a limited extent. Telemetric systems will allow more patient mobility than systems which require the patient to remain tethered to the monitor by the lead wires. ST segment trend records may show small abrupt changes with such patient mobility or change in patient position or posture. These changes are usually readily identified by the experienced observer (Drew and Krucoff, 1999).

Most false positive ST segment changes that occur during the course of monitoring are the result of electrical noise due to poor contact between the patient's skin and the electrode

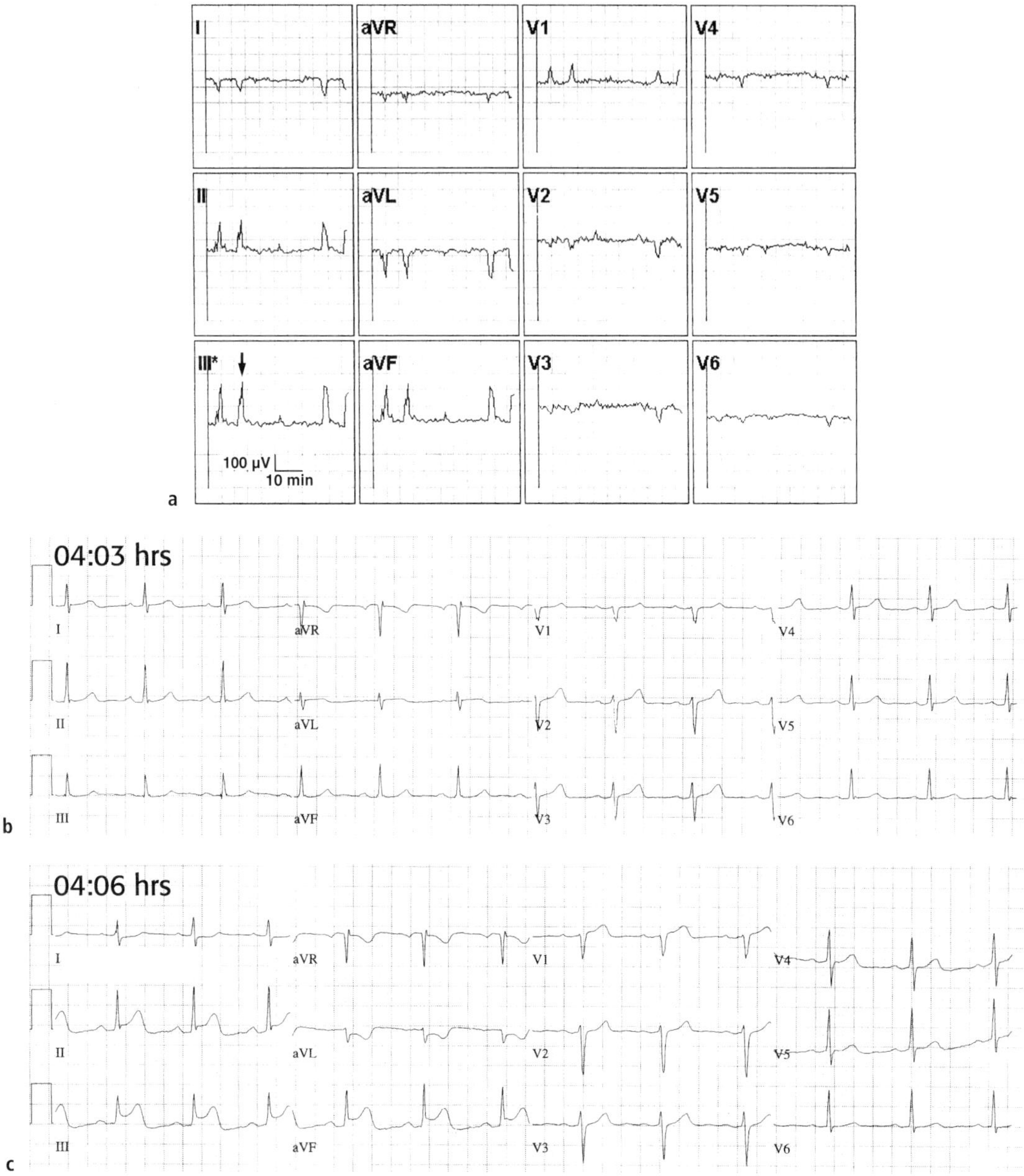

Fig. 28.2 (a) ST segment trend monitoring display with brief changes in ST amplitude reflecting transient ischaemic episodes. These changes did not reach threshold for alarm criteria (100 μV change in two or more contiguous leads for three consecutive ECGs). (b) Normal 12 lead EKG at 04:03. (c) Transiently abnormal 12 lead EKG (04:06 hours) showing ST elevation in leads III and aVF, and ST depression in aVL suggestive of acute injury (d) EKG changes have resolved 1 min later (04:07 hours). (e) Table of ST segment amplitude in each of the 12 leads. Values reflect the change (μV) from baseline ECG. These changes do not meet criteria for alarm violation, i.e. ST change ≥ 100 μV in two or more leads for two or more consecutively recorded EKGs.

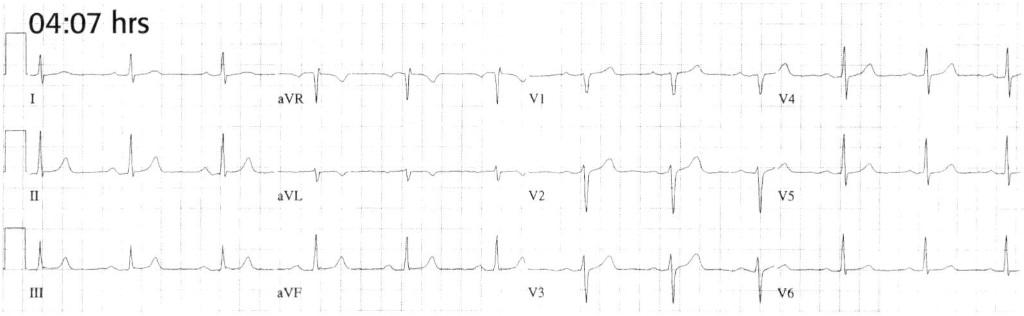

d

Change in ST Magnitude (μV) Relative to Initial EKG

	Lead:											
Time	**aVL**	**I**	**-aVR**	**II**	**aVF**	**III**	**V1**	**V2**	**V3**	**V4**	**V5**	**V6**
4:03	15	5	-10	-24	-24	-29	0	0	-20	-15	-9	-5
4:04	-68	-34	19	69	88	103	15	-49	-40	-5	0	0
4:05	-58	-39	0	40	59	78	54	-30	-35	-24	-19	-19
4:06	-127	-59	39	132	166	191	88	-44	-35	-63	-39	-24
4:07	-24	-25	-10	0	15	25	24	-5	-20	-19	-19	-5

e

Fig. 28.2 *Continued*

surface. Meticulous attention to skin preparation and electrode placement will minimize such electrical noise and false triggering of alarms.

As with the standard 12-lead ECG, the absence of a diagnostic change on ST segment monitoring does not necessarily rule out pathology. The exact predictive value of a period of normal ST segment monitoring in the acute chest pain patient is not yet fully understood. Once myocardial infarction and rest angina are excluded by serial serum markers of necrosis and electrocardiography, chest pain evaluation algorithms (Kontos 2001; Graff *et al.* 1995) recommend provocative testing for cardiac ischaemia.

ST vector magnitude

Some monitoring devices use the Frank lead-set of orthogonal electrodes to detect dynamic ischaemia by ST segment analysis. In such a system an index of ST amplitude, the ST Vector Magnitude (ST_{VM}), has been derived. $ST_{VM} = (ST_X^2 + ST_Y^2 + ST_Z^2)^{1/2}$ ST points are defined as discussed above, and the threshold for abnormality in ST_{VM} is typically set at 50 uV (Jensen *et al.* 1994). This method has been studied in the setting following angioplasty in patients with left bundle branch block, as well (Gurfinkel *et al.* 1994). A change in ST_{VM} of 100 μV was found to be a sensitive parameter for detection of ischaemia in these patients. Figure 28.3 shows the graphical display of such a device used for a patient monitored for several hours following successful treatment for ST elevation acute myocardial infarction.

Selection of leads for ischaemia monitoring

The technique of ST segment monitoring has evolved from the use of the typical 12-lead ECG. Most systems analyse all 12 leads to detect diagnostic changes suggestive of ischaemia or injury. However, ST segment monitoring may be accomplished with fewer than 12 leads. Within such systems, selection of the several leads to monitor should be based on an estimation of the area of myocardium felt to be most at risk. This area may be predicted based on prior ECGs or following interventional procedures (Horacek

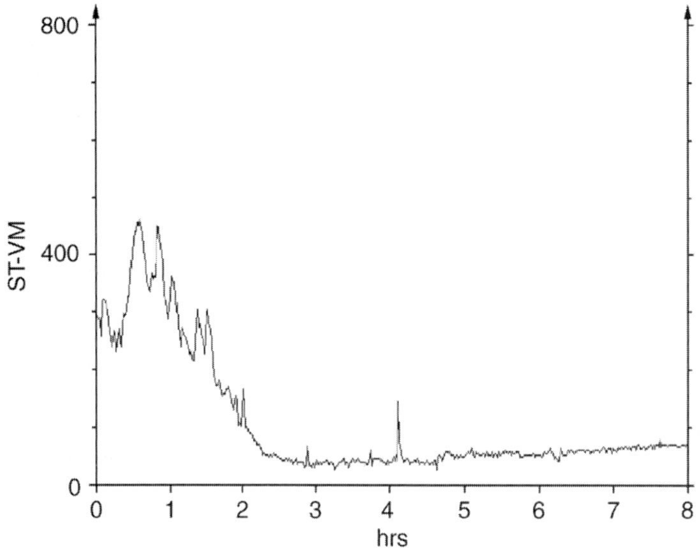

Fig. 28.3 ST vector magnitude (ST_{VM}) trend. Patient presented with ST elevation acute myocardial infarction. Trend shows resolution of ST_{VM} with treatment. A brief episode of ischaemia is noted shortly after the 4 h mark.

et al. 2001), but often the coronary anatomy is unknown at the time of evaluation of the acute chest pain patient. Drew *et al.* (Drew and Krucoff, 1999; Drew and Tisdale, 1993) suggest that optimal 3 lead monitoring for ST segment changes should include leads III, V3 and V5. If only two-lead monitoring is available, leads III and V3 are recommended for ST segment monitoring.

Detection of myocardial ischaemia

ST segment trend monitoring has been used in several situations in which the identification of myocardial ischaemia will alter the management of patients. Much of the experience with this application is derived from studies related to the prediction of coronary artery patency following percutaneous intervention (Gurfinkel *et al.* 1994; Krucoff *et al.* 1994; Eriksson *et al.* 1999) and thrombolytic therapy (Krucoff *et al.* 1986; French *et al.* 2002; Califf *et al.* 1988; Figueras and Cortadellas, 1995; Badir *et al.* 1995; Schroder *et al.* 1995). Perioperative ST segment monitoring for ischaemia detection has been compared to other techniques in the operating theatre (Jopling, 1996; Kotrly *et al.* 1984; Slogoff *et al.* 1990; London *et al.* 1988). This has not, however, been universally accepted (Proctor and Kingsley, 1996), and is probably best used in combination with other tools available to the anaesthesiologist (Ellis *et al.* 1992).

ST segment monitoring in the emergency department

A recent evaluation of technologies for identifying acute cardiac ischaemia in the ED reviewed prospective clinical trials conducted between 1966 and 1998 (Lau *et al.* 2001). This review had insufficient material to substantiate an evidence-based recommendation regarding the utility of ST segment trend monitoring in the acute chest pain patient. Both anecdotal reports and accumulating clinical trials now appear to suggest that there is a benefit of ST segment monitoring in the emergency department setting (Garvey, 1999). Published case reports (Velez *et al.* 2002; Fesmire and Smith, 1993; Finefrock, 1995; Fu *et al.* 1994; Di Chiara and Badano, 2002) illustrate the utility of ST segment trend monitoring in the evaluation of acute coronary syndrome patients.

Early identification of patients with myocardial ischaemia is a primary goal in the evaluation of emergency department patients with chest pain. ST segment trend monitoring as surveillance for acute myocardial ischaemia is applied to two ED patient populations. Patients with 'typical' symptoms of ischaemia, but otherwise few risk factors for CAD may be monitored. Patients known to have CAD, or those at high risk for CAD (diabetic, hypertensive, cigarette smoker, etc.) but with 'atypical' presentations for acute ischaemia are also monitored for electrocardiographic evidence of ischaemia. Gibler *et al.* (1993) studied a relatively low-risk ED population with presentations consistent with acute cardiac ischaemia but having normal or 'non-diagnostic' initial ECGs (Gibler *et al.* 1993). They found that continuous ST segment monitoring over a 9-h evaluation period identified 39% of individuals ultimately diagnosed with an acute myocardial ischaemic event. Often the diagnostic changes on the ST segment monitoring device were the first indication that the patient was experiencing an acute coronary syndrome. Such early identification of these patients can lead to earlier administration of appropriate treatments.

Ischaemia monitoring is applied to patients with undifferentiated chest pain, as well as those with obvious electrocardiographic evidence of myocardial infarction. This can be useful in identifying transient ischaemic episodes that otherwise may be missed, or in following the response to treatments. Figure 28.2 depicts an ST segment monitoring episode for a patient with chest pain. This monitoring occurred over a period of several hours, in which hundreds of ECGs were analysed by the ST segment trend monitor. Brief episodes of ischaemia were identified in this patient. The ECG changes manifested by this patient show the limit of detection of such devices, as the changes in ST segment amplitude were abnormal for only a minute or two.

In a series of 1000 patients Fesmire *et al.* (1998) showed that ST segment trend monitoring is useful to clinicians in the ED. When compared to the ECG obtained at the time of presentation, ST segment monitoring during the ED evaluation improved both the sensitivity (27.5 vs. 34.2; $P < 0.0001$) and specificity (97.1 vs 99.4; $P < 0.01$) in detecting acute coronary syndromes. This technique also improved the sensitivity in detecting acute myocardial infarction (55.4 vs. 68.1; $P < 0.0001$). Diagnostic changes during continuous ST segment monitoring of acute chest pain patients identifies patients for ICU admission, revascularization procedures, and long-term complications (Fesmire *et al.* 1998; Jernberg *et al.* 1999).

Advantage of ST segment monitoring

Current standard of care dictates that patients suspected of cardiac ischaemia should be monitored for significant arrhythmias. While this is certainly a crucially important goal in managing these patients, such arrhythmias portend extensive underlying myocardial damage and subsequent patient risk. If noninvasive electrocardiographic monitoring could detect abnormalities in cardiac function at a time before such significant damage, interventions may be initiated to abort the evolving pathophysiological course. Such a concept is illustrated by the case presented in Fig. 28.4. In this patient with known CAD and a presentation consistent with ACS, the ST segment monitoring alarm detected a change in her ECG that was diagnostic for injury several minutes before the arrhythmia monitor detected ventricular fibrillation. While the time course for these changes was quite rapid for the patient presented here, such a concept of ischaemia identification before progression to a potentially lethal arrhythmia identification suggests that there may be an opportunity for intervention identified by ST segment monitoring.

Static 12-lead ECGs are repeated when a patient experiences a change in symptoms. The usual scenario requires the patient to initiate a report to the staff, who then arrange for an electrocardiograph to be made available at the bedside and ultimately record the ECG for interpretation by the nurse and physician. The interval from symptom onset to ECG interpretation can easily be 20 min or more in this scenario. Often the patient's symptoms will have resolved by the time the repeat ECG can be obtained. Information that would be useful to the diagnostician is lost. While the incidence of truly silent ischaemia is thought to be an infrequent occurrence, mild symptoms may be present but of insufficient intensity or duration to cause a patient to summon help. With ST segment monitoring in place, consecutive ECGs can be reviewed on a minute to minute basis without the need for the patient to notify staff of a change in their condition, or for staff to physically acquire the ECGs at each instance.

The advantage of ST segment ischaemia monitoring is essentially 'time'. This technique brings the time dimension to the electrocardiogram. The dynamic nature of myocardial ischaemia pathophysiology is now matched by real-time monitoring for dynamic electrocardiographic

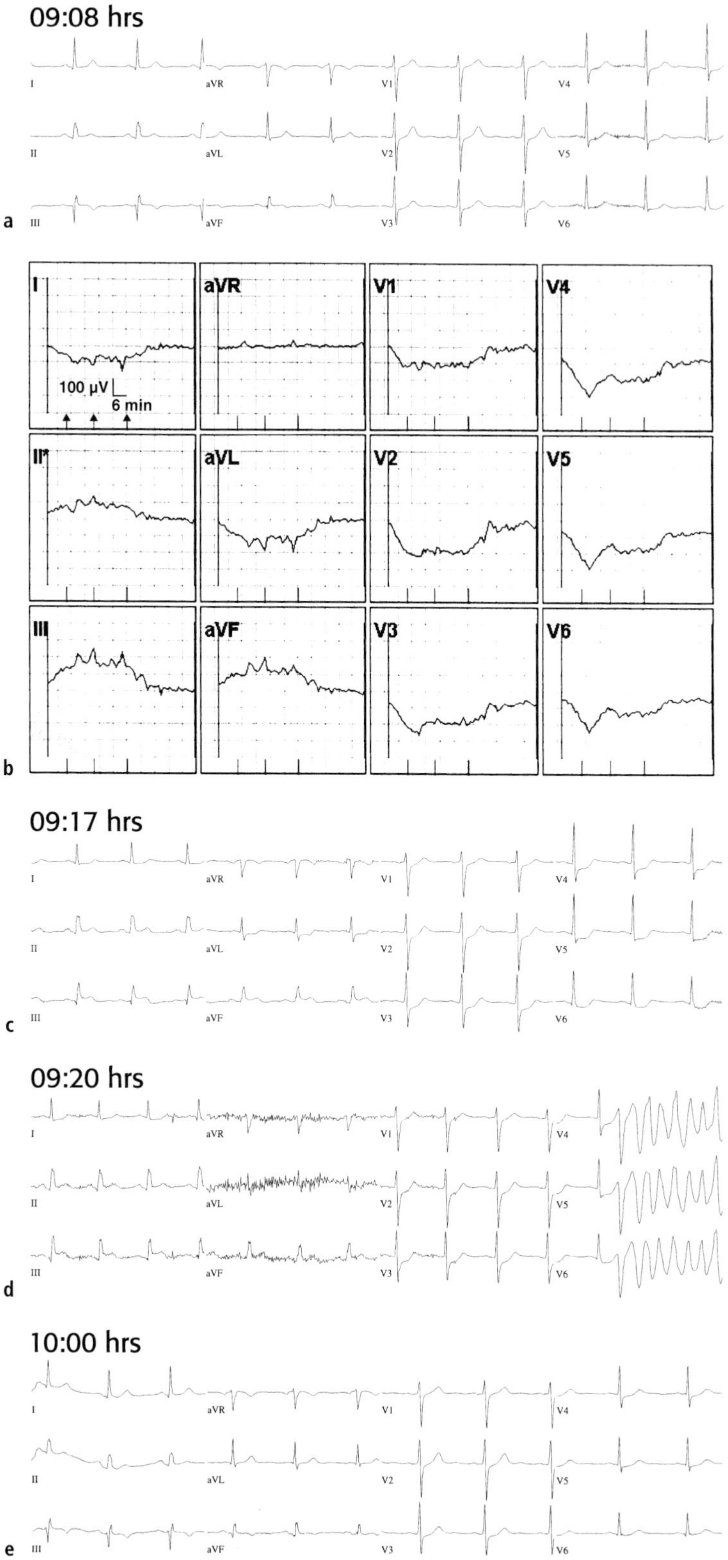

Fig. 28.4 ST segment trend monitoring display from a patient with acute myocardial infarction. (a) Initial 12-lead ECG is not diagnostic for infarction or ischaemia. (b) ST segment amplitude trends from 12 leads. ST elevation in inferior leads and ST depression in anterior septal leads is apparent. Arrow indicates visual marks on display at times of ST segment alarm violations. (c) 12-lead ECG at time of ST segment monitor alarm is now diagnostic for acute ischaemia, i.e. ST depression in precordial leads and aVL, ST elevation in leads III and aVF. (d) 12-lead ECG at time of arrhythmia alarm shows onset of ventricular fibrillation. (e) 12-lead ECG at time of transfer from ED to cardiac catheterization laboratory. Transient ST changes have nearly completely resolved. (Adapted from Velez *et al.* 2002, with permission.)

changes. When repeat electrocardiograms are scheduled at intervals of several hours or more, the dynamic nature of the underlying pathology may be manifest only by Q wave development, for example. While helpful in establishing the ultimate diagnosis, the opportunity to intervene – pharmacologically or mechanically – may have passed by the time such abnormalities are detected.

References

Aufderheide, T.P. & Brady, W.J. (1994) Electrocardiography in the patient with myocardial ischaemia or infarction. In: *Emergency Cardiac Care* (ed. L. Craven), pp. 169–216. Mosby, St Louis, MO.

Badir, B.F., Nasmith, J.B., Dutoy, J.L. *et al.* (1995) Continuous ST segment recording during thrombolysis in acute myocardial infarction: a report on orthogonal ECG monitoring. *Canadian Journal of Cardiology*, **11**, 545–552.

Califf, R.M., O'Neil, W., Stack, R.S. *et al.* (1988) Failure of simple clinical measurements to predict perfusion status after intravenous thrombolysis. *Annals of Internal Medicine*, **108**, 658–662.

Di Chiara, A. & Badano, L. (2002) ST segment monitoring of coronary reperfusion. *Heart*, 88, 334.

Drew, B.J. & Krucoff, M.W. (1999) Multilead ST segment monitoring in patients with acute coronary syndromes: a consensus statement for healthcare professionals. ST-Segment Monitoring Practice Guideline International Working Group. *American Journal of Critical Care*, **8**, 372–386.

Drew, B.J. & Tisdale, L.A. (1993) ST segment monitoring for coronary artery reocclusion following thrombolytic therapy and coronary angioplasty: identification of optimal bedside monitoring leads. *American Journal of Critical Care*, **2**, 280–292.

Ellis, J.E., Shah, M.N., Briller, J.E., Roizen, M.F., Aronson, S. & Feinstein, S.B. (1992) A comparison of methods for the detection of myocardial ischaemia during noncardiac surgery: automated ST segment analysis systems, electrocardiography, and transesophageal echocardiography. *Anesthesia & Analgesia*, **75**, 764–772.

Eriksson, P., Albertsson, P., Ekstrom, L. & Dellborg, M. (1999) Continuous vectorcardiographic monitoring of ischaemia during coronary angioplasty in patients with bundle-branch block. *Coronary Artery Disease*, **10**, 501–507.

Fesmire, F.M., Percy, R.F., Bardoner, J.B., Wharton, D.R. & Calhoun, F.B. (1998) Usefulness of automated serial 12-lead ECG monitoring during the initial emergency department evaluation of patients with chest pain. *Annals of Emergency Medicine*, **31**, 3–11.

Fesmire, F.M. & Smith, E.E. (1993) Continuous 12-lead electrocardiograph monitoring in the emergency department. *American Journal of Emergency Medicine*, **11**, 54–60.

Figueras, J. & Cortadellas, J. (1995) Further elevation of the ST segment during the first hour of thrombolysis. A possible early marker of reperfusion. *European Heart Journal*, **16**, 1807–1813.

Finefrock, S.C. (1995) Continuous 12-lead ST segment monitoring: an adjunct to identifying silent ischaemia and infarct in the emergency department. *Journal of Emergency Nursing*, **21**, 413–416.

French, J.K., Andrews, J., Manda, S.O.M., Stewart, R.A.H., McTigue, J.J.C. & White, H.D. (2002) Early ST segment recovery, infarct artery blood flow, and long-term outcome after acute myocardial infarction. *American Heart Journal*, **143**, 265–271.

Fu, G.Y., Joseph, A.J. & Antalis, G. (1994) Application of continuous ST segment monitoring in the detection of silent myocardial ischaemia. *Annals of Emergency Medicine*, **23**, 1113–1115.

Garvey, J.L. (1999) Can ST segment trend monitoring beat static twelve-lead ECGs? In: *Pushing the therapeutic envelope for emergency cardiac medicine: Acute coronary syndromes and beyond* (ed. B. Gibler), pp. 10–12. Health Science Communications, New York.

Gibler, W.B., Sayre, M.R., Levy, R.C. *et al.* (1993) Serial 12-lead electrocardiographic monitoring in patients presenting to the emergency department with chest pain. *Journal of Electrocardiology*, **26** (Suppl.), 238–243.

Gomez, M.A., Anderson, J.L., Karagounis, L.A., Muhlestein, J.B. & Mooers, F.B. (1996) An emergency department-based protocol for rapidly ruling out myocardial ischaemia reduces hospital time and expense: results of a randomized study (ROMIO). *Journal of the American College of Cardiology*, **28**, 25–33.

Graff, L., Joseph, T., Andelman, R., Bahr, R. *et al.* (1995) American College of Emergency Physicians information paper: chest pain units in emergency departments – a report from the Short-Term Observation Services Section. *American Journal of Cardiology*, **76**, 1036–1039.

Gurfinkel, E., Duronto, E., Manos, E. *et al.* (1994) ST segment computerized monitoring before and after angioplasty: clinical correlation with recurrent angina during the short-term follow-up. *Clinical Cardiology*, **17**, 433–436.

Horacek, B.M., Warren, J.W., Penney, C.J. *et al.* (2001) Optimal electrocardiographic leads for detecting acute myocardial ischaemia. *Journal of Electrocardiology*, **34** (Suppl.), 97–111.

Jensen, S., Johansson, G., Osterman, G., Reiz, S. & Naalund, U. (1994) On-line computerized vectorcardiography monitoring of myocardial ischaemia during coronary angioplasty: Comparison with 12 lead electrocardiography. *Coronary Artery Disease*, **5**, 507–514.

Jernberg, T., Lindahl, B. & Wallentin, L. (1999) ST segment monitoring with continuous 12-lead ECG improves early risk stratification in patients with chest pain and ECG nondiagnostic of acute myocardial infarction. *Journal of the American College of Cardiology*, **34**, 1413–1419.

Jopling, M.W. (1996) Pro: automated electrocardiogram ST segment monitoring should be used in the monitoring of cardiac surgical patients. *Journal of Cardiothoracic & Vascular Anesthesia*, **10**, 678–680.

Kontos, M.C. (2001) Evaluation of the emergency department chest pain patient. *Cardiology in Review*, **9**, 266–275

Kotrly, K.J., Kotter, G.S., Mortara, D. & Kampine, J.P. (1984) Intraoperative detection of myocardial ischaemia with an ST segment trend monitoring system. *Anesthesia & Analgesia*, **63**, 343–345.

Krucoff, M.W., Green, C.E., Satler, L.F. *et al.* (1986) Non-invasive detection of coronary artery patency using continuous ST segment monitoring. *American Journal of Cardiology*, **57**, 916–922.

Krucoff, M.W., Loeffler, K.A., Haisty, W.K.J. *et al.* (1994) Simultaneous ST segment measurements using standard and monitoring-compatible torso limb lead placements at rest and during coronary occlusion. *American Journal of Cardiology*, **74**, 997–1001.

Lau, J., Ioannidis, J., Balk, E. *et al.* (2001) *Evaluation of technologies for identifying acute cardiac ischaemia in emergency departments.* Evidence Report/Technology Assessment No. 26. 01-E006. Agency for Healthcare Research and Quality (AHRQ), Rockville MD.

London, M.J., Hollenberg, M., Wong, M.G., Levenson, L., Tubau, J.F., Browner, W. & Mangano, D.T. (1988) Intraoperative myocardial ischaemia: localization by continuous 12-lead electrocardiography. *Anesthesiology*, **69**, 232–241.

Proctor, L.T. & Kingsley, C.P. (1996) Con: ST segment analysis – who needs it? *Journal of Cardiothoracic & Vascular Anesthesia*, **10**, 681–682.

Sarko, J. & Pollack, C.V., Jr (1997) Beyond the twelve-lead electrocardiogram: diagnostic tests in the evaluation for suspected acute myocardial infarction in the emergency department, part I. *Journal of Emergency Medicine*, **15**, 839–847.

Schroder, R., Wegscheider, K., Schroder, K., Dissmann, R. & Meyer-Sabellek, W. (1995) Extent of early ST segment elevation resolution: a strong predictor of outcome in patients with acute myocardial infarction and a sensitive measure to compare thrombolytic regimens. A substudy of the International Joint Efficacy Comparison of Thrombolytics (INJECT) Trial. *Journal of the American College of Cardiology*, **26**, 1657–1664.

Slogoff, S., Keats, A.S., David, Y. & Igo, S.R. (1990) Incidence of perioperative myocardial ischaemia detected by different electrocardiographic systems [see comments]. *Anesthesiology*, **73**, 1074–1081.

Velez, J., Brady, W.J., Perron, A.D. & Garvey, L. (2002) Serial electrocardiography. *American Journal of Emergency Medicine*, **20**, 43–49.

CHAPTER 29

Circadian Patterns of Ischaemic Episodes

Shlomo Feldman

Introduction

The circadian variation in biological functions (chronobiology) plays an important role in the pathogenesis and exacerbation of different diseases. Circadian variation of the autonomic nervous system, together with the circadian variation of biochemical factors such as lipoprotein (a), cholesterol (total, high and low densities), triglycerides, cortisol, fibrinogen and platelets and the circadian variation of bioelectrical parameters such us the QT interval, have been published in the medical literature (Bremner *et al.* 2000). In the present review, the relationship between these circadian variations and pathological situations, methods of follow-up and clinical applications will be discussed.

Circadian variations of biological functions

Chronobiology

The sympathetic and parasympathetic branches of the autonomic nervous system (controlled by an area located in the anterior hypothalamus of the brain called the suprachiasmatic nucleus: SCN), with its direct effect on the sinus node of the heart (Sassone-Corsi 1998; Mathias & Alam 1995), shows a clear predominance of the sympathetic branch during day light hours, with increased activity of the parasympathetic branch during the night. This is reflected in changes of blood pressure, plasma epinephrine levels, heart rate, and heart rate variability with a special emphasis on the relationship between the low frequency/high frequency of the power spectrum, this relationship increasing during the day and decreasing at night (Malliani *et al.* 1991).

Together with the findings previously described, the lipoprotein metabolism, plasma cortisol levels, blood viscocity, and the coagulation mechanism (related to the endogenous tissue plasminogen activator (t-PA) and plasminogen activator inhibitor-1 (PAI-1)) have a tendency to hypercoagulability and hypofibrinolysis early in the morning, thus explaining the relative resistance to thrombolytic therapy at this time of the day (Braunwald 1995; Aronson 2001).

CLIF (cycle-like factor) a bHLH/PAS protein, together with the genes PER and CRY, regulates the circadian oscillation of PAI-I gene expression in endothelial cells (Maemura *et al.* 2001) (Fig. 29.1).

Bremner *et al.* (2000) describe an increase of cholesterol and platelets in the late afternoon that seems to coincide with late afternoon peak frequencies of sudden cardiac death and fatal stroke.

QT measurements and probably changes in QT dispersion, and the presence of QT alternans may present a circadian variation detected during Holter monitoring of the electrocardiogram (Yetkin *et al.* 2001).

There are gender differences in the risk of repolarization-related ventricular arrhythmias. Batchvarov *et al.* (2002) in their research based on 22 healthy men and 24 healthy women (age 27 ± 8 years) concluded that repolarization heterogeneity is greater in women, while depolarization heterogeneity is greater in men. Repolarization heterogeneity exhibits a circadian pattern, which might be linked to the gender differences in repolarization-related arrhythmias and to the circadian variation in the frequency of cardiac events. There was no detectable circadian variation in depolarization heterogeneity.

The normal circadian variation of biological

Oscillation of PAI-1 gene expression is regulated *by*

suprachiasmatic nucleus(SCN) (central clock)

through the endocrine and autonomic nervous systems

to the genes CLIF.PER.CRY(peripheral clock):

a feedback loop of the biological clock situated in the

endothelial cells.

Fig. 29.1 Circadian oscillation of PAI-1 gene expression. (Adapted from Maemura *et al.* 2001, with permission.)

functions can change according to our daily activities, with a rapid return to the usual pattern of the particular subject under normal conditions.

It can also change in shift workers (Garbarino *et al.* 2002) and in artificial situations such as space flights (Baevsky *et al.* 1997), geomagnetic disturbances and storms (Otsuka *et al.* 2001).

During situations related to stress, panic (Kloner & Leor 1999), exaggerated or inappropriate physical effort, and in many diseases, the normal circadian variation of the different parameters is altered (in particular the parasympathetic effect at night time), but able to return to normal either spontaneously with the disappearance of the factor involved, or with suitable treatment.

Circadian patterns of ischaemic episodes

Myocardial ischaemia

The use of isotope rubidium-82 and positron emission tomography (Fox *et al.* 1989) help to confirm the significance of the changes in the ST segment of the electrocardiogram, during both painful and silent ischaemia. Ischaemia is detected by a reduction in the uptake of the isotope in a region of the heart, reflecting a decrease in myocardial blood flow, coinciding with variations of the ST segment.

Episodes of ST segment depression and ischaemic events show a circadian rhythm similar to that seen for catecholamine release and heart rate circadian variation. A clear relationship exists between the episodes of coronary ischaemia and the drop of heart rate variability at arousal (06.00 to 11.00 hours) and during the day (18.00 to 23.00 hours) although the mechanisms may be different: during the early hours a high demand of oxygenated arterial blood to the heart is linked to daily activities outstripping supply; as opposed to the supply of blood at night in the absence of a change in demand (Benhorin *et al.* 1993); this situation at night may be related to a drop of vagal activity with increased sympathetic activity and coronary vasoconstriction without an increase on the demand of oxygenated arterial blood to the heart.

A sudden increase of the heart rate may be present and become an important parameter as a prognostic index for risk stratification. In the Angina and Silent Ischaemia Study Group (ASIS) (Andrews *et al.* 1993), mean minute heart rate activity during ambulatory electrogram was determined for 50 patients under different medications or placebo; the trial showed that 81% of ischaemic episodes were preceded by an increase in heart rate $\geq$ 5 beats/min. The likelihood of developing ischaemia associated with a heart rate increase was proportional to the magnitude and duration of the heart rate increase and the baseline heart rate: likelihood ranged from 4% when the heart rate increased from 5 to 9 beats/min and lasted for < 10 min, to 60% when the heart rate increased to $\geq$ 20 beats/min and lasted for $\geq$ 40 min.

Propranolol and nadolol therapy significantly reduced the magnitude and duration of heart rate increase and baseline rate compared with placebo, diltiazem or nifedipine ($P = 0.001$). Propranolol reduced the proportion of heart rate-related ischaemic episodes and increased the proportion of non heart-rate related episodes compared with placebo ($P < 0.02$); nifedipine exerted the opposite effect ($P = 0.005$) (Parker *et al.* 1994).

A minority of ischaemic episodes is not associated with preceding periods of increased heart rate, and may be caused by episodic coronary vasoconstriction, more effectively reduced by nifedipine than by propranolol. The combination therapy of nifedipine GITS (gastrointestinal therapeutic system) with a beta blocker is particularly efficacious in reducing coronary ischaemia (Parmley *et al.* 1992).

The European survey on circadian variation of angina pectoris (ESCVA) demonstrated a significant circadian variation ($P < 0.001$) with a primary morning peak from 09:00 to 12:00 (relative risk 3.0 compared with other times of the day) and a secondary afternoon peak from 15.00 to 18.00 hours. Fifty per cent of all attacks occurred within 6 h after awakening (Willich 1999).

The Prinzmetal syndrome may also be related to this possible sequence of events with a clear circadian rhythm of angina pectoris mostly in patients without severe coronary stenosis. But in a study published by Lanza *et al.* (1999), 26 patients had no significant circadian variation of ischaemia-related ventricular arrhythmias.

The presence of ischaemic episodes in subjects with normal coronary arteries and syndrome X is also explained by the mechanism of vasoconstriction due to an increased sympathetic effect (Fei *et al.* 1994).

Daily stress and various biochemical factors such us the renin–angiotensin system and endothelin, may alter the balance of the sympathetic and parasympathetic systems (predominantly the sympathetic system) and develop lethal arrhythmias (Shaw *et al.* 2001).

Impaired endothelium-dependent vasodilatation exists both in the coronary and peripheral circulation of post-menopausal women with angina and normal coronary angiograms. Flow-mediated dilation improves in these women after short and mid-term therapy with transdermal oestradiol, irrespective of concomitant progesterone use (Sitges *et al.* 2001)

In a small sample of 10 patients with coronary artery disease and 10 normal volunteers, Shaw *et al.* (2001) concluded that normal volunteers have a diurnal variation in their endothelium-dependent vasodilatation which may counteract other potential adverse diurnal variations linked to hemodynamic changes (vasoconstriction), to excessive coagulation and to other parameters. Conversely, coronary artery disease patients who presented with acute coronary syndromes showed a loss of this protective mechanism of endothelium-dependent vasodilatation.

Sudden cardiac death

Sudden cardiac death due to malignant arrhythmias such as sustained ventricular tachycardia and ventricular fibrillation, are recorded on Holter monitoring during the tragic event (Vybiral & Glasser 1995). The possible sequence of the mechanism of sudden cardiac death is ischaemia in a non-protected heart (without collateral circulation and proper treatment) with an increase in the tone of the sympathetic system, together with the secretion of catecholamines, hypercoagulation and a drop in activity of the parasympathetic system.

The sequence may be as follows:

A sudden increase in sympathetic activity (due to a trigger mechanism or transient precipitating risk factors with a withdrawal of the vagal tone) → production of catecholamines, blood pressure peak and vasoconstriction of the coronary arteries + hypercoagulability (Linsell *et al.* 1985; Tofler *et al.* 1987; Andreotti *et al.* 1988), with or without rupture of plaque (Stone 1990) → hypoxia (Keyl *et al.* 1996) → ischaemic event (Fox *et al.* 1989; Benhorin *et al.* 1993; Andrews *et al.* 1993) → angina pectoris, myocardial infarction, stroke or lethal arrhythmias (Schwartz 1998).

Reduced circadian variation of heart rate with marked blunting of the night-time heart rate decline, identifies survivors of sudden cardiac death (Molnar *et al.* 2002).

Myocardial infarction

A molecular mechanism may be responsible for the morning onset of the myocardial infarction. CLIF (cycle-like factor) regulates the circadian oscilla-tion of PAI-I gene expression in endothelial cells (Maemura *et al.* 2001).

The Autonomic Nervous System participates in the circadian variation of the myocardial infarction dynamics. Post myocardial infarction patients with or without Q waves have low heart rate variability, with a daily and a septadian circadian variation (Cornelissen *et al.* 1993). The circadian variation of ischaemic episodes is absent in patients developing myocardial infarction receiving previous ß blocker or aspirin treatment.

Myocardial damage can result in abolished, exaggerated or regionally discordant QT modulation, and this may generate arrhythmic vulnerability (Viitasalo *et al.* 1998).

According to Johanson *et al.* (2001) from their report on the ASSENT 2 monitoring sub-study, small variations in ST segment shift during the first 4 h of an acute myocardial infarction predict a worse outcome.

Episodes of paroxysmal dyspnoea and acute pulmonary oedema had a circadian variation with a definite increase during night h (Manfredini *et al.* 2000).

Circadian variation not related to ischaemia

Patients with Brugada syndrome have lethal ventricular tachyarrhythmias and sudden cardiac death at rest or during sleep. Wichter *et al.* (2002) investigated the presynaptic sympathetic function using ^{123}I-MIBG-SPECT; their study performed on 17 patients, demonstrated an abnormal uptake, indicating presynaptic sympathetic dysfunction. These findings may have a potential impact on the pathophysiology and arrhythmogenesis in patients with Brugada syndrome, apart from the genetic factors (Priori *et al.* 2002).

Grimm *et al.* (2000) showed in 29 patients with idiopathic dilated cardiomyopathy similar circadian distributions of ventricular tachycardia episodes as in patients with coronary disease. The majority of the episodes were preceded by a complex occurrence of ventricular premature beats like the classic short–long–short sequence. These findings may have important implications for the development of preventive pacing methods.

Sleep apnoea and sudden infant death syndrome are prone to circadian variation (Pincus *et al.* 1993).

It may be concluded that the presence of circadian variations could help significantly in finding suitable treatment for patients suffering from circadian ischaemic events (chronotherapy) (Burger *et al.* 1999).

As an exception to the circadian variation discussed in this review, it has been reported in the literature that the circadian variation may not be present in patients with an ischaemic heart linked to diabetes mellitus (Munger & Kenney 2000).

Follow-up

Together with the Holter monitoring and the systems developed to measure the heart rate and calculate the circadian variations of heart rate variability (such us the time domain and frequency domain calculated by Fast Fourier Transform Algorithm (Fig. 29.2); the multiple method using skewness and kurtosis (Bloch-Thomsen *et al.* 2002); the wavelet transform analysis using the orthogonal multiresolution pyramidal algorithm (Gamero *et al.* 2002), the approximate entropy (Pincus *et al.*1993), other methods may be utilized: heart rate turbulence (Schmidt *et al.* 1999; Schmidt 2002), baroreflex sensitivity (La Rovere *et al.* 2001), monitoring of the pulse rate, blood pressure, ST segment and QT measurements, are all indicated for improved follow-up and the identification of patients at risk from life-threatening arrhythmias, mostly in patients suffering from unstable angina pectoris, state post myocardial infarction and resuscitated patients after sudden cardiac death.

Automatic internal cardioverter defibrillator with the backing of a dual chamber pacemaker with a rate responsive program is advised in patients suffering from lethal arrhythmias (Van Hemel 2002). The memory incorporated in the device will detect the circadian changes of the heart rate (Lampert *et al.* 1994; Peters *et al.* 1996) and the heart rate variability, and adapt the treatment accordingly (Moss *et al.* 2002). To improve the results of heart rate variability, the addition of SDNN, and the low frequency/high frequency relationship are recommended (S. Feldman unpublished observations).

Periodic blood tests linked to lipoproteins, cortisol (Weitzman *et al.* 1971) and coagulation, are strongly advised; samples taken at different hours during day and night may be useful.

Clinical applications of the circadian patterns

Chronotherapy

Several publications have demonstrated the benefit of chronotherapy. The timing treatment in relation to the rhythm of diseases that have predictable circadian variations have been applied in arthritis, asthma, allergies, peptic ulcer, and cancer (Elliott 2001).

Pharmacological treatments based on β blockers, ACE inhibitors, calcium^{++} channels antagonists, statins, vasodilators, anticoagulants, and noninvasive and invasive procedures for revascularization like thrombolysis (Braunwald 1995; Goldhammer *et al.* 1999), percutaneous transluminal coronary angioplasty and

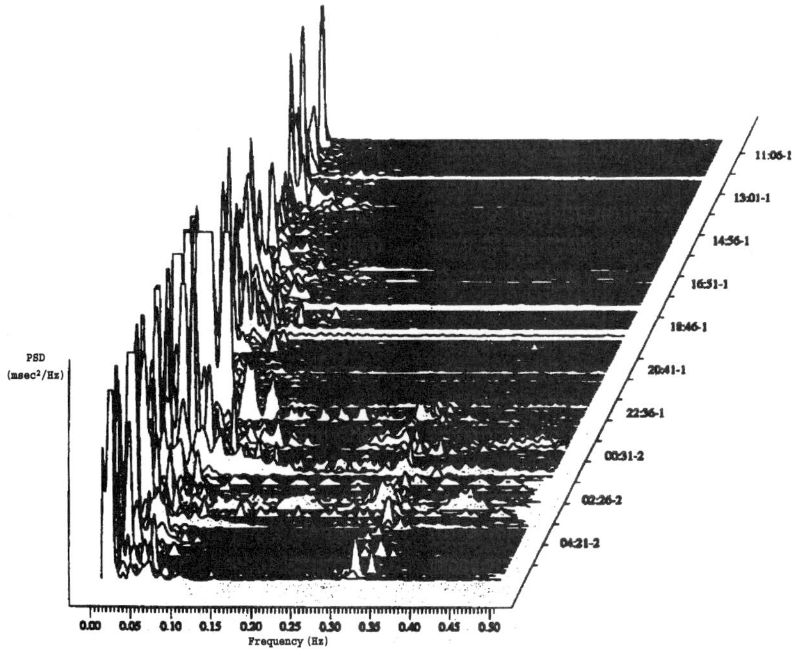

Fig. 29.2 Frequency-domain. Abnormal pattern of a syndrome X female patient. The sympathetic system (at left) in the low-frequency range is present during the 24 h, showing circadian variation. The parasympathetic system (at right) in the high-frequency range, shows a clear diminution during the day and the night hours. The LF/HF is 7,294 (S. Feldman unpublished observations).

insertion of stents or other protective devices (Temizhan *et al.* 2001), have increased the usefulness of these procedures taking in account the circadian patterns of cardiac ischaemic episodes and performing non-elective procedures at suitable hour. As in patients with diabetes mellitus, slow release medications with an increase of medication delivery during dangerous hours will avoid the appearance of ischaemic coronary episodes. Researches have begun to apply the science of chronotherapy, or the timing of drug effect with synchronized biological needs, in order to improve cardiovascular outcomes. This includes administering traditional agents at specific times throughout the day and developing new agents – chronotherapeutic formulations with special release mechanisms – targeted at inducing the greatest effect during morning surges. Chronotherapeutic agents are specifically designed to provide peak plasma concentrations during early morning hours, when effect seems to be most needed; lowest concentrations occur at night, when heart rate and blood pressure are lowest and, consequently, cardiovascular events are least likely to occur (Munger & Kenney 2000). One chronotherapeutic formulation that utilizes a unique drug-delivery system, controlled-onset extended-release (COER) verapamil, aligns peak plasma drug levels with times when blood pressure, heart rate, and myocardial oxygen demand are at their highest levels (Glasser 1999; Prisant *et al.* 2000).

Besides chronotherapy, the MADIT II trial, based on 1232 patients, concluded that in patients with a prior myocardial infarction and advanced left ventricular dysfunction, prophylactic implantation of a defibrillator improves survival and should be considered as a recommended therapy (Moss *et al.* 2002).

The recommendations presented have to be complemented with cardiac rehabilitation programs including progressive and controlled exercise, occupational therapy, early return to work and balanced diet avoiding large fatty meals, together with advice on the cessation of smoking.

Hereditary factors partially determine lipid profile responses to regular exercise. Maximal heritabilities were similar across ethnic groups and variables, except for higher heritabilities near 60% for ΔApoB in black people, ΔHDL 2-C in white people, and a lower estimate of zero for ΔLDL-C in black people. These factors are under investigation in the Health, Risk Factors, Exercise training and Genetics (HERITAGE) family study (Rice *et al.* 2002). Molecular markers and genes associated with these influences are currently underway.

There is also a need to study the role of *n*-3 fatty acids, vitamin E, vitamin C and the coenzyme Q10 (Singh *et al.* 2001).

The noninvasive treatment based on Enhanced External Counter Pulsation Therapy may offer a new chronotherapy method to decrease the episodes of angina pectoris (Arora *et al.* 2001).

Conclusion

Circadian variation of biological parameters have become an important factor in the understanding of ischaemic episodes occurring at different hours. It seems that increase of the sympathetic branch with a decrease of the parasympathetic branch of the autonomic nervous system, together with an exaggerated secretion of catecholamines and an increase of lipoproteins and hypercoagulability have a bimodal appearance with a peak at early morning hours and during the late afternoon (chronobiology).

This sequence of ischaemic events will enable better noninvasive and elective invasive treatment according to the circadian variation, timing recommended treatment to biological need, resulting in improvement of cardiovascular outcomes (chronotherapy).

References

Andreotti, F., Davies, G.J., Hacket, D.R. *et al.* (1998) Major circadian fluctuations in fibrinolytic factors and possible relevance to time of onset of myocardial infarction, sudden cardiac death and stroke. *American Journal of Cardiology*, **62**, 635–637.

Andrews, T.C., Fenton, T., Toyosaki, N. *et al.* (1993) Subsets of ambulatory myocardial ischaemia based on heart rate activity. Circadian distribution and response to anti-ischaemic medication. The Angina and Silent Ischaemia Study Group (ASIS). *Circulation*, **88**, 92–100.

Aronson, D. (2001) Impaired modulation of circadian rhythms in patients with diabetes mellitus: a risk factor for cardiac thrombotic events? *Chronobiology International*, **18** (1), 109–121.

Arora, R.R., Carlucci, M.L., Malone, A.M. *et al.* (2001) Acute and chronic hemodynamic effects of enhanced external counterpulsation in patients with angina pectoris. *Journal of Investigative Medicine*, **49** (6): 500–504.

Baevsky, R.M., Petrov, V.M., Cornelissen, G. *et al.* (1997) Meta-analysed heart rate variability, exposure to geomagnetic storms, and risk of ischaemic heart disease. *Scripta Medica (Brno)* **70** (4–5): 201–206.

Baevsky, R.M., Petrov, V.M. & Chernikova, A.G. (1998) Regulation of autonomic nervous system in space and magnetic storms. *Advances in Space Research*, **22** (2), 227–234.

Batchvarov, V., Smetana, P., Ghuran, A., Hnatkova, K., Camm, A.J. & Malik, M. (2002) Depolarization and repolarization heterogeneities differ between men and women. In: *XIII International Congress in Cardiac Electrophysiology* 19–22 June, Nice, France. *Europace*, Vol. 3, Suppl. A (ed. R. Sutton), p. 175, abstract 154/2. Elsevier Science, London.

Benhorin, J., Banai, S., Moriel, M. *et al.* (1993) Circadian variations in ischaemic threshold and their relation to the occurrence of ischaemic episodes. *Circulation*, **87**, 808–814.

Bloch-Thomsen, P.E., Saermark, K., Huikuri, H. *et al.* (2002) Multipole analysis predicts mortality after myocardial infarction. In: *NASPE, 23rd Annual Scientific Sessions*, 8–11 May. From *PACE (Pacing and Clinical Electrocardiography)*, **25** (4 Pt II), 692, abstract 678.

Braunwald, E. (1995) Morning resistance to thrombolytic therapy. *Circulation*, **91**, 1604.

Bremner, W.F., Sothern, R.B., Kanabrocki, E. *et al.* (2000) Relation between circadian patterns in levels of circulating lipoproteins (a), fibrinogen, platelets, and related lipid variables in men. *American Heart Journal*, **139** (1 Pt 1), 164–173.

Burger, A.J., Charlamb, M. & Sherman, H.B. (1999) Circadian patterns of heart rate variability in normals, chronic stable angina and diabetes mellitus. *International Journal of Cardiology*, **71** (1): 41–48.

Cornelissen, G., Breus, T.K., Bingham, C. *et al.* (1993) Beyond circadian chronorisk: worldwide circaseptan–circasemiseptan patterns of myocardial infarctions, other vascular events and emergencies. *Chronobiologia*, **20** (1–2), 87–115.

Elliott, W.J. (2001) Timing treatment to the rhythm of disease. A short course in chronotherapeutics. *Postgraduate Medicine*, **110** (2), 119–122.

Fei, L., Anderson, M.H., Katritsis, S. *et al.* (1994) Decreased heart rate variability in survivors of sudden cardiac death not associated with coronary artery disease. *British Heart Journal*, **71**, 16–21.

Fox, K., Mulcahy, D., Keegan, J., Wright, C. (1989) Circadian patterns of myocardial ischaemia. *American Heart Journal*, **118**, 1084–1086.

Gamero, L.G., Vila, J. & Palacios, F. (2002) Wavelet transform analysis of heart rate variability during myocardial ischaemia. *Medical & Biological Engineering & Computing*, **40** (1), 72–78.

Garbarino, S., Beelke, M., Costa, G. *et al.* (2002) Brain function and effects of shift work: implications for clinical neuropharmacology. *Neuropsychobiology*, **45** (1), 50–56.

Glasser, S.P. (1999) Circadian variations and chronotherapeutic implications for cardiovascular management: a focus on Coer verapamil. *Heart Disease*, **1** (4), 226–232.

Goldhammer, E., Kharash, L. & Abinader, E.G. (1999) Circadian fluctuations in the efficacy of thrombolysis with streptokinase. *Postgraduate Medicine Journal*, **75** (889), 667–671.

Grimm, W., Walter, M., Menz, V., Hoffmann, J. & Maisch, B. (2000) Circadian variation and onset mechanisms of ventricular tachyarrhthmias in patients with coronary disease vs. idiopathic dilated cardiomyopathy. *PACE (Pacing and Clinical Electrophysiology)*, **23** (11 Pt 2) 1939–1943.

Johanson, P., Svensson, A.M. & Dellborg, M. (2001) Clinical implications of early ST segment variability. A report from the second ASSENT (Assessment of Safety and Efficacy of a new Thrombolytic trial) ST-monitoring sub-study. *Coronary Artery Diseases* **12** (4), 277–283.

Keyl, C., Lemberger, P., Rodig, G. *et al.* (1996) Changes in cardiac autonomic control during nocturnal repetitive oxygen desaturation episodes in patients with coronary artery disease. *Journal of Cardiovascular Risk* **3** (2), 221–227.

Kloner, R.A. & Leor, J. (1999) Natural disaster plus wake-up time: a daily combination of triggers. *American Heart Journal*, **137**, 779–781.

Lampert, R., Rosenfeld, L., Batsford, W., Lee, F. & McPherson, C. (1994) Circadian variation of sustained ventricular tachycardia in patients with coronary artery disease and implantable cardioverter-defibrillators. *Circulation*, **90** (1), 242–247.

Lanza, G.A., Patti, G., Pasceri, V. *et al.* (1999) Circadian distribution of ischaemic attacks and ischaemia-related ventricular arrhythmias in patients with variant angina. *Cardiologia*, **44** (10), 913–919.

La Rovere, M., Pinna, G.D., Hohnloser, S.H. *et al.* (2001) Baroreflex sensitivity and heart rate variability in the identification of patients at risk for life-threatening arrhythmias. Implications for clinical trials. *Circulation*, **103**, 2072–2077.

Linsell, C.R., Lightman, S.L., Mullen, P.E. & Brown, M.J. (1985) Circadian rhythms of epinephrine and noradrenaline in man. *Journal of Clinical Endocrinology & Metabolism*, **60**, 1210–1215.

Maemura, K., Layne, M.D., Watanabe, M., Perrel, M.A., Nagai, R. & Mu-En, L. (2001) Molecular mechanisms of morning onset of myocardial infarction. *Annals of the New York Academy of Sciences*, **947**, 398–402.

Malliani, A., Pagani, M., Lombardi, F. & Cerutti, S. (1991) Cardiovascular neural regulation explored in the frequency domain. *Circulation*, **84**, 482–492.

Manfredini, R., Portaluppi, F., Boari, B., Salmi, R., Fersini, C. & Gallerani M. (2000) Circadian variation in onset of acute cardiogenic pulmonary oedema is independent of patients' features and underlying pathophysiological causes. *Chronobiology International*, **17** (5), 705–715.

Mathias, C.J. & Alam, M. (1995) Circadian changes of the cardiovascular system and the autonomic nervous system: observations in autonomic disorders. In: *Heart Rate Variability* (eds M. Malik & A.J. Camm), pp. 21–30. Futura Publishing, Armonk, NY.

Molnar, J., Weiss, J.S. & Rosenthal, J.E. (2002) Does heart rate identify sudden death survivors? Assessment of heart rate, QT interval and heart rate variability. *American Journal of Therapy*, **9** (2), 99–110.

Moss, A.J., Zareba W., Hall, W.J. *et al.* For the Multicentre Automatic Defibrillator Implantation Trial II (MADIT II) Investigators (2002). Prophylactic implantation of a defibrillator in patients with myocardial infarction and reduced ejection fraction. *New England Journal of Medicine*, **346**, 877–883.

Munger, M.A. & Kenney, J.K. (2000) A chronobiological approach to the pharmacotherapy of hypertension and angina. *Annals of Pharmacotherapy*, **34** (11), 1313–1319.

Otsuka, K., Oinuma, S., Cornelissen, G. *et al.* (2001) Alternating light–darkness-influenced human electrocardiographic magnetoreception in association with geomagnetic pulsations. *Biomedicine & Pharmacotherapy*, **55** (Suppl. 1), 63s–75s.

Parker, J.D., Testa, M.A., Jimenez, A.H. *et al.* (1994) Morning increase in ambulatory ischaemia in patients with stable coronary artery disease. Importance of physical activity and increased cardiac demand. *Circulation*, **89** (2), 604–614.

Parmley, W.W., Nesto, R.W., Singh, B.N. *et al.* (1992) Attenuation of the circadian patterns of myocardial ischaemia with nifedipine GITS in patients with chronic stable angina. N-CAP Study Group. *Journal of the American College of Cardiology*, **19** (7), 1380–1389.

Peters, R.W., McQuillan, S., Resnick, S.K. & Gold, M.R. (1996) Increased Monday incidence of life-threatening ventricular arrhythmias: experience with a third-generation implantable defibrillator. *Circulation*, **94**, 1346–1349.

Pincus, S.M., Cummins, T.R. & Haddad, G.G. (1993) Heart rate control in normal and aborted-SIDS infants. *American Journal of Physiology*, **264**, R638–R646.

Priori, S.G., Napolitano, C., Gaparini, M. *et al.* (2002) Natural history of Brugada syndrome. Insights for risk stratification and management. *Circulation*, **105**, 1342–1347.

Prisant, L.M., Devane, J.G. & Butler, J. (2000) A steady-state evaluation of the bioavailability of chronotherapeutic oral drug absorption system verapamil PM after night time dosing vs. immediate-acting verapamil dosed every eight hours. *American Journal of Therapy*, **7** (6): 345–351.

Rice, T., Després, J.-P., Pérusse, L. *et al.* (2002) Familial aggregation of blood lipid response to exercise training in the Health, Risk Factors, Exercise Training, and Genetics (HERITAGE) Family Study. *Circulation*, **105**, 1904–1908.

Sassone-Corsi, P. (1998) Molecular clocks: mastering time by gene regulation. *Nature (London)* **392**, 871–874.

Schmidt, G., Malik, M., Barthel, P. *et al.* (1999) Heart-rate turbulence after ventricular premature beats is a predictor of mortality after acute myocardial infarction. *Lancet*, **53**, 1390–1396.

Schmidt, G. (2002) *Results of the ISAR LVEF/HRT (Innovative Stratification of Arrhythmic Risk/By Means of LV Turbulence)*. Report submitted by P. Wang. Presented by G. Schmidt at the NASPE, 23rd Annual Scientific Sessions, 8–11 May. Late–Breaking Clinical Trials. http://www.naspe.org/library/naspe_on_clinical_trials/isar_ivef_hrt/

Schwartz, P.J. (1998) The autonomic nervous system and sudden death. *European Heart Journal*, **19** (Suppl, F), F72–F80.

Shaw, J.A., Chin-Dusting, J.P., Kingwell, B.A. & Dart, M. (2001) Diurnal variation in endothelium-dependent vasodilatation is not apparent in coronary artery disease. *Circulation*, **103** (6), 806–812.

Singh, R.B., Weydahl, A., Otsuka, K. *et al.* (2001) Can nutrition influence circadian rhythm and heart rate variability?. *Biomedicine & Pharmacotherapy*, **55** (Suppl. 1), 115s–124s.

Sitges, M., Heras, M., Roig, E. *et al.* (2001) Acute and mid-term combined hormone replacement therapy improves endothelial function in post-menopausal women with angina and angiographically normal coronary arteries. *European Heart Journal*, **22** (22), 2116–2124.

Stone, P.H. (1990) Triggers of transient myocardial ischaemia: circadian variation and relation to plaque rupture and coronary thrombosis in stable coronary artery disease. *American Journal of Cardiology*, **66** (16), 32G–36G.

Temizhan, A., Dincer, I., Pamir, G., Alpman, A. & Oral, D. (2001) Is there any effect of chronobiological changes on coronary angioplasty? *Journal of Cardiovasc Risk*, **8** (1), 15–19.

Tofler, G.H., Brezinski, D.A., Schafer, A.I. *et al.* (1987) Concurrent morning increase in platelet aggregability and the risk of myocardial infarction and sudden cardiac death. *New England Journal of Medicine*, **316**, 1514–1518.

Van Hemel N.M. (2002) Ambulatory rhythm recording with implanted devices: is arrhythmia analysis easier and treatment better? In: *Einthoven 2002. 100 Years of Electrocardiography* (eds M.J. Schalij, M.J. Janse, A. van Oosterom, H.J.J. Wellens & E. van der Wall), pp. 389–394. The Einthoven Foundation, Leiden.

Viitasalo, M., Karjalainen, J., Makijarvi, M. & Toivonen, L. (1998) Autonomic modulation of QT intervals in post-myocardial infarction patients with and without ventricular fibrillation. *American Journal of Cardiology*, **82** (2), 154–159.

Vybiral, T. & Glasser, D.H. (1995) Changes of heart rate variability preceding ventricular arrhythmias. In: *Heart Rate Variability* (eds M. Malik & A.J. Camm), pp. 421–428. Futura Publishing, Armonk, NY.

Weitzman, E.D., Fukushima, D., Nogeire, C. *et al.* (1971) Twenty-four hour pattern of the episodic secretion of cortisol in normal subjects. *Journal of Clinical Endocrinology & Metabolism*, **33**, 14–22.

Wichter, T., Matheja, P., Eckardt, L. *et al.* (2002) Cardiac autonomic dysfunction in Brugada syndrome. *Circulation*, **105**, 702–706.

Willich, S.N. (1999) European survey on circadian variation of angina pectoris (ESCVA): design and preliminary results. *Journal of Cardiovascular Pharmacology*, **34** (Suppl. 2), S9–S13.

Yetkin, E., Senen, K., Ileri, M. *et al.* (2001) Diurnal variation of QT dispersion in patients with and without coronary artery disease. *Angiology* **52** (5), 311–316.

CHAPTER 30

Electrocardiographic Findings in Patients with Cardiovascular Syndrome X

Juan Carlos Kaski and Juan Cosin-Sales

Introduction

Patients with cardiovascular 'syndrome X' have typical exertional chest pain, positive responses to stress testing and completely normal coronary arteriograms. These patients represent as many as 20% of those undergoing diagnostic coronary angiography for the assessment of angina (Kaski 1999).

Chest pain in patients with syndrome X is similar in character and radiation to that observed in patients with obstructive coronary artery disease (CAD). Nevertheless, the chest pain of cardiac syndrome X has several atypical characteristics, i.e. it occurs at rest in a large proportion of patients (41%) and tends to be long-lasting (> 10 min to hours) (Kaski *et al.* 1995).

The pathogenesis of cardiac syndrome X remains controversial and diverse mechanisms have been proposed. Due to the typical chest pain and ischaemic ECG changes, myocardial ischaemia has been suggested to play a role. However, only a proportion of cardiac syndrome X patients have documented evidence of ischaemia. In these patients myocardial ischaemia has been mainly related to endothelial dysfunction and microvascular abnormalities. Alterations of membrane ionic pumps have been also implicated (Fig. 30.1). Extracardiac mechanisms such as esophageal spasm and pain perception abnormalities, appear to be responsible for chest pain in at least some syndrome X patients. Other extracardiac causes of chest pain mimicking angina include the chest wall syndrome and psychological abnormalities. These conditions are normally excluded from the definition of syndrome X.

Prognosis is good regarding survival (Kemp 1986) but quality of life is poor in many patients with chest pain and normal coronary angiograms (CPNCA). This is mainly due to the occurrence of prolonged and recurrent chest pain episodes. Deterioration of left ventricular function over time is a rare event in these patients (Kaski *et al.* 1995), but is more common in patients with left bundle branch block (LBBB). The main clinical characteristics of syndrome X patients are summarized in Table 30.1.

In view of the good prognosis regarding survival, therapeutic goals in syndrome X should be the control of chest pain and the improvement in quality of life. The mechanisms underlying chest pain in syndrome X probably vary in different patient subgroups and there is no standard, off-the-shelf therapeutic protocol that can be used in these patients. Standard anti-anginal therapy with sublingual nitrates is often ineffective in controlling symptoms in CPNCA patients (Kaski *et al.* 1995). In contrast, other antianginal treatments such as beta blockers and calcium channel blockers are more effective treatments in a sizeable proportion of subjects (Kaski *et al.* 2001). Nonantianginal drugs, such as angiotensin-converting enzyme (ACE) inhibitors have offered good results in cardiac syndrome X and this is probably because the renin–angiotensin system plays an important role in the regulation of coronary vasomotion (Kaski *et al.* 1994). Imipramine, a tricyclic antidepressant, has been shown to significantly reduce the number of chest pain episodes in syndrome X

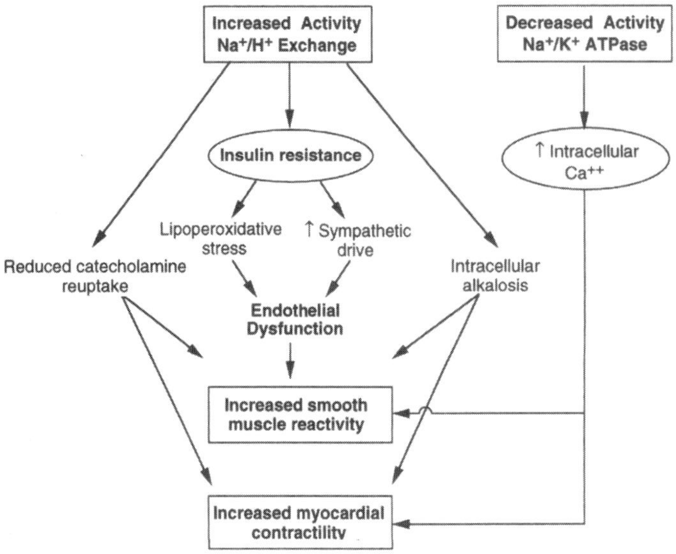

Fig. 30.1 Potential role of an alteration of membrane ionic pump in the pathogenesis of syndrome X.

Table 30.1 Main clinical characteristics of syndrome X patients

Poorly defined
Relatively common
High prevalence of women
Multifactorial pathogenesis
Good prognosis but poor quality of life
Major burden to health services
Empirical treatment

patients. However, imipramine was associated with a high incidence of side-effects that may lead to impaired quality of life (Cox *et al.* 1998). Finally, aminophylline, a competitive blocker of adenosine purinergic receptors, has been shown to reduce the magnitude of chest pain and ST segment changes in syndrome X patients (Elliott *et al.* 1997).

Baseline electrocardiographic features

The baseline ECG in patients with CPNCA is generally similar to that in the normal population. However, several abnormalities have been found in these patients, such as higher heart rate at baseline together with a prolonged *QTc*, when compared to healthy subjects (Mammana *et al.* 1997; Leonardo *et al.* 1997). These findings might be explained by sympathetic predominance (Rosano *et al.* 1994) in CPNCA patients. Also, in a small proportion of syndrome X patients, flat T waves and mild nonspecific ST segment depression have been observed in the baseline ECG (Fig. 30.2) (Kaski *et al.* 1995). Left bundle branch block, although uncommon in syndrome X patients, has been related to a deterioration of LV function over time (Opherk *et al.* 1989) in some studies but not in others (Cannon *et al.* 1991).

ECG responses during exercise stress testing

The ECG exercise response of patients with syndrome X is frequently indistinguishable from that of patients with CAD (Figs 30.3 and 30.4). Although, on average, syndrome X patients tend to develop typical ST segment changes at a higher rate-pressure product than patients with CAD, patterns of onset and offset of ST segment depression are similar in both groups of patients, as described by Pupita *et al.* (1990). Continuous plots of ST segment depression related to heart rate during exercise and recovery (heart rate-recovery loops) also followed counterclockwise loop rotations in both CAD and syndrome X patients (Gavrielides *et al.* 1991).

Interestingly, contrary to findings in CAD patients, an ischaemic response to exercise has not been associated with increased mortality or

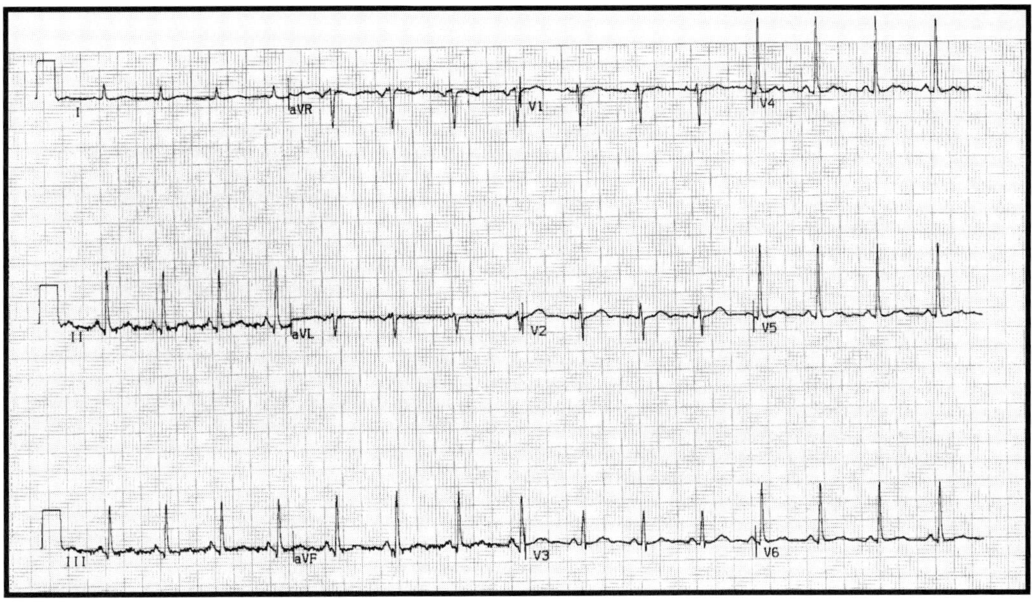

Fig. 30.2 Baseline ECG from a female 56 years old diagnosed as syndrome X. Increased heart rate (95 bpm) and flat T waves can be observed.

Table 30.2 Effects of pharmacological agents on exercise-induced ST segment changes in patients with cardiac syndrome X

Study	*Type study*	*Drug*	*Effect*
Radice *et al.* 1994	Not controlled	s.l. GTN	Variable effects on ET duration and time to ST segment depression
Bugiardini *et al.* 1989	Randomized	Propranolol	Improved angina and ET-induced ST depression
Fragasso *et al.* 1997	Randomized	Atenolol	Improved ET-induced ST depression and LV diastolic function
Cannon *et al.* 1985	Randomized	CCB	Beneficial effects on anginal pain and exercise capacity
Montorsi *et al.* 1990	Randomized	Nifedipine	Beneficial effects on anginal pain and exercise capacity
Elliott *et al.* 1997	Randomized	Aminophylline	Time to chest pain onset. No effect on ST segment depression
Kaski *et al.* 1994	Randomized	Enalapril	↓ (+) responses to ET and degree of ST segment depression
Bøtker *et al.* 1998	Randomized	Doxazosin	No effect on ST segment depression or angina onset

CCB, Calcium channel blocker; ET, exercise test; LV, left ventricular; ↓, decrease; (+) ischaemic.

worse long-term prognosis in patients with CPNCA (Kemp 1986).

Therapeutic interventions affect ECG responses during stress testing in a variety of ways (Kaski *et al.* 2001). Beta blockers (Bugiardini *et al.* 1989; Fragasso *et al.* 1997), calcium channel blockers (Cannon *et al.* 1985; Montorsi *et al.* 1990) and ACE-inhibitors (Kaski *et al.* 1994) have shown beneficial effects on ECG exercise stress testing responses, i.e. decreasing the degree of maximal ST segment depression or time to ST segment depression onset. In contrast, nitrates (Radice *et al.* 1994), aminophylline (Elliott *et al.* 1997) or doxazosin (Bøtker *et al.* 1998) have not been able to show objective beneficial effects on stress testing (Table 30.2).

Also, nonpharmacological approaches such as transcendental meditation (TM), a behavioural relaxation technique, can modify ST segment response to exercise stress testing. After 12 weeks practice, TM has been shown to increase the time to ST segment depression and to reduce maximal

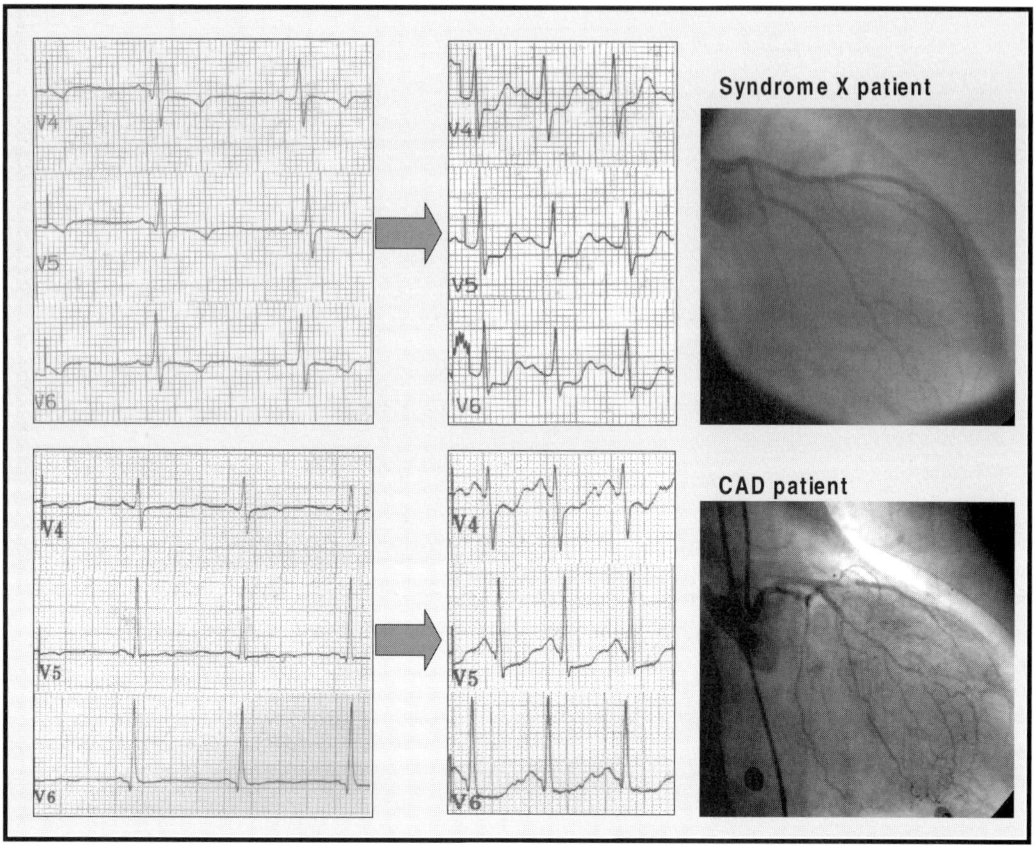

Fig. 30.3 Baseline and maximal heart rates ECG (leads V4–6) during an exercise stress test from syndrome X and CAD patients, alone with their coronary angiography. In the syndrome X patients, at baseline, typical T wave inversion and at peak exercise (heart rate:139 bpm), −1.8 mm ST segment depression can be observed. In the CAD patient, at peak exercise (heart rate 141 bpm), −1.9 mm ST segment depression can be observed.

ST segment depression (Cunningham *et al.* 2000). Possible explanations for these interesting findings include the beneficial effects that TM may have on blood pressure, sympathetic tone, and β-adrenergic receptor sensitivity.

The role of myocardial ischaemia

The cause of a positive response to stress testing in patients with cardiac syndrome X is controversial. Ischaemic and nonischaemic mechanisms have been postulated (Table 30.3). Myocardial ischaemia has been reported in early studies by Boudoulas *et al.* (1974) who showed that CPNCA patients in whom transmyocardial lactate production was demonstrated during atrial pacing had greater ST segment depression than those without. Later, Rosano *et al.* (1996) observed a decrease of pH and oxygen saturation in the coronary sinus blood of syndrome X patients during atrial pacing. This occurred in approximately 15% of patients in their study. More recently, Buffon *et al.* (2000), measured lipid hydroperoxides (ROOHs) and conjugated dienes (CDs), two sensitive and independent markers of ischaemia-reperfusion oxidative stress, in paired aortic and great cardiac vein blood samples before and after pacing-induced tachycardia in patients with syndrome X and normal controls. They observed that whilst controls subjects showed no increased in ROOH and CD levels after pacing, syndrome X patients consistently showed an increase in ROOH and CD levels in the great cardiac vein along with ischaemic ST segment changes during pacing. Zeiher *et al.* (1995)

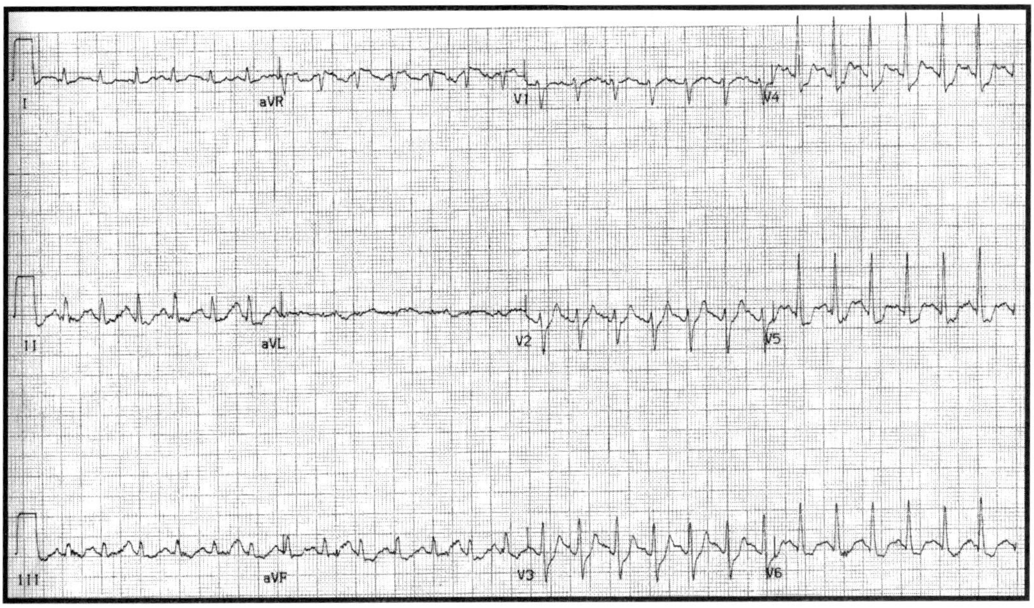

Fig. 30.4 Peak exercise 12-lead ECG from a syndrome X patient.

Table 30.3 Proposed pathogenetic mechanism in cardiac syndrome X

Myocardial ischaemia	*Nonischaemic mechanisms*
Microvascular dysfunction	Abnormal interstitial potassium
Microvascular spasm	Adenosine release
Endothelial dysfunction	Early cardiomyopathy
Estrogen deficiency	Increased pain perception
Increased sympathetic tone	Insulin resistance
Prearteriolar constriction	Myocardial metabolic abnormality
Endogenous peptides (endothelin)	(sympathetic tone)
Structural abnormalities in microvessels	
Diffuse epicardial and microvascular constriction	
Combined mechanisms: increased pain perception and microvascular dysfunction	

showed thallium[201] scintigraphy exercise-induced myocardial perfusion defects in 13 of 27 syndrome X patients. Of interest, these 13 patients exhibited a marked impairment of the endothelium-dependent dilatation of the coronary resistance vasculature. Further endorsing an ischaemic origin of chest pain and ECG changes in syndrome X, magnetic resonance studies showed the presence of myocardial ischaemia in approx. 20% of women with syndrome X (Buchtal *et al.* 2000). More recently, Panting *et al.* (2002) provided further evidence of the presence of subendocardial hypoperfusion during the intravenous administration of adenosine in patients with syndrome X. All these findings contrast with those obtained with dobutamine stress echocardiography (Zouridakis *et al.* 2000; Panza *et al.* 1997), which showed the absence of regional wall motion abnormalities despite positive ECG responses in syndrome X patients. The absence of regional wall motion abnormalities on stress-echocardiographic studies have been attributed to patchy or diffuse microvascular constriction (Maseri *et al.* 1991). Also, as proposed by Zouridakis *et al.* (2000), mild subendocardial myocardial ischaemia may be undetected by echocardiography due to limitations of the technique or the compensatory effect of hypercontractile normally perfused myocardium.

Nonischaemic mechanism

Despite the occurrence of myocardial ischaemia in some syndrome X patients, it is accepted that nonischaemic mechanisms may explain the development of ST segment changes and chest pain in a large proportion of syndrome X patients. ST segment changes may be due to minor intramyocardial conduction abnormalities and pain may be the consequence of uncoordinated myocardial contractions (Perin *et al.* 1991). A further possibility is that ST segment depression might be related to atrial repolarization changes affecting the QRS complex. Atrial repolarization waves are opposite in direction to P waves and have a magnitude ranging from 100 to 200 μV and may thus extend into the ST segment and the T wave. If exaggerated, this phenomenon could cause ST segment depression during exercise, mimicking myocardial ischaemia (Sapin *et al.* 1991).

Further explanations to nonischaemic ST segment changes include abnormalities in adenosine and potassium homeostasis. Release of adenosine in the extracellular compartment may alter electrical conduction, myocardial contractility, the duration of the action potential and also elicit pain (Maseri *et al.* 1991). Potassium is released from the human myocardium under stressful conditions or increased heart rate. On cessation of the tachycardia the small net loss of potassium is replaced, thus ensuring a steady state. If patients with syndrome X release greater amounts of potassium, take potassium up more slowly or have minor anatomical changes in the orientation of myocardial cells and capillaries, potassium could be retained in the myocardium. Such an occurrence may account for all features of syndrome X, including ECG changes, the presence of chest pain, the long-term good prognosis and abnormal coronary vasoconstriction. Indeed, Bøtker *et al.* (1998) reported that patients with syndrome X exhibit enhanced exercise-induced hyperkalemia, compared to healthy controls. Interestingly, adenosine may also alter potassium fluxes and this may represent yet another mechanism whereby adenosine may be implicated in the pathogenesis of syndrome X. An important point, however, needs to be considered in this context. Although high extracellular concentrations of potassium have been associated with ST segment depressions similar to those observed in syndrome X during exercise, the peak serum potassium concentrations observed by Botker *et al.* (1998) were much lower than serum concentrations required to cause ST segment depression (8–12 mmol/L).

Ambulatory electrocardiography

Episodes of diagnostic ST segment depression during 24 h ECG monitoring is a common finding in syndrome X patients (Kaski *et al.* 1986). The circadian distribution of these episodes is similar to that observed in CAD patients and opposite to that seen in variant angina patients. In syndrome X patients, the ischaemic episodes occur predominantly during day time and are, on average, similar in duration and magnitude to episodes in CAD patients. The ischaemic threshold has been shown to be lower during the night and early morning hours, progressively increasing in the early afternoon hours and decreasing again in the evening (Lanza *et al.* 1995). Prolonged ST segment depression associated with anginal symptoms is not infrequent in these patients (Fig. 30.5). Both painful and silent ischaemic episodes have been equally described in syndrome X patients. Kaski *et al.* (1986) showed that 52% of Holter ST segment depression episodes in syndrome X patients were asymptomatic. Moreover, Frobert *et al.* (1996) found up to 90% of silent ST segment depression episodes in CPNCA patients. The large majority of ischaemic episodes during ambulatory ECG monitoring are heart rate related although a significant proportion are not preceded by an increase of heart rate (Kaski *et al.* 1995).

Twenty-four-hour ECG Holter monitoring has also been used to assess possible anomalies of autonomic control (heart rate variability, HRV, analysis) in syndrome X patients. Rosano *et al.* (1994) were the first to report that, compared with healthy controls patients with syndrome X had an imbalance of the autonomic nervous system, with a shift to-wards sympathetic predominance. The Rosano study (1994) showed that syndrome X patients had lower values of SDRR and pNN50, which are sensitive markers

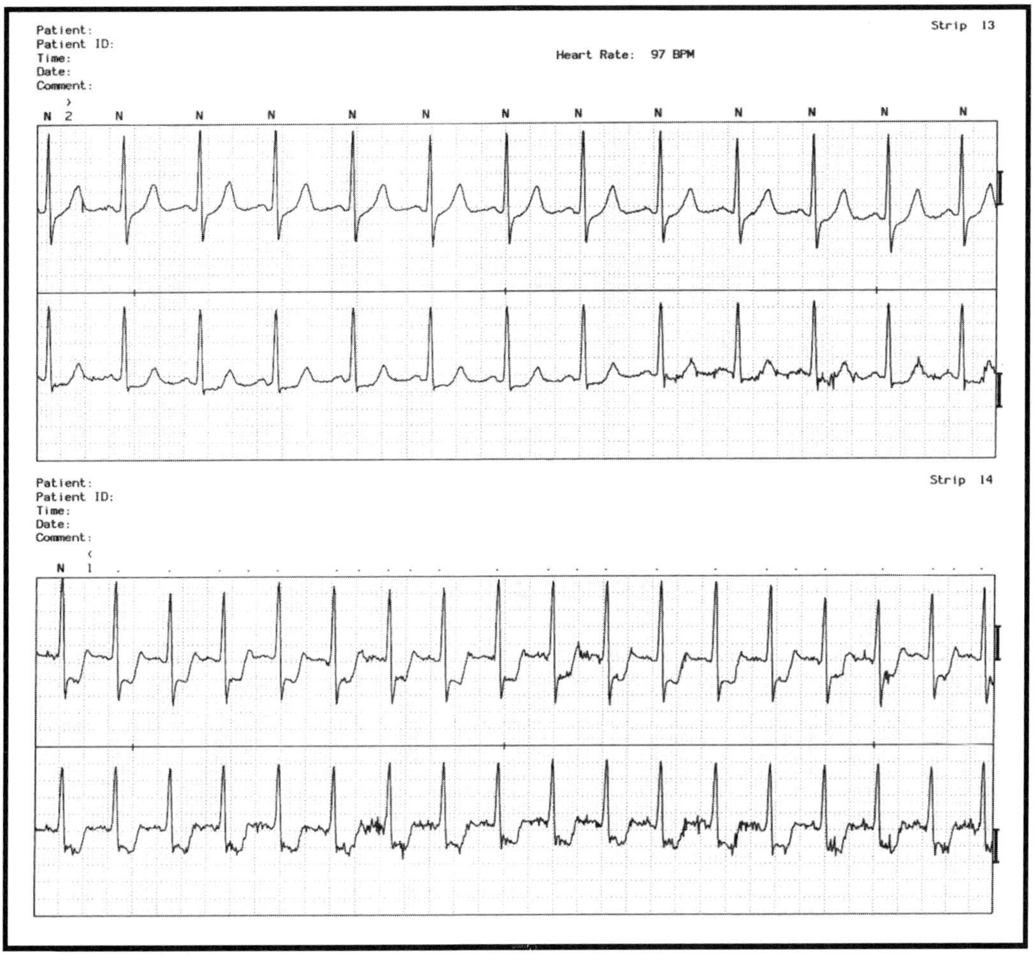

Fig. 30.5 ECG ambulatory monitoring trace during a daily life chest pain episode in a syndrome X patient.

of parasympathetic activity. The same group of investigators (Ponikowski *et al.* 1996) later showed that transient ST segment depression was associated with an imbalance of the autonomic nervous system. They found that episodes of ST segment depression accompanied by an increase in heart rate were preceded by a reduction of high-frequency power and an increase in low- to high-frequency ratio. No changes in these parameters were found preceding episodes of ST segment depression that were not associated with an increased heart rate. Among frequency-domain measures of HRV, the high-frequency power is considered to be a pure index of parasympathetic activity because it reflects the influence of respiratory sinus arrhythmia. Low-frequency power, however, is more controversial, as it seems to be related to both the sympathetic and parasympathetic systems. Ponikowski *et al.* (1996) concluded that in patients with syndrome X, a sympatho-vagal imbalance (sympathetic predominance due to vagal tone withdrawal) precedes episodes of ST segment depression that are associated with an increased heart rate. Finally, studies from the same group of researchers evaluated baroreceptor sensitivity in cardiac syndrome X patients by calculating the regression line relating phenylephrine-induced increases in systolic blood pressure to the attendant changes in the *RR* interval. They also studied sympatho-vagal balance by using HRV in the time and frequency domains and measuring plasma noradrenaline at rest and during incremental bicycle exercise in patients with: syndrome X, stable angina patients and healthy controls. Baroreceptor sensitivity was found to be significantly reduced in syndrome X and was associated with a lower percentage of adjacent normal *RR* intervals differing by >50 ms, lower root-mean-square of the difference of adjacent *RR* intervals, and lower logarithmic value of the high-frequency component in patients with syndrome X compared with normal subjects. No difference was detected in noradrenaline levels at rest or during exercise or between the three groups. Adamopoulos *et al.* (1998) concluded that patients with syndrome X have an im-paired baroreceptor sensitivity and a reduced HRV, without increased plasma levels of catecholamines. The latter finding is not concordant with results of a previous study (Ishihara *et al.* 1990) but the reasons for the discrepancy are not clear.

Holter monitoring studies have also shown significantly longer duration of both *QT* and *QTc* intervals in patients with syndrome X compared with age-matched controls (Mammana *et al.* 1997). Rosen *et al.* (1994) suggested that *QT* prolonga-tion was due to increased sympathetic activity. Mammana *et al.* (1997), however, found that the difference in the duration of *QT* and *QTc* between syndrome X patients and controls persisted even after strict heart rate matching, and was not associated with indirect markers of sympathetic activation, refuting Rosen *et al.* findings.

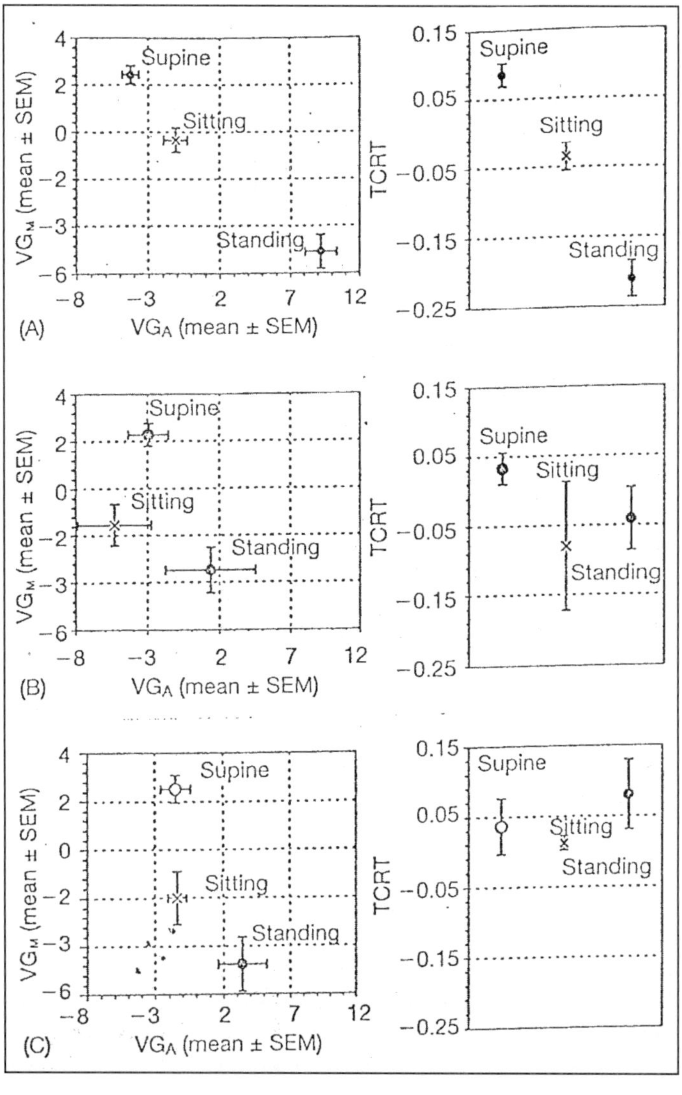

Fig. 30.6 Effect of posture in ventricular gradient (VG) and total RT cosine (TCRT) in healthy subjects (A), patients with syndrome X (B), and patients with syndrome X and normal T waves. (C) VG_A: angle of ventricular gradient (°), VG_M: magnitude of ventricular gradient (ms.mV), SEM: standard error of the mean.

Increased ventricular repolarization inhomogeneity in response to different manoeuvres has also been studied using Holter monitoring in syndrome X patients. Lee *et al.* (1998), showed that postural change from supine to standing position in syndrome X patients induced a higher increase in heart rate, a longer maximal *QTc* interval, and higher *QT* and *QTc* values when compared to controls and CAD patients. The authors explained these differences due to the activation of both sympathetic efferent input to the heart and adrenal gland as well as inhibition of the parasympathetic efferent input to the heart. Recently, Batchvarov *et al.* (2002) studied two descriptors of ventricular repolarization in syndrome X patients, the classical ventricular gradient (VG), which provides a global estimation of spatial heterogeneity of ventricular repolarization and the newly described TCRT (total *r* to T cosine) that quantifies the difference between the global direction of depolarization and repolarization, as expressed as an average cosine of the angles between the QRS and T vectors in a mathematically derived three-dimensional space. When compared to healthy controls, syndrome X patients had an attenuated response of VG and TCRT to postural changes and the Valsalva manoeuvre, which was independent of the presence of baseline T wave abnormalities (Fig. 30.6). They also found that syndrome X patients, but not control subjects, had a significantly increased QT dispersion during Valsalva manoeuvre. These findings taken together confirm the previously reported presence of abnormal autonomic control in syndrome X patients.

Conclusions

Cardiac syndrome X is heterogeneous in presentation and pathogenesis. Patients with syndrome X have ECG changes during exercise stress testing and during their daily life, as assessed by ambulatory ECG monitoring. ST segment shifts in these patients are similar to those found in CAD patients. Although myocardial ischaemia, mainly due to coronary microvascular dysfunction, may cause ST segment changes in some patients, other nonischaemic causes are likely to be responsible for the rest of syndrome X patients. Finally, syndrome X patients also have a reduced heart rate variability and an altered autonomic control of the cardiovascular system as shown in a large number of studies.

References

Adamopoulos, S., Rosano, G.M., Ponikowski, P. *et al.* (1998) Impaired baroreflex sensitivity and sympathovagal balance in syndrome X. *American Journal of Cardiology*, **82**, 862–868.

Batchvarov, V., Kaski, J.C., Parchure, N. *et al.* (2002) Comparison between ventricular gradient and a new descriptor of the wavefront of ventricular activation and recovery. *Clinical Cardiology*, **25**, 230–236.

Botker, H.E., Sonne, H.S., Frøbert, O. & Andreasen, F. (1999) Enhanced exercise-induced hyperkalemia in patients with syndrome X. *Journal of the American College of Cardiology*, **33**, 1056–1061.

Botker, H.E., Sonne, H.S., Schmitz, O. & Nielsen, T.T. (1998) Effects of doxazosin on exercise-induced angina pectoris, ST segment depression, and insulin sensitivity in patients with syndrome X. *American Journal of Cardiology*, **82**, 1352–1356.

Boudoulas, H., Cobb, T.C., Leighton, R.F. & Wilt, S.M. (1974) Myocardial lactate production in patients with angina-like chest pain and angiographically normal coronary arteries and left ventricle. *American Journal of Cardiology*, **84**, 501–505.

Buchtal, S., Den Hollander, J., Merz, B. *et al.* (2000) Abnormal myocardial phosphorus-31 nuclear magnetic resonance spectroscopy in women with chest pain but normal coronary angiograms. *New England Journal of Medicine*, **342**, 829–835.

Buffon, A., Rigattieri, S. & Santini, S.A. (2000) Myocardial ischaemia-reperfusion damage after pacing-induced tachycardia in patients with cardiac syndrome X. *American Journal of Physiology and Heart Circulatory Physiology*, **279**, H2627–H2633.

Bugiardini, R., Borghi, A., Biagetti, L., Puddu, P. (1989) Comparison of verapamil vs. propranolol therapy in syndrome X. *American Journal of Cardiology*, **63**, 286–290.

Cannon, R.O., III, Watson, R.M., Rosing, D.R. & Epstein, S.E. (1985) Efficacy of calcium channel blocker therapy for angina pectoris resulting from small-vessel coronary artery disease and abnormal vasodilator reserve. *American Journal of Cardiology*, **56**, 242–246.

Cannon, R.O., Dilsizian, V., Correa, R., Epstein, S.E. & Bonow, R.O. (1991) Chronic deterioration in left ventricular function in patients with microvascular angina. *Journal of the American College of Cardiology*, **17**, 28A.

Cunningham, C., Brown, S. & Kaski, J.C. (2000) Effects of transcendental meditation on symptoms and electrocardiographic changes in patients with cardiac syndrome X. *American Journal of Cardiology*, **85**, 653–655.

Cox, I.D., Hann, C.M., Kaski, J.C. (1998) Low dose imipramine improves chest pain but not quality of life in patients with angina and normal coronary angiograms. *European Heart Journal*, **19**, 250–254.

De Ambroggi, L. Bertoni, T., Breghi, M.L., Marconi, M. & Mosca, M. (1988) Diagnostic value of body surface potential mapping in old anterior non-Q myocardial infarction. *Journal of Electrocardiology*, **21**, 321–329.

Egashira, K., Inou, T., Hirooka, Y. *et al.* (1993) Evidence of impaired endothelium-dependent coronary vasodilatation in patients with angina pectoris and normal coronary angiograms. *New England Journal of Medicine*, **328**, 1659–1664.

Elliott, P.M., Krzyzowska-Dickinson, K., Calvino, R., Hann, C. & Kaski, J.C. (1997) Effect of oral aminophylline in patients with angina and normal coronary arteries (cardiac syndrome X). *Heart*, **77**, 523–526.

Fragasso, G., Chierchia, S.L., Pizzetti, G. *et al.* (1997) Impaired left ventricular filling dynamics in patients with angina and angiographically normal coronary arteries: effect of beta adrenergic blockade. *Heart*, **77**, 32–39.

Frobert, O., Funch-Jensen, P. & Bagger, J.P. (1996). Diagnostic value of esophageal studies in patients with angina-like chest pain and normal coronary angiograms. *Annals of Internal Medicine*, **11**, 959–969.

Gavrielides, S., Kaski, J.C., Galassi, A.R. *et al.* (1991) Recovery-phase patterns of ST segment depression in the heart rate domain cannot distinguish between anginal patients with coronary artery disease and patients with syndrome X. *American Heart Journal*, **122**, 1593–1598.

Green, L.S., Lux, R.L. & Haws, C.W. (1987) Detection and localization of coronary artery disease with body surface mapping in patients with normal electrocardiograms. *Circulation*, **76**, 1290–1297.

Ishihara, T., Seki, I., Yamada, Y.S. *et al.* (1990) Coronary circulation, myocardial metabolism and cardiac catecholamine flux in patients with syndrome X. *Journal of Cardiology*, **20**, 267–274.

Kaski, J.C. (1999) Cardiac syndrome X and microvascular angina. In: *Chest pain with normal coronary angiograms. Pathogenesis, diagnosis, and management* (ed. J.C. Kaski), 2nd edn, pp. 1–12. Kluwer Academic Publishers, Massachusetts.

Kaski, J.C., Crea, F., Nihoyannopoulos, P., Hackett, D. & Maseri, A. (1986) Transient myocardial ischaemia during daily life in patients with syndrome X. *American Journal of Cardiology*, **58**, 1242–1247.

Kaski, J.C., Rosano, G., Gavrielides, S. & Chen, L. (1994) Effects of angiotensin-converting enzyme inhibition on exercise induced angina and ST segment depression in patients with microvascular angina. *Journal of the American College of Cardiology*, **23**, 652–657.

Kaski, J.C., Rosano, G.M., Collins, P., Nihoyannopoulos, P., Maseri, A. & Poole-Wilson, P.A. (1995) Cardiac syndrome X: clinical characteristics and left ventricular function. Long-term follow-up study. *Journal of the American College of Cardiology*, **25**, 807–814.

Kaski, J.C., Valenzuela Garcia, L.F. (2001) Therapeutic options for the management of patients with cardiac syndrome X. *European Heart Journal*, **22**, 283–293.

Kemp, H.G., Kronmal, R.A., Vliestra, R.A. *et al.* (1986) Seven year survival of patients with normal or near normal coronary arteriograms: a CASS registry study. *Journal of the American College of Cardiology*, **7**, 479–485.

Kemp, H.G. (1973) Left ventricular function in patients with the anginal syndrome and normal coronary arteriograms. *American Journal of Cardiology*, **32**, 375–376.

Kornreich, F., Montaque, T.J. & Rautaharju, P.M. (1991) Identification of first acute Q wave and non-Q wave myocardial infarction by multivariate analysis of body surface potential maps. *Circulation*, **84**, 2442–2453.

Lanza, G.A., Stazi, F., Colonna, G. *et al.* (1995). Circadian variation of ischaemic threshold in syndrome X. *American Journal of Cardiology*, **75**, 683–686.

Lee, T.M., Su, S.F., Wang, T.D. *et al.* (1998) Increased ventricular repolarization inhomogeneity during postural changes in patients with syndrome X. *American Journal of Cardiology*, **82**, 615–620.

Leonardo, F., Fragasso, G., Rosano, G., Pagnotta, P. & Chierchia, S. (1997) Effect of atenolol on *QT* interval and dispersion in patients with Syndrome X. *American Journal of Cardiology*, **80**, 789–790.

Mammana, C., Salomone, O.A., Kautzner, J., Schwartzman, R.A. & Kaski, J.C. (1997) Heart rate-independent prolongation of *QTc* interval in women with syndrome X. *Clinical Cardiology*, **20**, 357–360.

Maseri, A., Crea, F., Kaski, J.C. & Crake, T. (1991) Mechanisms of angina pectoris in syndrome X. *Journal of the American College of Cardiology*, **17**, 499–506.

Montorsi, P., Cozzi, S., Loaldi, A. *et al.* (1990) Acute coronary vasomotor effects of nifedipine and therapeutic correlates in syndrome X. *American Journal of Cardiology*, **66**, 302–307.

Opherk, D., Schuler, G., Wetterauer, K., Manthey, J., Schwarz, F. & Kubler, W. (1989) Four-year follow-up in patients with angina pectoris and normal coronary arteriograms (syndrome X). *Circulation*, **80**, 1610–1616.

Panting, J., Gatehouse, P., Yang, G.Z. *et al.* (2002) Abnormal subendocardial perfusion in cardiac syndrome X detected by cardiovascular magnetic resonance imaging. *New England Journal of Medicine*, **346**, 1948–1953.

Panza, J.A., Laurienzo, J.M., Curiel, R.V. *et al.* (1997) Investigation of the mechanism of chest pain in patients with angiographically normal coronary arteries using transesophageal dobutamine stress echocardiography. *Journal of the American College of Cardiology*, **29**, 293–301.

Perin, E., Petersen, F. & Massuni, A. (1991) Rate-related left bundle branch block as a cause of a nonischaemic chest pain. *Catheterization and Cardiovascular Diagnosis*, **22**, 45–46.

Ponikowski, P., Rosano, G.M., Amadi, A.A. *et al.* (1996) Transient autonomic dysfunction precedes ST segment depression in patients with syndrome X. *American Journal of Cardiology*, **77**, 942–947.

Pupita, G., Kaski, J.C., Galassi, A.R., Gavrelides, S., Crea, F. & Maseri, A. (1990) Similar time course of ST depression during and after exercise in patients with coronary artery disease and syndrome X. *American Heart Journal*, **120**, 848–854.

Radice, M., Giudici, V., Albertini, A. & Mannarini, A. (1994) Usefulness of changes in exercise tolerance induced by nitroglycerin in identifying patients with syndrome X. *American Heart Journal*, **127**, 531–535.

Rosano, G.M., Kaski, J.C., Arie, S. *et al.* (1996) Failure to demonstrate myocardial ischaemia in patients with angina and normal coronary arteries. Evaluation by continuous coronary sinus pH monitoring and lactate metabolism. *European Heart Journal*, **17**, 1174–1179.

Rosano, G.M., Ponikowski, P., Adamopoulos, S. *et al.* (1994) Abnormal autonomic control of the cardiovascular system in syndrome X. *American Journal of Cardiology*, **73**, 1174–1979.

Rosen, S.D., Dritsas, A., Bourdillon, P.J. & Camici, P.G. (1994) Analysis of the electrocardiographic *QT* interval in patients with syndrome X. *American Journal of Cardiology*, **73**, 971–972.

Sapin, P.M., Koch, G., Blauwet, M.B., McCarthy, J.J., Hinds, S.W. & Gettes, L.S. (1991) Identification of false positive exercise tests with use of electrocardiographic criteria: a possible role for atrial repolarization waves. *Journal of the American College of Cardiology*, **18**, 127–135.

Zeiher, A., Krause, T., Schechinger, V., Minners, J. & Moser, E. (1995) Impaired endothelium dependent vasodilatation of coronary resistance vessels is associated with exercise induced myocardial ischaemia. *Circulation*, **91**, 2345–2352.

Zouridakis, E.G., Cox, I.D., Garcia-Moll, X., Brown, S., Nihoyannopoulus, P. & Kaski, J.C. (2000) Negative stress echocardiographic responses in normotensive and hypertensive patients with angina pectoris, positive exercise stress testing, an normal coronary arteriograms. *Heart*, **83**, 141–146.

SECTION IV
Ventricular Repolarization

CHAPTER 31

Cellular Basis for the Repolarization Waves of the ECG

Charles Antzelevitch*

Introduction

Willem Einthoven first recorded the electrocardiogram (ECG) at the turn of the century (Einthoven 1903; Einthoven 1912). Despite the span of 100 years, physicians and scientists are still learning how to extract valuable information from the ECG and continue to debate the cellular basis for the various waves of the ECG. Our focus in this chapter will be on the cellular basis for repolarization waves of the ECG, the J, T and U waves. The J wave and T wave are thought to arise as a consequence of voltage gradients that develop as a result of the electrical heterogeneities that exist within the ventricular myocardium. The basis for the U wave has long been a matter of debate. Three predominant theories prevail: one attributing the U wave to mechano-electrical feedback, another ascribing it to voltage gradients within ventricular myocardium, and a third to voltage gradients between the ventricular myocardium and the His–Purkinje system.

A brief description of the electrical heterogeneities intrinsic to ventricular myocardium is provided in order to facilitate our understanding of the heterogeneities responsible for the inscription of the ECG. Over the past decade and half, studies from several laboratories have demonstrated that ventricular myocardium is not homogeneous as previously thought. A number of studies have highlighted regional differences in electrical properties of ventricular cells as well as differences in the response of the different cell types to pharmacological agents and pathophysiological states (for reviews see Antzelevitch *et al.* 1999; Antzelvitch & Dumaine 2001). Among the heterogeneities uncovered are electrical and pharmacological distinctions between endocardium and epicardium of the canine, feline, rabbit, rat and human heart as well as differences in the electrophysiological characteristics and pharmacological responsiveness of M cells located in the deep structures of the ventricles of the heart.

Ventricular epicardial and M, but not endocardial, action potentials display a prominent phase 1, owing to a prominent transient outward current (I_{to}), giving rise to a spike and dome or notched configuration. Regional differences in I_{to} have been demonstrated in canine, feline, rabbit, rat, and human ventricular myocytes (for references see Antzelvitch & Dumaine 2002). Important differences also exist in the magnitude of I_{to} and action potential notch between right and left ventricular epicardial and M cells with right ventricular cells displaying a much greater I_{to} (Di Diego *et al.* 1996; Volders *et al.* 1999).

M cells are distinguished by the ability of their action potential to prolong more than those of epicardial and endocardial cells in response to a slowing of rate and/or in response to drugs with *QT*-prolonging actions (Sicouri & Antzelvitch 1991). The ionic basis for these characteristics features include the presence of a smaller slowly activating delayed rectifier current (I_{Ks}), a larger late sodium current (late I_{Na}), and a larger electrogenic sodium–calcium exchange current ($I_{Na\text{-}Ca}$). Cells with M cell characteristics have been reported in the canine,

Supported by grants from the National Institutes of Health (HL 47678), the American Heart Association, Northeast Affiliate, and the Masons of New York State and Florida.

guinea pig, rabbit, pig and human ventricles (for references see Antzelvitch & Shimizu 2002).

J wave

A prominent action potential notch in epicardium but not endocardium gives rise to a transmural voltage gradient during ventricular activation that manifests as a late delta wave following the QRS or what more commonly is referred to as a J wave (Yan & Antzelvitch 1996) or Osborn wave. A distinct J wave is often observed under baseline conditions in the ECG of some animal species, including dogs and baboons. Humans more commonly display a J point elevation rather than a distinct J wave. A prominent J wave in the human ECG is considered pathognomonic of hypothermia (Clements & Hurst 1972; Thompson *et al.* 1977; Eagle 1994) or hypercalcaemia (Kraus 1920; Sridharan & Horan 1984).

A transmural gradient in the distribution of I_{to} is responsible for the transmural gradient in the magnitude of phase 1 and action potential notch, which gives rise to a voltage gradient across the ventricular wall responsible for the inscription of the J wave or J point elevation in the ECG (Antzelevitch *et al.* 1995; Litovsky & Antzelevitch 1988; Liu *et al.* 1993). Direct evidence in support of the hypothesis that the J wave is caused by a transmural gradient in the magnitude of the I_{to}-mediated action potential notch derives from experiments conducted in the arterially-perfused right ventricular wedge preparation (Fig. 31.1) (Yan & Antzelevitch 1996) showing a correlation between the amplitude of the epicardial action potential notch and that of the J wave recorded during interventions that alter the appearance of the electrocardiographic J wave, including hypothermia, premature stimulation (restitution), and block of I_{to} by 4-AP (Fig. 31.2). The molecular basis for the transmural distribution of I_{to} was recently demonstrated to be due to the distribution of KChIP2, a subunit that coassembles with Kv4.3 product to form the I_{to} channel (Rosati *et al.* 2001).

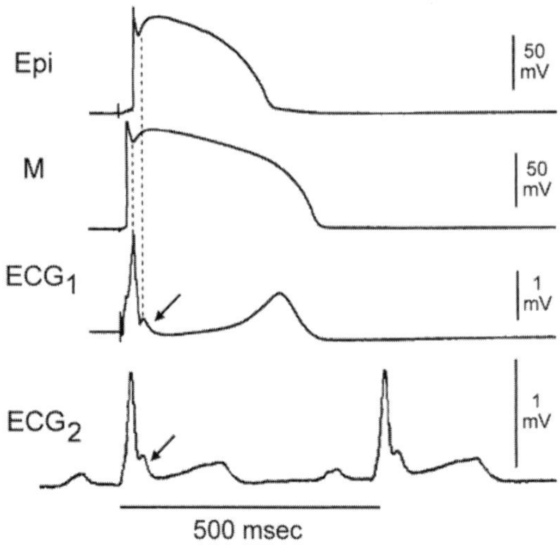

Fig. 31.1 Relationship between the spike-and-dome morphology of the epicardial action potential and the appearance of the J wave. ECG_2 is a lead V5 ECG recorded from the dog *in vivo*. ECG_1 is a transmural ECG recorded across the bath in which the arterially perfused left ventricular wedge isolated from the heart of the same dog was placed. Both display a prominent J wave (arrows). The two upper traces are transmembrane action potentials simultaneously recorded from the epicardial (Epi) and M regions with floating microelectrodes. The preparation was paced at a basic cycle length of 4000 ms. The sinus cycle length at the time ECG_2 was recorded was 500 ms. The J wave is temporally coincident with the notch of the epicardial action potential. (From Yan & Antzelevitch 1996, with permission.)

Because the right ventricular wall is relatively thin, transmural activation may be so rapid as to cause the J wave to be buried inside the QRS. Thus, although the action potential notch is most prominent in right ventricular epicardium, right ventricular myocardium would be expected to contribute relatively little to the manifestation of the J wave. These observations are consistent with the manifestation of the J wave in ECG leads in which the mean vector axis is transmurally oriented across the left ventricle and septum. Accordingly, the J wave in the dog is most prominent in leads II, III, aVR, aVF, and mid to left precordial leads V3 to V6. A similar picture is seen in the human ECG (Sridharan & Horan 1984; Eagle 1994). In addition, vectorcardiography indicates that the J wave forms an extra loop that occurs at the junction of the QRS and T loops (Emslie-Smith *et al.* 1959). It is directed leftward and anteriorly, which explains its prominence in leads associated with the left ventricle.

The first description of the J wave was in animal experiments involving hypercalcemia conducted in the 1920s (Kraus 1920). The first

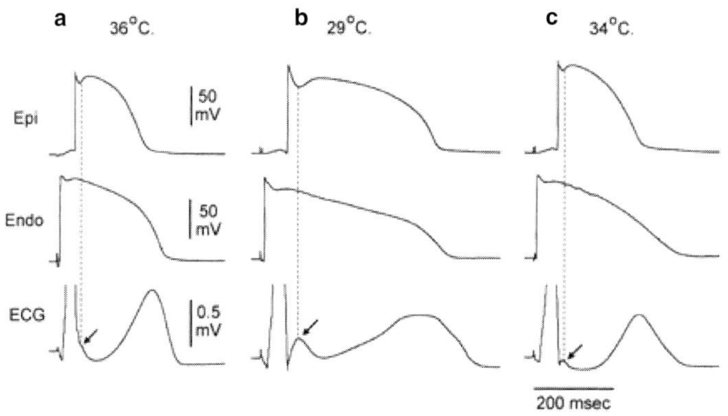

Fig. 31.2 Effect of hypothermia on action potential and ECG morphology. Each panel shows transmembrane recordings obtained from the epicardial (Epi) and endocardial (Endo) regions of an arterially perfused canine left ventricular wedge and a transmural ECG recorded simultaneously. (a) A small but distinct action potential notch in epicardium but not in endocardium is associated with an elevated J point at the R–ST junction (arrow) at 36°. (b) A decrease in the temperature of the perfusate and bath to 29°C results in an increase in the amplitude and width of the action potential notch in epicardium but not in endocardium, leading to a prominent J wave on the transmural ECG (arrow). (c) Re-warming to a temperature of 34°C is attended by a parallel reduction in the amplitude and width of the J wave and epicardial action potential notch. (From Yan & Antzelevitch 1996, with permission.)

extensive description and characterization appeared 30 years later by Osborn in a study involving experimental hypothermia in dogs (Osborn 1953).

The appearance of a prominent J wave in the clinic is typically associated with pathophysiological conditions, including hypothermia (Clements & Hurst 1972; Eagle 1994) and hypercalcemia (Kraus 1920; Sridharan & Horan 1984). The prominent J wave induced by hypothermia is the result of a marked accentuation of the spike-and-dome morphology of the action potential of M and epicardial cells (i.e. an increase in both width and magnitude of the notch) as illustrated in Fig. 31.2. In addition to inducing a more prominent notch, hypothermia produces a slowing of conduction which permits the epicardial notch to clear the QRS so as to manifest a distinct J wave.

Association of hypercalcemia with the appearance of the J wave (Kraus 1920; Sridharan *et al.* 1983; Sridharan & Horan 1984) may also be explained on the basis of an accentuation of the epicardial action potential notch, possibly as a result of an augmentation of the calcium-activated chloride current and a decrease in I_{Ca} (Di Diego & Antzelevitch 1994).

The presence of a prominent action potential notch predisposes canine ventricular epicardium to all-or-none repolarization and phase 2 re-entry. Under ischaemic conditions and in response to sodium channel blockers, parasympathetic agonists, potassium channel blockers and a variety of other drugs, canine ventricular epicardium exhibits an all-or-none repolarization at the end of phase 1 of the action potential, leading to a marked (40–70%) abbreviation of the action potential. Failure of the action potential dome to develop at some epicardial sites but not others, gives rise to a marked dispersion of repolarization. Propagation of the action potential dome from sites at which it is maintained to sites at which it is abolished can cause local re-excitation of the preparation. This mechanism, called phase 2 re-entry, produces a very closely coupled extrasystole, which can in turn initiate one or more cycles of circus movement re-entry (Antzelevitch & Dumaine 2002). Because the J wave provides an index of the prominence of the spike-and-dome morphology of the epicardial response, it can be of diagnostic value in iden-tifying subjects predisposed to phase 2 re-entry or individuals who may be inclined to develop life-threatening arrhythmias such as the Brugada syndrome and other forms of idiopathic ventricular fibrillation (Yan & Antzelevitch 1999; Antzelevitch 2001). The accentuation of epicardial action potential and eventual loss of the dome is thought to underlie the *ST* segment elevation and arrhythmogenic substrate associ-

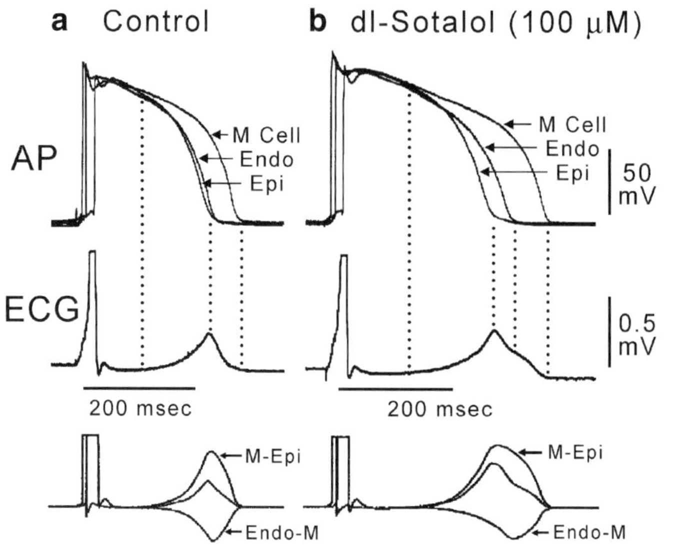

Fig. 31.3 Voltage gradients on either side of the M region are responsible for inscription of the electrocardiographic T wave. Top: Action potentials simultaneously recorded from endocardial, epicardial and M region sites of an arterially-perfused canine left ventricular wedge preparation. Middle: ECG recorded across the wedge. Bottom: Computed voltage differences between the epicardium and M region action potentials ($\Delta V_{M\text{-}Epi}$) and between the M region and endocardium responses ($\Delta V_{Endo\text{-}M}$). If these traces are representative of the opposing voltage gradients on either side of the M region, responsible for inscription of the T wave, then the weighted sum of the two traces should yield a trace (middle trace in bottom grouping) resembling the ECG, which it does. The voltage gradients are weighted to account for differences in tissue resistivity between M and Epi and Endo and M regions, thus yielding the opposing currents flowing on either side of the M region. (a) Under control conditions the T wave begins when the plateau of epicardial action potential separates from that of the M cell. As epicardium repolarizes, the voltage gradient between epicardium and the M region continues to grow giving rise to the ascending limb of the T wave. The voltage gradient between the M region and epicardium ($\Delta V_{M\text{-}Epi}$) reaches a peak when the epicardium is fully repolarized – this marks the peak of the T wave. On the other end of the ventricular wall, the endocardial plateau deviates from that of the M cell, generating an opposing voltage gradient ($\Delta V_{Endo\text{-}M}$) and corresponding current that limits the amplitude of the T wave and contributes to the initial part of the descending limb of the T wave. The voltage gradient between the endocardium and the M region reaches a peak when the endocardium is fully repolarized. The gradient continues to decline as the M cells repolarize. All gradients are extinguished when the longest M cells are fully repolarized. (b) dl-sotalol (100 μM) prolongs the action potential of the M cell more than those of the epicardial and endocardial cells, thus widening the T wave and prolonging the *QT* interval. The greater separation of epicardial and endocardial repolarization times also gives rise to a notch in the descending limb of the T wave. Once again, the T wave begins when the plateau of epicardial action potential diverges from that of the M cell. The same relationships as described for panel (a) are observed during the remainder of the T wave. The sotalol-induced increase in dispersion of repolarization across the wall is accompanied by a corresponding increase in the T_{peak}–T_{end} interval in the pseudo-ECG. (Modified from Yan & Antzelevitch 1998, with permission.)

ated with the Brugada syndrome (Antzelevitch *et al.* 2002).

T wave

Studies involving the arterially-perfused wedge have provided new insights into the cellular basis of the T wave showing that currents flowing down voltage gradients on either side of the M region are in large part responsible for the T wave (Fig. 31.3) (Yan & Antzelevitch 1998). The interplay between these opposing forces establishes the height and width of the T wave and the degree to which either the ascending or descending limb of the T wave is interrupted, leading to a bifurcated or notched appearance of the T wave. The voltage gradients result from a more positive plateau potential in the M region than in epicardium or endocardium and from differences in the time-course of phase 3 of the action potential of the three predominant ventricular cell types. Under normal and long *QT* conditions, the epicardial response is the earliest to repolarize and the M cell action potential is often the last. Full repolarization of the epicardial action potential is coincident with peak of the T wave and repolarization of the M cells coincides with the end of the T wave. Under these conditions, the T_{peak}–T_{end} interval provides an index of transmural dispersion of repolarization, which may prove to be a valuable prognostic tool (Antzelevitch 1997; Yan & Antzelevitch 1998).

Validation of the T_{peak}–T_{end} interval as an index of transmural dispersion and as an arrhythmogenic risk factor has been provided in several reports demonstrating a prolongation of this parameter under a variety of conditions known to predispose to Torsade de Pointes arrhythmias (Antzelevitch & Shimizu 2002; Lubinski *et al.* 1998; Sarubbi *et al.* 1999; Tun *et al.* 1999; Tanabe *et al.* 2001; Pietila *et al.* 2002; Viitasalo *et al.* 2002; Yoshiga *et al.* 2002). Further studies are needed to assess the value of these noninvasive indices of electrical heterogeneity and their prognostic value in the assignment of arrhythmic risk.

More recent investigations involving the wedge suggest that the area between the peak and end of the T wave may provide an index of TDR over a wider set of conditions (M. Tsuboi & C. Antzelevitch unpublished observations). It is noteworthy that van Opstal and co-workers recently reported that in the chronic AV block dog, the JT area (area of the entire T wave) correlates well with interventricular dispersion of repolarization, another index of risk for the development of TdP (van Opstal *et al.* 2002).

Transmural dispersion of repolarization should not be confused with QT dispersion of repolarization, another proposed risk factor, which remains somewhat controversial (Antzelevitch *et al.* 1998; Batchvarov & Malik 2000; Malik *et al.* 2000).

Apico-basal repolarization gradients measured along the epicardial surface have been suggested to play a role in the registration of the T wave (Cohen *et al.* 1976). In contrast, more recent studies involving the perfused wedge suggest little or no contribution, owing to the fact that the ECG recorded along the apico-basal axis fails to display a T wave (Fig. 31.4) (Yan & Antzelevitch 1998). These findings suggest that in this part of the canine left ventricular wall (anterior, mid apico-basal) the inscription of the T wave is largely the result of voltage gradients along the transmural axis.

U wave

Since the original description of the U wave by Einthoven (1912), various theories have been proposed to explain its origin: (a) ventricular septum (Zuckerman *et al.* 1947); (b) papillary muscles (Furbetta *et al.* 1956); (c) negative afterpotentials (Nahum & Hoff 1939; Lepeschkin 1957); (d) Purkinje system (Hoffman & Cranefield 1960; Watanabe 1975); (e) early or delayed afterdepolarizations (Lepeschkin 1957); or (f) 'mechano-electrical feedback' (Lab 1982; Choo & Gibson 1986).

The most popular hypothesis ascribes the U wave to delayed repolarization of the His–Purkinje system (Hoffman & Cranefield 1960; Watanabe 1975). The small mass of the specialized conduction system is difficult to reconcile with the sometimes very large U wave deflections reported in the literature, especially in cases of acquired and congenital long QT syndrome. In 1996, we suggested that the M cells, more abundant in mass and possessing delayed repolarization characteristics similar to those of Purkinje fibres, may be responsible for the inscription of the pathophysiological U wave (Antzelevitch *et al.* 1996). More recent findings derived from the wedge clearly indicate that what many clinicians refer to as an accentuated or inverted U wave is not a U wave, but rather a component of the T wave whose descending or ascending limb (especially during hypokalemia) is interrupted (Fig. 31.5) (Shimizu & Antzelevitch 1997; Yan & Antzelevitch 1998). A transient reversal in current flow across the ventricular wall due to shifting voltage gradients between epicardium and the M region and endocardium and the M region underlies this phenomenon. The data suggest that the 'pathophysiological U wave' that develops under conditions of acquired or congenital LQTS is part of the T wave and that the various hump morphologies represent different levels of interruption of the ascending limb of

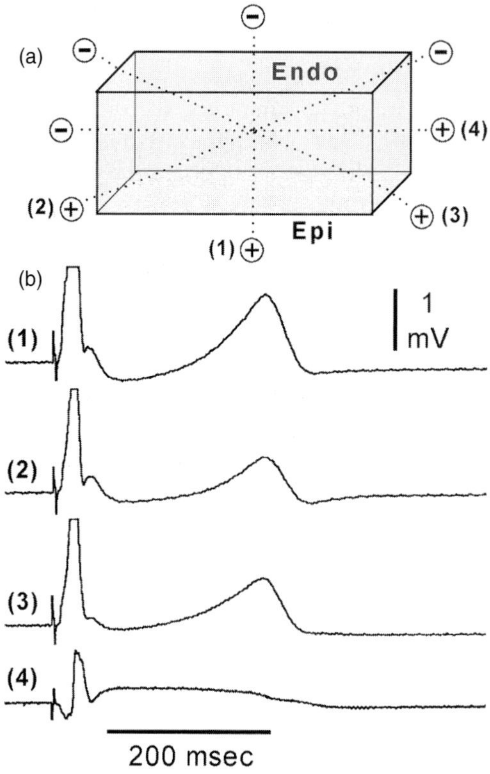

Fig. 31.4 Transient shift of voltage gradients on either side of the M region results in T wave bifurcation. The format is the same as in Fig. 31.3. All traces were simultaneously recorded from an arterially perfused left ventricular wedge preparation. (a) Control. (b) In the presence of hypokalemia ($[K^+]_o$ = 1.5 mM), the I_{Kr} blocker dl-sotalol (100 μM) prolongs the *QT* interval and produces a bifurcation of the T wave, a morphology some authors refer to as TU complex. The rate of repolarization of phase 3 of the action potential is slowed giving rise to smaller opposing transmural currents that cross over producing a low amplitude bifid T wave. Initially the voltage gradient between the epicardium and M regions (M-Epi) is greater than that between endocardium and M region (Endo-M). When endocardium pulls away from the M cell, the opposing gradient (Endo-M) increases, interrupting the ascending limb of the T wave. Predominance of the M-Epi gradient is restored as the epicardial response continues to repolarize and the Epi-M gradients increases, thus resuming the ascending limb of the T wave. Full repolarization of epicardium marks the peak of the T wave. Repolarization of both endocardium and the M region contribute importantly to the descending limb. BCL = 1000 ms. (Modified from Yan & Antzelevitch 1998, with permission.)

the T wave, arguing for use of the term T2 in place of U to describe these events, as previously suggested by Lehmann *et al.* (Yan & Antzelevitch 1998; Lehmann *et al.* 1994).

While delayed repolarization of the M cells contributes to the inscription of T2 (pathophysiological U wave), it is unlikely that it is responsible for the normal U wave, the very small distinct deflection following the T wave. The repolarization of the His–Purkinje system as previously suggested by Hoffman, Cranfield and Lepeshkin (Hoffman & Cranefield 1960) and by Watanabe and coworkers (Watanabe 1975) remains a most plausible hypothesis. Repolarization of the Purkinje system is temporally aligned with the expected appearance of the U wave in the perfused wedge preparation (Fig. 31.6) (Yan & Antzelevitch 1998). The lack of a U wave in the wedge may be related to a low density of the Purkinje system in the dog. A test of this hypothesis awaits the availability of an experimental model displaying a prominent U wave (most animal species do not manifest a U wave).

Support for the Purkinje hypothesis derives from the recent finding that isoproterenol-induced changes in the repolarization of Purkinje fibres parallel those of the U wave (Burashnikov & Antzelevitch 1999). In healthy humans, isoproterenol abbreviates both *QT* and *QU* intervals, whereas in LQT1 patients (defective I_{Ks}) isoproterenol remarkably prolongs the *QT* interval but apparently abbreviates the *QU* interval (Zhang *et al.* 1999). Experimental studies involving canine left ventricular M cell preparations and Purkinje fibres demonstrate that isoproterenol abbreviates the action potential of both cell types under normal conditions, but that under conditions mimicking LQT1 (use of chromanol 293B to block I_{Ks}) isoproterenol abbreviates the Purkinje fibre action potential, but markedly prolongs that of the M cell (Burashnikov & Antzelevitch 1999). The isoproterenol-induced changes in the action potential duration (APD) of Purkinje parallel those of the QU interval, thus providing indirect support for the hypothesis that repolarization of the Purkinje system is responsible for the inscription of the U wave.

A second hypothesis that endures despite lack of direct experimental and clinical evidence is that the normal U wave is associated with the

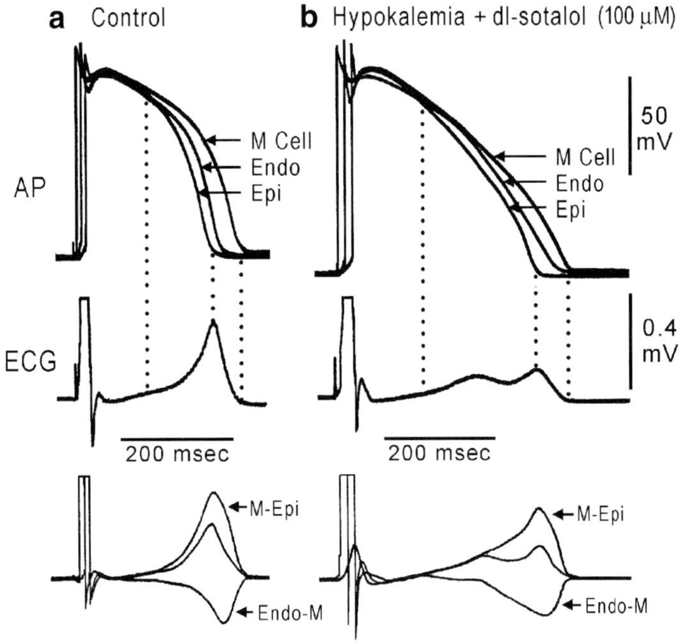

Fig. 31.5 Contribution of transmural vs. apico-basal and anterior–posterior gradients to the registration of the T wave. The four ECG traces were simultaneously recorded at 0°, 45°, −45°, and 90° (apico-basal) angles relative to the transmural axis of an arterially-perfused left ventricular wedge preparation. Inscription of the T wave is largely the result of voltage gradients along the transmural axis. (Modified from Yan & Antzelevitch 1998, with permission.)

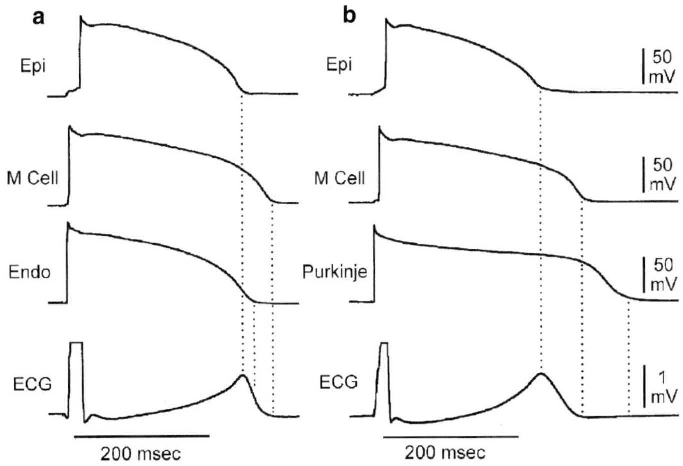

Fig. 31.6 Correlation of transmembrane and electrocardiographic activity. Transmembrane potentials and a transmural ECG recorded from two different arterially-perfused canine left ventricular wedge preparations. (a) Action potentials from epicardial (Epi), mid myocardial (M) and endocardial (Endo) sites were simultaneously recorded using floating glass microelectrodes. A transmural ECG was recorded concurrently across the bath. (b) Action potentials from epicardium (Epi), midmyocardium (M) and subendocardial Purkinje were recorded simultaneously together with a transmural ECG. In both cases, repolarization of epicardium is coincident with the peak of the T wave of the ECG, whereas repolarization of the M cells is coincident with the end of the T wave. The endocardial APD is intermediate (a). Note that although repolarization of the Purkinje fibre occurs after that of the M cell (b), it does not register on the ECG. BCL = 2000 ms. (Modified from Yan & Antzelevitch 1998, with permission.)

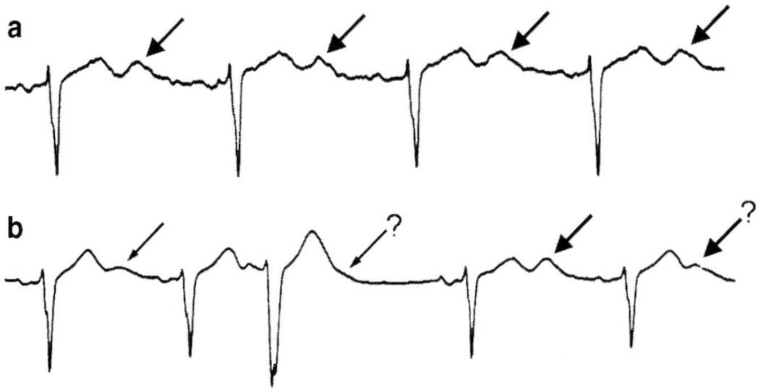

Fig. 31.7 Spectrum of TU transitions recorded in the 71-year-old male on amiodarone (for atrial fibrillation). Lead II. (a) The U wave (thick arrows) is completely separated from the T wave and may be erroneously excluded in measurement of the *QT* interval. The *QTc* (without the U) is 400 ms, too short for a patient on amiodarone, whereas the *QTc* (with the U) is 600 ms, very long even for a patient on amiodarone. In this case, the U wave is pathologic (T2) and the *QT* is abnormally prolonged. (b) ECG recorded the next day in the same patient. The U waves are greatly diminished (thin arrows) but seem to become much more prominent (thick arrows) following a postextrasystolic compensatory pause. The postpause T2 augmentation suggests that, regardless of their origin, these pathophysiological waves reflect early afterdepolarizations (EADs), increased dispersion of repolarization or both. Question marks indicate intermediate TU configurations that are very difficult to classify as either T2 or U.

mechanical activity of the heart (mechano-electrical feed-back). Initially proposed by Lepeshkin (Lepeschkin 1957) and more recently advocated by Surawicz (1998), this hypothesis emphasizes the coincidence between the start of the U wave and the second heart sound, suggesting that mechanical mechanisms associated with the opening of the AV valves generate afterpotentials that are responsible for the appearance of the normal U wave.

The distinction between a T2 and U wave is critically important from the standpoint of identifying potential risk of agents that prolong the *QT* interval. A continuous spectrum of TU transitions can make distinction of the two difficult at times. Such distinction however becomes paramount when studying the effects of agents with class III antiarrhythmic actions. *QTc* may be grossly underestimated if a T2 is judged to be a U wave and excluded from the measurement of the *QT* interval. Figure 31.7 shows a clinical example in a patient receiving amiodarone, illustrating how such confusion can arise. The prominent apparent U waves are actually T2 waves. If excluded from the measurement of *QT*, a value of 400 ms would be obtained, far shorter than the actual *QT* interval of 600 ms (Sami Viskin persomal communication).

References

Antzelevitch, C., Brugada, P., Brugada, J. *et al.* (2002) Brugada syndrome: a decade of progress. *Circulation Research*, **91**, 1114–1118.

Antzelevitch, C. & Dumaine R. (2001) Electrical heterogeneity in the heart: physiological, pharmacological and clinical implications. In: *Handbook of Physiology. The Heart* (eds E. Page, H.A. Fozzard & R.J. Solaro), pp. 654–692. Oxford University Press, New York.

Antzelevitch, C., Nesterenko, V.V. & Yan, G.X. (1996) The role of M cells in acquired long QT syndrome, U waves and torsade de pointes. *Journal of Electrocardiology*, **28**, 131–138.

Antzelevitch, C., Shimizu, W., Yan, G.X. *et al.* (1999) The M cell. Its contribution to the ECG and to normal and abnormal electrical function of the heart. *Journal of Cardiovascular Electrophysiology*, **10**, 1124–1152.

Antzelevitch, C., Shimizu, W., Yan, G.X. *et al.* (1998) Cellular basis for QT dispersion. *Journal of Electrocardiology*, **30**, 168–175.

Antzelevitch, C. & Shimizu, W. (2002) Cellular mechanisms underlying the long QT syndrome. *Current Opinion in Cardiology*, **17**, 43–51.

Antzelevitch, C., Sicouri, S., Lukas, A. *et al.* (1995) Regional differences in the electrophysiology of ventricular cells: Physiological and clinical implications. In: *Cardiac Electrophysiology: From Cell to Bedside* (eds D.P. Zipes & J. Jalife), pp. 228–245. W.B. Saunders, Philadelphia.

Antzelevitch, C. (1997) The M cell. Invited editorial comment. *Journal of Cardiovascular Pharmacology and Therapeutics*, **2**, 73–76.

Antzelevitch, C. (2001) The Brugada syndrome: ionic basis and arrhythmia mechanisms. *Journal of Cardiovascular Electrophysiology*, **12**, 268–272.

Batchvarov, V. & Malik M. (2000) Measurement and interpretation of *QT* dispersion. *Progress in Cardiovascular Diseases*, **42**, 325–344.

Burashnikov, A. & Antzelevitch, C. (1999) Is the Purkinje system the source of the electrocardiographic U wave? *Circulation*, **100**, II-386 (abstract).

Choo, M.H. & Gibson, D.G. (1986) U waves in ventricular hypertrophy: possible demonstration of mechanoelectrical feedback. *British Heart Journal*, **55**, 428–433.

Clements, S.D. & Hurst, J.W. (1972) Diagnostic value of ECG abnormalities observed in subjects accidentally exposed to cold. *American Journal of Cardiology*, **29**, 729–734.

Cohen, I.S., Giles, W.R. & Noble, D. (1976) Cellular basis for the T wave of the electrocardiogram. *Nature (London)*, **262**, 657–661.

Di Diego, J.M. & Antzelevitch, C. (1994) High [Ca^{2+}]-induced electrical heterogeneity and extrasystolic activity in isolated canine ventricular epicardium: Phase 2 re-entry. *Circulation*, **89**, 1839–1850.

Di Diego, J.M., Sun, Z.Q. & Antzelevitch, C. (1996) I_{to} and action potential notch are smaller in left vs. right canine ventricular epicardium. *American Journal of Physiology*, **271**, H548–H561.

Eagle, K. (1994) Images in clinical medicine. Osborn waves of hypothermia. *New England Journal of Medicine*, **10**, 680.

Einthoven, W. (1903) The galvanometric registration of the human electrocardiogram, likewise a review of the use of the capillary electrometer in physiology. *Pfluegers Archiv*, **99**, 472–480.

Einthoven, W. (1912) Über die Deutung des Electrokardiogramms. *Pfluegers Archiv*, **149**, 65–86.

Emslie-Smith, D., Sladden, G.E., Stirling, G.R. (1959) The significance of changes in the electrocardiogram in hypothermia. *British Heart Journal*, **21**, 343–351.

Furbetta, D., Bufalari, A., Santucci, F. *et al.* (1956) Abnormality of the U wave and the T–U segment of the electrocardiogram: the syndrome of the papillary muscles. *Circulation*, **14**, 1129–1137.

Hoffman, B.F. & Cranefield, P.F. (1960) *Electrophysiology of the Heart*. McGraw-Hill, New York.

Kraus, F. (1920) Ueber die Wirkung des Kalziums auf den Kreislauf. *Deutsche Mediziniche Wochenschrift*, **46**, 201–203.

Lab, M.J. (1982) Contraction–excitation feedback in myocardium: physiological basis and clinical relevance. *Circulation Research*, **50**, 757–766.

Lehmann, M.H., Suzuki, F., Fromm, B.S. *et al.* (1994) T wave 'humps' as a potential electrocardiographic marker of the long QT syndrome. *Journal of the American College of Cardiology*, **24**, 746–754.

Lepeschkin, E. (1957) Genesis of the U wave. *Circulation*, **15**, 77–81.

Litovsky, S.H. & Antzelevitch, C. (1988) Transient outward current prominent in canine ventricular epicardium but not endocardium. *Circulation Research*, **62**, 116–126.

Liu, D.W., Gintant, G.A. & Antzelevitch, C. (1993) Ionic bases for electrophysiological distinctions among epicardial, midmyocardial, and endocardial myocytes from the free wall of the canine left ventricle. *Circulation Research*, **72**, 671–687.

Lubinski, A., Lewicka-Nowak, E., Kempa, M. *et al.* (1998) New insight into repolarization abnormalities in patients with congenital long QT syndrome: the increased transmural dispersion of repolarization. *PACE (Pacing and Clinical Electrophysiolgy)*, **21**, 172–175.

Malik, M., Acar, B., Gang, Y. *et al.* (2000) QT dispersion does not represent electrocardiographic interlead heterogeneity of ventricular repolarization. *Journal of Cardiovascular Electrophysiology*, **11**, 835–843.

Nahum, L.H. & Hoff, H.E. (1939) The interpretation of the U wave of the electrocardiogram. *American Heart Journal*, **17**, 585–598.

van Opstal, J.M., Verduyn, S.C., Winckels, S.K. *et al.* (2002) The JT-area indicates dispersion of repolarization in dogs with atrioventricular block. *Journal of Interventional Cardiac Electrophysiology*, **l6**, 113–120.

Osborn, J.J. (1953) Experimental hypothermia: respiratory and blood pH changes in relation to cardiac function. *American Journal of Physiology*, **175**, 389–398.

Pietila E., Fodstad, H., Niskasaari, E. *et al.* (2002) Association between HERG K897T polymorphism and *QT* interval in middle-aged Finnish women. *Journal of the American College of Cardiology*, **40**, 511–514.

Rosati, B., Pan, Z., Lypen, S. *et al.* (2001) Regulation of KChIP2 potassium channel beta subunit gene expression underlies the gradient of transient outward current in canine and human ventricle. *Journal of Physiology*, **533**, 119–125.

Sarubbi, B., Pacileo, G., Ducceschi, V. *et al.* (1999) Arrhythmogenic substrate in young patients with repaired tetralogy of Fallot: role of an abnormal ventricular repolarization. *International Journal of Cardiology*, **72**, 73–82.

Shimizu, W., Antzelevitch, C. (1997) Sodium channel block with mexiletine is effective in reducing dispersion of repolarization and preventing Torsade de Pointes in LQT2 and LQT3 models of the long-QT syndrome. *Circulation*, **96**, 2038–2047.

Sicouri, S. & Antzelevitch, C. (1991) A subpopulation of cells with unique electrophysiological properties in the deep subepicardium of the canine ventricle: the M cell. *Circulation Research*, **68**, 1729–1741.

Sridharan, M.R. & Horan, L.G. (1984) Electrocardiographic J wave of hypercalcemia. *American Journal of Cardiology*, **54**, 672–673.

Sridharan, M.R., Johnson, J.C., Horan, L.G. *et al.* (1983) Monophasic action potentials in hypercalcemic and hypothermic 'J' waves-a comparative study. *American Federation of Clinical Research*, **31**, 219.

Surawicz, B. (1998) U wave: facts, hypotheses, misconceptions, and misnomers. *Journal of Cardiovascular Electrophysiology*, **9**, 1117–1128.

Tanabe, Y., Inagaki, M., Kurita, T. *et al.* (2001) Sympathetic stimulation produces a greater increase in both transmural and spatial dispersion of repolarization in LQT1 than LQT2 forms of congenital long QT syndrome. *Journal of the American College of Cardiology*, **37**, 911–919.

Thompson, R., Rich, J., Chmelik, F. *et al.* (1977) Evolutionary changes in the electrocardiogram of severe progressive hypothermia. *Journal of Electrocardiology*, **10**, 67–70.

Tun, A., Khan, I.A., Wattanasauwan, N. *et al.* (1999) Increased regional and transmyocardial dispersion of ventricular repolarization in end-stage renal disease. *Canadian Journal of Cardiology*, **15**, 53–56.

Viitasalo, M., Oikarinen, L., Swan, H. *et al.* (2002) Ambulatory electrocardiographic evidence of transmural dispersion of repolarization in patients with long-QT syndrome type 1 and 2. *Circulation*, **106**, 2473–2478.

Volders, P.G., Sipido, K.R., Carmeliet, E. *et al.* (1999) Repolarizing K^+ currents ITO1 and IKs are larger in right than left canine ventricular midmyocardium. *Circulation*, **99**, 206–210.

Watanabe, Y. (1975) Purkinje repolarization as a possible cause of the U wave in the electrocardiogram. *Circulation*, **51**, 1030–1037.

Yan, G.X. & Antzelevitch, C. (1996) Cellular basis for the electrocardiographic J wave. *Circulation*, **93**, 372–379.

Yan, G.X. & Antzelevitch, C. (1998) Cellular basis for the normal T wave and the electrocardiographic manifestations of the long QT syndrome. *Circulation*, **98**, 1928–1936.

Yan, G.X. & Antzelevitch, C. (1999) Cellular basis for the Brugada Syndrome and other mechanisms of arrhythmogenesis associated with *S–T* segment elevation. *Circulation*, **100**, 1660–1666.

Yoshiga, Y., Shimizu, A., Yamagata, T. *et al.* (2002) Beta blocker decreases the increase in QT dispersion and transmural dispersion of repolarization induced by bepridil. *Circulation Journal*, **66**, 1024–1028.

Zhang, L., Compton, S. J., Antzelevitch, C. *et al.* (1999) Differential response of *QT* and *QU* intervals to adrenergic stimulation in long *QT* patients with IKs defects. *Journal of the American College of Cardiology*, **33**, 138A (abstract).

Zuckerman, R. & Cabrera-Cosio, E. (1947) La ondu U. [The U wave.] *Archivos del Instituto de Cardiologia de Mexico*, **17**, 521–532.

CHAPTER 32

Individual QT/RR Relationships

Velislav Batchvarov and Marek Malik

Introduction

The heart rate-corrected *QT* interval (*QTc*) is a recognized marker of cardiac and arrhythmic death in various patient populations (Schwartz & Wolf 1978; Elming *et al.* 1998; De Bruyne *et al.* 1999; Okin *et al.* 2000). In recent years, the measurement of *QTc* interval has gained additional importance because of the increased awareness that many cardiac as well as noncardiac drugs have the potential of affecting ventricular repolarization and inducing a potentially lethal torsades de pointes ventricular arrhythmia (Report on a Policy Conference of the European Society of Cardiology 2000). With most drugs, the induction of torsades de pointes tachycardia is rather rare and is believed to occur exclusively in the presence of predisposing conditions, such as heart failure, bradycardia or electrolyte imbalance and/or in susceptible individuals (i.e. asymptomatic carriers of 'silent' mutations of genes underlying the long QT syndrome) (Priori *et al.* 1999; Roden 2002). Therefore the absence of cases of torsades de pointes induction in clinical programmes of drug development is not reassuring. With some drugs that were later withdrawn from the market because of clear proarrhythmic toxicity, the initial postmarketing surveillance was both substantial and signal-free (Walker *et al.* 1999). Consequently, the assessment of drug-induced changes of cardiac repolarization need to be based on surrogate markers, of which practically the most important is the prolongation of the *QTc* interval. If the investigated drug changes heart rate, either directly or indirectly through therapeutic actions, the appropriate heart rate correction for the calculation of *QTc* becomes very important.

The precision requirements of the *QTc* interval measurement are different in clinical practice and in risk stratification and/or drug studies. In clinical practice, an imprecision of 10 to 20, or perhaps even 30 ms is unlikely to lead to an incorrect decision about the management of individual patients since all borderline findings are not only checked but also considered within the context of other clinical findings. On the contrary, errors of 10 ms or even lower may be misleading in drug studies and risk stratification trials (e.g. when selecting patients for a prospective intervention), especially when introduced in a biased way owing to systematic differences in heart rate.

The observations that the duration of cardiac systole is heart rate dependent have been made even before the invention of electrocardiography (Waller 1887). For example, Thurston (1876) used sphygmographical tracings of the radial pulse to measure the length of the cardiac systole at different heart rates. He confirmed that 'the length of the systole of the heart, as indicated in the radial artery, is constant for any given pulse rate, and varies as the cube root of the rapidity.' Even earlier, Garrod analysed sphygmographic recordings of the apex beat in healthy subjects and came to the conclusion that 'In health, the length of the first part of the heart beat varies . . . inversely as the square root of the rapidity' (Garrod 1871). In other publications the same author observed that 'the length of the interval between the commencement of the primary and dicrotic rises (of the sphygmogram) is constant for any given pulse rate, and varies as the cube root of the pulse rate . . .' (Garrod 1870).

Following the introduction of electrocardiography, the relationship between mechanical systole and the *QT* interval (called, at that time, the electrical systole) was studied extensively and the relationship between the *QT* and *RR* intervals has been researched ever since.

Unfortunately, in spite of all the research work spanned over a whole century, the problem of finding an appropriate heart rate-correction of the *QT* interval has not been solved. Tens of heart rate correction formulae have been proposed (Malik 2001) – by 1949 about 30 such formulae had already been described (Ljung 1949), but none of these has been found to be universally applicable (Hodges *et al.* 1983; Rautaharju *et al.* 1990; Funck-Brentano & Jaillon 1993; Aytemir *et al.* 1999; Malik 2001, 2002). It has been repeatedly pointed out that the validity of any formula expressing the *QT* interval as a function of the simultaneously measured *RR* interval is limited by physiological factors, such as the extra-heart rate influences on the *QT* interval duration (Fig. 32.1) (Rickards & Norman 1981; Browne *et al.* 1983; Cappato *et al.* 1991) and the 'lag hysteresis' of the *QT* interval (Fig. 32.2) (Franz *et al.* 1988; Lau *et al.* 1988). Significantly

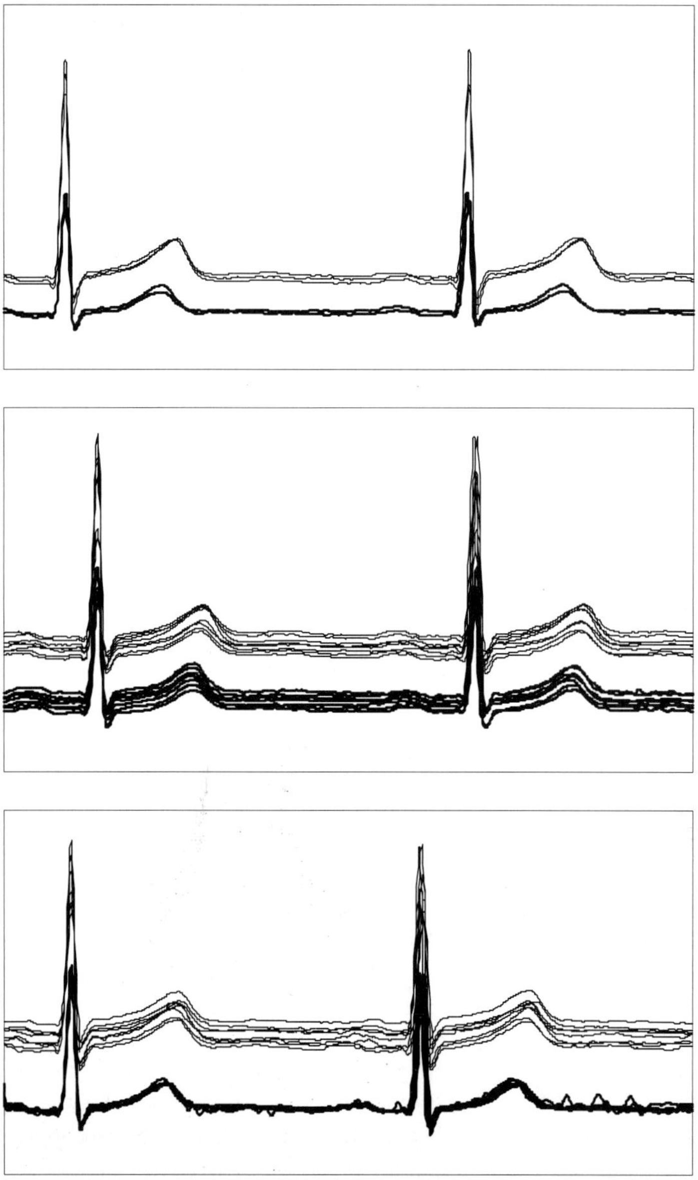

Fig. 32.1 Direct effect of the autonomic nervous system on the *QT* interval duration. Each panel shows *QT* intervals recorded during the night (top thin lines) and during the day (bottom thick lines) at identical heart rates of 61 beats/min (top panel), 65 beats/min (middle panel) and 70 beats/min (bottom panel). *QT* intervals recorded during the night are clearly longer than those recorded during the day despite identical heart rates.

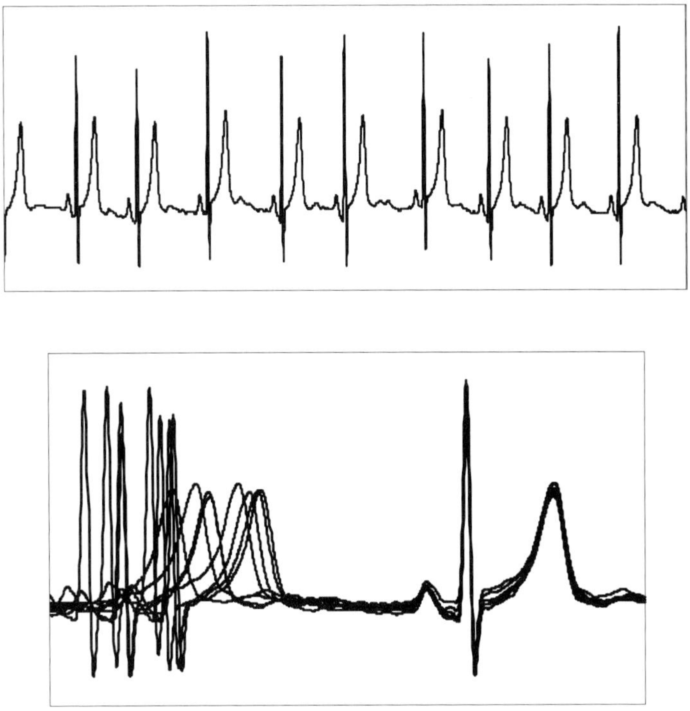

Fig. 32.2 An example of hysteresis of the *QT* interval. Top: 10-second ECG recording during which 8 *RR* intervals are visibly variable. Bottom: all 8 *RR* intervals have been overlapped and aligned by the R-peak of the second QRS complex. It can be seen that *QT* intervals preceded by very different *RR* intervals are almost identical, i.e. they have not yet adapted to the changes in the *RR* interval.

less attention has been paid to the errors resulting from interindividual variations of the QT/RR relationship.

Intersubject variability of the QT/RR relationship

While studying different groups of cardiac patient and/or healthy subjects, different authors often reported substantially variable results even when using the same form of generic formula to describe the QT/RR relationship. For instance, with the frequently popular parabolic formula $QTc = QT/RR^{\alpha}$ (*RR* interval expressed in s), the reported values of optimum parameter α ranged from 0.25 (Kawataki *et al.* 1984) to 0.6 (Mayeda 1934), and included the widely known formulae of Bazett ($\alpha = 0.5$) (Bazett 1920) and of Fridericia ($\alpha = 0.33$) (Fridericia 1920). Similar disagreement exists between the results of studies using the linear formula $QTc = QT + \alpha \times (1 - RR)$ (Larsen & Skulason 1941; Schlamowitz 1946; Ljung 1949; Sagie *et al.* 1992) as well as studies using other types of generic heart rate correction formulae (Hodges *et al.* 1983; Karjalainen *et al.* 1994; Wohlfart & Pahlm 1994). Previously, the discrepancies have mainly been attributed to different types of databases (pooled data of different subjects, multiple recordings in each subject, or mixture of both), different physiological conditions (rest, exercise electrocardiograms, continuous ambulatory recordings), various heart rate ranges, and different number of ECG samples in the different studies. At the same time, all studies seeking the 'true' heart rate correction formula have assumed that there is a 'physiologically correct' relationship between *QT* and *RR* intervals that is common to all healthy subjects (and perhaps also to patients with various cardiac diseases) and that the problem of finding the correct formula just lies in establishing the proper mathematical description of such a relationship. The possibility that the QT/RR relationship might be different in different individuals even when they are recorded under comparable conditions has been systematically overlooked.

At the same time, substantial variability in QT/RR relationship has been repeatedly observed in different studies that have collected sufficient data to characterize individual QT/RR patterns. To reliably investigate the individual QT/RR relationship, multiple serial ECGs recorded in the same subject over a wide range of heart rate are needed, either in the form of frequently repeated recordings or in the form of continuous ambulatory ECG recordings (in both cases, accurate *QT* interval measurement in multiple cardiac cycles is also needed).

Several studies demonstrated the advantages of an 'individualised' approach to the heart rate-correction of the *QT* interval. Davey (1999) estimated the slope of the individual *QT*/heart rate linear regressions from multiple QT/RR data points during exercise stress tests in healthy subjects and patients with hypertrophic cardiomyopathy and heart failure. Separately in each participant, he obtained corrected *QT* intervals by extrapolating the *QT*/heart rate regression to the heart rate of 60 beats/min. These 'individual' *QTc* values separated the three study groups better than the Bazett corrected *QTc* interval and, unlike the latter, were not correlated to heart rate.

Using multiple QT/RR data from standard Holter recordings in 21 healthy subjects, Molnar *et al.* (1996) compared five correction formulae with individually optimized formulae derived from the data of each patient. They found that the individual optimizations were superior to conventional heart rate corrections.

A systematic analysis of the interindividual variations of the QT/RR relationship was published by Malik *et al.* (2002). The authors investigated ECG data of 25 healthy women (age 31.1 ± 9.9 years) and 25 men (age 36.0 ± 8.6 years). In each subject, one 10-s 12-lead ECG was obtained every 2 min over 24 h (671 ± 58 recordings per subject) using 12-lead ambulatory digital ECG recorder (SEER MC, GE Medical Systems, Milwaukee, WI). In each individual, the 24-h sequence of QT/RR data points was fitted with six different two-parameter regression models included the linear ($QT = \beta + \alpha \times RR$), hyperbolic ($QT = \beta + \alpha/RR$) and parabolic ($QT = \beta + RR^{\alpha}$) model. The individually optimized values of the α coefficient of each regression model were used to derive individually optimized formulae for heart rate-correction of the *QT* interval.

The pattern of QT/RR scatterplots differed significantly between different subjects (Fig. 32.3). With all models, both coefficients α and β varied substantially between the participants. With the parabolic model, for example, the coefficient α varied between 0.23 and 0.49, i.e. some subjects followed the prediction of the Kawataki formula ($\alpha = 0.25$), some subjects the prediction of the Fridericia formula ($\alpha = 0.33$), and one extreme subject was near to the prediction of the Bazett formula ($\alpha = 0.5$). The study clearly showed that no 'physiological' QT/RR relationship exists that is common to all subjects. Consequently, no 'optimum' heart rate correction can be derived that would permit accurate comparisons of *QT* intervals recorded in different individuals over a wide range of heart rates. For example, correcting a *QT* interval of 360 ms recorded at 75 beats/min with a parabolic formula $QTc = QT/RR^{\alpha}$, the range of exponent α of 0.23–0.49 represents a range of *QTc* interval values of 379–401 ms, i.e. differences of up to 22 ms. At 85 and 95 beats per min, these *QTc* differences increase to 36 and 49 ms, respectively (Fig. 32.4).

Stability of the individual QT/RR relationship

The concept of an individually optimized heart rate-correction formula derived separately for each subject from the particular QT/RR relationship is only valid if the relationship is stable over time, that is if it varies significantly less within each individual than between different individuals. While methods for individual correction of the *QT* interval have been proposed previously (Molnar *et al.* 1996), the problem of the stability of the individual QT/RR pattern has not been investigated or even formulated until very recently.

Lecocq *et al.* (1989) studied the QT/RR relationship of 11 subjects at rest, during exercise and after intravenous isoproterenol, and in 12 subjects at rest and after oral propranolol. An exponential model $QT = A - B \times e^{-k \times R-R}$ was fitted to the individual QT/RR data. Four of the subjects participated in different parts of the study (10 months apart). When comparing the individual equations from both parts of the study, the authors briefly mentioned that they '. . . could not find any significant change between the 2 periods.'

In a most recent study, we have further investigated the individual QT/RR relationship in healthy volunteers (Batchvarov *et al.* 2002).

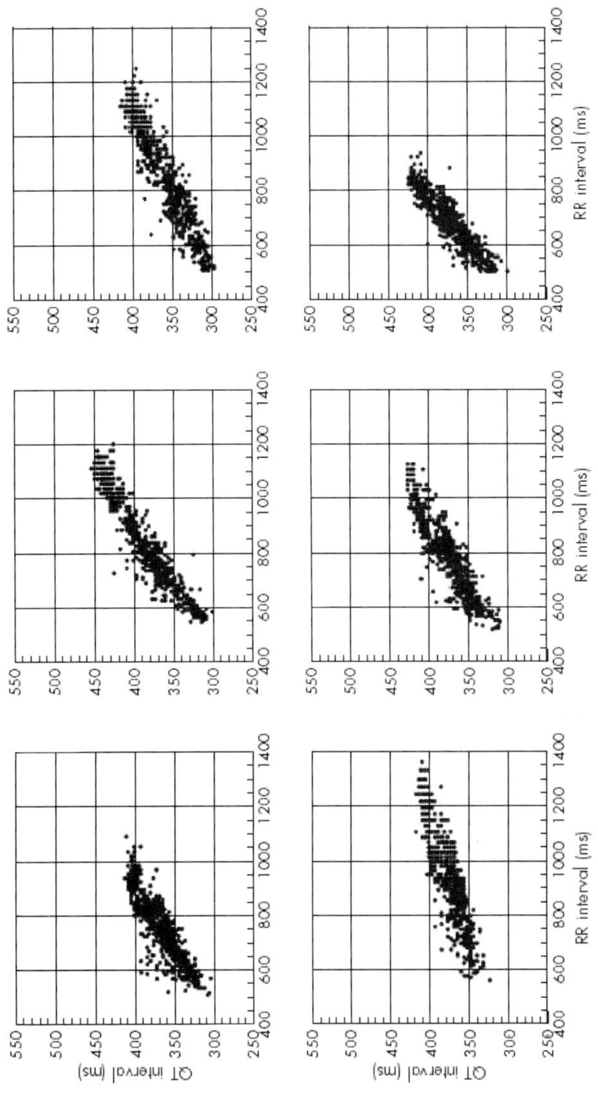

Fig. 32.3 Examples of 24-h QT/RR relationship patterns in six healthy subjects. Note the individual differences. See the text for details. (Reproduced from Malik *et al.* 2002, with permission.)

Twenty-four h 12-lead digital ECG recordings were obtained at baseline, after 24 ± 0 h, 7.7 ± 2.0 days, and 31.2 ± 3.9 days in 46 healthy subjects (22 men, 24 women, aged 26.8 ± 7.3 years and 27.3 ± 8.1 years, respectively, P = NS). In each 24-h recording, one 10-s ECG was obtained every 30 s (1504 ± 283 ECGs per recording). To improve the accuracy of automatic *QT* measurement, each *QT* interval was measured using six different algorithms. The *QT* measurement was accepted if the results with the six algorithms differed by ″ 40 ms. In such a case, the mean of the six measurements was taken as the true value of the *QT* interval (automatic measurement without any visual control and/or manual editing was necessary since the study involved > 750 000 individual ECGs). In each recording of each individual, the QT/RR relationship was investigated using 10 different two-parameter regression models, including the linear ($QT = \beta + \alpha \times RR$), hyperbolic ($QT = \beta + \alpha/RR$), parabolic log/log ($QT = \beta + RR^{\alpha}$), logarithmic ($QT = \beta + \alpha \times \ln(RR)$) and exponential ($QT = \beta + \alpha \times e^{-RR}$) models.

To compare the intra- and intersubject variability of the regression parameters, the standard deviations of curvature-describing parameter (α) and the slope-describing parameter (β) of the four consecutive recordings in each participant were compared with the standard

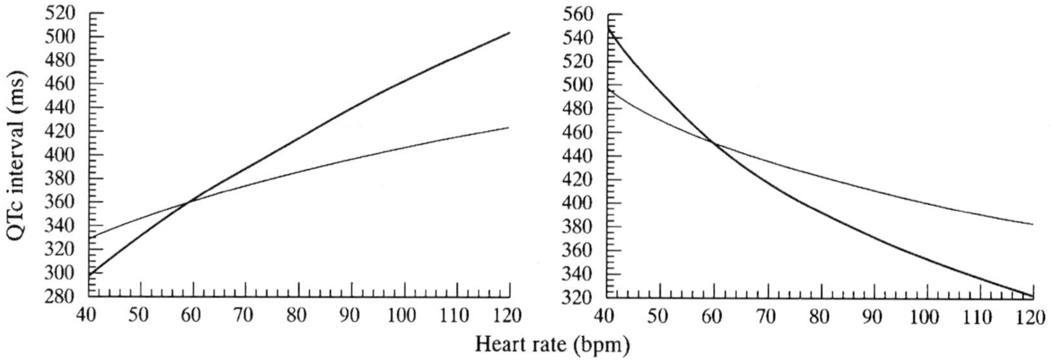

Fig. 32.4 Effect of different values of the curvature coefficient (of the generic correction formula *QTc* = QT/RR (on the heart rate-corrected *QT* (*QTc*) interval. This study found coefficient in a group of healthy subjects ranging from 0.233 to 0.485. The figure shows the differences between the correction formulae *QTc* = *QT/RR*0.233 (grey lines) and *QTc* = *QT/RR*0.485 (black lines). For both formulas, the left panel shows the *QTc* values corresponding to a *QT* interval of 360 ms measured at different heart rates. The right panel shows 'normality limits,' that is, *QT* interval durations that, when measured at different heart rates, correspond to *QTc* = 450 ms. See text for details. (Reproduced from Malik *et al.* 2002, with permission.)

deviation of the subject-specific mean values of α and β with a nonparametric one-sample Wilcoxon test.

The shape of the 24-h QT/RR scatter plots clearly suggested that the QT/RR relationship exhibits substantial intrasubject stability and intersubject variability both in women as well as in men (Fig. 32.5).

With all QT/RR regression models, the individual standard deviations of both regression parameters were highly significantly smaller than the standard deviations of the means of the individual subjects ($P = 10^{-5} - 10^{-9}$, Fig. 32.6).

In order to assess the long-term stability of the individual QT/RR relationship, an additional (fifth) 24-h ECG recording was acquired in 16 of the participants in the original study (8 men, mean age 26.1 ± 7.4 years) after 21.5 ± 5.6 months using the same recording technique (unpublished data). Automatic *QT* measurement and analysis of the QT/RR relationship was performed using the same methods as in the original study. Figure 32.7 shows examples of QT/RR relationship patterns from recordings taken at baseline, after 1 month and after approximately 2 years in two women and two men. The long-term stability of the individual QT/RR relationship pattern is clearly visible. The individual standard deviations (from five consecutive recordings) of the regression parameters were again significantly smaller ($P < 0.01$) than the standard deviations of the means of the individual subjects. Figure 32.8 shows the comparison of the inter- and intrasubject variability of the regression parameters with the linear and parabolic models. It is shown that although the parameters of the fifth recording are different from the first four, the intersubject variability (lower panels) is substantially higher than the intrasubject variability (top panels).

Individualized heart rate-correction of the *QT* interval: clinical application

The goal of the application of any heart rate-correction formula is to provide *QTc* interval values that are independent of heart rate.

As already mentioned, when analysing a standard clinical ECG with only few ECG complexes recorded at physiological heart rates (e.g. 50–70 beats per min), most published heart rate correction formulae provide clinically satisfactory results (Hodges 1997). Our data suggest that in such a scenario Fridericia formula is superior to Bazett formula, since in most healthy subjects the optimum curvature coefficient (parameter α) with the parabolic QT/RR model ($QT = \beta + RR^{\alpha}$) is close to 0.33 (Batchvarov *et al.* 2002a; Malik *et al.* 2002) (Fig. 32.6).

However, when precise estimation of *QTc* interval is required, such as in drug trials or risk-stratification studies, an arbitrarily chosen heart

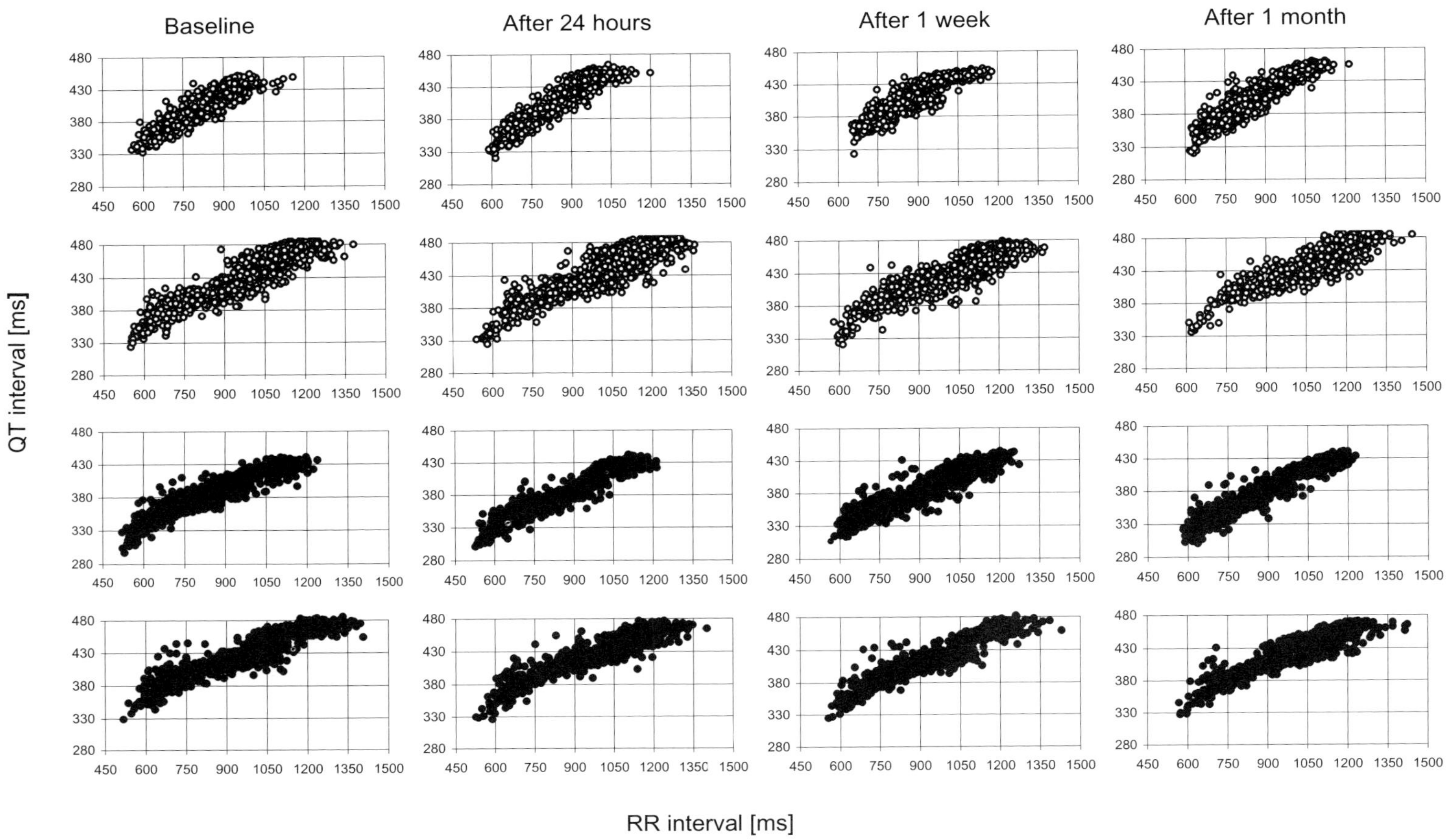

Fig. 32.5 Examples of QT/RR patterns of the four recordings in two female (top two rows, open circles) and two male subjects (bottom two rows, closed circles). Each row presents the four recordings of one subject, while the four columns present the first and the subsequent recordings of all subjects, respectively. Note the stability of the QT/RR pattern in each subject and the variability of the patterns in different subjects. (Reproduced from Batchvarov *et al.* 2002, with permission.)

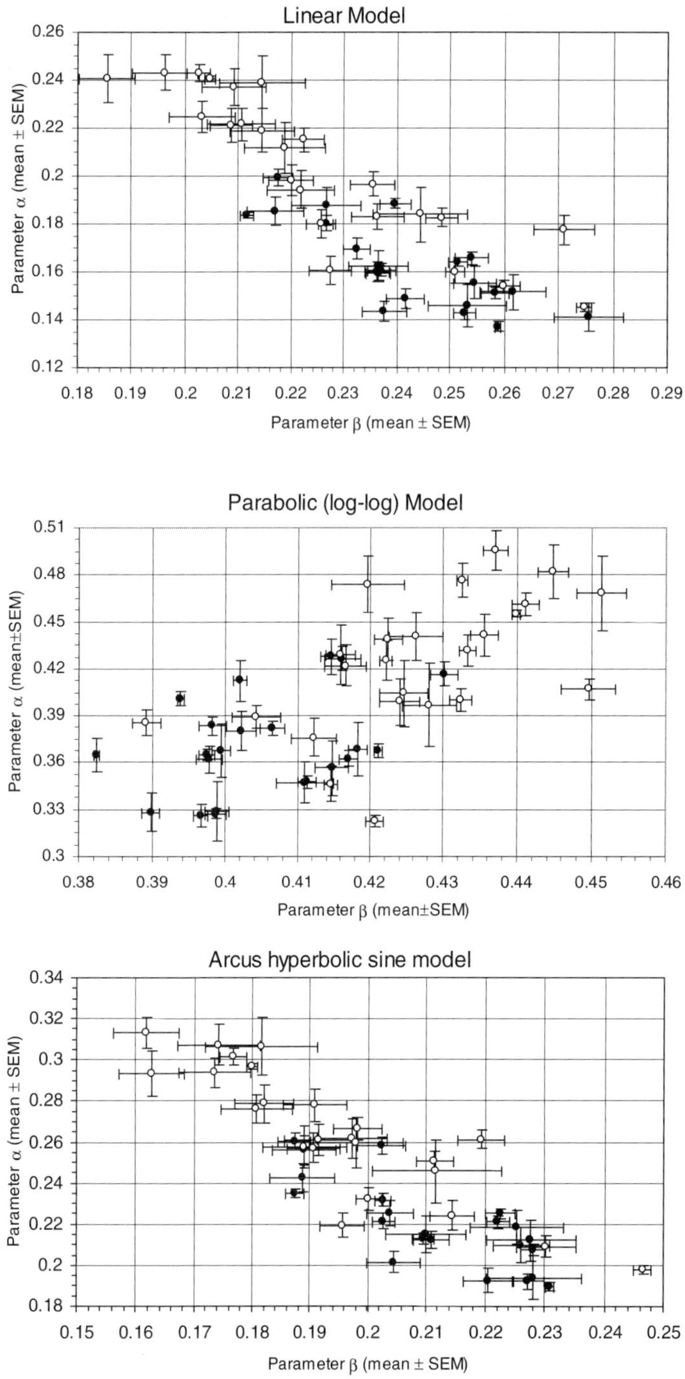

Fig. 32.6 Mean ± SEM from the four recordings of the α and β parameters of each male (closed circles) and female (open circles) subject with the linear (top panel), parabolic (middle panel) and arcus hyperbolic sine (bottom panel) QT/RR regression model. Note that the standard errors of the individual means are substantially smaller than the range of the individual means. See text for details. (Reproduced from Batchvarov *et al.* 2002, with permission.)

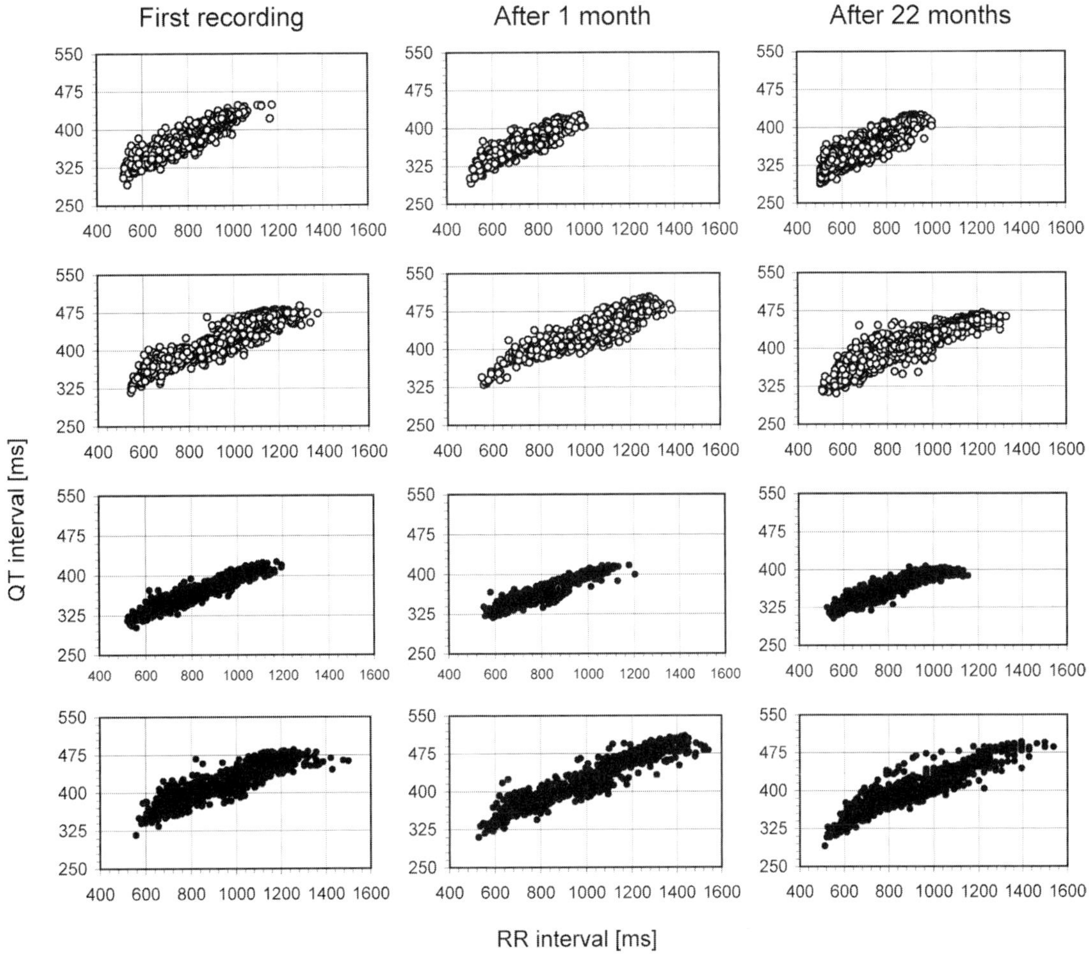

Fig. 32.7 Examples of QT/RR patterns of recordings acquired at baseline (left column), after 1 month (middle column) and after approximately 22 months (right column) in two women (top 2 rows, open circles) and two men (bottom 2 rows, closed circles). The intersubject variability and the intrasubject stability of the QT/RR relationship are clearly visible.

rate correction formula will not respect the individual QT/RR patterns of the majority of patients and/or healthy subjects. It is important to realise that in such cases, Bazett or Fridericia formulae may provide misleading results even at physiological resting heart rates (e.g. 60–90 beats/min) (Batchvarov *et al.* 2002b) (Fig. 32.9).

The resulting under- or overcorrection of the *QT* intervals may lead to substantially misleading results. In such studies, an individually optimized heart rate-correction formula should be derived in each subject from multiple ECG recordings taken in baseline state. Moreover, in drug studies, the individual baseline and/or placebo QT/RR pattern may be compared with the on-treatment pattern in the same subject.

This concept was applied in a recent study by Malik who investigated data from a phase I study of the nonsedating antihistamines ebastine and terfenadine in healthy volunteers (Malik 2001). The effectiveness of three different rate-correction methods to detect drug-induced *QT* interval prolongation was compared. The *QT* intervals were first corrected using 20 previously published heart rate-correction formulae, including the formulae of Bazett (1920), Fridericia (1920), Hodges *et al.* (1983), Sarma *et al.*

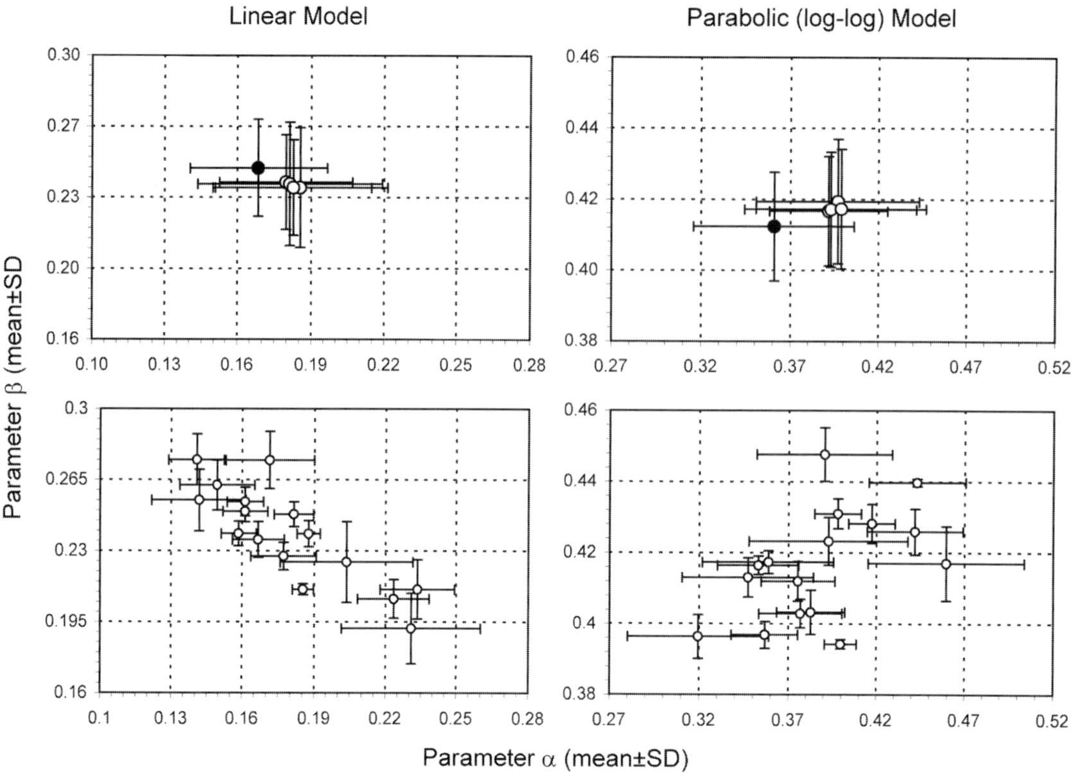

Fig. 32.8 Comparison of the inter- and intrasubject variability of the regression parameters α and β with the linear (left column) and logarithmic (right column) models. The upper panels present the mean ± SD of α and β of all subjects of the first four (open circles) and of the fifth recording (closed circle). The bottom panels present mean ± SD of α and β of the five recordings in each subject. It is visible that while the parameters of the fifth recording are different from the first four, the intersubject variability (lower panels) is substantially higher than the intrasubject variability (top panel). Note that unlike Fig. 32.6, data in this figure are presented as mean ± SD.

(1984), the Framingham study (Sagie *et al.* 1992), and others. Secondly, an optimized correction formula was derived by QT/RR regression modelling of the pooled drug-free data of all participants. Finally, individually optimized formulae were derived for each participant from available 41 QT/RR data points obtained in the drug-free state. While the pooled drug-free regression found an optimized correction $QTc = QT/RR^{0.314}$, the correction coefficient α varied between 0.161 and 0.417 in individually optimized corrections $QTc = QT/RR^{\alpha}$.

While all the results with terfenadine confirmed previous findings that the drug prolongs *QT* interval (Honig *et al.* 1993; Benton *et al.* 1996; Clifford *et al.* 1997), the results with ebastine were hugely different with different previously published formulae and ranged from statistically significant prolongation to statistically significant shortening of *QTc*. Moreover, the results obtained with previously published formulae were significantly dependent on the success of each formula to correct *QT* interval for heart rate (i.e. to provide *QTc* values that are heart rate independent) (Fig. 32.10). The individually optimized rate-correction formulae were superior to both the conventional rate-correction formulae, as well as to the group-optimized formula. (The study showed that unlike terfenadine, ebastine did not prolong *QTc* interval.) This study also suggested that the individual QT/RR relationship could be estimated from several tens of QT/RR data points.

This study also suggested that although inferior to the individualized rate-correction approach, optimising the heart rate-correction formula for the pooled data of all subjects is supe-

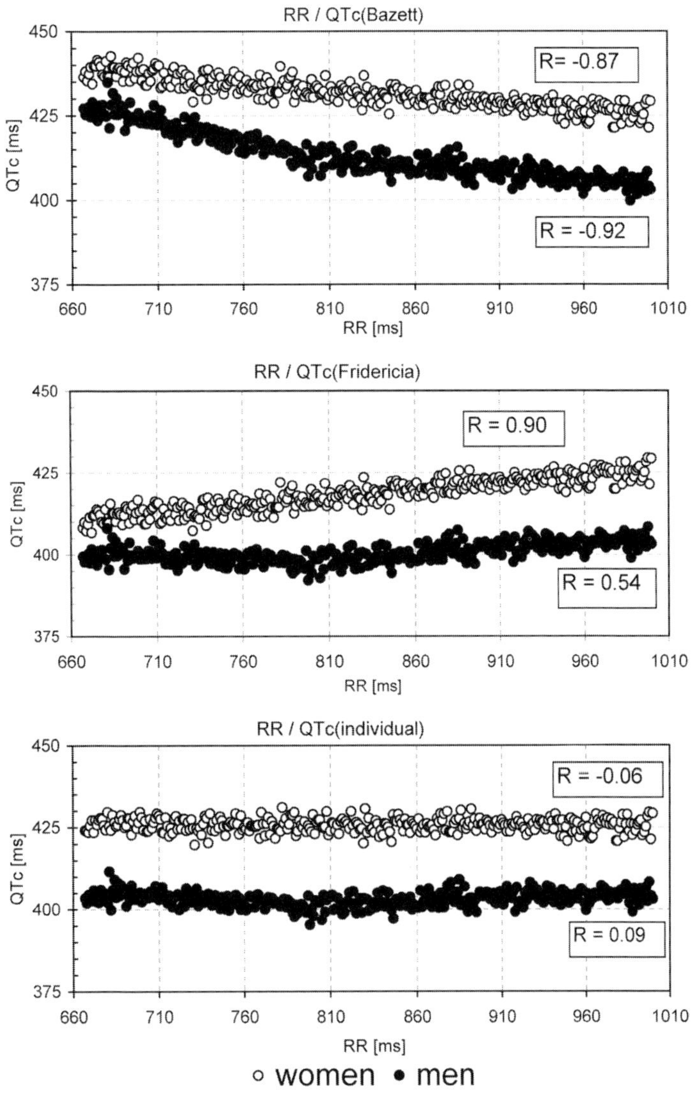

Fig. 32.9 Correlation between the *RR* interval and *QT* interval corrected for heart rate with Bazett formula (top panel), Fridericia formula (middle panel) and individualized formulae (bottom panel). Pooled data from 24-h ECG recordings in 24 healthy women (open circles) and 22 healthy men (closed circles). Only QT/RR data at heart rate of 60–90 beats/min are presented. Note that even within this physiological range of resting heart rates, the *QT* interval corrected by Bazett formula (top panel) is strongly negatively correlated to the *RR* interval (R = −0.92 and −0.87 in men and women, respectively), rendering artificial *QTc* differences of about 20 ms. Although Fridericia formula (middle panel) renders better results in men, only the individualized *QT* correction formulae (bottom panel) produce *QTc* intervals that are practically heart rate-independent.

rior to the application of any correction formula with fixed parameters. The regression analysis of the pooled QT/RR data therefore should be used only as an approximate heart rate-correction approach when sufficient QT/RR data are not available for each patient in a drug-free state to estimate their individual QT/RR relationship. Molnar *et al.* (1996) also demonstrated the superiority of the individualized over the group-based approach for heart-rate correction of the *QT* interval.

Similarly to drug studies, the application of arbitrarily chosen formula for heart rate correction of the *QT* interval in prospective studies assessing the prognostic value of *QTc* interval prolongation should be strongly discouraged. The practice of comparing the *QTc* interval in patient groups with different outcome without even reporting their heart rates seems even less acceptable (Okin *et al.* 2000; Wong *et al.* 2003). Since estimation of the individual QT/RR relationship in such studies is usually not possible, a group-based heart rate-correction approach should be applied (Fauchier *et al.* 2000; Malik 2001). At the very least, the heart rate could be entered as an independent variable in addition to the *QTc* interval in multivariate regression analysis (Brendorp *et al.* 2001).

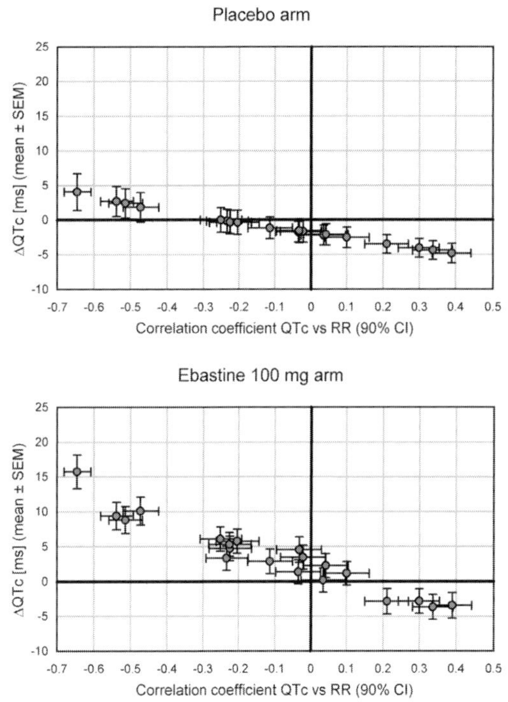

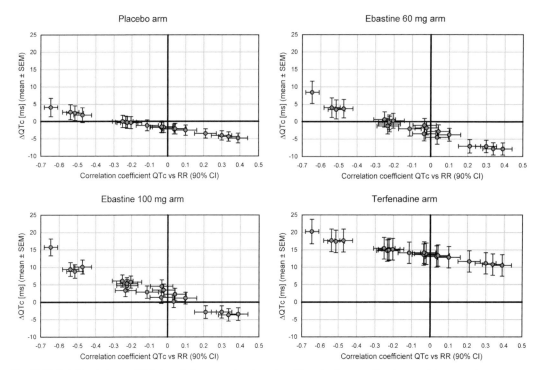

Fig. 32.10 Relation between *QTc* interval change on treatment and heart rate correction 'success' (expressed as correlation coefficient between *QTc* and corresponding *RR* intervals in the drug-free data) of 20 published heart rate-correction formulae. Note that the results lead practically to straight lines, demonstrating that results by the different formulas are grossly determined by their correction success. Note also that the bands of the results of the placebo and ebastine arms practically pass through the points of zero *QTc* difference and zero correlation coefficient. (Reproduced from Malik, M., *Journal of Cardiovascular Electrophysiology* (2001), **12**, 411–420, with permission.)

Conclusions

The use of *QTc* interval in clinical practice should be clearly distinguished from *QTc* measurement in clinical investigations when substantially higher precision is required. The application of individually optimized heart rate-correction formulae should be adopted as a standard approach in studies of drug effects or in interventions that change both the *QT* interval, as well as the heart rate. In such cases, it is crucial to obtain a sufficient number of ECGs in each subject over a significant physiological range of heart rates.

References

Aytemir, K., Maarouf, N., Gallagher, M.M., Yap, Y.G., Waktare, J.E.P. & Malik M. (1999) Comparison of formulae for heart rate correction of QT interval in exercise electrocardiograms. *PACE (Pacing and Clinical Electrophysiology)*, **22**, 1397–1401.

Batchvarov, V.N., Ghuran, A., Smetana, P. *et al.* (2002) QT/RR relationship in healthy subjects exhibits substantial intersubject variability and high intrasubject stability. *American Journal of Physiology (Heart Circulation Physiology)* **282**, H2356–H2363.

Batchvarov, V.N., Smetana, P., Ghuran, A., Hnatkova, K., Camm, A.J. & Malik, M. (2002) Comparison of Bazett, Fridericia, and an individually derived formula for heart rate correction of the QT interval. *PACE (Pacing and Clinical Electrophysiology)*, **24** (Pt II), 606 (abstract).

Bazett, H.C. (1920) An analysis of the time-relations of electrocardiograms. *Heart*, **vii**, 353–370.

Benton, R.E., Honig, P.K., Zamani, K., Cantilena, L.R. & Woosley, R.L. (1996) Grapefruit juice alters terfenadine pharmacokinetics, resulting in prolongation of repolarization on the electrocardiogram. *Clinical Pharmacology and Therapeutics*, **59**, 383–388.

Brendorp, B., Elming, H., Jun, L. *et al.* for the DIAMOND Study Group. (2001) QTc interval as a guide to select those patients with congestive heart failure and reduced left ventricular systolic function who will benefit from antiarrhythmic treatment with dofetilide. *Circulation*, **103**, 1422–14 27.

Browne, K.F., Prystowsky, E., Heger, J.J. & Zipes, D.P. (1983) Modulation of the QT interval by the autonomic nervous system. *PACE (Pacing and Clinical Electrophysiology)*, **6**, 1050–1056.

De Bruyne, M.C., Hoes, A.W., Kors, J.A., Hofman, A., van Bemmel, J.H. & Grobbee, D.E. (1999) Prolonged QT interval predicts cardiac and all-cause mortality in the elderly. The Rotterdam Study. *European Heart Journal*, **20**, 278–284.

Cappato, R., Alboni, P., Pedroni, P., Gilli, G. & Antonioli, G.E. (1991) Sympathetic and vagal influences on rate-dependent changes of QT interval in healthy subjects. *American Journal of Cardiology*, **68**, 1188–1193.

Clifford, C.P., Adams, D.A., Murray, S. *et al.* (1997) The cardiac effects of terfenadine after inhibition of its metabolism by grapefruit juice. *European Journal of Clinical Pharmacology*, **52**, 311–315.

Davey, P. (1999) A new physiological method for heart rate correction of the QT interval. *Heart*, **82**, 183–186.

Elming, H., Holm, E., Jun, L. *et al.* (1998) The prognostic value of the QT interval and QT interval dispersion in all-cause and cardiac mortality in a population of Danish citizens. *European Heart Journal*, **19**, 1391–1400.

Fauchier, L., Maison-Blanche, P., Forhan, A. *et al.* and the DESIR Study Group. (2000) Association between heart rate-corrected QT interval and coronary risk factors in 2,894 healthy subjects (the DESIR Study). *American Journal of Cardiology*, **86**, 557–559.

Franz, M.R., Swerdlow, C.D., Liem, L.B. & Schaefer, J. (1988) Cycle length dependence of human action potential duration *in vivo*: effects of single extrastimuli, sudden sustained rate acceleration and deceleration, and different steady-state frequencies. *Journal of Clinical Investigation*, **82**, 972–979.

Fridericia, L.S. (1920) Die Systolendauer im Elektrokardiogramm bei normalen Menschen und bei Herzkranken. *Acta Medica Scandinavica*, **53**, 469–486.

Funck-Brentano, K. & Jaillon, P. (1993) Rate-corrected QT interval: techniques and limitations. *American Journal of Cardiology*, **72**, 17B–22B.

Garrod, A.H. (1870) *Proceedings of the Royal Society, London*, p.351.

Garrod, A.H. (1871) On cardiograph tracings from the human chest-wall. *Journal of Anatomical Physiology*, **5**, 2–27.

Hodges, M. (1997) Rate correction of the QT interval. *Cardiac Electrophysiology Review*, **3**, 360–363.

Hodges, M., Salerno, D. & Erlien, D. (1983) Bazett's QT correction reviewed: Evidence that a linear QT Correction for heart rate is better. *Journal of the American College of Cardiology*, **1**(2), 694 (abstract).

Honig, P.K., Wortham, D.C., Zamani, K., Conner, D.P., Mullin, J.C. & Cantilena, L.R. (1993) Terfenadine–ketoconazole interaction: pharmacokinetic and electrocardiographic consequences. *JAMA (Journal of the American Medical Association)*, **269**, 1513–1518.

Karjalainen, J., Viitasalo, M., Manttari, M. & Manninen, V. (1994) Relation between QT intervals and heart rates from 40 to 120 beats/min in rest electrocardiograms of men and a simple method to adjust QT interval values. *Journal of the American College of Cardiology*, **23**, 1547–1553.

Kawataki, M., Kashima, T., Toda, H. & Tanaka, H. (1984) Relation between QT interval and heart rate. Applications and limitations of Bazett's formula. *Journal of Electrocardiology*, **17**, 371–375.

Larsen, K. & Skulason, T. (1941) Det normale Elektrocardiogram. I. Analyse af Ekstremitetsafledningerne hos 100 sunde Mennesker I Alderen fra 30 til 50 Aar. *Nordisk Medicin* **9**, 350–358.

Lau, C.P., Freedman, A.R., Fleming, S., Malik, M., Camm, A.J. & Ward, D.E. (1988) Hysteresis of the ventricular paced QT interval in response to abrupt changes in pacing rate. *Cardiovascular Research*, **22**, 67–72.

Lecocq, B., Lecocq, V. & Jaillon, P. (1989) Physiologic relation between cardiac cycle and QT duration in healthy volunteers. *American Journal of Cardiology*, **63**, 481–486.

Ljung, O. (1949) A simple formula for clinical interpretation of the QT interval data. *Acta Medica Scandinavica*, **CXXXIV**, 79–86.

Malik, M. (2001) Problems of heart rate correction in assessment of drug-induced QT interval prolongation. *Journal of Cardiovascular Electrophysiology*, **12**, 411–420.

Malik, M. (2002) The Imprecision in heart rate correction may lead to artificial observations of drug-induced QT interval changes. *PACE (Pacing and Clinical Electrophysiology)*, **25**, 209–216.

Malik, M., Färbom, P., Batchvarov, V., Hnatkova, K. & Camm, A.J. (2002) Relation between QT and *R–R* intervals is highly individual among healthy subjects: implications for heart rate correction of the QT interval. *Heart*, **87**, 220–228.

Mayeda, I. (1934) On time relation between systolic duration of heart and pulse rate. *Acta Scholae Medicinalis Universitatis in Kyoto*, **17**, 53–55.

Molnar, J., Weiss, J., Zhang, F. & Rosenthal, J.E. (1996) Evaluation of five QT correction formulas using a software assisted method of continuous QT measurement from 24-h Holter recordings. *American Journal of Cardiology*, **78**, 920–926.

Okin, P.M., Devereux, R.B., Howard, B.V., Fabsitz, R.R., Lee, E.T. & Welty, T.K. (2000) Assessment of QT interval and QT dispersion for prediction of all-cause and cardiovascular mortality in American Indians. The Strong Heart Study. *Circulation*, **101**, 61–66.

Priori, S.G., Napolitano. C. & Schwartz, P.J. (1999) Low penetrance in the long QT syndrome. Clinical impact. *Circulation*, **99**, 529–533.

Rautaharju, P.M., Warren, J.W. & Calhoun, H.P. (1990) Estimation of QT prolongation. A persistent, avoidable error in computer electrocardiography. *Journal of Electrocardiology*, **23** (Suppl.), 111–117.

Report on a Policy Conference of the European Society of Cardiology. (2000) The potential for QT prolongation and proarrhythmia by non-antiarrhythmic drugs: clinical and regulatory implications. *European Heart Journal*, **21**, 1216–1231.

Rickards, A.F. & Norman, J. (1981) Relation between QT interval and heart rate. New design of physiologically adaptive cardiac pacemaker. *British Heart Journal*, **45**, 56–61.

Roden, D.M. (2002) The genetics of the long-QT syndrome. *American College of Cardiology Current Journal Review*, Mar/Apr 70–73.

Sagie, A., Larson, M.G., Goldberg, R.J., Bengtson, J.R. & Levy, D. (1992) An improved method for adjusting the QT interval for heart rate (the Framingham study). *American Journal of Cardiology*, **70**, 797–801.

Sarma, J.S.M., Sarma, R.J., Bilitch, M., Katz, D. &, Song, S.L. (1984) An exponential formula for heart rate dependence of QT interval during exercise and cardiac pacing in humans: reevaluation of Bazett's formula. *American Journal of Cardiology*, **54**, 103–108.

Schlamowitz, I. (1946) An analysis of the time relationships within the cardiac cycle in electrocardiograms of normal men. I. The duration of the QT interval and its relationship to the cycle length (*R–R* interval). *American Heart Journal*, **31**, 329–342.

Schwartz, P.J. & Wolf, S. (1978) QT interval prolongation as predictor of sudden death in patients with myocardial infarction. *Circulation*, **57**, 1074–1077.

Thurston, E. (1876) The length of the systole of the heart, as estimated from sphygmographic tracings. *Journal of Anatomy and Physiology*, **10**, 494–501.

Walker, A.M., Szneke, P., Weatherby, L.B. *et al.* (1999) The risk of serious cardiac arrhythmias among cisapride users in the United Kingdom and Canada. *American Journal of Medicne*, **107**, 356–362.

Waller, A.D. (1887) A demonstration on man of electromotive changes accompanying the heart's beat. *Journal of Physiology*, **8**, 229–235.

Wohlfart, B. & Pahlm O. (1994) Normal values for QT interval in ECG during ramp exercise on bicycle. *Clinical Physiology* **14**, 371–377.

Wong, K.Y.K, Mac Walter, R.S., Douglas, D., Fraser, H.W., Ogston, S.A. & Struthers, A.D. (2003) Long QT*c* predicts future cardiac death in stroke survivors. *Heart* **89**, 377–381.

CHAPTER 33

Circadian Patterns of *QTc* Interval

Peter Smetana, Esther Pueyo, Katerina Hnatkova and Marek Malik

Introduction

Rhythmic variations of metabolic processes and physiological events have been appreciated for centuries. Since their average frequency often is one cycle in 24 h the term circadian, derived from the Latin phrase *circa dies*, meaning about a day was introduced. Influenced or driven by factors such as light and activity, these rhythms provide insight into the regulatory mechanisms of organism adaptation to the environment (Moore-Ede *et al.* 1983; Panda *et al.* 2002).

The diurnal variation of uncorrected *QT* interval closely resembles the circadian rhythm of *RR* interval. Longest values are observed during the night with an abrupt shortening to daytime level in the early morning, followed by a slow increase during the late afternoon and evening (Fig. 33.1).

After correcting for the influence of heart rate, the circadian pattern of *QTc* is supposed to reveal the heart rate independent diurnal variations of ventricular repolarization. Nevertheless, reports on the circadian pattern of the *QTc* interval are inconsistent. Different studies reported a non-existent (Morganroth *et al.* 1991), blunted (Molnar *et al.* 1996), or marked (Sarma *et al.* 1990) circadian pattern of *QTc* interval in normal subjects. Thus, before discussing the potential value of changes in diurnal variation of *QTc*, this discrepancy needs to be clarified.

In addition to heart rate, it is mainly the autonomic tone that affects diurnal modulation of *QT* interval. The impacts of other factors like cyclic changes in hormone and electrolyte metabolism are still to be investigated.

RR interval – technical considerations

Every heart rate correction formula assumes that QT/RR relationship can be described by a mathematical model which can be converted to a formula that normalizes the measured *QT* interval to that associated with a standard heart rate, usually 60 beats/min. The resulting *QTc* interval should be independent of heart rate making measurements obtained at different heart rates comparable. However, shortcomings of any universal heart rate correction formula have been discussed repeatedly (Funck-Brentano & Jaillon 1993; Aytemir *et al.* 1999, Malik *et al.* 2002) and have recently been explained by the marked inter-individual variability and intra-individual stability of the QT/RR relationship (Molnar *et al.* 1996; Batchvarov *et al.* 2002). For the assessment of the diurnal pattern of a truly heart rate independent *QT* interval, proper heart rate correction is essential to avoid over- and/or underestimation of the circadian changes. Inconsistency in previous reports on the circadian variation of *QTc* is likely to be at least partly caused by differences in correction models. Comparing the circadian pattern of *QTc* derived by four frequently used correction formulae with that obtained by individually optimized heart rate correction models (Smetana *et al.* 2003) we found that the extent of the circadian pattern of *QTc* is substantially influenced by the formulae for heart rate correction (Fig. 33.2).

The use of continuous ambulatory 24-h recordings instead of steady-state resting ECGs creates another problem. It is known that the changes in the *QT* interval lag behind changes in heart rate – the phenomenon termed QT/RR hys-

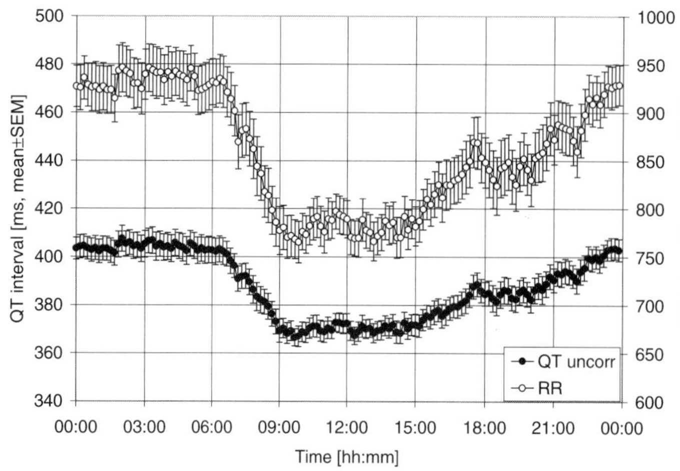

Fig. 33.1 Circadian pattern of RR (open circles) and uncorrected *QT* intervals (closed circles).

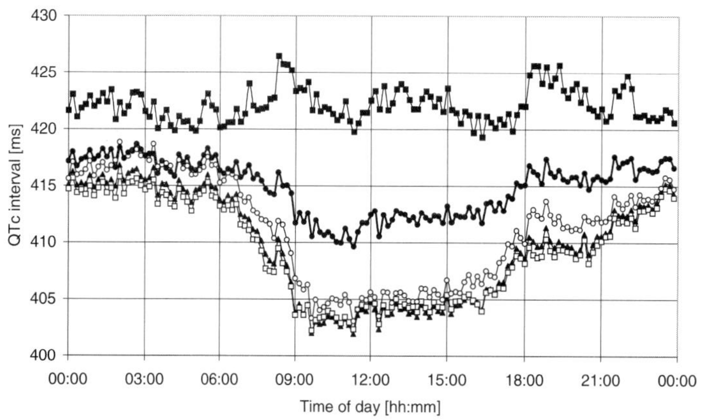

Fig. 33.2 Circadian pattern of *QTc* interval obtained by the Bazett (closed squares), Fridericia (closed triangles), Framingham (open squares), Hodges (open circles), and individually optimized (closed circles, bold) heart rate corrections. (Redrawn from Smetana *et al.* 2003, with permission.)

teresis (Arnold *et al.* 1982; Lau *et al.* 1988). However with automatic *QT* interval analysis from continuous 24-h Holter recordings, the QT hysteresis is usually ignored and frequently, only the preceding *RR* interval is taken for analysis or a constant duration of the hysteresis lag is assumed in all patients. This might result in significant errors in the *QTc* estimate. Using 24-h Holter recordings of 404 post myocardial infarction patients we found a mean length of hysteresis adaptation of 3.9 ± 2.4 min. However, in > 50% of the patients it took more than 3 min for the 90% *QT* interval adaptation to changes in *RR* interval (Fig. 33.3). Thus, the QT hysteresis adaptation is highly individual and any generalized approach tends to over- or underestimate the individual QT/RR relationship and leads to potentially incorrect *QTc* values (Coumel *et al.* 1994; Lang *et al.* 2001).

Finally the finding of diurnal changes of QT/RR relationship (Anselme *et al.* 1996; Badilini *et al.* 1999; Extramiana *et al.* 1999; Lande *et al.* 2000) might also be of some impact. Significant differences in QT/RR slopes between day and night in some individuals suggest that using the same formula over 24 h might lead to inappropriate results (Fig. 33.4).

This all suggests that measurements of circadian variations of heart rate corrected *QT* interval might be strongly influenced by inappropriate methodology.

QT interval and autonomic tone

Circadian variations in the autonomic nervous system (Boas & Weiss 1929) and in circulating catecholamines (Barnes *et al.* 1980) have been appreciated for a long time. Thus findings of cir-

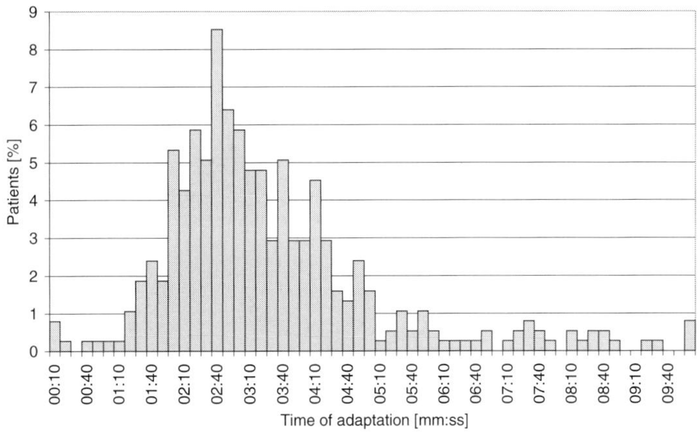

Fig. 33.3 Distribution of individual adaptation times of QT/RR hysteresis in postinfarction patients.

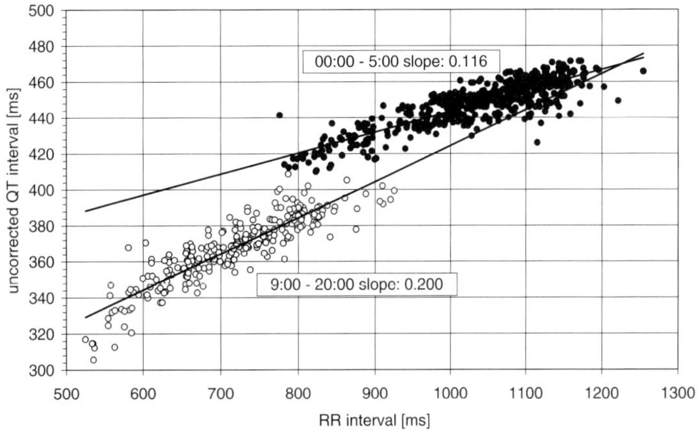

Fig. 33.4 Differences in QT/RR relationship and linear slope values in one individual during day and night.

cadian variations of *QTc* (Browne *et al.* 1983; Bexton *et al.* 1986) have been immediately considered to reflect the autonomic modulations of ventricular repolarization. This was supported by findings of a blunted circadian variation of *QTc* intervals in denervated hearts of heart transplant recipients (Bexton *et al.* 1986; Alexopoulos *et al.* 1988) (Fig. 33.5). Various experimental studies provided further evidence of direct autonomic effects on ventricular repolarization.

Under various combinations of artificial autonomic cardiac stimulation resulting in identical heart rates, it was shown in dogs that the effects of the sympatho-vagal interactions differ at the level of the sinus node and the ventricular myocardium (Inoue & Zipes 1987). A direct influence of cholinergic activity on ventricular repolarization was also described in studies evaluating the effect of sympathetic and parasympathetic blockade in patients in whom heart rate was kept at a constant level by atrial pacing. No significant effect on *QT* interval was found after beta blockade but when atropine was added, *QT* interval shortened significantly (Ahnve & Vallin 1982; Browne *et al.* 1982; Cappato *et al.* 1991). Others (Sarma 1993; Kowallik *et al.* 2000) used spectral analysis of beat-to-beat *RR* and *QT* intervals to assess autonomic effects on the sinus node and ventricular myocardium to confirm the differences in autonomic modulations. Further confirmation (Diedrich *et al.* 2002) of autonomic influence on ventricular repolarization was obtained very recently by showing that interruption of sympathetic and parasympathetic nerve traffic by ganglionic blockade results in *QTc* prolongation (Fig. 33.6).

Taken together, these results provide strong evidence for modulation of ventricular repolarization by the autonomic nervous system.

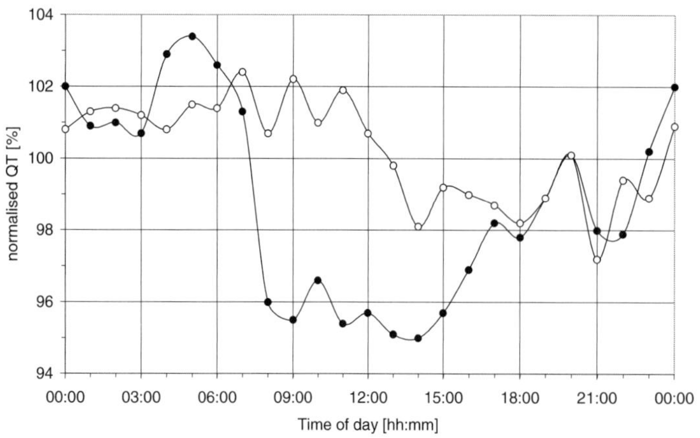

Fig. 33.5 Normalized *QT* interval plotted against time of day for paced patients (open circles) and transplant patients (closed circles). (Redrawn from Bexton *et al.* 1986, with permission.)

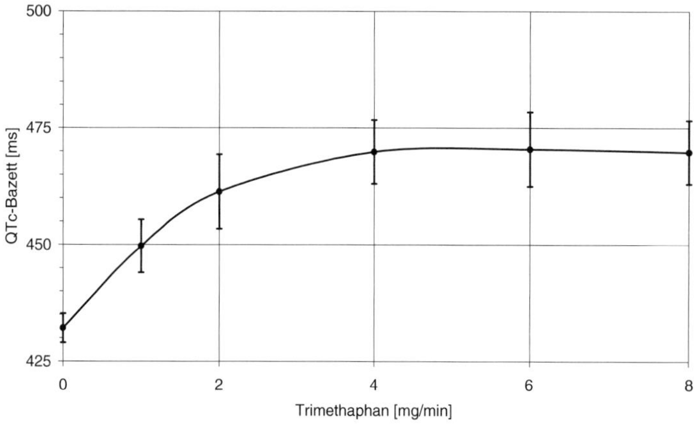

Fig. 33.6 Changes in *QTc* interval with incremental infusion of a ganglionic blocker (trimethapan). (Redrawn from Diedrich *et al.* 2002, with permission.)

Circadian pattern of *QTc* in normal subjects

The circadian pattern of *QTc* was investigated repeatedly in healthy subjects. As shown by examples in Table 33.1, results of these studies were inconsistent, as was their methodology (Fig. 33.7).

Studies investigating the effect of sleep deprivation (Ahnve *et al.* 1981) or activity (Cinca *et al.* 1986; Gillis *et al.* 1988) gave additional information on the dependence of the diurnal variation of *QTc* on external factors. Ahnve *et al.* (1981) showed that sleep deprivation and isolation from external time keeping attenuated the rhythmicity of *QT* interval, and thus suggested that the circadian rhythm measured under normal conditions is caused by the alternation between sleep and awake stages. Using 24-h bedside electrophysiological testing, Cinca *et al.* (1986) confirmed nocturnal lengthening of *QT* but did not find any difference between *QT* interval values obtained during nocturnal sleep and nocturnal awake states. Gillis *et al.* (1988) described a clear decrease in the variation of *QT* interval in subjects kept inactive and supine for 24 h. They also found *QT* interval during awake inactivity to be longer than during awake activity and those during non-rapid eye movements (NREM) sleep to be longer than those during REM sleep.

Risk stratification and the circadian pattern of *QTc*

Based on the assumption that differences in the extent of circadian pattern of *QTc* reflect autonomic modulation of ventricular repolarization and the finding of a morning surge in cardiovas-

Table 33.1 Studies on the circadian pattern of *QTc* in healthy subjects

Study	*n**	*QTc†*	*Measurement‡*	*Calculation§*	*Presentation*	*Circadian pattern*
Sarma *et al.* 1990	6	Exponential	Continuous	Beat-to-beat	3-h mean	Yes
Morganroth *et al.* 1991	20	Bazett	3×/h	1 beat	8-h mean	No
Rasmussen *et al.* 1991	60	Bazett	3 beats/4 h	3 beats	4-h mean	Yes
Ong *et al.* 1993	13	Exponential	Continuous	Beat-to beat	1-h mean	Yes
Molnar *et al.* 1996	21	Framingham	Continuous	5-min	1-h mean	No
Ishida *et al.* 1997	17	Bazett	First 6 min/h	6-min	1-h mean	No
Yi *et al.* 1998	14	Bazett	Continuous	Beat-to-beat	1-h mean	No
Smetana *et al.* 2002	51	Individual	2 × 10-s/min	10-s	10-min mean	Yes

* Number of subjects included, † heart rate correction used, ‡ number of ECG samples taken, § segment on which analysis was performed.

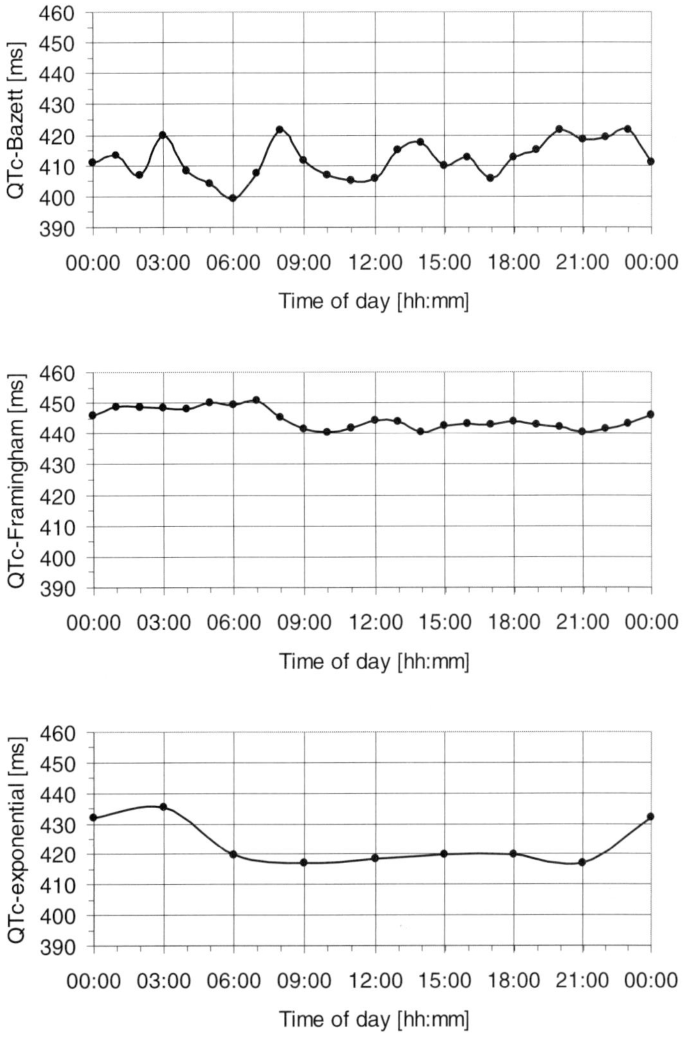

Fig. 33.7 Circadian variation of *QTc* interval in healthy subjects obtained by Bazett's formula (upper panel, from Ishida 1997), the Framingham formula (middle panel, from Molnar 1996), and an exponential formula (lower panel, from Sarma *et al.* 1990). (All redrawn with permission.)

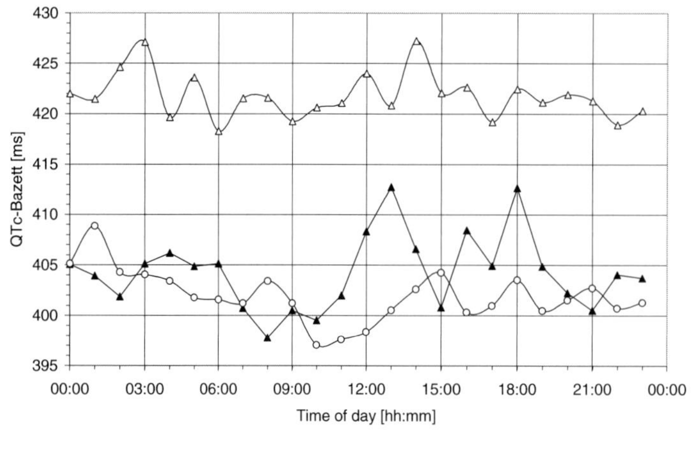

Fig. 33.8 Mean hourly *QTc* intervals for normal subjects (open circles), myocardial infarction survivors (closed triangles), and victims of sudden cardiac death (open triangles). (Redrawn from Yi *et al.* 1998, with permission.)

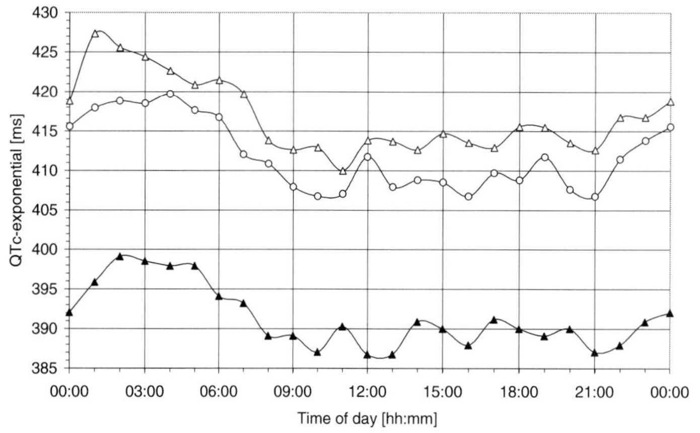

Fig. 33.9 Circadian variation of *QTc* intervals in diabetic patients with (closed triangles) and without (open triangles) diabetic autonomic neuropathy and in healthy controls (open circles). (Redrawn from Ong *et al.* 1993, with permission.)

cular (Muller 1991) and arrhythmic events (Willich *et al.* 1987), some studies evaluated circadian pattern of *QTc* in respect to risk stratification.

Comparing patients with complicated and uncomplicated outcome after myocardial infarction, variations in the circadian pattern of *QTc* seem to provide little prognostic information for risk stratification. Brüggemann *et al.* (1997) found no circadian variation of *QTc* and no significant difference in *QTc* duration in high and low risk patients. Others (Homs *et al.* 1997; Yi *et al.* 1998) also found no significant diurnal variation of *QTc* in different risk groups, though *QTc* duration was significantly longer in the group with complicated outcome (Fig. 33.8). Finally, comparing *QT* intervals at the same heart rate at day and night, Extramiana *et al.* (1999) showed larger diurnal variations and shorter *QT* intervals in the group with uncomplicated outcome.

In contrast, comparing survivors of sudden cardiac death with matched controls, Molnar *et al.* (1997) found significant differences between day and night *QTc* in survivors but not in the control group.

Some studies (Ong *et al.* 1993; Valensi *et al.* 2002) investigated diabetic patients with and without autonomic neuropathy. Whereas one study (Ong *et al.* 1993) found significantly shorter *QTc* values in the neuropathy group but no differences in the circadian pattern (Fig. 33.9), another study (Valensi *et al.* 2002) described *QTc* not differing between both groups with a reversed day night pattern and an increased nocturnal rate dependence in the neuropathy group.

Long QT syndrome (LQTS) and circadian pattern of *QTc*

One of the main diagnostic criteria of LQTS remains the *QTc* interval (Schwartz *et al.* 1993). Reports suggesting that the autonomic nervous system has an important role in modulating repolarization abnormalities in LQTS (Zipes 1991) indicate that it might be appropriate to investigate repolarization characteristics during day and night.

Comparing *QT* variables during day and night in LQT1 patients and controls Neyroud *et al.* (1998) found increased rate dependence at night to be a valuable diagnostic marker of LQTS. Lande *et al.* (2001) confirmed steeper night time than daytime slopes in genetically uniform LQT1 patients even when the *QTc* interval was normal. The authors further reported LQTS patients to have a similar *QT* interval at the same cycle length during day and night whereas controls showed longer *QT* intervals at night. These differences in circadian pattern, especially the reversed pattern of QT/RR relation might simplify diagnosis of LQTS in gene carriers with normal *QTc* values.

Studying 26 patients with different genotypes of LQTS (11 LQT1, 9 LQT2, and 6 LQT3), Stramba-Badiale *et al.* (2000) also found significant differences in the circadian variation of *QTc* interval. Whereas there was no circadian variation in LQT2 patients and LQT1 patients only showed a modest decrease during the night, the night-time *QTc* interval was markedly prolonged in LQT3 patients (Fig. 33.10). The authors suggested this to be an explanation for the higher risk for sudden death during sleep in LQT3 patients.

Drugs and circadian pattern of *QTc*

Investigation of the circadian pattern of *QTc* during drug therapy may bear valuable information additional to findings from single resting ECGs. Changes in circadian variation of *QTc* as result of drug treatment may suggest drug-related changes in autonomic modulation of ventricular repolarization.

For example, in patients with ischaemic heart disease, 3 weeks of nadolol treatment was shown to have no effect on the circadian variation of *QTc* (Sarma *et al.* 1994) (Fig. 33.11). This is consistent with experimental findings of just little effect of beta blockade alone on *QT* interval. Atenolol was shown (Viitasalo & Karjalainen 1992) to have no effect on *QT* intervals at night but, dependent of heart rate, *QT* was lengthened or shortened during the day. Sotalol therapy was also reported (Kantelip *et al.* 1986; Hohnloser *et al.* 1993; Sharma *et al.* 1999) to maintain the circadian rhythm of *QTc*. On the other hand, long-term treatment (>1 year) with amiodarone resulted in a virtual loss of circadian periodicity of *QTc* (Antimisiaris *et al.* 1994) suggesting suppression of direct autonomic modulation of ventricular repolarization.

Investigating the effect of hypothyroidism and thyroxine therapy on repolarization, Sarma *et al.* (1990) described longer *QTc* intervals and

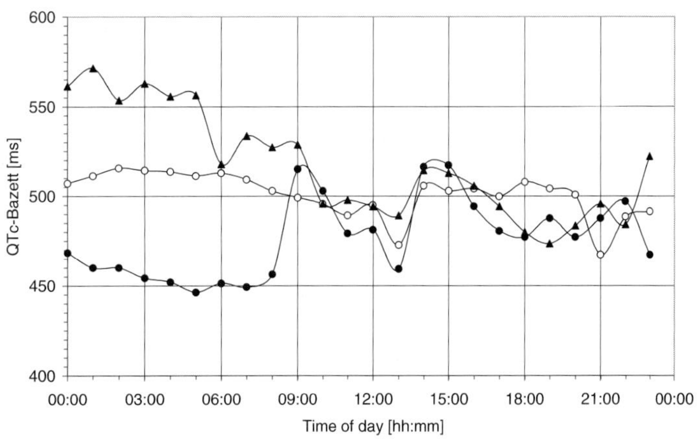

Fig. 33.10 Circadian variation of *QTc* of three patients representative of the three different LQTS subgroups: LQT1, closed circles; LQT2, open circles; LQT3, closed triangles. (Redrawn from Stramba-Badiale *et al.* 2000, with permission.)

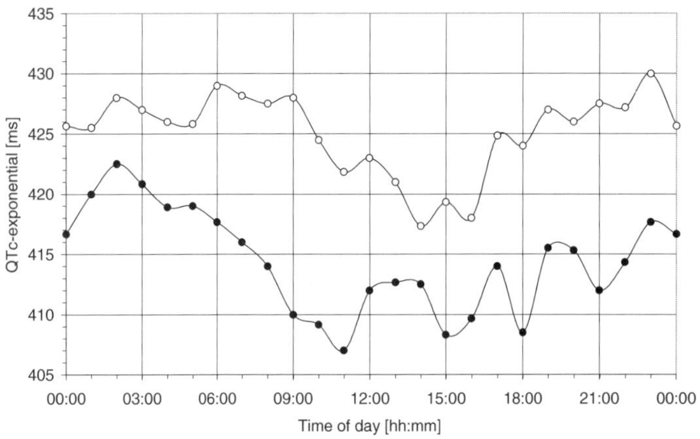

Fig. 33.11 Mean hourly *QTc* intervals plotted against hour of the day before (open circles) and after (closed circles) 3 weeks of nadolol therapy. (Redrawn from Sarma *et al.* 1994, with permission.)

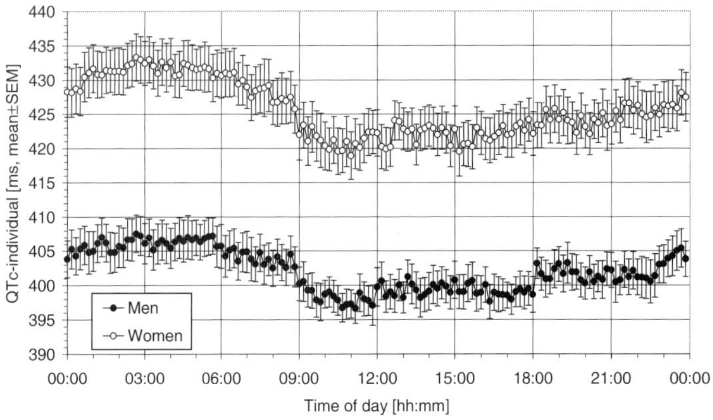

Fig. 33.12 Circadian pattern of individually rate corrected *QTc* intervals in women (open circles) and men (closed circles). (Redrawn from Smetana 2002, with permission.)

a less marked pattern in hypothyroid patients compared to controls. Thyroxine therapy did not influence the circadian pattern and only decreased the disease-related *QTc* prolongation.

Diurnal variations in the extent of any drug-related *QTc* prolongation (whether intended or otherwise) might also have direct implications on dosage regimes and arrhythmic risk assessment. However, we are not aware of studies using this approach.

Gender and circadian pattern of *QTc*

Appreciation of the higher risk of women to develop torsades de pointes in different settings of *QT* prolongation recently focused the interest on sex differences in *QT* interval duration and QT/RR relation. However, besides the well-appreciated longer *QTc* intervals (Bazett 1920) and steeper QT/RR slopes (Kligfield *et al.* 1996) in women, studies on the differences in the circadian modulation of the *QT* interval between women and men are sparse.

Most studies were performed only in men (Browne *et al.* 1983). One study (Anselme *et al.* 1996) comparing daytime and night-time QT_{apex} intervals at similar heart rates found nocturnal prolongation to be not significantly larger in women than in men. However, due to the use of QT_{apex} instead of *QT* interval, the results are difficult to compare with other investigations. Studying repolarization properties in healthy young women and men (Smetana 2002) we found *QTc* intervals obtained by individually optimized heart rate correction to be significantly longer in women over the entire 24 h, with the circadian variation also being more marked in women (Fig. 33.12).

Summary

Properly corrected *QTc* interval shows a circadian pattern with longer intervals during the night and shorter intervals during the day. This is likely to reflect diurnal changes in autonomic modulation of ventricular repolarization as well as influence from cyclic fluctuations in the metabolism of hormones and electrolytes. The extent of the circadian variation of *QTc* depends on technical factors like the heart rate correction model. Thus, the use of variations in the circadian pattern of *QTc* to assess risk, diagnosis, or drug effects is dependent on proper individualised heart rate correction and individualised quantification of QT/RR hysteresis.

References

Ahnve, S., Theorell, T., Akerstedt, T., Froberg, J.E. & Halberg, F. (1981) Circadian variations in cardiovascular parameters during sleep deprivation. A noninvasive study of young healthy men. *European Journal of Applied Physiology and Occupational Physiology*, **46**, 9–19.

Ahnve, S. & Vallin, H. (1982) Influence of heart rate and inhibition of autonomic tone on the QT interval. *Circulation*, **65**, 435–439.

Alexopoulos, D., Rynkiewicz, A., Yusuf, S., Johnston, J.A., Sleight, P. & Yacoub, M.H. (1988) Diurnal variations of QT interval after cardiac transplantation. *American Journal of Cardiology*, **61**, 482–485.

Antimisiaris, M., Sarma, J.S., Schoenbaum, M.P., Sharma, P.P., Venkataraman, K. & Singh, B.N. (1994) Effects of amiodarone on the circadian rhythm and power spectral changes of heart rate and QT interval: significance for the control of sudden cardiac death. *American Heart Journal*, **128**, 884–891.

Anselme, F., Maison-Blanche, P., Cheruy, P., Saoudi, N., Letac, B. & Coumel, P. (1996) Absence of gender difference in circadian trends of QT interval duration. *Annals of Noninvasive Electrocardiology*, **1**, 278–286.

Arnold, L., Page, J., Attwell, D., Cannell, M. & Eisner, D.A. (1982) The dependence on heart rate of the human ventricular action potential duration. *Cardiovascular Research*, **16**, 547–551.

Aytemir, K., Maarouf, N., Gallagher, M.M., Yap, Y.G., Waktare, J.E. & Malik, M. (1999) Comparison of formulae for heart rate correction of QT interval in exercise electrocardiograms. *PACE (Pacing and Clinical Electrophysiology)*, **22**, 1397–1401.

Barnes, P., FitzGerald, G., Brown, M. & Dollery, C. (1980) Nocturnal asthma and changes in circulating epinephrine, histamine, and cortisol. *New England Journal of Medicine*, **303**, 263–267.

Badilini, F., Maison-Blanche, P., Childers, R. & Coumel, P. (1999) QT interval analysis on ambulatory electrocardiogram recordings: a selective beat averaging approach. *Medical & Biological Engineering & Computing*, **37**, 71–9.

Batchvarov, V.N., Ghuran, A., Smetana, P. *et al.* (2002) QT/RR relationship in healthy subjects exhibits substantial intersubject variability and high intrasubject stability. *American Journal of Physiology (Heart Circulation Physiology)* **282**, H2356–H2363.

Bazett, H. (1920) An analysis of the time-relations of electrocardiograms. *Heart*, **vii**, 353–370.

Bexton, R.S., Vallin, H.O. & Camm, A.J. (1986) Diurnal variation of the QT interval – influence of the autonomic nervous system. *British Heart Journal*, **55**, 253–258.

Boas, E.P. & Weiss, M.M. (1929) The heart rate during sleep as determined by the cardiotachometer. Its clinical significance. *JAMA (Journal of the American Medical Association)*, **92**, 2162–2168.

Browne, K.F., Zipes, D.P., Heger, J.J. & Prystowsky, E.N. (1982) Influence of the autonomic nervous system on the QT interval in man. *American Journal of Cardiology*, **50**, 1099–1103.

Browne, K.F., Prystowsky, E., Heger, J.J., Chilson, D.A. & Zipes, D.P. (1983) Prolongation of the QT interval in man during sleep. *American Journal of Cardiology*, **52**, 55–59.

Brüggemann, T., Eisenreich, S., Behrens, S., Ehlers, C., Müller, D. & Andresen, D. (1997) Continuous QT interval measurements from 24-hour electrocardiography and risk after myocardial infarction. *Annals of Noninvasive Electrocardiology*, **2**, 264–273.

Cappato, R., Alboni, P, Pedroni, P., Gilli, G. & Antonioli, G.E. (1991) Sympathetic and vagal influences on rate-dependent changes of QT interval in healthy subjects. *American Journal of Cardiology*, **68**, 1188–1193.

Cinca, J., Moya, A., Figueras, J., Roma, F. & Rius, J. (1986) Circadian variations in the electrical properties of the human heart assessed by sequential bedside electrophysiological testing. *American Heart Journal*, **112**, 315–321.

Coumel, P., Fayn, J., Maison-Blanche, P. & Rubel, P. (1994) Clinical relevance of assessing QT dynamicity in Holter recordings. *Journal of Electrocardiology*, **27** (Suppl.), 62–66.

Diedrich, A., Jordan, J., Shannon, J.R., Robertson, D. & Biaggioni, I. (2002) Modulation of QT interval during autonomic nervous system blockade in humans. *Circulation*, **106**, 2238–2243.

Extramiana, F., Maison-Blanche, P., Badilini, F., Pinoteau, J., Deseo, T. & Coumel, P. (1999a) Circadian modulation of QT rate dependence in healthy volunteers: gender and age differences. *Journal of Electrocardiology*, **32**, 33–43.

Extramiana, F., Neyroud, N., Huikuri, H.V., Koistinen, M.J., Coumel, P. & Maison-Blanche, P. (1999b) QT interval and arrhythmic risk assessment after myocardial infarction. *American Journal of Cardiology*, **83**, 266–269.

Funck-Brentano, C. & Jaillon, P. (1993) Rate-corrected QT interval: techniques and limitations. *American Journal of Cardiology*, **72**, 17B–22B

Gillis, A.M., MacLean, K.E. & Guilleminault, C. (1988) The QT interval during wake and sleep in patients with ventricular arrhythmias. *Sleep*, **11**, 333–339.

Hohnloser, S.H., Zabel, M., Just, H. & Raeder, E.A. (1993) Relation of diurnal variation of ventricular repolarization to ventricular ectopic activity and modification by sotalol. *American Journal of Cardiology*, **71**, 475–478.

Homs, E., Marti, V., Guindo, J. *et al.* (1997) Automatic measurement of corrected QT interval in Holter recordings: Comparison of its dynamic behaviour in patients after myocardial infarction with and without live-threatening arrhythmias. *American Heart Journal*, **134**, 181–187.

Inoue, H. & Zipes, D.P. (1987) Changes in atrial and ventricular refractoriness and in atrioventricular nodal conduction produced by combinations of vagal and sympathetic stimulation that result in a constant spontaneous sinus cycle length. *Circulation Research*, **60**, 942–951.

Ishida, S., Nakagawa, M., Fujino, T., Yonemochi, H., Saikawa, T. & Ito, M. (1997) Circadian variation of QT interval dispersion: correlation with heart rate variability. *Journal of Electrocardiology*, **30**, 205–210.

Kantelip, J.P., Trolese, J.F., Cadilhac, M., Pechadre, J.C. & Duchene-Marullaz, P. (1986) Effects of sotalol on ambulatory electrocardiography in volunteers. *Clinical Pharmacology and Therapeutics*, **40**, 554–560.

Kligfield, P., Lax, K.G. & Okin, P.M. (1996) QT interval–heart rate relation during exercise in normal men and women: definition by linear regression analysis. *Journal of the American College of Cardiology*, **28**, 1547–1555.

Kowallik, P., Braun, C. & Meesmann, M. (2000) Independent autonomic modulation of sinus node and ventricular myocardium in healthy young men during sleep. *Journal of Cardiovascular Electrophysiology*, **11**, 1063–1070.

Lande, G., Funck-Brentano, C., Ghadanfar, M. & Escande, D. (2000) Steady-state vs. non-steady-state QT/RR relationships in 24-h Holter recordings. *PACE (Pacing and Clinical Electrophysiology)*, **23**, 293–302.

Lande, G., Kyndt, F., Baro, I. *et al.* (2001) Dynamic analysis of the QT interval in long QT1 syndrome patients with a normal phenotype. *European Heart Journal*, **22**, 410–422.

Lang, C.C., Flapan, A.D. & Neilson, J.M. (2001) The impact of QT lag compensation on dynamic assessment of ventricular repolarization, reproducibility and the impact of lead selection. *PACE (Pacing and Clinical Electrophysiology)*, **24**, 366–373.

Lau, C.P., Freedman, A.R., Fleming, S., Malik, M., Camm, A.J. & Ward, D.E. (1988) Hysteresis of the ventricular paced QT interval in response to abrupt changes in pacing rate. *Cardiovascular Research*, **22**, 67–72.

Malik, M., Färbom, P., Batchvarov, V., Hnatkova, K. & Camm, A.J. (2002) Relation between QT and RR intervals is highly individual among healthy subjects: implications for heart rate correction of the QT interval. *Heart*, **87**, 220–228.

Molnar, J., Weiss, J., Zhang, F. & Rosenthal, J.E. (1996a) Evaluation of five QT correction formulas using a software-assisted method of continuous QT measurement from 24-h Holter recordings. *American Journal of Cardiology*, **78**, 920–926.

Molnar, J., Zhang, F., Weiss, J., Ehlert, F.A. & Rosenthal, J.E. (1996b) Diurnal pattern of QT*c* interval: how long is prolonged? Possible relation to circadian triggers cardiovascular events. *Journal of the American College of Cardiology*, **27**, 76–83.

Molnar, J., Rosenthal, J.E., Weiss, J.S. & Somberg, J.C. (1997) QT interval dispersion in healthy subjects and survivors of sudden cardiac death: circadian variation in a twenty-four-hour assessment. *American Journal of Cardiology*, **79**, 1190–1193.

Moore-Ede, M.C., Czeisler, C.A. & Richardson, G.S. (1983a) Circadian timekeeping in health and disease. Part 1. Basic properties of circadian pacemakers. *New England Journal of Medicine*, **309**, 469–476.

Moore-Ede, M.C., Czeisler, C.A. & Richardson, G.S. (1983b) Circadian timekeeping in health and disease. Part 2. Clinical implications of circadian rhythmicity. *New England Journal of Medicine*, **309**, 530–536.

Morganroth, J., Brozovich, F.V., McDonald, J.T. & Jacobs, R.A. (1991) Variability of the QT measurement in healthy men, with implications for selection of an abnormal QT value to predict drug toxicity and proarrhythmia. *American Journal of Cardiology*, **67**, 774–776.

Muller, J.E., Stone, P.H., Turi, Z.G. *et al.* (1985) Circadian variation in the frequency of onset of acute myocardial infarction. *New England Journal of Medicine*, **313**, 1315–1322.

Neyroud, N., Maison-Blanche, P., Denjoy, I. *et al.* (1998) Diagnostic performance of QT interval variables from 24-h electrocardiography in the long QT syndrome. *European Heart Journal*, **19**, 158–165.

Ong, J.J., Sarma, J.S., Venkataraman, K., Levin, S.R. & Singh, B.N. (1993) Circadian rhythmicity of heart rate and QT*c* interval in diabetic autonomic neuropathy: implications for the mechanism of sudden death. *American Heart Journal*, **125**, 744–752.

Panda, S., Hogenesch, J.B. & Kay, S.A. (2002) Circadian rhythms from flies to human. *Nature (London)*, **417**, 329–335.

Rasmussen, V., Jensen, G. & Hansen, J.F. (1991) QT interval in 24-h ambulatory ECG recordings from 60 healthy adult subjects. *Journal of Electrocardiology*, **24**, 91–95.

Sarma, J.S., Venkataraman, K., Nicod, P. *et al.* (1990) Circadian rhythmicity of rate-normalized QT interval in hypothyroidism and its significance for development of class III antiarrhythmic agents. *American Journal of Cardiology*, **66**, 959–963.

Sarma, J.S., Singh, N., Schoenbaum, M.P., Venkataraman, K. & Singh, B.N. (1994) Circadian and power spectral changes of RR and QT intervals during treatment of patients with angina pectoris with nadolol providing evidence for differential autonomic modulation of heart rate and ventricular repolarization. *American Journal of Cardiology*, **74**, 131–136.

Schwartz, P.J. & Wolf, S. (1978) QT interval prolongation as predictor of sudden death in patients with myocardial infarction. *Circulation*, **57**, 1074–1077.

Schwartz, P.J., Moss, A.J., Vincent, G.M. & Crampton, R.S. (1993) Diagnostic criteria for the long QT syndrome. An update. *Circulation*, **88**, 782–784.

Sharma, P.P., Sarma, J.S. & Singh, B.N. (1999) Effects of sotalol on the circadian rhythmicity of heart rate and QT intervals with a index of reverse-use dependency. *Journal of Cardiovascular Pharmacology and Therapeutics*, **4**, 15–21.

Smetana, P., Batchvarov, V., Hnatkova, K., Camm, A.J. & Malik, M. (2003) Circadian rhythm of *QTc* interval: impact of different heart rate correction models. *PACE (Pacing and Clinical Electrophysiology)*, **26**, 383–386.

Smetana, P., Batchvarov, V.N, Hnatkova, K., Camm, A.J. & Malik, M. (2002) Sex differences in repolarization homogeneity and its circadian pattern. *American Journal of Physiology (Heart Circulation Physiology)* **282**, H1889–H1897.

Stramba-Badiale, M., Priori, S.G., Napolitano, C. *et al.* (2000) Gene-specific differences in the circadian variation of ventricular repolarization in the long QT syndrome: a key to sudden death during sleep? *Italian Heart Journal*, **1**, 323–328.

Valensi, P.E., Johnson, N.B., Maison-Blanche, P., Extramania, F., Motte, G. & Coumel, P. (2002) Influence of cardiac autonomic neuropathy on heart rate dependence of ventricular repolarization in diabetic patients. *Diabetes Care*, **25**, 918–923.

Viitasalo, M. & Karjalainen, J. (1992) QT intervals at heart rates from 50 to 120 beats/min during 24-h electrocardiographic recordings in 100 healthy men. Effects of atenolol. *Circulation*, **86**, 1439–1442.

Willich, S.N., Levy, D., Rocco, M.B., Tofler, G.H., Stone, P.H. & Muller, J.E. (1987) Circadian variation in the incidence of sudden cardiac death in the Framingham Heart Study population. *American Journal of Cardiology*, **60**, 801–806.

Yi, G., Guo, X.H., Reardon, M. *et al.* (1998) Circadian variation of the QT interval in patients with sudden cardiac death after myocardial infarction. *American Journal of Cardiology*, **81**, 950–956.

Zipes, D.P. (1991) The long QT interval syndrome. A Rosetta stone for sympathetic related ventricular tachyarrhythmias. *Circulation*, **84**, 1414–1419.

CHAPTER 34

QT Dispersion

Velislav Batchvarov and Marek Malik

Introduction

The recovery times vary throughout ventricular myocardium as a result of differences in both activation times and action potential duration and morphology (Franz *et al.* 1987). The exact mechanisms and magnitude of regional and transmural dispersion of repolarization in the beating heart under normal and abnormal conditions as opposed to experimental preparations are still not clear and are subject to an ongoing debate (Anyukhovsky *et al.* 1996; Yan & Antzelevitch 1998; Antzelevitch 2001; Taggart *et al.* 2001) (Figs 34.1 and 34.2). However, experimental studies repeatedly demonstrated that abnormal augmentation of ventricular repolarization dispersion creates a substrate for the development of re-entrant arrhythmias (Wiggers 1940; Han & Moe 1964; Allessie *et al.* 1976; Kuo *et al.* 1983; Shimizu & Antzelevitch 1997, 1998) (Fig. 34.3). These results, as well as the increased awareness of clinicians, researchers, drug developers and regulators of the role of repolarization abnormalities in spontaneous and drug-inducedventricular arrhythmogenesis led to intensive search of methods to quantify dispersion of ventricular repolarization from the standard 12-lead electrocardiogram (ECG).

The variations of the shape, duration and timing of action potentials are summarily represented in the ECG by the T wave (Surawicz 1989). Nevertheless, the relation between dispersion of repolarization and the T wave is too complex to allow quantitative analysis of the former by simple visual inspection or manual measurement of the latter. Abnormally dispersed repolarization is also often abnormally prolonged which explains the well-documented link between prolongation of the *QT* interval and cardiac and arrhythmic mortality in the general population and different patient groups (Karjalainen *et al.* 1997; De Bruyne *et al.* 1999; Okin *et al.* 2000). Unfortunately, *QT* interval durations in survivors and victims are largely overlapping, in addition (and partially also due to) the well-known problems with the measurement of the *QT* interval and its correction for heart rate. There is no easy way to discern 'good' (homogeneous, therapeutically beneficial) from 'bad' (heterogeneous, potentially arrhythmogenic) or 'indifferent' *QT* interval prolongation (Surawicz 1999), unless it is excessive, and the dichotomy values from the epidemiological studies are of very little use for individual risk assessment.

The variations in ventricular recovery times are summarily represented in the concept of ventricular gradient (or 'net' QRST area) proposed Frank Wilson and colleagues in the 1930's (Wilson *et al.* 1931, 1934). Since then many authors have pointed out that ventricular gradient is a global index of the heterogeneity of ventricular repolarization (Ashman & Byer 1948; Plonsey 1979; Abildskov *et al.* 1980) but instead of being further investigated the concept became largely forgotten.

Triggered by the publication by Day *et al.* in 1990, many researchers were fascinated by the idea to quantify dispersion of ventricular repolarization from the interlead differences of *QT* interval durations of the standard 12-lead ECG (QT dispersion) in basically the same way as with monophasic action potential durations (MAP) directly recorded from the heart. The idea was not new and QT dispersion in the six precordial leads could be regarded as a simplification of similar earlier studies with multiple electrode body surface maps (Mirvis 1985). No justifica-

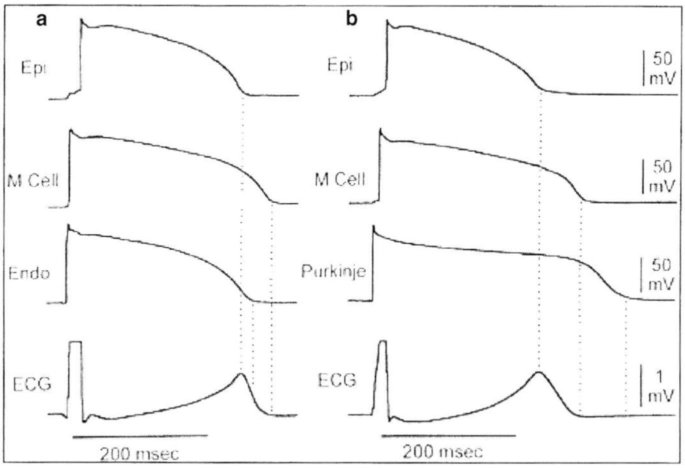

Fig. 34.1 Transmural dispersion of repolarization underlying the normal T wave. Transmembrane potentials and a transmural ECG recorded from 2 different arterially perfused canine LV wedges. A. Action potentials from epicardial (Epi), midmyocardial (M), and endocardial (Endo) sites have been simultaneously recorded using floating glass microelectrodes. A transmural ECG has been recorded concurrently. B. Action potentials from epicardium (Epi), midmyocardium (M), and subendocardial Purkinje fibers have been recorded simultaneously together with a transmural ECG. In both cases, repolarization of epicardium is coincident with the peak of the T wave of the ECG, whereas repolarization of the M cells is coincident with the end of the T wave. The endocardial APD is intermediate (A). Although repolarization of the Purkinje fiber occurs after that of the M cell (B), it does not register on the ECG. BCL = 2000 ms. (Reproduced from Yan & Antzelevitch *Circulation* (1998), **98**, 1928–1936, with permission.)

tion, however, was proposed for the extension of the same idea to the six peripheral leads which express the potential differences between three body surface points! Despite all criticism of its physiological background (Lee *et al.* 1998; Kors *et al.* 1999; Malik *et al.* 2000), the number of studies on QT dispersion increased dramatically, many of them reporting positive correlation between increased dispersion and various symptoms, adverse clinical events, markers of myocardial damage, lack of therapeutic success with drugs or interventions, etc. Most of the published literature on QT dispersion has been summarized in previous reviews (Surawicz 1996; Malik & Batchvarov 2000a, b).

Physiology and measurement

QT dispersion and dispersion of ventricular recovery times

Three early studies showed a correlation between QT dispersion and the dispersion of ventricular recovery times measured with MAPs.

Higham *et al.* (1992) found high positive correlation between dispersion of ventricular recovery times measured from epicardial MAPs recorded during cardiac surgery and QT dispersion during sinus rhythm and ventricular pacing.

Using a custom-build rabbit heart set-up with simultaneous recording of MAP and 12-lead ECGs, Zabel *et al.* showed that the dispersion of *QT* and JT intervals was significantly correlated with the dispersion of MAP duration recovery times (Zabel *et al.* 1995). Later the same authors confirmed their findings in patients with 12-lead ECGs recorded within 24 h of the MAPs (Zabel *et al.* 1998).

The high correlation between direct measures of dispersion of repolarization and QT dispersion, however, were questioned by more recent studies. Punske *et al.* (1999) compared the spatial distribution of the *QT* intervals from high-resolution maps on (a) human body surface, (b) the surface of a tank containing an isolated canine heart, and (c) the surface of exposed canine hearts, with the potential distributions on cardiac and body surfaces, and with recovery times on cardiac surfaces. They showed that on the body and tank surface, as well as on the epicardium, the 'zero potential line' (no potential difference relative to a reference electrode) sta-

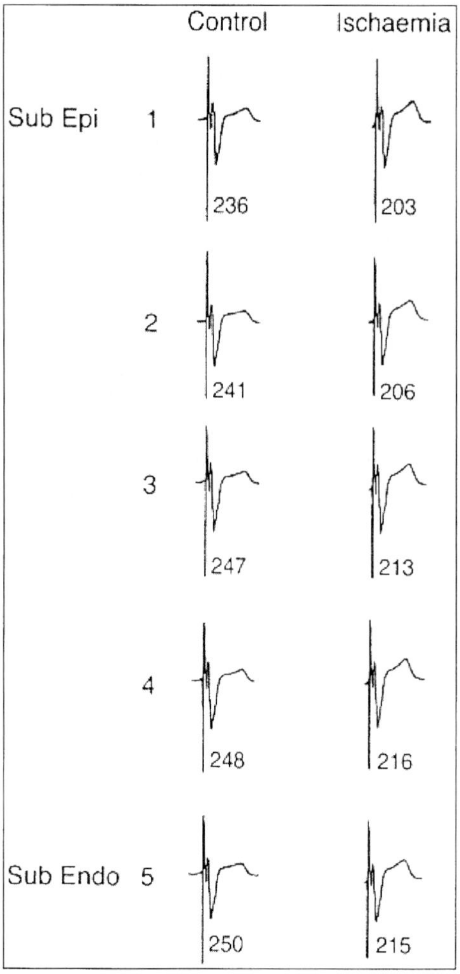

Fig. 34.2 Electrograms recorded at five intramural sites between subepicardium (sub epi) and subendocardium (sub endo) from the mid left ventricular wall during right ventricular pacing with a cycle length of 750 ms (80 beats per minute) in a patient with coronary heart disease, no previous MI, good ventricular function and no haemodynamically significant stenosis of the coronary vessel supplying the recording site. Values for activation recovery intervals (ARI) are shown for each electrogram. During control only a small ARI gradient is present (transmural dispersion of 14 ms, left-hand column). During ischemia ARIs shorten but the transmural gradient remains similar to control (13 ms). Compare these results obtained in beating human heart with the experimental results in Figure 1. (Reproduced from Taggart *et al. Cardiovascular Research* (2001), **50**, 454–462, with permission.)

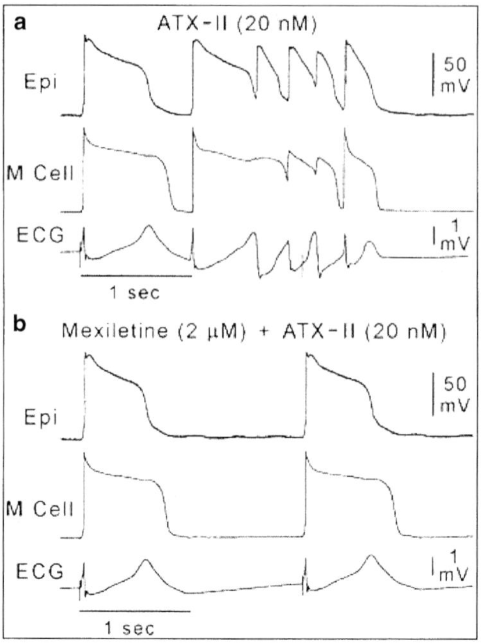

Fig. 34.3 Spontaneous occurrence of a short episode of torsades de pointes induced by ATX-II (an agent that slows the inactivation of the sodium channel and thus mimics long QT syndrome type III) and effect of mexiletine on this activity in canine left ventricular arterially perfused wedge preparation. Each trace shows action potentials simultaneously recorded from epicardial (Epi) and M cells together with a transmural ECG. Basic cycle length 2000 ms. ATX-II 20 nmol/L markedly prolonged action potential duration at both recording sites and increased transmural dispersion of repolarisation due to a greater prolongation of APD in M cell. A spontaneous ventricular premature beat is seen to initiate a short episode of TdP. Mexiletine 2 μmol/L added in continued presence of ATX-II completely suppressed spontaneous torsades de pointes. (Reproduced from Shimizu & Antzelevitch *Circulation* (1997), **96**, 2038–2047, with permission.)

bilises for 10–30 ms at the end of repolarization. This stabilisation of the 'zero line' in a given location leads to isoelectric terminal portions of the T wave for leads in the vicinity. Regions of shortest *QT* intervals always coincided with the location of the zero line. In addition, there were no consistent regions of earliest recovery times on the cardiac surface that coincided with the location of the zero potential line or shortest *QT* intervals.

Fuller *et al.* (2000) used isolated, perfused

canine hearts suspended in a torso-shaped electrolytic tank to record simultaneously electrograms from 64 epicardial sites and ECGs from 192 'body surface' sites. QT dispersion and a new surface ECG measure of dispersion of repolarization, root-mean-square (RMS) of the ECG curve were derived from four lead sets: epicardial, body surface, precordial, and a 6-lead optimal set. Repolarization was altered by changing cycle length, temperature, and activation sequence. Repolarization dispersion, calculated directly from recovery times of the 64 epicardial potentials, was then compared with the width of the T wave of the RMS curve and with QTd for each of these four lead sets. The correlation between T wave width and Rd for each lead set, respectively, was epicardium, 0.91; body surface, 0.84; precordial, 0.72; and optimal leads, 0.81. In contrast, the correlation between QTd and Rd for each lead set was 0.46 for epicardium, 0.47 for body surface and only 0.17 and 0.11 for the precordial and optimal leads, respectively (Figs 34.4 and 34.5).

Other arguments against the concept of QT dispersion as a valid index of dispersion of repolarization originated from the electrocardiographic lead theory. If the majority of the information about the ventricular electrical activity is contained in the spatial QRS and T loops (the heart vector), the major reason for the differences between separate leads has to be the loss of information from the projection of the loop into the separate leads (Coumel *et al.* 1998). Several studies supported this idea.

Macfarlane *et al.* (1998) and Lee *et al.* (1998) showed independently that QT dispersion can also be found in the so-called 'derived' 12-lead ECGs, i.e. ECGs reconstructed from the XYZ leads which, naturally, contain no regional information. In both studies the QT dispersion in the originally recorded and in the 'derived' 12 leads was surprisingly similar (29.1 ± 10.2 vs. 27.5 ± 10.8 ms and 41 ± 18 vs. 40 ± 20 ms, respectively).

Kors *et al.* (1999) found that QT dispersion was significantly different between patients with narrow (54.2 ± 27.1 ms) and wide T loops (69.5 ± 33.5 ms, $P < 0.001$). They also showed that in each of the six limb, as well as six precordial leads, the difference between the *QT* interval in a lead and the maximum *QT* interval was dependent on the angle between the axis of the lead and the axis of the terminal part of the T loop (Fig. 34.6).

Another and different approach provided an argument against the validity of QT dispersion as an index of dispersion of ventricular repolarization. Malik *et al.* (2000) proposed an ECG processing technique to distinguish the T wave signals representing the 3D movement of the ECG dipole from the non-dipolar components likely to be related to regional heterogeneity of myocardial repolarization. Although the non-dipolar components differed between the different clinical groups, there was very little correlation between the relative amount of the non-dipolar components and QT dispersion calculated automatically (QT Guard Program, GE Marquette Medical Systems, Milwaukee, WI) in the same ECGs ($r = -0.046$, 0.2805, −0.1531, and 0.0771, in normal subjects, HCM patients, DCM patients, and survivors of acute MI, respectively, $P = 0.03$ for HCM, others NS).

Rautaharju (2002) analysed digital 12-lead ECGs of 966 patients with coronary artery disease (CAD) and 3844 subjects considered free of CAD. A computer program (ECG Morphology Program, Novaheart Inc., Winston-Salem, NC) was used to calculate the non-dipolar voltage (NDPV) of the T wave and of its terminal 40 ms, the ratio of the first two eigenvalues (E1/E2) and an ECG estimate of left ventricular (LV) mass. QT dispersion was calculated automatically (QT Guard, GE Marquette). NDPV alone explained only 6% and NDPV, E1/E2 and LV mass combined 13% of QTd variance. There was a modest but significant increase in the fraction of subject with QTd > 60 ms among subjects with NDPV in the terminal part of the T wave > 7 μV compared to those with NDPV ≤ 7 μV (15% vs. 10%, $P < 0.001$). In contrast, the proportion of patients with QTd > 60 ms was 3 times higher among those with abnormal axis of the terminal part of the T wave compared to those with normal T axis (36.7 vs. 12%). It was concluded that QTd was unlikely to be a meaningful representation of local myocardial electrical events and was rather mainly determined by the main repolarization dipole (i.e. the terminal T wave axis). It is also worth reminding that, at least theoretically,

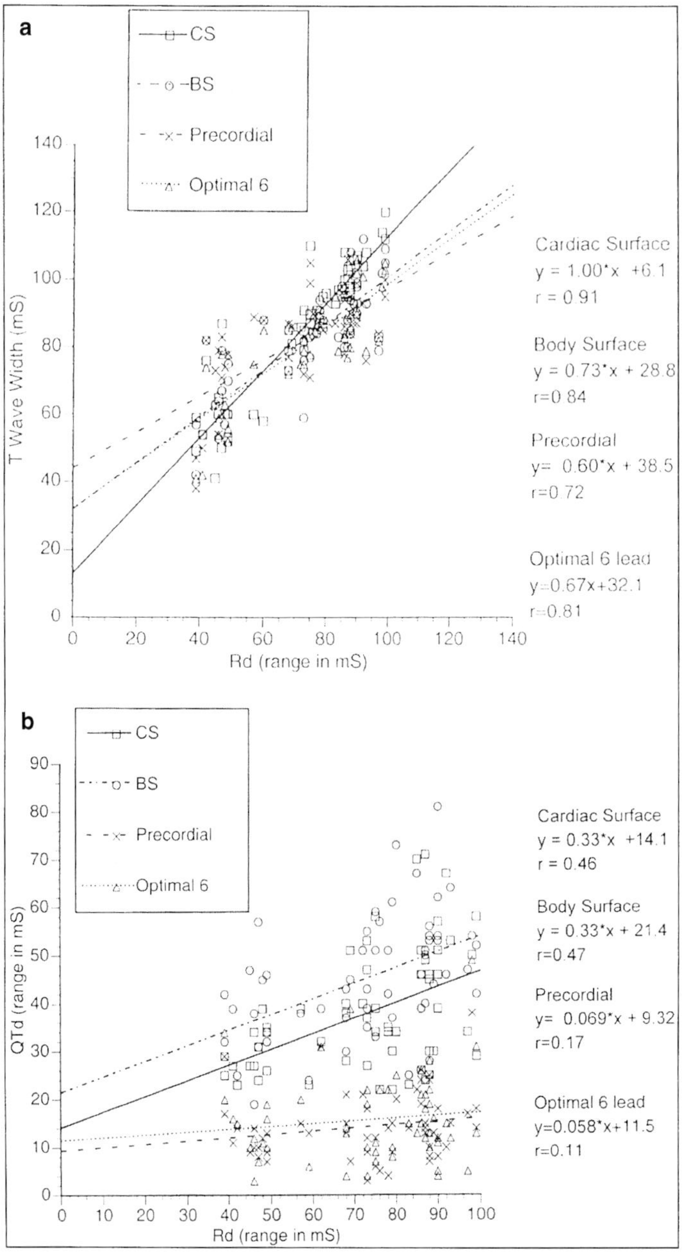

Fig. 34.4 Correlation of dispersion of ventricular repolarisation (Rd) directly measured from 64 epicardial sites of isolated, perfused canine hearts with QT dispersion (QTd) (bottom panel) and the width of the T wave of the root mean square (RMS) curve of an ECG lead set (top panel). In each panel, QTd and the RMS curve were calculated for 4 lead sets: the 64 epicardial sites ('Cardiac Surface'), 'Body Surface' (i.e. torso-shaped electrolytic tank), the precordial leads, and a 6-lead optimal set. Note the low to moderate correlation between QTd and Rd, especially for the precordial and 6 optimal leads, as opposed to the high correlation between the width of the T wave of the RMS curve, which was proposed by the authors as a new surface ECG measure of dispersion of repolarization (see also Fig. 34.6). (Reproduced from Fuller *et al.* *Circulation* (2000), **102**, 685–691, with permission.)

increased noise in the terminal part of the T wave could increase both the error of automatic QT measurement (and hence QTd) as well as the non-dipolar components of the ECG signal, without any physiological link between the two.

It is reasonable to conclude that presently no serious scientific argument has been presented against (whilst substantial evidence has been presented in favour of) the contention that QTd of the standard 12-lead ECG mainly results from projection effects of the main cardiac dipole (heart vector) onto the separate ECG leads. It is worth remembering that the presentation of the electrical activity of the heart as a single dipole not only justifies the application of the orthogonal XYZ leads and vectorcardiography, but also provides the very basis of the visual interpretation of the standard ECG. However, the localization of the site of myocardial infarction (accessory pathway, chamber hypertrophy, etc.)

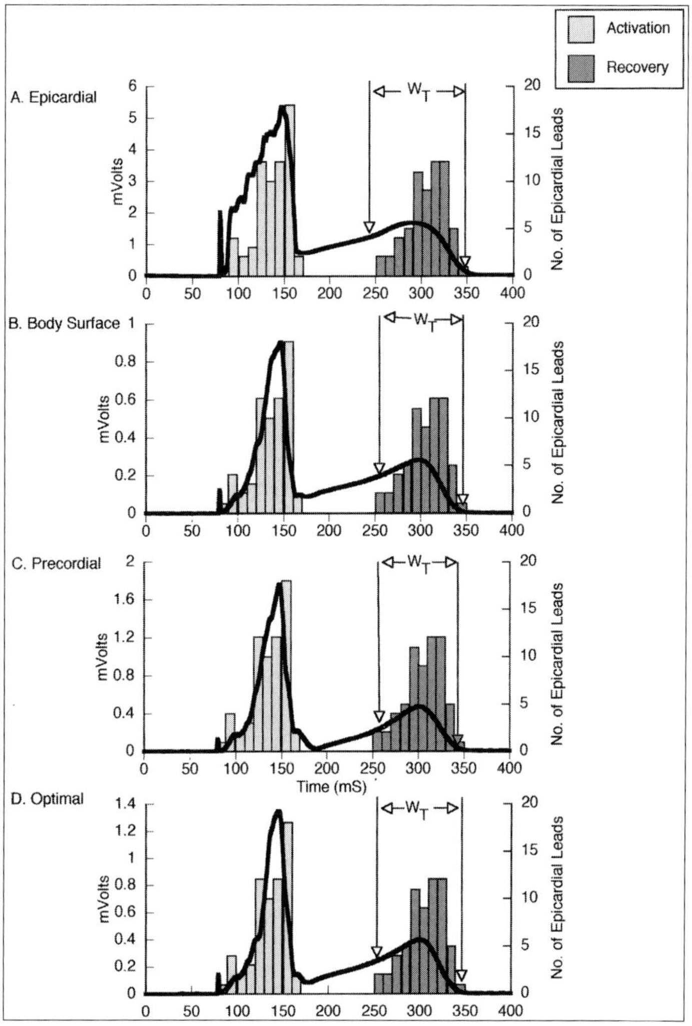

Fig. 34.5 RMS curves from epicardium (A), body surface (B), precordial leads (C), and 'optimal' leads (D) recorded simultaneously during ventricularly paced beat. Histograms of activation and recovery times from 64 epicardial electrograms are overlaid with each curve (bin width 10 ms so that relation between actual activation and recovery time distributions and curves is apparent). Note that the T-wave width (W_T) of the RMS curve closely corresponds to the dispersion of recovery times. (Reproduced from Fuller *et al. Circulation* (2000), **102**, 685–691, with permission.)

by visual inspection of the standard 12-lead ECG, is made possible by the effects of these local lesions on the direction and magnitude of the heart vector, and not by selective sensitivity of different leads to particular cardiac areas' (Abildskov *et al.* 1977).

General abnormalities of ventricular repolarization, not only those leading to regional dispersion of recovery times, modify the spatial T wave loop. As a result of any abnormality, projections of the loop into the individual ECG leads may become less normal and the terminal points of the T wave in the ECG tracings more difficult to be localized. The effect of local dispersion of repolarization on the morphology of the T wave loop, explain the (indirect) link between MAP recordings and QT dispersion. Thus, T wave loop dynamics and the variable projections of the loop into individual ECG leads seem to be the true mechanistic background of QT dispersion. At present, it seems hardy possible to exactly quantify the proportions of the 'projection effect' the and 'measurement error effect' on QT dispersion (Fig. 34.7).

Technical problems with the measurement of QT dispersion

The technical problems with the measurement of QT dispersion, which stem from difficulties with both automatic, as well as manual determination of the T wave end, are well known and have

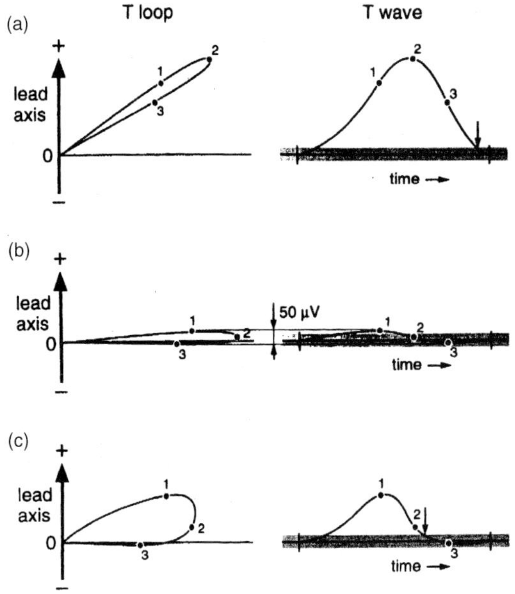

Fig. 34.6 Effect of the shape of the T loop on the *QT* interval measurement in a hypothetical lead. Projections of T loops with different shapes and at different angles to the axis of the lead results in T waves with different amplitude and morphology. Only insignificant proportion of the final part of a T wave with high amplitude may be unmeasurable because of falling into the noise band (a); T waves with smaller amplitude as a result of wider T loop (c) or elongated loop at different angle (b), have greater proportion of their final parts falling into the noise band. Thus, the measurable *QT* interval can almost coincide with the real end of repolarization (a), or be significantly smaller (b,c). Points 1, 2 and 3 indicate three time instants of the T loop and of the T wave. (Reproduced from Kors *et al. Circulation* (1999), **99**, 1458–1463, with permission.)

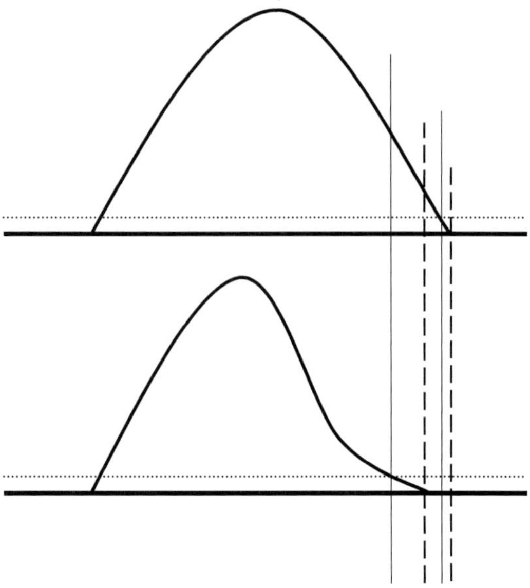

Fig. 34.7 *QT* dispersion as a result of both different real duration and different measurable duration of *QT* intervals. Two hypothetical T waves of the same amplitude have different offset (dashed lines) when the heart vector becomes perpendicular to the axis of one of the leads. This results in 'real' dispersion of the *QT* intervals (vertical dashed lines). In addition, different proportion of the final part of the two T waves is below the threshold level (e.g. with an automatic threshold method). This leads to the measured dispersion of the *QT* intervals (vertical solid line) which is different from the real dispersion.

studied extensively (for review see Kautzner & Malik 1997; Malik & Batchvarov 2000). The main sources of error, both for human observer and computer, continue to be low T wave amplitude (Murray *et al.* 1994; McLaughlin *et al.* 1995), abnormal T wave morphology and merging of T wave with U and/or P wave (Lepeschkin & Surawicz 1952; Surawicz 1998).

Some of the basic algorithms for automatic determination of the T wave end are presented in Fig. 34.8. The threshold methods localize the T offset as an intercept of the T wave or of its derivative with a threshold above the isoelectric line, usually expressed as a percentage of the T wave amplitude. The tangent methods determine the T offset as an intercept between the slope of the descending part of the T wave and the isoelectric line, or a threshold line above it. The slope can be the steepest tangent computed by various line fitting algorithms or a straight line through the inflex point and the peak of the T wave. The amplitude of the T wave strongly influences the reliability of both automatic (McLaughlin *et al.* 1995, Kors *et al.* 1998) and manual (Murray *et al.* 1994) measurement.

The origin of the U wave remains disputed. The theories that attributed the U wave to the delayed repolarization of the His–Purkinje fibres (Watanabe 1975) or to mechanoelectrical mechanism (Lepeschkin 1972) were superseded by the M-cell theory by Antzelevitch *et al.* (1996). However, later experiments by the same group showed that what is often interpreted as a 'pathologically augmented U wave' or 'TU complex' is in fact a prolonged biphasic T wave with an inter-

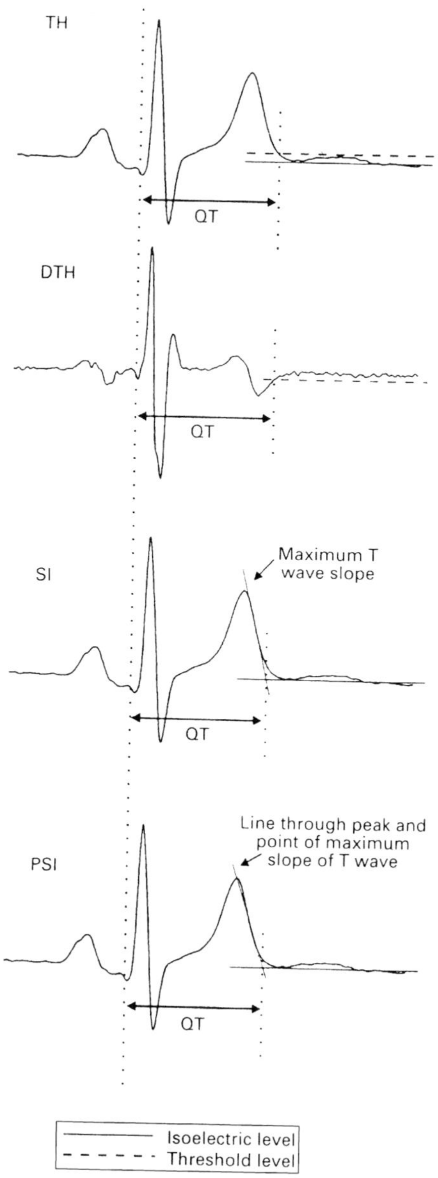

Fig. 34.8 Main automatic QT measurement techniques. From top to bottom: threshold method applied to the original T wave (TH), or to its differential (DTH), tangent method with a tangent to the steepest point of the descending limb of the T wave (SI), tangent method with a line through the T wave peak and the maximum slope point (PSI). (Reproduced from McLaughlin *et al. British Heart Journal* (1995), **74**, 84–89, with permission.)

rupted ascending or descending limb (Yan & Antzelevitch 1998). Manual measurement is even less reliable for certain TU patterns, e.g. when the T wave is flat or inverted and the U wave augmented. Repolarization patterns of complex morphology are frequently classified differently by different observers leading to substantial variability of the measurement (Kautzner *et al.* 1996).

Probably, mechanisms responsible for usual the 'physiological' U wave are different from those leading to abnormal gross U waves, for instance those seen in congenital and acquired long QT syndrome. In our view, all repolarization signals originating from repolarization of ventricular myocardium should belong to the T wave. In this sense, we agree that the concept of biphasic and other unusually shaped T waves is more appropriate than a distinction between the T wave and an augmented U wave which may lead to serious underestimation of *QT* interval.

A pattern resembling a U wave may also originate from slow after-depolarization of ventricular myocytes. Distinction of such a pattern from bizarre T waves may be very difficult. At the same time, in practical *QT* interval measurements (e.g. for the assessment of acquired long QT syndrome) signs of afterdepolarizations indicate the same proarrhythmic danger as bizarre T wave shapes and prolonged *QT* interval. Thus, in all cases, which are difficult, to reconcile augmented U waves should be preferably included into the T wave. Only distinction between T wave and clearly physiological U waves of small amplitude should be attempted when measuring *QT* interval.

The various patterns of T and U wave merging were described by Lepeschkin & Surawicz in 1952 (Lepeschkin & Surawicz 1952) (Fig. 34.9) and since then very little of substance has been added to their classical study (Surawicz 1997).

In experimental (Zabel *et al.* 1995) and clinical (Zabel *et al.* 1998) studies, Zabel *et al.* showed that the QT dispersion values reflect better the dispersion of the recovery times, than of the action potential duration. On the other hand, the JT dispersion reflected better the dispersion of APD90. Consequently, some authors suggested the QT and JT dispersions to be used as separate entities rather than mutual surrogates (Spodick 1992; Zhou *et al.* 1992). However, neither the QT dispersion nor the JT dispersion reflects directly the dispersion of the ventricular recovery time or of the action potential duration. As already discussed, the dispersion of various repolarization duration intervals is merely an indirect measure

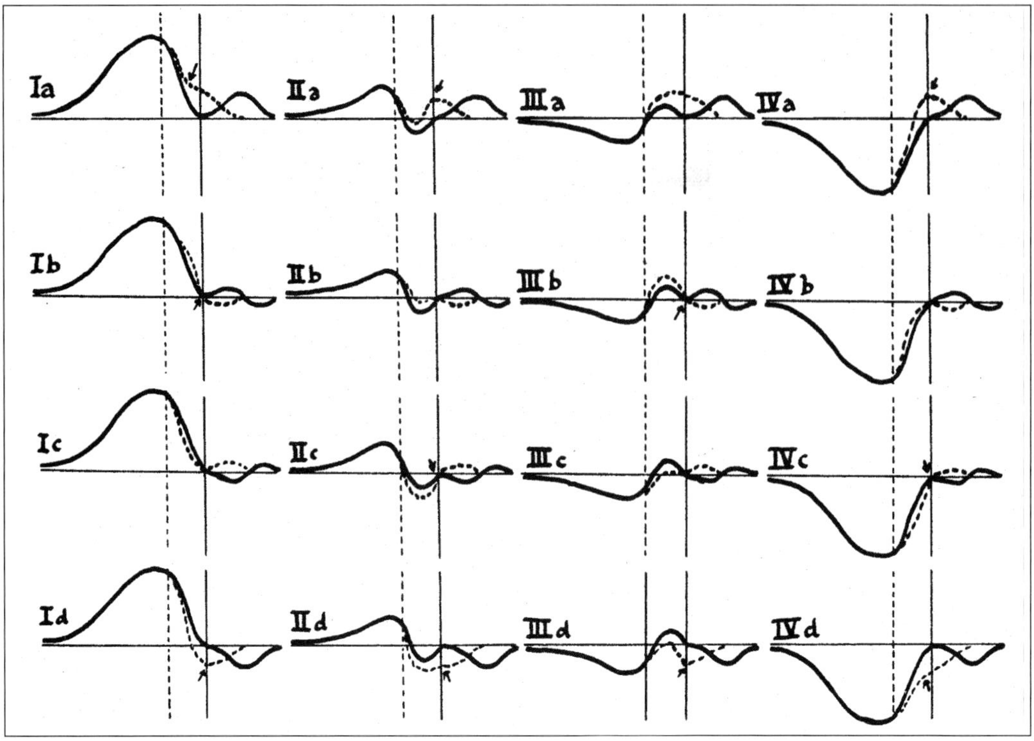

Fig. 34.9 Schematic representation of 16 possible combinations of separate (full curves) and partially merged (dotted curves) T and U waves. The vertical lines indicate the end of the T wave. (Reproduced from Lepeschkin & Surawicz *Circulation* (1952) **VI**, 378–388, with permission.)

of general repolarization abnormalities. It is therefore questionable whether JT dispersion offers any real complement to the QT dispersion, except, possibly, in cases of conduction abnormalities such as bundle branch block.

The Q wave dispersion, although significantly smaller than the T wave offset dispersion, may also influence QT dispersion (Cowan *et al.* 1988; Mirvis 1985). Traditional manual measurement, as well as some computer algorithms, assesses the Q wave onset separately in each lead (Macfarlane *et al.* 1990), while other computer algorithms use a common, lead independent Q onset (Xue & Reddy 1996; Van Bemmel *et al.* 1990). This may account for part of the variability between different algorithms.

Theoretically, an accurate assessment of QT dispersion requires all 12 leads of the ECG to be re-corded simultaneously in order to avoid the effect of *QT* dynamicity due to heart rate changes. Therefore, simultaneous 12-lead recordings have been proposed as 'gold standard' for QT dispersion measurement. On the other hand, it is possible that the slow dynamicity of the *QT* interval (Lau *et al.* 1987) renders QT dispersion measurements based on simultaneous recording of six or even only three recordings during ectopic-free sinus rhythm acceptable for practical purposes. This approach, however, has never been properly validated.

Influence of heart rate

Many studies, including large prospective evaluations (De Bruyne *et al.* 1988; Okin *et al.* 2000) used the so-called 'corrected QT dispersion', i.e. the dispersion of the *QT* intervals corrected for heart rate by some correction formula. While the application of additive formulae for heart-rate correction, such as those proposed by Hodges *et al.* (Hodges 1997) and in the Framingham Study (Sagie *et al.* 1992) renders identical values for QT dispersion and QTc dispersion, this is not true for the multiplicative formulae which include the Bazett correction. Although experimental and clinical data show that the rhythmicity and the site of impulse origin can influence the dispersion of the ventricular recovery times (Han *et al.* 1966; Mitchell *et al.* 1986; Morgan *et al.* 1992), this has never been shown for QT dispersion. Clinical (Maarouf *et al.* 1999) and experimental (Zabel *et al.* 1997) studies failed to find correlation between heart rate and the dispersion of ventricular recovery times measured with MAPs or QT dispersion.

The exact relation between the heart rate and the dispersion of recovery times is still an unresolved issue. It is certain, however, that QT dispersion measured in the standard 12-lead ECG does not depend on heart period in the same way as the *QT* interval. Even more importantly, it has been demonstrated that the dispersion of the corrected *QT* intervals may differ between different clinically defined groups simply as a result of the application of Bazett formula in the presence of different heart rates (Malik & Camm 1997).

Meanwhile, many studies including large prospective ones, such as the Rotterdam (De Bruyne *et al.* 1998) and the Strong Heart Study (Okin *et al.* 2000) continue to report statistically significant and physiologically meaningful differences in the 'corrected' QT dispersion between different clinical groups, somewhat contributing to the artificial 'credit' of this parameter. The inappropriateness of such approaches should clearly be recognized, especially since the observation of these studies that increased QT dispersion (i.e. repolarization abnormality) predicts adverse outcome in general population seems to be independent of the heart rate correction. We believe that it is in principle incorrect to apply any heart rate-correction formula to a parameter, the dependence of which on heart rate, let alone a mathematical model of such dependence, has never been demonstrated.

Influence of the number of ECG leads and of the ECG lead system

In addition to the original expression of QT dispersion as the range of *QT* interval duration in all measurable ECG leads, many other measurement possibilities have been proposed. To mitigate the effect of outliers in the *QT* interval data, standard deviation of the *QT* interval duration in all leads (Hnatkova *et al.* 1994) or coefficient of variation (SD of *QT*/*QT* average (100, the so-called 'relative QT dispersion'; Hailer *et al.* 1999) have been used. However, the range and standard deviation values have been shown to correlate very closely (Hnatkova *et al.* 1994; Yi *et al.* 1998).

The number of measurable leads in the standard ECG clearly influences the range of *QT* interval durations. Some researchers proposed a correction factor dividing *QT* interval range by the square root of the number of measurable ECG leads, leading to the so-called 'adjusted QT dispersion' (Day *et al.* 1991). Hnatkova *et al.* (1994) showed that this formula results in a reasonable correction of mean values of QT dispersion in normal ECGs. They also showed, however, that the individual errors caused by omitting separate leads are very substantial. Consequently, it is not appropriate to compare results based on *QT* interval values obtained from ECGs with very different numbers of measurable leads.

Many clinical studies have measured QT dispersion only in the six precordial leads. In addition, other lead combinations, such as the orthogonal XYZ or 'quasi-orthogonal' I, aVF, V2 leads, have also been studied. It was reported that although, as one would expect, QT dispersion is decreased when a smaller number of leads is used for QT measurement, QT dispersion differences between different patients groups can still be detected with the three leads (aVF, V1, V4) that are most likely to contribute to QT dispersion (Glancy *et al.* 1995), the limb leads (Zareba *et al.* 1995), the orthogonal (X,Y,Z) (Saint Beuve *et al.* 1999; Macfarlane *et al.* 1998) or the 'quasi-orthogonal leads' (I, aVF, V2) (Glancy *et al.* 1995; Zareba *et al.* 1995; Saint Beuve *et al.* 1999). Clearly, practically any lead combination may detect abnormalities in the morphology of the T loop and translate them into increased values of QT dispersion. On the other hand, the more projections of the T loop into different leads with different axes are used, the more sensitive the measurement becomes. Unfortunately, as already mentioned, none of these directly translates into an increased regional heterogeneity of recovery times. Therefore there is little point in continuing the quest for the 'perfect lead combination' for QT dispersion measurement.

Reliability of QT dispersion assessment

Many studies have shown high inter- and intraobserver variability of manually measured QT dispersion. The errors reach the order of the differences between normal subjects and cardiac patients. Relative errors of 25–40% of interobserver and intraobserver variability of manual measurement of QT dispersion have been reported (Lepeschkin & Surawicz 1952; Kautzner *et al.* 1994), as opposed to relative errors < 6% for manual measurement of the *QT* interval (Kautzner *et al.* 1994). Occasionally, substantially better reproducibility of manual measurement of QT dispersion has also been reported, with interobserver variability of 13–18% (Perkiömäkki *et al.* 1995) and even < 5% (Halle *et al.* 1999). Explanations of these discrepancies can only be very speculative. Since a 'majority consensus' clearly agrees on poor reproducibility of QT dispersion measurement, a wishful bias was likely involved in some reports presenting the very low measurement errors.

In addition to the differences in the investigated populations, the variations of the results can be attributed to differences in the measurement method (manual measurement with calliper or ruler (Tran *et al.* 1998), application of a digitising board with or without magnification, on screen measurement with electronic callipers, etc.), the noise level, and the paper speed at which the ECGs were recorded (Murray *et al.* 1994). In a technical study, Malik & Bradford (1998) showed that even the 'gold standard' manual measurement using the digitising board, can produce intraobserver variations corresponding to purely error-related QT dispersion >40 ms and >60 ms, in 20% and 10% of observers, respectively.

The available automatic methods for QT measurement have not shown a superior reproducibility. For example, Yi *et al.* (1998) reported that the immediate reproducibility (in sequentially recorded ECGs) of various QT dispersion indices measured with a downslope tangent method in healthy volunteers varied between 16% and 44%. Variations of computer algorithms for T wave offset determination (McLaughlin *et al.* 1995) include signal processing options, the way in which the tangent is characterized, the definition of the isoelectric line, the threshold level, etc. Some software packages offer a great variety of parameter settings. For instance, one of the versions of the QT Guard software package by GE Marquette (Xue & Reddy 1996) offers > 100 programmable options for the T wave end localization.

Many studies tried to validate automatic algorithms against manual measurement by experienced ECG readers. The results were disappointing showing large difference (Kors & van Herpen 1998; Murray *et al.* 1997; Savelieva *et al.* 1998; Vloka *et al.* 1999). Savelieva *et al.* (1998) investigated the agreement between automatic (downslope tangent) and manual QT measurement in normal subjects and patients with HCM. The agreement between the two methods of *QT* interval measurement was poor and lower in normal subjects (r^2 = 0.10 to 0.25 in the separate leads) than in HCM patients (r^2 = 0.46 to 0.67). The agreement between automatic and manual measurement of QT dispersion was even much worse (r^2 = 0.06 in HCM patients and r^2 = 0.00 in normal subjects).

Relatively few studies compared different algorithms for automatic QT measurement. McLaughlin *et al.* (1995) compared two threshold and two slope based techniques, and a validated manual measurement. The results of the mean measurements with different algorithms varied up to 62 ms, which was greater than the manual interobserver variability. The threshold algorithm demonstrated largest variability and its results depended on filtering and algorithm parameters. In another study (McLaughlin *et al.* 1996) the same authors showed that the variability of automatic QT measurement in cardiac patients was twice that in normal subjects and that it was significantly increased with the decrease of the T wave amplitude. In a study only part of which was published, Batchvarov *et al.* (1998) evaluated the multiple parameter options in the QT Guard package. The differences between the downslope tangent method using different number of samples around the inflex point used for the tangent computation and the modifications of the threshold method were substantial. Changes in the permissible range of the settings of the package led to differences of up to 60 ms in normal subjects and up to 70 ms in HCM patients. Hence, only comparison of results obtained with the same automatic methods and with the same parameter setting is appropriate.

Unfortunately, no systematic experience exists which would allow an optimum algorithmic setting to be selected. Moreover, it seems even reasonable to speculate that all present algorithmic approaches to *QT* interval measurement are too simplistic and superficial and that a truly successful algorithm for automatic *QT* interval measurement will eventually need to be based on a completely different mathematical approach reflecting a deep electrocardiographic knowledge.

Clinical studies

A review of the extreme abundance of studies on QT dispersion published over the past decade reveals an amazingly wide range of QT dispersion values in both 'positive' and 'negative' studies, and a complete lack of any tendency towards establishing reference values. For example, large studies (Zaidi *et al.* 1997) or literature reviews (Surawicz 1996) suggesting QT dispersion of 65 ms as an upper normal limit in healthy subjects were published alongside a report claiming QT dispersion > 40 ms to have 88% sensitivity and 57% specificity for prediction of inducibility of sustained ventricular tachycardia during an electrophysiology study (Goldner *et al.* 1995). Many of the studies with 'positive' results published QT dispersion data well within the demonstrated measurement error of both manual and automatic measurement.

QT dispersion in normal subjects and in the general population

Literature reviews found the QT dispersion to vary mostly between 30 and 60 ms in normal subjects (Statters *et al.* 1994; Kautzner & Malik 1997), although average values around 70 ms were also reported. In 51 studies, in which QT dispersion was measured in 56 groups with total of 8455 healthy subjects of various ages (including three large studies of healthy children (Berul *et al.* 1998; Tutar *et al.* 1998; Macfarlane *et al.* 1994)), we found mean QT dispersion values (*QT* maximum – *QT* minimum) to range from 10.5 ± 10.0 ms (Shah *et al.* 1998) to 71 ± 7 ms (Davey *et al.* 1994). The weighted mean ± SD from all these studies is 33.4 ± 20.3 ms, while the median is 37 ms. Moreover, most researchers reported a wide overlap of values between normal individuals and different patient groups. Thus, all values proposed for upper normal limit in healthy subjects are unreliable.

Published reports show either no statistically significant difference in QT dispersion between the genders (Macfarlane *et al.* 1998; Tutar *et al.* 1998), or marginally greater values in men (Challapalli *et al.* 1998; Savelieva *et al.* 1999). Age-related differences < 10 ms were reported and seemed to be statistically significant in some studies (Savelieva *et al.* 1999; Zhang *et al.* 1999) but not in others (Berul *et al.* 1998; Tutar *et al.* 1998).

Several large prospective studies have assessed the predictive value of QT dispersion for cardiac and all-cause mortality in the general population. In the Rotterdam study (De Bruyne *et al.* 1998) QT dispersion was found to predict cardiac mortality in a general population of 5812 adults of 55 years or older, followed-up for 3–6.5 (mean 4) years.

In the Strong Heart Study (Okin *et al.* 2000) the predictive value of the 'corrected' QTc dispersion was assessed in 1839 American Indians followed up for 3.7 ± 0.9 years. *QTc* assessed as a continuous variable remained significant and independent predictor of cardiovascular mortality in both univariate and multivariate Cox proportional hazard models, with 34% increase of cardiovascular mortality for each 17 ms increase in QTc dispersion in multivariate analysis. In multivariate analysis QTc dispersion > 58 ms (the upper 95th percentile in a separate population of normal subjects) were associated with a 3.2-fold increased risk of cardiovascular mortality (95% confidence interval (CI) 1.8–5.7). Unfortunately, neither values for the uncorrected QT dispersion, or for the simple resting heart rate were provided. Thus, the possibility of the strong predictive power being maintained by the differences in heart rate cannot be excluded.

The West of Scotland Coronary Prevention Study (WOSCOPS) (Macfarlane 1998) included 6595 middle-aged men with moderately raised cholesterol but no previous myocardial infarction. In a multivariate analysis, an increment of 10 ms in QT dispersion increased risk for death of coronary heart disease or nonfatal myocardial infarction by 13% (95% CI 4%–22%, P = 0.0041). QT dispersion > 44 ms carried an increased risk of 36% (95% CI 2%–81%, P = 0.034) compared to QT dispersion < 44 ms. On the other hand, this cut-off level of 44 ms had a sensitivity of only 8.8% with a specificity of 93.8%. The area under the receiver operator characteristic curve was only 54% indicating an almost complete lack of predictive power of QT dispersion.

QT dispersion in cardiac disease

The majority of studies have shown increased QT dispersion in various cardiac diseases. We have pooled data from 18 studies with a total of 2525 post-MI patients, 16 studies with 855 patients with LVH of various origin, excluding HCM, 8 studies with 1082 patients with heart failure, including idiopathic DCM, 11 studies with 635 patients with HCM, 16 studies with a total of 1578 patients with acute MI, and 10 studies with 208 patients with long QT syndrome of various genotype (Malik & Batchvarov 2000).

There was a clear tendency towards increase of QT dispersion in various cardiac disease, with highest mean values reported in the long QT syndrome. On the other hand, the overlap of values between patients with different cardiac diseases, between patients and normal subjects, as well as the wide variation of values within each cardiac disease renders any attempt at establishing reference values fruitless. However, patients with various clinical symptoms, with and without arrhythmias, and on various medications have been included in these pooled studies, which probably accounts for a part of the variation.

Generally, QT dispersion is increased in acute MI, although mean values from 40±18 (Shah *et al.* 1998) to 162.3 ± 64.8 ms (Glancy *et al.* 1996) have been reported. Although QT dispersion is increased in the chronic phase of MI and in other chronic forms of ischaemic artery disease, there seems to be a trend towards lower values compared to the acute phase of MI, possibly owing to the spontaneous dynamicity or to revascularization procedures. Some authors did not find significant differences in QT dispersion between patients with chronic MI or other forms of chronic CAD and normal subjects (Sporton *et al.* 1997; Ashikaga *et al.* 1999).

Compared to healthy controls, an increased QT dispersion has been reported in heart failure and left ventricular dysfunction of various aetiology (Pye *et al.* 1994; Fei *et al.* 1996; Zaidi *et al.* 1997; Bonnar *et al.* 1999), including highly trained athletes (Simoncelli *et al.* 1998; Muir *et al.* 1999), in LVH of various origin (Davey *et al.* 1994; Ichkhan *et al.* 1997; Perkiömäki *et al.* 1996; Maheshwari *et al.* 1998; Tomiyama *et al.* 1998), and even in patients with arterial hypertension irrespective of the presence or absence of hypertrophy (Özerkan *et al.* 1999), in HCM patients compared to healthy controls (Dritsas *et al.* 1992; Zaidi *et al.* 1996; Yi *et al.* 1998), in the long QT syndrome (Gayrilescu & Luca 1978; Bonatti *et al.* 1983; Priori *et al.* 1994) and in many other cardiac and even noncardiac diseases. However, some studies have found QT dispersion values not significantly different between healthy subjects and patients with heart failure (Yap *et al.* 1999), LVH as a result of physical training (Halle *et al.* 1999; Mayet *et al.* 1999; Zoghi *et al.* 1999), or between patients with and without LVH (Bugra *et al.* 1998).

Many studies tried to correlate QT dispersion with the extent or the localization of the pathological process of various diseases. Some studies have shown greater QT dispersion in anterior compared to inferior MI (Bennemeier *et al.* 1999; Paventi *et al.* 1999; Yap *et al.* 1999), correlation between QT dispersion in MI and indirect measures of infarct size, such as ejection fraction (Puljevic *et al.* 1998), or the amount of viable myocardium in the infarct region (Schneider *et al.* 1997). Similarly, significant correlation between QT dispersion and left ventricular mass index in hypertensive patients with LV hypertrophy was found in some studies (Clarkson *et al.* 1995; Kohno *et al.* 1998), but not in others (Bugra *et al.* 1998).

Changes of QT dispersion have been shown to follow the spontaneous or induced dynamicity of the pathological process in some cardiac diseases. For instance, QT dispersion seems to undergo dynamic changes during the first day (Higham *et al.* 1995), as well as during the following days (Glancy *et al.* 1996; Yap *et al.* 1999) of acute MI. It increases significantly during ischaemia induced by balloon inflation during angioplasty (Okishige *et al.* 1996; Tarabey *et al.* 1998; Aytemir *et al.* 1999), by exercise stress testing (Yi *et al.* 1998) or atrial pacing (Sporton *et al.* 1997), or during reperfusion following angioplasty (Michelucci *et al.* 1996). It has also been shown to correlate with the improvement of left ventricular contractility on the echocardiogram after the infarction (Gabrielli *et al.* 1997) and with the degree of improvement of left ventricular function after revascularization (Schneider *et al.* 1997; Nakajima *et al.* 1998).

Treatment has been shown to decrease QT dispersion, e.g. after successful reperfusion after thrombolysis (Moreno *et al.* 1994; Karagounis *et al.* 1998), revascularization with angioplasty (Kelly *et al.* 1997; Szydlo *et al.* 1998; Choi *et al.* 1999) or coronary artery bypass grafting (Schneider *et al.* 1997). Treatment of heart failure patients with losartan (Brooksby *et al.* 1999), successful antihypertensive treatment of hypertensive patients with LV hypertrophy (Mayet *et al.* 1996; Gonzalez-Juanatey *et al.* 1998; Karpanou *et al.* 1998; Lim *et al.* 1999), or successful beta blocker treatment of patients with the long-QT syndrome (Priori *et al.* 1994) have also been shown to decrease QT dispersion.

Prognostic value of QT dispersion

Many studies aimed at investigating the value of QT dispersion for the prediction of ventricular arrhythmias or other adverse events in various cardiac diseases. The results are again controversial.

Several studies, most of them retrospective, have found that patients with acute (Zaputovic *et al.* 1997; Papandonakis *et al.* 1999) or chronic MI (Pye *et al.* 1994; Zareba *et al.* 1994; Shulan *et al.* 1998) with ventricular arrhythmias have significantly higher QT dispersion than patients without arrhythmias. However, the first prospectively analysed study in post-MI patients reported by Zabel *et al.* (1998) showed that none of the 26 ventricular dispersion indices that were tested had any predictive value for an adverse outcome in 280 consecutive MI survivors followed-up for 32 ± 10 months. Newer studies (Moenning *et al.* 1999; Tavernier & Jordeans 1999) provided controversial findings.

Some studies showed that QT dispersion could predict inducibility of ventricular arrhythmias during electrophysiology study (Lee *et al.* 1997; Gillis *et al.* 1998; Berul *et al.* 1999), while others failed to observe this (Armoundas *et al.* 1998; Zabel *et al.* 1998; De Sutter *et al.* 1999).

Several studies (Fu *et al.* 1997; Galinier *et al.* 1998; Anastasiou-Nana *et al.* 1999) showed significant correlation between QT dispersion and outcome in patients with heart failure. Analysis (Brooksby *et al.* 1999b) from the ELITE heart failure study in which heart failure patients treated with the angiotensin-II antagonist, losartan, had reduction of sudden cardiac death compared to those treated with captopril (Pitt *et al.* 1997) showed that captopril but not losartan increased QT dispersion. However, the results of ELITE were not confirmed by the much larger double-blind, randomized controlled ELITE-II trial (Pitt *et al.* 2000), in which patients treated with losartan showed no significant differences in all-cause mortality, sudden death or resuscitated cardiac arrest compared to those treated with captopril.

Substudies of the DIAMOND-CHF Study (Brendorp *et al.* 1999), the UK-HEART study (Brooksby *et al.* 1999a) as well as other large prospective study (Radmanabhan *et al.* 1999) failed to show any power of QT dispersion for predicting outcome in heart failure patients. Available studies also failed to show independent predictive value of QT dispersion for sudden cardiac death and cardiac mortality in patients with LV hypertrophy (Galinier *et al.* 1997).

Several authors reported significantly higher QT dispersion in HCM patients with ventricular arrhythmias compared to those without arrhythmias (Buja *et al.* 1993; Miorelli *et al.* 1994; Baranowski *et al.* 1998). Larger studies, however, did not confirm these findings (Yi *et al.* 1998; Maron *et al.* 1999).

In the long QT syndrome, the diagnostic value of increased QT dispersion seems undisputed. On the other hand, although Priori *et al.* (Priori *et al.* 1994) reported that patients not responding to beta blockers had a significantly higher QT dispersion than responders (137 ± 52 vs. 75 ± 38 ms, $P < 0.05$), no other presently available data suggest that QT dispersion has any prognostic value in long QT syndrome patients.

Generally, the positive results of small retrospective studies conducted in the years of initial enthusiasm were later confirmed only in some very large prospective studies. However, even in the large studies, patient groups with adverse outcomes had often QT dispersion values well within both the measurement error and the range of values in healthy subjects reported in other studies. Thus, as phrased by Surawicz *et al.* (1999), the positive results can be interpreted as indicating an 'indifferent' QT dispersion. This does not necessarily signify lack of clinical importance. In the majority of the cases, the abnormality is already visible from abnormal T wave morphology and/or increased *QT* interval. At present, this does not necessitate a specific therapeutic action and, in practice, does not help in the risk stratification of individual patients.

Effect of drugs on QT dispersion and the risk of torsades de pointes tachycardia

The limitations of both the presence and the degree of *QT* interval prolongation for prediction of torsades de pointes are well known (Moss 1999). Consequently, the potential role of QT dispersion for the prediction of drug-induced torsades de pointes has been addressed in several studies.

Quinidine increases QT dispersion (Hii *et al.* 1992; Hohnloser *et al.* 1995) and unlike the corrected *QTc* interval, increased QT dispersion seems to have some predictive value for development of torsades de pointes during quinidine therapy (Hii *et al.* 1992; Hohnloser *et al.* 1995). Sotalol has been shown to decrease (Day *et al.* 1991) or not to change (Cui *et al.* 1994) QT dispersion in patients with ischaemic heart disease. However, Dancey *et al.* (Hohnloser *et al.* 1993) observed increased QT dispersion in 4 cases of torsades de pointes caused by low-dose sotalol in patients with renal failure.

In clinical studies, amiodarone has been reported to decrease (Dritsas *et al.* 1992; Cui *et al.* 1994) or not to change (Hii *et al.* 1992; Grimm *et al.* 1997; Meierhenrich *et al.* 1997) QT dispersion. It is known that amiodarone can be administered relatively safely in patients who had experienced torsades de pointes during antiarrhythmic therapy with other drugs (Van de Loo *et al.* 1994) and this effect is paralleled by a decrease of QT dispersion (Hii *et al.* 1992). However, cases of an excessive increase of QT dispersion and induction of torsades de pointes by amiodarone have also been reported (Tran *et al.* 1997). On the other hand, it has been demonstrated that increase of *QTc* and QT dispersion during chronic amiodarone treatment does not affect survival and is independent of the decrease in arrhythmia risk (Yadav *et al.* 1999).

Propafenone (Faber *et al.* 1997), disopyramide (Trusz-Gluza *et al.* 1998) and almokalant (blocker of the rapid component of the delayed rectifier, I_{Kr}) (Houltz *et al.* 1998) has been shown to increase QT dispersion, while in one study dofetilide infusion did not produce increase of the dispersion of repolarization between two right ventricular endocardial sites (Sedwick *et al.* 1992). A decrease of QT dispersion after treatment with azimilide (Brum *et al.* 1999) and magnesium have also been reported (Parikka *et al.* 1999). In addition to the long QT syndrome (Priori *et al.* 1994), beta blockers have been shown to decrease QT dispersion in patients with syndrome X (Leonardo *et al.* 1997), heart failure (Bonnar *et al.* 1999), but not in HCM (Yi *et al.* 1998).

Conclusions

Contrary to the initial expectations, QT dispersion did not evolve into a useful clinical tool. Although this simple ECG parameter is probably not (only) a result of measurement error, it does not reflect directly and in a quantifiable way the dispersion and the heterogeneity of the ventricular recovery times. The standard 12-lead ECG contains information about regional electrical phenomena but this information can not be extracted by such a simple technique as QT dispersion assessment.

In addition, not only the magnitude of dispersion of recovery times, but the distance over which they are dispersed is important for arrhythmogenesis. In a similar way as we distinguish, though arbitrarily, 'micro re-entry' from 'macro re-entry', it seems logical to distinguish dispersion of recovery times of adjacent areas (local dispersion), from dispersion over large areas (global dispersion) and, possibly, from dispersion between both ventricles (interventricular dispersion). Such a scale is clearly beyond the resolution of the standard surface ECG. Local dispersion of recovery times created by MI is no more visible on the standard surface ECG, than the delayed conduction caused by the same infarct.

The very idea of detecting and quantifying only the dispersion of the end of repolarization, i.e. the dispersion of the complete recovery times, seems also questionable. Action potentials of different duration usually have very different shape, particularly during phase 3. Such a 'phase 3 dispersion', i.e. the dispersion of the partial recovery times, has direct relation to arrhythmogenesis. While it is reflected in the shape of the T wave, it does not contribute to the dispersion of the ends of the MAPs, let alone the dispersion of the *QT* intervals.

In a recently published experimental study, Shimizu *et al.* (1999) showed that the T wave alternans induced by rapid pacing was a result of alterations in the APD of the M-cells, leading to exaggeration of transmural dispersion of repolarization during alternate beats, and thus to the potential for development of torsades de pointes. The result of the study clearly emphasized that spatial dispersion of the recovery times can not be estimated without the analysis of the morphology of the T wave, as well as without taking into account its dynamicity.

Despite all limitations, the decade of investigation of QT dispersion emphasized the clinical importance of the repolarization abnormalities. We have to understand that QT dispersion is nothing more (and nothing less) than an approximate and simplistic expression of repolarization abnormality. At the same time, the technology clearly suffers from serious methodological problems, from the lack of any direct link to a pathophysiological background, and from complete absence of any reference values. The technological limitations and methodological problems also impose serious restrictions on the interpretation of the results of any study, including those already published. The poor reproducibility and substantial dependence of the measurement on the operator make the results of different studies not easily comparable. Group differences of only few ms even when statistically significant, should always be interpreted with caution and scepticism because they are unlikely to be reproducible. Similarly, the lack of a difference in QT dispersion values does not prove the absence of the involvement of myocardial repolarization. The technology is clearly too crude to depict minor repolarization changes.

In clinical practice concerning individual patients, only grossly abnormal values of QT dispersion, that are clearly outside the possible measurement error, e.g. 100 ms, may have a significance by signalling that the repolarization is abnormal. However, it is unlikely that such a gross repolarization abnormality would occur in ECGs with normal T wave morphology and normal *QT* duration. Even in the long QT syndrome, i.e. in the case of the 'pure global repolarization disease', QT dispersion failed to add substantial additional information to that provided by the general observation of abnormal TU complexes.

Thus, it seems reasonable to conclude that future studies of QT dispersion should be strongly discouraged. Still, classification and quantification of the regional information in the 12-lead ECG remains a challenging problem. Despite initial hopes, it is now obvious that it has not been addressed by QT dispersion, which is more about global than localized repolarization abnormality.

Older concepts of quantification of repolarization abnormalities, as well as newer ideas, deserve more attention than parameters based on duration of repolarization intervals. Principal component analysis (PCA) has been used for decades in the analysis of ECG signals from body surface potential mapping for reduction of the redundancy of the data (Horan *et al.* 1964). Recently, it has also been implemented to assess the complexity of the T wave from standard 12-lead ECG and from 12-lead digital Holter recordings. The method has been shown to differentiate between normal subjects and patients with the long QT syndrome from 12-lead Holter ECGs (Priori *et al.* 1997), in patients with HCM (Yi *et al.* 1998) and arrhythmogenic right ventricular dysplasia (De Ambroggi *et al.* 1997). In general, the method defines the principal, non-redundant spatial components (or 'factors'), into which the T wave is decomposed and which contribute (in descending order of significance) to the morphology of the T wave. The significance of each component is measured by its eigenvalue. When the repolarization is uniform, i.e. the T wave is smooth, without notches, most of the information about its morphology is contained in the first, main principal component. When the T wave becomes more complex, the relative value of the next, smaller components of T wave increases (i.e. their eigenvalues increase). Although PCA has already been included in some commercially available programs for automatic repolarization analysis, its clinical role is still not well defined.

Frontal and horizontal T wave axis has also been demonstrated to be predictive of cardiac mortality (Kors *et al.* 1998). Most probably, other wavefront direction parameters, based on measurement of vector time integrals (i.e. QRST areas) will also be studied in the near future.

Most recently, a concept of measuring the T wave 'morphology dispersion' in surface electrocardiograms has been proposed by Acar *et al.* (1999). Based on single value decomposition of simultaneously recorded 12-lead ECGs and on the computation of the eigenvalues of the signal, they proposed several indices characterizing the sequence of repolarization changes through the ventricular myocardium, including parameters describing the dissimilarities of the shape of the T wave in individual ECG leads. Comparison of normal and abnormal ECG of HCM patients showed that indices of T wave morphology separated these two groups more powerfully than both QT dispersion and rate corrected *QT* interval duration. The concept was subsequently applied to the ECGs database of the first prospective study on QT dispersion in survivors of myocardial infarction by Zabel *et al.* (1998). They showed that unlike QT dispersion selected indices of T wave morphology characteristics obtained from single beat resting 12-lead ECGs are powerful and independent predictors of adverse events during follow-up.

Only after more experience has accumulated with these and other descriptors of repolarization 'morphology', it will be possible to address their relationship to the expressions of repolarization dynamicity, such as T wave alternans or QT/RR relationship and adaptation. The present approaches to the assessment of repolarization dynamics are also rather simplistic and in need of further improvement. Studies of the dynamics of repolarization morphology are an obvious step forward. It is therefore reasonable to expect that the distinction between 'static' and 'dynamic' repolarization assessment will gradually be suppressed and that a 'comprehensive' spectrum of repolarization characteristics will eventually appear.

References

Abildskov, J.A., Burgess, M.J., Urie, P.M., Lux, R.L. & Wyatt R.F. (1977) The unidentified information content of the electrocardiogram. *Circulation Research*, **40**, 3–7.

Abildskov, J.A., Evans, A.K., Lux, R.L. & Burgess, M.J. (1980) Ventricular recovery properties and QRST deflection area in cardiac electrograms. *American Journal of Physiology*, **239**, H227–H231.

Acar, B., Yi, G., Hnatkova, K. *et al.* (1999) Spatial, temporal and wavefront direction characteristics of 12-Lead T wave morphology. *Medical & Biological Engineering & Computing*, **37**, 574–584.

Allessie, M.A., Bonke, F.I.M. & Schopman, F.J.G. (1976) Circus movement in rabbit atrial muscle as a mechanism of tachycardia. II: The role of nonuniform recovery of excitability in the occurrence of unidirectional block, as studied with multiple microelectrodes. *Circulation Research*, **39**, 168–177.

Anastasiou-Nana, M.I., Nanas, J.N., Karagounis, L.A. *et al.* (1999) Dispersion of QRS and QT in patients with advanced congestive heart failure: relation to cardiac and sudden cardiac death mortality. *European Heart Journal*, **20** (Suppl.), 117 (abstract).

Antzelevitch, C. (2001) Transmural dispersion of repolarization and the T wave. *Cardiovascular Research*, **50**, 426–431.

Antzelevich, C., Nesterenko, V.V. & Yan, G.X. (1996) The role of M cells in acquired long QT syndrome, U waves and torsade de pointes. *Journal of Electrocardiology*, **28** (Suppl.), 131–138.

Anyukhovsky, E.P., Sosunov, E.A. & Rosen, M.R. (1996) Regional differences in electrophysiological properties of epicardium, midmyocardium and endocardium: *in vitro* and *in vivo* correlations. *Circulation*, **94**, 1981–1988.

Armoundas, A.A., Osaka, M., Mela, T. *et al.* (1998) T wave alternans and dispersion of the *QT* interval as risk stratification markers in patients susceptible to sustained ventricular arrhythmias. *American Journal of Cardiology*, **82**, 1127–1129.

Ashikaga, T., Nishizaki, M., Arita, M. *et al.* (1999) Effect of dipyridamole on QT dispersion in vasospastic angina pectoris. *American Journal of Cardiology*, **84**, 807–810.

Ashman, R. & Byer. E. (1948) The normal human ventricular gradient. II. Factors which affect its manifest area and its relationship to the manifest area of the QRS complex. *American Heart Journal*, **25**, 36–57.

Aytemir, K., Bavafa, V., Ozer, N. *et al.* (1999) Effect of balloon inflation-induced acute ischaemia on QT dispersion during percutaneous transluminal coronary angioplasty. *Clinical Cardiology*, **22**, 21–24.

Baranowski, R., Malecka, L., Poplawska, W. *et al.* (1998) Analysis of QT dispersion in patients with hypertrophic cardiomyopathy – correlation with clinical data and survival. *European Heart Journal*, 19 (Suppl.), 428 (abstract).

Batchvarov, V., Yi, G., Guo, X.-H. *et al.* (1998) *QT* interval and QT dispersion measured with the threshold method depend on threshold level. *PACE (Pacing and Clinical Electrophysiolgy)*, **21**, 2372–2375.

Bennemeier, H., Hartmann, F., Giannitsis, E. *et al.* (1999) Effects of primary angioplasty on the course of QT dispersion after myocardial infarction and its association with infarct size. *PACE (Pacing and Clinical Electrophysiolgy)*, **22**, A19 (abstract).

Berul, C.I., Michaud, G.F., Lee, V.C. *et al.* (1999) A comparison of T wave alternans and QT dispersion as noninvasive predictors of ventricular arrhythmias. *Annals of Noninvasive Electrocardiology*, **4**, 274–280.

Berul, C.I., Sweeten, T.L., Hill, S.L. *et al.* (1998) Provocative tests in children with suspect congenital long QT syndrome. *Annals of Noninvasive Electrocardiology*, **3**, 3–11.

Bonatti, V., Rolli, A. & Botti, G. (1983) Recording of monophasic action potentials of the right ventricle in long QT syndromes complicated by severe ventricular arrhythmias. *European Heart Journal*, **4**, 168–179.

Bonnar, C.E., Davie, A.P., Caruana, L. *et al.* (1999) QT dispersion in patients with chronic heart failure: beta blockers are associated with a reduction in QT dispersion. Heart **81**, 297–302.

Brendorp, B., Elming, H., Køber, L., Malik, M., Jun, L. & Torp-Pedersen, C., for the DIAMOND Study Group. (1999) Prognostic implications of *QT* interval and dispersion in patients with congestive heart failure. *European Heart Journal*, **20** (Suppl.), 89 (abstract).

Brooksby, P., Batin PD, Nolan J *et al.* (1999a) The relationship between *QT* intervals and mortality in ambulant patients with chronic heart failure. The United Kingdom Heart Failure Evaluation and Assessment of Risk Trial (UK-HEART). *European Heart Journal*, **20**, 1335–41.

Brooksby, P., Robinson, P.J., Segal, R., Klinger, G., Pitt, B. & Cowley, A.J.C. on behalf of the ELITE study group (1999b) Effects of losartan and captopril on QT dispersion in elderly patients with heart failure. *Lancet*, **534**, 395–396.

Brum, J., Alkhalidi, H., Karam, R. *et al.* (1999) Effects of azimilide, an IKs/IKr blocking anti-arrhythmic on *QT* and QTc dispersion, in patients with ventricular tachycardia (VT). *PACE (Pacing and Clinical Electrophysiolgy)*, **22**, A13 (abstract).

Bugra, Z., Koylan, N., Vural, A. *et al.* (1998) Left ventricular geometric patterns and QT dispersion in untreated essential hypertension. *American Journal of Hypertension*, **11**, 1164–1170.

Buja, G., Miorelli, M., Turrini, P. *et al.* (1993) Comparison of QT dispersion in hypertrophic cardiomyopathy between patients with and without ventricular arrhythmias and sudden death. *American Journal of Cardiology*, **72**, 973–976.

Challapalli, S., Lingamneni, R., Horvath, G. *et al.* (1998) Twelve-lead QT dispersion is smaller in women than in men. *Annals of Noninvasive Electrocardiology*, **3**, 25–31.

Choi, K.-J., Lee, C.-W., Kang, D.-H. *et al.* (1999) Change of QT dispersion after PTCA in angina patients. *Annals of Noninvasive Electrocardiology*, **4**, 195–199.

Clarkson, P.B.M., Naas, A.A.O., McMahon, A. *et al.* (1995) QT dispersion in essential hypertension. *Quarterly Journal of Medicine*, **88**, 327–332.

Coumel, P., Maison-Blanche, P. & Badilini, F. (1998) Dispersion of ventricular repolarization. Reality? Illusion? Significance? *Circulation*, **97**, 2491–2493.

Cowan, J.C., Yusoff, K., Moore, M. *et al.* (1988) Importance of lead selection in *QT* interval measurement. *American Journal of Cardiology*, **61**, 83–87.

Cui, G., Sen, L., Sager, P. *et al.* (1994) Effects of amiodarone, sematilide, and sotalol on QT dispersion. *American Journal of Cardiology*, **74**, 896–900.

Davey, P.P., Bateman, J., Mulligan, I.P. *et al.* (1994) *QT* interval dispersion in chronic heart failure and left ventricular hypertrophy: relation to autonomic nervous system and Holter tape abnormalities. *British Heart Journal*, **71**, 268–273.

Day, C.P., McComb, J.M. & Campbell, R.W.F. (1990) QT dispersion: an indication of arrhythmias risk in patients with long *QT* intervals. *British Heart Journal*, **63**, 342–344.

Day, C.P., McComb, J.M., Mathews, J. *et al.* (1991) Reduction of QT dispersion by sotalol following myocardial infarction. *European Heart Journal*, **12**, 423–427.

De Ambroggi, L.D., Aime, E., Ceriotti, C. *et al.* (1997) Mapping of ventricular repolarization potentials in patients with arrhythmogenic right ventricular dysplasia. Principal component analysis of the ST–T waves. *Circulation*, **96**, 4314–4318.

De Bruyne, M.C., Hoes, A.W., Kors, J.A., Hofman, A., van Bemmel, J.H. & Grobbee, D.E. (1999) Prolonged *QT* interval predicts cardiac and all-cause mortality in the elderly. The Rotterdam Study. *European Heart Journal*, **20**, 278–284.

De Bruyne, M.C., Hoes, A.W., Kors, J.A., Hofman, A., van Bemmel, J.H. & Grobbee, D.E. (1998) QTc dispersion predicts cardiac mortality in the elderly. The Rotterdam study. *Circulation*, **97**, 467–472.

De Sutter, J., Tavernier, R., van de Wiele, C. *et al.* (1999) QT dispersion is not related to infarct size or inducibility in patients with coronary artery disease and life threatening ventricular arrhythmias. *Heart*, **81**, 533–538.

Dritsas, A., Gilligan, D., Nihoyannopoulos, P. *et al.* (1992a) Amiodarone reduces QT dispersion in patients with hypertrophic cardiomyopathy. *International Journal of Cardiology*, **36**, 345–349.

Dritsas, A., Sbarouni, E., Gilligan, D. *et al.* (1992b) *QT*-interval abnormalities in hypertrophic cardiomyopathy. *Clinical Cardiology*, **15**, 739–742.

Faber, T.S., Zehender, M., Krahnfeld, O. *et al.* (1997) Propafenone during acute myocardial ischaemia in patients: A double-blind, randomized, placebo-controlled study. *Journal of the American College of Cardiology*, **29**, 561–567.

Fei, L., Goldman, J.H., Prasad, K. *et al.* (1996) QT dispersion and *RR* variations on 12-lead ECGs in patients with congestive heart failure secondary to idiopathic dilated cardiomyopathy. *European Heart Journal*, **17**, 258–263.

Franz, M.R., Bagheer, K., Rafflenbeul, W., Haverich, A., Lichtlen, P.R. (1987) Monophasic action potential mapping in human subjects with normal electrocardiograms: direct evidence for the genesis of the T wave. *Circulation*, **75**, 379–386.

Fu, G.-S., Meissner, A. & Simon, R. (1997) Repolarization dispersion and sudden cardiac death in patients with impaired left ventricular function. *European Heart Journal*, **18**, 281–289.

Fuller, M.S., Sándor, G., Punske, B. *et al.* (2000) Estimates of repolarization dispersion from electrocardiographic measurements. *Circulation*, **102**, 685–691.

Gabrielli, F., Balzotti, L. & Bandiera, A. (1997) QT dispersion variability and myocardial viability in acute myocardial infarction. *International Journal of Cardiology* **61**, 61–67.

Galinier, M., Balanescu, S., Fourcade, J. *et al.* (1997) Prognostic value of arrhythmogenic markers in systemic hypertension. *European Heart Journal*, **18**, 1484–1491.

Galinier, M., Vialette, J.-C., Fourcade, J. *et al.* (1998) *QT* interval dispersion as a predictor of arrhythmic events in congestive heart failure. Importance of aetiology. *European Heart Journal*, **19**, 1054–1062.

Gavrilescu, S. & Luca, C. (1978) Right ventricular monophasic action potentials in patients with long QT syndrome. *British Heart Journal*, **40**, 1014–1018.

Gillis, A.M., Traboulsi, M., Hii, J.T.Y. *et al.* (1998) Antiarrhythmic drug effects on *QT* interval dispersion in patients undergoing electropharmacologic testing for ventricular tachycardia and fibrillation. *American Journal of Cardiology*, **81**, 588–593.

Glancy, J.M., Garrat, C.J., de Bono DP. (1996) Dynamics of QT dispersion during myocardial infarction and ischaemia. *International Journal of Cardiology*, **57**, 55–60.

Glancy, J.M., Garratt CJ, Woods KL *et al.* (1995) Three-lead measurement of QTc dispersion. *Journal of Cardiovascular Electrophysiology*, **6**, 987–992.

Goldner, B., Brandspiegel, H.Z., Horwitz, L. *et al.* (1995) Utility of QT dispersion combined with the signal-averaged electrocardiogram in detecting patients susceptible to ventricular tachyarrhythmia. *American Journal of Cardiology*, **76**, 1192–1194.

Gonzalez-Juanatey, J.R., Garcia-Acuna, J.M., Pose, A. *et al.* (1998) Reduction of *QT* and QTc dispersion during long-term treatment of systemic hypertension with enalapril. *American Journal of Cardiology*, **81**, 170–174.

Grimm, W., Steder, U., Menz, V. *et al.* (1997) Effect of amiodarone on QT dispersion in the 12-lead standard electrocardiogram and its significance for subsequent arrhythmic events. *Clinical Cardiology*, **20**, 107–110.

Hailer, B., Van Leeuwen, P., Lange, S. *et al.* (1999) Corornary artery disease may alter the spatial dispersion of the *QT* interval at rest. *Annals of Noninvasive Electrocardiology*, **4**, 267–273.

Halle, M., Huonker, M., Hohnloser, S.H. *et al.* (1999) QT dispersion in exercise-induced myocardial hypertrophy. *American Heart Journal*, **138**, 309–312.

Han, J., Millet, D., Chizzonitti, B. *et al.* (1966) Temporal dispersion of recovery of excitability in atrium and ventricle as a function of heart rate. *American Heart Journal*, **71**, 481–487.

Han, J. & Moe, G.K. (1964) Nonuniform recovery of excitability in ventricular muscle. *Circulation Research*, **14**, 44.

Higham, P.D., Furniss, S.S. & Campbell, R.W.F. (1995) QT dispersion and components of the *QT* interval in ischaemia and infarction. *British Heart Journal*, **73**, 32–36.

Higham, P.D., Hilton, C.J., Aitcheson, J.D., Furniss, S.S., Bourke, J.P. & Campbell, R.W.F. (1992) Does QT dispersion reflect dispersion of ventricular recovery? *Circulation*, **86** (Suppl. I), 392 (abstract).

Hii, J.T.Y., Wyse, D.G., Gillis, A.M. *et al.* (1992) Precordial *QT* interval dispersion as a marker of torsades de pointes. Disparate effects of class Ia antiarrhythmic drugs and amiodarone. *Circulation*, **86**, 1376–1382.

Hnatkova, K., Malik, M., Yi, G. *et al.* (1994) Adjustment of QT dispersion assessed from 12 lead electrocardiograms for different number of analysed electrocardiographic leads: comparison of stability of different methods. *British Heart Journal*, **72**, 390–396.

Hodges, M. (1997) Rate correction of the *QT* interval. *Cardiac Electrophysiology Review*, **3**, 360–363.

Hohnloser, S.H., van de Loo, A. & Baedeker, F. (1995) Efficacy and proarrhythmic hazards of pharmacologic cardioversion of atrial fibrillation: Prospective comparison of sotalol versus quinidine. *Journal of the American College of Cardiology*, **26**, 852–858.

Hohnloser, S.H., van de Loo, A., Kalusche, D. *et al.* (1993) Does sotalol-induced alteration of *QT*-dispersion predict drug effectiveness or proarrhythmic hazards? *Circulation*, **88** (Suppl. I), 397 (abstract).

Horan, L.G., Flowers, N.C. & Brody, D.A. (1964) Prinicipal factor waveforms of the thoracic QRS complex. *Circulation Research*, **XV**, 131–145.

Houltz, B., Darpö, B., Edvardsson, N. *et al.* (1998) Electrocardiographic and clinical predictors of torsades de pointes induced by almokalant infusion in patients with chronic atrial fibrillation of flutter: A prospective study. *PACE (Pacing and Clinical Electrophysiolgy)*, **21**, 1044–1057.

Ichkhan, K., Molnar, J. & Somberg, J. (1997) Relation of left ventricular mass and QT dispersion in patients with systemic hypertension. *American Journal of Cardiology*, **79**, 508–511.

Karagounis, L.A., Anderson, J.L., Moreno, F.L. & Sorensen, S.G. for the TEAM-3 Investigators (1998) Multivariate associates of QT dispersion in patients with acute myocardial infarction: primacy of patency status of the infarct-related artery. *American Heart Journal*, **135**, 1027–1035.

Karjalainen, J., Reunanen, A., Ristola, P. & Viitasalo, M. (1997) *QT* interval as a cardiac risk factor in a middle aged population. *Heart*, **77**, 543–548.

Karpanou, E.A., Vyssoulis, G.P., Psichogios, A. *et al.* (1998) Regression of left ventricular hypertrophy results in improvement of QT dispersion in patients with hypertension. *American Heart Journal*, **136**, 765–768.

Kautzner, J. & Malik, M. (1997) *QT* interval dispersion and its clinical utility. *PACE (Pacing and Clinical Electrophysiology)*, **20** (Pt II), 2625–2640.

Kautzner, J., Yi, G., Camm, A.J. & Malik, M. (1994) Short- and long-term reproducibility of *QT*, *QTc*, and QT dispersion measurement in healthy subjects. *PACE (Pacing and Clinical Electrophysiolgy)*, **17**, 928–937.

Kautzner, J., Yi, G., Kishore, R. *et al.* (1996) Interobserver reproducibility of *QT* interval measurement and QT dispersion in patients after acute myocardial infarction. *Annals of Noninvasive Electrocardiology*, **1**, 363–374.

Kelly, R.F., Parillo, J.E. & Hollenberg, S.M. (1997) Effect of coronary angioplasty on QT dispersion. *American Heart Journal*, **134**, 399–405.

Kohno, I., Takusagawa, M., Yin, D. *et al.* (1998) QT dispersion in dipper- and nondipper-type hypertension. *American Journal of Hypertension*, **11**, 280–285.

Kors, J.A., de Bruyne, M.C., Hoes, A.W. *et al.* (1998) T axis as an indicator of risk of cardiac events in elderly people. *Lancet*, **352**, 601–604.

Kors, J.A. & van Herpen, G. (1998) Measurement error as a source of QT dispersion: a computerised analysis. *Heart*, **80**, 453–458.

Kors, J.A., van Herpen, G. & van Bemmel, J.H. (1999) QT dispersion as an attribute of T-loop morphology. *Circulation*, **99**, 1458–1463.

Kuo, C.-S., Munakata, K., Reddy, P. *et al.* (1983) Characteristics and possible mechanism of ventricular arrhythmia dependent on the dispersion of action potential durations. *Circulation*, **67**, 1356–1367.

Lau, C.P., Freedman, A.R., Fleming, S. *et al.* (1987) Hysteresis of the ventricular paced *QT* interval in response to abrupt changes in pacing rate. *Cardiovascular Research*, **22**, 67–72.

Lee, K.W., Kligfield, P., Okin, P.M. & Dower, G.E. (1998) Determinants of precordial QT dispersion in normal subjects. *Journal of Electrocardiology*, **31** (Suppl.), 128–133.

Lee, K.W., Okin, P.M., Kligfield, P. *et al.* (1997) Precordial *QT* Dispersion and inducible ventricular tachycardia. *American Heart Journal*, **134**, 1005–1013.

Leonardo, F., Fragasso, G., Rosano, G.M.C. *et al.* (1997) Effect of atenolol on *QT* interval and dispersion in patients with syndrome X. *American Journal of Cardiology*, **80**, 789–790.

Lepeschkin, E. (1972) Physiologic basis of the U wave. In: *Advances in Electrocardiography* (eds R. C. Schlant & J. W. Hurst), pp. 431–447. Grune & Stratton, New York.

Lepeschkin, E. & Surawicz, B. (1952) The measurement of the *QT* interval of the electrocardiogram. *Circulation*, **VI**, 378–88.

Lim, P.O., Nys, M., Naas, A.A.O. *et al.* (1999) Irbesartan reduces QT dispersion in hypertensive individuals. *Hypertension*, **33**, 713–718.

Maarouf, N., Aytemir, K., Gallagher, M. *et al.* (1999) Is *QT* Dispersion heart rate dependent? What are the values of correction formulas for *QT* interval? *Journal of the American College of Cardiology*, **33** (Suppl. A): 113A–114A (abstract).

Macfarlane, P.W. on behalf of the WOSCOPS. (1998) QT dispersion – lack of discriminating power. *Circulation*, **98** (Suppl.):I-81 (abstract).

Macfarlane, P.W., Devine, B., Latif, S. *et al.* (1990) Methodology of QRS interpretation in the Glasgow program. *Methods of Information in Medicine*, **29**, 354–361.

Macfarlane, P.W., McLaughlin, S.C. & Rodger, C. (1998) influence of lead selection and population on automated measurement of QT dispersion. *Circulation*, **98**, 2160–2167.

Macfarlane, P.W., McLaughlin, S.C., Devine, B. *et al.* (1994) Effects of age, sex, and race on ECG interval measurements. *Journal of Electrocardiology*, **27**, 14–19.

McLaughlin, N.B., Campbell, R.W.F. & Murray, A. (1995) Influence of T wave amplitude on automatic *QT* measurement. In: *Computers in Cardiology 1995*, pp. 777–780. IEEE Computer Society Press, New York.

McLaughlin, N.B., Campbell, R.W.F. & Murray, A. (1996) Accuracy of four automatic QT measurement techniques in cardiac patients and healthy subjects. *Heart*, **76**, 422–426.

Maheshwari, V.D. & Girish, M.P. (1998) QT dispersion as a marker of left ventricular mass in essential hypertension. *Indian Heart Journal*, **50**, 414–417.

Malik, M. (2000) QT dispersion: Time for an obituary? *European Heart Journal*, **21**, 955–957.

Malik, M., Acar, B., Yap, Y.-G. *et al.* (2000) QT dispersion does not represent electrocardiographic interlead heterogeneity of ventricular repolarization. *Journal of Cardiovascular Electrophysiology*, **11** (8), 835–843

Malik, M. & Batchvarov, V. (2000a) Measurement, interpretation and clinical potential of QT dispersion. *Journal of the American College of Cardiology*, **36**, 1749–1766.

Malik, M. & Batchvarov, V. (2000b) *QT Dispersion*. Futura Publishing, Armonk, NY.

Malik, M. & Bradford A. (1998) Human precision of operating a digitizing board: Implications for electrocardiogram measurement. *PACE (Pacing and Clinical Electrophysiolgy)*, **21**, 1656–1662.

Malik, M. & Camm, A.J. (1997) Mystery of *QTc* interval dispersion. *American Journal of Cardiology*, **79**, 785–787.

Mandecki, T., Szulc, A., Kastelik, J. *et al.* (1998) The observation of the QT dispersion in left ventricular hypertrophy in weight lifters. *Annals of Noninvasive Electrocardiology*, **3**, S18 (abstract).

Maron, B.J., Leyhe, M.J., Gohman, T.E. *et al.* (1999) QT dispersion is not a predictor of sudden cardiac death in hypertrophic cardiomyopathy as assessed in an unselected patient population. *Journal of the American College of Cardiology*, **33** (Suppl. A), 128A (abstract).

Mayet, J., Kanagaratnam, P., Shahi, M. *et al.* (1999) *QT* Dispersion in athletic left ventricular hypertrophy. *American Heart Journal*, **137**, 678–681.

Mayet, J., Shahi, M., McGrath, K. *et al.* (1996) Left ventricular hypertrophy and QT dispersion in hypertension. *Hypertension*, **28**, 791–796.

Meierhenrich, R., Helguera, M.E., Kidwell, G.A. *et al.* (1997) Influence of amiodarone on QT dispersion in patients with life-threatening ventricular arrhythmias and clinical outcome. *International Journal of Cardiology*, **60**, 289–294.

Michelucci, A., Padeletti, L., Frati, M. *et al.* (1996) Effects of ischaemia and reperfusion on QT dispersion during coronary angioplasty. *PACE (Pacing and Clinical Electrophysiolgy)*, **19**, 1905–1908.

Miorelli, M., Buja, G., Melacini, P. *et al.* (1994) *QT*-interval variability in hypertrophic cardiomyopathy patients with cardiac arrest. *International Journal of Cardiology*, **45**, 121–127.

Mirvis, D.M. (1985) Spatial variation of *QT* intervals in normal persons and patients with acute myocardial infarction. *Journal of the American College of Cardiology*, **5**, 625–631.

Mitchell LB, Wyse DG, Duff HJ. (1986) Programmed electrical stimulation for ventricular tachycardia induction in humans. I. The role of ventrcular functional refractoriness in tachycardia induction. *Journal of the American College of Cardiology*, **8**, 567–575.

Moenning, G., Haverkamp, W., Schulte, H. *et al.* (1999) Prognostic value of *QT*-interval and -dispersion in apparently healthy individuals. Results from the Münster heart study (PROCAM). *Journal of the American College of Cardiology*, **33** (Suppl. A), 333A (abstract).

Moreno, F.L., Villanueva, T., Karagounis, L.A. *et al.* (1994) Reduction of *QT* interval dispersion by successful thrombolytic therapy in acute myocardial infarction. TEAM-2 study investigators. *Circulation*, **90**, 94–100.

Morgan, J.M., Cunningham, D. & Rowland, E. (1992) Dispersion of monophasic action potential duration: demonstrable in humans after premature ventricular extrastimulation but not in steady state. *Journal of the American College of Cardiology*, **19**, 1244–1253.

Moss, A.J. (1999) Drugs that prolong the *QT* interval: regulatory and QT measurement issues from the United States and European perspectives. *Annals of Noninvasive Electrocardiology*, **4**, 255–256.

Muir, D.F., Love, M.W.A., MacGregor, G.D. *et al.* (1999) Athletic left ventricular hypertrophy is associated with increased QT dispersion: An observational study. *Journal of the American College of Cardiology*, **33** (Suppl. A), 510A (abstract).

Murray, A., McLaughlin, N.B., Bourke, J.P., Doig, J.C., Furniss, S.S. & Campbell R.W.F. (1994) Errors in manual measurement of *QT* intervals. *British Heart Journal*, **71**, 386–390.

Murray, A., McLaughlin, N.B. & Campbell, R.W.F. (1997) Measuring QT dispersion: man versus machine. *Heart*, **77**, 539–542.

Nakajima, T., Fujimoto, S., Uemura, S. *et al.* (1998) Does increased QT dispersion in the acute phase of anterior myocardial infarction predict recovery of left ventricular wall motion? *Journal of Electrocardiology*, **31**, 1–8.

Okin, P., Devereux, R.B., Howard, B.V., Fabsitz, R.R., Lee, E.T. & Welty, T.K. (2000) Assessment of *QT* interval and QT dispersion for prediction of all-cause and cardiovascular mortality in American Indians The Strong Heart Study. *Circulation*, **101**, 61–66.

Okishige, K., Yamashita, K., Yoshinaga, H. *et al.* (1996) Electrophysiological effects of ischaemic preconditioning on QT dispersion during coronary angioplasty. *Journal of the American College of Cardiology*, **28**, 70–73.

Özerkan, F., Zoghi, M., Gürgün, C. *et al.* (1999) QT dispersion in hypertensive patients who had normal coronary angiogram with or without left ventricular hypertrophy. *European Heart Journal*, **20** (Suppl.), 85 (abstract).

Papandonakis, E., Tsoukas, A. & Christakos, S. (1999) QT dispersion as a noninvasive arrhythmogenic marker in acute myocardial infarction. *Annals of Noninvasive Electrocardiology*, **4**, 35–38.

Parikka, H., Toivonen, L., Naukkarinen, V. *et al.* (1999) Decreases by magnesium of QT dispersion and ventricular arrhythmias in patients with acute myocardial infarction. *European Heart Journal*, **20**, 111–120.

Paventi, S., Bevilacqua, U., Parafati, M.A. *et al.* (1999) QT dispersion and early arrhythmic risk during acute myocardial infarction. *Angiology* **50**, 209–215.

Perkiömäki, J.S., Ikäheimo, M.J., Pikkujämsä, S.M. *et al.* (1996) Dispersion of the *QT* interval and autonomic modulation of heart rate in hypertensive men with and without left ventricular hypertrophy. *Hypertension*, **28**, 16–21.

Perkiömäki, J.S., Kiostinen, M.J., Yli-Mäyry, S. *et al.* (1995) Dispersion of the *QT* interval in patients with and without susceptibility to ventricular tachyarrhythmias after previous myocardial infarction. *Journal of the American College of Cardiology*, **26**, 174–179.

Pitt, B., Poole-Wilson, P.A., Segal, R. *et al.* on behalf of the ELITE II Investigators (2000) Effect of losartan compared with captopril on mortality in patients with symptomatic heart failure: randomized trial – the Losartan Heart Failure Survival Study ELITE II. *Lancet*, **355**, 1582–1587.

Pitt, B., Segal, R., Martinez, F.A. *et al.* (1997) Randomised trial of losartan versus captopril in patients over 65 with heart failure. *Lancet*, **349**, 747–752.

Plonsey, R. (1979) A contemporary view of the ventricular gradient of Wilson. *Journal of Electrocardiology*, **12**, 337–341.

Priori, S.G., Mortara, D.W., Napolitano, C. *et al.* (1997) Evaluation of the spatial aspects of T wave complexity in the long-QT syndrome. *Circulation*, **96**, 3006–3012.

Priori, S.G., Napolitano, C., Diehl, L. *et al.* (1994) Dispersion of the *QT* interval. A marker of therapeutic efficacy in the idiopathic long QT syndrome. *Circulation*, **89**, 1681–1689.

Puljevic, D., Smalcelj, A., Durakovic, Z. *et al.* (1998) Effects of postmyocardial infarction scar size, cardiac function, and severity of coronary artery disease on *QT* interval dispersion as a risk factor for complex ventricular arrhythmia. *PACE (Pacing and Clinical Electrophysiology)*, **21**, 1508–1516.

Punske, B.B., Lux, R.L., MacLeod, R.S. *et al.* (1999) Mechanisms of the spatial distribution of *QT* intervals on the epicardial and body surfaces. *Journal of Cardiovascular Electrophysiology*, **10**, 1605–1618.

Pye, M., Quinn, A.C. & Cobbe, S.M. (1994) *QT* interval dispersion: a noninvasive marker of susceptibility to arrhythmia in patients with sustained ventricular arrhythmias? *British Heart Journal*, **71**, 511–514.

Radmanabhan, S., Amin, J., Silvet, H. *et al.* (1999) QT dispersion has no impact on mortality in patients with moderate and severe left ventricular dysfunction: Results from a cohort of 2263 patients. *Journal of the American College of Cardiology*, **33** (Suppl. A), 107A (abstract).

Rautaharju, P.M. (1999) *QT* and dispersion of ventricular repolarization: the greatest fallacy in electrocardiography in the 1990s. *Circulation*, **18**, 2477–2478.

Rautaharju, P.M. (2002) Why did QT dispersion die? *Cardiac Electrophysiology Review* **6**, 295–301.

Sagie, A., Larson, M.G., Goldberg, R.J. *et al.* (1992) An improved method for adjusting the *QT* interval for heart rate (The Framingham Heart Study). *American Journal of Cardiology*, **70**, 797–801.

Saint Beuve, C., Badilini, F., Maison-Blanche, P. *et al.* (1999) QT dispersion: comparison of orthogonal, quasi-orthogonal, and 12-lead configurations. *Annals of Noninvasive Electrocardiology*, **4**, 167–175.

Savelieva, I., Camm, A.J. & Malik, M. (1999a) Do we need age-adjustment of QT dispersion? Observations from 1096 normal subjects. *Heart*, **81** (Suppl. 1), P47 (abstract).

Savelieva, I., Camm, A.J. & Malik, M. (1999b) Gender-specific differences on QT dispersion measured in 1100 healthy subjects. *PACE (Pacing and Clinical Electrophysiolgy)*, **22**, 885 (abstract).

Savelieva, I., Yi, G., Guo, X.-H. *et al.* (1998) Agreement and reproducibility of automatic versus manual measurement of *QT* interval and QT dispersion. *American Journal of Cardiology*, **81**, 471–477.

Schneider, C.A., Voth, E., Baer, F.M. *et al.* (1997) QT dispersion is determined by the extent of viable myocardium in patients with chronic Q wave myocardial infarction. *Circulation*, **96**, 3913–3920.

Sedwick, M.L., Rasmussen, H.S. & Cobbe, S.M. (1992) Effects of the class III antiarrhythmic drug dofetilide on ventricular monophasic action potential duration and the *QT* interval dispersion in stable angina pectoris. *American Journal of Cardiology*, **70**, 1432–1437.

Shah, C.P., Thakur, R.K., Reisdorff, E.J. *et al.* (1998) QT dispersion may be a useful adjunct for detection of myocardial infarction in the chest pain centre. *American Heart Journal*, **136**, 496–498.

Shimizu, W. & Antzelevitch, C. (1997) Sodium channel block with mexiletine is effective in reducing dispersion of repolarization and preventing torsades de pointes in LQT2 and LQT3 models of the long-QT syndrome. *Circulation*, **96**, 2038–2047.

Shimizu, W. & Antzelevitch, C. (1998) Cellular basis for the ECG features of the LQT1 form of the long-QT syndrome. Effects of β-adrenergic agonists and antagonists and sodium channel blockers on transmural dispersion of repolarization and torsades de pointes. *Circulation*, **98**, 2314–2322.

Shimizu, W. & Antzelevitch, C. (1999) Cellular and ionic

basis for T wave alternans under long-*QT* conditions. *Circulation*, **99**, 1499–1507.

Shulan, Z., Yin'an, S. & Huixian, H. (1998) Prediction value of ventricular arrhythmia of patients with acute myocardial infarction by QT dispersion. *Journal of the Xi'An Medical University*, **19**, 616–617.

Simoncelli, U., Rusconi, C., Nicosia, F. *et al.* (1998) QT dispersion in endurance athletes. *International Journal of Sports Cardiology* **7**, 63–67.

Spodick, D.H. (1992) Reduction of *QT*-interval imprecision and variance by measuring the JT interval (editorial). *American Journal of Cardiology*, **72**, 103.

Sporton, S.C., Taggart, P., Sutton, P.M. *et al.* (1997) Acute ischaemia: a dynamic influence on QT dispersion. *Lancet*, **349**, 306–309

Statters, D.J., Malik, M., Ward, D.E. *et al.* (1994) QT dispersion: problems of methodology and clinical significance. *Journal of Cardiovascular Electrophysiology*, **5**, 672–685.

Surawicz, B. (1996) Will QT dispersion play a role in clinical decision-making? *Journal of Cardiovascular Electrophysiology*, **7**, 777–784.

Surawicz, B. (1998) U wave: facts, hypotheses, misconceptions, and misnomers. *Journal of Cardiovascular Electrophysiology*, **9**, 1117–1128.

Surawicz, B. (1999) Long *QT*: good, bad, indifferent and fascinating. *ACC Current Journal Review* **8**, 19–21.

Surawicz, B. ST–T abnormalities. T wave. (1989) In: *Comprehensive Electrocardiography. Theory and Practice in Heath and Disease* (eds P. W. Macfarlane & T. D. Vetch Lawries), pp. 521–550. Pergamon Press, Oxford.

Szydlo, K., Trusz-Gluza, M., Drzewiecki *et al.* (1998) Correlation of heart rate variability parameters and *QT* interval in patients after PTCA of infarct related coronary artery as an indicator of improved autonomic regulation. *PACE (Pacing and Clinical Electrophysiolgy)*, **21**, 2407–2410.

Taggart, P., Sutton, P.M.I., Opthof, T. *et al.* (2001) Transmural repolarization in the left ventricle in humans during normoxia and ischaemia. *Cardiovascular Research*, **50**, 454–462.

Tarabey, R., Sukenik, D., Milnar, J. *et al.* (1998) Effect of intracoronary balloon inflation at percutaneous transluminal coronary angioplasty on QT dispersion. *American Heart Journal*, **135**, 519–522.

Taran, L. & Szilagyi, N. (1951) The measurement of the *Q–T* interval in acute heart disease. *Bulletin of the St Francis Sanatorium*, **8**, 13.

Tavernier, R. & Jordaens, L. (1999) Repolarization characteristics and sudden death after myocardial infarction: A case control study. *Journal of the American College of Cardiology*, **33** (Suppl. A), 146A (abstract).

Tomiyama, H., Doba, N., Fu, Y. *et al.* (1998) Left ventricular geometric patterns and QT dispersion in borderline and mild hypertension: Their evolution and regression. *American Journal of Hypertension*, **11**, 286–292.

Tran, H.T., Chow, M.S., Kluger, J. (1997) Amiodarone induced torsades de pointes with excessive QT dispersion following quinidine induced polymorphic ventricular tachycardia. *PACE (Pacing and Clinical Electrophysiology)*, **20**, 2275–2278.

Tran, H.T., Fan, C., Tu, W.Q. *et al.* (1998) *QT* measurement: a comparison of three simple methods. *Annals of Noninvasive Electrocardiology*, **3**, 228–231.

Trusz-Gluza, M, Świderska, E., Śmieja-Jaroczynska, B. *et al.* (1998) Factors influencing dispersion of repolarization under antiarrhythmic treatment. *Annals of Noninvasive Electrocardiology*, **3**, S18 (abstract).

Tutar, H., Öcal, B., Imamoglu, A. *et al.* (1998) Dispersion of *QT* and *QTc* interval in healthy children, and effects of sinus arrhythmia on QT dispersion. *Heart*, **80**, 77–79.

Van Bemmel, J.H., Kors, J.A. *et al.* (1990) Methodology of the modular ECG analysis system MEANS. *Methods of Information in Medicine*, **29**, 346–353.

Van de Loo, A., Klingenheben, T. & Hohnloser, S.H. (1994) Amiodarone therapy after sotalol-induced torsades de pointes: prolonged *QT* interval and QT dispersion in differentiation of proarrhythmic effects. *Zeitschrift für Kardiologie*, **83**, 887–890.

Vloka, M.E., Babaev, A., Ehlert, F.A. *et al.* (1999) Poor correlation of automated and manual QT dispersion measurements in patients and normal subjects. *Journal of the American College of Cardiology*, **33** (Suppl. A), 350A (abstract).

Watanabe, Y. (1975) Purkinje repolarization as a possible cause of the U wave in the electrocardiogram. *Circulation*, **51**, 1030–1037.

Wiggers, C.J. (1940 The mechanism and nature of ventricular fibrillation. *American Heart Journal*, **20**, 399.

Wilson, F.N., Macleod, A.G. & Barker, P.S. (1931) The T deflection of the electrocardiogram. *Transactions of the Association of American Physicians*, **46**, 29–38.

Wilson, F.N., Macleod, A.G., Barker, P.S. & Johnston, F.D. (1934) The determination and the significance of the areas of the ventricular deflections of the electrocardiogram. *American Heart Journal*, **10**, 46–61.

Xue, Q. & Reddy, S. (1996) New algorithms for QT dispersion analysis. In: *Proceedings of the Marquette 14th ECG Analysis Seminar*, pp. 20–23.

Yadav, A., Paquette, M., Newman, D. *et al.* (1999) Amiodarone is associated with increased QT dispersion but low mortality in a CIDS cohort. *PACE (Pacing and Clinical Electrophysiolgy)*, **22**, 896 (abstract).

Yan, G.X. & Antzelevitch, C. (1998) Cellular basis for the normal T wave and the electrocardiographic manifestations of the long QT syndrome. *Circulation*, **98**, 1928–1936.

Yap, Y.G., Yi, G., Aytemir, K. *et al.* (1999) Comprehensive assessment of QT dispersion in various at risk groups including acute myocardial infarction, unstable angina, hypertrophic cardiomyopathy, idiopathic dilated cardiomyopathy, and healthy controls. *PACE (Pacing and Clinical Electrophysiology)*, **22**, A38 (abstract).

Yap, Y.G., Yi, G., Guo, X.-H. *et al.* (1999) Dynamic changes of QT dispersion and its relationship with clinical variables and arrhythmic events after myocardial infarction. *Journal of the American College of Cardiology*, **33** (Suppl. A), 107A (abstract).

Yi, G., Crook, R., Guo, H. *et al.* (1998a) Exercise-induced changes in the *QT* interval duration and dispersion in patients with sudden cardiac death after myocardial infarction. *International Journal of Cardiology*, **63**, 271–279.

Yi, G., Elliott, P., McKenna, W.J. *et al.* (1998b) QT dispersion and risk factors for sudden cardiac death in patients with hypertrophic cardiomyopathy. *American Journal of Cardiology*, **82**, 1514–1519.

Yi, G., Guo, X.-H., Crook R *et al.* (1998c) Computerised measurements of QT dispersion in healthy subjects. *Heart*, **80**, 459–466.

Yi, G., Prasad K, Elliott P *et al.* (1998d) T wave complexity in patients with hypertrophic cardiomyopathy. *PACE (Pacing and Clinical Electrophysiology)*, **21**, 2382–2386.

Zabel, M., Klingenheben, T., Franz, M.R. *et al.* (1998a) Assessment of QT dispersion for prediction of mortality or arrhythmic events after myocardial infarction. *Circulation*, **97**, 2543–2550.

Zabel, M., Klingenheben, T., Sticherling C *et al.* (1998b) *QT*-dispersion does not predict inducibility or adequate device treatment in patients with malignant ventricular tachyarrhythmias. *European Heart Journal*, **19** (Suppl.), 600 (abstract).

Zabel, M., Lichtlen P.R., Haverich A. & Franz M.R. (1998c) Comparison of ECG variables of dispersion of ventricular repolarization with direct myocardial repolarization measurements in the human heart. *Journal of Cardiovascular Electrophysiology*, **9**, 1279–1284.

Zabel, M., Portnoy, S. & Franz, M.R. (1995) Electrocardiographic indexes of dispersion of ventricular repolarization: an isolated heart validation study. *Journal of the American College of Cardiology*, **25**, 746–752.

Zabel, M., Woosley, R.L. & Franz, M.R. (1997) Is dispersion of ventricular repolarization rate dependent? *PACE (Pacing and Clinical Electrophysiology)*, **20**, 2405–2411.

Zaidi, M., Robert, A., Fesler, R. *et al.* (1996) Dispersion of ventricular repolarization in hypertrophic cardiomyopathy. *Journal of Electrocardiology*, **29** (Suppl.), 89–94.

Zaidi, M., Robert, A., Fesler, R. *et al.* (1997a) Dispersion of ventricular repolarization: a marker of ventricular arrhythmias in patients with previous myocardial infarction. *Heart*, **78**, 371–375.

Zaidi, M., Robert, A., Fesler, R. *et al.* (1997b) Dispersion of ventricular repolarization in dilated cardiomyopathy. *European Heart Journal*, **18**, 1129–1134.

Zaputovic L, Mavric Z, Zaninovic-Jurjevic T *et al.* (1997) Relationship between QT dispersion and the incidence of early ventricular arrhythmias in patients with acute myocardial infarction. *International Journal of Cardiology*, **62**, 211–6.

Zareba, W. & Moss, A. (1995) Dispersion of repolarization evaluated in three orthogonal-type electrocardiographic leads: L1, aVF, V2. *PACE (Pacing and Clinical Electrophysiology)*, **18**, 895 (abstract).

Zareba, W., Moss, A.J. & le Cessie, S. (1994) Dispersion of ventricular repolarization and arrhythmic cardiac death in corornary artery disease. *American Journal of Cardiology*, **74**, 550–553.

Zhang, N., Ho, T.F., Yip, W.C.L. (1999) *QT* Dispersion in healthy Chinese children and adolescents. *Annals of Noninvasive Electrocardiology*, **4**, 281–285.

Zhou, S.H., Wong, S., Rautaharju, P.M. *et al.* (1992) Should the JT rather than the *QT* interval be used to detect prolongation of ventricular repolarization? An assessment in normal conduction and in ventricular conduction defects. *Journal of Electricardiology* **25** (Suppl.), 131–136.

Zoghi, M., Gürgün, C., Ercan, E. *et al.* (1999) QT dispersion in patients with different aetiology of left ventricular hypertrophy. *European Heart Journal*, **20** (Suppl.): 335 (abstract).

CHAPTER 35

Morphological Assessment of T Wave Patterns

Markus Zabel and Marek Malik

Introduction

To overcome the methodological shortcomings of QT dispersion (QTd), a marker derived from the 12-lead electrocardiogram (ECG) for stratification of patients at risk for sudden cardiac death, novel ECG variables of T wave morphology and the so-called T wave residua have been proposed. The total cosine *r*-to-T (TCRT), T wave morphology dispersion, T wave loop dispersion, normalized T wave loop area, as well as the absolute and relative T wave residuum evaluating non-dipolar ECG signal contents were prospectively studied in two clinical trials involving post myocardial infarction (MI) patients and US veterans with cardiovascular disease. In the first study in 280 post MI patients with 27 events over a mean follow-up of 32 months, TCRT and T wave loop dispersion were independent predictors of mortality. In the second study which enrolled 813 male US veterans with cardiac disease and with a long-term follow-up of >10 years the absolute and relative T wave residua were independent predictors of patient risk. This study therefore was the first to demonstrate that a novel parameter characterizing heterogeneity of ventricular repolarization within the 12-lead surface ECG permits risk stratification of sudden death in patients with cardiovascular disease. All novel ECG variables of T wave morphology as well as the T wave residua are easily accessible from digital 12-lead surface ECG recordings using custom computer programs. They may prove useful to easily and prospectively identify risk patients that benefit from the implantable cardioverter-defibrillator (ICD).

Need for novel ECG variables of ventricular repolarization

Noninvasive identification of patients with increased risk of sudden cardiac death using measurements of ventricular repolarization derived from the 12-lead surface ECG had received new interest about a decade ago when the method of QT dispersion (QTd) was proposed for electrocardiographic assessment of heterogeneity of ventricular repolarization (Day *et al.* 1990, 1992). Following encouraging early reports (Day *et al.* 1990; Hii *et al.* 1992; Barr *et al.* 1994) QTd was evaluated in a large body of clinical studies (for review see Batchvarov & Malik 2000) until it became obvious that QTd identified rather crude features of pathological ventricular repolarization (Kors & van Herpen, 1998; Savelieva *et al.* 1998; Kors *et al.* 1999). Moreover, carefully conducted prospective studies – despite or because of the application of digital analysis techniques (Zabel *et al.* 1998; Brendorp *et al.* 2001) – did not confirm the predictive value of QTd for clinical risk assessment as suggested by the earlier studies. Following the necessary search for innovative ECG markers detecting *the arrhythmogenic substrate of pathological repolarization*, it was recently hypothesized that *new temporo-spatial measures* of T wave morphology and T wave heterogeneity could provide a valid clinical tool as initially intended for the earlier simpler ECG variables.

Methodology of novel T wave morphology variables and the T wave residua

Detecting and quantifying distinct pathological features of ventricular repolarization, a set of different T wave morphology variables was proposed by Acar *et al.* (1999). These variables can be computed applying a custom-developed fully automatic software program to the 12-lead digital ECG signal of a single steady-state beat. As a first analysis step, singular value decomposition of the ECG signal generates vectors defining a space of eight dimensions. Next, based on defined algorithms (Acar *et al.* 1999), several descriptors of temporo-spatial variations of T wave morphology and repolarization wavefront direction (Acar *et al.* 1999; Zabel *et al.* 2000) are calculated. These novel 12-lead ECG variables of T wave morphology are the total cosine r-to-T (TCRT), the T wave morphology dispersion, the T wave loop dispersion, and the normalized T wave loop area (see Fig. 35.1). The TCRT determines the cosine of the 3D angle between the depolarization and the repolarization vectors, extending the concept of the ventricular gradient proposed by Wilson over 60 years ago (Wilson *et al.* 1934). T wave morphology dispersion measures dissimilarities of the T wave shapes between the different leads and reconstruction vectors of the individual ECG leads and is calculated as the average of angles between pairs of reconstruction vectors. T wave loop dispersion is a descriptor of the normalized T wave loop length; it measures spatial irregularities of the T wave loop during its time course. The normalized T wave loop area determines the area of the normalized T wave loop as a unitless fraction of a rectangular area encompassing it.

Similar to the above described T wave morphology variables, the relative and absolute T wave residuum are also derived from the digital 12-lead ECG subsequent to singular value decomposition (Malik *et al.* 2000). In the eight-dimensional vector space, the first three orthogonal components correspond to the traditional 3D T wave vector. This vector can be visualized as a dipole in an X–Y–Z coordinate graphical plot (see Fig. 35.1) and by definition contains the so-called dipolar signal energy. In contrast, the signal energy in the remaining fourth to eighth leads reflects the non-dipolar ECG signal contents. The latter components represent repolarization signals that are contained within the ECG but are not reflected in the globally reconstructed dipolar T wave vector (as shown in Fig. 35.1). For this reason, they are expected to measure the true heterogeneity of ventricular repolarization within the ECG. By definition, the absolute T wave residuum quantifies the absolute energy of the non-dipolar ECG signals while the relative T wave residuum expresses the nondipolar contents as a percentage of the overall signal contents.

All T wave morphology variables as well as the T wave residua can be instantly calculated from digital 12-lead ECG recordings. The speed of automatic calculation is a dramatic improvement over previously required operator-dependent interactive analyses even of digitally acquired ECG data, and more so as compared to the time-consuming manual QTd measurement techniques. Reproducibility of results with the new methodology is evidently superior, as automatic calculation by a predefined algorithm ensures 100% reproducibility. In contrast, interactive analyses have been prone to multiple sources of inaccuracies including the analyser's subjectivity. Both immediate calculation and fully automatic analysis of T wave morphology and T wave residua therefore offered straight solutions for the methodological shortcomings of QTd.

Prognostic value of ECG variables of T wave morphology and the T wave residua

The prognostic value of the new T wave morphology variables and the T wave residua was assessed in two large clinical studies (Zabel *et al.* 2000, 2002). Both unequivocally demonstrated that for the first time reliable risk assessment from a single beat ECG repolarization variable was possible. Testing the initial hypothesis that temporo-spatial measures of ECG repolarization dispersion improve post-MI risk stratification a post-hoc digital analysis of a prospectively enrolled patient population was conducted (Zabel *et al.* 2000). During long-term follow-up over a mean of 32 months, 27 clinical events defined as death or nonfatal VT/VF were observed. A 12-lead ECG had been recorded on

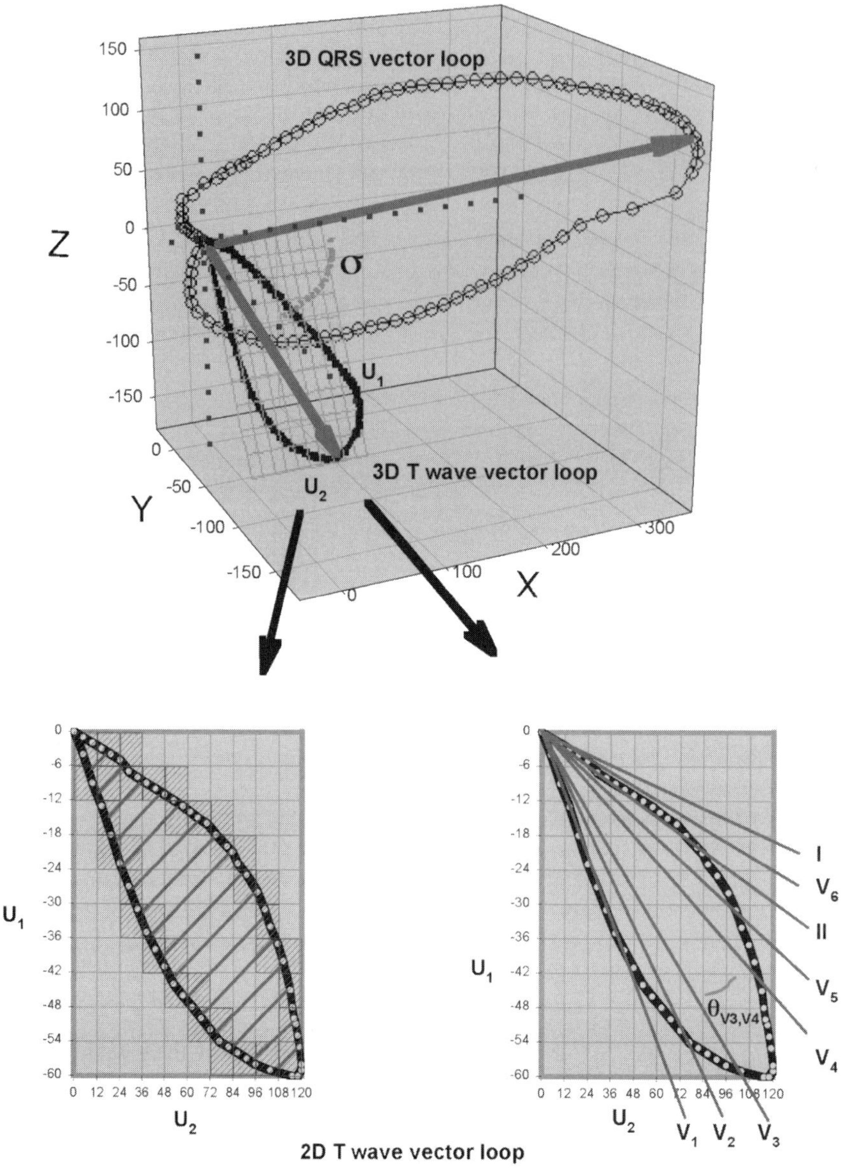

Fig. 35.1 Schematic view of the QRS and T wave vector loops. The 3D angle determines the total cosine *r* to T (TCRT). On the lower left panel, the T wave loop is shown in its two-dimensional plane. The loop passes 35 marked subdivisions of a rectangle encompassing the loop and divided into 100 subdivisions, i.e. T wave loop dispersion is 35. The normalized T wave loop area is calculated as the fraction of the loop area (marked by stripes) to the encompassing rectangle. The right lower panel plots the reconstruction vectors of the different ECG leads onto the T wave loop, T wave morphology dispersion is then calculated by averaging the angle between all possible reconstruction vector pairs. (Adapted from Zabel *et al.* 2000, with permission.)

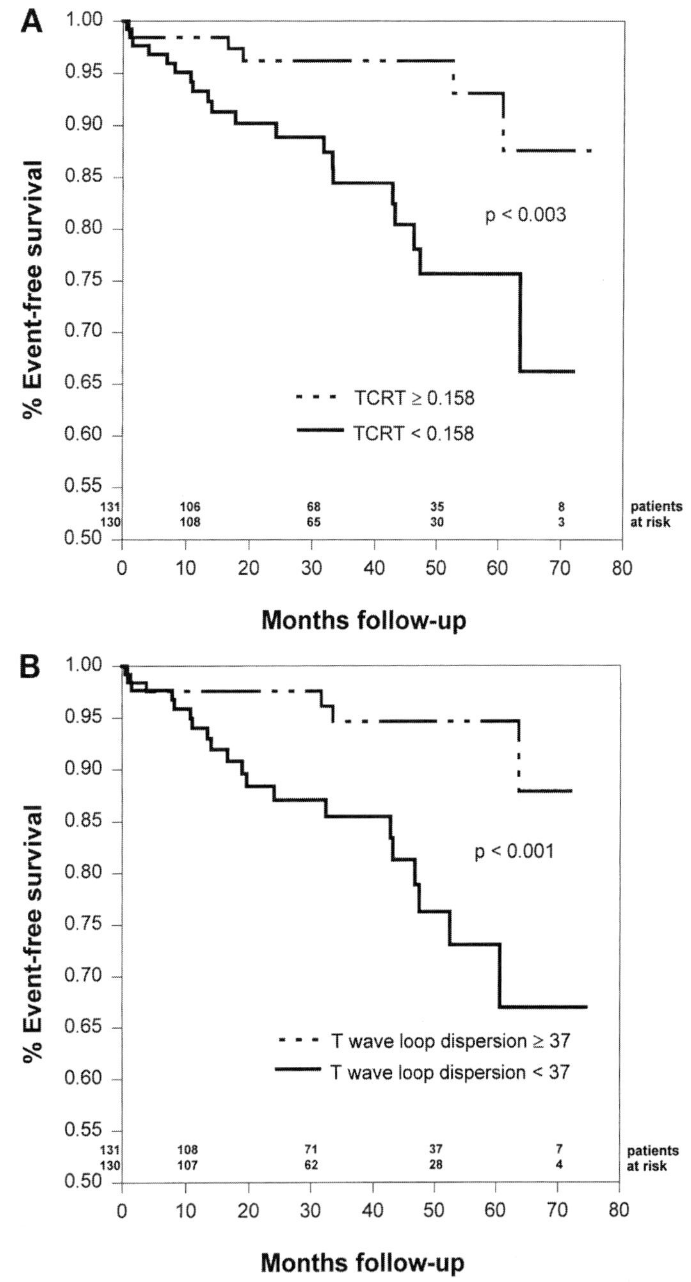

Fig. 35.2 Kaplan–Meier event probability curves for 280 post myocardial infarction patients stratified by the median value of the total cosine *r* to T (TCRT) ($P < 0.003$ by log-rank test) and T wave loop dispersion ($P < 0.001$ by log-rank test). (From Zabel *et al.* 2000, with permission.)

paper before discharge and converted into digital format. The above described T wave morphology variables TCRT, T wave loop dispersion, T wave morphology dispersion, and normalized T wave loop area were computed and their prognostic value was assessed. TCRT and T wave loop dispersion were univariately associated ($P = 0.0002$ and $P < 0.002$) with events. The discrimination of risk by these two variables was confirmed by the comparison of Kaplan–Meier curves for patient strata above and below the median ($P < 0.003$ and $P < 0.001$, Fig. 35.2). On multivariate Cox regression analysis entering other univariately predictive risk stratifiers including age, LVEF, heart rate, reperfusion therapy, beta adrenergic blocker treatment, and SDNN from Holter, TCRT ($P < 0.03$) yielded independent predictive value for overall events while T wave loop dispersion was of borderline independence (P = 0.064). Heart rate ($P < 0.02$), LVEF ($P < 0.02$), and reperfusion therapy ($P < 0.02$) also remained in the final model. T wave loop dispersion was, however, a significant independent predictor of arrhythmic events ($P = 0.008$), when considering patients without left bundle branch block (LBBB).

Assessing possible interactions between T wave morphology variables, conventional repolarization variables, and clinical variables, the only clinically relevant relationship was the influence of LBBB on TCRT. In nine patients with LBBB the average TCRT was – 0.77 ± 0.25 as compared to 0.11 ± 0.12 in 252 patients without LBBB ($P = 0.005$). Other T wave morphology variables were not significantly influenced. Moreover, the prognostic value of TCRT was maintained in patients without LBBB. None of the clinical variables were univariately related to the T wave morphology variables. In addition, no relevant correlation was found among T wave morphology variables ($r < 0.25$).

For the second clinical study digital 12-lead ECGs were recorded between 1984 and 1991 in 813 male US veterans treated at the VA Medical Centre Washington, DC with cardiovascular disease. This patient series was retrospectively compiled in 1991, follow-up was prospectively assessed until 2000. T wave morphology variables (TCRT, T wave loop dispersion, T wave morphology dispersion, and normalized T wave loop area) as well as the absolute and relative T wave residuum were analysed. Of 772 patients with technically analysable data, 252 patients (32.6%) died after a mean follow-up of 10.4 ± 3.8 years. Direct comparison between deceased and alive patients showed that the T wave residua predicted mortality (111900 ± 164700 vs. 85600 ± 144800 between dead and alive patients, $P < 0.0002$; and 0.43 ± 0.62% vs. 0.33 ± 0.56%, $P < 0.0005$ for the absolute and relative T wave residuum, respectively). Kaplan–Meier analysis dichotomizing patient groups by the median of a given ECG variable revealed a significantly worse survival for patients with a relative T wave residuum above the median (i.e. >0.15%) as compared to patients with values below ($P < 0.0002$, Fig. 35.3). Similarly, patients with an absolute T wave residuum above the median (i.e. >51042) had a worse survival than those patients with values below ($P < 0.0004$, Fig. 35.3). On multivariate regression analysis entering age, LVEF, echocardiographic LVH and either of the T wave residua, risk prediction was independent for the absolute ($P = 0.022$) and for the relative ($P = 0.006$) T wave residuum, respectively, with age ($P < 0.0001$), presence of LVH ($P = 0.002$), and LVEF ($P = 0.004$) also being predictors of survival. This study in a large cohort of US veterans was the first to demonstrate that a novel parameter characterizing heterogeneity of ventricular repolarization within the 12-lead surface ECG permits risk stratification in patients with cardiovascular disease over a long-term follow-up of >10 years. Deceased patients exhibited significantly higher heterogeneity of repolarization as compared to patients alive at the end of the follow-up period. Also useful for comparison, much smaller T wave residuum values (0.029%) were reported in normal subjects (Malik *et al.* 2000).

Pathophysiology of novel T wave morphology variables and the T wave residua

With regard to the assessment of the already mentioned arrhythmogenic substrate of pathological ventricular repolarization, the early concepts stemming from experimental (Kuo *et al.* 1985, 1983) and body-surface mapping studies (Abildskov *et al.* 1977, 1982) proved their validity – as demonstrated by the above prognostic studies utilizing novel ECG variables of T wave morphology. The array of these four variables was designed to quantify different facets of abnormal repolarization that may play a role in the genesis of malignant ventricular tachyarrhythmias, such as wavefront direction between repolarization and depolarization (TCRT), abnormalities of the shape and size of the T wave loop (T wave loop dispersion, normalized T wave loop area), as well as differences between the reconstructed T wave loop and the various leads of the 12-lead ECG (T wave morphology dispersion).

TCRT reflects a three-dimensional comparison between repolarization and depolarization wavefronts. TCRT therefore is akin to the concept of the ventricular gradient introduced by Wilson as early as 1934 (Wilson *et al.* 1934) later expanded

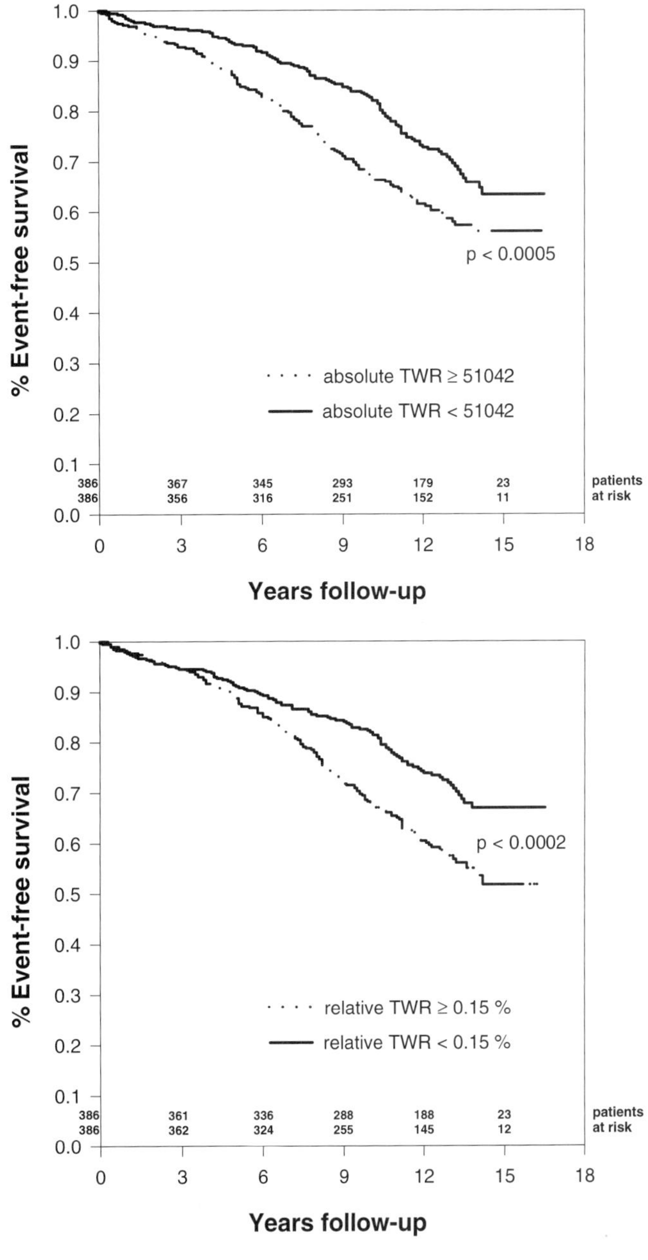

Fig. 35.3 Kaplan–Meier event probability curves for 772 US veterans with long-term follow-up stratified by the median value of the absolute T wave residuum ($P < 0.0005$ by log-rank test) and the relative T wave residuum ($P < 0.003$ by log-rank test). (From Zabel *et al.* 2002, with permission.)

by QRST area distributions (Abildskov *et al.* 1977, 1982; Tsunakawa *et al.* 1985) from the above-mentioned technique of body surface potential mapping. It is important to note that TCRT does not consider the amplitude of both depolarization and repolarization processes but only the difference in their direction and thus represents a modification of the earlier concepts. When comparing values found in the post MI population (Zabel *et al.* 2000) with established normal values reported by Acar *et al.* (1999) (0.52 ± 0.27 for TCRT, 36.4 ± 1.1 for T wave loop dispersion, 0.67 ± 0.09 for the normalized T wave loop area, and 10.7 ± 4.8 for T wave morphology dispersion, respectively), increased T wave morphology dispersion as well as lowered values for TCRT, T wave loop dispersion and normalized T wave area are pathological as such and differentiate event and non-event patients. While a low TCRT relates to a large deviation between the QRS and T wave loops, a large T wave morphology dispersion is associated with increased dissimilarities among the T waves in various ECG leads, a low value in normalized T wave area as well as T wave loop dispersion may be explained as arrhythmogenic by a pathologically compressed and narrowed T wave loop. Furthermore, irregularity of the loop and deviation from an ellipsoid would also result in a decreased normalized T wave area. Beyond these considerations and due to the novelty of the algorithms used in this study, a more detailed experimental basis on the electrophysiological mechanisms involved is necessary. However, other ECG approaches to noninvasive risk stratification for sudden cardiac death, such as principal component analysis, T wave alternans or *QT* variability, also fell short of a precise pathophysiological explanation during their initial clinical evaluation.

The concept of T wave residua relates to a methodological concern previously raised regarding QTd. The study by Kors *et al.* (1999) revealed that QTd could be explained by different projections of the T wave loop onto the surface ECG leads, and thus concluded that it was impossible to link QTd to regional repolarization information. Kors *et al.* (1999) assumed an entirely dipolar nature of the T wave which is true only for a very substantial portion but not for the entire ECG signal (Tsunakawa *et al.* 1985; Brody *et al.* 1977). To study the genesis of QTd in more detail, Malik *et al.* (2000) compared QTd with the 3D T wave vector from the 12-lead ECG in several clinically well-defined patient populations and quantified the nondipolar signal contents, i.e. the signal extent not explained by the 3D T wave vector. It was found that these nondipolar signal contents did not correlate with QTd. Technically this demonstrated that QTd was not measuring heterogeneity of ventricular repolarization but instead and as a new concept of 12-lead ECG assessment, it was now proposed that the non-dipolar signal contents might quantify the heterogeneity of repolarization. Consistent with the expectation that heterogeneity of ventricular repolarization increases with myocardial disease states, significantly higher values were found for the T wave residua in patients after myocardial infarc-tion (MI). While the values of the relative T wave residuum appear small, the differences between post MI patients and normal subjects are more than sixfold with almost no overlap between the values (Malik *et al.* 2000). Similar as for the above T wave morphology variables, a better pathophysiological understanding will be provided by ongoing experimental studies.

Summary

The previously widely used QTd is now considered an unspecific and indirect marker of pathological ventricular repolarization. It should be replaced by more precise descriptors of repolarization pathophysiology which are now readily available to computerized analyses of any 12-lead ECG. As summarized in this text, automatic analysis of various T wave morphology variables from the 12-lead resting ECG permits independent risk assessment in two large populations at risk for sudden cardiac death. The TCRT which is measuring the 3D angle between the QRS and the T wave vector loop is particularly useful in post MI risk assessment. The T wave residua demonstrate particular strength in risk stratifying US veterans over a long-term follow-up. Both markers may prove useful to detect patients with intermediate to high sudden death risk that will benefit from ICDs. The exact pathophysiological mechanisms as to how abnormalities in these variables translate into clinical events are currently being investigated in experimental studies.

References

Abildskov, J.A., Burgess, M.J., Urie, P.M. *et al.* (1977) The unidentified information content of the electrocardiogram. *Circulation Research*, **40**, 3–7.

Abildskov, J.A., Green, L.S., Evans, A.K. *et al.* (1982) The QRST deflection area of electrograms during global alterations of ventricular repolarization. *Journal of Electrocardiology*, **15**, 103–107.

Acar, B., Yi, G., Hnatkova, K. *et al.* (1999) Spatial, temporal and wavefront direction characteristics of 12-lead T-wave morphology. *Medical & Biological Engineering & Computing*, **37**, 574–584.

Barr, C.S., Naas, A., Freeman, M. *et al.* (1994) QT dispersion and sudden unexpected death in chronic heart failure. *Lancet*, **343**, 327–329.

Batchvarov, V. & Malik, M. (2000) Measurement and interpretation of QT dispersion. *Progress in Cardiovascular Disease*, **42**, 325–344.

Brendorp, B., Elming, H., Jun, L. *et al.* (2001) QT dispersion has no prognostic information for patients with advanced congestive heart failure and reduced left ventricular systolic function. *Circulation*, **103**, 831–835.

Brody, D.A., Mirvis, D.M., Ideker, R.E. *et al.* (1977) Relative dipolar behaviour of the equivalent T wave generator: quantitative comparison with ventricular excitation in the rabbit heart. *Circulation Research*, **40**, 263–268.

Day, C.P., McComb, J.M. & Campbell, R.W. (1990) QT dispersion: an indication of arrhythmia risk in patients with long QT intervals. *British Heart Journal*, **63**, 342–344.

Day, C.P., McComb, J.M. & Campbell, R.W. (1992) QT dispersion in sinus beats and ventricular extrasystoles in normal hearts. *British Heart Journal*, **67**, 39–41.

Hii, J.T., Wyse, D.G., Gillis, A.M. *et al.* (1992) Precordial QT interval dispersion as a marker of torsades de pointes. Disparate effects of class Ia antiarrhythmic drugs and amiodarone. *Circulation*, **86**, 1376–1382.

Kors, J.A., van Herpen, G. & van Bemmel, J.H. (1999) QT dispersion as an attribute of T-loop morphology. *Circulation*, **99**, 1458–1463.

Kors, J.A. & van Herpen, G. (1998) Measurement error as a source of QT dispersion: a computerised analysis. *Heart*, **80**, 453–458.

Kuo, C.S., Munakata, K., Reddy, C.P. *et al.* (1983) Characteristics and possible mechanism of ventricular arrhythmia dependent on the dispersion of action potential durations. *Circulation*, **67**, 1356–1367.

Kuo, C.S., Reddy, C.P., Munakata, K. *et al.* (1985) Mechanism of ventricular arrhythmias caused by increased dispersion of repolarization. *European Heart Journal*, **6**, 63–70.

Malik M., Acar, B., Gang, Y. *et al.* (2000) QT dispersion does not represent electrocardiographic interlead heterogeneity of ventricular repolarization. *Journal of Cardiovascular Electrophysiology*, **11**, 835–843.

Savelieva, I., Yi, G., Guo, X. *et al.* (1998) Agreement and reproducibility of automatic vs. manual measurement of QT interval and QT dispersion. *American Journal of Cardiology*, **81**, 471–477.

Tsunakawa, H., Hoshino, K., Kanesaka, S. *et al.* (1985) Dipolarity and dipole location during QRS and T waves in normal men estimated from body surface potential distribution. *Japanese Heart Journal*, **26**, 319–334.

Wilson, F.N., Macleod, A.G., Barker, P.S. *et al.* (1934) Determination and the significance of the areas of the ventricular deflections of the electrocardiogram. *American Heart Journal*, **10**, 46.

Zabel, M., Acar, B., Klingenheben, T. *et al.* (2000) Analysis of 12-lead T wave morphology for risk stratification after myocardial infarction. *Circulation*, **102**, 1252–1257.

Zabel, M., Klingenheben, T., Franz, M.R. *et al.* (1998) Assessment of QT dispersion for prediction of mortality or arrhythmic events after myocardial infarction: results of a prospective, long-term follow-up study. *Circulation*, **97**, 2543–2550.

Zabel, M., Malik, M., Hnatkova, K. *et al.* (2002) T wave morphology analysis from the 12-lead ECG predicts long-term prognosis in male US veterans. *Circulation*, **105**, 1066–1070.

CHAPTER 36

Circadian Pattern of T Wave Morphology

Velislav Batchvarov

Introduction

In recent years, a growing interest appeared in the circadian variations (i.e. rhythms with a period of approximately 24 h, e.g. 24 ± 4 h; Cugini 1993) of parameters of ventricular repolarization, which could be attributed to the coincidence of two important groups of observations. First, there is an increased awareness of the clinical significance of repolarization abnormalities. During the last decade, several large studies demonstrated that prolonged *QT* interval, reflecting prolonged (and presumably abnormally heterogeneous) repolarization was associated with increased sudden and cardiac mortality in several patient and population groups (Karjalainen *et al.* 1997; de Bruyne *et al.* 1999; Okin *et al.* 2000). In addition, there is a growing evidence that a large number of antiarrhythmic, other cardiovascular and noncardiovascular drugs can prolong repolarization and increase its heterogeneity and cause in certain individuals and/or under certain conditions potentially lethal ventricular arrhythmia torsades de pointes (Policy Conference of the European Society of Cardiology 2000) (Fig. 36.1).

Secondly, these observations approximately coincided with the publication of multiple reports of circadian variations with morning peaks, or less frequently, with an additional afternoon or evening peak in the frequency of many cardiovascular, including arrhythmic events. Examples include sudden cardiac death (SCD) and malignant ventricular arrhythmias (Muller *et al.* 1987; Willich *et al.* 1987; Behrens *et al.* 1995, 1997), out of hospital cardiac arrest (Soo *et al.* 2000), sustained monomorphic ventricular tachycardia (Twindale 1989; Lampert *et al.* 1994), paroxysmal atrial fibrillation (Yamashita *et al.* 1997; Viskin *et al.* 1999; Gillis *et al.* 2001), idiopathic ventricular tachycardia (Hayashi *et al.* 1999), ventricular premature beats (Canada *et al.* 1983; Raeder *et al.* 1988), paroxysmal supraventricular tachycardia (Lee *et al.* 1999), and others (Fig. 36.2).

Many researchers hypothesized a link between repolarization heterogeneity and the circadian fluctuation of arrhythmic risk. This was indirectly supported by the well-documented link between increased cardiac sympathetic activity – the most likely culprit for the increased morning risk of many arrhythmic events, and increase of ventricular heterogeneity. In addition, circadian pattern has been demonstrated for many electrocardiographical and electrophysiological parameters, as discussed elsewhere in this book (Fig. 36.3).

This hypothesis was tested in many studies examining the diurnal pattern of the *QT*, heart rate-corrected *QT* and other repolarization intervals and their dispersion (see Chapter 33), invasively or noninvasively measured ventricular recovery periods (Fig. 36.4) (Huikuri *et al.* 1995; Kong *et al.* 1995; Simantirakis *et al.* 2001), pacing and defibrillation threshold, T wave alternans (Fig. 36.5) (Cruz Filho *et al.* 2000; Guo & Stein 2002; Chapters 44–46 of this book), as well as the morphology of the T wave.

The T wave: the most changeable part of the electrocardiogram

The T wave is the surface ECG expression of transmural, apex-base and interventricular dif-

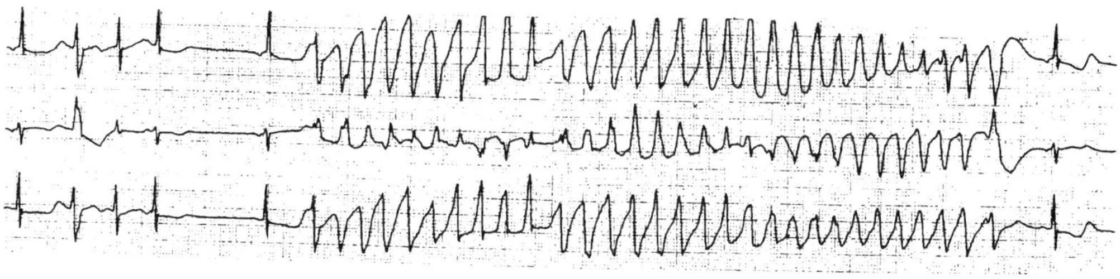

Fig. 36.1 Induction of torsades de pointes in a patient with long QT syndrome. Note the marked QT prolongation of the first sinus complex and the typical short–long–short sequence preceding the onset of the tachycardia. (Reproduced from Chiang & Roden, *Journal of the American College of Cardiology* (2000), **36**, 1–12, with permission.)

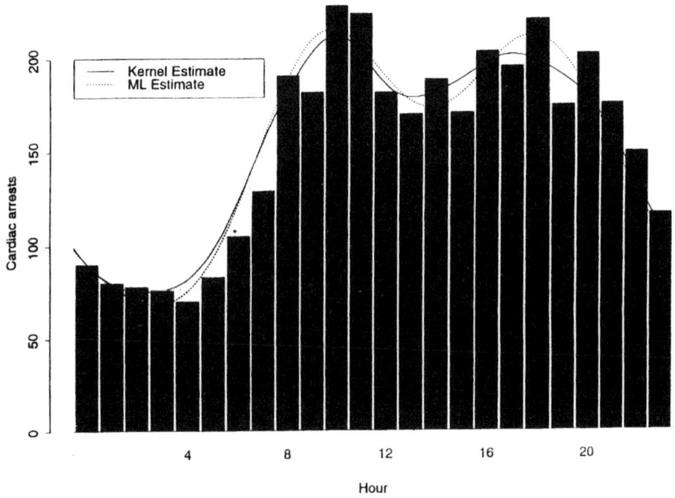

Fig. 36.2 Distribution of time of 3690 episodes of out-of-hospital cardiac arrests that were witnessed or treated with advanced life support. A clear circadian pattern of incidence of cardiac arrest is visible: low incidence at night, sharp increase between 08.00 and 12.00 hours with peaking at ≈10.00 hours, relatively high incidence during the day, and another peak between 17.00 and 20.00 hours. The presence of circadian pattern is confirmed by the histogram, by the Kernel estimate (a nonparametric technique to fit a smooth line), and the maximum likelihood harmonic polynomial estimate (ML estimate). (Reproduced from Peckova M *et al. Circulation* (1998) **98**, 31–39, with permission.)

ferences in the duration, shape and timing of ventricular action potentials (Autenrieth *et al.* 1975; Franz *et al.* 1987; Yan & Antzelevitch 1998). It has been estimated that the uncancelled potentials created by these differences represent only 1–8% or less of the total time-voltage product of the heart (Surawicz 1989). None the less, the pathological augmentation of these differences, the so-called 'abnormal spatial repolarization heterogeneity', is an important and common factors for ventricular arrhythmogenesis (Han & Moe 1963). This is one of the main reasons for the unabiding interest in the T wave, which is rightfully considered to be a 'window on ventricular repolarization' (Gettes 2001).

The clinically meaningful interpretation of the T wave has always been hampered by its variability, by the lack of understanding of the specific mechanisms of its changes, and by the lack of methods for its quantitative analysis. The ST–T segment is the most sensitive, but least specific part of the electrocardiogram (ECG). The effect of local action potential differences on the amplitude, shape and polarity of the T wave is complex and is influenced by various factors,

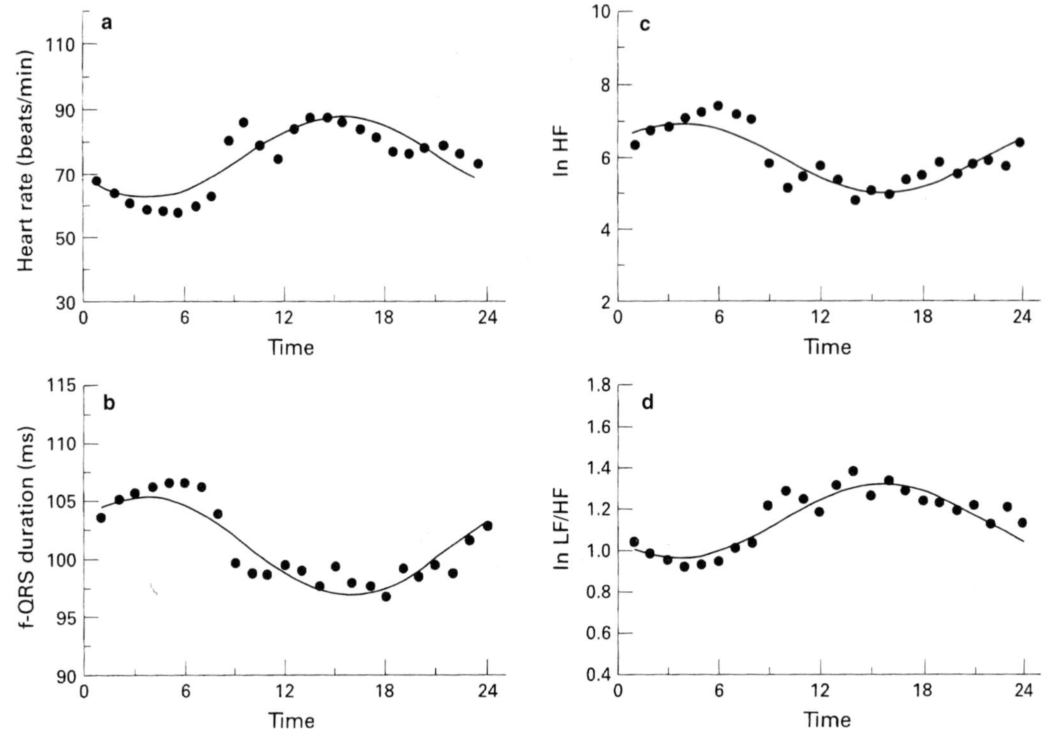

Fig. 36.3 Circadian rhythm of the hourly means of heart rate (a), filtered QRS duration of the signal-averaged ECG (b), logarithm of the high-frequency (c), and logarithm of the ratio low-frequency/high frequency components of heart rate variability (d) in 20 healthy subjects. Solid lines represent curves fitted to the data by the single cosinor method. (Reproduced from Nakagawa *et al. Heart* (1998) **79**, 493–496, with permission.)

such as heart rate, temperature, autonomic tone, extracellular K^+, catecholamines, various geometrical factors, etc. Significant changes in the T wave amplitude in orthogonal leads have been demonstrated to follow shortening of monophasic action potentials (MAP) by 18 ± 8 ms in a portion of the left ventricle comprising only about 8% of ventricular myocardium (Autenrieth *et al.* 1975). This suggests that repolarization heterogeneity cannot be reliably quantified by simple T wave parameters. The T wave amplitude, shape and polarity can be visibly affected by eating, smoking, change in body position, hyperventilation, drinking cold water, Valsalva manoeuvre, and even emotions (Rosen & Gardberg 1957; Karjalainen 1983; Mirvis & Goldberger, 2001). Therefore, the study of the dynamic changes (including circadian and other rhythmical variations) of simple T wave parameters can provide meaningful results only when performed under strictly controlled (and hardly compatible with ambulatory electrocardiography) conditions (Fig. 36.6).

As a result of this, the ECG literature is abundant with descriptions of various 'functional' or 'neurogenic' (i.e. presumably normal), as well as apparently abnormal but with unknown diagnostic/prognostic value T wave patterns (e.g. the so-called 'nonspecific ST–T changes'). Although some descriptive patterns, such as, for example, 'symmetrical and pointed T waves' during acute myocardial ischaemia, 'broad-based' or 'low-amplitude and notched' T waves in congenital long-QT syndrome type 1 and 2, respectively (Lupoglazoff *et al.* 2001), have proven clinical value, they lack significant prognostic power.

Circadian variation of the visually assessed T wave morphology

De Leonardis *et al.* (1985) found significant circadian T wave amplitude variation with acrophase (timing of the maximum value of cosinor function describing the data, Cugini 1993) in the early morning hours (around

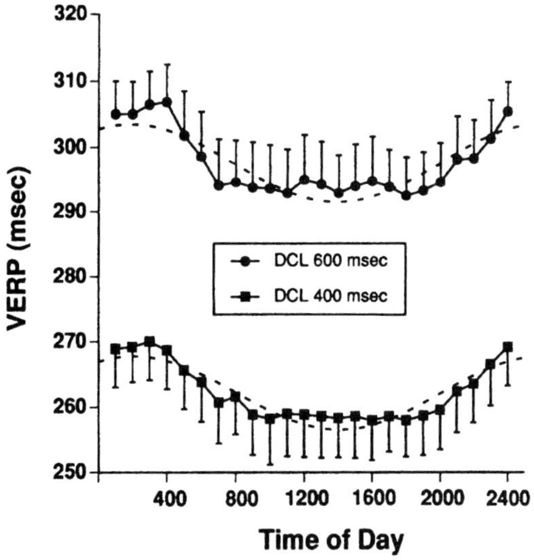

Fig. 36.4 Circadian variation of ventricular effective refractory periods determined by noninvasive programmed ventricular stimulation in nine subjects with primary conduction abnormalities, no structural heart disease and implanted pacemakers. Curves show mean (and standard error) hourly ventricular effective refractory periods (VERP) at drive cycle lengths (DCL) of 600 ms and 400 ms. Curves fitted to the data by harmonic regression analysis are shown as dashed lines. A significant circadian variation exists in mean ventricular refractory periods at both drive cycle lengths, with the longest refractory periods observed during sleep and the shortest refractory periods observed in the morning hours. (Reproduced from Kong *et al. Circulation* (1995) **92**, 1507–1516, with permission.)

05:00) in healthy subject and a similar circadian pattern in the majority of a group of patients with risk factors for coronary artery disease. On the other hand, Koch *et al.* (1999) reported maximum T wave amplitudes at 12 pm in a group of healthy male subjects. Myrtek *et al.* (1990) also reported maximum T wave amplitude around midday in a group of 31 male cardiac patients (81% of them with myocardial infarction) with and without ventricular arrhythmias and ischaemic episodes. Diurnal variations in the amplitude of negative giant T waves in patients with apical hypertrophic cardiomyopathy have also been described (Iida *et al.* 1990).

The T wave amplitude and, hence, its circadian variation cannot be used as a meaningful index of the level of cardiac sympathetic activity (Schwartz & Weiss 1983), as has been once suggested (Scher *et al.* 1984).

At present, it is difficult to see any clinical application of the circadian variation of the T wave amplitude except for the possibility that it might exacerbate (at least theoretically) the problem of T wave over-sensing and inappropriate activation of implanted antiarrhythmic devices (Barold *et al.* 1985; Kelly *et al.* 1994; Weretka *et al.* 2003).

At present, it is still unclear whether the circadian variation of QT dispersion (Molnar *et al.* 1997; Ishida *et al.* 1997; Batur *et al.* 1999; Yee *et al.* 2001; Yetkin *et al.* 2001) (Fig. 36.7)

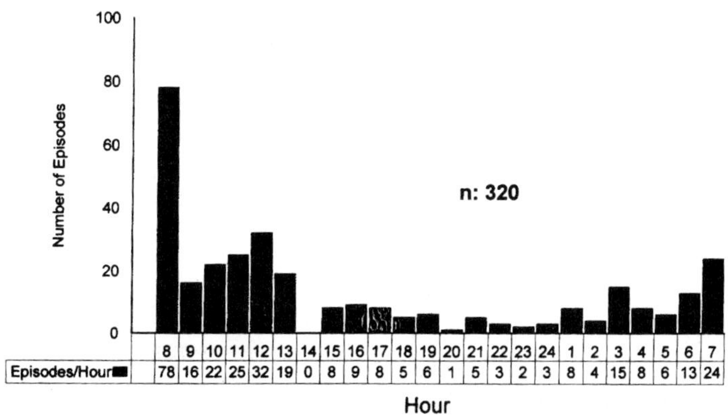

Fig. 36.5 Hourly distribution of the beat-to-beat alternans of the polarity of the T wave over a 24-h period in 11 patients with congenital long QT syndrome. Note that the incidence of episodes of T wave alternans is higher during the daytime period (from 08.00 to 20.00 hours) and especially during the morning (08.00 to 12.00 hours). (Reproduced from Cruz Filho *et al.*, *Journal of the American College of Cardiology* (2000) **36**, 167–173, with permission.)

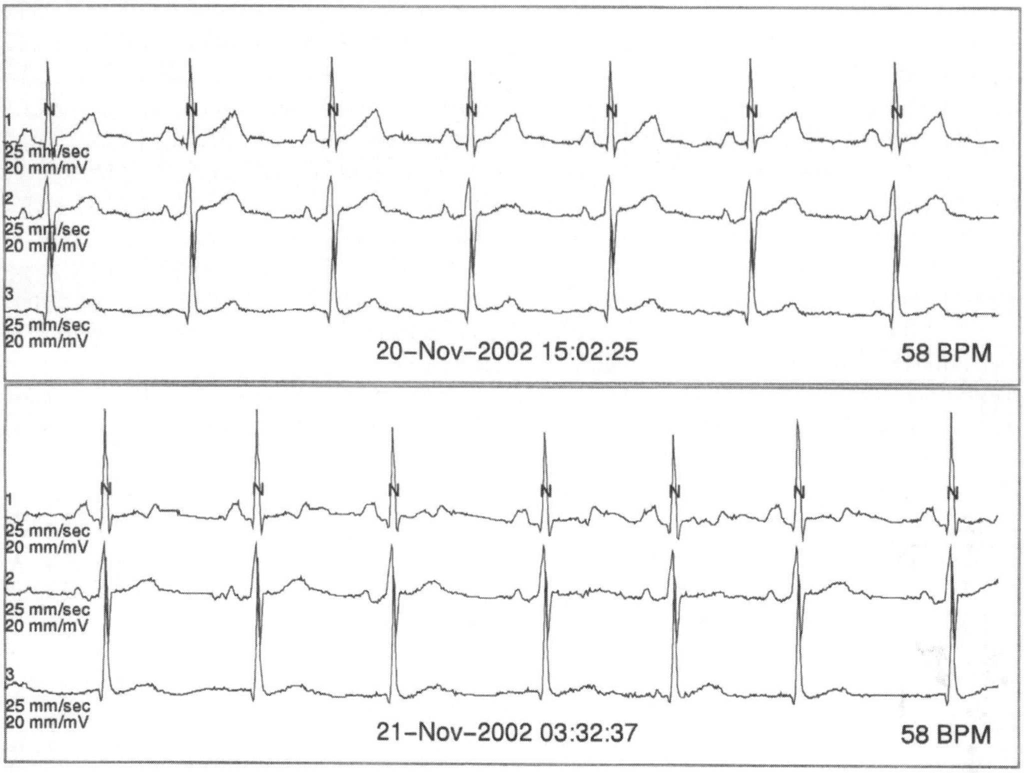

Fig. 36.6 An example illustrating the variability of the T wave in ECGs recorded under uncontrolled conditions. Ambulatory 24-hour three-channel ECG recording in a 54-year-old man with no heart disease. From top: leads II, V1 and V6. Note the difference in the T waves between ECG recorded at identical average heart rates at 15.00 hours (top panel) and approximately 12 hours later, at about 03.30 hours (bottom panel). In the bottom panel, note also the difference in the T wave shape between consecutive beats which all seem to be of sinus origin. It is not clear whether the variations in the T wave shape are due to differences in the autonomic tone, body position, respiration, slight variations in the *RR* interval, changes in the QRS amplitude, or other factors.

does indeed reflect variation in the properties of ventricular repolarization, and if so, whether it has a link to the frequency of arrhythmic events.

Ventricular gradient and the nondipolar content of the T wave as indices of repolarization heterogeneity

Ventricular gradient (VG) and TCRT

Approximately 70 years ago Wilson *et al.* (1931, 1934) formulated the concept of ventricular gradient (VG), or 'manifest QRST area', and pointed out that this parameter is a measure of the local variations in the excitatory process. If all ventricular action potentials had the same shape and duration and were only displaced in time, the

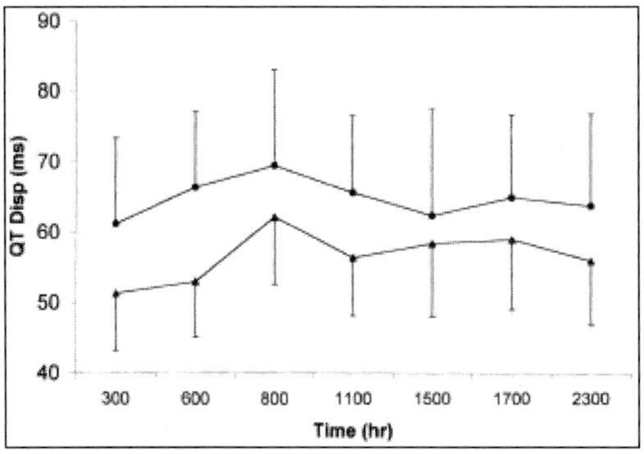

Fig. 36.7 Circadian variation of QT dispersion (mean ± SEM) in 28 patients with congestive heart failure. QT dispersion is significantly higher during the day compared to the night. (Reproduced from Yee *et al.*, *Journal of the American College of Cardiology* (2001) **37**, 1800–1807, with permission.)

algebraic sum of the QRS and T wave areas (and, respectively, VG) would be zero. Therefore, the magnitude of VG quantifies the global variation of action potential duration, while its direction points to the direction along which this variation is greatest. The possible value of VG as an index of arrhythmia vulnerability has been suggested repeatedly (Abildskov *et al.* 1977), but has never been tested in a prospective study.

The concept of VG was revived with the introduction of the method of computerised analysis of T wave morphology (Acar *et al.* 1999). In general, the method is based on singular value decomposition, which removes the redundant information contained in the standard 12-lead ECG. It transforms its eight independent leads (i.e. any two peripheral plus the six precordial leads) into a system of eight truly independent (i.e. containing no redundant information) lead S_1, S_2, . . . , S_8, in which the information is distributed in descending order. The first three leads, $S_1S_2S_3$, which contain >95% of the ECG information, correspond to vectorcardiographic XYZ leads that are oriented (rotated) in the direction of the greatest variation of the ECG signal. Thus, while the orientation of the XYZ leads is anatomically the same in all subjects, the $S_1S_2S_3$ orthogonal leads are differently rotated in each individual dependent on the vectorial direction of the ECG signal.

A parameter, analogous to VG, quantifies the average cosine of the angles between the main QRS and T vectors of the ECG in the $S_1S_2S_3$-lead system (TCRT, total cosine R-to-T). Lower (and more negative) values signify increased difference between the wavefronts of depolarization and repolarization, and is an index of the global variations in the duration and shape of the action potentials (for computational details see Malik *et al.* 2000: appendix; Smetana *et al.* 2002.).

Nondipolar components of the T wave (T wave residua)

The ECG in leads $S_1S_2S_3$ corresponds to the movements of the heart vector (cardiac dipole), while the information contained in leads S_4–S_8 corresponds to the nondipolar components of the 12-lead ECG. Although the latter represent only a small proportion of the whole ECG content, their clinical importance has been suspected long ago (Abildskov *et al.* 1977). Malik *et al.* (2000) quantified the proportion of the nondipolar components within the whole T wave signal (dipolar + nondipolar components). This proportion, termed relative T wave residua (TWR) differed significantly between healthy subjects and patients with hypertrophic cardiomyopathy, dilated cardiomyopathy and acute myocardial infarction. TWR were only moderately correlated to QT dispersion in patients with hypertrophic cardiomyopathy (r = 0.28, P = 0.03), but not in the other 3 groups.

Very recently, Rautaharju (2002) reported that the nondipolar voltage (NDPV) of the T wave was 12 ± 4.9 μV in patients with coronary artery disease (CAD) and 11 ± 36 μV in patients without CAD (P < 0.0001, one-tailed t-test). The NDPV of the T wave was about twice smaller (6 ± 1.3 μV and 6 ± 1.5 μV). NDPV of the T wave was only modestly correlated to QT dispersion (r = 0.25) and weakly correlated (r = 0.11) to the ratio between the eigenvalues of the first and second principal components of the T wave, a measure of the relation between the length and the width of the spatial T loop.

TCRT yielded independent predictive value for all-cause mortality, sustained ventricular tachycardia or resuscitated ventricular fibrillation in a study of 280 post-myocardial infarction patients followed up for 32 ± 10 months (Zabel *et al.* 2000). In another study, TCRT calculated from XYZ leads was independently predictive of total cardiac and arrhythmic mortality in 1047 survivors of acute MI (Batchvarov *et al.* 2002b). Recently it was reported that both the absolute (P = 0.022), as well as the relative TWR (P = 0.006) were independently predictive of all-cause mortality in 813 male US veterans with cardiovascular disease followed up for 10 ± 4 years (Zabel *et al.* 2002).

It has been suggested that TCRT and TWR reflect different aspects of repolarization heterogeneity (Smetana *et al.* 2002). TCRT reflects the degree of departure of the sequence of repolarization from that of depolarization, i.e. global repolarization heterogeneity. TWR, on the other hand, reflects local repolarization dipoles, i.e. local repolarization heterogeneity. These local dipoles are cancelled out when summed up into the global cardiac dipole (i.e. TCRT).

Circadian variation of TCRT and TWR

A very recently published study (Smetana *et al.* 2002), for the first time addressed the possibility to quantify heterogeneity of ventricular repolarization from 24-h digital 12-lead ECGs, its circadian pattern and gender differences.

Patient population

The study was conducted on 60 volunteers (27 men aged 26.7 ± 7.3 years, and 33 women aged 27.1 ± 9.6 years, P = NS) with normal medical history and physical examination, and a normal 12-lead electrocardiogram. None of the participants was taking any medication and they all had a normal day–night activity profile.

Data acquisition

In each participant, four 24-h 12-lead digital ECG recordings were obtained at baseline, after 1 day, 1 week, and 1 month using SEER MC recorders (GE Marquette Medical Systems, Milwaukee, WI). During each 24-h recording, 10-s 12-lead ECG samples were obtained every 30 s (2880/24h). Subjects were asked to adhere to a standard daily routine without any physical or mental excesses during the recording days.

Data analysis

Analysis of all ECG parameters was performed on the basis of median beats constructed in all leads of each 10-s ECG sample using the QT Guard research software of GE Marquette (Xue & Reddy 1988). The *QT* interval was measured automatically using 6 different algorithms and the mean value of the 6 measurements was taken for analysis if the range of the 6 *QT* measurements was ≤40 ms (Batchvarov *et al.* 2002a). The *QT* interval was corrected for heart rate using individually optimised heart rate-correction formulae of the generic type $QTc = QT/RR^{\alpha}$, where the optimum value of α for each patient was estimated from their four 24-h ECG recordings (Malik *et al.* 2001, 2002). The mean *RR* interval of each 10-s sample was also calculated using the QT Guard software.

Calculation of TCRT and TWR

TCRT and TWR were calculated from the median beat constructed from each 10-s sample of each 24-h recording in each individual.

Data analysis and estimation of the circadian pattern

In each subject, repeated 24-h recordings were pooled and *RR*, *QT*, and *QTc* intervals, as well as TCRT, and TWR obtained in separate ECG samples were correlated using Pearson correlation coefficients.

For the investigation of the circadian profile *RR* interval, *QTc* interval, TCRT, and TWR values were calculated for each 10-s ECG sample and averaged over 10-min time-bands from day (09.00–20.00) and night (01.00–05.00), as well as averages of individual measures were calculated from the averaged 10-min values. The averaged values of individual measures in women and men were compared within individual 10-min bands. Early morning dynamics were characterized by linear slope of the values between 06.00 and 09.30 hours. Inter-sex comparisons were performed by Student's *t*-test. Data are presented as mean ± SD. Statistical significance was considered as $P < 0.05$.

Results

The average values for day and night, day–night differences, morning slope of *RR* interval, TCRT and TWR in men and women are presented in Table 36.1.

There were significant differences in the pattern of repolarization heterogeneity between men and women. Whilst global repolarization heterogeneity was greater in men (i.e. lower values of TCRT), local repolarization heterogeneity was greater in women (greater TWR). However, in both sexes TCRT and TWR exhibited marked circadian pattern with an increase in repolarization heterogeneity (i.e. decrease in TCRT and increase in TWR) during the morning (Figs 36.8 and 36.9). The slope of morning increase of TWR was significantly steeper in women (Table 36.1).

The pattern of circadian variation and sex differences of TCRT and TWR were remarkably similar in all four recordings (Figs 36.8 and 36.9).

Whilst the circadian pattern of TCRT and TWR was similar to the well-known circadian pattern of the *RR* interval, there was only a moderate correlation between *RR* interval and TCRT (0.55 ± 0.21 in men, 0.46 ± 0.21 in women), and between *RR* and TWR (−0.51 ± 0.08 in men, −0.52 ± 0.06 in women).

Table 36.1 Circadian variation and sex differences of *RR* interval, TCRT and TWR

	Day	*Night*	*Day–night difference*	*Morning slope*
RR interval (ms)				
Men	835 ± 137	982 ± 152	147 ± 221	−55 ± 70
Women	798 ± 137	888 ± 175	89 ± 154	−54 ± 65
P value	0.073	1.7×10^{-4}	0.048	0.91
TCRT				
Men	0.29 ± 0.41	0.44 ± 0.39	0.15 ± 0.29	−0.052 ± 0.09
Women	0.63 ± 0.2	0.71 ± 0.2	0.08 ± 0.19	−0.046 ± 0.07
P value	2.1×10^{-10}	1.9×10^{-8}	0.061	0.65
TWR (%)				
Men	0.18 ± 0.09	0.11 ± 0.09	0.07 ± 0.11	0.03 ± 0.05
Women	0.34 ± 0.14	0.21 ± 0.15	0.13 ± 0.19	0.08 ± 0.14
P value	1.7×10^{-17}	4.4×10^{-8}	0.011	5.4×10^{-4}

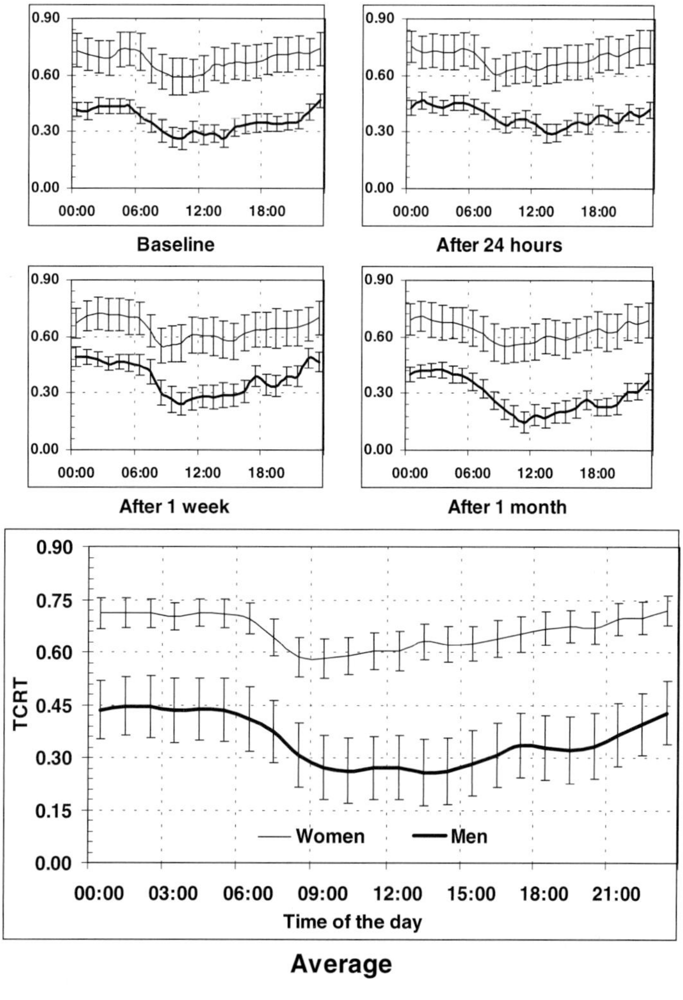

Fig. 36.8 Circadian pattern of TCRT in men and women. Top small panels: hourly means of TCRT from each of the 4 recordings. Bottom large panel: averaged hourly means of TCRT.

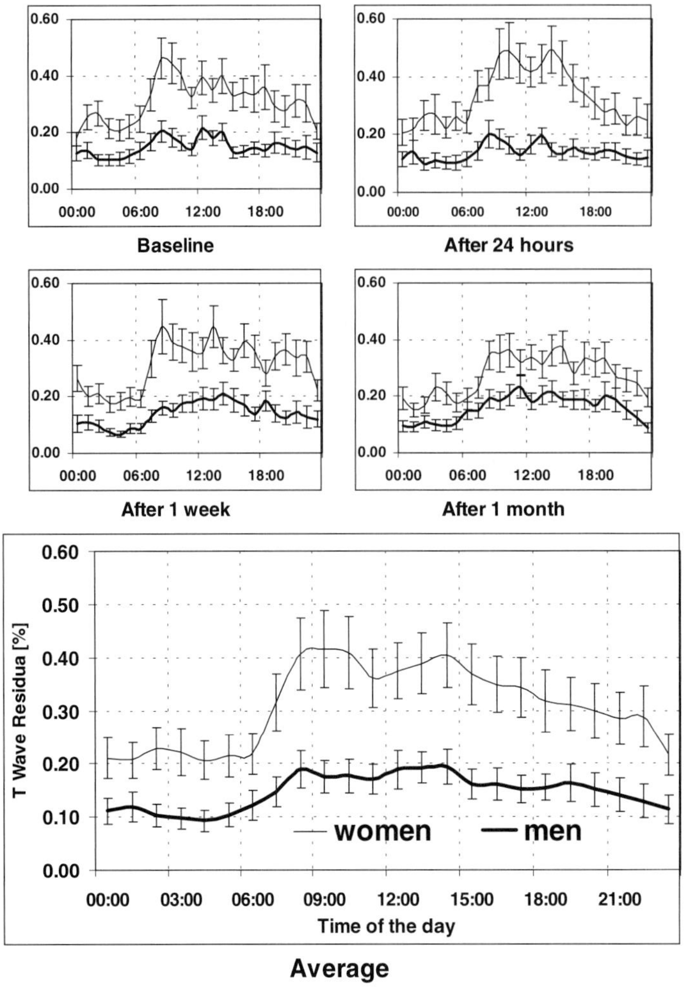

Fig. 36.9 Circadian pattern of relative T wave residua in men and women. Top small panels: hourly means of TWR from each of the 4 recordings. Bottom large panel: averaged hourly means of TWR. See the text for details.

Discussion

This study demonstrated that computerised analysis of the T wave of ambulatory 24-h digital 12-lead ECGs can quantify heterogeneity of ventricular repolarization and its diurnal variations. Whilst the pattern of repolarization heterogeneity is different in men and women, in both sexes it exhibits diurnal variations similar to the circadian variations in the frequency of arrhythmic events.

Ventricular refractory periods, determined both invasively (Cinca *et al.* 1986), as well as noninvasively (using the telemetry function of implanted pacemakers) (Huikuri *et al.* 1995; Kong *et al.* 1995; Simantirakis *et al.* 2001) have been found to be shortest during daytime and longest during the night. Simantirakis *et al.* (2001) also provided evidence for autonomic involvement in these variations by reporting that the refractory periods were shorter when the low-frequency power of heart rate variability (HRV) was increased, and were prolonged (during the night) when the high frequency power of HRV was increased. Studies of circadian (or other periodic) variations of direct measures of repolarization heterogeneity (e.g. with recordings of MAPs or programmed stimulation), to our knowledge, have not been performed, for obvious technical reasons.

Today, no direct link has yet been established between increased heterogeneity of repolarization and the circadian variation in arrhythmia risk. One of the reasons is the absence of reliable noninva-sive markers of abnormal heterogeneity. Before TCRT and TWR are more widely used,

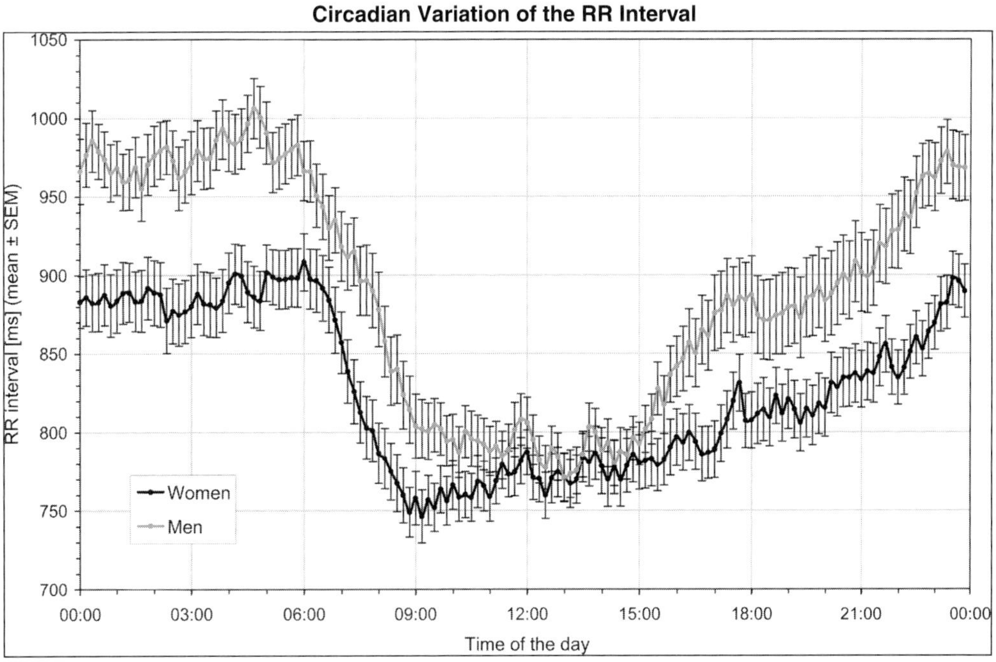

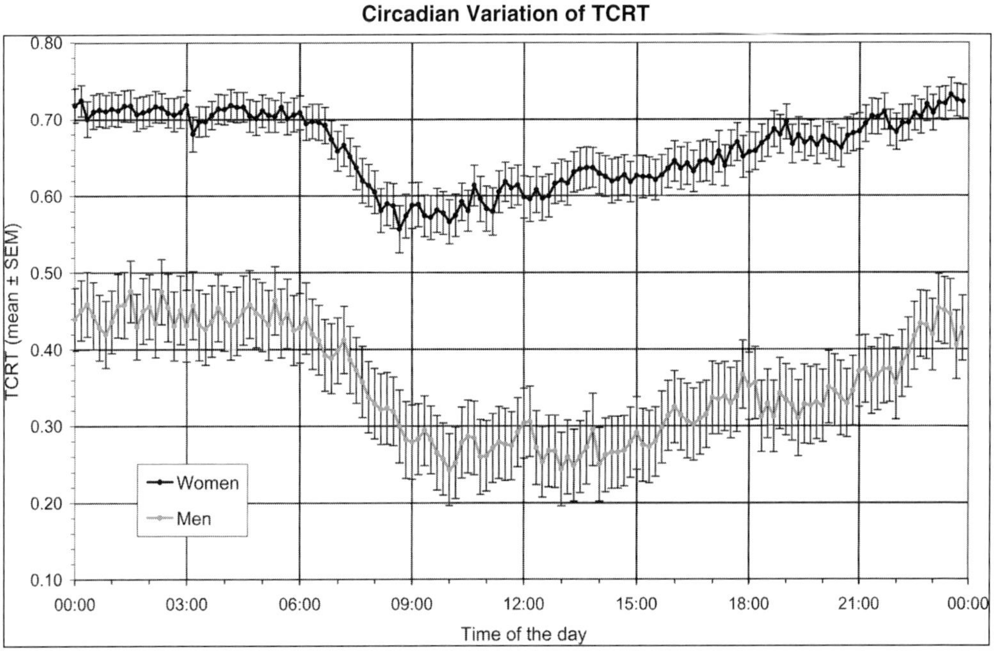

Fig. 36.10 Circadian variation of the *RR* interval l (top panel) and of TCRT (bottom panel) in 60 healthy subjects. Both parameters follow similar circadian pattern and there is a significant linear correlation between them ($r = 0.46 \pm 21$ and $r = 0.55 \pm 0.21$ in women and men, respectively). Note, however, that there is also a substantial difference: while the differences in the *RR* interval between women and men diminish during the day (when they are not statistically significant), the sex differences in TCRT are increased during the day (and remain statistically significant throughout the whole 24-hour period). This suggests that in addition to heart rate, other factors also influenced the circadian pattern of TCRT. (Reproduced from Smetana *et al.*, *American Journal of Physiology* **282**, H1889–H1897, with permission.)

important methodological and technical issues need to be clarified. Postural changes and respiration (Batchvarov *et al.* 2002c, unpublished data), heart rate and autonomic effects are all likely to influence TCRT (Batchvarov *et al.* 2000c) and TWR (Fig. 36.10). The relative contribution of each of these factors needs to be determined in physiological studies under strictly controlled conditions before the circadian pattern of TCRT and TWR can have a clinically meaningful interpretation. The nondipolar ECG content is not constant throughout depolarization and repolarization (Harumi *et al.* 1986) and therefore it is not clear whether they should be averaged over the whole T wave or measured in separate windows. The effect of noise level of signals of such small amplitude also should be investigated.

Conclusions

Spatial heterogeneity of ventricular repolarization exhibits circadian pattern similar to the circadian frequency pattern of many arrhythmic events. The pattern of repolarization heterogeneity seems to differ significantly between men and women, although in both genders the circadian pattern is present. Visual assessment of T wave morphology or amplitude cannot provide reliable information about the circadian variation of the ventricular repolarization segment of the standard 12-lead ECG. Spatial heterogeneity repolarization of its temporal variability can be quantified using computerised analysis of the T wave of ambulatory recorded 24-h digital 12-lead ECGs. The technical aspects and the clinical application of TCRT and T wave residua from digital ambulatory ECGs needs further study.

References

Abildskov, J.A., Burgess, M.J., Urie, P.M., Lux, R.L. & Wyatt, R.F. (1977) The unidentified information content of the electrocardiogram. *Circulation Research*, **40**, 3–7.

Acar, B., Yi, G., Hnatkova, K. & Malik, M. (1999) Spatial, temporal and wavefront direction characteristics of 12-lead T wave morphology. *Medical & Biological Engineering & Computing*, **37**, 574–584.

Autenrieth, G., Surawicz B. & Kuo C.S. (1975) Sequence of repolarization on the ventricular surface in the dog. *American Heart Journal*, **89**, 463–469.

Barold, S.S., Falkoff, M.D., Ong, L.S. & Heinle, R.A. (1985) Oversensing by single-chamber pacemakers: mechanisms, diagnosis, and treatment. *Clinical Cardiology*, **3**, 565–585.

Batchvarov, V.N., Ghuran, A., Smetana, P. *et al.* (2002a) QT/RR relationship in healthy subjects exhibits substantial intersubject variability and high intrasubject stability. *American Journal of Physiology Heart and Circulatory Physiology* **282**, H2356–H2363.

Batchvarov, V.N., Hnatkova, K., Ghuran, A. *et al.* (2002b) Ventricular gradient is an independent risk factor in survivors of acute myocardial infarction. *Europace*, **3** (Suppl.), A44 (abstract).

Batchvarov, V.N., Kaski, J.C., Parchure, N. *et al.* (2002c) Comparison between ventricular gradient and a new descriptor of the wavefront direction of ventricular activation and recovery. *Clinical Cardiology* **25**, 230–236.

Batur M.K., Aksoyek S., Oto A. *et al.* (1999) Circadian variations of QTc dispersion: is it a clue to morning increase of sudden cardiac death? *Clinical Cardiolology*, **22**:103–106.

Behrens, S., Galecka, M., Bruggemann, T. *et al.* (1995) Circadian variation of sustained ventricular tachyarrhythmias terminated by appropriate shocks in patients with an implantable defibrillator. *American Heart Journal*, **130**, 79–84.

Behrens, S., Ney, G., Fisher, S.G., Fletcher, R.D., Franz, M.R. & Singh, S.N. (1997) Effect of amiodarone on the circadian pattern of sudden cardiac death (Department of Veterans Affairs Congestive Heart Failure-Survival Trial of Antiarrhythmic Therapy). *American Journal of Cardiology*, **80**, 45–48.

De Bruyne, M.C., Hoes, A.W., Kors, J.A., Hofman, A., van Bemmel, J.H. & Grobbee, D.E. (1999) Prolonged QT interval predicts cardiac and all-cause mortality in the elderly. The Rotterdam Study. *European Heart Journal*, **20**, 278–284.

Canada, W.B., Woodward, W., Lee, G. *et al.* (1983) Circadian rhythm of hourly ventricular arrhythmia frequency in man. *Angiology*, **34**, 274–282.

Cinca, J., Moya, A., Figueras, J., Roma, F. & Ruis, J. (1986) Circadian variations in the electrical properties of the human heart assessed by sequential bedside electrophysiological testing. *American Heart Journal*, **112**, 315–321.

Cruz Filho, F.E. S., Maia, I.G., Fagundes, M.L.A. *et al.* (2000) Electrical behaviour of T-wave polarity alternans in patients with congenital long QT syndrome. *Journal of the American College of Cardiology*, **36**:167–173.

Cugini, P. (1993) Chronobiology: principles and methods. Medical semiology and methodology. *Annali Istituto Superiore Sanità*, **29**, 483–500.

Franz, M.R., Bargheer, K., Rafflenbeul, W., Haverich, A.

& Lichlen, P.R. (1987) Monophasic action potential mapping in human subjects with normal electrocardiograms: direct evidence for the genesis of the T wave. *Circulation*, **75**, 379–386.

Gettes, L.S. (2001) The T wave: a window on ventricular repolarization? *Journal of Cardiovascular Electrophysiology*, **12**, 1326–1328.

Gillis, A.M., Connolly, S.J., Dubuc, M. *et al.* (2001) PA3. Atrial Pacing Peri-ablation for Prevention of Atrial Fibrillation Trial. Circadian variation of paroxysmal atrial fibrillation. *American Journal of Cardiology*, **87**, 794–798.

Guo, Y.-F. & Stein, P. (2002) Circadian rhythm in the cardiovascular system: considerations in noninvasive electrophysiology. *Cardiac Electrophysiology Review*, **6**, 267–272.

Han, J. & Moe, G.K. (1963) Nonuniform recovery of excitability in ventricular muscle. *Circulation Research*, **XIV**, 44–60.

Harumi, K., Tsunakawa, H., Kanesaka, S. & Nishiyama, G. (1986) Moving dipole analysis in normal and myocardial infarction. In: *Electrocardiographic Body Surface Mapping* (eds R. T. van Dam & A. van Oosterom), pp. 283–288. Martinus Nijhoff Publishers, Dordrecht.

Hayashi, H., Fujiki, A., Tani, M. *et al.* (1999) Circadian variation of idiopathic ventricular tachycardia originating from right ventricular outflow tract. *American Journal of Cardiology*, **84**, 99–101.

Huikiri, H., Yli-Mäyry, S., Linnaluoto, M.K. & Ikäheimo, M. (1995) Diurnal fluctuations in human ventricular and atrial refractoriness. *PACE (Pacing and Clinical Electrophysiology)*, **18**, 1362–1368.

Iida, K., Sugishita, Y., Yukisada, K. & Ito, I. (1990) Diurnal change of giant negative T wave in patients with hypertrophic cardiomyopathy. *Clinical Cardiology*, **13**, 272–278.

Ishida, S., Nakagawa, M., Fujino, T., Yonemochi, H., Saikawa, T. & Ito, M. (1997) Circadian variation of QT interval dispersion: correlation with heart rate variability. *Journal of Electrocardiology*, **30**, 205–210.

Karjalainen, J. (1983) Functional and myocarditis-induced T wave abnormalities. Effect of orthostasis, beta-blockade, and epinephrine. *Chest*, **83**, 868–874.

Karjalainen, J., Reunanen, A., Ristola, P. & Viitasalo, M. (1997) QT interval as a cardiac risk factor in a middle aged population. *Heart*, **77**, 543–548.

Kelly, P.A., Mann, D.E., Damle, R.S. & Reiter, M.J. (1994) Oversensing during ventricular pacing in patients with a third-generation implantable cardioverter-defibrillator. *Journal of the American College of Cardiology*, **23**, 1531–1534.

Koch, H.J., Raschka, C. & Banzer, W. (1999) Diurnal variations of ECG intervals and R or T amplitudes in healthy male subjects assessed by means of spectral and cosinor analysis. *Japanese Heart Journal*, **40**, 45–53.

Kong, T.O., Jr, Goldberger, J.J., Parker, M., Wang, T. & Kadish, A.H. (1995) Circadian variation in human ventricular refractoriness. *Circulation*, **92**, 1507–1516.

Lampert, R., Rosenfeld, L., Batsford, W., Lee, F. & McPherson, C. (1994) Circadian variation of sustained ventricular tachycardia in patients with coronary artery disease and implantable cardioverter-defibrillators. *Circulation*, **90**, 241–247.

Lee, S.H., Chang, P.C., Hung H.F., Kuan, P., Cheng, J.J. & Hung, C.R. (1999) Circadian variation of paroxysmal supraventricular tachycardia. *Chest*, **115**, 674–678.

De Leonardis, V., de Scalzi, M., Fabiano, F.S. & Cinelli, P. (1985) A chronobiologic study on some circadian parameters. *Journal of Electrocardiology*, **18**, 385–394.

Lupoglazoff, J.M., Denjoy, I., Berthet, M. *et al.* (2001) Notched T waves on Holter recordings enhance detection of patients with LQT2 (HERG) mutations. *Circulation*, **103**, 1095–1101.

Malik, M., Acar, B., Yi, G., Yap, Y.G., Hnatkova, K. & Camm, A.J. (2000) QT dispersion does not represent electrocardiographic interlead heterogeneity of ventricular repolarization. *Journal of Cardiovascular Electrophysiology*, **11**, 835–843.

Malik, M., Färbom, P., Batchvarov, V.N., Hnatkova, K. & Camm, A.J. (2002) Relation between QT and *RR* intervals is highly individual among healthy subjects: implications for heart rate correction of the QT interval. *Heart*, **87**, 220–228.

Mirvis, D.M. & Goldberger, A.L. (2001) Electrocardiography. In: *Heart Disease: A Textbook of Cardiovascular Medicine* (ed. E. Braunwald), 6th edn., p. 93. W. B. Saunders, Philadelphia.

Molnar, J., Rosenthal, J.E., Weiss, J.S. & Somberg, J.C. (1997) QT interval dispersion in healthy subjects and survivors of sudden cardiac death: circadian variation in a twenty-four-hour assessment. *American Journal of Cardiology*, **79**, 1190–1193.

Muller, J.E., Ludmer, P.L., Willich, S.N. *et al.* (1987) Circadian variation in the frequency of sudden cardiac death. *Circulation*, **75**, 131–138.

Myrtek, M., Brügner, G. & Fichtler, A. (1990) Diurnal variations of ECG parameters during 23-h monitoring in cardiac patients with ventricular arrhythmias or ischaemic episodes. *Psychophysiology*, **27**, 620–626.

Okin, P.M., Devereux R.B., Howard, B.V., Fabsitz, R.R., Lee, E.T. & Welty, T.K. (2000) Assessment of QT interval and QT dispersion for prediction of all-cause and cardiovascular mortality in American Indians. The Strong Heart Study. *Circulation*, **101**, 61–66.

Raeder, E.A., Hohnloser, S.H., Graboys, T.B., Podrid, P.J., Lampert, S. & Lown, B. (1988) Spontaneous variability and circadian distribution of ectopic activity in patients with malignant ventricular arrhythmia. *Journal of the American College of Cardiology*, **12**, 656–661.

Rautaharju, P.M. (2002) Why did QT dispersion die? *Cardiac Electrophysiology Review*, **6**, 295–301.

Report on a Policy Conference of the European Society of Cardiology (2000) The potential for QT prolongation and proarrhythmia by non-antiarrhythmic drugs: clinical and regulatory implications. *European Heart Journal*, **21**, 1216–1231.

Rosen, I.L. & Gardberg, M. (1957) The effects of nonpathologic factors on the electrocardiogram. *American Heart Journal*, **53**, 494–734.

Scher, H., Furedy, J.J. & Heslegrave, R.J. (1984) Phasic T wave amplitude and heart rate changes as indices of mental effort and task incentive. *Psychophysiology*, **21**, 326–333.

Schwartz, P.J., La Rovere, M.T. & Vanoli, E. (1992) Autonomic nervous system and sudden cardiac death: experimental basis and clinical observations for post-myocardial infarction risk-stratification. *Circulation*, **85** (Suppl I), I77–I91.

Schwartz, P.J. & Weiss, T. (1983) T wave amplitude as an index of sympathetic activity: a misleading concept. *Psychophysiology*, **20**, 696–701.

Simantirakis, E.N., Chrysostomakis, S.I., Marketou, M.E. *et al.* (2001) Atrial and ventricular refractoriness in paced patients. Circadian variation and its relation to autonomic nervous system activity. *European Heart Journal*, **22**, 2192–2200.

Smetana, P., Batchvarov, V.N., Hnatkova, K., Camm, A.J. & Malik, M. (2002) Sex differences in repolarization homogeneity and its circadian pattern. *American Journal of Physiology Heart and Circulatory Physiology* **282**, H1889–H1897.

Soo, L.H., Gray, D., Young, T. & Hampton, J.R. (2000) Circadian variation in witnessed out of hospital cardiac arrest. *Heart*, **84**, 370–376.

Surawicz, B. (1989) ST-T abnormalities. T wave. In: *Comprehensive Electrocardiography. Theory and Practice in Heath and Disease* (eds P. W. Macfarlane & T. D. Vetch Lawries), pp. 521–550. Pergamon Press, Oxford.

Twindale, N., Taylor, S., Heddle, W.F., Ayres, B.F. & Tonkin, A.M. (1989) Morning increase in the time of onset of sustained ventricular tachycardia. *American Journal of Cardiology*, **64**, 1204–1206.

Viskin, S., Golovner, M., Malov, N. *et al.* (1999) Circadian variation of symptomatic paroxysmal atrial fibrillation. Data from almost 10 000 episodes. *European Heart Journal*, **20**, 1429–1434.

Weretka, S., Michaelsen, J., Becker, J. *et al.* (2003) Ventricular oversensing: a study of 101 patients implanted with dual chamber defribrillators and two different lead systems. *PACE (Pacing and Clinical Electrophysiology)*, **26** (Pt 1), 65–70.

Willich, S.N., Levy, D., Rocco, M.B., Tofler, G.H., Stone, P.H. & Muller, J.E. (1987) Circadian variation in the incidence of sudden cardiac death in the Framingham Heart Study Population. *American Journal of Cardiology*, **60**, 801–806.

Wilson, F.N., Macleod, A.G. & Barker, P.S. (1931) The T deflection of the electrocardiogram. *Transactions of the Association of American Physicians*, **46**, 29–38.

Wilson, F.N., Macleod, A.G., Barker, P.S. & Johnston, F.D. (1934) The determination and the significance of the ventricular deflections of the electrocardiogram. *American Heart Journal*, **10**, 46–61.

Xue, Q. & Reddy, S. (1988) Algorithms for computerised QT analysis. *Journal of Electrocardiology*, **30**, 181–186.

Yamashita, T., Murakawa, Y., Sezaki, K. *et al.* (1997) Circadian variation of paroxysmal atrial fibrillation. *Circulation*, **96**, 1537–1541.

Yan, G.X. & Antzelevitch, C. (1998) Cellular basis for the normal T wave and the electrocardiographic manifestations of the long-QT syndrome. *Circulation*, **98**, 1928–1936.

Yee, K.-M., Pringle, S.D. & Struthers, A.D (2001) Circadian variation in the effects of aldosterone blockade on heart rate variability and QT dispersion in congestive heart failure. *Journal of the American College of Cardiology*, **37**, 1800–1807.

Yetkin, E., Senen, K., Ileri, M. *et al.* (2001) Diurnal variation of QT dispersion in patients with and without coronary artery disease. *Angiology*, **52**, 311–316.

Zabel, M., Acar, B., Klingenheben, T., Franz, M.R., Hohnloser, S.H. & Malik, M. (2000) Analysis of 12-lead T wave morphology for risk stratification after myocardial infarction. *Circulation*, **102**, 1252–1257.

Zabel, M., Malik, M., Hnatkova, K. *et al.* (2002) Analysis of T wave morphology from the 12-lead electrocardiogram for prediction of long-term prognosis in male US veterans. *Circulation*, **105**, 1066–1070.

CHAPTER 37

QT Interval Dynamics During Exercise

Paul Kligfield and Peter M. Okin

Prolongation of the rate-adjusted *QT* interval on the resting electrocardiogram has been identified as a sign of disordered repolarization that can serve as a surrogate marker for potential arrhythmogenic events (De Ponte *et al.* 2002). A number of technical problems influence *QT* measurement, including lead selection for *QT* determination, definition of the end of the T wave, and the relationship of *QT* measurement to heart rate (Locati 2001). Shortening of the *QT* interval with increasing heart rate is a consequence of the interval–duration relationship (Seed *et al.* 1987), but the *QT* interval is modulated by additional rate-independent factors (Laakso *et al.* 1987; Cappato *et al.* 1991; Zaza *et al.* 1991). The adequacy of different methods for adjusting resting repolarization for cycle length has been controversial since the early work of Bazett (1920) (Ahnve 1985; Sagie *et al.* 1992).

Problems relating to adjustment of the *QT* interval at rest are further increased during activities of daily living, including exercise, because variable autonomic and neurohumoral responses to cardiovascular adaptation may also affect the manner of *QT* interval shortening (Rickards & Norman 1981; Sarma *et al.* 1984; Coghlan *et al.* 1992). During dynamic recording of the ECG under these conditions, *QT* intervals can be plotted against corresponding heart rates (or cycle lengths). From these data, individual or group *QT*–heart rate relationships can be quantified by a number of algorithms that include calculation of the slope of the regression between variables (Extramiana *et al.* 1999; Locati 2001). Investigation of *QT* interval behaviour in relation to heart rate by ambulatory electrocardiography has revealed diurnal variability of the QT–heart rate relationship, with greater slopes during the day than during the night (Fayn & Rubel 1988; Coumel & Maison-Blanche 1992; Tavernier *et al.* 1995). These findings are consistent with different effects of sympathetic and parasympathetic predominance on the underlying interval–duration relationship.

Regression-based methods also can be applied to evaluation of the *QT* interval during exercise electrocardiography, as suggested by the work of Vincent *et al.* (1991) in patients with the Romano-Ward syndrome and by and Gill *et al.* (1993) in patients with ischaemic heart disease and exercise-induced ventricular tachycardia, among others (Rickards & Norman 1981; Akhras & Rickards 1981; Coghlan *et al.* 1992). During exercise, sympathetic tone increases while parasympathetic tone is withdrawn, so the dynamics of QT–heart rate behaviour might provide insight into neurohumoral balance. Abnormalities of the QT responses to exercise have been associated with various forms of long QT syndrome (Vincent *et al.* 1991; Tobe *et al.* 1992), with a predisposition to proarrhythmic effects of drugs (Kadish *et al.* 1990), and with coronary artery disease (Egloff *et al.* 1987). Clarification of effort-related repolarization behaviour is therefore of clinical importance, and findings in normal subjects are needed to define criteria for test abnormality in cardiac conditions.

Definition and description of repolarization must extend beyond the simple Bazett correction alone. It has become evident that the Bazett corrected *QT* (*QTc*) is not linear with respect to heart rate (or cycle length) during exercise, and as a consequence, end-exercise *QTc* is dependent on the peak workload that is achieved (Lax *et al.*

1994; Kligfield *et al.* 1995). In contrast, group mean unadjusted *QTo* (QRS onset to T wave offset) and *QT*peak (QRS onset to T wave peak) have been observed to vary linearly with mean heart rate, and also with corresponding cycle length, under conditions of gently graded treadmill exercise (Kligfield *et al.* 1995). Accordingly, we examined the linear regression characteristics of the *QT* interval–heart rate relationships in individuals to describe and to define the 'dynamic' features of repolarization during exercise in normal men and women. The complementary and methodologically challenging issue of QT dispersion behaviour during exercise will not be considered here.

Dynamic behaviour of repolarization during exercise in normal subjects

The underlying relationships between unadjusted *QTo* (Q to T wave offset) interval and heart rate and cycle length, and between unadjusted *QT*peak (Q to T wave peak) have been examined by linear regression during submaximal exercise in 50 normal men (mean age was 48 years) and in 30 normal women (mean age 51 years) (Kligfield *et al.* 1996). All subjects were asymptomatic, without clinical evidence of valvular or myopathic disease, and all had normal resting 12-lead electrocardiograms. Submaximal exercise was performed using the gently graded Cornell treadmill protocol, which produces small heart rate increments between two minute equilibrated stages. Linear regression used only submaximal exercise test data to minimize measurement ambiguity due to T-P fusion at fast heart rates. Including the upright control tracing, 8 end-stage data points were available at a work-load of approximately 11 METs, corresponding to 14 min of graded exercise to a maximum 3.4 mph on a 14% grade. At this level of exercise, mean heart rate in the group of 50 men was 135 ± 18 beats/min and in the group of 30 women was 142 ± 21 beats/min.

All rest and exercise measurements (to the nearest 10 ms) were made from digitized precordial V5 complexes that were averaged by computer over 20-s periods at upright control and at the end of each stage of exercise. *QTo* in ms was measured from the onset of the QRS deflection to the end of the T wave in V5. The effect of exercise on subintervals of the overall *QT* interval was also examined, with the duration of the terminal component of the T wave defined by *QTo* – *QT*peak.

The *QTo*–heart rate relationship was examined at upright control and during submaximal exercise as defined by:

$$QTo = b - mHR$$

where unadjusted *QTo* is measured in ms, *HR* is the heart rate (beats/min), *m* is the slope of the linear relationship, and *b* is the intercept (ms). Since the linear regression intercept *b* represents a theoretically impractical heart rate of 0, the intercept at a physiological heart rate of 60 was defined as the QTo_{60} and calculated as ($b - 60m$). Similar equations were used to define the comparable relationships involving QTpeak and heart rate, and the relationships of both *QTo* and *QT*peak to cycle length (*RR* interval) in ms.

Results of the regression analyses of *QT* (ms) against heart rate (bpm) are shown in Table 37.1, and results of the regression analyses against cycle length(s) are shown in Table 37.2. Group data for slopes, intercepts, and correlation coefficients are presented with the standard deviation of the mean as the index of dispersion and with the 5–95% range of individual values for each variable. These values represent the range of repolarization behaviour in response to gently graded treadmill exercise in normal men and women.

With respect to the linear regressions against heart rate, the strength of correlation is similarly high in men and women, but the *QTo* and *QT*peak changes with heart rate are more 'dynamic' in women than in men, as indicated by the larger negative mean slope values. In men, the mean intercept and slope in men result in a mean calculated QTo_{60} of 403 ± 21 ms, with a 5 to 95% range of 365–431 ms. In women, the mean intercept and slope result in a greater mean QTo_{60} of 426 ± 23 ms, with a 5 to 95% range of 392 to 462 ms. Similarly more dynamic slopes for *QTo* and *QT*peak are found for women than for men when the data are analysed with respect to cycle length.

The *QT* subintervals (*QT*peak and *QT*peak – *QT*end, measured as *QTo* – *QT*peak) shorten proportionally during exercise in the 50 normal men. Regression of the ratio *QT*peak/*QTo* against

Table 37.1 The *QT*/heart rate relationship in men and women defined by linear regression analysis

	Mean	*SD*	*5th percentile*	*95th percentile*
QT_0/heart rate relationship				
Men				
Slope	−1.45	0.34	−1.96	−0.90
Intercept	490	38	415	539
r value	−0.93	0.06	−0.99	−0.81
Women				
Slope	−1.74	0.32	−2.18	−1.23
Intercept	531	41	468	598
r value	−0.95	0.05	−0.99	−0.84
QT_{peak}/heart rate relationship				
Men				
Slope	−1.24	0.38	−1.89	−0.74
Intercept	386	43	327	455
r value	−0.94	0.06	−0.99	−0.85
Women				
Slope	−1.33	0.31	−1.85	−0.99
Intercept	401	38	354	463
r value	−0.95	0.05	−0.99	−0.90

Table 37.2 The *QT*/cycle length relationship in men and women defined by linear regression analysis

	Mean	*SD*	*5th percentile*	*95th percentile*
QT_0/cycle length relationship				
Men				
Slope	237	71	109	351
Intercept	199	42	130	270
r value	0.90	0.09	0.72	0.98
Women				
Slope	333	127	167	574
Intercept	154	65	31	245
r value	0.91	0.06	0.79	0.98
QT_{peak}/cycle length relationship				
Men				
Slope	205	59	101	288
Intercept	137	34	91	191
r value	0.93	0.06	0.82	0.99
Women				
Slope	256	65	159	331
Intercept	112	37	65	172
r value	0.96	0.05	0.88	0.99

heart rate revealed a mean slope of only −0.0004 ± 0.0010 (5 to 95% range −0.0022 to 0.0010), indicating a relatively proportional change of early and late *QTo* subintervals at this level of generally submaximal effort. To further explore the proportional shortening of the *QT* subintervals, the ratios of the 14 min measured intervals to the corresponding upright control measured intervals were calculated. Overall mean and standard deviation, with 5 to 95% values, for the ratio of shortening of the *QTo* during moderate treadmill exercise (the measured *QTo* at 14 min

The *QT* interval varies with exercise according to both rate-dependent and rate-independent factors. Several observations document the wide range in which repolarization behaviour of clinically normal individuals can be expected to vary during the neurohumoral activation provoked by slowly graded exercise. Although regression data using different exercise test protocols might vary as a consequence of altered restitution of the *QT* interval to different patterns of change in workload and heart rate (Seed *et al.* 1987; Zaza *et al.* 1991; Coghlan *et al.* 1992), there appears to be directional consistency in these and other reports. A recent study by Mayuga *et al.* (2001) has confirmed the more dynamic values of *QT*–heart rate slopes in women compared with men using the standard Bruce protocol, and in their normal subjects signficant *QTo* and *QTpeak* differences between men and women were not present above heart rates of 100–110.

Regression analysis by Magnano *et al.* (2002) also has confirmed sex differences with similar slope values during bicycle exercise as in our subjects during treadmill testing. Of note, the QT–heart rate slopes during exercise were similar to those resulting from an increase in heart rate caused by atropine injection, but less dynamic during isoproterenol infusion, demonstrating that the *QT* response to rate change in normal subjects is dependent on neurohumoral conditions and not just on rate alone. These findings extend previous observations by Cuomo *et al.* (1997) that parasympathetic influence may be more important than sympathetic influence in rate-independent modulation of the *QT* interval. However, reduced dynamic behaviour of the *QT* interval in response to catecholamine stimulation, and increased dynamic behaviour during beta blockade, appears to be a feature of patients with some forms of congenital abnormalities of repolarization (Furushima *et al.* 2001; Krahn *et al.* 2002).

It should be noted that linearity of unadjusted *QT* interval duration with changing heart rate during exercise may not occur during all conditions and in all subjects. Adaptation of the *QT* interval to changing heart rate in humans is not an instantaneous consequence of varying cycle length alone, but rather depends on rate and the additional influence of duration of rate as further modified by the complex neurohumoral changes that accompany exercise. A presumption of inverse linearity between *QTo* and heart rate may not be entirely accurate in the very earliest exercise phases of treadmill testing. Coughlin *et al.* (1992) reported a paradoxical increase in unadjusted *QT* interval during the first minute of exercise in patients with *QT* dependent rate responsive ventricular pacemakers, and we observed small increases in unadjusted *QTo* from upright control recordings through the first few stages of exercise in approximately 20% of our normal subjects (Kligfield *et al.* 1996).

Findings in our normal subjects suggest that the decrease in *QTpeak* is proportional to, or at most only very slightly proportionally less than, the overall decrease in *QTo* during submaximal exercise in normal subjects. This is consistent with prior observations by O'Donnell *et al.* (1985) that the terminal T wave subinterval *QTo-QTpeak* (defined as aT-eT in that report) is relatively unchanged or slightly increased as a fraction of *QTo* in normals but may be significantly decreased in the presence of myocardial ischaemia. The relative proportion and range of the terminal T wave calculated at rest from observed *QTpeak/QTo* in our normal men are nearly identical with the findings of Murray *et al.* (1995) in a smaller group of semi-supine subjects studied by routine electrocardiography.

Clinical correlates of repolarization behaviour during exercise

QT prolongation during exercise has been examined as a marker for myocardial ischaemia in patients with coronary artery disease (Maceira-Cuelho *et al.* 1983; Egloff *et al.* 1987). However, a major consequence of the wide range of *QTc* behaviour during exercise in normal subjects is that mere prolongation of the *QTc* may not be a useful marker for disease at the relatively lower peak exercise heart rates at which cardiac patients may be limited. Thus, we also found greater *QTo* at peak exercise in patients with coronary artery disease than in normal men (Lax *et al.* 1994), suggesting that an end-exercise *QTo* partition with high specificity in normal subjects could have high sensitivity for the detection of myocardial ischaemia. Because the patients with coronary disease had substantially lower peak exercise heart rates than the normal subjects, this finding was almost entirely dependent on heart rate differences between groups and the non-linear behaviour of the Bazett corrected *QTo* within these rates. When compared at comparable heart rate levels during exercise, the ability of Bazett rate-corrected *QTo* to separate patients with disease from normal subjects was markedly reduced.

Vincent *et al.* (1991) suggested that exercise can unmask subtle cases of the Romano-Ward inherited long *QT* syndrome in which the *QT* interval is borderline at rest. These investigators found a linear decrease in *QTo* with heart rate in normal subjects, but not in Romano-Ward patients in whom the absolute *QTo* failed to shorten normally with exercise. This corresponds to very reduced 'dynamic' behaviour (low slope) of the *QT* response to exercise in this disorder. In a small group of patients with the long QT syndrome, Furushima *et al.* (2001) demonstrated that addition of alpha-adrenergic blockade to β-adrenergic blockade increased the steepness of the exercise QT–heart rate slope and attenuated the associated prolongation of Bazett corrected *QTc* in this population.

In this context, it is apparent from the behaviour of the *QTc*–heart rate relationship in normal men and women that mere prolongation of *QTc* with exercise cannot be used as a specific marker for occult long QT syndrome in otherwise normal subjects. However, recent evaluation of *QT* interval recovery patterns with respect to slowing heart rates after exercise may provide useful additional insight. Thus, for example, Krahn *et al.* (2002) found that beta-blockade in patients with the long QT syndrome reduced the magnitude of *QT* hysteresis, defined as the difference between recovery *QT* interval at 1 min of recovery compared with the *QT* interval at the corresponding heart rate during exercise, to levels found in normal subjects.

Clinical implications

These observations suggest that it can be useful to describe repolarization behaviour by reference to the statistical distribution of slopes and intercepts from regression of unadjusted *QT* intervals and heart rate during exercise in normal subjects. These parameters may provide insights that complement currently available data that can be obtained from the resting tracing and from the ambulatory electrocardiogram. Because exercise repolarization can be influenced by both rate-dependent and rate-independent phenomena, careful attention to details of protocol are required to assure reliable standardization of these methods in normal subjects and in patients with a variety of disorders. Under these conditions, characterization of repolarization during exercise might facilitate identification of otherwise subtle forms of the long QT syndrome, and it also might assist in the detection of subjects at increased risk of complex arrhythmias or for proarrhythmic effects of drugs. While it appears unlikely that regression based analysis of *QT* intervals will be useful for improving the detection of coronary obstruction during exercise testing, findings in other forms of heart disease remain to be investigated.

References

Ahnve, S. (1985) Correction of the QT interval for heart rate: review of different formulas and the use of Bazett's formula in myocardial infarction. *American Heart Journal*, **109**, 568–573.

Akhras, F. & Rickards, A.F. (1981) The relationship between QT interval and heart rate during physiological exercise and pacing. *Japanese Heart Journal*, **22**, 345–351.

Aytemir, K., Maarouf, N., Gallagher, M.M., Yap, Y.G., Waktare, J.E. & Malik, M. (1999) Comparison of formulae for heart rate correction of QT interval in exercise electrocardiograms. *Pacing and Clinical Electrophysiology*, **22**, 1397–1401.

Bazett, H.C. (1920) An analysis of the time relationship of electrocardiograms. *Heart* **7**, 353–370.

Benatar, A., Decraene, T. (2001) Comparison of formulae for heart rate correction of QT interval in exercise ECGs from healthy children. *Heart* **86**, 199–202.

Cappato, R., Alboni, P., Pedroni, P., Gilli, G. & Antonioli, G. (1991) Sympathetic and vagal influences on rate-dependent changes of QT interval in healthy subjects. *American Journal of Cardiology*, **68**, 1188–1193.

Coghlan, J.G., Madden, B., Norell, M.N., Ilsley, C.D. & Mitchell, A.G. (1992) Paradoxical early lengthening and subsequent linear shortening of the QT interval in response to exercise. *European Heart Journal*, **13**, 1325–1328.

Coumel, P. & Maison-Blanche, P. (1992) Electrocardiography and computers. *Journal of Ambulatory Monitoring*, **4**, 265–272.

Cuomo, S., De Caprio, L., Di Palma, A., Lirato, C., Lombardi, L., De Rosa, M.L., Vetrano, A. & Rengo, F.

(1997) Influence of autonomic tone on QT interval duration. *Cardiologia*, **42**, 1071–1076.

Davey, P. (1999) A new physiological method for heart rate correction of the QT interval. *Heart*, **82**, 183–186.

De Ponti, F., Poluzzi, E., Vaccheri, A. *et al.* (2002) Non-antiarrhythmic drugs prolonging the QT interval: considerable use in seven countries. *British Journal of Clinical Pharmacology*, **54**, 171–177.

Egloff, C., Merola, P., Schiavon, C. *et al.* (1987) Sensitivity, specificity and predictive accuracy of Q wave, QX/QT ratio, QT*c* interval and *S–T* depression during exercise testing in men with coronary artery disease. *American Journal of Cardiology*, **60**, 1006–1008.

Extramiana, F., Maison-Blanche, P., Badilini, F., Pinoteau, J., Deseo, T. & Coumel, P. (1999) Circadian modulation of QT rate dependence in healthy volunteers: gender and age differences. *Journal of Electrocardiology*, **32**, 33–43.

Fayn, J., Rubel, P. (1988) CAVIAR, a serial ECG processing system for the comparative analysis of VCGs and their interpretation with autoreference to the patient. *Journal of Electrocardiology*, **21** (Suppl), S173–S176.

Furushima, H., Chinushi, M., Washizuka, T. & Aizawa, Y. (2001) Role of alpha1-blockade in congenital long QT syndrome: investigation by exercise stress test. *Japanese Circulation Journal*, **65**, 654–658.

Gill, J.S., Baszko, A., Xia, R., Ward, D.E. & Camm, A.J. (1993) Dynamics of the QT interval in patients with exercise-induced ventricular tachycardia in normal and abnormal hearts. *American Heart Journal*, **126**, 1357–1363.

Kadish, A.H., Weisman, H.F., Veltri, E.P., Epstein, A.E., Slepian, M.J. & Levine, J.H. (1990) Paradoxical effects of exercise on the QT interval in patients with polymorphic ventricular tachycardia receiving type Ia antiarrhythmic agents. *Circulation*, **81**, 14–19.

Kligfield, P., Lax, K.G. & Okin, P.M. (1995) QT*c* behaviour during treadmill exercise as a function of underlying QT–heart rate relationship. *Journal of Electrocardiology*, **28**(Suppl), 206–210.

Kligfield, P., Lax, K.G. & Okin, P.M. (1996) The QT interval–heart rate relationship during exercise in normal men and women: definition by linear regression analysis. *Journal of the American College of Cardiology*, **28**, 1547–1555.

Krahn, A.D., Yee, R., Chauhan, V. *et al.* (2002) Beta blockers normalize QT hysteresis in long QT syndrome. *American Heart Journal*, **143**, 528–534.

Laakso, M., Aberg, A., Savola, J., Pentikainen, P.J. & Pyorala, K. (1987) Diseases and drugs causing prolongation of the QT interval. *American Journal of Cardiology*, **59**, 862–865.

Lax, K.G., Okin, P.M., Kligfield, P. (1994) Electrocardiographic repolarization measurements at rest and during exercise in normal subjects and in patients with coronary artery disease. *American Heart Journal*, **128**, 271–280.

Locati, E.H. (2001) QT interval duration and adaptation to heart rate. In: Zareba, W., Maison-Blanche, P, Locati, E.H. eds., *Noninvasive Electrocardiology in Clinical Practice*. Armonk, New York: Futura Publishing Company, 2001, pp. 71–96.

Maceira-Cuelho, E., Monteiro, F., DaConceicao, J.M. *et al.* (1983) Post-exercise changes of the QTc interval in coronary heart disease. *Journal of Electrocardiology*, **16**, 345–350.

Magnano, A.R., Holleran, S., Ramakrishnan, R., Reiffel, J.A. & Bloomfield, D.M. (2002) Autonomic nervous system influences on QT interval in normal subjects. *Journal of the American College of Cardiology*, **39**, 1820–1826.

Mayuga, K.A., Parker, M., Sukthanker, N.D., Perlowski, A., Schwartz, J.B. & Kadish, A.H. (2001) Effects of age and gender on the QT response to exercise. *American Journal of Cardiology*, **87**, 163–167.

Merri, M., Benhorin, J., Alberti, M., Locati, E. & Moss, A.J. (1989) Electrocardiographic quantitation of ventricular repolarization. *Circulation*, **80**, 1301–1308.

Murray, A, McLaughlin, N.B. & Campbell, R.W.F. (1995) Errors associated with assuming that the complete QT duration can be estimated from QT measured to the peak of the T wave. *Journal of Ambulatory Monitoring*, **8**, 265–270.

O'Donnell, J., Lovelace, D.E., Knoebel, S.B. & McHenry, P.L. (1985) Behaviour of the terminal T wave during exercise in normal subjects, patients with symptomatic coronary artery disease and apparently healthy subjects with abnormal *S–T* segment depression. *Journal of the American College of Cardiology*, **5**, 78–84.

Rickards, A.F., Norman, J. (1981) Relation between QT interval and heart rate: new design of physiologically adaptive cardiac pacemaker. *British Heart Journal*, **45**, 56–61.

Sagie, A., Larson, M.G., Goldberg, R.J., Bengtson, J.R. & Levy, D. (1992) An improved method for adjusting the QT interval for heart rate (the Framingham heart study). *American Journal of Cardiology*, **70**, 797–801.

Sarma, J.S.M., Sarma, R.J., Bilitch, M., Katz, D. & Song, S.L. (1984) An exponential formula for heart rate dependence of QT interval during exercise and cardiac pacing in humans: reevaluation of Bazett's formula. *American Journal of Cardiology*, **54**, 103–108.

Seed, W.A., Noble, M.I.M., Oldershaw, P. *et al.* (1987) Relation of human cardiac action potential duration to the interval between beats: implications for the validity of rate corrected QT interval (QT*c*). *British Heart Journal*, **57**, 32–37.

Tavernier, R., Jordaens, L., Schiettekatte, V., DeBacker, G. & Clement, D.L. (1995) Relation of dynamic QT behaviour and baseline QT measurements. *Journal of Ambulatory Monitoring*, **8**, 207–218.

Tobe, T.J.M., de Langen, C.D.J., Bink-Boelkens, M.Th.E. *et al.* (1992) Late potentials in a bradycardia-dependent long QT syndrome associated with sudden death during sleep. *Journal of the American College of Cardiology*, **19**, 541–549.

Viitasalo, M., Rovamo, L., Toivonen, L., Pesonen, E. & Heikkila, J. (1996) Dynamics of the QT interval during and after exercise in healthy children. *European Heart Journal* **17**, 1723–1728.

Vincent, G.M., Jaiswal, D. & Timothy, K.W. (1991) Effects of exercise on heart rate, QT, QTc, and QT/QS2 in the Romano-Ward inherited long QT syndrome. *American Journal of Cardiology*, **68**, 498–503.

Zaza, A., Malfatto, G. & Schwartz, P.J. (1991) Sympathetic modulation of the relation between ventricular repolarization and cycle length. *Circulation Research*, **68**, 1191–1203.

CHAPTER 38

T Wave and *QT* Interval Changes Related to Myocardial Ischaemia

Juha Hartikainen

Myocardial ischaemia results from mismatch of myocardial oxygen supply and demand. It is most often related to coronary atherosclerosis. In stable coronary artery disease, myocardial ischaemia develops if an increase in myocardial oxygen demand caused physiological challenges of everyday life, such as physical or psychological stress, cannot be compensated by an adequate increase in coronary blood flow and oxygen supply. The mechanism responsible for flow restriction can be anatomical (coronary artery stenoses) and/or functional (impaired coronary vasodilatation). In the vasospastic angina (Prinzmetal's angina) and, particularly in a more severe form of coronary artery disease – acute coronary syndrome – an abrupt rupture or erosion of an atherosclerotic plaque results in superimposed thrombosis, distal microembolisation and coronary vasoconstriction reducing myocardial blood flow and oxygen supply at rest and provokes myocardial ischaemia, injury or infarction without any increase in myocardial oxygen consumption (Davies 1995).

Recording of the depolarization and the repolarization

The electrocardiogram mirrors electrical events associated with the activation (depolarization) and recovery (repolarization) of myocardial cells. These are due to ionic fluxes, mainly potassium, sodium and calcium across the myocardial cell membrane. The effects of ischaemia on the electrocardiogram are also mediated via its effects on the ionic fluxes and the subsequent changes in the potentials across the cell membranes. Thus, understanding of the mechanisms of normal depolarization and repolarization constitutes the basis for understanding the effects of ischaemia on the electrocardiogram.

Transmembrane action potential

Usually, depolarization and repolarization events are described as recordings from a single cardiac myocyte. The potentials from a cell can be measured by means of a bipolar electrode in which an intracellular microelectrode represents one pole and the other pole being a surface electrode. The recording of the changes of potentials obtained from a single cell is termed the transmembrane action potential (Fig. 38.1). The pattern of the transmembrane action potential can be divided into slow and fast types. Slow types are typical for P cells of the sinoatrial node and N cells of the atrioventricular nodes, whereas fast forms are typical for atrial internodal cells, other atrial myocytes, Purkinje cells and ventricular myocytes.

The transmembrane action potential is characterized with four phases. Phase 4 represents the resting phase of the cell. At rest, the inside of the cell has negative potential of approximately −90 mV when compared with the outside of the cell. The normal, resting myocardial cell has a positive surface charge and a negative intracellular charge. On the other hand, there is no change in the potential between the adjacent cells, and no current flows. The resting potential is maintained by an energy dependent transport of sodium out from the cell and potassium into the cell by means of a sodium–potassium pump located in the cell membrane. Phase 0 represents the depolarization, i.e. activation of the cell. Depolarization is associated with an abrupt rise in the intracellular potential. This is caused by opening of sodium channels and a rapid influx of sodium into the cell. At the end of this phase the inside of the cell becomes positive with reference to the outside of the cell by approximately 10 mV. At the end of Phase 0, the sodium channels begin to close and potassium channels to open. This is followed by a slower period of repolarization, i.e. recovery of the transmembrane potential back to the resting state. The repolarization period can be further divided into three phases: Phase 1 is an early, rapid phase which is caused by slow inflow of sodium into the cell and outflow of potassium from the cell. This is followed by a relatively slow phase 2, during which there is inflow of sodium and calcium into the cell as well as potassium outflow from the cell.

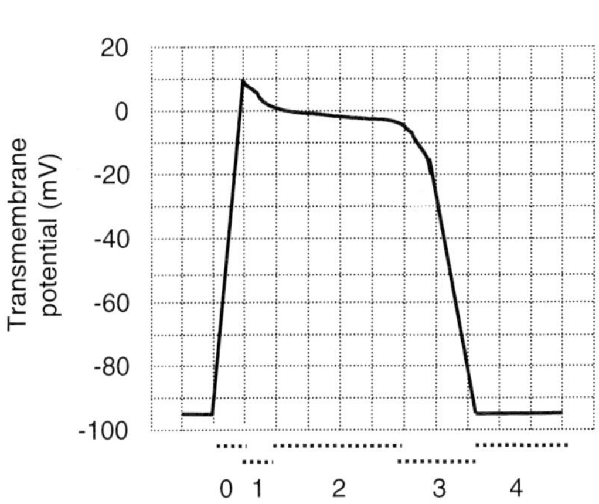

Fig. 38.1 Normal transmembral action potential. For details, see text.

During phase 2, the sodium and calcium channels are closed and the potassium outflow is increased resulting in speeding up the repolarization and returning the transmembrane potential back to the resting state.

Electrocardiographic recording

When applying the above into interpretation of an electrocardiogram one has to remember that the transmembrane action potential is caused by events recorded from a single cardiac cell, whereas the clinical electrocardiogram is recorded from outside of the heart. In addition, electrocardiogram reflects depolarization and repolarization events caused by not only a single cardiac myocyte but multiple myocytes from different parts of the heart.

During the resting phase (phase 4) the outside of the myocardial cells in the endocardium as well as in the epicardium have positive charge. Thus, no potential exists between the endocardium and the epicardium and no currents are generated. The electrocardiogram shows isoelectric line (TP segment, Fig. 38.2a). Depolarization starts from the endocardium and directs transversely through the ventricular wall towards the epicardium. The outside of the endocardial myocytes become negative with reference to the inside of the cells (phase 0). At this time point, the epicardial cells are still repolarized, i.e. their outside is positive with reference to the inside of the cells. This potential difference between the endocardium and epicardium generates an elec-

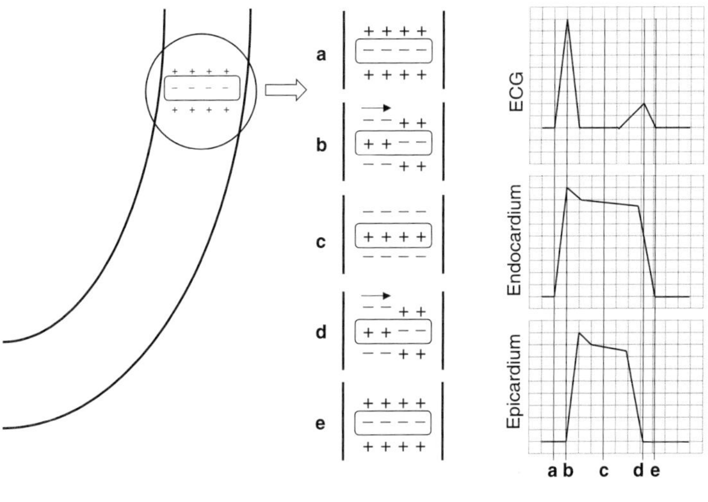

Fig. 38.2 Electrocardiographic recording of the ventricular wall. Electrocardiographic recording and the transmembral action potential curves of the endocardium and epicardium are shown: (a) resting phase, (b) depolarization phase, (c) plateau of the repolarization phase, (d) end of repolarization phase in the epicardium and (e) in the endocardium. For details, see text.

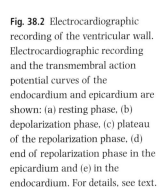

trical current directed from the negative pole (endocardium) to the positive pole (epicardium) and results in a positive deflection (QRS complex, Fig. 38.2b) in an electrode facing towards the epicardium. During the phases 1–2 of repolarization both the endocardial and epicardial myocytes are depolarized and no potential exists between the endocardium and the epicardium. Thus, no currents are generated and the electrocardiogram records isoelectric line (ST segment, Fig. 38.2c).

During repolarization, the change in the transmembral potential is opposite to that of the depolarization. The outside of the myocytes becomes positive as compared to the inside (phase 3). However, the also direction of the repolarization is opposite to that of the depolarization, occurring transversally from the epicardium to the endocardium. As soon as repolarization has occurred in the epicardium the outside of epicardial cells become positive while the endocardium is still negative giving rise to an electrical current directed from the negative pole (endocardium) to the positive pole (epicardium) and positive deflection of the T wave in an electrode facing towards the epicardium (Fig. 38.2 d). Thus, normally, the polarities of the QRS complex and the T wave are the same. At the end of repolarization both the endocardial and epicardial myocardial cells have resumed the resting state and no currents are generated between the endocardium and the epicardium (phase 4).

The normal T wave

A normal T wave has typical shape and pattern (Fig. 38.2). As mentioned above, the normal T wave is inscribed in the same direction as the QRS complex. It has asymmetrical limbs, the proximal limb being shallower than the distal limb. In addition, it has relatively blunt apex. As a result, the normal T wave merges smoothly with the distal part of the ST segment, making it difficult to determine where the ST segment ends and the T wave starts.

The T wave is followed by the U wave. The normal U wave is a small, rounded deflection with the same polarity as the T wave. The amplitude of the U wave is approximately 10% of the T wave. Usually, the T wave can be separated from the U wave for the assessment of the *QT* interval. However, in situations where the U wave becomes large or inverted it can merge smoothly with the preceding T wave and make the accurate measurement of the *QT* interval difficult.

Effects of mismatch of myocardial oxygen supply and demand on the repolarization and depolarization

The effects of mismatch of myocardial oxygen supply and consumption on the depolarization and repolarization are caused by their effects on the transmembrane ionic fluxes and intracellular concentration of ions, mainly potassium. Depending on severity and duration the mismatch of myocardial oxygen supply and demand can lead to different clinical conditions, namely ischaemia, injury or infarction. Pathophysiologically, all these are presentations of the same continuous process with different degree of severity. However, from clinical point of view myocardial ischaemia, injury and infarction have to be differentiated from each other because they have different implications on the patient management and prognosis.

In addition, one has to keep in mind that although later the different manifestation of mismatch of myocardial oxygen supply and demand are discussed separately, in real life the patient usually presents with combinations rather than isolated patterns of ischaemia, injury and infarction. An infarct zone is surrounded by an injury zone, which is surrounded by an ischaemic zone (Fig. 38.3) each giving rise to a typical pattern of electrocardiogram abnormality. In addition, usually the ischaemic process starts from the subendocardium and spreads towards the epicardium with the progression of the ischaemia and finally gives rise to transmural ischaemia. Thus, often a subepicardial or transmural ischaemia shares the characteristics of subendocardial as well as subepicardial ischaemia.

Finally, one has to recognize that the electrocardiogram may be normal in the presence of severe ischaemic heart disease. Less than half of the patients with an acute myocardial infarction present with typical and diagnostic changes in the first electrocardiography recording and almost one fifth of the patients present with com-

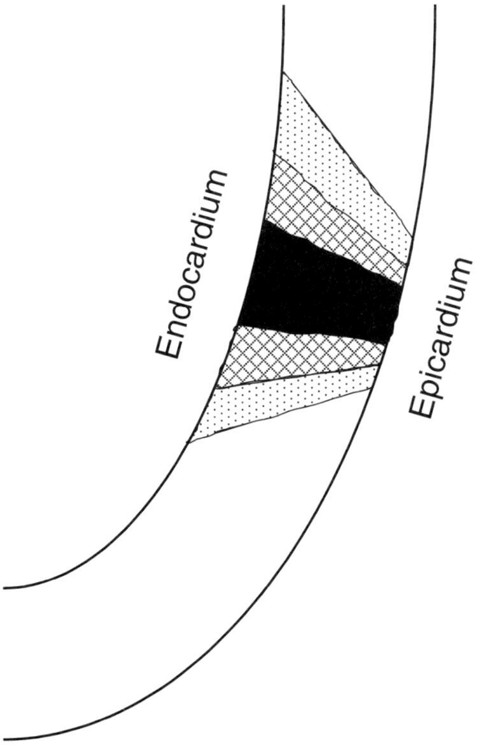

Fig. 38.3 Myocardial infarction. The infarcted zone (shadowed area) is surrounded by the injury zones (hatched area) and ischaemic zones (dotted area).

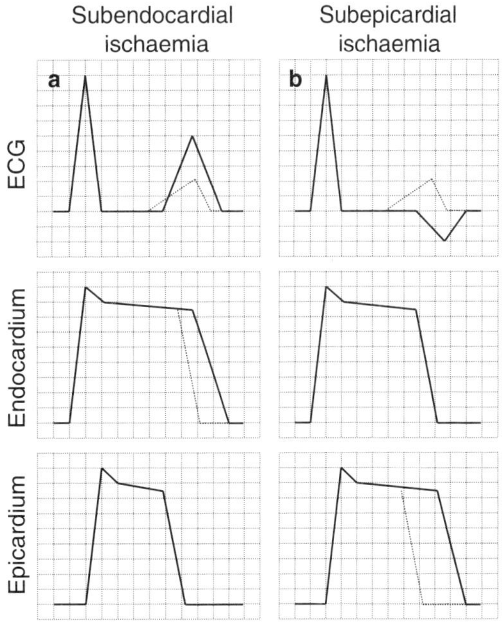

Fig. 38.4 Effects of myocardial ischaemia on the electrocardiogram and transmembrane action potential. Myocardial ischaemia causes prolongation of the repolarization resulting in (a) positive T waves with increased amplitude in the case of subendocardial ischaemia and (b) inverted T waves in the case of subepicardial ischaemia. The dotted line represents normal pattern.

pletely normal or near normal electrocardiogram (Woods *et al.* 1963; Cannon *et al.* 1997; Task Force Report 2000; Channer & Morris 2002).

The effects of myocardial ischaemia on the T wave and the *QT* interval

The earliest signs of the mismatch of myocardial oxygen supply and demand are evident in the repolarization process manifested as abnormalities in the T wave, the U wave and the *QT* interval. Myocardial ischaemia causes a loss of intracellular potassium concentration resulting in a slight, subtle diminution of the resting potential. The major effect of ischaemia is, however, a delay in the repolarization, especially phase 3 of the transmembral action potential in the ischaemic myocardium. The delay and the imbalance of repolarization, i.e. the disturbance in the sequence of repolarization of the ischaemic myocardium, manifests as typical ischaemic changes of the T wave and *QT* interval (Fig. 38.4, Table 38.1).

Table 38.1 The effects of myocardial ischaemia and injury on the T wave and the *QT* interval

	T wave	*QT interval*
Ischaemia	Symmetricity Narrowness Sharper apex Increased magnitude Directed away from the ischaemic region	Prolonged
Injury	Increased magnitude Directed towards the ischaemic region	Shortened

The T wave

The delay in the repolarization caused by myocardial ischaemia influences the shape, the magnitude and the direction of the T wave.

Myocardial ischaemia contributes to the symmetrical, narrow and sharper appearance of the T wave. As a result of myocardial ischaemia the angle between the proximal T wave and the ST segment becomes more obvious. This is partly due to the direct effects of ischaemia on the T wave shape, partly due the effect of ischaemia on the ST segment. The ST segment tends to be more isoelectric and as a result, the angle between the ST segment and the proximal limb of the T wave becomes steeper. In addition, the apex of the T wave becomes sharper. An ischaemic T wave is also usually increased in magnitude, which further contributes to the symmetrical, arrowhead appearance of the T wave.

Because of delayed repolarization, the ischaemic myocardium presents with a positive internal charge (negative external charge) at the time the normal myocardium has already repolarized completely and resumed a negative internal charge (positive external charge). The repolarization vector tends to flow from an area of negative charge to an area of positive charge. Thus, the vector of the T wave in association with ischaemia is directed away from the surface of the ischaemic region. The leads orientated to the ischaemia (ischaemic zone between the healthy myocardium and the recording electrode) will record inverted T waves, whereas the leads orientated to the healthy myocardium (healthy myocardium between the ischaemic zone and the recording electrode) will record upright T waves. For example, an electrode in the lateral frontal plane position (V5–V6) records a T wave with increased amplitude in the case of true subendocardial ischaemia of the lateral wall of the left ventricle (Figs 38.4a and 38.5a), but an inverted T wave in the case of true subepicardial ischaemia (Figs 38.4b, and 38.5b). On the other hand, depending on the extent of ischaemia cross the ventricular wall, ischaemia may present with different combinations of T wave changes, including a biphasic T wave (Fig. 38.5c). An isolated tall, positive T wave is not a very common finding, but usually associated with other findings of ischaemia and injury (see Fig. 38.8a). In addition, when interpreting the effects of ischaemia on the polarity of the T wave one has to bear in mind that the above principles refer to the recording leads orientated to the surface of the abnormality. The recording lead orientated to the opposite surface record a mirror image, i.e. reciprocal changes of ischaemia Fig. 38.7b).

The *QT* interval

A delay in the repolarization process becomes manifests as prolongation of the *QT* interval. Indeed, a prolongation of the *QT* interval may be

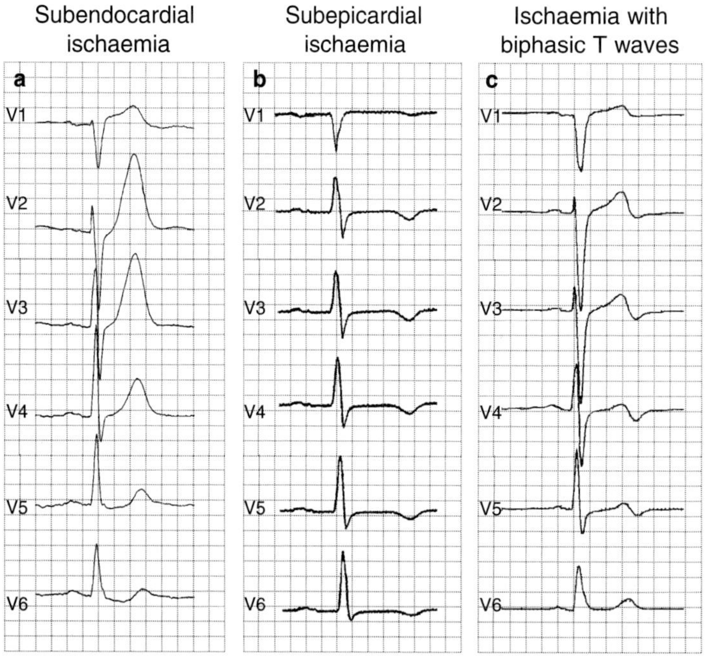

Fig. 38.5 Typical electocardiographic patterns of (a) subendocardial ischaemia resulting in increased amplitude of the T waves and (b) subepicardial ischaemia resulting in inverted T waves. (c) Combined subendocardial and subepicardial ischaemia resulting in biphasic T waves (V3–V5).

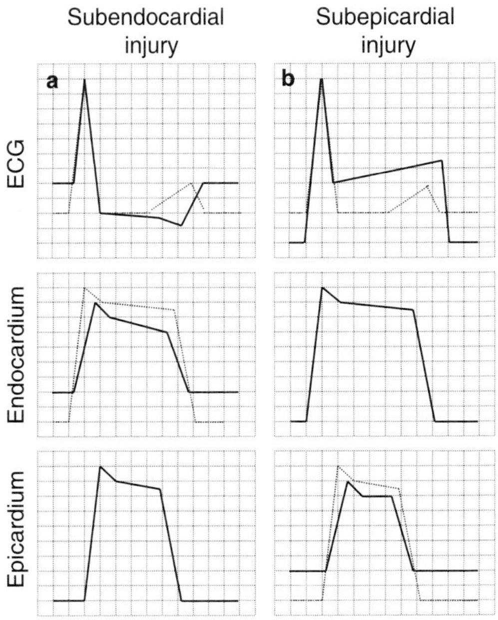

Fig. 38.6 Effects of myocardial injury on the electrocardiogram and transmembrane action potential. Myocardial injury causes a shift of the isoelectric baseline and shortening of the repolarization resulting in (a) depression of the ST segment with inverted T waves in the case of subendocardial injury and (b) elevation of the ST segment with positive T waves in the case of subepicardial injury. The dotted line represents normal pattern.

the earliest presentation of myocardial ischaemia and evolving infarction.

The effects of myocardial injury on the T wave and the *QT* interval

Prolongation or deterioration of mismatch of myocardial oxygen supply and demand results in progression of myocardial ischaemia to myocardial injury. With the progression of the ischaemia the level of intracellular potassium is further decreased and leads to an increase in the resting potential of the myocardium. The development of a difference in the transmembrane resting potential between the ischaemic and normal myocardium manifests in the repolarization pattern primarily as an abnormality of the ST segment (depression or elevation of the ST segment) (see Section III). However, also the T wave becomes involved in the setting is injury.

The T wave

An early injury phase is gives rise to a paradoxical shortening of the refractory period. This is due to three reasons. First, the depolarization amplitude of the injured myocardial cells does not reach the level of the healthy myocytes (phase 0). Secondly, the transmembral potential of the injured

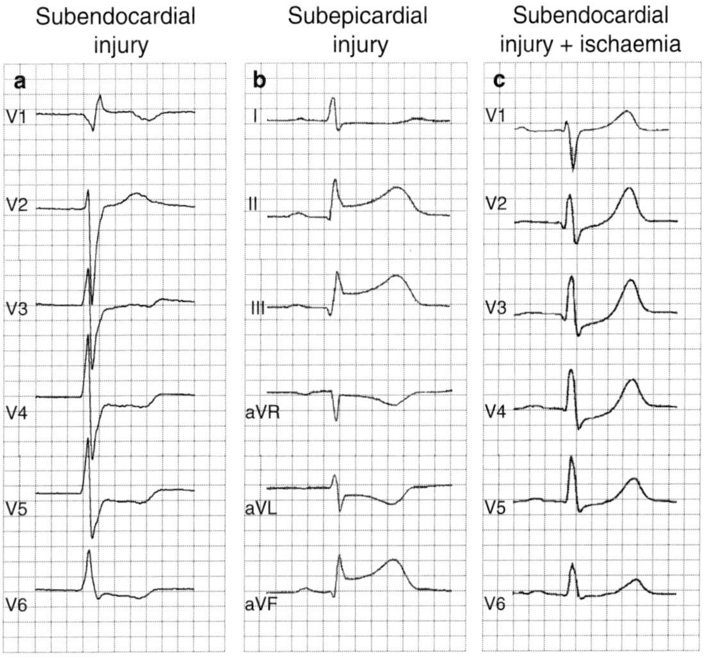

Fig. 38.7 Typical electocardiographic patterns of (a) subendocardial injury resulting in depression of the ST segment and negative T wave (V4–V6), (b) subepicardial ischaemia resulting in elevation of the ST and positive T wave (II, III, aVF) and reciprocal changes in leads aVR and aVL (c) combined subendocardial injury and ischaemia resulting in depression of the ST segment and positive T wave.

myocardial cells start to decrease earlier than in the healthy cells (phase 2). Thirdly, as a consequence of the above, the injured myocardial cells reach the resting potential earlier than the healthy cells (phase 3) (Fig. 38.6). The injured myocardium reaches repolarization earlier than the healthy myocardium, i.e. at the time the injured myocardium presents with a negative internal charge (positive external charge) the healthy myocardium presents still with a positive internal charge (negative external charge). A current directed from the negative charge (healthy myocardium) towards the positive charge (injured myocardium) is generated at the end of the repolarization. This influences both the magnitude and the shape of the T wave.

The myocardial injury is characterized by an increase in the magnitude of the T wave. In addition, the T wave becomes more symmetrical and pointed. The T wave morphology is also influenced by the abnormality of the preceding ST segment. Especially, the transition of the ST segment to T wave becomes straightened resulting in indirect wider appearance of the proximal part of the T wave.

The main effect of myocardial injury is related to the direction of the T wave. Because of shortening of the refractory period the recovery (repolarization) of the injured myocardial zone occurs faster than that of the adjacent normal myocardium. The negative internal charge (positive external charge) of the injured myocardium while the normal myocardium has still negative internal charge (positive external charge) results in a repolarization current directed from the normal myocardium towards the injured myocardium. Thus, the effect of injury on the repolarization vector is reversal of that associated with less severe myocardial ischaemia and directed to the same direction as the preceding ST segment deviation. For example, an electrode facing towards the injured segment of the left ventricular wall will record depression of the ST segment and inverted T wave in the case of subendocardial injury (Figs 38.6a and 38.7a), and elevation of the ST segment and positive T wave in the case of subepicardial or transmural injury (Figs 38.6b and 38.7b).

Myocardial injury may occur as an isolated manifestation, but more often it occurs in association with surrounding myocardial ischaemia. As a consequence, the electrocardiographic pattern of injury is usually a combination of injury and ischaemia. This does not influence the ST segment but it does influence the T wave because the effects of ischaemia and injury on the T wave are opposite. Thus, subendocardial injury often manifests with depression of the ST segment associated with positive or inverted T wave depending on the extent of the surrounding ischaemia (Fig. 38.7c).

The *QT* interval

A shortening of the refractory period associated with myocardial injury phase results in a shortening of the *QT* interval. This, however, is often transient lasting only a few minutes. In addition, as mentioned above, the injury zone is usually surrounded by ischaemic zone with prolonged refractory period and *QT* interval. Thus, during the course of myocardial ischaemia and injury, the *QT* interval may fluctuate between shortened and prolonged.

The effects of acute myocardial infarction and myocardial necrosis on the T wave and the *QT* interval

The process of myocardial infarction presents with two phases, the hyperacute phase and the fully evolved phase of myocardial infarction.

The very early stage of developing myocardial infarction, the hyperacute phase, starts with a pattern of myocardial ischaemia influencing the T waves (see above) (Fig. 38.8a). If ischaemia does not subside the change in the T waves is usually present for less than 30 min and it is followed by the change of myocardial injury influencing the ST segment (see above). The presentation of the hyperacute phase lasts but a few hours and usually less than 24 h. However, the time scale and degree of severity of the hyperacute phase depends on recanalisation of the occlusion and the extent of existing collateral circulation.

A severe and/or prolonged injury leads to the fully evolved phase of myocardial infarction characterized by further reduction of the intracellular potassium concentration and resting potential to the inertial potential and the cell

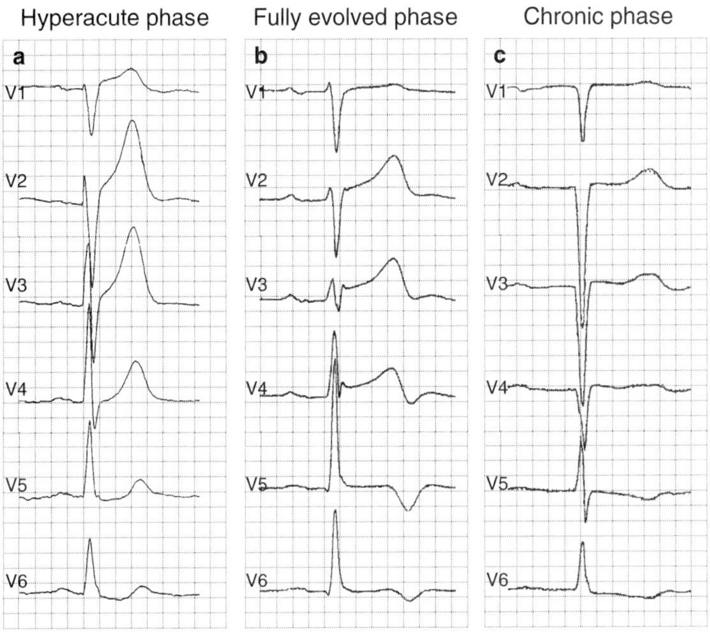

Fig. 38.8 Typical electrocardiographic patterns of myocardial infarction. (a) hyperacute phase with elevation of the ST segment and positive, tall T waves (V2–V4), (b) fully evolved phase showing a decrease in the R wave amplitude (V2–V4), elevation of the ST segment (V2–V4) and inversion of the T waves (V4–V6) and (c) chronic phase with deep Q waves but no repolarization abnormalities.

becomes electrically dead. This is mirrored by abnormalities in the myocardial depolarization, the QRS complex, a reduction of the R wave amplitude and/or development of pathological Q waves. The changes in the QRS complex occur within one or two hours after the occlusion of a coronary artery, though often they take 12–24 h to appear. In addition, the changes in the depolarization abnormalities are associated with abnormalities in the repolarization; elevated ST segments and inverted, symmetrical T waves (Fig. 38.8b).

The acute phase and fully evolved phases of myocardial infarction are followed by development of the chronic phase of myocardial infarction. During this, there is gradual resolution of the repolarization changes – the ST segment and the T wave – towards normal (Fig. 38.8c). After an inferior myocardial infarction the resolution of the repolarization abnormalities occurs usually within 2–3 weeks. The polarisation abnormalities associated with an anterior infarction persist longer and occasionally – especially the T wave inversion – remains as a permanent sign of myocardial infarction (Mills *et al.* 1975). Persistent abnormalities in the ST segment and the T wave may also indicate the presence of a left ventricular aneurysm.

Clinical implications related to T wave and *QT* interval changes of myocardial ischaemia

In a patient with acute chest pain the presence of abnormalities in the repolarization can be used to predict the development of myocardial infarction. The likelihood that a patient experiences an acute myocardial infarction is approximately 30% in a patient with isolated T wave abnormalities, approximately 50% in a patient with depression of the ST segment and reaches 80% in a patient with elevation of the ST segment (Savonitto *et al.* 1999).

Electrocardiographic abnormalities confer also long-term prognostic information in patients with acute chest pain. In patients with unstable angina pectoris or a non-Q wave myocardial infarction and repolarization abnormalities restricted to the T wave (T wave inversion) the occurrence of death or a new myocardial infarction during a one-year follow-up was 7%. Indeed, it did not differ from the occurrence of death or myocardial infarction (8%) of patients with no electrocardiographic changes during hospital admission (Cannon *et al.* 1997). In contrast, the rate of death or development of new myocardial infarction was 1.5- to 2-fold in patients present-

Table 38.2 Differential diagnosis of abnormalities of the T wave

Normal variants
Persistent juvenile pattern
Early repolarization (athlete's heart)
Vagal stimulation
Anxiety or fear
Orthostatic response
Postprandial response
Hyperventilation
Alcoholism
Extracardiac causes
Abdominal disorders (appendicitis, pancreatitis, cholecystitis, peritonitis)
Cerebrovascular accident
Hypothyroidism
Hypoadrenalism
Hypopituitarism
Phaeochromocytoma
Cardiac nonischaemic causes
Myocarditis
Pericarditis
Cardiomyopathies
Ventricular hypertrophy
Mitral valve prolapse
Cor pulmonale
Bundle branch block
Wolff–Parkinson–White syndrome
Cardiac pacing
Post-tachycardia syndrome

ing with depression or elevation of the ST segment (Schwartz & Wolf 1978; Cannon *et al.* 1997).

The long-term risk associated with myocardial ischaemia is mainly due to occurrence of reinfarctions. However, myocardial ischaemia renders the injured myocardium also vulnerable to ventricular arrhythmias. The increase in the resting potential (diastolic depolarization) favours ventricular automaticity, ventricular extrasystoles and ventricular tachycardia. This is particularly prone to occur at the peri-infarcted zone. A prolongation of repolarization protects from ventricular arrhythmias. However, the prolongation of repolarization caused by ischaemia and infarction is not homogeneous, but results in differences in the depolarization and repolarization between the ischaemic/injured and normal myocardium. The temporal and spatial fragmentation and out-of-phase state of the ventricular depolarization and repolarization becomes manifested as dispersion of refractoriness, i.e. *QT* dispersion. Indeed, both prolongation of the *QT* interval and QT dispersion have been found to be associated with vulnerability for ventricular tachycardia and ventricular fibrillation (Schwartz & Wolf, 1978; Ward, 1988; Perkiömäki *et al.* 1997).

Table 38.3 Differential diagnosis of abnormalities of the *QT* interval

Prolonged *QT* interval
Congenital long QT syndrome
Acquired *QT* prolongation
Drug induced
Bradycardia
Myocarditis
Hypertrophic cardiomyopathy
Cardiac trauma
Hypocalcaemia
Hypothermia
Hypothyroidism
Sleep
Shortened *QT* interval
Hypercalcaemia
Hyperkalaemia
Hyperthermia
Vagal stimulation
Digitalis

Differential diagnosis of abnormal T wave and *QT* interval

The abnormalities in the repolarization – especially those related to the T wave and the *QT* interval – seen in patient with coronary artery disease are far from being specific for myocardial ischaemia and injury. They can be normal variants or they can occur in association with several cardiac and non-cardiac diseases and conditions (Tables 38.2 and 38.3). Therefore, the diagnosis of ischaemic heart disease should not be solely based on electrocardiographic findings but must be set in the light of patients' symptoms and clinical manifestations.

References

Cannon, C.P., McCabe, C.H., Stone, P.H. *et al.* (1997) The electrocardiogram predicts one-year outcome of patients with unstable angina and non-Q wave myocardial infarction: results of the TIMI III Registry ECG Ancillary Study. *Journal of the American College of Cardiology*, **30**, 133–40.

Channer, K. & Morris, F. (2002) ABC of clinical electrocardiography. *British Medical Journal*, **321**, 1023–1026.

Davies, M. (1995) Acute coronary thrombosis; the role of plaque disruption and its initiation and prevention. *European Heart Journal*, **16**, 3–7.

Mills, R.M., Young, E., Grolin, R. *et al.* (1975) Natural history of ST segment elevation after acute myocardial infarction. *American Journal of Cardiology*, **35**, 609–616.

Perkiömäki, J.S., Huikuri, H.V., Koistinen, J.M. *et al.* (1997) Heart rate variability and dispersion of QT interval in patients with vulnerability to ventricular tachycardia and ventricular fibrillation after previous myocardial infarction. *Journal of the American College of Cardiology*, **30**, 1331–1338.

Savonitto, S., Ardissino, D., Granger, C.B. *et al.* (1999) Prognostic value of the admission electrocardiogram in acute coronary syndromes *JAMA (Journal of the American Medical Association)*, **281**, 707–713.

Schwartz, P.J. & Wolf, S. (1978) QT interval prolongation as predictor of sudden death in patients with myocardial infarction. *Circulation*, **57**, 1074–1077.

Task Force Report (2000) Management of acute coronary syndromes: acute coronary syndromes without persistent ST segment elevation. *European Heart Journal*, **21**, 1406–1432.

Ward, D.E. (1988) Prolongation of the QT interval as an indicator of risk of a cardiac event. *European Heart Journal*, **9**, 139–144.

Woods, J.D., Laurie, W. & Smith, WG. (1963) The reliability of the electrocardiogram in myocardial infarction. *Lancet*, **ii**, 265–9.

CHAPTER 39

Influence of Rhythm Abnormalities on Ventricular Repolarization

Rory Childers

Introduction

The impact of rhythm abnormalities on ventricular repolarization comprises instances where a change in rate or rhythm induces alteration of ST or T wave polarity, contour, duration, T descent or U wave morphology. Such events may be extrinsic: without change in the physiology of ventricular recovery, or intrinsic: with major change. Not dealt with here are the converse: those instances where changes in repolarization generate arrhythmia (syndromes of Brugada, congenital long QT, etc.; Childers 2001).

Extrinsic influence: the atrial impact

Both depolarization and repolarization of the atrium can impose on T wave configuration. Recognition of the 'buried' P wave, sinus or ectopic, within the T wave, enables the diagnosis of blocked PACs, atrial bigemini, QRS aberration, and ventricular tachycardia. More subtle is the impact of atrial repolarization. The negative T_a wave of sinus rhythm is quite shallow or even invisible in clinical tracings with marked PR interval delay, or complete heart block. But it often imposes on the ST segment in exercise tests. Signified by PR segment depression in the inferolateral leads during stress-induced sinus tachycardia, it can help to achieve ST depression suggestive of ischaemia. As shown in Fig. 39.1, the pause following a PAC, by eliminating PR segment depression, can demonstrate true – as opposed to extrinsically influenced – ST depression (especially in II, aVF, and V4).

More interesting is the T_a wave of low atrial ectopic rhythm or the retrograde P wave (axis: *c.* −90°). The voltage of this T_a wave, a positive hump, greatly exceeds that of the aforesaid negative T_a wave of sinus rhythm. It can inflict ST elevation suggestive of early acute inferior myocardial infarction (Fig. 39.2a). Restoration of sinus rhythm normalizes the ST segment (Fig. 39.2b). The first premature ventricular complexes (PVC) in Fig. 39.3 shows sinus rhythm undisturbed. The second achieves retrograde conduction: the T_a wave of this inverted P creates a shelf on the T wave descent of the PVC, reminiscent of the U-on-T phenomenon. A like infliction is shown in strips 1 and 3 of Fig. 39.4 where the inverted retrograde P wave falls to the right of the junctional QRS. The amplitude of the junctional T wave is enhanced, and a U wave seems to have been unmasked at A. It is absent at B and C which show sinus Ps. Since this sequence follows a postectopic pause, the T-U changes should not be mistaken for the pause-related T amplification and U wave unmasking typifying the electrocardiographic climate of torsades de pointes (see below).

Intrinsic influence: cardiac memory

This name, first coined by M. B. Rosenbaum *et al.* (1982), is associated with a distinct T wave abnormality. After prolonged periods of abnormal ventricular activation, the restored normal sinus beat shows new T wave inversions. The latter display the same spatial directionality as the previously abnormal QRS, as though the latter was *remembered* by the heart. This phenomenon is sometimes called anamnestic inversion of the T wave (anamnesis: recalling to memory, recollection; New Latin from Greek *ana-*, back + *mimneskin*, to call to mind).

Anamnestic T inversion was first noted in repetitive or 'incessant' ventricular tachycardia by Gallavardin (1922). The T wave inversions were also seen following a single bout of ventricular tachycardia, provided it lasted long enough [days, not hours]. The T wave changes lasted days to weeks, according to a review of 26 cases (Smith 1946), and showed the same lead for lead polarity as the tachycardic QRS. Most patients were free of serious heart disease.

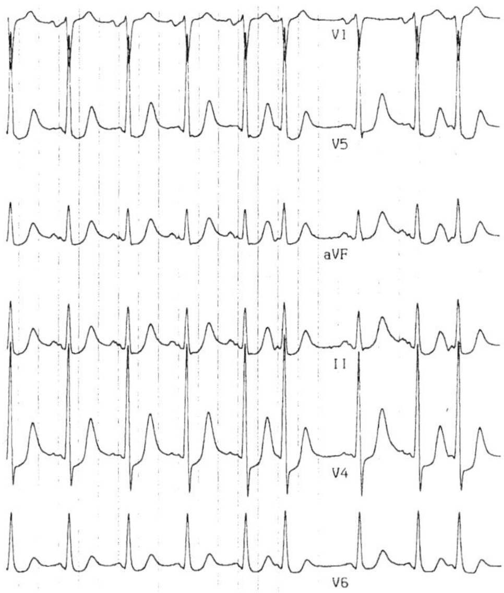

Fig. 39.1 Impact of atrial repolarization on inferolateral ST segment during stress test. The pause after the PAC allows recession of the PR segment depression. The subsequent ST deviation is unencumbered and less depressed.

Cossio *et al.* (1944) noted the same phenomenon with paroxysmal long-duration supraventricular tachycardia provided the latter showed sustained aberration (especially functional bifascicular block) (Kernohan, 1969). The tenacious T wave inversions are sometimes 'giant'. Such cases are not now reported because tachycardias of either sort are not allowed to continue for days, the means for arresting them being substantial.

Chatterjee *et al.* (1969a) noted that 'massive T wave inversion and ST depression occur in the unpaced electrocardiogram subsequent to ventricular pacing, and persist for a varying length of time'. The inversions appeared in those leads, the previously paced QRS of which, was negatively inscribed. Thus with standard transvenous right ventricular apical artificial pacing, spontaneous supraventricular beats like the fourth and fifth beat of Fig. 39.5 will show T inversion in II,

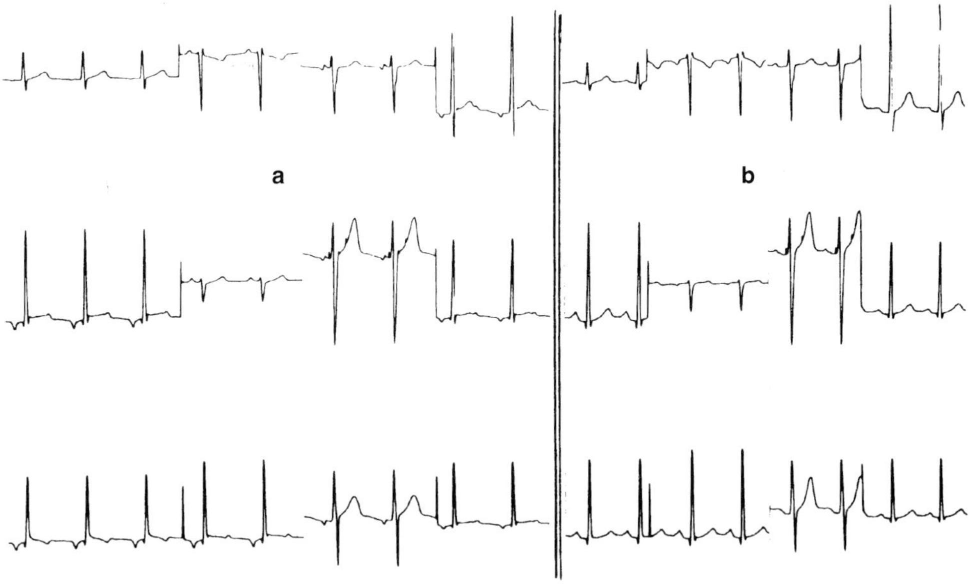

Fig. 39.2 ST elevation due to imposition of atrial repolarization on inferior leads (a); ST normalized by return of NSR (b).

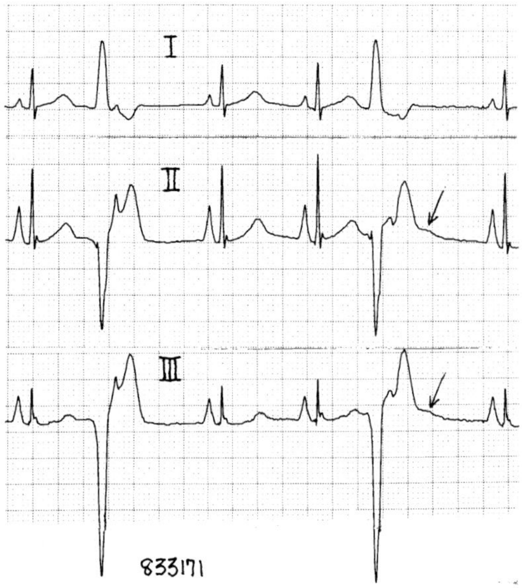

Fig. 39.3 Left, PVC with no disturbance of sinus function; right, PVC with retrograde P. The positive T_a wave of this retrograde emerges as a slanting interruption of the PVCs T wave descent (arrow).

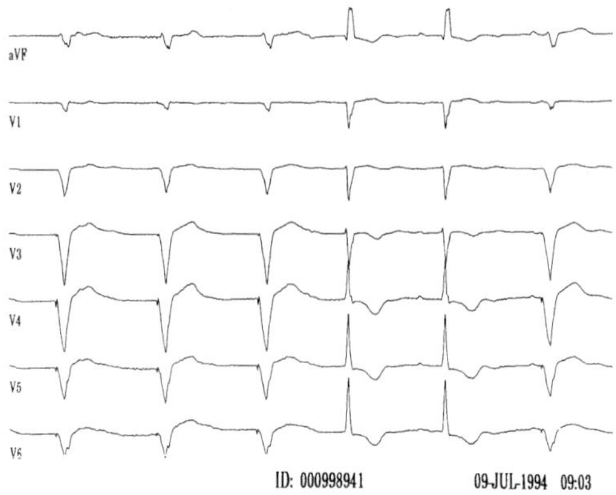

Fig. 39.5 Post-pacing anamnestic T inversion in supraventricular captures. The T wave follows the polarity of the paced QRS.

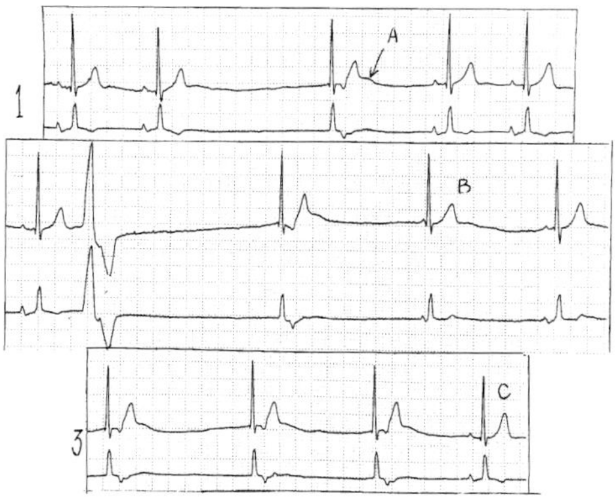

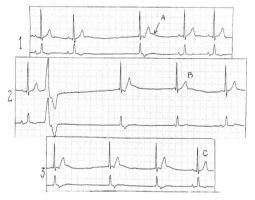

Fig. 39.4 Type II second degree SA block with junctional escape. The retrograde P of the latter has a T_a wave powerful enough to augment the T wave amplitude and simulate the unmasking of a U wave at A. The escape at B, and the sinus beat at C show none of these features.

III, aVF, and V1–V5, and sometimes V6 (Wirtzfeld & Baedeker 1972). Pacing the apex of the right ventricle M. B. Rosenbaum *et al.* (1982) showed that the evolution of the anamnestic T wave could be accelerated by faster pacing rates. The inversion process was very far from complete even after 60 h of pacing. The recovery process of the T wave could likewise be hurried by faster rates. Recovery took 8–38 days. When the outflow tract of the right ventricle, rather than the apex, was paced, creating a 'left bundle branch block (LBBB) morphology' with a vertical, or rightward frontal plane axis, the unpaced T wave showed such an axis, instead of the commoner leftward orientation. Left ventricular pacing sites also showed a concordance of paced QRS with the subsequent unpaced T wave (Lorincz *et al.* 1981).

The post-pacing T wave change is optimally revealed when the unpaced sinus rhythm QRS is of normal duration. The post-pacing T wave change does not have to compete with the secondary T wave changes of bundle branch or bifascicular block. Still to be evaluated (Alves *et al.* 1991): does the push for anamnestic T wave alteration eventually flatten or squash the secondary T waves of ventricular pacing, or execute the frequent massive T wave inversion of idioventricular rhythm in unpaced third degree atrio-ventricular (AV) block (Ippolito *et al.* 1954; Jacobson & Schrire 1966; Warenbourg *et al.* 1969)?

Rosenbaum (M. B. Rosenbaum *et al.* 1968) had noted and Denes *et al.* (1974) confirmed that chronic intermittent LBBB was often associated with right precordial T wave inversion when the QRS normalized (Fig. 39.6). The biplanar directionality of these T waves mirrored that of the QRS during the LBBB, another example of anamnestic T wave. In intermittent right bundle branch block (RBBB), normalization of the QRS

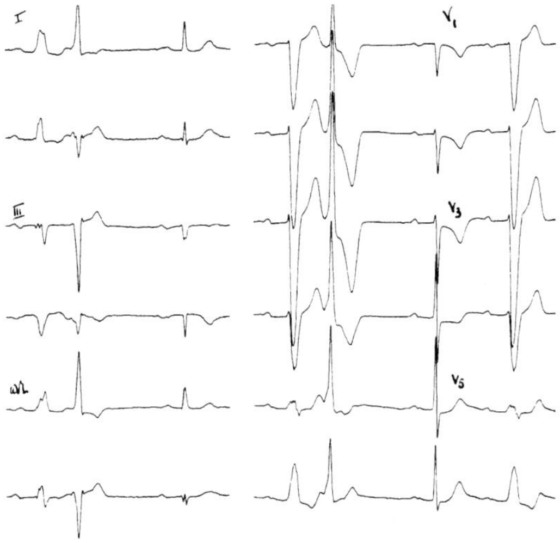

Fig. 39.6 Anamnestic T inversion with intermittent LBBB. The QRS is normalized after the postectopic pauses, but the T follows the polarity of the LBBB QRS complexes.

does not reveal T inversion, but often the positivity of the normal T in $V1_{/2}$ is exaggerated.

In intermittent pre-excitation, whether random or rate-related, antegrade conduction through the accessory pathway becomes functionally blocked, the delta wave disappearing in single, or alternate beats (2/1 pre-excitation), or even for minutes or hours. Nicolai (1966) and Apostolov (1966) noted that T wave inversion was often seen in the normalized beats, specifically in those leads which showed negative delta waves. The same T wave inversion continues to be present 1–3 months after ablation or surgical division (Fig. 39.7) of the accessory tract (Kalbfleisch *et al.* 1991).

To summarize: ectopic stimulation, or eccentric ventricular depolarization, if maintained for a long enough period (or more probably, for some hypothetically critical number of beats), can induce a revision in the values assigned to the basic determinants of the normal upright T wave: the repolarization gradients in action

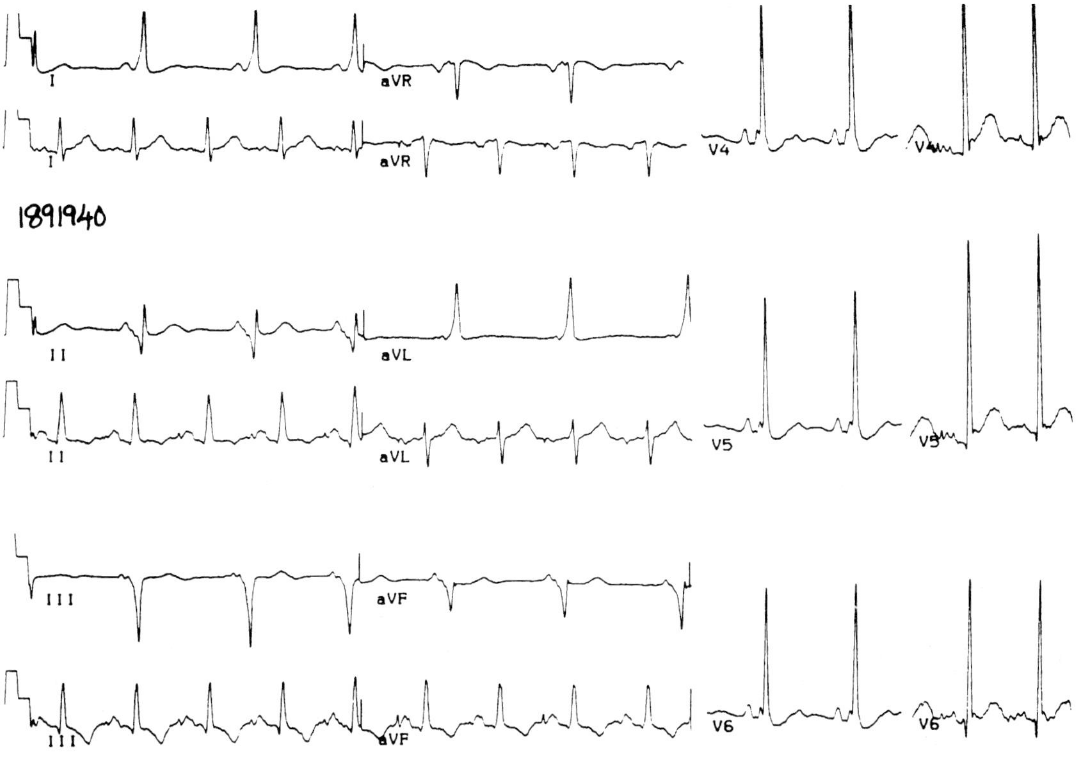

Fig. 39.7 Wolff–Parkinson–White syndrome: nine lead ECG before and after surgical division of the accessory tract. The T of the normalized QRS follows the polarity of the former delta wave, negative in inferior leads.

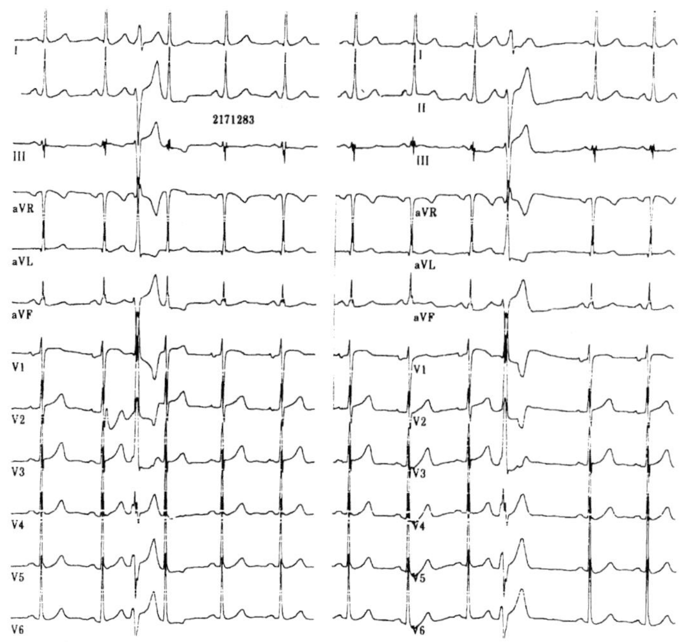

Fig. 39.8 Interpolated PVC: postextrasystolic T wave change obedient to the directionality of the ectopic QRS. The pause after the second PVC disallows change.

potential duration, whether endo-epicardial (Higuchi & Nakaya 1984), or apico-basal (Burgess *et al.* 1972; Spach & Barr 1975) in action potential duration (see below). This revision is sustained *after* the removal of its cause.

Atrial memory

Wijffels *et al.* (1995, 1997) has shown that not only are the atrial action potentials foreshortened during atrial fibrillation, the longer the arrhythmia persists the greater will be the degree and persistence of a shortened atrial refractory period with the return of sinus rhythm. Parenthetically: this physiological state is often associated with a failure in the rate-adaptation of atrial refractoriness (Attuel *et al.* 1982). This phenomenon, termed 'atrial remodelling' in contemporary literature, is essentially an example of atrial memory.

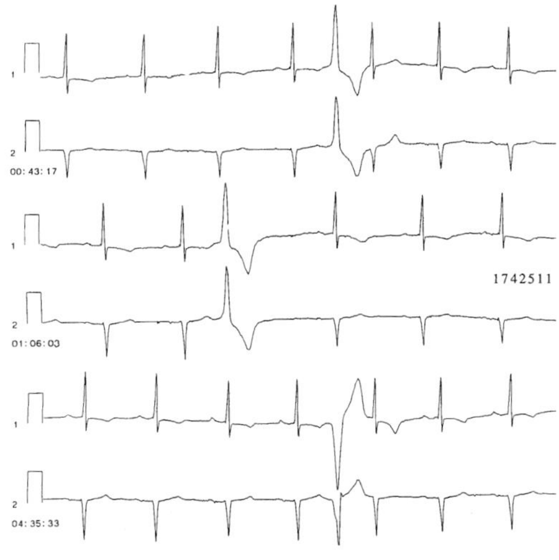

Fig. 39.9 Twin channel Holter. Top and bottom: interpolated PVCs from two foci produce obedient T wave inversion. Middle: PVC with pause has no effect on T wave.

Postextrasystolic T wave inversion or change

First observed by P. D. White in 1915 it is not rare for PVCs to be followed by T inversion in the subsequent sinus beat (Mann & Burchell 1954). It exists in two forms: the T wave subsequent to the PVC may be obedient or nonobedient to the directionality of the ectopic QRS (Meyer & Schmidt 1949; Fagin & Guidot 1958; Edmands & Bailey 1971). The obedient form mirrors, in extraordinary singularity, the postpacing T wave change described above; the two phenomena have been constantly linked, in the literature. Rosenbaum (M. B. Rosenbaum *et al.* 1990) was careful to apply the link only to 'some cases'. The

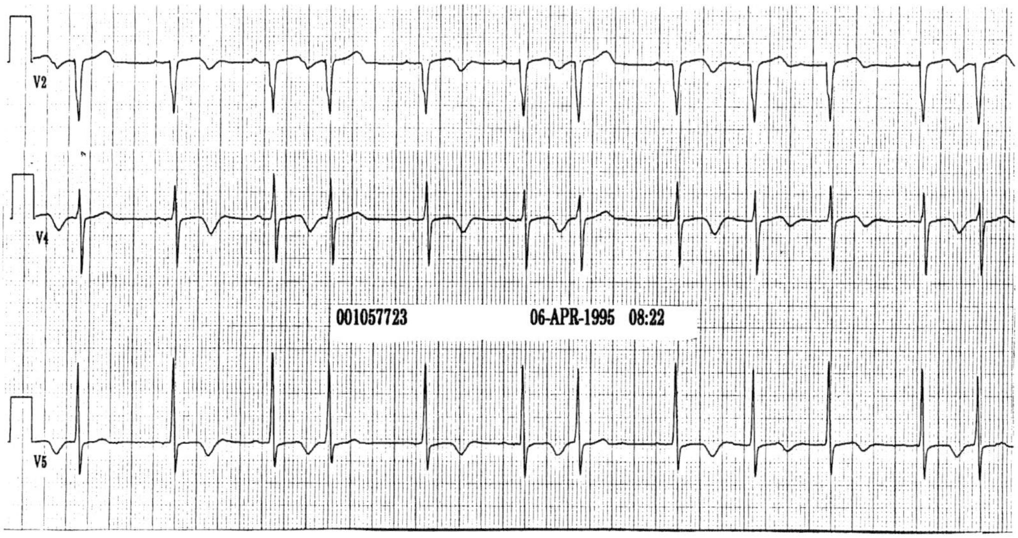

Fig. 39.10 Pause-related T inversion T positive in PACs; depth of inversion varies with previous cycle length.

anamnestic T wave change (Fig.39.8) is seen when the PVC is interpolated, but not when it is followed by a pause (suggesting a short memory span). Rhythm strips may show T waves obedient to more than one ectopic ventricular focus (Fig. 39.9). T wave inversion – obedient or not – is never seen when the ventricular ectopic shows no prematurity as with escapes or fusion beats.

If T wave change after a PVC is nonobedient, failing to show concordance lead for lead with the ectopic QRS, but *does* follow a long postectopic pause, then the T wave inversion is either: (1) purely pause-related (Fig. 39.10), such as those seen after PACs or any long cycle (Scherf 1944); or (2) purely postextrasystolic, where the depth of inversion depends not on the length of the pause but on the prematurity of the preceding single or multiple extrasystole(s). T inversion can sometimes be seen in the wake of both PVCs and PACs, in the same rhythm strip. In Fig. 39.11 the postectopic T inversion is more marked after the PAC than the PVC because the PAC is more closely coupled (the pauses are of equal length). If T inversion is seen after a PVC, but not after any other similar pause, it may be purely postextrasystolic. In the Holter, pause-related T inversion generally appears and then disappears, sometimes even when the cycle structure or heart rate, remains the same. It suggests that the phenomenon may somehow require to be 'turned on' or facilitated,by other influences, such as vagal tone (Litovsky & Antzelevitch 1991). Pause-related T inversion has probably been ignored in the Holter literature because the inversions are modest; and there is sometimes uncertainty as to whether T change is the result of an alteration in the R/S ratio of the QRS. The T wave changes can be quite striking: in the atrial fibrillation of Fig. 39.12, the longer the cycle, the deeper the inversion.

Although *in vitro* studies in the past have addressed the issue of abrupt change in cycle length (Greenspan *et al.* 1967) the focus has been on the impact of the acutely altered cycle length on subsequent AP duration, and alternans, There has not as yet been any study of the differential effect of closely coupled premature depolarization(s) on subsequent endo-epicardial repolarization gradients.

In examining the nature of anamnestic or pause-related T wave change, one must first examine the reasons for its normal concordancy with the QRS.

T wave positivity: the endo-epicardial gradient

Although bilateral activation of the Purkinje network by the sinus impulse causes endocardial action potentials to be initiated in advance of the epicardial, the latter finish first, because they are shorter in duration (Burgess *et al.* 1972; Spach & Barr 1975). Endocardial action potentials are longer because of the electrotonic influence of the anastomosing Purkinje fibres (which have

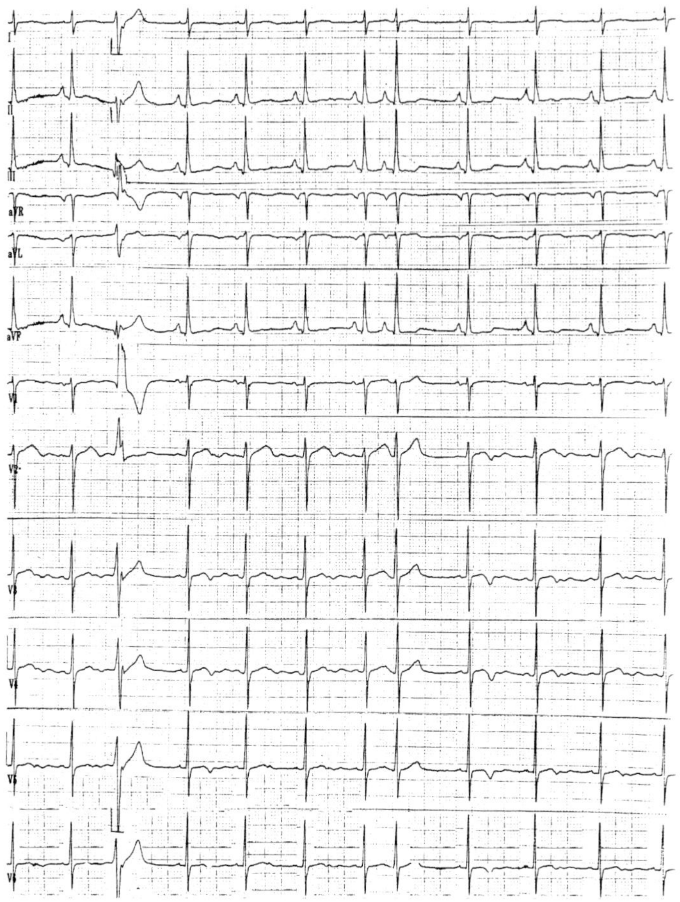

Fig. 39.11 Postextrasystolic T inversion more marked after PAC than PVC because of tighter coupling.

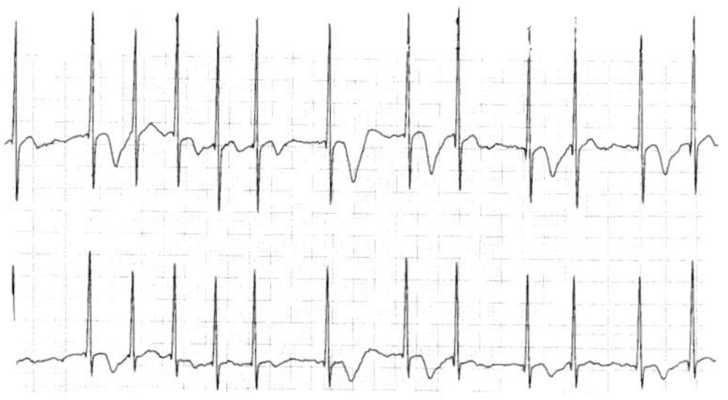

Fig. 39.12 Pause-related T inversion in atrial fibrillation: the longer the cycle the deeper the T wave.

the longest repolarization phase of any cardiac tissue) and the 0.6° cooler temperature in the left ventricular cavity (Reynolds & Yu 1964). Cooling dog epicardium so lengthens the *surface* action potentials that the T wave inverts (Higuchi & Nagaya 1984). Endocardial action potentials have to be longer than epicardial by a time interval equal (at least) to the transmural conduction time, and approximating 10% of the action potential duration (Barr 1989). The greater the disparity between epicardial and endocardial action potential termination, the taller the T wave, especially in V4/5. The amplitude of the latter can be increased thus by shortening the epicardial or lengthening the endocardial action potentials, or by a reduction in the transmural conduction time, or by combinations of these. In simple terms, maintenance of the endo-epicardial gradient requires epicardial repolarization to start last, and finish first (Reynolds & Vander Ark 1959).

T wave positivity: the apico-basal gradient

While the apex is activated early, and the basal muscle activated last, repolarization is completed first at the base, and last at the apex (Spach & Barr 1975). Muscle is thickest at the base, thinnest at the apex. Purkinje fibres are absent at the base, and dense at the apex. The sequence of repolarization is achieved, in the face of these anatomic strictures, by the Purkinje-rich apex having the longest of all endocardial and epicardial action potentials; the short transmural conduction time effectively maintains the endo-epicardial gradient. Intraoperative data show the same apico-basal gradient in humans (Cowan *et al.* 1988).

T wave amplitude and polarity: summary

The amplitude and polarity of the sinus T wave (as examined in V5) can thus be altered by: (1) exaggeration or minimising of physiological repolarization gradients; (2) by rearranging the sequence in which regional locations in the ventricle finish repolarization. Such rearrangements occur when local depolarization is late in starting, when repolarization is locally prolonged, or both (e.g. with ischaemia/infarction).

Previous cycle length and AP duration: usual presumptions

Postponing the issue of 'cumulative effect' of frequency, the duration of ventricular action potentials varies directly with previous cycle length, or the previous diastolic period (Vick 1971). The majority of studies have assumed that the slopes relating endocardial and epicardial action potential duration to rate or previous cycle length are approximately parallel, thus maintaining, at a wide range of heart rates or cycle lengths, the endo-epicardial gradient. In most normal and abnormal 12-lead ECGs, this assumption finds support in the striking constancy of the T wave, which retains the same amplitude and polarity in the face of abrupt change in cycle length (with fidelity greater than might be anticipated by *in vitro* studies of such) (D. S. Rosenbaum *et al.* 1991)

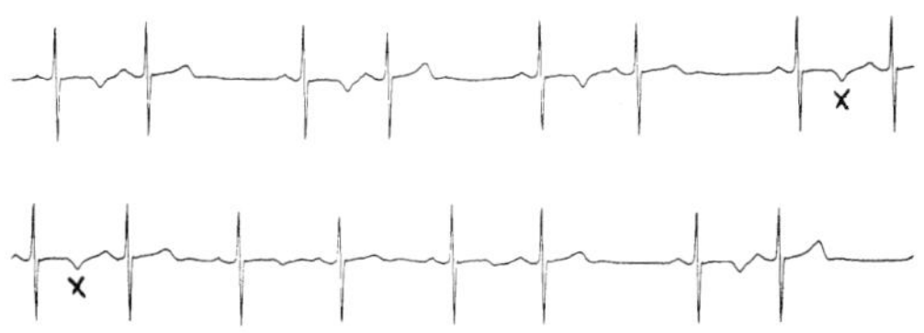

Fig. 39.13 Pause-related T inversion. X marks the same beat continued in bottom strip.

Clinical pause-related T inversion

In pause-related T inversion, the inversion is often seen in every sinus beat, restitution being immediate and inevitable in every PAC (Fig. 39.13). Almost postulating the inversion as a variant physiological state, the explanation for it was demonstrated by the Utica group (Litovsky & Antzelevitch 1988, 1989; Sicouri & Antzelevitch 1991). They showed, in endocardium and subepicardium (Fig. 39.14), that the respective curves relating cycle length to action potential duration, far from remaining parallel, intersect or 'cross-over' at the upper right slow or 'long cycle' end of the slope. The epicardial and subepicardial curves show the spike and dome shape characteristic of the transient outward current (It_o) and retain greater linearity of slope than that of endocardium, which without It_o flattens out at long cycles, enabling the cross-over.

Canine vs. clinical pause-related T inversion

The relative infrequency in humans of a phenomenon found quite regularly in the tissues of the dog heart (the aforementioned cross-over) suggests that the transient outward current, which drives these physiological gradients, may clinically be (1) physiologically blocked or not 'turned on', or (2) only demonstrable following

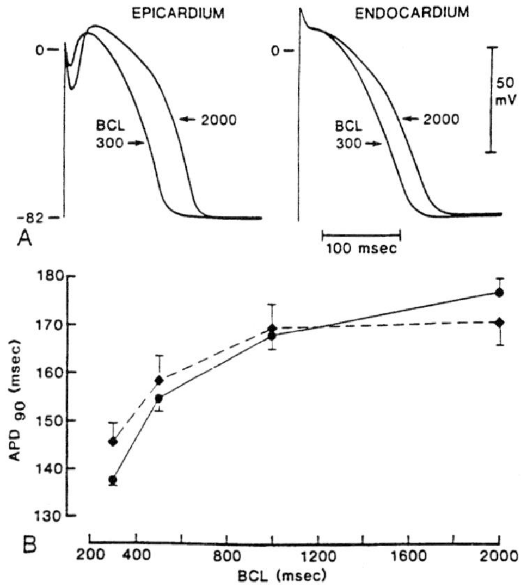

Fig. 39.14 Endo- and epicardial action potential durations plotted against cycle length. (From Litovsky & Antzelevitch 1989, with permission.)

exceptionally long pauses (e.g. > 2000 ms), or (3) precociously evident in this particular canine tissue preparation (which among other features, has no tonic autonomic influence). On the other hand monophasic APs with phase 1 notches and spike-and-dome shape have demonstrated the presence of It_o in human epicardium during cardiac surgery (Cowan *et al.* 1988). It_o is less active with fast rates and completely inactive with markedly premature depolarization. Hence in labile T wave states restitution is common with tachycardia and T inversion rare in PACs. Since It_o activity lowers the amplitude of phase 0 of the AP, PACs may show taller R waves and increased T wave voltage as in Fig. 39.11, yet another means by which rhythm can influence repolarization. There are no studies regarding cardiac status or outcome in cases where either postextrasystolic or pause-related T wave change have been demonstrated.

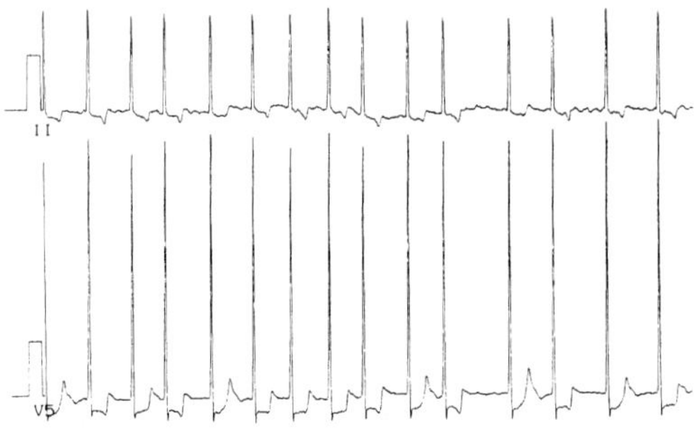

Fig. 39.15 Atrial fibrillation: longer cycles show terminal T wave restitution. J point depression is unchanged.

Other cycle length or rate-related changes in repolarization

Uncommonly one sees: (1) T wave normalization after long pauses (Fig. 39.15); (2) T wave inversions or less overt abnormalities exaggerated by ordinary or accelerated rates; (3) very rare T inversions exaggerated by PACs, and labelled 'the Ashman phenomenon of the T wave' by Akiyama *et al.* (1989); (4) T wave alternation, generally transient, following a PVC (Childers 1966); (5) pure tachycardia-related ST depression: often the cause of false positive stress tests, the diagnosis is secured when the arrest of a paroxysmal tachycardia is recorded (Fig. 39.16). The ST depression is seen to acutely diminish or disappear in the first and second sinus escape beats (ischaemic ST depression would take 12 beats to 30 s to clear).

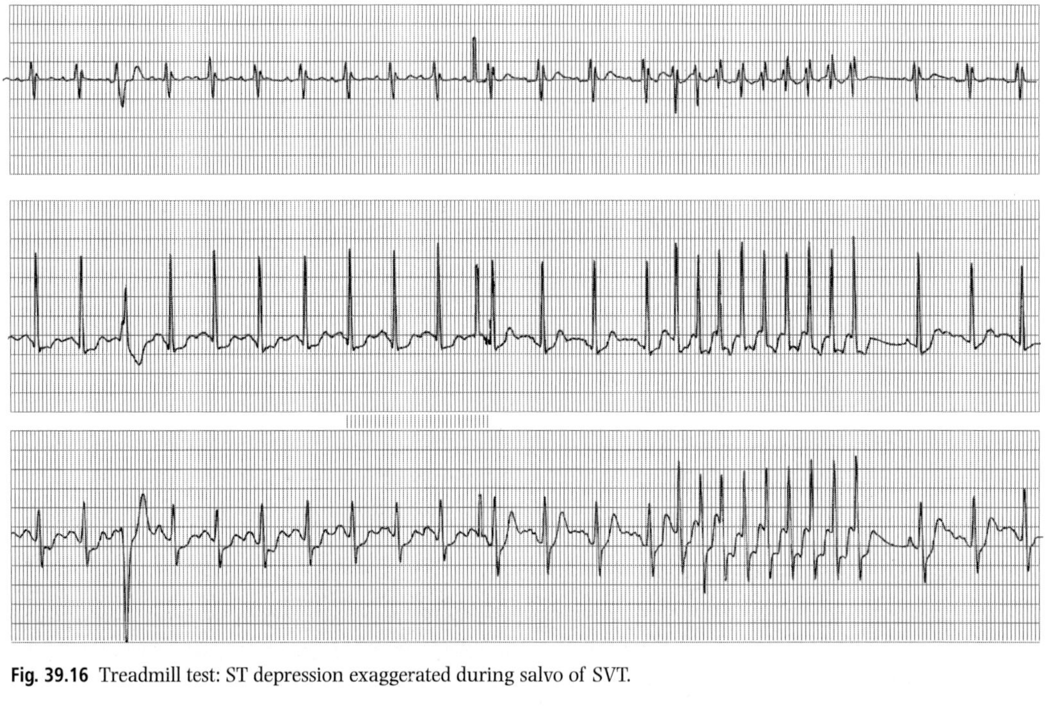

Fig. 39.16 Treadmill test: ST depression exaggerated during salvo of SVT.

Recognizable causes of rate or cycle-related ST–TU change

In atrial fibrillation the ST segment depression of digitalis effect becomes more marked with rapid rates (Fig. 39.17). In hypokalaemia (K^+ = 2.4 mEq/L in Fig. 39.18) U wave amplitude is markedly augmented following a pause, often rendering it larger than the T itself. The paroxysmal tachycardia in Fig. 39.18 shows ST depressions with slope reversal which would otherwise – for example in a treadmill stress test – be counted as 'positive for ischaemia'; this hypokalaemia-related depression is absent in the sinus escape beat. Unstudied is the clinical significance of postextrasystolic ST segment depression during a treadmill exercise test (Fig. 39.19). With the gross QT prolongation of severe hypocalcaemia sustained T wave alternans may be instigated by a premature beat, or by a pause. One may see variable depth of inversion in the deeper of the alternating T waves (Fig. 39.20). These in turn may give rise to spontaneous PVCs, to torsades de pointes, to monomorphic or polymorphic ventricular tachycardia, or to fibrillation and death.

Possible mechanisms of anamnestic repolarization

The ability of the ventricle to remember previous depolarizations can be demonstrated by measuring the refractory period generated by a programmed pause, and comparing the values obtained when this pause is preceded first by slow then by rapid pacing, and by pacing at the same cycle length as the pause. If previous cycle length was the sole determinant of action potential duration all three values would be the same. But actually rapid pacing hysteretically shortens refractoriness. The ventricle in fact remembers a remarkable number of depolarizations; final stabilization may require 100 or more beats (Janse *et al.* 1969). This example is the nearest likeness to anamnestic depolarization. But the memory extends for minutes, not weeks.

Rosen's group have invoked the transient outward current as the major participant in the mechanism of cardiac memory (Del Balzo & Rosen 1992; Geller & Rosen 1993). Costard-Jackle *et al.* (1989), using the monophasic action potential recordings, demonstrated the 'remembered' downstream shortening of the refractory period at distanced remote from the site of stimulation

Clinical impact of the anamnestic T wave

The anamnestic T wave often confounds the possibility of recognizing injury, acute pericar-

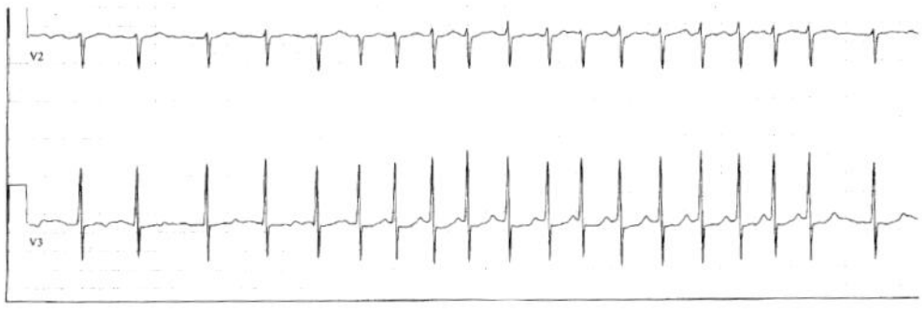

Fig. 39.17 Atrial fibrillation. Digitalis effect accentuated with increased rates.

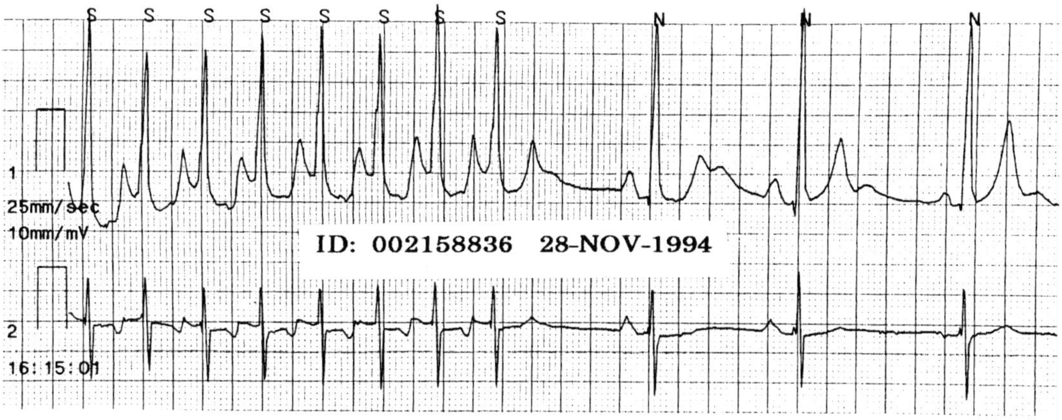

Fig. 39.18 Arrest of paroxysmal SVT; hypokalaemia (K^+ 2.3 mEq/L.). U wave accentuation in first sinus beat: instantaneous disappearance of ST depression

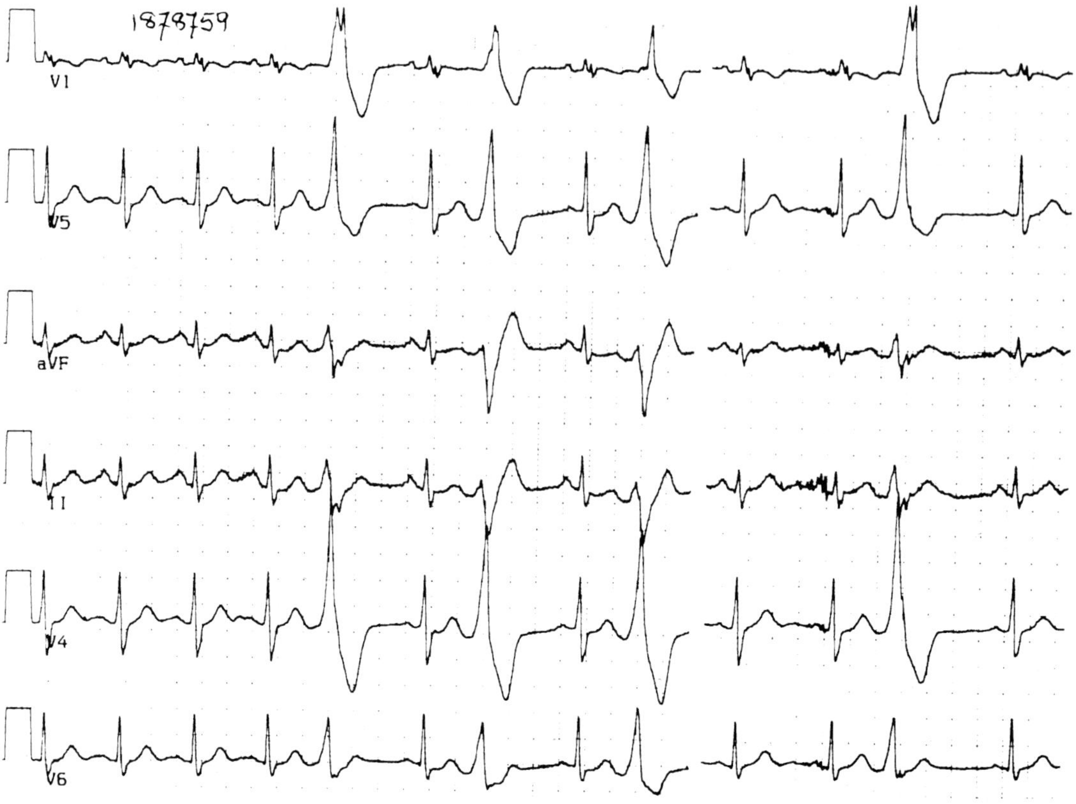

Fig. 39.19 Treadmill stress test: postextrasystolic ST depression during exercise. Absent during rest at right.

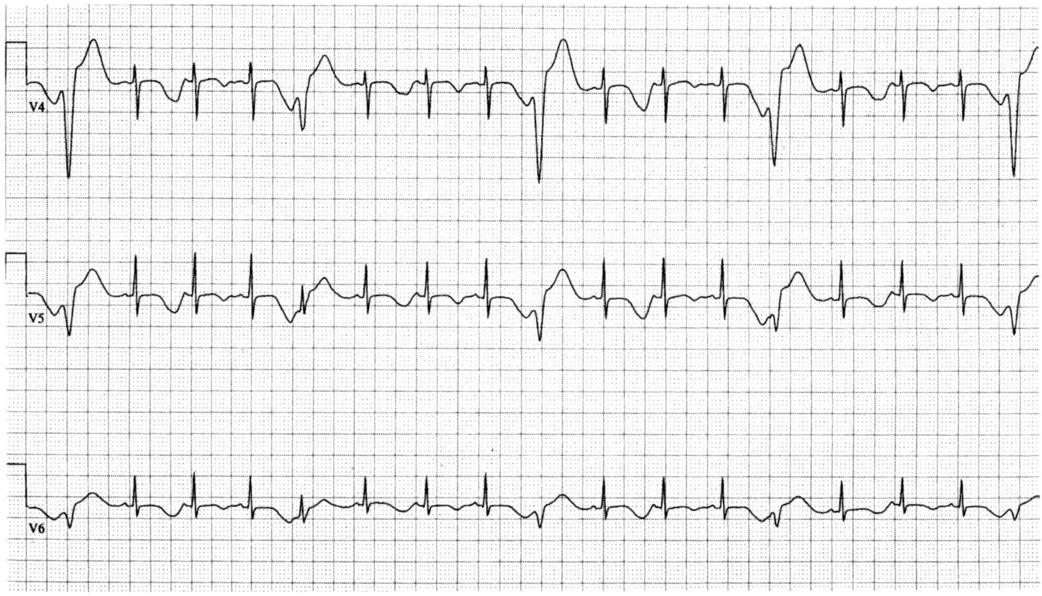

Fig. 39.20 T wave alternans: terminal liver failure with severe hypocalcaemia. The deeper of the T wave inversions in II and V5 show a longer *QT* and generate PVCs.

ditis, ischaemia and acute non-Q wave MI in paced patients, or those with intermittent pre-excitation or LBBB. The T inversions may be of the 'giant' type, but generally without QT prolongation.

Pause-related perturbations of repolarization: climate of torsades de pointes

The triggering event in the common form of torsades is a pause, often induced by a PAC or PVC. The voltage of the T wave (Fig. 39.21) or U wave of the subsequent (generally sinus) beat becomes exaggerated (Jackman *et al.*1988). Figure 39.22 shows in the top two single lead rhythm strips a quinidine-prolonged *QT* interval and a post-PVC enhancement of the depth of T wave inversion. In the bottom twin channel, arrows show the unmasking of a U wave. In a minority of cases, exclusively in the wake of the said pauses, the U wave appears for the first time (Jackman *et al.* 1984). This U wave is probably an early afterdepolarization or EAD (EADs are the hallmark of one type of *triggered automaticity* in which a hump or upward deflection emerges out of the action potential phase 3 descent before it reaches the baseline). A freshly lengthened *QT* interval in this context is the collective expression at the body surface of nonthreshold-attaining EADs developing in a sufficiently large number of myocytes (Childers 1995). In the patient illus-

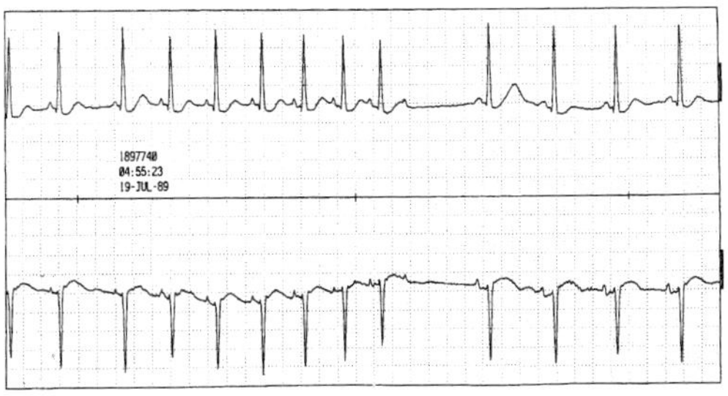

Fig. 39.21 Electrocardiographic climate of torsades de pointes. Arrest of salvo of atrial tachycardia: short-long structure augments T wave.

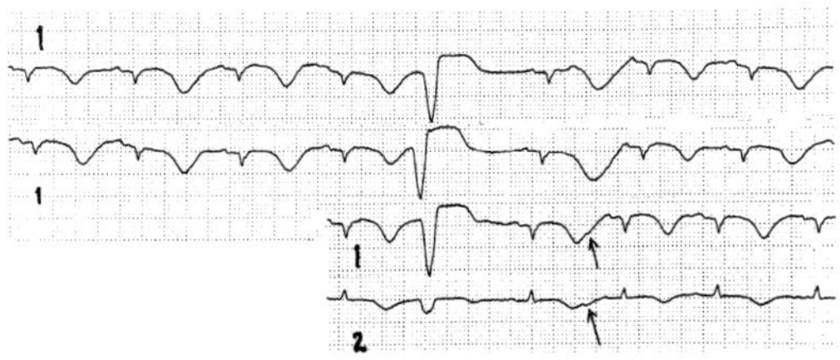

Fig. 39.22 Postectopic pause-related T wave enhancement and U wave unmasking during quinidine administration

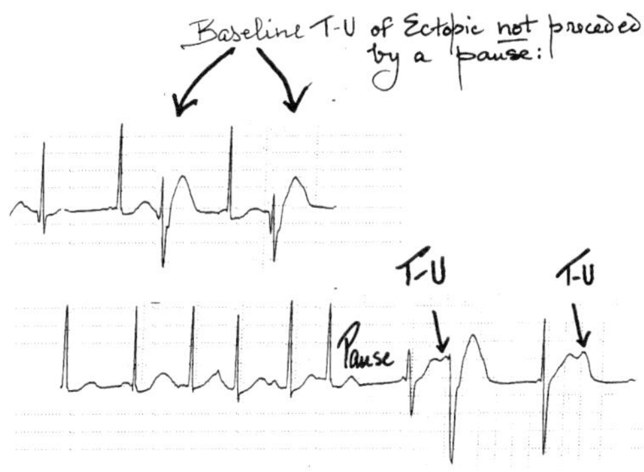

Fig. 39.23 Electrocardiographic climate of torsades de pointes. Baseline PVCs with suggestion of U wave on T descent of 2nd. As a ventricular escape, the same ectopic after a pause shows prominent U wave (T–U arrows)

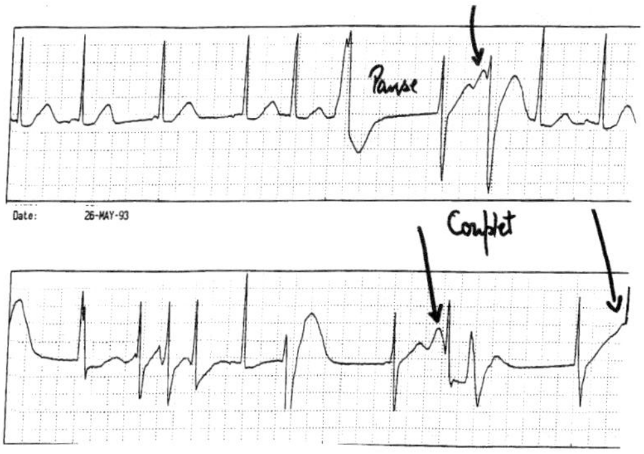

Fig. 39.24 Same case as Fig. 39.23. Arrows indicate pause-related grotesque exaggeration of the U wave of the ectopic triggering singlet or couplet PVCs.

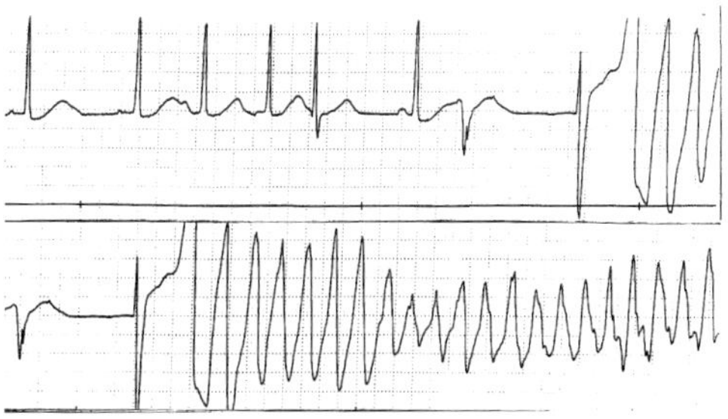

Fig. 39.25 Same case as Fig. 39.24. Pause-related triggering of torsades de pointes.

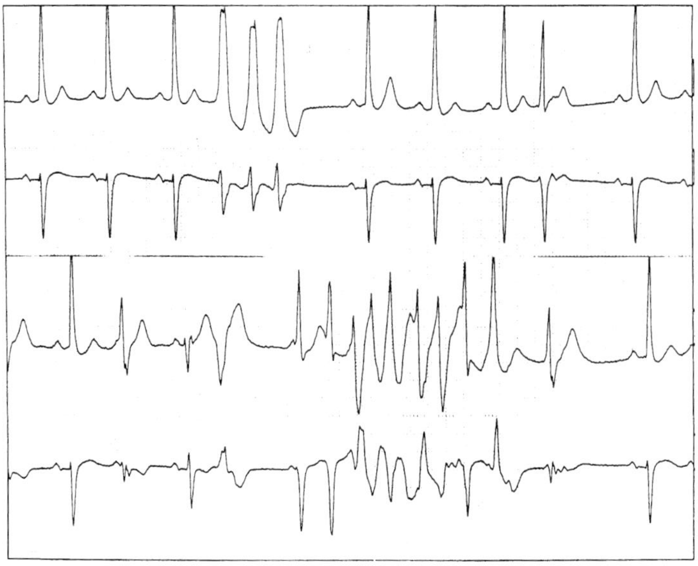

Fig. 39.26 Climate of torsades de pointes in twin-channel Holter. Top, pause-related T wave augmentation is greater after the triplet than the singlet; bottom, short torsade.

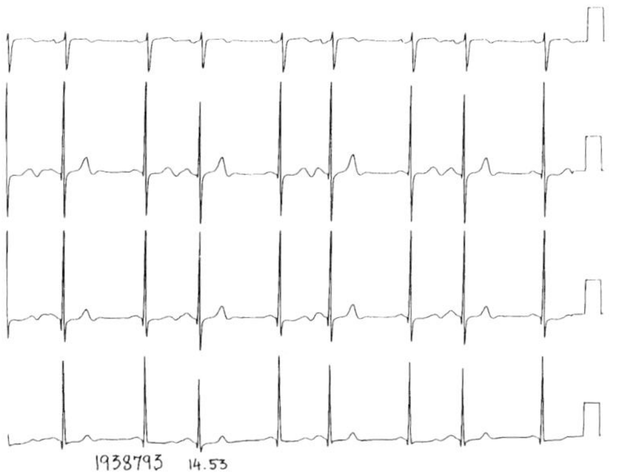

Fig. 39.27 3/2 second degree SA block type I. Pause-related amplification of U at the expense of T. Rectification of T follows the short cycle.

trated in Fig. 39.23 a ventricular ectopic is, at baseline, seen twice as a PVC; the second one displays a slight U wave hump on the T descent. As a ventricular escape after pauses, this same ectopic develops gross unmasking of a U wave (T-U arrows). In Fig. 39.24 the U wave (arrows) is in places enormous and grotesque, often generating another ectopic or couplet. In Fig. 39.25 torsades de pointes finally develops. The patient was on quinidine and had hypokalaemia.

Often both T and U are enhanced but optimally seen in different leads. Pause-dependent T or U enhancement does not presage torsades, even though it appears to be a requisite for its advent. As phenomena adjacent to salvos of torsades, they constitute the electrocardiographic climate of the tachycardia. If an EAD reaches threshold, a PVC will appear. If this process becomes regenerative, each ectopic producing yet another threshold-attaining EAD, torsades de pointes is the result (Coumel 1990). Torsades de pointes is more likely to appear when QT prolongation is attended by some degree of rounded ST depression.

Assuming a constant pre-pause rate, the amplitude of TU enhancement varies directly with the length of the pause. The longer the pause the greater the amplitude of the EAD and the U. For a given long pause after a PVC U wave growth is increased by the prematurity of the PVC. Figure 39.26 shows that two or three tightly coupled ectopy are more provocative than the one on the right These factors – ectopic prematurity and length of pause – spell out the essential *short–long* recipe for T-U enhancement and torsades de pointes (Locati 1996). These features have been emphasized in acquired QT syndrome, but are also sometimes seen in the congenital long QT syndrome. In a given lead the U may be enhanced at the expense of the T (Fig. 39.27). The major difference between

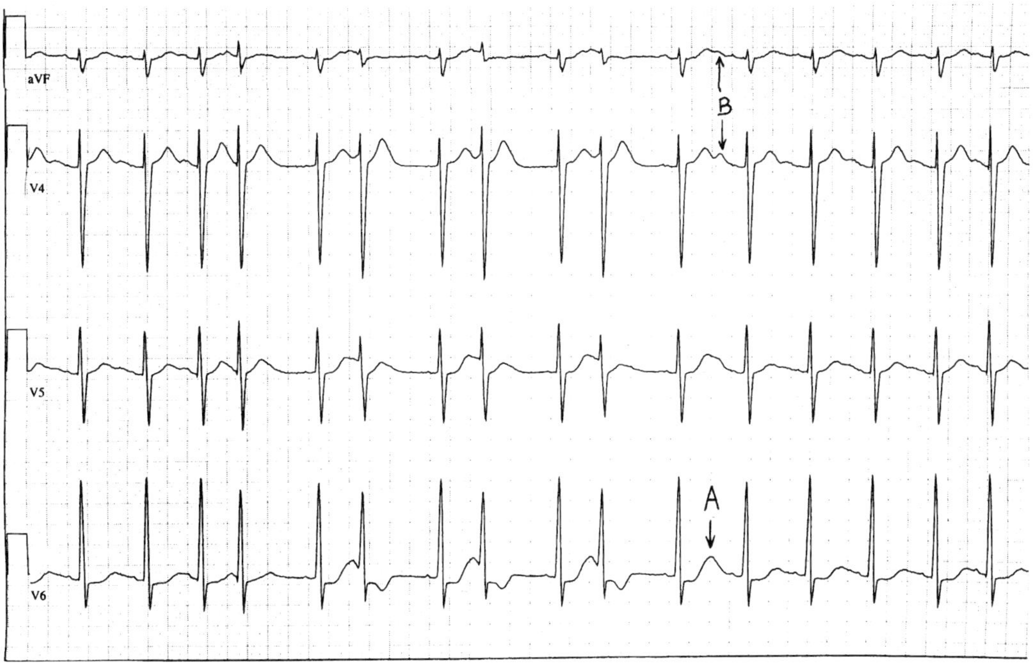

Fig. 39.28 Climate of torsades de pointes; leads II, V2–V4. The baseline T and U waves are seen in the first 2 and last 3 beats. The pauses following the PACs cause gross T wave augmentation and unmask the U wave (arrows). Patient on i.v. erythromycin with a K^+ of 2.4 mEq/L and a calcium of 7.0 mg/dL.

pre-tachycardic augmented T-U of acquired and congenital long QT is in the shape and energy distribution of the repolarization segment. In the latter the voltage is often greater in the post-pause beat towards the termination of its long *QT* interval; in the former the *QT* is less prolonged and the maximal amplitude is in the middle of the interval.

Figure 39.28 shows four leads of a routinely taken tracing which exhibits the typical electrocardiographic climate of torsades de pointes. The ECG has all the warning features of impending torsades de pointes. The control T and U waves are seen in the first two and the last three beats. The pauses following the PACs cause gross T wave augmentation and U wave unmasking (arrows). The recipe for torsades de pointes was very completely satisfied: a patient being treated for pneumonia with intravenous erythromycin, had depletion of both potassium and calcium. The tracing permitted the service to be warned.

In Fig. 39.29 there is a gross increment of T wave voltage following the long cycles. The pauses marked 'B' are terminated with the inverted P of a low atrial escape. The explanation for T enhancement might be attributed entirely to superpositioning or elision of the atrial escape's repolarizing hump or T_a wave. However, pause A is terminated by a different P wave – a fusion of atrial escape and sinus P – and the sub-

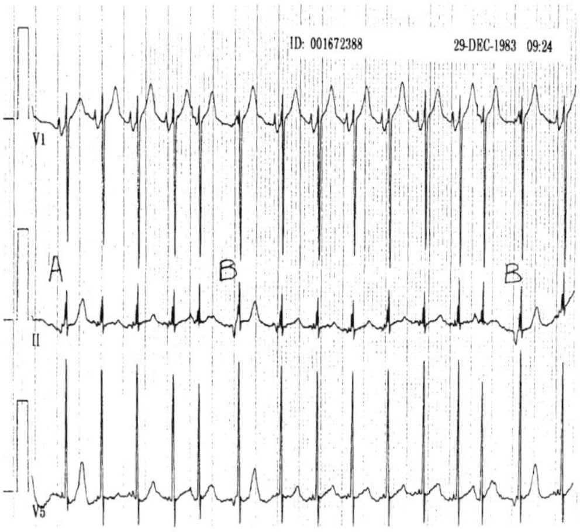

Fig. 39.29 Large T waves after pauses generated by PACs. The pauses are terminated by low atrial escapes. T enhancement due to atrial repolarization *and* pause-related T wave enhancement.

sequent T is enhanced like all the others suggesting a second additive influence on repolarization: the climate of torsades.

Pause-related TU boosting vs. pause-related T wave inversion

In the climate of torsades de pointes the augmentation of T or U in the wake of a pause is always in the same direction as the nonaugmented deflection. Inversions will get deeper but fresh inversions are not induced. The main potential source of confusion is with obedient postextrasystolic T wave change. Any lead in which the QRS of the PVC is positive will command enhanced subsequent T wave voltage augmentation. But if the PVC is interpolated it excludes the torsades context because no pause has been generated. The presence of *QT* prolongation favours the latter, particularly in the beat enhanced by the pause. Additionally, obedient postextrasystolic change does not unmask U waves or cause them to grow.

References

Akiyama, T., Richeson, J.F., Faillace, R.T., Lockhart, J. & Scherer, J.C. (1989) Ashman phenomenon of the T wave. *American Journal of Cardiology*, **63**, 886.

Alves, P.A., Ribeiro, J.C., Sabino, M., De Souza, O. & Maia, I.G. (1991) Cardiac memory in patients with permanent artificial pacemakers. *Arquivos Brasileiros de Cardiologia*, **57**, 207.

Apostolov, L. (1966) Su una nuova prova farmacologica nella sindrome di Wolff–Parkinson–White. *Minerva Medica*, **58**, 216

Attuel, P., Childers, R., Cochenez, B., Poveda, J., Mugica, J. & Coumel, P. (1982). Failure in the rate-adaptation of the atrial refractory period: its relationship to vulnerability. *International Journal of Cardiology*, **2**, 179–197.

Barr, R.C. (1989) Genesis of the electrocardiogram. In: *Comprehensive Electrocardiology*, Vol. 1 (eds P. W. MacFarlane & T. D. V. Lawrie), p.145. Pergamon, New York.

Burgess, M.J., Green, L.S., Millar, K., Wyatt, R. & Abildskov, J.A. (1972) The sequence of normal ventricular recovery. *American Heart Journal*, **84**, 660

Chatterjee, K., Harris, A., Davies, G. & Leatham, A. (1969) Electrocardiographic changes subsequent to artificial ventricular depolarization. *British Heart Journal*, **31**, 770.

Chatterjee, K., Harris, A.M. & Davies, J.G. (1969) T wave changes after artificial pacing. *Lancet*, **1**, 759.

Childers, R.W (1966) Usefulness of extrasystoles in cardiac diagnosis and prognosis. *Medical Clinics of North America*, **50**, 51–71.

Childers, R.W (1995) Time related perturbations in repolarization. *Journal of Electrocardiology*, **28**, 124.

Childers, R.W (2001) Arrhythmia risk assessment: the 12 lead electrocardiogram. In: *Risk of Arrhythmia and Sudden Death* (ed. M. Malik). BMJ Books, London

Cossio, P., Vodoya, R. & Borconsky, L. (1944) Modificaciones del electrocardiograma despues de ciertas crisis de taquicardia paroxistica. *Revista Argentina de Cardiologia*, **11**, 164.

Costard-Jackle, A., Goetsch, B., Antz, M. & Franz, M.R. (1989) Slow and long-lasting modulation of myocardial repolarization produced by ectopic activation in isolated rabbit hearts. Evidence for cardiac 'memory'. *Circulation*, **80**, 1412.

Coumel, P. (1990) Early after-depolarization and triggered activity in clinical arrhythmias. In: *Cardiac Electrophysiology. A Textbook* (eds M. J. Rosen, M. J. Janse, & A. L. Wit), p.387. Futura Publishing, Mount Kizko, NY.

Cowan, J.C., Hilton, C.J., Griffiths, C.J. *et al.* (1988) Sequence of epicardial repolarization and configuration of the T wave. *British Heart Journal*, **60**, 424: fig. 2.

Del Balzo, U. & Rosen, M.R. (1992) T wave changes persisting after ventricular pacing in canine heart are altered by 4-aminopyridine but not by lidocaine, *Circulation*, **85**, 1464.

Denes, P., Pick, A., Miller, R.H., Pietras, R.J. & Rosen, K.M. (1978) A characteristic precordial repolarization abnormality with intermittent left bundle branch block. *Annals of Internal Medicine*, **89**, 55.

Edmands, R.E., Bailey, J.C. (1971) The post-extrasystolic T wave change. *American Journal of Cardiology*, **28**, 536–540.

Fagin, I.D. & Guidot, J.M. (1958) Post-extrasystolic T wave changes. *American Journal of Cardiology*, **1**, 597.

Gallavardin, L. (1922) Extrasystolie ventriculaire à paroxysmes taquicardiques prolongés. *Archives des Maladies du Coeur et des Vaisseaux*, **15**, 298.

Geller, J.C. & Rosen, M.R. (1993) Persistent changes after alteration of the ventricular activation sequence. *Circulation*, **88**, 1811–1819.

Greenspan, K., Edmands, R.E. & Fisch, C. (1967) Effects of cycle length alteration on canine cardiac action potentials. *American Journal of Physiology*, **212**, 1416.

Higuchi, T. & Nakaya, Y. (1984) T wave polarity related to the repolarization process of epicardial and endocardial ventricular surfaces. *American Heart Journal*, **108**, 290.

Ippolito, T.L., Blier, J.S. & Fox, T.T. (1954) Massive T wave inversion. *American Heart Journal*, **48**, 88.

Jackman, W.M., Clark, M., Friday, K.J. *et al.* (1984) Ventricular tachyarrhythmias in the long QT syndrome. *Medical Clinics or North America*, **68**, 1079.

Jackman, W.M., Friday, K.J., Anderson, J.L., Aliot, E.M., Clark, M. & Lazzara, R. (1988) The long QT syndrome a critical review, new clinical observations and a unifying hypothesis. *Progress in Cardiovascular Diseases*, **31**, 115.

Jacobson, D. & Schrire, V. Giant T wave inversion associated with Stokes–Adams syncope. *South African Medical Journal*, 1966;31:206.

Janse, M.J., van der Steen, A.B.M., van Dam, R. Th. & Durrer, D. (1969) Refractory period of the dog's ventricular myocardium following sudden changes in frequency. *Circulation Research*, **24**, 251.

Kalbfleisch, S.J., Sousa, J., El-Atassi, R., Calkins, H., Langberg, J. & Morady, F. (1991) Repolarization abnormalities after catheter ablation of accessory atrioventricular connections with radiofrequency current. *Journal of the American College of Cardiology*, **18**, 1761.

Kernohan, R.J. (1969) Post-paroxysmal tachycardia syndrome. *British Heart Journal*, **31**, 803.

Litovsky, S.H. & Antzelevitch, C. (1988) Transient outward current prominent in canine ventricular epicardium but not endocardium. *Circulation Research*, **62**, 116.

Litovsky, S.H. & Antzelevitch, C. (1989) Rate-dependence of action potential duration and refractoriness in canine ventricular endocardium differs from that of epicardium role of the transient outward current. *Journal of the American College of Cardiology*, **14**, 1053.

Litovsky, S.H. & Antzelevitch, C. (1991) Differences in the electrophysiological response of canine ventricular subendocardium and subepicardium to acetylcholine and isoproterenol. *Circulation Research*, **67**, 615.

Locati, E.H. (1996) Torsades de pointes In: *Noninvasive Electrocardiology* (eds A. J. Moss & S. Stern), p.59. W. B. Saunders, Philadelphia.

Lorincz, I., Worum, F., Kovacs, P., Polgar, P., Worum, I. & Gomory, A. (1981) Different localization of ST segment and T wave abnormalities during permanent pacing. In: *Electrocardiology '81, Proceedings of the Eighth International Congress on Electrocardiology* (ed. P. L. Antoloczy), p.393. Akademiai Kiado, Budapest.

Mann, R.H. & Burchell, H.B. (1954) The significance of T wave inversion following ventricular extrasystoles. *American Heart Journal*, **47**, 504.

Meyer, P. & Schmidt, C.L. (1949) Troubles post-extrasystoliques de la repolarization. *Archives des Maladies du Coeur et des Vaisseaux*, **42**, 1175.

Nicolai, P. (1966) Le syndrome de Wolff–Parkinson–White. In: *Les Cahiers de Medicographie*, p. 35. Servier, Suresnes.

Reynolds, E.W., Jr & Yu, P.N. (1964) Transmural temperature gradient in dog and man. *Circulation Research*, **15**, 110.

Reynolds, E.W. & Vander Ark, C.R. (1959) An experimental study on the origin of T waves based on determinations of effective refractory period from epicardial and endocardial aspects of the ventricle. *Circulation Research*, **7**, 943.

Rosenbaum, D.S., Kaplan, D.T., Kanai, A. *et al.* (1991) Repolarization inhomogeneities in ventricular myocardium change dynamically with abrupt cycle length shortening. *Circulation* **84**, 1333.

Rosenbaum, M.B., Blanco, H.H. & Elizari, M.V. (1990) Electrocardiographic characteristics and main causes of pseudoprimary T wave changes. *Annals of the New York Academy of Sciences*, **601**, 35.

Rosenbaum, M.B., Blanco, H.H., Elizari, M.V., Lazzari, J.O. & Davidenko, J.M. (1982) Electrotonic modulation of the T wave and cardiac memory. *American Journal of Cardiology*, **50**, 213.

Rosenbaum, M.B.,Elizari, M.V. & Lazzari, J.O. (1968) *Los Hemibloqueos*, 464. Paidos, Buenos Aires.

Scherf, D. (1944) Alterations in the form of the T waves with changes in heart rate. *American Heart Journal*, **28**, 332.

Sicouri, S. & Antzelevitch, C. (1991) A subpopulation of cells with unique electrophysiological properties in the deep subepicardium of the canine ventricle; The M cell. *Circulation Research*, **68**, 1729.

Smith, L.B. (1946) Paroxysmal ventricular tachycardia followed by electrocardiographic syndrome. *American Heart Journal*, **32**, 257.

Spach, M. & Barr, R.C. (1975) Ventricular intramural and epicardial potential distributions during ventricular activation and repolarization in the intact dog. *Circulation Research*, **37**, 243.

Vick, R.L. (1971) Action potential duration in canine Purkinje tissue effects of preceding excitation. *Journal of Electrocardiology*, **4**, 105.

Warenbourg, H., Pauchant, M., Ducloux, G. *et al.* (1969) Les troubles de repolarization ventriculaire des blocks auriculo-ventriculaires complets. Les inversions 'massives' de l'onde T. *Archives des Maladies du Coeur et des Vaisseaux*, **62**, 1219.

White, P.D. (1915) Alternation of the pulse: a common clinical condition. *American Journal of Medicine, Science*, **150**, 82.

Wijffels, M.C., Kirchhof, C.J, Dorland, R. & Allessie, M.A. (1995) Atrial fibrillation begets atrial fibrillation. A study in awake chronically instrumented goats. *Circulation*, **92**, 1954.

Wijffels, M.C., Kirchhof, C.J., Dorland, R., Power, J. & Allessie, M.A. (1997) Electrical remodeling due to atrial fibrillation in chronically instrumented conscious goats: roles of neurohumoral changes, ischaemia, atrial stretch, and high rate of electrical activation. *Circulation*, **96**, 3710

Wirtzfeld, A. & Baedecker, W. (1972) T-Wellen-Negativierung nach Schrittmacherimplantation *Zeitschrift für Kreislaufforchung*, **61**, 828.

CHAPTER 40

Dynamics of Acquired long QT Syndrome

Elijah R. Behr and A. John Camm

Introduction

The acquired long QT syndrome (LQTS) is defined as abnormal prolongation of ventricular repolarization as manifested on the surface electrocardiogram (ECG) by *QT* prolongation, T wave abnormalities and/or ventricular arrhythmias (specifically torsades de pointes [TdP]). It must not be solely due to the mutations responsible for congenital long QT syndrome. It is most commonly secondary to certain cardiac and non-cardiac drugs with myocardial electrophysiological side effects (Table 40.1). Pharmacological blockade of the rapid inward rectifying current (I_{Kr}) is the usual mechanism responsible for drug-induced prolongation of repolarization (Viskin 1999) but blockade of the slow rectifier (I_{Ks}) or activation of the inward sodium current may also be responsible.

The impact on cardiac electrophysiology of arrhythmogenic (or torsadogenic) agents then depends on their concentration and potency as well as other properties such as concomitant channel blockade or effects on autonomic function. Drug concentration is increased either due to excess intake (e.g. overdose) and/or decreased elimination (e.g. renal and/or liver failure) (Yap & Camm 1999). The presence of hepatic enzyme inhibitors (e.g. ketoconazole, erythromycin and grapefruit juice) decreases drug metabolism and hence increases concentrations and the attendant risk of cardiac side effects (Yap & Camm 1999). Drug-induced *QT* prolongation and TdP can occur either alone or in conjunction with other pathologies that may also be responsible for acquired LQTS in their own right. These include structural cardiac disease (e.g. left ventricular hypertrophy, cardiomyopathies and ischaemic heart disease), metabolic abnormalities (e.g. hypokalaemia, hypomagnesaemia and hypocalcaemia), ECG abnormalities (e.g. bradycardia and conduction disease) and specific conditions (e.g. liver disease, diabetes mellitus, obesity and anorexia nervosa) (Table 40.2) (Ben-David & Zipes 1993; Viskin 1999). There may also be an underlying genetic predisposition to acquired LQTS secondary to mutations and polymorphisms of the cardiac ion channels implicated in the congenital long QT syndrome (Donger *et al.* 1997; Napolitano *et al.* 1997; Wei & *et al.* 1999a,b; Makita *et al.* 2002; Yang *et al.* 2002). Due to reduced expression, these patients' electrocardiograms do not demonstrate abnormalities of repolarization (the 'forme fruste') until exposure to an appropriate agent (Donger *et al.* 1997; Priori *et al.* 1999) and/or the occurrence of other cofactors such as bradycardia or hypokalaemia (Yap & Camm 1999).

This chapter deals with the ECG changes associated with acquired LQTS, particularly drug-induced, by describing T/U wave features (changes in T/U wave morphology and T wave alternans), rate-related features of the *QT* interval itself (*QT* prolongation and the QT/RR relationship), the short–long–short initiation of TdP and delayed events ('late' proarrhythmia).

T/U wave morphology

Changes in T wave morphology, sometimes without any *QT* prolongation, are common in acquired LQTS (Fig. 40.1). Novel measures of T wave morphology such as the total cosine R-to-T (TCRT), T wave loop dispersion and T wave

Table 40.1 A list of potentially proarrhythmic agents that prolong the *QT* interval to varying degrees with or without documented torsades de pointes

Antiarrhythmics	Class I: quinidine, procainamide, disopyramide, ajmaline, encainide*, flecainide, propafenone, pirmenol, cibenzoline, dihydroquinidine
	Class III: amiodarone, sotalol, *d*-sotalol*, bretylium, dofetilide, almokalant*, azimilide, ibutilide, nifekalant, dronedarone, ersentilide, E4031, terikalant, sematilide.
Anti-anginals/ vasodilators	Prenylamine*, terodiline*, lidoflazine*, ranolazine Bepridil, tedisamil
Anti-hypertensives	Nicardipine, isradipine
	Moexipril/hydrochlorthiazide, indapamide
Antihistamines	Terfenadine*, astemizole*, diphenhydramine, hydroxyzine, azelastine (loratadine, ebastine, and cetirizine uncertain)
Serotonin agonists and antagonists	Cisapride*, ketanserin*
	Ondansetron, granisetron, dolasetron
Antimicrobials	Erythromycin, clarithromycin, spiramycin, telithromycin
	Cotrimoxazole
	Ketoconazole, fluconazole (caution with itraconazole)
	Trimethoprim sulphamethoxazole (bactrim), pentamidine
	Sparfloxacin, gatifloxacin, grepafloxacin*, levofloxacin, moxifloxacin
Antiviral	Foscarnet (HIV)
Antimalarials	Quinine, chloroquine, halofantrine, amantidine
Psychiatric drugs	Tricyclic antidepressants: amitriptyline, nortriptyline, desipramine, clomipramine, imipramine, doxepin, protriptyline, trimipramine
	Phenothiazines: thioridazine*, chlorpromazine, trifluoperazine, prochlorperazine, fluphenazine
	Others: haloperidol, droperidol*, pericycline, sertindole, pimozide, fluoxetine, venlafaxine, trazodone, mesoridazine, quetiapine, risperidone, citalopram, ziprasidone, zimelidine, maprotiline, chloral hydrate, lithium, paroxetine
Anticonvulsant	Felbamate, fosphenytoin (prodrug of phenytoin)
Anti-migraine	Naratriptan, sumatriptan, zolmitriptan
Anti-cancer	Arsenic trioxide, tacrolimus, tamoxifen,
Others	Organophosphates, probucol, vasopressin, domperidone, levomethadyl, octreotide, salmeterol, tizanidine, ritodrine, cocaine, methadone, midodrine

* Withdrawn or suspended.

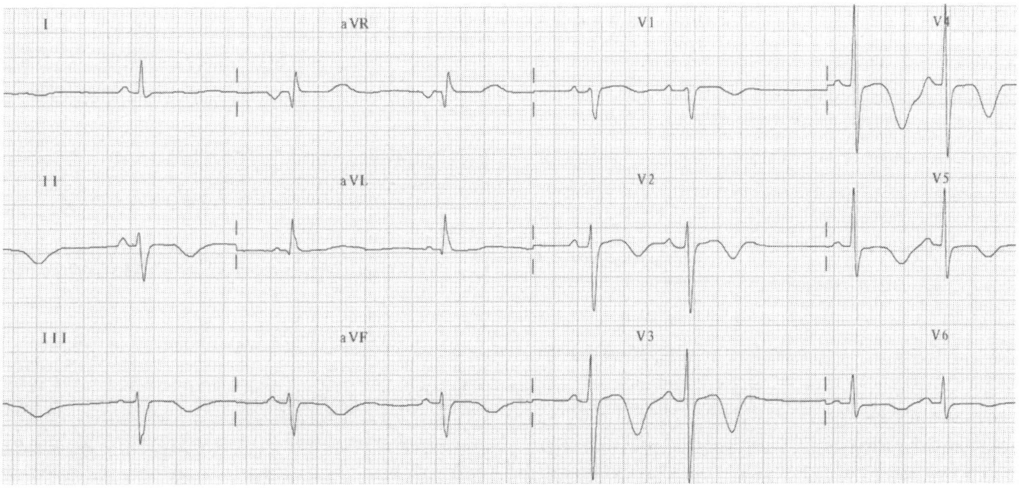

Fig. 40.1 12-lead electrocardiogram of 65-year-old man with thioridazine associated torsades de pointes. The *QT* interval is significantly prolonged and associated with marked T wave inversion throughout the precordial leads accompanied by some changes in morphology consistent with T wave alternans.

Table 40.2 Structural causes and cofactors in acquired LQTS*

Patient profile	*Female*
Electrolyte abnormalities	Hypokalaemia Hypomagnesaemia Hypocalcaemia
Drugs	See Table 40.1 Imidazole antifungals Macrolide antibiotics Grapefruit juice
Cardiac disease	'forme fruste' LQTS Bradycardias: sinus and AV block Ischaemic heart disease Cardiomyopathy Hypertension Myocarditis Myocardial hypertrophy Valvular disease
Cerebrovascular diseases	Intracranial haemorrhage Subarachnoid haemorrhage Stroke
Systemic conditions	Liver disease Renal disease Hypothyroidism Diabetes Obesity
ECG parameters on drug therapy	QT prolongation T/U wave abnormality Increased QT dispersion Sequential bilateral bundle branch block Ventricular ectopics

* Derived from Yap & Camm (1999).

residuum have been suggested as useful independent predictors of sudden death probably secondary to acquired abnormal repolarization in post-myocardial infarction patients and US veterans with cardiovascular disease (Zabel & Malik 2002). Changes in T wave morphology are often associated with U waves (Fig. 40.2; see also Fig. 40.4) the presence of which is thought to be a better predictor of the onset of TdP in acquired LQTS than the *QT* interval itself (Jackman *et al.* 1988; Roden 1993). The U wave may blend with the T wave to form a T/U wave particularly in the precordial leads, which may confuse measurement of the *QT* interval. The amplitude of the T wave tends to decrease as the amplitude of the associated U wave increases (Jackman *et al.* 1988). The end of the U wave is then used to mark the end of the *QT/U* interval. Otherwise the U wave should be ignored in *QT* interval measurement (Jackman *et al.* 1988).

T wave alternans

Changes in T wave morphology, axis and even reversal of polarity can occur from beat-to-beat in acquired LQTS in a similar fashion to the congenital form (Tan & Wilde 1998). This is known as T wave alternans (TWA) (Figs 40.3 and 40.4) and is thought to warn of impending TdP. A study of the cardioversion of atrial fibrillation by almokalant, a class III antiarrhythmic and I_{Kr} blocker, suggested that T wave alternans both before infusion and during infusion was a significant predictor of the development of TdP (Houltz *et al.* 1998). TWA can also occur with minimal variation in T wave amplitude and morphology that cannot be visualized (microvolt TWA) but can be evaluated using specific analyses of Holter monitoring or high fidelity ECG recordings. Patients with coronary artery disease can demonstrate this feature with a similar frequency to congenital long QT syndrome patients but with lower amplitudes, shorter associated *RR* intervals and more transient patterns (Burattini *et al.* 1998).

Sometimes the amplitude of the U wave that forms part of the T/U wave complex can oscillate demonstrating sudden bizarre changes in T/U wave morphology (Fig. 40.4) and manifesting as gross U wave alternans, also a predictor of risk of TdP development (Jackman *et al.* 1988). The circumstances associated usually include metabolic disturbance (hypokalaemia, hypocalcaemia and hypomagnesaemia) with background cardiac and/or renal disease (Jackman *et al.* 1988).

QT prolongation and QT/RR behaviour

The *QT* interval in acquired LQTS classically demonstrates 'significant prolongation' despite correction for heart rate (*QTc*) and is associated with an increased risk of the development of TdP. For example, patients developing TdP early in an infusion of almokalant exhibit greater *QT* prolongation compared to unaffected drug-exposed individuals (Houltz *et al.* 1998). This risk is usually only appreciable in drug-induced LQTS if

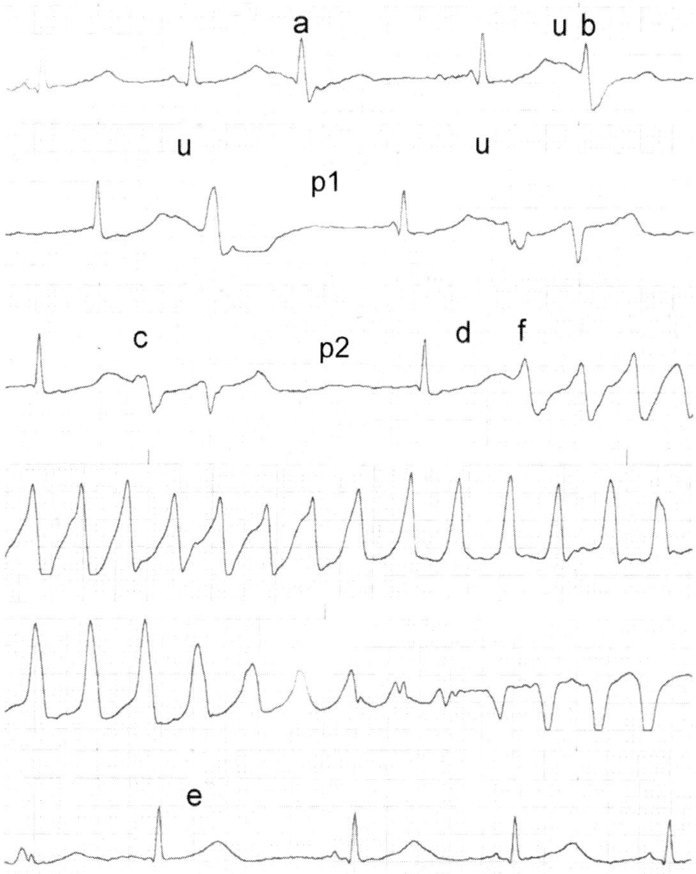

Fig. 40.2 Electrocardiographic trace of 60-year-old man with renal failure and receiving intravenous erythromycin. The 'cascade phenomenon' is shown with an initial supraventricular ectopic (a) inducing a pause followed by late-coupled ventricular extrasystoles (b). More complex arrhythmia are generated (c) until torsades de pointes intervenes (f) when the preceding post-pause supraventricular extrasystole reaches a critically prolonged *QT* interval (d). Once the tachycardia settles the *QT* interval appears to normalise (e). Abnormal U waves are marked with (u). The increasing prolongation of pauses preceding TdP is demonstrated by (p1) and (p2).

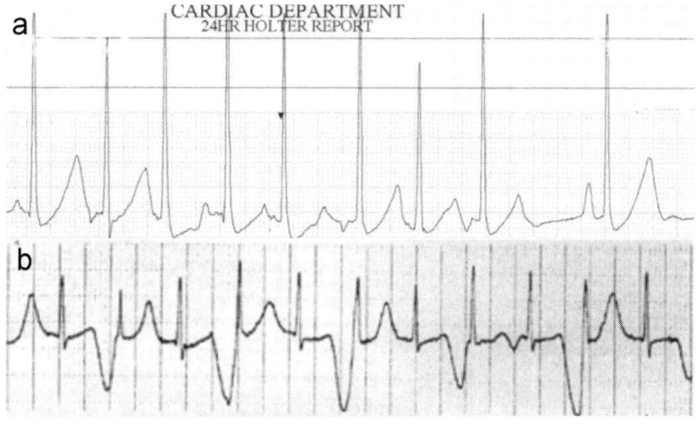

Fig. 40.3 Examples of T wave alternans (a) moderate variation of T wave morphology during a run of supraventricular tachycardia. (b) gross alternans with reversal of T wave polarity. (Part (b) reproduced from Roden *et al.* 1996, with permission of AHA Publishing.)

the *QTc* is >500 ms (Bednar *et al.* 2001). Different agents, however, have different propensities for causing TdP. For example, amiodarone is well known to cause *QT* prolongation, similar to quinidine. It, however, has a significantly lower incidence of TdP (Hohnloser *et al.* 1994) probably due to its additional actions that include non-competitive adrenergic antagonism as well as I_{Ks}, sodium and calcium channel blockade (Nattel 2000). A study of patients who were receiving

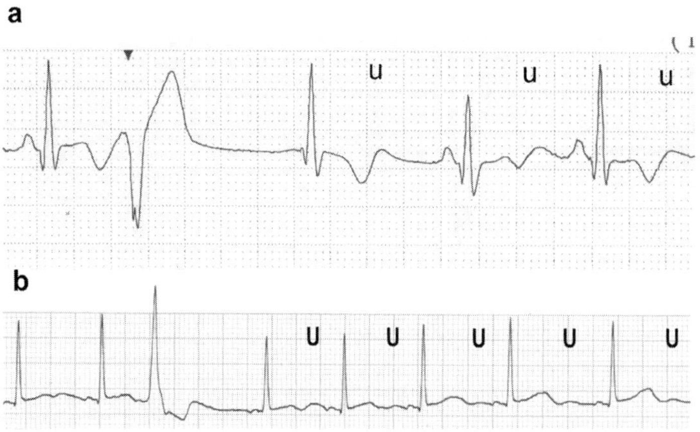

Fig. 40.4 (a) Combined T and U wave alternans associated with a ventricular extrasystole. (b) More subtle U wave variation induced by a ventricular extrasystole. (u) indicates the U wave.

class Ia antiarrhythmics and amiodarone consecutively for arrhythmia suppression demonstrated comparable drug-induced increases in *QTc* interval. Class Ia agents, however, also caused increases in QT dispersion and the incidence of TdP that were not apparent when amiodarone was prescribed in the same patients (Hii *et al.* 1992).

Often, though, *QT* and/or *QTc* prolongation will not be evident on a resting ECG even though myocardial repolarization may be abnormal. Prolongation of the *QT* interval can be precipitated, however, in the first spontaneous sinus complex after an ectopic beat that causes a pause (Fig. 40.2a), the basis for the short–long–short sequence (Roden 1993). Rate correction of the *QT* interval (see later) can be difficult owing to the presence of such ectopics but the absolute value will be prolonged abnormally. The abnormal beat is usually accompanied by T wave abnormalities (Roden 1993).

Because the absolute *QT* interval varies with heart rate it must be corrected, as mentioned above, to establish whether prolongation is drug-related or rate-related. This is most commonly performed using Bazett's and occasionally Fridericia's formulae that adjust the *QT* to a standardized value when the *RR* interval is 1 s (rate = 60 beats/min). Unfortunately the *QTc* when calculated in this manner is not a constant, Bazzet's formula resulting in an overcorrection for bradycardia and an undercorrection for tachycardia (Fig. 40.5) (Sheridan 2000). The limitations of this commonly used methodology must be appreciated until more accurate algorithms replace it.

Other methods for detecting subtle abnormalities of repolarization have been used including analysis of the *QT* interval at different heart rates to uncover inappropriate prolongation. This has become increasingly sophisticated with the use of beat to beat analysis on Holter monitoring and QT/RR regression curves to examine the dynamics of ECG changes. Dofetilide, a potent I_{Kr} blocker, has been examined in this way by comparing Holter monitor data in patients on and off the drug (Lande *et al.* 1998). The QT/RR regression curve demonstrated an increase in slope as well as a general increase in *QT* interval associated with the presence of the drug whether at low or high dose. Thus at shorter *RR* intervals the increase in the *QT* interval was present and significant but not as great as at longer *RR* intervals, i.e. associated with bradycardia. This is described as reverse rate dependence (Lande *et al.* 1998). Halofantrine, an antimalarial with known I_{Kr} blocking effects and a cause of TdP, has been studied in patients with uncomplicated *Plasmodium falciparum* malaria. Holter monitors provided beat-to-beat *QT* and *RR* data and this was compared to Holters from control patients. The *QTc* correlated to drug concentration and the QT/RR regression slope was significantly increased, also demonstrating reverse rate dependence (Touze *et al.* 2002). Quinidine, an antiarrhythmic with I_{Kr}, I_{Ks} and sodium current blocking characteristics, also has similar QT/RR properties (Cappato *et al.* 1993). Figure 40.6

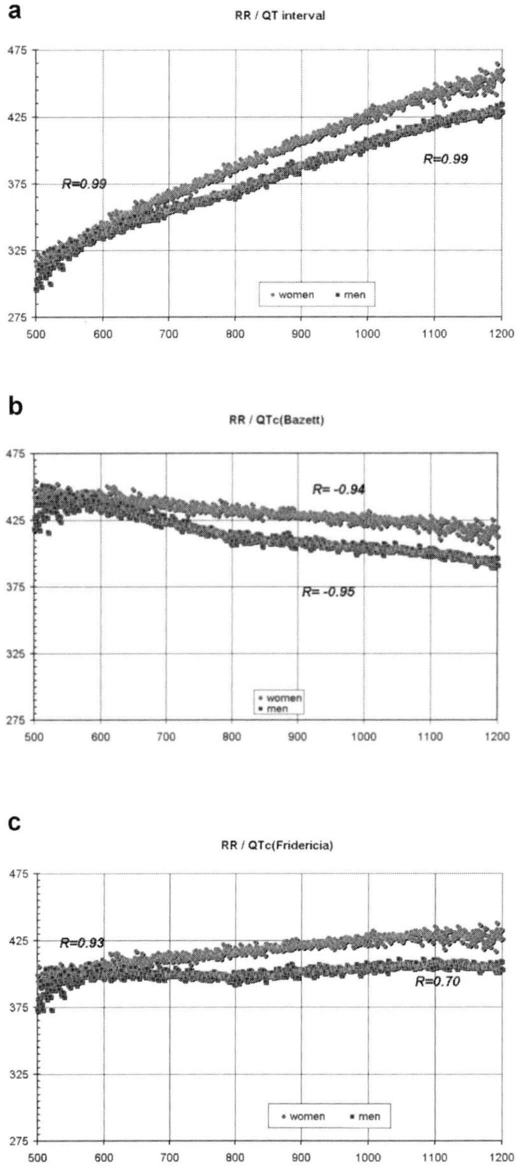

Fig. 40.5 Linear regression between *RR* interval and *QT* interval (a) and *QTc* interval calculated with Bazett's formula (b) and Fridericia's formula (c) in men and women showing positive correlation in (a), negative correlation in (b) and less strong positive correlation in (c). *QTc* is therefore not a constant when calculated with either formula although Fridericia's formula appears a more ideal correction method. Unpublished data courtesy of Dr V Batchvarov, Cardiological Sciences, St. George's Hospital Medical School, London.

demonstrates the increase in slope of the QT/RR regression curve associated with antihistamine-induced acquired LQTS in a 58-year-old woman compared to the drug-free state a few days later (Maison-Blanche & Coumel 1997).

Patients with hypertrophic cardiomyopathy (HCM) taking amiodarone have been studied compared to a mixed population of HCM patients (half high risk and half low risk) not taking amiodarone (Fei *et al.* 1994). Amiodarone caused significant *QT* and *QTc* prolongation but the slope of the QT/RR regression line was not affected (Fei *et al.* 1994). Analysis of the HCM patient group not on amiodarone demonstrated significant prolongation of *QTc* intervals and increased QT/RR regression slopes in comparison with normal subjects. The HCM patients therefore exhibited acquired LQTS secondary to structural disease.

Circadian rhythmicity of *QT* interval

Sotalol, an I_{Kr} blocker with beta blocker properties, has been studied in Holter monitor recordings and as expected causes significant prolongation of the *QT*, *QTc* and *RR* intervals although the circadian pattern of *QT* and *RR* behaviour is maintained (Sharma *et al.* 1999). Chronic amiodarone therapy abolishes such variation (Antimisiaris *et al.* 1994), probably due to its additional cardiac effects. Yi *et al.* (1998) examined a postinfarct group derived from a prospective survey cohort. Fifteen individuals were selected randomly from a subgroup that suffered a sudden cardiac death (SCD) within 1 year of infarction. Their Holters were compared with those of 15 patients who survived >3 years after infarction but were matched for age, sex, infarct characteristics, left ventricular function and therapy. An additional comparison was made with age- and gender-matched healthy controls. While the 24 h mean *QTc* intervals of SCD victims were increased compared to normal subjects and post-MI survivors, the circadian variation of *QT* interval was blunted and *QTc* variation abolished completely (Fig. 40.7) (Yi *et al.* 1998). The alteration of *QT* circadian rhythmicity is therefore inconsistent depending upon aetiology but it may support the presence of acquired LQTS and an increased risk of ventricular arrhythmias.

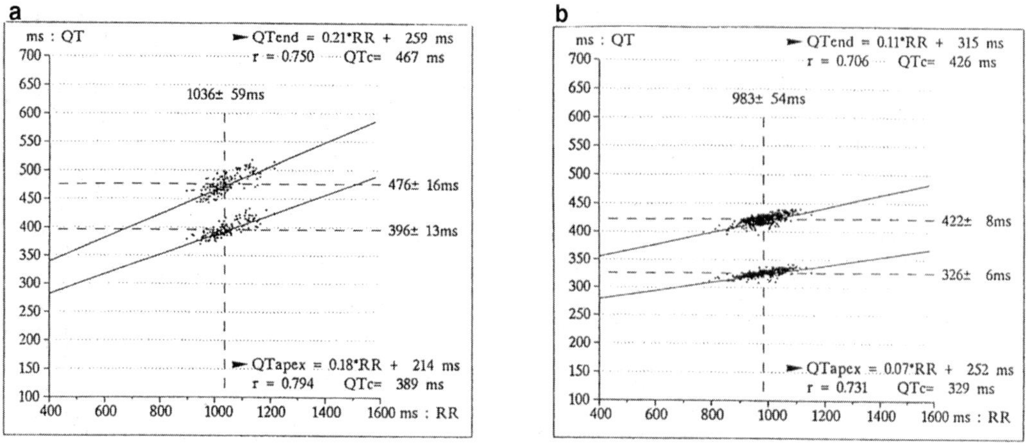

Fig. 40.6 QT/RR and *QT*-apex/*RR* curves derived from Holter data in a 58-year-old woman with syncope and documented TdP due to an antihistamine. (a) Regression curve during medication and compared to off therapy (b), demonstrates increased *QT* intervals for the same *RR* values and with a steeper curve, i.e. reverse rate dependence. (Reproduced from Maison-Blanche & Coumel 1997, with permission of Blackwell Publishing.)

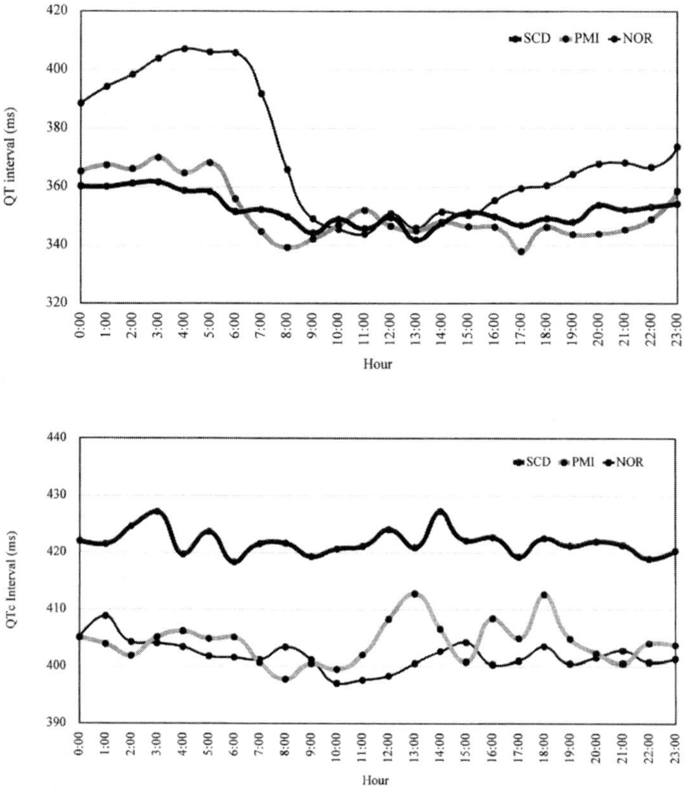

Fig. 40.7 Mean hourly *QT* and *QTc* intervals plotted with time of day demonstrating loss of *QT* circadian rhythmicity of sudden death victims (SCD) compared to post-MI survivors (PMI) and normal individuals (NOR) and persistent *QTc* elevation with blunting of variation in SCD compared to PMI and NOR. (Reproduced from Yi *et al. American Journal of Cardiology*, **81**, 950–956, copyright 1998, with permission of Excerpta Medica Inc.)

Short–long–short initiation

Kay and coworkers (1983) first described the short–long–short initiation pattern to TdP, detecting it in around 90% of their cohort, which consisted of 31 patients with acquired LQTS and one with the congenital syndrome (Fig. 40.2). More recent research has suggested a 98% prevalence in acquired LQTS patients with TdP (Locati *et al.* 1995). Jackman *et al.* postulated a distinct form of LQTS known as 'pause dependent' that is typical of the acquired condition and some forms of congenital LQTS. It is characterized by TdP occurring after a pause or rapid deceleration in heart rate (e.g. after a run of supraventricular tachycardia) (Jackman *et al.* 1988). Pauses have been described as induced by either a preceding ventricular (Fig. 40.2b) or supraventricular extrasystole (Fig. 40.2a) or a salvo of ventricular beats (Fig. 40.2c) (Locati *et al.* 1995). Rarely a sudden sinus pause without an extrasystole can be seen to induce TdP with the loss of the initial short-long component (Locati *et al.* 1995). Heart rate increases in the minute before the onset of TdP are also commonly seen before the short–long–short sequence (Locati *et al.* 1995).

Kay also observed that all the documented episodes of TdP were preceded by complexes demonstrating abnormally prolonged and labile *Q–T* intervals with variable T wave morphology, despite the presence of normal baseline *QTc* values in more than half of their patient group (Kay *et al.* 1983). It has subsequently been demonstrated that critical prolongation of the *QT* interval is associated with the generation of the extrasystole that initiates the short–long–short sequence preceding TdP (Fig. 40.2d) although not every critical *QT* interval results in this outcome (Gilmour *et al.* 1997). Other factors such as changes in potassium and drug concentrations may be involved (Gilmour *et al.* 1997). The development of the critical *QT* interval is a function not only of the immediately preceding *RR* interval but also previous *RR* intervals. The varying rates of *QT* adaptation associated with the sudden onset of bradycardia support the complexity of this dynamic behaviour (Gilmour *et al.* 1997). Figure 40.8 demonstrates the *RR* and *QT* intervals of normal sinus rhythm associated with runs of TdP, each arrhythmia being preceded by a gently increasing *QT* interval despite relatively stable *RR* intervals until a relatively consistent critical length is seen. This is immediately preceded by increased *RR* intervals (i.e. bradycardia). The *QT* interval of the first spontaneous complex after a run of ventricular tachycardia then shorten dramatically (Figs 40.2e and 40.5) (Gilmour *et al.* 1997). These features of *QT* interval behaviour are consistent with experimental models that incorporate early afterdepolarizations as the initiation of ectopic activity that leads to TdP (Gilmour *et al.* 1997).

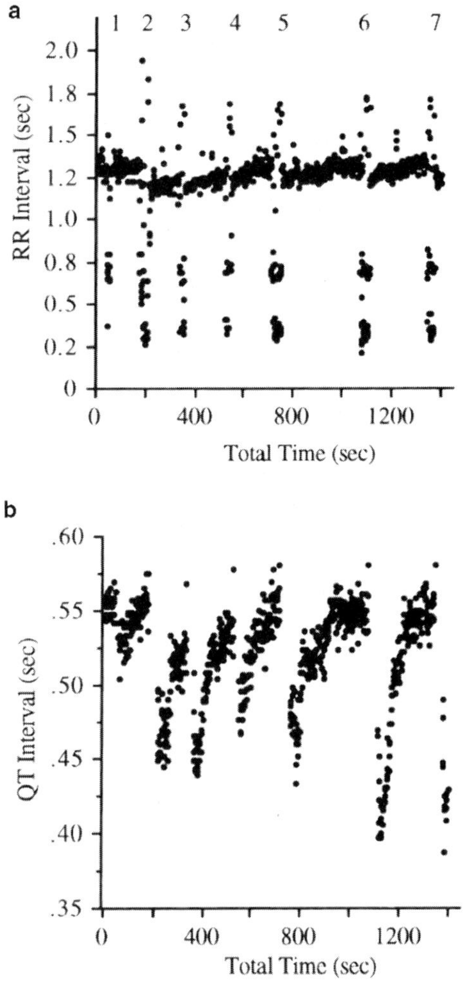

Fig. 40.8 *RR* and *QT* intervals during periods of normal sinus rhythm interrupted by 6 episodes of TdP in a patient with acquired LQTS. (a) *RR* intervals during 7 periods of sinus rhythm. (b) *QT* intervals corresponding to the *RR* intervals in (a). *QT* intervals during the ventricular arrhythmias are excluded. The *QT* interval increases in a similar manner after each episode of TdP while the *RR* intervals remain relatively stable. When a similar *QT* interval is reached TdP ensues. The *QT* interval then normalizes once the arrhythmia resolves spontaneously. (Reproduced from Gilmour *et al.*, the American College of Cardiology Foundation *Journal of the American College of Cardiology* (1997), **30** (1), 209–217, with permission.)

The first complex of TdP is coupled with the first spontaneous post-pause complex and arises from the significantly abnormal T/U wave exhibited by the post-pause complex (Fig. 40.2(f)) (Kay *et al.* 1983; Jackman *et al.* 1988). The coupling of the post-pause complex is usually late ('late coupled') in relation to the preceding normal beat so that the initiation is consistent with the post-pause U wave (Kay *et al.* 1983; Jackman *et al.* 1988). Kay noted coupling intervals that varied from 270ms to 880ms with a mean of 490 ms (Kay *et al.* 1983). The amplitude and duration of the post-pause T/U wave increases if faster preceding tachycardias and longer preceding pauses are present (Jackman *et al.* 1988). The amplitude of the U wave is also thought to correlate positively with the length of the subsequent ventricular tachycardia but it does not depend upon the associated *QT* interval (Jackman *et al.* 1988). Thus the U wave seems to be 'arrhythmogenic' and is probably the surface ECG representation of early after-depolarizations (Jackman *et al.* 1988; Locati *et al.* 1995; Gilmour *et al.* 1997). If TdP does not initiate and normal rhythm persists then the U wave amplitude tends to decrease and may oscillate for several cycles after the pause resulting in U wave alternans (Jackman *et al.* 1988).

Ventricular ectopic activity is a common feature of acquired LQTS (Jackman *et al.* 1988; Locati *et al.* 1995). Its presence before the introduction of a torsadogenic agent is a predictor of the development of TdP (Houltz *et al.* 1998). In acquired LQTS a stable bigeminal rhythm is frequent and establishes in a mechanism similar to TdP. It occurs when an extrasystole late coupled with an abnormal preceding T/U wave generates a pause that causes a subsequent spontaneous beat with an abnormal T/U wave (Jackman *et al.*1988; Locati *et al.*1995). This in turn associates with another late-coupled extrasystole inducing another pause. This can self-perpetuate as a stable rhythm based on repetitive short–long–short sequences (Jackman *et al.* 1988; Locati *et al.* 1995). When it occurs spontaneously on administration of a potentially torsadogenic drug it is a predictor of the subsequent occurrence of TdP (Houltz *et al.* 1998; Jackman *et al.* 1988) as is post-pause accentuation of the U wave causing U wave alternans (Jackman *et al.* 1988). They are specific but not sensitive indicators (Houltz *et al.* 1998; Jackman *et al.* 1988). Short salvos and runs of TdP can also commonly be seen in this context and are also initiated by the short–long–short sequence (Jackman *et al.* 1988; Locati *et al.* 1995). Alternatively the ectopic activity may enter an accelerated phase with larger U waves forming and longer runs of tachycardias that become more sustained causing ventricular fibrillation (VF). Locati *et al.* defined this escalation of arrhythmic activity preceding TdP as a 'cascade phenomenon' (Fig. 40.2) with two characteristic features: (1) an initial supraventricular ectopic causing a short–long sequence (Fig. 40.2a) followed by a first ventricular beat, and (2) a sequence of short–long–short oscillations with shorter short intervals and longer long intervals generating increasingly complex arrhythmia and eventually TdP (Locati *et al.* 1995). In their series, this latter feature of shorter short intervals and longer long intervals (see Fig. 40.2, p1and p2) was the best predictor of the onset of TdP.

Once such a run of TdP or VF develops then subsequent recurrence is frequent (Jackman *et al.* 1988). The tachycardia itself may seem relatively slow and monomorphic initially particularly if there are brief salvos but the longer the duration and the greater the frequency the more rapid and polymorphic it becomes (Jackman *et al.* 1988). A retrospective multivariate analysis of a large group of patients with acquired LQTS and pause dependent TdP revealed three significant predictors for the development of VF. These were the presence of structural heart disease, depressed left ventricular ejection fraction and the relative dispersion of *QTc* (Da Costa *et al.* 2000). No other ECG features were of significant predictive value for the onset of VF. Locati *et al.* noted however that the degeneration of TdP to VF was associated with a more rapid tachycardia of longer duration than self-terminating TdP (Locati *et al.* 1995).

'Late' proarrhythmia

QT prolongation and TdP induced by potent torsadogenic drugs such as quinidine is usually seen soon after initiation of drug therapy. An excess of unexpected sudden deaths had been seen amongst patients on chronic quinidine therapy and it has become apparent that a minority of those who suffer consequent TdP do so late after initiation. One series suggested a mean duration of therapy of 4.7 ± 5.7 years with a median of 2.5 years (Oberg *et al.* 1994) before onset of TdP in delayed cases. Other factors (metabolic, pharmacodynamic and structural) may be responsible for this 'late' proarrhythmia but the need for observation of the patient prescribed such drugs is emphasized.

Conclusion

The acquired long QT syndrome is defined as the abnormal prolongation of repolarization as manifested on the surface electrocardiogram (ECG) by *QT* prolongation, T wave abnormalities and/or torsades de pointes. Changes in T wave morphology, sometimes without any *QT* prolongation, are common. The QT/RR regression slope usually demonstrates reverse rate dependence, reflecting abnormal repolarization, but as with *QT* circadian rhythmicity this can be inconsistent depending on the agent involved. These measures of ECG dynamicity may still support the presence of acquired LQTS and an increased risk of ventricular arrhythmias. The short–long–short sequence that initiates torsades de pointes is characteristic of the acquired condition and is 'pause-dependent'. The pause is usually initiated by a late coupled ectopic that generates a post-pause beat with *QT* prolongation and an abnormal T/U wave from which torsades de pointes arises. The onset of ventricular ectopic activity with accompanying T/U wave alternans therefore predicts the risk of torsades de pointes. This risk is usually apparent early after initiation of torsadogenic drug therapy but in a minority may develop years later probably due to intervening metabolic, electrolytic or structural influences.

Further research is required into the effects of drugs on *QT* adaptation as the delays of hysteresis associated with exercise, recovery, stress and sudden changes in heart rate demonstrated in LQT1 and LQT2 forms of the congenital syndrome (Paavonen *et al.* 2001; Swan *et al.* 1998, 1999) may represent an arrhythmogenic mechanism in the acquired condition.

References

Antimisiaris, M., Sarma, J.S., Schoenbaum, M.P., Sharma, P.P., Venkataraman, K. & Singh, B.N. (1994) Effects of amiodarone on the circadian rhythm and power spectral changes of heart rate and QT interval: significance for the control of sudden cardiac death. *American Heart Journal*, **128** (5), 884–891.

Bednar, M.M., Harrigan, E.P., Anziano, R.J., Camm, A.J. & Ruskin, J.N. (2001) The QT interval. *Progress in Cardiovascular Diseases*, **43** (5 Suppl. 1), 1–45.

Ben-David, J. & Zipes, D.P. (1993) Torsades de pointes and proarrhythmia. *Lancet*, **341** (8860), 1578–1582.

Burattini, L., Zareba, W., Rashba, E.J., Couderc, J.P., Konecki, J. & Moss, A.J. (1998) ECG features of microvolt T wave alternans in coronary artery disease and long QT syndrome patients. *Journal of Electrocardiology*, **31** (Suppl.), 114–120.

Cappato, R., Alboni, P., Codeca, L., Guardigli, G., Toselli, T. & Antonioli, G.E. (1993) Direct and autonomically mediated effects of oral quinidine on RR/QT relation after an abrupt increase in heart rate. *Journal of the American College of Cardiology*, **22** (1), 99–105.

Da Costa, A., Chalvidan, T., Belounas, A. *et al.* (2000) Predictive factors of ventricular fibrillation triggered by pause-dependent torsades de pointes associated with acquired long QT interval: role of QT dispersion and left ventricular function. *Journal of Cardiovascular Electrophysiology*, **11** (9), 990–997.

Donger, C., Denjoy, I., Berthet, M. *et al.* (1997) KVLQT1 C-terminal missense mutation causes a forme fruste long-QT syndrome. *Circulation*, **96** (9), 2778–2781.

Fei, L., Slade, A.K., Grace, A.A., Malik, M., Camm, A.J. & McKenna, W.J. (1994) Ambulatory assessment of the QT interval in patients with hypertrophic cardiomyopathy: risk stratification and effect of low dose amiodarone. *PACE (Pacing and Clinical Electrophysiology)*, **17** (11 Pt 2), 2222–2227.

Gilmour, R.F., Jr, Riccio, M.L., Locati, E.H., Maison-Blanche, P., Coumel, P. & Schwartz, P.J. (1997) Time- and rate-dependent alterations of the QT interval precede the onset of torsades de pointes in patients with acquired QT prolongation. *Journal of the American College of Cardiology*, **30** (1), 209–217.

Hii, J.T., Wyse, D.G., Gillis, A.M., Duff, H.J., Solylo, M.A. & Mitchell, L.B. (1992) Precordial QT interval dispersion as a marker of torsades de pointes. Disparate effects of class Ia antiarrhythmic drugs and amiodarone. *Circulation*, **86** (5), 1376–1382.

Hohnloser, S.H., Klingenheben, T. & Singh, B.N. (1994) Amiodarone-associated proarrhythmic effects. A review with special reference to torsades de pointes tachycardia. *Annals of Internal Medicine*, **121** (7), 529–535.

Houltz, B., Darpo, B., Edvardsson, N. *et al.* (1998) Electrocardiographic and clinical predictors of torsades de pointes induced by almokalant infusion in patients with chronic atrial fibrillation or flutter: a prospective study. *PACE (Pacing and Clinical Electrophysiology)*, **21** (5), 1044–1057.

Jackman, W.M., Friday, K.J., Anderson, J.L., Aliot, E.M., Clark, M. & Lazzara, R. (1988) The long QT syndromes: a critical review, new clinical observations and a unifying hypothesis. *Progress in Cardiovascular Diseases*, **31** (2), 115–172.

Kay, G.N., Plumb, V.J., Arciniegas, J.G., Henthorn, R.W. & Waldo, A.L. (1983) Torsades de pointes: the long-short initiating sequence and other clinical features: observations in 32 patients. *Journal of the American College of Cardiology*, **2** (5), 806–817.

Lande, G., Maison-Blanche, P., Fayn, J., Ghadanfar, M., Coumel, P. & Funck-Brentano, C. (1998) Dynamic analysis of dofetilide-induced changes in ventricular repolarization. *Clinical Pharmacology and Therapeutics*, **64** (3), 312–321.

Locati, E.H., Maison-Blanche, P., Dejode, P., Cauchemez, B. & Coumel, P. (1995) Spontaneous sequences of onset of torsades de pointes in patients with acquired prolonged repolarization: quantitative analysis of Holter recordings. *Journal of the American College of Cardiology*, **25** (7), 1564–1575.

Maison-Blanche, P. & Coumel, P. (1997) Changes in repolarization dynamicity and the assessment of the arrhythmic risk. *PACE (Pacing and Clinical Electrophysiology)*, **20** (10 Pt 2), 2614–2624.

Makita, N., Horie, M., Nakamura, T. *et al.* (2002) Drug-induced long-QT syndrome associated with a subclinical SCN5A mutation. *Circulation*, **106** (10), 1269–1274.

Napolitano, C., Civile, O., Priori, S. & *et al.* (1997) Identification of a long QT syndrome molecular defect in drug-induced torsades de pointes. *Circulation*, **96**, I-211 (abstract).

Nattel, S. (2000) Class III drugs: amiodarone, bretylium, ibutilide, and sotalol. In: *Cardiac Electrophysiology: From Cell to Bedside* (eds D. P. Zipes & J. Jalife), 3rd edn, pp. 921–932. W.B. Saunders, Philadelphia.

Oberg, K.C., O'Toole, M.F., Gallastegui, J.L. & Bauman, J.L. (1994) Late proarrhythmia due to quinidine. *American Journal of Cardiology*, **74** (2), 192–194.

Paavonen, K.J., Swan, H., Piippo, K. *et al.* (2001) Response of the QT interval to mental and physical stress in types LQT1 and LQT2 of the long QT syndrome. *Heart*, **86** (1), 39–44.

Priori, S.G., Napolitano, C. & Schwartz, P.J. (1999) Low penetrance in the long-QT syndrome: clinical impact. *Circulation*, 99 (4), 529–533.

Roden, D.M. (1993) Torsades de pointes. *Clinical Cardiology*, **16** (9), 683–686.

Roden, D.M., Lazzara, R., Rosen, M., Schwartz, P.J., Towbin, J. & Vincent, G.M. (1996) Multiple mechanisms in the long-QT syndrome: current knowledge, gaps, and future directions. *Circulation*, **94** (8), 1996–2012.

Sharma, P.P., Sarma, J.S. & Singh, B.N. (1999) Effects of sotalol on the circadian rhythmicity of heart rate and QT intervals with a noninvasive index of reverse-use dependency. *Journal of Cardiovascular Pharmacology and Therapeutics*, **4** (1), 15–21.

Sheridan, D.J. (2000) Drug-induced proarrhythmic effects: assessment of changes in QT interval. *British Journal of Clinical Pharmacology*, **50** (4), 297–302.

Swan, H., Toivonen, L. & Viitasalo, M. (1998) Rate adaptation of QT intervals during and after exercise in children with congenital long QT syndrome. *European Heart Journal*, **19** (3), 508–513.

Swan, H., Viitasalo, M., Piippo, K., Laitinen, P., Kontula, K. & Toivonen, L. (1999) Sinus node function and ventricular repolarization during exercise stress test in long QT syndrome patients with KvLQT1 and HERG potassium channel defects. *Journal of the American College of Cardiology*, **34** (3), 823–829.

Tan, H.L. & Wilde, A.A. M. (1998) T wave alternans after sotalol: evidence for increased sensitivity to sotalol after conversion from atrial fibrillation to sinus rhythm. *Heart*, **80** (3), 303–306.

Touze, J.E., Heno, P., Fourcade, L. *et al.* (2002) The effects of antimalarial drugs on ventricular repolarization. *American Journal of Tropical Medicine and Hygiene*, **67** (1), 54–60.

Viskin, S. (1999) Long QT syndromes and torsades de pointes. *Lancet*, **354** (9190), 1625–1633.

Wei, J., Abbott, G.W., Sesti, F. *et al.* (1999a) Prevalence of KCNE2 (Mirp1) mutations in acquired long QT syndrome. *Circulation*, **100** (18 Pt I), I-495 (abstract).

Wei, J., Yang, I., Tapper, A. *et al.* (1999b) KCNE1 polymorphism confers risk of drug-induced long QT syndrome by altering kinetic properties of I_{KS} potassium channels. *Circulation*, **100** (18 Pt I), I-495 (abstract).

Yang, P., Kanki, H., Drolet, B. *et al.* (2002) Allelic variants in long-QT disease genes in patients with drug-associated torsades de pointes. *Circulation*, **105** (16), 1943–1948.

Yap, Y.G. & Camm, A.J. (1999) Arrhythmogenic mechanisms of non-sedating antihistamines. *Clinical and Experimental Allergy*, **29** (Suppl. 3), 174–181.

Yi, G., Guo, X.H., Reardon, M. *et al.* (1998) Circadian variation of the QT interval in patients with sudden cardiac death after myocardial infarction. *American Journal of Cardiology*, **81** (8), 950–956.

Zabel, M. & Malik, M. (2002) Practical use of T wave morphology assessment. *Cardiac Electrophysiology Review*, **6** (3), 316–322.

CHAPTER 41

Electrocardiogram of Brugada Syndrome and its Dynamic Patterns

Maximo Rivero-Ayerza, Ramon Brugada, Josep Brugada, Peter Geelen and Pedro Brugada

Introduction

The syndrome of right bundle branch block, ST segment elevation in the right precordial leads and sudden death was described 10 years ago (Brugada & Brugada 1992). Individuals with this syndrome have, by definition, a structurally normal heart. The ECG findings (Fig. 41.1) are unrelated to ischaemia, electrolyte disturbances or any other transient, reversible, or acquired known cause. This syndrome is genetically determined and caused by mutations in the cardiac sodium channel gene SCN5A. The pattern of transmission is autosomal dominant with incomplete penetrance. Approximately 60% of patients with aborted sudden death and the typical ECG have a family history of sudden death or a relative with the characteristic ECG pattern. In contrast to other arrhythmic syndromes, one of the main characteristics of Brugada syndrome is the marked variability of the ECG pattern.

Cellular basis of the Brugada ECG pattern

Available data suggests that the ST segment elevation (or also called J point elevation) in the right precordial leads is the result of depression or loss of the action potential dome in the right ventricular epicardium. That occurs by recently uncovered mechanisms (Yan & Antzelevitch 1996). The action potential of ventricular epicardial cells has a characteristic spike and dome morphology, as a consequence of an outward potassium current (I_{to}) that causes the notch (phase 1). A prominent action potential notch in the right ventricular epicardium but not endocardium gives rise to a transmural voltage gradient that is responsible for the J point elevation observed in the ECG. This transient outward current is much more prominent in the epicardial than in endocardial ventricular cells of many species including man (Langer *et al.* 1975; Furukawa *et al.* 1990; Fedida & Giles 1991; Clark *et al.* 1993; Wettwer *et al.* 1994; Nabauer *et al.* 1996; Antzelevitch *et al.* 1998) and more prominent in right ventricular than left ventricular myocytes (Zygmunt 1993). In Brugada syndrome, a reduction in the density of the sodium channel current (I_{Na}) accentuates the action potential notch and prevents the dome ('plateau') from developing, resulting in a marked abbreviation of the action potential duration in the epicardium. This phenomenon leads to ST segment elevation in the right precordial leads, as a consequence of the voltage gradient generated between the right ventricular epicardium and endocardium. This voltage gradient is also responsible for the triggering of the first extrasystole that may lead to polymorphic ventricular tachycardia, ventricular fibrillation and eventually to sudden arrhythmic death.

The prevalence of Brugada ECG in the asymptomatic, apparently healthy population

A prospective study of an adult Japanese population (22 027 subjects) showed an incidence of 1:2000 (Tohyou *et al.* 1995) of electrocardio-

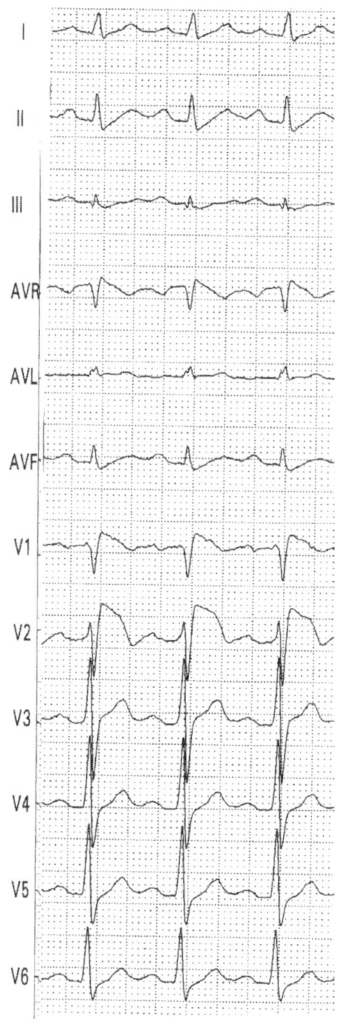

Fig. 41.1 The characteristic ECG pattern in Brugada syndrome. Twelve-lead ECG showing the 'coved' type ST segment elevation pattern, followed by a negative T wave. Paper speed 25 mm/s.

grams compatible with the syndrome (12 subjects). A second study (Namiki *et al.* 1995) of adults in Awa (Japan) showed an incidence of 6:1000 (66 cases out of 10 420). However, a third study in children from Japan (Hata *et al.* 1997) showed an incidence of electrocardiograms compatible with the syndrome of only 6:1 000 000 (1 case in 163 110). These results suggest that the phenotype may become manifest in adulthood, which is in accordance to the mean age of the sudden death victims (35–40 years).

As previously mentioned the syndrome is a clinical-electrocardiographic diagnosis based on the occurrence of syncopal or sudden death episodes in patients without demonstrable structural heart disease and a characteristic ECG pattern of apparent right bundle branch block and ST segment elevation in leads V1–V3.

The presence of a J point elevation of >2 mm or 0.2 mV giving rise to an elevated ST segment that gradually descends and is followed without isoelectric separation by a negative T wave determines the characteristic 'coved' type ECG pattern (Fig. 41.1) which is diagnostic of this disease. There is a second ECG morphology, the 'saddle back' type pattern, that is characterized also by an elevated ST segment that gradually descends but in this case is followed by a positive or biphasic T wave determining an image that resembles a saddle (Fig. 41.2). Patients can present with the coved type pattern and another time the ECG can show the saddle-back type of ST segment elevation or even normalize completely (Fig. 41.3). It is unknown whether this behaviour is expression of different genotypes or is the consequence of variations in the degree of sodium channel dysfunction due to the propensity of the sodium channel to be influenced by different factors. Depending on anatomical variations or on different sites of ventricular affectation ST segment elevation can also be observed in the inferior leads or in aVL (Fig. 41.4).

We would like to stress that in all series of patients studied by us, a diagnosis of Brugada syndrome is only made when the 'coved' type ST segment elevation is recognized at one or another moment (spontaneously or after the administration of antiarrhythmic drugs). We do not accept an ECG with only the 'saddle-back' type of ST segment elevation as diagnostic of Brugada syndrome.

Conduction disturbances in Brugada syndrome

Besides the previously discussed ST segment elevation, another important component of the characteristic ECG is the presence of conduction disturbances. There exist typical ECGs where no conduction abnormalities are observed (Fig. 41.5). When conduction disturbances occur in Brugada syndrome, the most common are right bundle branch block (RBBB) and prolongation of the *PR* interval (Fig. 41.4). In some ECGs the elevated J point and the consequent high ST

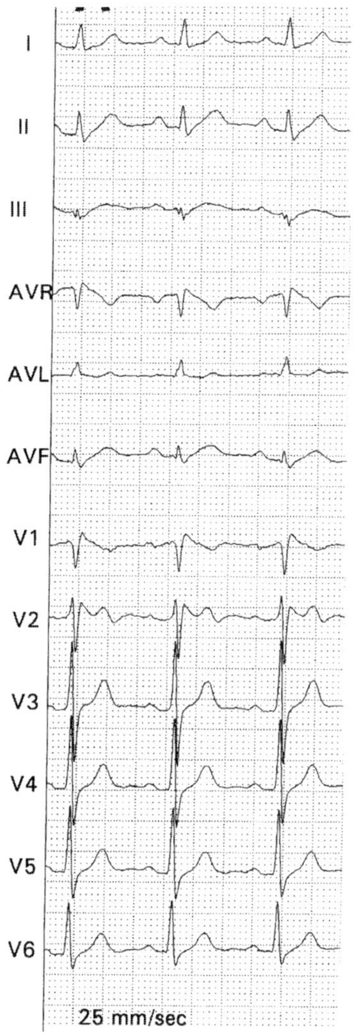

Fig. 41.2 Twelve lead ECG showing in lead V2 the 'saddle-back' type ST segment elevation pattern. The elevated J point and the gradually descending ST segment are followed by a positive-negative T wave. Paper speed 25 mm/s.

segment take-off, resembling the presence of an r′ deflection and broad QRS in the right precordial leads may mimic an incomplete RBBB pattern (Fig. 41.2). However, no prolongation of the QRS can be observed in other leads and there is lack of the characteristic broad S wave in the lateral leads excluding a true RBBB. The prolongation of the *PR* interval is usually caused by a prolongation of the HV interval, confirming the presence of subnodal conduction disturbances. The association of conduction disturbances and repolarization abnormalities caused by mutations in the sodium channel gene SCN5A does not come as a surprise. It has been shown that certain mutations in this gene cause exclusively conduction disturbances (Tan *et al.* 2001), others only repolarization abnormalities (Chen *et al.* 1998) and others a combination of both (Kyndt *et al.* 2001). In most cases the *QT* interval is normal, though it can be slightly prolonged. However, some mutations affecting the same gene SCN5A that link the Brugada syndrome to its 'mirror image' the LQT3 syndrome have been described (Bezzina *et al.* 1999; Priori *et al.* 2000).

Variability of the ECG pattern

Chen *et al.* (1998) first described a mutation in the SCN5A gene that codifies for the α subunit of the sodium channels as being responsible for this syndrome. This dysfunction alters the cardiac cells' action potential and is evidenced by the ECG changes previously described. It is expected that different endogenous or exogenous stimuli that in physiological conditions modulate the action potential, will be expressed in carriers of this disease as different ECG patterns. Despite the fact that the syndrome was initially described as a persistent ECG condition, it was soon recognized that it is variable over time (Miyazaki *et al.* 1996). Transient normalization has been observed in as many as 40% of patients who had once documentation of the 'coved' type pattern. The sodium channel in Brugada syndrome is sensitive to many factors like autonomic interactions, different antiarrhythmic drugs, temperature variations and other unknown conditions that modify the ECG exaggerating the typical pattern or normalizing it.

Influence of the autonomic nervous system, heart rate and temperature

As previously mentioned, an increase in the Ito current and a consequent loss of the action potential dome in epicardial cells is the cause of both the characteristic ECG pattern and the substrate for the occurrence of arrhythmias (phase 2 re-entry). Miyazaki *et al.* (1996) were the first to show the variability of the ECG pattern. Beta-adrenergic stimulation decreases the ST segment elevation by increasing the ICa, a transient calcium current that restores the action potential dome. At the same time transient α-adrenergic stimulation normalizes the ECG.

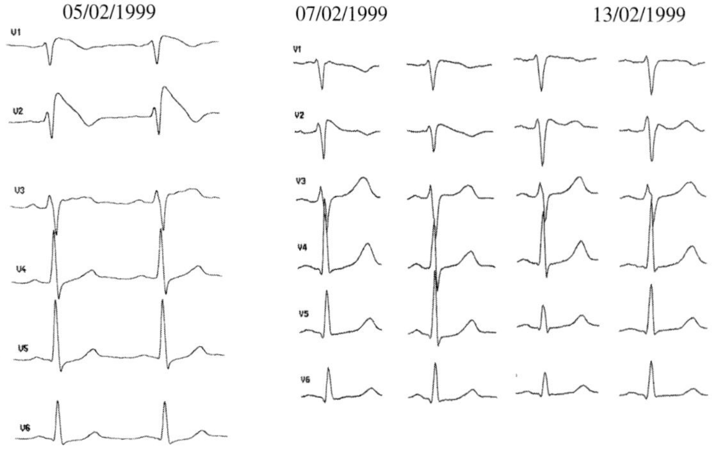

Fig. 41.3 Spontaneous and gradual normalization of the characteristic ECG pattern over a one week period. Note how from the 'coved' type pattern (left side) the ECG gradually changes to the 'saddle back' type to then normalise. Paper speed 25 mm/s.

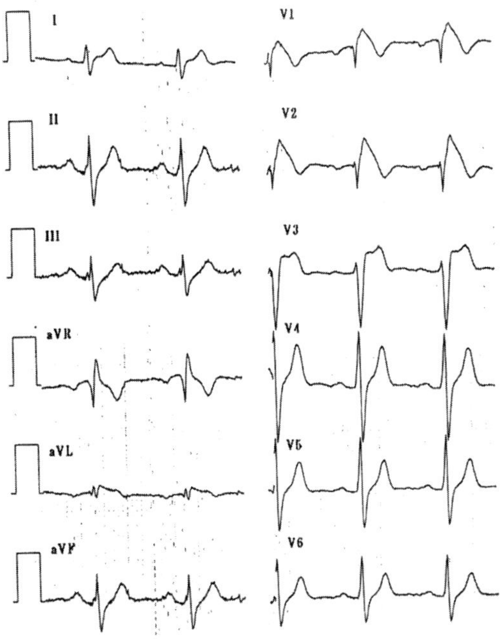

Fig. 41.4 Anatomic variations or different sites of ventricular affectation can determine ST segment elevation in leads different from the right precordial leads. Note in this case, besides the 'coved' type ST segment elevation in leads V1–V3, the ST segment elevation in lead aVL. The PR interval is slightly prolonged. Paper speed 25 mm/s.

For this reason β-adrenergic agonists like isoproterenol tend to normalize the ECG pattern, and have been shown to prevent spontaneous arrhythmias and their induction during programmed ventricular stimulation. β-adrenergic blockers and β-adrenergic agonists have an opposite effect.

A frequent finding is that during exercise the ST segment normalizes because both an increase in heart rate and adrenergic stimulation decrease ST segment elevation.

An artificial increase in heart rate (by atrial pacing) decreases ST segment elevation, while a decrease in heart rate increases it. These data are again in agreement with the loss of the dome of the action potential at epicardial level as the cause of ST segment elevation. Ito becomes more prominent at slow rates increasing heterogeneity and ST segment elevation. On the other hand, vagal stimulation through the muscarinic receptors, increases ST segment elevation by facilitating the loss of dome due to ICa suppression. These data are also in agreement with the clinical observations documenting a bradycardia dependency and a higher incidence of sudden death during sleep in patients with this syndrome.

The ionic mechanism responsible for the Brugada syndrome have been shown to be temperature dependent (Dumaine *et al.* 1999). Some patients develop the overt form of the electrocardiogram and even ventricular arrhythmias when they develop fever. For this reason fever should be avoided or aggressively treated in carriers of the disease.

Influence of drugs on the ECG

Class Ia, Ic and class III drugs increase ST segment elevation and the propensity for arrhythmias. For this reason they should be avoided as a therapeutic option in carriers of this disease. Other medications like antibiotics, anti-

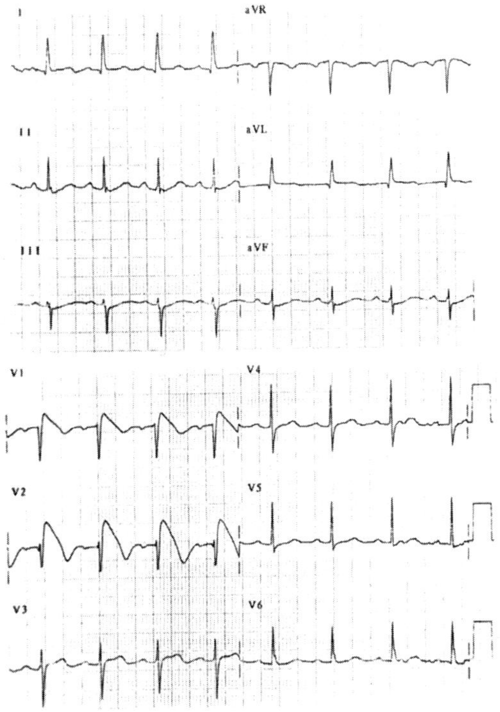

Fig. 41.5 Characteristic ECG without RBBB. J point and ST segment elevation in leads V1–V3 resembles a RBBB. However, note that there is no prolongation of the QRS in other leads and no broad S wave in the lateral leads. Paper speed 25 mm/s.

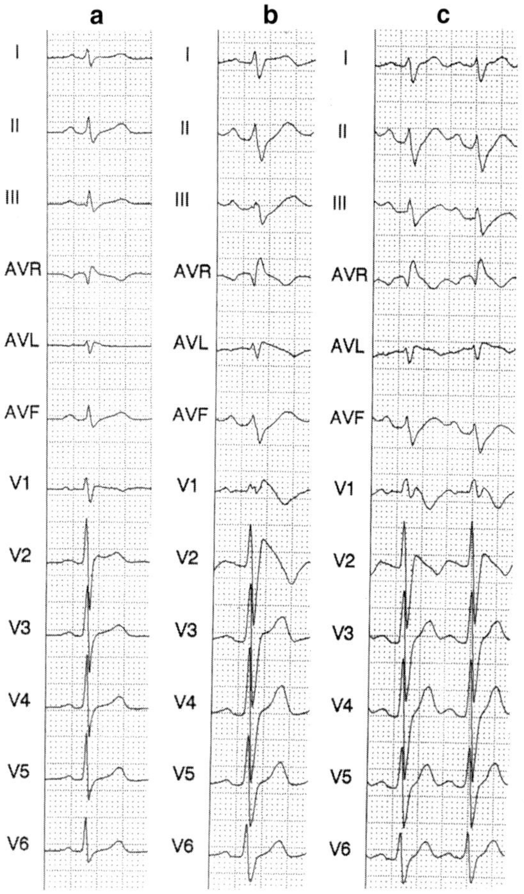

Fig. 41.6 Effect of intravenous administration of sodium channel blockers. (a) ECG of a patient with a concealed form of the disease. (b) A 'coved' type ST segment elevation developing after intravenous administration of ajmaline. (c) Administration of an adrenergic agonist like isoproterenol can improve ECG changes. Paper speed 25 mm/s.

depressants and antimalarial agents can also be arrhythmogenic and should be avoided.

Antiarrhythmic drugs as a diagnostic test in Brugada syndrome

Sodium channel blockers like flecainide (2 mg/kg in 10 min), procainamide (10 mg/kg in 10 min) and ajmaline (1 mg/kg in 5 min) have been used to unmask Brugada syndrome in individuals with a normal ECG or an ECG of the 'saddle-back' type. Although much more data are required, the use of these drugs promises to have sufficient sensitivity and specificity (Brugada *et al.* 2000).

Intravenous administration of these drugs can exacerbate the characteristic ECG changes or most importantly can unmask concealed forms the disease (Fig. 41.6).

Considering that even asymptomatic carriers of this disease are at considerable risk of dying suddenly, there are some clinical situations that make the provocative test mandatory. In patients with syncope or symptoms that could be due to Brugada syndrome and have no evident ECG changes, a provocative test is indicated. Family members of affected individuals should also be screened in order to evaluate the need of further risk stratification. The test is also useful in those individuals who don't have a clear ECG pattern, mostly those with a 'saddle-back' type ST segment elevation. In these cases the development of a coved type ECG pattern after drug administration is diagnostic of the disease. The test is considered positive when a coved type ST segment elevation appears after drug administration or when a >2 mm rise in the J point is observed in patients with a previously normal ECG. Patients should be monitored until the ECG normalizes because ventricular fibrillation or polymorphic ventricular tachycardia can spontaneously occur while there is still effect of the drug. The characteristic ECG changes induced by this provocative tests can be reversed by the administration of isoproterenol (Fig. 41.6).

Electrocardiographic differential diagnosis

Other conditions may result in electrocardiograms simulating Brugada syndrome: arrhythmogenic right ventricular dysplasia, Steinert's disease, pectus excavatum, early repolarization, athlete's heart, mediastinal tumors and even the classical RBBB. In these cases the response to drug challenge is different to that of patients with Brugada syndrome. In carriers of arrhythmogenic right ventricular dysplasia, early repolarization, athlete's heart and or a classic RBBB no modifications in the level of the ST segment are observed after drug administration (Fig. 41.7).

Conclusions

Variability of the ECG pattern, the clinical presentation and a variable prognosis are characteristic of this syndrome as is the RBBB-like morphology and ST segment elevation. The

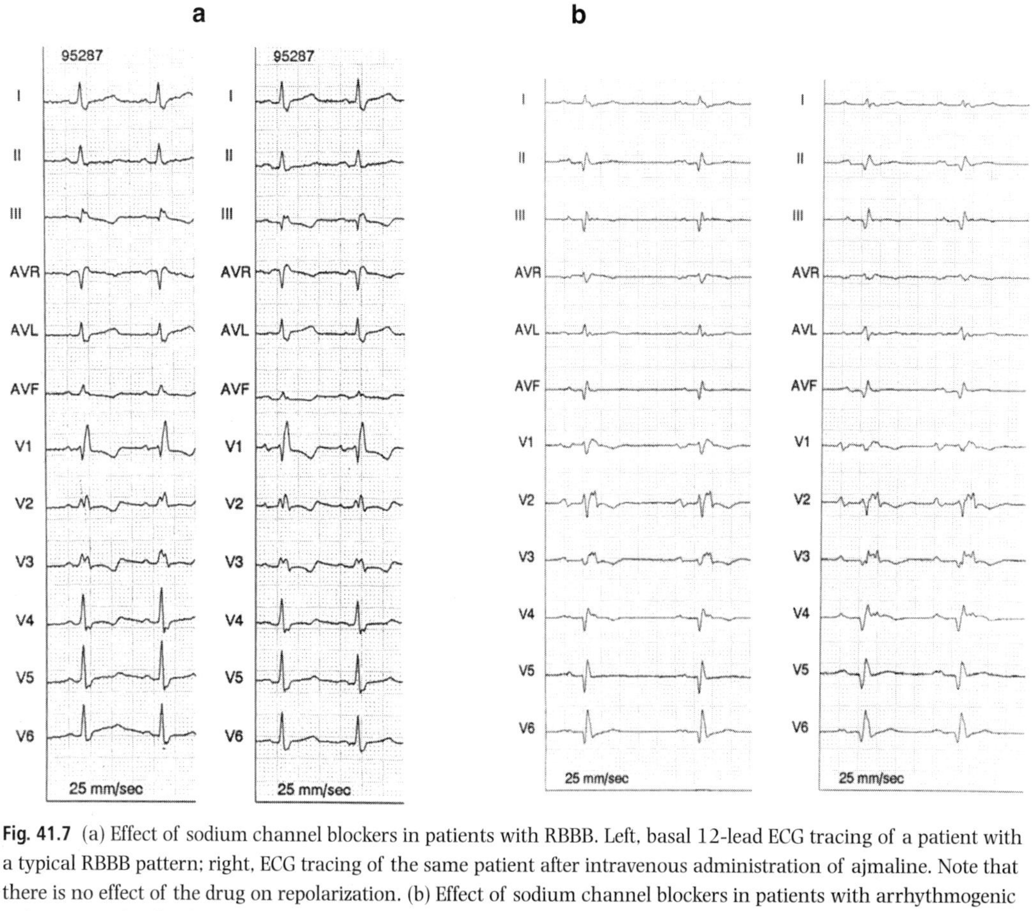

Fig. 41.7 (a) Effect of sodium channel blockers in patients with RBBB. Left, basal 12-lead ECG tracing of a patient with a typical RBBB pattern; right, ECG tracing of the same patient after intravenous administration of ajmaline. Note that there is no effect of the drug on repolarization. (b) Effect of sodium channel blockers in patients with arrhythmogenic right ventricular dysplasia (ARVD). Note the prominent epsilon wave after the QRS complex. Left, basal ECG tracing of a patient with ARVD; right, ECG tracing of the same patient recorded after intravenous administration of ajmaline showing only a broader QRS complex.

disease is caused by mutations affecting channel physiology, and particularly the sodium channel. It may very well be that the clinical manifestations and prognosis relate to the degree of damage to the sodium current. Accepting an autosomal dominant mode of inheritance of the disease, the normal individual has no affectation at all of the sodium current. However, we may obtain a 'Brugada' ECG in a normal individual if we decrease sodium channel function by toxic means: suicide attempts with flecainide, extreme hypothermia and compression of the right ventricular wall. At the other site of the spectrum, the full-blown syndrome occurs because of a 50% spontaneous affectation of sodium channels. Many of these individuals may develop intrauterine death (early abortions). Those who survive have the typical ECG and may develop sudden infant death around 6 months of age when I_{to} (transient outward potassium current) becomes prominent in humans. Those less affected survive to adulthood and develop the ventricular arrhythmias around 40 years of age, the fascinating age where many other genetically determined diseases manifest their phenotypes for the first time. Less affectation of the sodium channels may lead to the group of patients who develop repeated episodes of syncope because of self-limited ventricular arrhythmias. Asymptomatic individuals with a spontaneously abnormal ECG and inducible may constitute a group with less affectation of the sodium channels, but according to recent data are still at an important risk of developing the spontaneous arrhythmias. In those asymptomatic individuals in whom the 'Brugada' ECG is only uncovered by drugs, the degree of damage to the sodium channel is so low, that they may never manifest the ECG spontaneously and will probably never develop ventricular arrhythmias unless exposed to potentially harmful circumstances (drugs, fever).

References

Antzelevitch, C., Yan, G.X., Shimizu, W. *et al.* (1998) Electrical heterogeneity, the ECG, and cardiac arrhythmias. In: *Cardiac Electrophysiology: From Cell to Bedside* (eds D. P. Zipes & J. Jalife), pp. 1–34. W. B. Saunders, Philadelphia.

Bezzina, C., Veklkamp, M., Van den Berg, M.P. *et al.* (1999) A single sodium channel mutation causing both long-*Q–T* and Brugada syndromes. *Circulation Research*, **85**, 1206–1213

Brugada, P. & Brugada, J. (1992) Right bundle branch block, persistent ST segment elevation and sudden cardiac death; a distinct clinical and electrocardiographic syndrome: a multicentre report. *Journal of the American College of Cardiology*, **20**, 1391–1396.

Brugada, R., Brugada, J., Antzelevitch, C. *et al.* (2000) Sodium channel blockers identity risk for sudden death in patients with ST segment elevation and right bundle branch block but structurally normal hearts. *Circulation*, **101**, 510–515.

Chen, Q., Kirsch, G.E., Zhang, D. *et al.* (1998) Genetic basis and molecular mechanisms for idiopathic ventricular fibrillation. *Nature (London)*, **392**, 293–296.

Clark, R.B., Bouchard, R.A., Salinas-Stefanon, E., Sanchez-Chapula, J. & Giles, W.R. (1993) Heterogeneity of action potential waveforms and potassium currents in rat ventricle. *Cardiovascular Research*, **27**, 1795–1799.

Dumaine, R., Towbin, J.A., Brugada, P. *et al.* (1999) Ionic mechanism responsible for the electrocardiographic phenotype of the Brugada syndrome are temperature dependent. *Circulation Research*, **85**, 872–874.

Fedida, D. & Giles, W.R. (1991) Regional variations in action potentials and transient outward current in myocytes isolated from rabbit left ventricular. *Journal of Physiology, (London)* **442**, 191–209.

Furukawa, T., Myerburg, R.J., Furukawa, N., Bassett, A.L. & Kimura, S.(1990) Differences in transient outward currents of feline endocardial and epicardial myocytes. *Circulation Research*, **67**, 1287–1291.

Hata, Y., Chiba, N., Hotta, K. *et al.* (1997) Incidence and clinical significance of right bundle branch block and ST segment elevation in leads V1–V3 in 6 to 11 year old school children in Japan. *Circulation*, **95**, 2310.

Kyndt, F., Probst, V., Potet, F. *et al.* (2001) Novel SCN5A mutation leading either to isolated cardiac conduction defect or Brugada syndrome in a large French family. *Circulation*, **104**, 3081–3086.

Langer, G.A., Brady, A.J., Tan, S.T. & Serena, S.D. (1975) Correlation of the glucoside reponse, the force staircase, and the action potential configuration in the neonatal rat heart. *Circulation Research*, **36**, 744–752.

Miyazaki, T., Mitamura, H., Miyoshi, S. *et al.* (1996) Autonomic and antiarrhythmic modulation of ST segment elevation in patients with Brugada syndrome. *Journal of the American College of Cardiology*, **27**, 1061–1070.

Nabauer, M., Beuckelman, G.J., Posival, H. *et al.* (1996) Regional differences in current density and rate-dependent properties of the transient outward current in subepicardial and subendocardial myocytes of human left ventricle. *Circulation*, **93**, 168–177.

Namiki, T., Ogura, T., Kuwabara, Y. *et al.* (1995) Five-year mortality and clinical characteristics of adult subjects with right bundle branch block and *S–T* elevation. *Circulation*, **93**, 334.

Priori, S.G., Napolitano, C., Schwartz, P.J. *et al.* (2000) The elusive link between LQT3 and Brugada syndrome: the role of flecainide challenge. *Circulation*, **102**, 945–947.

Tan, H.L., Bink-Boelkens, M.T., Bezzina, C.R. *et al.* (2001) A sodium-channel mutation causes isolated cardiac conduction disease. *Nature (London)*, **409**, 1043–1047.

Tohyou, Y., Nakazawa, K., Ozawa, A. *et al.* (1995) A survey in the incidence of right bundle branch block with ST segment elevation among normal population. *Japanese Journal of Electrocardiology*, **15**, 223–226.

Wettwer, E., Amos, G.J., Posival, H. & Ravens, U. (1994) Transient outward current in human ventricular myocytes of subepicardial and subendocardial origin. *Circulation Research*, **75**, 473–482.

Yan, G.X. & Antzelevitch, C. (1996) Cellular basis for the electrocardiographic J wave. *Circulation* **93**, 372–379.

Zygmunt, A.C. (1993) The calcium activated conductance. Ito2, in canine ventricle is a chloride current. *Biophysical Journal*, **64**, A389 (abstract).

CHAPTER 42

Electrocardiographic T Wave Changes in Left Ventricular Hypertrophy

Michael R Franz

Introduction

Electrocardiographically, left ventricular hypertrophy (LVH) is characterized by augmented depolarization voltage (R wave or S wave amplitude) and/or by abnormal repolarization (altered T wave morphology). These two changes do not necessarily appear at the same time. Augmented QRS voltage is sometimes noted without T wave changes, and T wave changes suggesting LVH are not necessarily accompanied by increased R or S wave amplitude. QRS voltage may be attenuated by emphysema, pericardial effusion and obesity or increased by skinny or emaciated body types. Variability based on ethnicity has also been documented (Oopik *et al.* 1996; Okin *et al.* 2002). Augmented R and S wave voltage in septal or right ventricular leads may alert to septal or right ventricular hypertrophy. In most cases of LVH, however, the vast majority of which are caused by chronic hypertension or aortic valve disease, QRS voltage alone is not very reliable or specific. It is more useful, in this author's view, to diagnose LVH on the basis of T wave alterations, also known as 'strain pattern'.

The most common T wave abnormalities associated with LVH are inverted T waves or biphasic T waves whose initial deflection is opposite to the main QRS vector. LVH-related T wave abnormalities often include J point elevation in right precordial leads and J point depression in left precordial leads, mimicking ischaemic ST segment changes (Fig. 42.1). Inverted T waves and depressed S-T segments are the main reasons why LVH is a common cause of misdiagnosed myocardial ischaemia.

A mechanistic evaluation of LVH-associated T wave abnormalities requires to first consider the cellular basis of the genesis of the normal T wave.

Genesis of the normal T wave

The paradox of the concordant T wave

The normal human ECG is characterized by a concordance between an upright R wave and an upright T wave in the majority of leads. This phenomenon has been called 'The Paradox of the Concordant T wave' because it contradicts depolarization and repolarization directions at the cellular level. The transmembrane action potential has a depolarization phase in one direction (by definition upright) and a repolarization phase that has an opposite (downward) direction. Likewise, in the myocardial surface electrogram, the main activation defection is upward while the initial repolarization deflection is downward. Why, then, does the body surface ECG show concordance between R wave or S wave (depolarization) and T wave (repolarization)?

This apparent paradox was explained by postulating that in the heart, as a whole, ventricular sites that depolarize earlier than others, repolarize later than ventricular sites with early activation. On average, this would invert the relationship between dominant depolarization and repolarization vectors and bring the T wave in line with the R wave. Initially, this assumption was based on topography and nurtured by the observation (Cohen *et al.* 1976) that action potentials recorded from the base and apex of the sheep heart were of different durations and that this difference corresponded inversely to the assumed difference in activation times (AT).

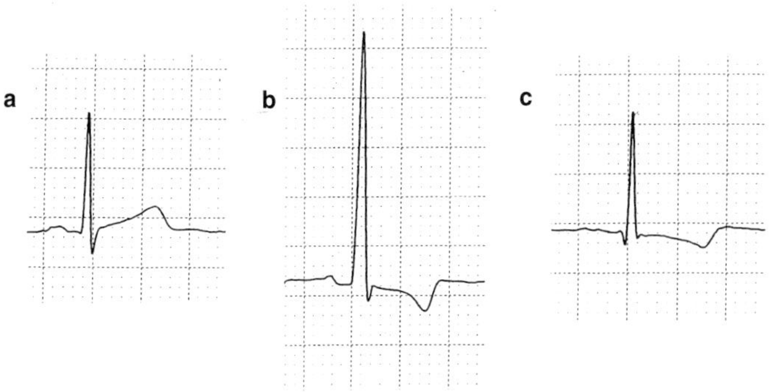

Fig. 42.1 ECG lead V5 in (a) normal (b) hypertrophy with voltage increase and (c) hypertrophy without voltage increase.

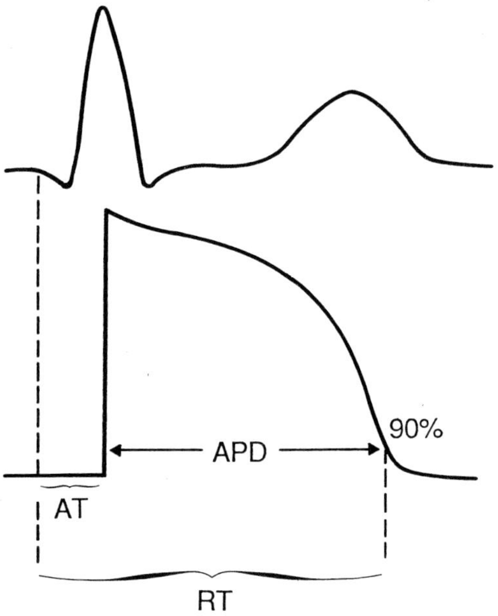

Fig. 42.2 Method of analysis of MAP signal for activation time (AT), action potential duration at 90% repolarization (APD) and total repolarization time (RT = AT + APD). (Reproduced from Franz *et al.* 1987, with permission.)

Because recordings were made from excised tissue preparation an inverse relationship between activation and repolarization could not be verified directly.

In-vivo exploration of left ventricular activation and repolarization became possible with the invention of the monophasic action potential (MAP) contact electrode catheter and probe that allow the electrophysiologist to map the endocardial and epicardial surface of the left ventricle in humans. Franz *et al.* (1987) recorded MAPs in 10 patients with electrocardiographically normal T waves and *QT* intervals. Seven patients had MAP recordings done at the left ventricular endocardium during routine catheterization and 5 patients had left ventricular epicardial MAP recordings performed during coronary artery bypass grafting, before initiation of heart–lung bypass. Figure 42.2 shows how the MAP recordings were analysed for AT, action potential duration (APD) and repolarization time (RT), and referenced to the surface ECG. Using similar methods, Cowan *et al.* (Cowan *et al.* 1988) recorded MAPs from the left ventricular epicardium in 10 patients undergoing coronary artery bypass grafting. MAPs were recorded from 10 sites in each patient during normothermic cardiopulmonary bypass. In both studies, a marked dispersion of AT and APD was measured at both the endocardial and epicardial surface of the human left ventricle. However, when APD was plotted as a function of AT (for either the endocardial or epicardial surface), a highly significant inverse relation was found in both studies (Fig. 42.3) (Franz *et al.* 1987; Cowan *et al.* 1988).

Activation occurred earlier at the endocardium than at the epicardium, yet epicardial repolarization occurred significantly earlier than endocardial repolarization (epicardial repolarization times ranged from 70.8 to 87.4 (mean 80.7 ± 3.9) per cent of the *QT* interval and endocardial repolarization times ranged from 80 to 97.8 (mean 87.1 ± 4.4) of the *QT* interval ($P < 0.001$)). Thus, there also is a transmural gradient of repolarization that is oriented opposite to that of transmural activation. These data do not prove but are consistent with the view that local repolarization is governed by local activation, regardless of the activation pathway or topology. The fact that 97.8% of body surface repolariza-

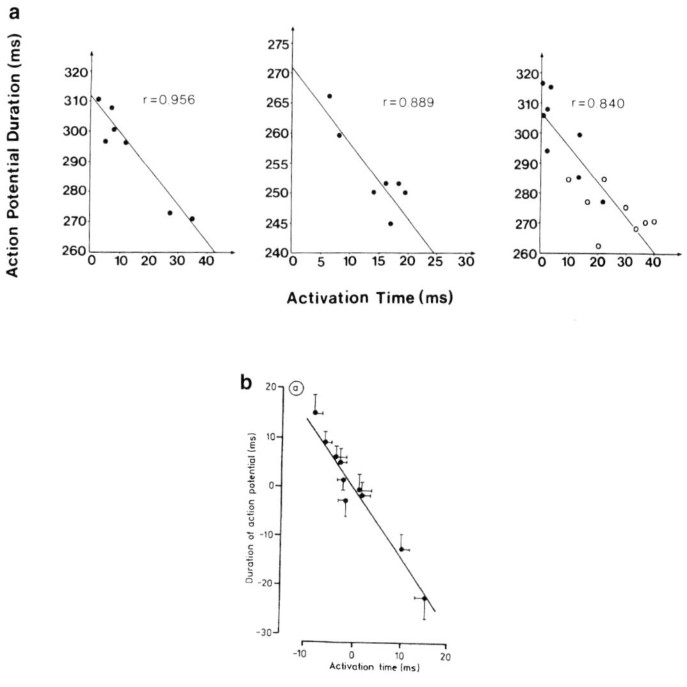

Fig. 42.3 (a) Individual linear regression analysis of the relationship between endocardial AT and APD in three patients with normal electrocardiograms. (Reproduced from Franz *et al.* 1987, with permission.) (b) Epicardial relation between AT and APD for 10 patients with upright T waves. (Reproduced from Cowan *et al.* 1988, with permission.)

tion (end of T wave) was accounted for by endocardial LV-MAP duration makes the existence of even longer repolarization intramurally (M-cells) unnecessary.

Dispersion of repolarization

At both the endocardial and the epicardial surface of the human left ventricle, the distribution of repolarization times was more uniform than the distribution of APD. Franz *et al.* (1987) reported 41.4 ms dispersion for APD and 26.4 ms dispersion for repolarization time. Cowan *et al.* (Cowan *et al.* 1988) reported 23 ms dispersion for (epicardial) activation, 35 ms dispersion for APD and 14 ms dispersion for repolarization. Given the greater duration of the T wave as compared to the QRS duration, it seems surprising at first that in the human left ventricle repolarization times are more evenly distributed than either AT or APD. This may be explained on the basis of the inverse relation between AT and APD (Fig. 42.3). The linear regression slopes of such plots typically have a value of slightly greater than negative unity: average −1.32 ± 0.45 in the study by Franz *et al.* (1987) and −1.44 in the study by Cowan *et al.* (1988). Although the AT-dependent shortening of APD slightly overcompensated for the activation delay, this inverse relationship is close enough to negative unity to help synchronize the repolarization in the entire ventricle. A more recent study in swine left ventricles using the CARTO mapping system and activation recovery intervals (ARI) as an index of local repolarization also showed less dispersion of repolarization than that of activation (Gepstein *et al.* 1997).

Why is the T wave longer than the QRS complex?

The greater duration of the T wave as compared to the QRS complex has been construed to indicate greater dispersion of repolarization than that of depolarization. This is true for the time domain but not for the voltage domain (Behrens *et al.* 1998). The QRS complex is caused by voltage gradients produced during successive ventricular cellular depolarizations whose upstrokes last only 1 ms. Repolarization, in contrast, may last well over 50 ms during phase 3 alone (the phase with the largest repolarizing voltage drop). Therefore, the entire QRS duration (upper limit of normal is 100 ms in humans) must be accounted for by the propagation time of activation through the ventricles. Repolarization, due to its much flatter slope, can produce a long-lasting deflection despite the fact that it occurs more uniformly across the ventricles (Fig. 42.4).

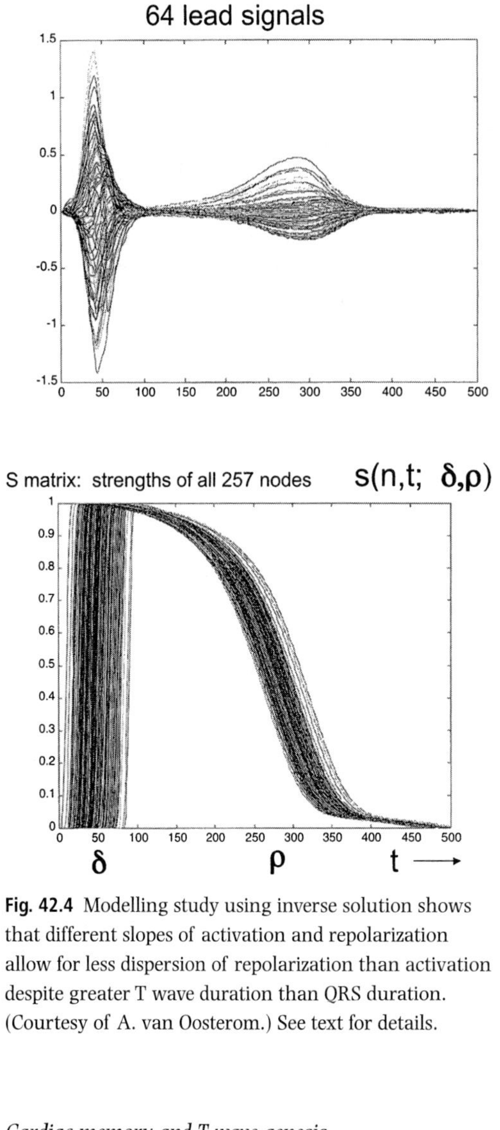

Fig. 42.4 Modelling study using inverse solution shows that different slopes of activation and repolarization allow for less dispersion of repolarization than activation despite greater T wave duration than QRS duration. (Courtesy of A. van Oosterom.) See text for details.

Cardiac memory and T wave genesis

The finding that APD seems dependent on AT yet independent of the anatomical location in the heart from which the measurements are obtained, has raised the intriguing question of whether regional differences in APD are due to intrinsic electrophysiological differences between myocardial cells, or whether they are secondary to the sequence of activation. Does a myocardial cell 'know' when to repolarize, just because of its site within the ventricle, or does an overriding mechanism 'tell' the cell when to repolarize?

One mechanism by which myocardial cells can be 'told' when to repolarize is electrotonic modulation. Electrically coupled cells may interact electrotonically which may produce an APD-shortening effect when neighbouring cells repolarize earlier and an APD-lengthening effect when neighbouring cells repolarize later. While electrotonic modulation by itself should exert its effect on repolarization without delay, several clinical and experimental observations suggest the involvement of a very slow, time-dependent mechanism in the modulation of ventricular repolarization.

On the basis of a meticulous analysis of ECGs recorded at various times during and after a period of right ventricular pacing, Rosenbaum *et al.* (1982) noted that T wave changes caused by ectopic ventricular pacing develop with a very slow time course of several hours and require an even longer time of normal activation to dissipate. These authors further noted that prolonged ventricular pacing modulates ventricular repolarization such that the T wave becomes again concordant to the R wave, as previously was the case during normal supraventricular activation. They interpreted this intriguing finding by attributing to the myocardium the properties of accumulation or 'memory' by which the heart 'learns' to adjust its repolarization to an altered activation sequence and by which it retains the adapted state long after the activation sequence is normalized.

Costard-Jäckle *et al.* (1989) were first to validate cardiac memory as an intrinsic myocardial property. Using MAP recordings in isolated Langendorff-perfused rabbit hearts, AT, APD, and RT were mapped in both the right and left ventricle, first during 45 min of right atrial pacing, then during 120 min of right ventricular pacing, and then again during 60 min of right atrial pacing. During the initial atrial pacing phase, APD was inversely related to AT (slope = –1.63; $r = 0.76$), indicating that sites with earlier activation repolarized later. With the onset of ventricular pacing, the inverse correlation between AT and APD disappeared (slope = –0.19; $r = 0.31$). Continuing ventricular pacing produced slow changes in APD that restored the inverse relation (slope = –0.71; $r = 0.68$ at 120 min; $P < 0.0002$ vs. 5 min). Switching back from ventricular to atrial pacing again perturbed the inverse correlation (slope = 0.28; $r = 0.35$), but at 60 min of atrial pacing a significant inverse correlation was re-established (S = –1.25; $r = 0.53$; $P < 0.01$ vs. 5 min).

This isolated heart study (Costärd-Jäckle *et al.* 1989) confirmed that cardiac muscle is capable of adjusting its repolarization sequence to a lasting change in activation sequence. Once adjusted, it retains this new repolarization sequence even when the original activation sequence is resumed. This conspicuous phenomenon, which was observed in the absence of innervation, suggests that the myocardium possesses some form of information retention ('memory'). The cellular and molecular mechanisms underlying this phenomenon are currently under intense investigation by the lab of Rosen (Geller & Rosen, 1993; Rosen, 2000).

Clinical implications of electrotonic modulation and cardiac memory

The dependence of APD on AT, and the long time required to establish this relationship, has several important implications. First, the inverse correlation between AT and APD tends to compensate for the successive delay along the ventricular activation pathway and, consequently, tends to synchronize ventricular repolarization. In support of the human heart data, Costard-Jäckle *et al.* (1989) found in the isolated rabbit heart *less* dispersion of repolarization after prolonged pacing from the same site, when the inverse correlation between AT and APD was highly significant, than shortly after a change in ventricular activation sequence, when the inverse correlation disappeared. Thus, a heart which is activated along the same activation pathway over a long time (as is the normal heart with supraventricular impulse origin and conduction over the His–Purkinje system), can be expected to have a more synchronized global repolarization of the ventricular myocardium than hearts shortly after a change in activation sequence, as in ventricular extrasystoles or short runs of ventricular tachycardia.

T wave inversion in LVH

Ventricular hypertrophy often is characterized not only by augmented QRS voltage but also by typical repolarization abnormalities ('strain pattern') (Surawicz, 1986). Hypotheses advanced to explain these repolarization abnormalities include secondary T wave changes due to changes in ventricular activation and primary T wave changes due to changes in APD independent of activation disturbances (Autenrieth *et al.* 1975; Surawicz, 1986). Results from intracellular action potential recordings in tissue preparations excised from animals with experimentally induced LVH showed disparate changes in APD between different areas of the ventricle (Cameron *et al.* 1986; Aronson & Ming 1993). Subendocardial ischaemia also has been implicated as a cause of electrocardiographic 'strain' (Pringle *et al.* 1992) although direct evidence for myocardial ischaemia in human LVH is lacking.

MAP data from patients with LVH

In contrast to non-hypertrophied left ventricles, in which the T wave is upright and in which APD is inversely related to AT, hypertrophied left ventricles with inverted negative T waves do not exhibit an inverse relationship between AT and APD. Rather, APD seems to be randomly distributed across the left ventricle, with no apparent relationship to AT. In the study of Franz *et al.* (1991) the pooled linear regression slope was slightly positive, but the regression did not attain statistical significance. Cowan *et al.* (1988) found that the epicardial APD were distributed randomly and followed the epicardial repolarization sequence rather than being inversely related to it (Fig. 42.5). This direct data is compatible with discordant T waves, as is further explained in Fig. 42.6. In both studies, the direction and dispersion of ventricular *activation* in patients with left ventricular hypertrophy were essentially similar to that in patients with normal, upright T waves. Thus, the T wave inversion associated with left ventricular hypertrophy cannot be labelled 'secondary T wave changes', but seems to result from a 'primary' change in repolarization.

Possible cellular mechanisms underlying T wave alterations in LVH

Is T wave inversion in LVH a sign of myocardial ischaemia?

LVH-related T wave inversions in left lateral leads are often misjudged as evidence of ischaemia. MAP recordings have been shown to be highly sensitive markers of ischaemia (Donaldson *et al.*

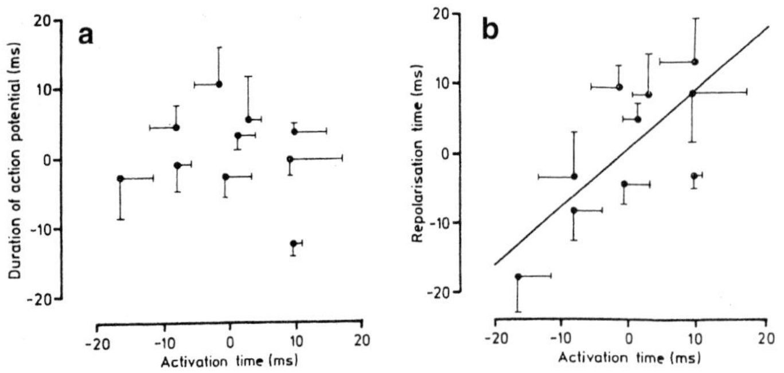

Fig. 42.5 (a) Lack of inverse relation between AT and APD in eight patients with aortic stenosis and LVH. (b) Owing to lack of inverse correlation, repolarization time was no longer opposite to activation but followed it. Data are derived from epicardial MAP recordings. (Reproduced from Cowan *et al.* 1988, with permission.)

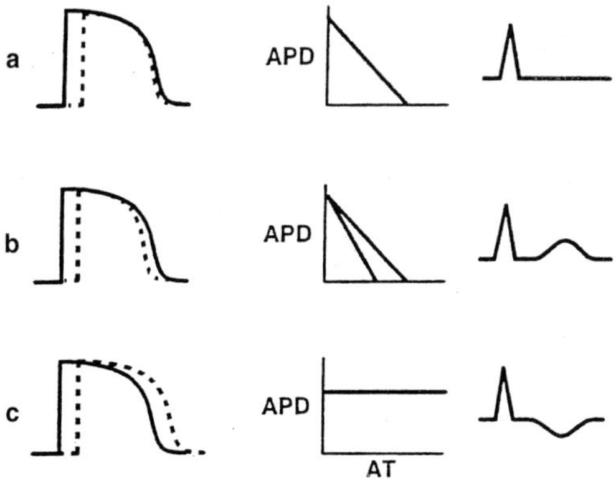

Fig. 42.6 Explanation of T wave polarity on the basis of the relationship between AT and APD. (a) A theoretical relationship in which each increment in AT is matched precisely by a corresponding decrement in APD. In this case, repolarization would occur simultaneously at all ventricular sites, the linear regression would have a slope of −1.0 and a correlation coefficient of 1.0, and the ECG would exhibit no T wave at all but rather an isoelectric line. (b) The relationship between AT and APD in subjects with normal T waves. APD is inversely related to AT, with a slope slightly greater than negative unity. This renders the direction of the repolarization wave opposite to that of depolarization, a situation which is consistent with, and which can explain the paradox of, T wave concordance. (c) Situation encountered in patients with LVH. With a correlation coefficient near zero, it might be said that ventricular APD is distributed at random, with no significant slope in either positive or negative direction. On average then, repolarization would travel in the same direction as depolarization, and in the ECG would cause a deflection opposite to that of depolarization.

1984; Franz *et al.* 1984). MAP recordings from hypertrophied human left ventricles (Cowan *et al.* 1988; Franz *et al.* 1991) were qualitatively normal, with sharp upstrokes, distinct plateau phases and steep final repolarization slopes. Although MAPs were recorded from a limited number of sites, ischaemia, if present, should not have gone undetected (especially in endocardial recordings). Also, endocardial AT did not differ significantly between LVH and control groups, while endocardial mapping studies in patients with coronary artery disease have reported significantly longer AT (Vassallo *et al.* 1988). Thus, it seems unlikely that myocardial ischaemia is the cause for T wave inversion in left ventricular hypertrophy. Lack of an inverse relation between AT and APD suffices to explain an altered ventricular gradient and T wave inversion without the assumption of myocardial ischaemia.

Deficiency of electrotonic modulation

If T wave concordance in the normal ECG is due to electrotonic modulation of ventricular repolarization by the sequence of ventricular activation, one must ask why such concordance is lost in patients with advanced LVH and inverted T waves. LVH is associated with a variety of cellular or histological alterations, including changes in fibre orientation (Maron *et al.* 1975), marked connective tissue infiltration, loss or thickening of gap junctions, and increase in basal membrane thickness (Hatt *et al.* 1974), all of which may decrease cellular electrical coupling (Cooklin *et al.* 1997). It is possible that some or all of these alterations diminish or alter electrotonic interaction in the heart so that APD no longer is influenced by AT. The random distribution of APD in the hypertrophied ventricle, with no apparent negative or positive correlation to AT, may therefore result from a lack of intercellular electrical communication that in normal hearts permits activation to modulate repolarization. This is further supported by the observation that the epicardial to endocardial repolarization process (as in normal hearts) is reversed in LVH in rats (Shipsey *et al.* 1997).

Channels and receptors involved in the transition to LVH

Progression of LVH is marked not only by changes in myocyte size (Campbell *et al.* 1991) and altered contractile proteins expression (Yamazaki *et al.* 1995) but also by changes in membrane ion channels and membrane receptors (Nuss & Houser *et al.* 1993; Sadoshima & Izumo, 1993; Gidh-Jain *et al.* 1995). The role of these mediators for intracardiac electrophysiology and body surface ECG has not yet been established. With respect to cardiac memory, data from the lab of Rosen suggest that calcium channels and angiotensin receptors play a role (Rosen & Plotnikov, 2002).

Arrhythmia implications of repolarization 'strain' in LVH

The correlation, or lack thereof, between AT and APD not only helps explain the T wave concordance in the normal ECG and T wave inversion in LVH patients but may also be relevant for the greater arrhythmia propensity reported for patients with LVH. As illustrated in Figs 42.3 and 42.5, the normal *inverse* correlation between AT and APD has a synchronizing effect on overall ventricular repolarization. Conversely, lack of an inverse correlation between AT and APD, as found in LVH, allows for a more random distribution of APD and, consequently, greater dispersion of repolarization time. This has been shown to be the case in patients and in experimental studies of LVH (Kowey *et al.* 1991; Shipsey *et al.* 1997).

It is well recognized that uniformity of ventricular repolarization is important for protecting the ventricle from re-entrant arrhythmias. Greater dispersion of repolarization in LVH patients may thus be a factor contributing to the increased arrhythmia susceptibility and the positive predic-tive value of electrocardiographic left ventricular hypertrophy for sudden death (McLenachan *et al.* 1987). Under this aspect, it is particularly noteworthy that left ventricular hypertrophy is associated with an increased risk for arrhythmias and sudden cardiac death only when T wave inversion ('strain') is present, alone or in company with voltage criteria of LVH (Okin *et al.* 2000, 2002).

References

Aronson, R.S. & Ming, Z. (1993) Cellular mechanisms of arrhythmias in hypertrophied and failing myocardium. *Circulation*, **83**, VII76–VII83.

Autenrieth, G., Surawicz, B., Kuo, C.S. & Arita, M. (1975) Primary T wave abnormalities caused by uniform and regional shortening of ventricular monophasic action potential in dog. *Circulation*, **51**, 668–676.

Behrens, S., Li, C., Knollmann, B.C. & Franz, M.R. (1998) Dispersion of ventricular repolarization in the voltage domain. *PACE (Pacing and Clinical Electrophysiology)*, **21**, 100–107.

Cameron, J.S., Miller, L.S., Kimura, S. *et al.* (1986) Systemic hypertension induces disparate localized left ventricular action potential lengthening and altered sensitivity to verapamil in left ventricular myocardium. *Journal of Molecular Cell Cardiology*, **18**, 169–175.

Campbell, S.E., Korecky, B. & Rakusan, K. (1991) Remodeling of myocyte dimensions in hypertrophic and atrophic rat hearts. *Circulation Research*, **68**, 984–996.

Cohen, I., Giles, W. & Noble, D. (1976) Cellular basis for the T wave of the electrocardiogram. *Nature (London)*, **262**, 657–661.

Cooklin, M., Wallis, W.R., Sheridan, D.J. & Fry, C.H. (1997) Changes in cell-to-cell electrical coupling associated with left ventricular hypertrophy. *Circulation Research*, **80**, 765–771.

Costard-Jäckle, A., Goetsch, B., Antz, M. & Franz, M.R. (1989) Slow and long-lasting modulation of myocardial repolarization produced by ectopic activation in isolated rabbit hearts. Evidence for cardiac 'memory'. *Circulation*, **80**, 1412–1420.

Cowan, J.C., Hilton, C.J., Griffiths, C.J. *et al.* (1988) Sequence of epicardial repolarization and configuration of the T wave. *British Heart Journal*, **60**, 424–433.

Donaldson, R.M., Taggart, P., Swanton, H., Fox, K., Rickards, A.F. & Noble, D. (1984) Effect of nitroglycerin on the electrical changes of early or subendocardial ischaemia evaluated by monophasic action potential recordings. *Cardiovascular Research*, **18**, 7–13.

Franz, M.R., Bargheer, K., Costard-Jäckle, A., Miller, D.C. & Lichtlen, P.R. (1991) Human ventricular repolarization and T wave genesis. *Progress in Cardiovascular Diseases*, **33**, 369–384.

Franz, M.R., Bargheer, K., Rafflenbeul, W., Haverich, A. & Lichtlen, P.R. (1987) Monophasic action potential mapping in human subjects with normal electrocardiograms: direct evidence for the genesis of the T wave. *Circulation*, **75**, 379–386.

Franz, M.R., Flaherty, J.T., Platia, E.V., Bulkley, B.H. & Weisfeldt, M.L. (1984) Localization of regional myocardial ischaemia by recording of monophasic action potentials. *Circulation*, **69**, 593–604.

Geller, J.C. & Rosen, M.R. (1993) Persistent T wave changes after alteration of the ventricular activation sequence. New insights into cellular mechanisms of 'cardiac memory'. *Circulation*, **88**, 1811–1819.

Gepstein, L., Hayam, G. & Ben-Haim, S.A. (1997) Activation–repolarization coupling in the normal swine endocardium. *Circulation*, **96**, 4036–4043.

Gidh-Jain M., Huang, B., Jain, P., Battula, V. & el-Sherif, N. (1995) Reemergence of the fetal pattern of L-type calcium channel gene expression in non infarcted myocardium during left ventricular remodeling. *Biochemical and Biophysical Research Communications*, **216**, 892–897.

Hatt, P.Y., Jouannot, P., Moravec, J. & Swynghedauw, B. (1974) Current trends in heart hypertrophy. *Basic Research in Cardiology*, **69**, 479–483.

Kowey, P.R., Friechling, T.D., Sewter, J. *et al.* (1991) Electrophysiological effects of left ventricular hypertrophy. Effect of calcium and potassium channel blockade. *Circulation*, **83**, 2067–2075.

Maron, B.J., Ferrans, V.J. & Roberts, W.C. (1975) Ultrastructural features of degenerated cardiac muscle cells in patients with cardiac hypertrophy. *American Journal of Pathology*, **79**, 387–434.

McLenachan, J.M., Henderson, E., Morris, K.I. & Dargie, H.J. (1987) Ventricular arrhythmias in patients with hypertensive left ventricular hypertrophy. *New England Journal of Medicine*, **317**, 787–792.

Nuss, H.B. & Houser, S.R. (1993) T-type Ca^{2+} current is expressed in hypertrophied adult feline left ventricular myocytes. *Circulation Research*, **73**, 777–782.

Okin, P.M., Devereux, R.B., Jern, S., Kjeldsen, S.E., Julius, S. & Dahlof, B. (2000) Baseline characteristics in relation to electrocardiographic left ventricular hypertrophy in hypertensive patients: the Losartan intervention for endpoint reduction (LIFE) in hypertension study. The Life Study Investigators. *Hypertension*, **36**, 766–773.

Okin, P.M., Wright, J.T., Nieminen, M.S. *et al.* (2002) Ethnic differences in electrocardiographic criteria for left ventricular hypertrophy: the LIFE study. Losartan Intervention For Endpoint. *American Journal of Hypertension*, **15**, 663–671.

Oopik, A.J., Dorogy, M., Devereux, R.B. *et al.* (1996) Major electrocardiographic abnormalities among American Indians aged 45 to 74 years (the Strong Heart Study). *American Journal of Cardiology*, **78**, 1400–1405.

Pringle, S.D., Dunn, F.G., Tweddel, A.C. *et al.* (1992) Symptomatic and silent myocardial ischaemia in hypertensive patients with left ventricular hypertrophy. *British Heart Journal*, **67**, 377–382.

Rosen, M.R. (2000) What is cardiac memory? *Journal of Cardiovascular Electrophysiology*, **11**, 1289–1293.

Rosen, M. & Plotnikov, A. (2002) The pharmacology of cardiac memory. *Pharmacology & Therapeutics*. **94**, 63–75.

Rosenbaum, M.B., Blanco, H.H., Elizari, M.V., Lazzari, J.O. & Davidenko, J.M. (1982) Electrotonic modulation of the T wave and cardiac memory. *American Journal of Cardiology*, **50**, 213–222.

Sadoshima, J. & Izumo, S. (1993) Molecular characterization of angiotensin II-induced hypertrophy of cardiac myocytes and hyperplasia of cardiac fibroblasts. Critical role of the AT1 receptor subtype. *Circulation Research*, **73**, 413–423.

Shipsey, S.J., Bryant, S.M. & Hart, G. (1997) Effects of hypertrophy on regional action potential characteristics in the rat left ventricle: a cellular basis for T wave inversion? *Circulation*, **96**, 2061–2068.

Surawicz, B. (1986) Electrocardiographic diagnosis of chamber enlargement. *Journal of the American College of Cardiology*, **8**, 711–724.

Vassallo, J.A., Cassidy, D.M., Kindwall, K.E., Marchlinski, F.E. & Josephson, M.E. (1988) Nonuniform recovery of excitability in the left ventricle. *Circulation*, **78**, 1365–1372.

Yamazaki, T., Komuro, I., Kudoh, S. *et al.* (1995) Angiotensin II partly mediates mechanical stress-induced cardiac hypertrophy. *Circulation Research*, **77**, 258–265.

CHAPTER 43

Macro T Wave Alternans

Robert L. Lux and Konrad Brockmeier

Introduction

T wave alternans (TWA) is the systematic alternation or variation of ST–T waveform in one or more leads of the electrocardiogram and has been associated with the presence of heart disease or abnormal cardiac conditions and as a harbinger of serious cardiac arrhythmias. The phenomenon of TWA is subdivided into two classes, microvolt TWA and macro TWA.

• Microvolt TWA refers to tiny alternations of ST–T waveform that are revealed by complex signal processing (spectral analysis) of continuous recordings (Adam *et al.* 1984; Smith *et al.* 1988; Nearing *et al.* 1991; Rosenbaum *et al.* 1994; Pastore *et al.* 1999). Microvolt TWA is heavily rate dependent and therefore dependent on its acquisition protocol, which is noninvasively performed under controlled exercise testing conditions or invasively by atrial pacing to maintain constant heart rates (Hohnloser *et al.* 1997; Turitto *et al.* 2001). The evidence of this alternation appears as a spectral spike at half the frequency of the heart rate and reflects a microvolt or submicrovolt but significant alternation of ST–T voltage. In general, microvolt TWA is not observable on standard ECGs, a consequence of its miniscule magnitude compared to the ECG signal and any noise or artefact present in the signals.

• In contrast, Macro TWA refers to beat-to-beat alternation or systematic variation of ST–T waveform that is easily observed in electrocardiographic leads without enhancement, filtering, or special signal processing. The ECG in Fig. 43.1 is from a patient with LQT syndrome and shows marked TWA.

Microvolt TWA has been shown to reflect abnormal electrophysiological function and has been implicated as a marker of risk in patients with coronary artery disease (Nearing *et al.* 1991; Rosenbaum *et al.* 1996; Ikeda *et al.* 2002; Pires 2002), dilated cardiomyopathy (Adachi *et al.* 1999), myocardial hypertrophy (Kon-No *et al.* 2001), and hypertension (Hennersdorf *et al.* 2001). Macro TWA can be observed in normal animal hearts that are being paced at rapid rates, but its occurrence at physiological heart rates has been associated with presence of disease and abnormal electrophysiology. Specifically, macro TWA has been observed in patients with long QT syndrome, Brugada's syndrome, and Prinzmetal's angina (Schwartz & Malliani 1975; Zareba *et al.* 1994; Brockmeier *et al.* 2001; Morita *et al.* 2002). The mechanisms of microvolt TWA and macro TWA remain elusive and it is not clear whether or not they are both just subclasses of a broader phenomenon relating to repolarization dynamics in the setting of heterogeneous repolarization. In the next sections, we shall review the electrophysiology of repolarization, discuss mechanisms that might explain these phenomena, and present a few provocative examples that illustrate the complexity of the problem.

Electrophysiology of repolarization – factors that influence repolarization

As for the entire ECG signal, the ST–T wave of the electrocardiogram results from the flow of ionic currents generated by each cardiac cell. The primary currents of repolarization relate to calcium, potassium and sodium channel function and reflect the plateau and downstroke phases of the action potential elicited from each

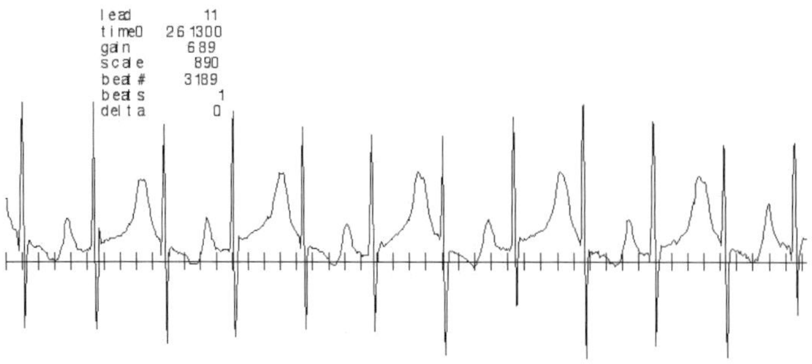

Fig. 43.1 Lead V5 of a young male with LQT3 syndrome showing gross macro TWA. The morphology of alternans varied over time and seemed to be related to cycle length. Adjacent tick marks are 100 ms apart.

cell during each heart beat. The summation of effects of all extracellular currents inscribe the ST–T wave of the electrocardiogram and the ultimate waveform observed in a particular ECG lead at arbitrary body surface site depends upon the sequence of activation (depolarization) of the heart and on the distribution of intrinsic repolarization properties (action potential durations). In addition, repolarization currents are influenced by heart rate, autonomic nerve tone, presence of global or regional disease or abnormal condition, and dynamic (memory) considerations.

The sequence with which heart cells depolarize determines the QRS waveform of the ECG. Importantly, the sequence of depolarization, and consequently, the time of depolarization for each cell dictates the time when each cell will repolarize (time of recovery) based on the action potential duration of the cell and on its electrotonic modulation by repolarization currents from neighbouring cells. Thus ST–T waveform is highly dependent upon activation sequence. Since action potential durations in the ventricles are heterogeneous (shorter on the epicardium and base, longer on the endocardium and apex) and clearly different in normal and diseased myocardium, the timing sequence of repolarization currents and hence the ST–T wave will be heavily dependent upon both the distribution of action potential characteristics and the sequence of activation.

Historically, rate dependency of repolarization, as evident in prolongation or shortening of the *QT* interval with decrease or increase of heart rate, respectively, reflects dependency of action potentials on cycle length. Although the gross morphology of ST–T waves generated by normal hearts does not change substantially over a range of physiological heart rates, *QT* interval and T wave width shorten with increased heart rate. Important to note is the fact that rate dependency itself is heterogeneous in the sense that sites having the longest repolarization (action potential duration) change more with increased heart rate than do sites of shortest repolarization. Although rate dependency of repolarization may not play a direct role in the establishment of TWA, it provides a substrate for facilitating TWA (Verrier *et al.* 2002).

Autonomic nerve fibres innervate the heart in a heterogeneous manner. Thus nerve tone, which is dynamic and regional in nature, leads to heterogeneous neural modulation of action potential characteristics. The influence of the cardiac sympathetic nerves in long QT syndrome as a modulator of arrhythmogenicity is well established. Furthermore, heterogeneous repolarization remains a likely candidate for explaining the increased risk of arrhythmia occurrence in these patients if not implicated as a secondary means of facilitating arrhythmia triggering mechanisms (Schwartz 2001).

Finally, the phenomenon of cardiac memory or the dynamics of cardiac repolarization, whether short term (several beats or minutes) or long term (hours, or longer), should be considered when describing repolarization heterogeneity and its relevance to repolarization phenomena. The changes of cardiac repolarization induced by changes in cycle length are systematic but complex. A rapid change of heart rate between two stable rates results in a rapid component of repolarization change (one or two beats) followed by a longer change (hundreds of beats). These repolarization time constants are themselves heterogeneous in the heart and suggest the potential for contributing to

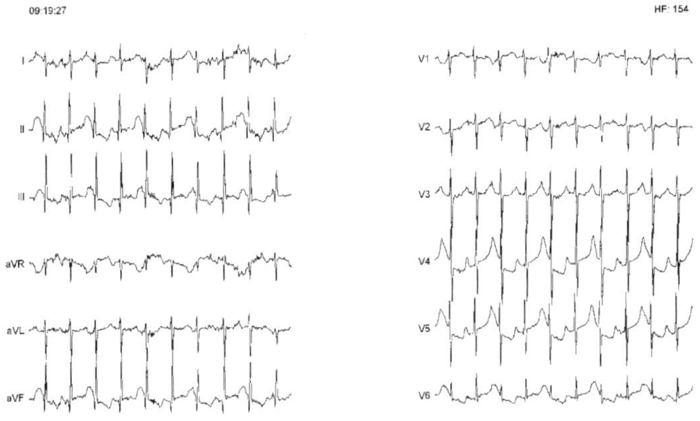

Fig. 43.2 Clinical 12-lead ECG in the same patient shown in Fig. 43.1. Note the varying extent of macro TWA across leads.

increased risk of arrhythmias (Libbus & Rosenbaum 2002; Rosen & Plotnikov, 2002).

Possible mechanisms of TWA

The observation that macro TWA usually does not appear in all ECG leads, even in densely sampled experimental preparations, suggests the presence of local or regional alternation of electrophysiology. The 12-lead ECG in Fig. 43.2 shows TWA in some but not all leads of a patient with LQT3. One potential explanation is that microvolt or macro TWA could result as a secondary consequence of regional alternation of activation sequence. For example a localized region that exhibited conduction block on alternate beats would contribute different repolarization currents on alternate beats. Furthermore, when conduction blocks in the region, the activation sequence downstream from the region would result in altered repolarization currents in the active tissue. Such a mechanism would require that there be QRS alternation in some ECG leads and, in fact, this has been observed and represents evidence that this is a viable explanation for TWA. A variation of this mechanism would be the existence of localized regions of alternating conduction, slow on one beat and fast (super-conduction) on the next. This mechanism is fundamentally not different than the one described for complete block and reflects a repolarization affect that is secondary to regional alternation of conduction, whether complete block or slowing and acceleration.

The obvious mechanism implicated in microvolt TWA observed during mild exercise in patients with coronary artery disease is the imposed hypoxia in localized regions that are ischaemic. The underlying changes in ion channel function on alternate beats may simply be a consequence of the ischaemic load or may reflect a combination of the above regional alternations of conduction in addition to primary changes to repolarization currents. However, the hypoxia/ischaemia mechanism does not explain occurrence of the phenomenon in patients without ischaemia or coronary artery disease.

Observation of TWA in patients with ion channel disorders such as long QT syndrome, Brugada's syndrome or idiopathic VT or VF suggest a mechanism that is a primary repolarization defect, e.g. a regional, primary alternation in the function of one or more of the repolarization ion currents or channels. The exact location within the ST–T interval over which the alternation is seen may offer a clue as to which of the many possible currents might be involved.

A final possibility relates to the fact that the heart is innervated regionally by parasympathetic fibres and that regional neural mediation of action potential duration heterogeneity, in conjunction with heterogeneous rate dependency of repolarization may offer a substrate favourable for the occurrence of TWA. Although the rate of change of nerve tone on repolarization may be too small to explain beat-to-beat alternation in T waveform, the potential contribution of regional nerve tone to influence repolarization regionally, may facilitate occurrence of TWA under abnormal conditions or in the presence of disease.

Examples of macro TWA

TWA preceding onset of episode of torsades de pointes

The data in Fig. 43.3 show an ECG strip obtained from a patient with long QT syndrome (LQT3) that followed an episode of macro TWA. The alternation of ST–T waveform was clear and there was no obvious QRS alternation or rate variation that could explain the TWA. The data in this figure show the onset of torsades de pointes, a ventricular tachyarrhythmia associated with long QT syndrome that can degenerate into ventricular fibrillation. In this instance the torsades de pointes resolved to sinus rhythm. The data in Fig. 43.4 show the superposition of ten successive beats in lead V5, time aligned to QRS onset, and clearly shows the two families of waveforms. This simple technique of superimposing ECG signals provides a quick means to asses macro TWA.

TWA during fixed rate pacing

In Fig. 43.5 we show several seconds of a body surface ECG recorded on a patient with an

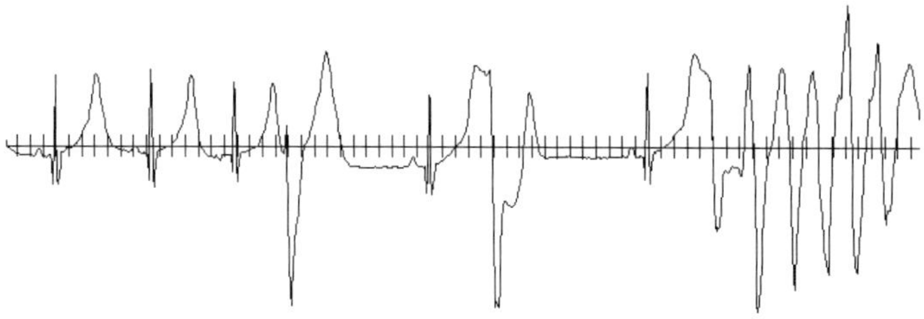

Fig. 43.3 Onset of torsades de pointes in a patient who exhibited macro TWA in a 12-lead Holter recording.

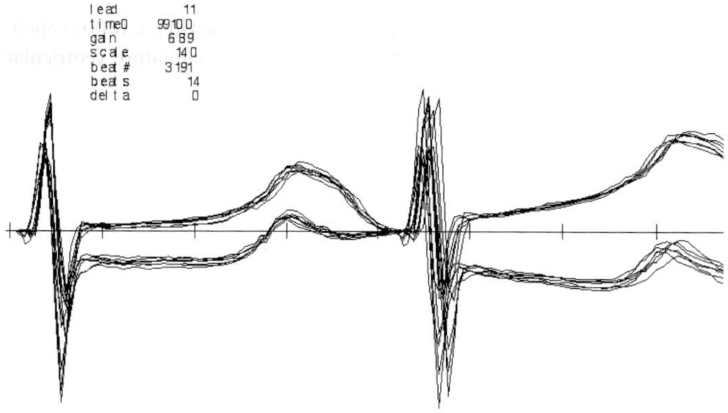

Fig. 43.4 Superposition of 10 consecutive beats from ECG lead V5 in a patient with long QT syndrome (LQT3). The data clearly show two families of ST–T morphology. Clearly, cycle lengths of these 10 beats were very stable. In this patient, the TWA morphologies changed over time and with rate.

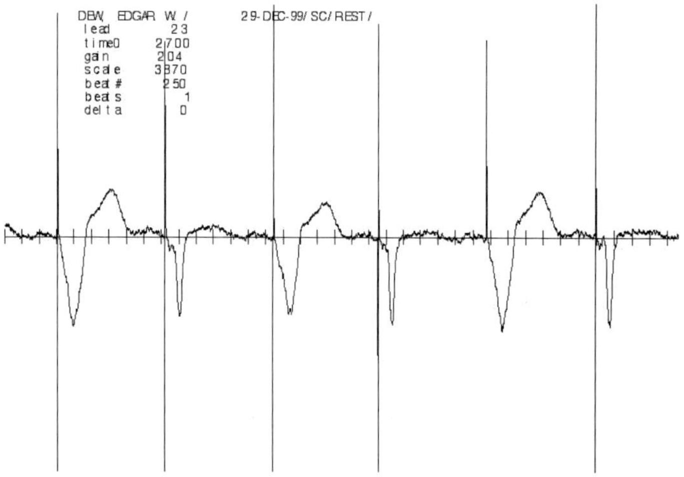

Fig. 43.5 ECG (lead V4) of a patient, post infarction, with fixed rate pacing. Note the obvious QRS alternans, which explains the observation of TWA as an effect secondary to alteration in activation sequence.

implanted pacemaker who had recently had a myocardial infarction. The alternation of ST–T waveform is highly visible and easily observed in the recording. Note that the patient was being paced at a fixed rate throughout the duration of the recording. On further examination, a systematic variation in QRS width and morphology can be seen which suggests that the ST–T alternation may be a consequence of activation sequence alternation. Thus in this patient, one might conclude that the TWA is strictly a secondary consequence of alternation or variation of activation sequence.

Summary

In summary, we have described the phenomenon of TWA as an alternation in the ST–T wave of the electrocardiogram, focusing on the 'visible' or macro TWA class of this phenomenon. The examples shown clearly implicate occurrence of macro TWA as a marker of impending arrhythmia or presence of precarious arrhythmia substrate. The association of TWA with specific cardiac diseases and conditions suggest its utility as a marker of disease, as a harbinger of impending arrhythmia, and as a potential means to monitor pharmacological or pacing efficacy designed to reduce risk of arrhythmia. The complexity of repolarization electrophysiology, in general, with its dependency on activation sequence, intrinsic repolarization properties, heart rate, nerve tone, memory, and pathologic condition or disease reflect the difficulty in accepting one mechanism or another to explain the observed phenomena. However, alternation of conduction and/or intrinsic repolarization, hypoxia induced alterations, and neural influences, either individually or in combination, remain likely candidates for causing if not facilitating occurrence of TWA.

References

Adachi, K., Ohnishi, Y., Shima, T. *et al.* (1999) Determinant of microvolt-level T-wave alternans in patients with dilated cardiomyopathy. *Journal of the American College of Cardiology*, **34**, 374–380.

Adam, D.R., Smith, J.M., Akselrod, S., Nyberg, S., Powell, A.O. & Cohen, R.J. (1984) Fluctuations in T-wave morphology and susceptibility to ventricular fibrillation. *Journal of Electrocardiology*, **17**, 209–218.

Brockmeier, K., Aslan, I., Hilbel, T., Eberle, T., Ulmer, H.E. & Lux, R.L. (2001) T-wave alternans in LQTS: repolarization-rate dynamics from digital 12-lead Holter data. *Journal of Electrocardiology*, **34** (Suppl.), 93–96.

Hennersdorf, M.G., Niebch, V., Perings, C. & Strauer, B.E. (2001) T wave alternans and ventricular arrhythmias in arterial hypertension. *Hypertension*, **37**, 199–203.

Hohnloser, S.H., Klingenheben, T., Zabel, M., Li, Y.G., Albrecht, P. & Cohen, R.J. (1997) T wave alternans during exercise and atrial pacing in humans. *Journal of Cardiovascular Electrophysiology*, **8**, 987–993.

Ikeda, T., Saito, H., Tanno, K. *et al.* (2002) T-wave alternans as a predictor for sudden cardiac death after myocardial infarction. *American Journal of Cardiology*, **89**, 79–82.

Kon-No, Y., Watanabe, J., Koseki, Y. *et al.* (2001) Microvolt T wave alternans in human cardiac hypertrophy: electrical instability and abnormal myocardial arrangement. *Journal of Cardiovascular Electrophysiology*, **12**, 759–763.

Libbus, I. & Rosenbaum, D.S. (2002) Remodeling of cardiac repolarization: mechanisms and implications of memory. *Cardiac Electrophysiology Review*, **6**, 302–310.

Morita, H., Nagase, S., Kusano, K. & Ohe, T. (2002) Spontaneous T wave alternans and premature ventricular contractions during febrile illness in a patient with Brugada syndrome. *Journal of Cardiovascular Electrophysiology*, **13**, 816–818.

Nearing, B.D., Huang, A.H. and Verrier, R.L. (1991) Dynamic tracking of cardiac vulnerability by complex demodulation of the T wave. *Science*, **252**, 437–440.

Pastore, J.M., Girouard, S.D., Laurita, K.R., Akar, F.G. & Rosenbaum, D.S. (1999) Mechanism linking T-wave alternans to the genesis of cardiac fibrillation. *Circulation*, **99**, 1385–1394.

Pires, L.A. (2002) T wave alternans and ventricular arrhythmia risk stratification: uses and limitations. *Journal of Cardiovascular Electrophysiology*, **13**, 776–777.

Rosen, M. & Plotnikov, A. (2002) The pharmacology of cardiac memory. *Pharmacology & Therapeutics*, **94**, 63–75.

Rosenbaum, D.S., Albrecht, P. & Cohen, R.J. (1996) Predicting sudden cardiac death from T wave alternans of the surface electrocardiogram: promise and pitfalls. *Journal of Cardiovascular Electrophysiology*, **7**, 1095–1111.

Rosenbaum, D.S., Jackson, L.E., Smith, J.M., Garan, H., Ruskin, J.N. & Cohen, R.J. (1994) Electrical alternans and vulnerability to ventricular arrhythmias. *New England Journal of Medicine*, **330**, 235–241.

Schwartz, P.J. (2001) QT prolongation, sudden death, and sympathetic imbalance: the pendulum swings. *Journal of Cardiovascular Electrophysiology*, **12**, 1074–1077.

Schwartz, P.J. & Malliani, A. (1975) Electrical alternation of the T-wave: clinical and experimental evidence of its relationship with the sympathetic nervous system and with the long QT syndrome. *American Heart Journal*, **89**, 45–50.

Smith, J.M., Clancy, E.A., Valeri, C.R., Ruskin, J.N. & Cohen, R.J. (1988) Electrical alternans and cardiac electrical instability. *Circulation*, **77**, 110–121.

Turitto, G., Caref, E.B., El-Attar, G. *et al.* (2001) Optimal target heart rate for exercise-induced T-wave alternans. *Annals of Noninvasive Electrocardiology*, **6**, 123–128.

Verrier, R.L., Nearing, B.D. & Stone, P.H. (2002) Optimizing ambulatory ECG monitoring of T-wave alternans for arrhythmia risk assessment. *Cardiac Electrophysiology Review*, **6**, 329–333.

Zareba, W., Moss, A.J., le Cessie, S. & Hall, W.J. (1994) T wave alternans in idiopathic long QT syndrome. *Journal of the American College of Cardiology*, **23**, 1541–1546.

CHAPTER 44

Microscopic T Wave Alternans

Otto Costantini

Historical background and definitions

Macroscopic electrical alternans on the surface electrocardiogram (ECG) is defined as a change in the amplitude, width, and/or shape of the ECG signal that repeats on an every-other beat basis. Hering (1909) first reported it in an experimental animal. Its correlation with cardiac pathology was soon made by Lewis (1910) in a patient with a paroxysmal supraventricular tachycardia: 'alternation occurs either when the heart muscle is normal but the heart rate is very fast or when there is serious heart disease and the heart rate is normal'. Others subsequently recorded alternans on the surface ECG, but the reported incidence of visible electrical alternans was only 0.1% (Kalter & Schwartz 1948). Since then, there have been numerous anecdotal reports of electrical alternans visible on the surface ECG in association with a wide variety of clinical situations. Electrical alternans can occur in any part of the ECG complex, including the QRS complex (with pericardial effusions), the ST segment (with acute ischaemia), and the *RR* interval (with some supraventricular tachycardias). These phenomena have not been shown to correlate with vulnerability to ventricular arrhythmias. In contrast, recent data have confirmed that T wave alternans (TWA), or repolarization alternans, is a heart rate dependant phenomenon associated with vulnerability to ventricular arrhythmias in a variety of clinical disease states including ischaemia, electrolyte abnormalities, long QT syndrome, mitral valve prolapse, and cardiomyopathies. In this chapter we will focus on microscopic TWA, alternans invisible on the surface ECG, but measurable through spectral analysis techniques. We will review the mechanisms underlying its development, its measurement, and its potential use as a clinical tool for screening and identifying patients at risk for sudden cardiac death.

Mechanism

The association of TWA with increased vulnerability to ventricular arrhythmias has been described in several clinical studies. However, our understanding of the electrophysiological mechanism by which TWA leads to ventricular arrhythmias and the cellular processes responsible for the initiation of alternans have lagged behind our clinical recognition of this phenomenon. Alternation of action potential durations in dog hearts (Saitoh *et al.* 1989) and heterogeneities of repolarization across the myocardium, from epicardium to endocardium (Liu & Antzelevitch 1995) have been shown in the past, but their relation to the generation of TWA and the vulnerability to ventricular arrhythmias has remained obscure. Recently, more insight into the mechanism of TWA was achieved applying optical mapping techniques to an experimental model of TWA in guinea-pig hearts (Pastore *et al.* 1999). During ventricular pacing, cellular action potentials were measured across the epicardial surface with the aid of optical mapping techniques employing voltage sensitive dyes. Above a critical heart rate threshold, alternation of the repolarization phase of the action potential was induced and coincided with the appearance of TWA on the surface ECG. Interestingly, the magnitude of repolarization alternans was several orders of magnitude greater at the cellular level, possibly explaining why even microvolt levels of TWA are clinically relevant on

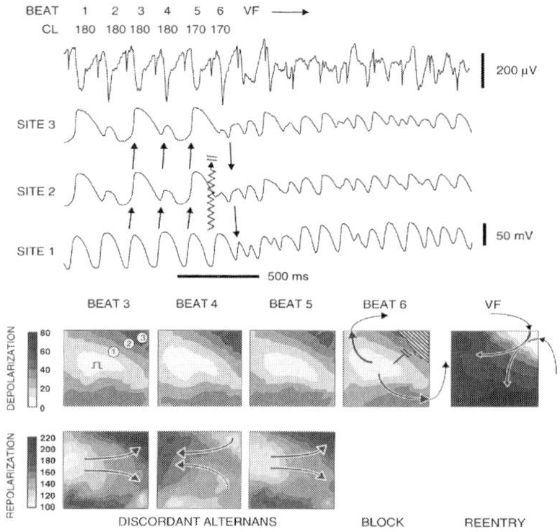

Fig. 44.1 Mechanism of initiation of VF during discordant alternans. Shown are 10-ms isochrone plots of depolarization and repolarization for beats that immediately preceded VF. ECG and action potentials (top) recorded from three ventricular sites marked on the isochrone map (bottom) from beat 3. Depolarization and repolarization times are referenced to stimulus artefact during pacing and to earliest activation time during the first beat of VF. On beats 1–5, the depolarizing wavefront propagated uniformly from the site of stimulation. However, patterns of repolarization differed substantially but reproducibly on alternating beats (compare beats 3 and 5). Pacing cycle length was decreased by 10 ms with beat 5. During beat 6, block occurred, as represented by hatched area in depolarization map. Block is shown in top panel by failure of propagation from site 1 to site3. After block occurred, pattern of depolarization reversed from (site 1 → site 2 → site 3) to (site 3 → site2 → site 1), indicating first re-entrant beat that led to VF. First beat of VF occurred 120 ms after pacing artefact of beat 6. (From Pastore *et al.* 1999, with permission.)

the surface ECG. This seminal study also demonstrated that as the heart rate is elevated, a threshold is reached where the repolarization of the membrane of neighbouring cells alternates in opposite phase (i.e. discordant alternans) creating large spatial gradients of repolarization. These heterogeneities were responsible for regional dispersion of ventricular repolarization, which is a necessary substrate for re-entrant ventricular arrhythmias. In fact, when discordant TWA was present at the cellular level it created the substrate for unidirectional block and re-entry propagation, and it was necessary for the initiation of ventricular fibrillation (Fig. 44.1). This mechanism could be applicable to patients at risk for ventricular arrhythmias, in whom TWA is present at lower heart rates than healthy controls and in whom ventricular ectopic beats may precipitate sustained ventricular tachycardia or ventricular fibrillation at critical times when discordant alternans is present. When discordant alternans is produced in the presence of a structural barrier, guinea-pigs are more likely to exhibit monomorphic ventricular tachycardia, rather than ventricular fibrillation, as the barrier acts as an anchor around which a stable circuit can form (Pastore *et al.* 2000). This could be relevant to patients in whom an old myocardial infarction acts as a structural barrier to cause stable monomorphic ventricular tachycardia rather than ventricular fibrillation. It could also explain why patients with dilated cardiomyopathies are more likely to develop ventricular fibrillation rather than monomorphic ventricular tachycardia. The weight of experimental evidence suggests that TWA arises from alternation of repolarization at the level of the single myocyte and that the mechanisms of TWA arise from alternation in the activity of sarcolemmal ion channels or from alternations in intracellular calcium handling which secondarily affects the ion channels (Walker & Rosenbaum 2003). Which calcium handling proteins and ion channels are directly involved and whether heterogeneous expression of such proteins and channels across the ventricular wall can explain the presence of TWA remains to be studied. Other areas that need further investigation include the influence of the autonomic nervous system on TWA and the effect of antiarrhythmic drugs. With regards to the former, studies have yielded conflicting results. Rashba *et al.* (2002a) showed a significant reduction in TWA by the acute administration of intravenous beta blockade. On the other hand, Kaufman *et al.* (2000) demonstrated that the initiation of TWA was related to heart rate and not adrenergic stimulation. With regards to the latter, although one study suggests a beneficial effect of amiodarone in terms of reducing the incidence of TWA (Groh *et al.* 1999), larger trials need to be performed.

Detection and measurement

As mentioned previously, TWA can rarely be identified on clinical ECG recordings, yet it may be present, and physiologically important, on a microscopic level. Therefore, digital processing techniques were developed to detect microscopic and electrocardiographically 'invisible' TWA from patients' ECGs. Smith *et al.* (1988) reported on a spectral method for detecting microvolt-level alternans, which was sensitive to morphological variations in the T wave. The technique distinguished beat-to-beat fluctuations occurring at the alternans frequency (every other beat or 0.5 cycles/beat) from other, nonalternating fluctuations caused by noise (myopotentials, respirations, etc). This proved to be a very sensitive tool for measuring subtle beat-to-beat alternation of T wave amplitude, even in the presence of noise sources commonly encountered in the clinical environment. The technique measures the T wave at a fixed point from the offset of the QRS in sequential beats. The time-series of fluctuations created in such a way is then transformed into a power spectrum, which reveals the frequencies at which that point of the T wave fluctuates from beat-to beat. The measurement is then repeated for each point on the T wave with a different offset from the QRS. The power spectra created in such a way are then averaged to form a composite power spectrum for the entire T wave (Fig. 44.2). The sensitivity and reliability of this technique is derived from its ability to distinguish and isolate alternans-type T wave fluctuations from much larger fluctuations caused by noise. TWA is measured in microvolts, and, generally speaking, a value of 1.9 μV or more is considered to be a positive finding. Of note, TWA is a threshold phenomenon related to heart rate. The threshold onset heart rate must be ≤110 beats/min and the TWA must be sustained above that heart rate in order for the test to be considered positive. TWA elicited only above a heart rate of 110 bpm can occur in normal individuals, and is therefore considered a nonspecific finding. Another important feature of this analysis is that the spectrum not only measures the magnitude of alternans, but it also provides a means for establishing the statistical confidence of the alternans measurement. This is determined by measuring the alternans ratio, which is obtained by dividing the noise-corrected alternans voltage by the standard deviation of the noise (Bloomfield *et al.* 2002). This value repre-

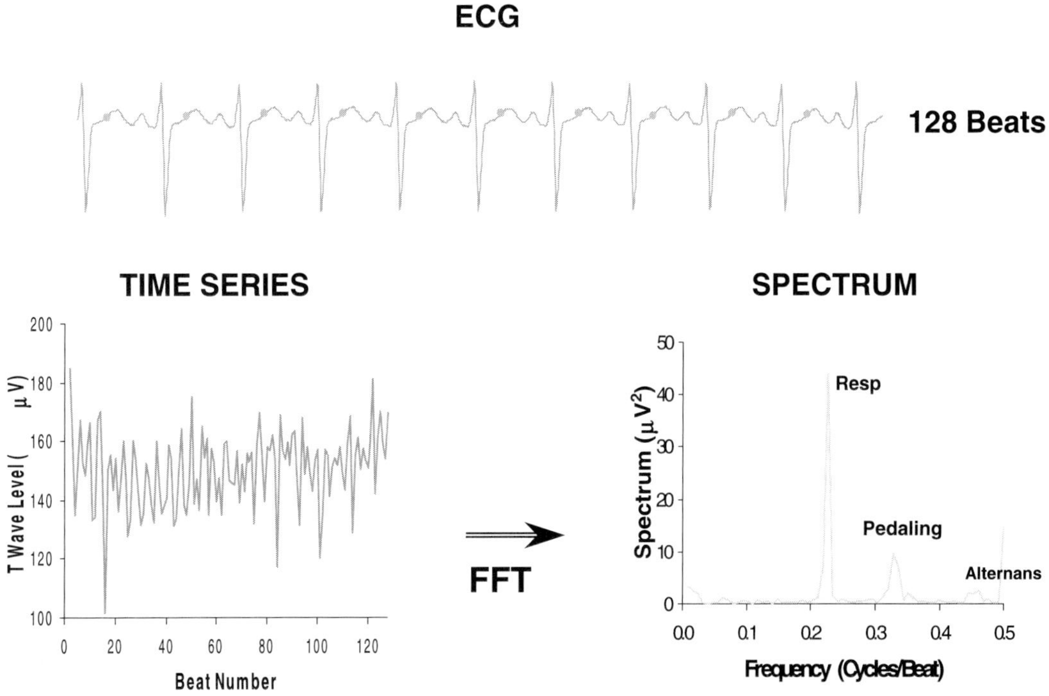

Fig. 44.2 Spectral method for the measurement of T wave alternans (TWA). See text for discussion. FFT, fast Fourier transform; Resp, respirations.

sents the number of standard deviations by which the alternans magnitude exceeds the noise level, and it is positive if it is ≥3. In earlier studies, TWA was measured during fixed rate atrial pacing (Rosenbaum *et al.* 1994). More recently, techniques have been developed to measure TWA noninvasively with treadmill or bicycle exercise stress testing and specialized noise reduction hardware and software (Bloomfield *et al.* 2002). These techniques correlate closely with alternans measured via the use of atrial pacing (Hohnloser *et al.* 1997) and have obviated the need for an invasive approach to measure TWA. The measurement of TWA can now be done on any standard exercise treadmill, making it possible for physicians to assess both the patient's ischaemic risk and potentially the risk of sudden cardiac death. Therefore, it is now feasible to noninvasively screen large populations for the presence of TWA and its association with sudden cardiac death.

Limitations of the TWA test include the fact that the test cannot be administered in patients with atrial fibrillation and in those who cannot exercise to achieve a target heart rate of at least 110 beats/min. Also, TWA could be masked, or falsely created in patients in whom the noise level is too high or in whom premature ventricular contractions are too frequent. The above limitations render the test uninterpretable (i.e. 'indeterminate') in approximately 20% of all patients. Finally, a recent study has called into question the validity of TWA testing for risk stratification of cardiac death in patients with QRS prolongation (Rashba *et al.* 2002b).

Clinical use and implications

Sudden cardiac death strikes 300 000–400 000 lives in the USA alone each year. In the minority of patients who are fortunate enough to have survived a cardiac arrest or a near-fatal ventricular tachyarrhythmia, studies such as the Antiarrhythmics vs. Implantable Defibrillator (AVID) trial (AVID Investigators 1997), support the clinical practice of implanting an implantable cardioverter defibrillator (ICD) to reduce total mortality. In light of these results, the focus has shifted to the primary prevention of sudden cardiac death, i.e. in patients who are at risk of, but have not yet suffered, a ventricular tachyarrhythmic event (Huikuri *et al.* 2001).

The majority of such patients are not routinely screened for, or even made aware of this risk. Traditional noninvasive risk stratifying measures, which may lead to further investigation, have included a family history of sudden death, near-syncope or syncope, a depressed left ventricular function (Bigger *et al.* 1984), non-sustained ventricular tachycardia on a 24-h ambulatory recording (Winkle 1980), or during in-patient monitoring, and signal averaged electrocardiography (Cain *et al.* 1996). However, when taken by themselves, none of these measures have a sufficiently high positive predictive value for the risk of a tachyarrhythmic event to justify therapy with an ICD. The 'gold standard' for risk stratification has been the invasive EPS. To identify the patients at highest risk, trials like the Multicentre Automatic Defibrillator Implantation Trial (MADIT) (Moss *et al.* 1996) and the Multicentre Unsustained Tachycardia Trial (MUSTT) (Buxton *et al.* 1999) have combined some of the traditional noninvasive risk stratification measures with the EPS. These seminal studies have shown that in patients with an ischaemic cardiomyopathy, a left ventricular ejection fraction ≤0.40, non-sustained ventricular tachycardia, and inducible ventricular arrhythmias, the use of an ICD improved survival compared to conventional medical therapy. Although these important studies established an effective paradigm for primary prevention, it is only applicable to a small minority of patients at risk for sudden death. Moreover, data from the MUSTT trial registry group (Buxton *et al.* 2000) indicate that patients with a negative EPS have a 12% risk of sudden death at 2-year follow-up. This suggests that even an EPS can miss a significant minority of patients at risk. The issue is further complicated by the fact that an EPS cannot reliably predict future arrhythmic events in patients with nonischaemic cardiomyopathies (Das *et al.* 1986; Poll *et al.* 1986). Therefore, a significant number of patients remain at risk for potentially lethal ventricular arrhythmias without a widely accepted method of risk stratification.

This has led to the design and recent publication of MADIT II (Moss *et al.* 2002), a randomized trial which demonstrated that survival is improved by implanting ICDs in all patients with an ischaemic cardiomyopathy and a depressed ejection fraction ("0.30) alone. However, the absolute reduction in mortality was only 5.6% and somewhat offset by a higher risk of technical complications and hospitalizations for congestive heart failure in the group with an implanted ICD. In addition, the cost effectiveness of this strategy is dubious, as one would have to implant ~17 ICDs for each life saved at a cost of approximately $400 000/life saved.

TWA, by itself or in combination with newer methods of noninvasive risk stratification, such as heart rate variability (La Rovere *et al.* 1998), may represent a viable alternative to depressed ejection fraction alone, non-sustained ventricular tachycardia or even EPS in identifying the patients at highest risk for sudden cardiac death. After several clinical and experimental studies had shown a consistent relationship between electrical alternans and cardiac electrical instability (Schwartz & Malliani 1975; Smith & Cohen 1984), Rosenbaum *et al.* (1994) measured TWA prospectively with the spectral technique using fixed-rate atrial pacing in a population of patients referred for EPS. The investigators showed for the first time that, in 83 patients referred to the EP laboratory for accepted clinical indications, when TWA was compared to the outcome of EPS and to arrhythmia-free survival, it was an independent and statistically significant marker of susceptibility to inducible ventricular tachyarrhythmias. The risk of a positive EPS was increased five-fold in the patients with a positive TWA test. A positive TWA test was also associated with a markedly reduced arrhythmia free survival, which was evident as early as four months post testing. The risk of developing life-threatening arrhythmias was increased 13 fold in the group with a positive TWA test. TWA and EPS were almost identical in predicting arrhythmia free survival (Fig. 44.3). Estes *et al.* (1997) supported these findings by studying 27 patients who presented with sustained ventricular tachyarrhythmias and underwent EPS. In this study, a new method of measuring TWA noninvasively during an exercise bicycle test had a sensitivity of 89% and a specificity of 75% and an overall clinical accuracy of 80% in predicting inducibility during EPS. More recently, in a multicentre trial, Gold *et al.* (2000) performed TWA testing and signal averaged ECGs in 313 patients undergoing EPS for clinically accepted indications. Though this was a heterogeneous population, with 30% of patients without structural heart disease and 19% with either a cardiac arrest or sustained ventricular tachycardia, the authors showed that TWA test positivity predicted the primary endpoint of sudden death or a ventricular tachyarrhythmic event with a relative risk of 10.9. EPS had a relative risk of 7.1 and signal averaged ECG had a relative risk of 4.5. TWA testing was a strong independent predictor of event free survival at one year and slightly better than EPS. Event-free survival was 0.81 for TWA positive patients and 0.77 for EP positive patients. Event free survival was 0.98 for TWA negative patients and 0.93 for EP negative patients.

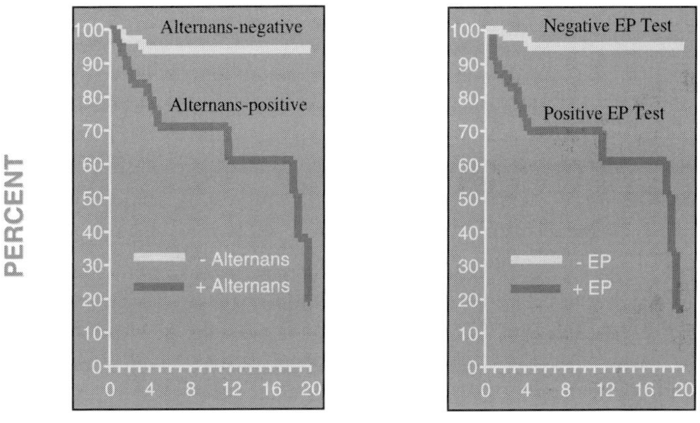

Fig. 44.3 Kaplan–Meier survival plots for T wave alternans (TWA) and electrophysiological (EP) testing. Left panel, arrhythmia-free survival is compared in patients with TWA and those without it. Note that TWA is a strong predictor of reduced survival. Right panel, patients with inducible ventricular arrhythmias (positive EP test) are compared to those without inducible ventricular arrhythmias (negative EP test).The predictive value of TWA and EP test was essentially equivalent. (From Rosenbaum *et al.* 1994, with permission)

Subsequent studies have shown the usefulness of this test in predicting the likelihood of spontaneous ventricular arrhythmic events in more homogeneous populations. Specifically, Ikeda *et al.* (2002) showed that in patients with coronary artery disease who underwent testing at least 2 weeks after a myocardial infarction, TWA predicted SCD or resuscitated ventricular fibrillation with a relative hazard ratio of 11 and a negative predictive value of 99%. In a study of 58 patients with a nonischaemic cardiomyopathy, Adachi *et al.* (1999) reported an association between ventricular tachycardia measured by 24-h ambulatory recording (non-sustained and sustained) and TWA positivity. Klingenheben *et al.* (2000) studied 107 patients with congestive heart failure from either an ischaemic or nonischaemic cardiomyopathy, and found that none of the patients with a negative TWA test experienced a ventricular tachyarrhythmic event as opposed to 21% of those with a positive TWA test. In all of the above-mentioned trials, an important recurrent theme is the outstanding negative predictive value of TWA testing, usually between 97–99%. Other patients where TWA may be useful, though the number of patients studied is small, are those with the long QT syndrome (Platt *et al.* 1996; Zareba *et al.* 1994), and those with hypertrophic cardiomyopathy (Momiyama *et al.* 1997; Kuroda *et al.* 2002).

In all studies, TWA has outperformed other established noninvasive markers in identifying patients at risk for sudden death. In a study by Armoundas *et al.* (1998) TWA was a highly significant predictor of the outcome of EPS and of the risk of spontaneous arrhythmic events in 43 patients undergoing EPS, while a signal averaged ECG offered no predictive value. Other studies comparing TWA to signal averaged ECG have supported these results (Gold *et al.* 2000; Ikeda *et al.* 2002). TWA also compares favourably with other noninvasive markers used for the assessment of the risk of sudden death. In a study of ICD recipients Hohnloser *et al.* (1998), showed that TWA and left ventricular ejection fraction were the only univariate predictors of a first defibrillation shock. Baroreflex sensitivity, signal averaged ECG, 24 h ambulatory ECG monitoring, and QT dispersion did not predict shock occurrence. Interestingly, in this study, EPS predicted events with a *P* value of only 0.2 in a univariate analysis and was not a significant predictor in a Cox regression model. The multicentre trial of Gold *et al.* (2000) supported these results, as the EPS was a weaker predictor of spontaneous ventricular events than TWA. The relative risk of the combined endpoint of a ventricular tachyarrhythmic event or death was 12.2 for TWA positive patients vs. 3.0 for EP positive patients. In addition, the study by Ikeda *et al.* (2002), demonstrated that TWA alone is at least as good, and in fact slightly better, than ejection fraction alone, in predicting the combined end point of sudden death or resuscitated ventricular fibrillation (relative hazard 5.9 vs. 4.4)

Based on available clinical data, our centre's current approach to patients at risk for sudden death is presented in Fig. 44.4. We excluded from the diagram patients with class IV congestive heart failure, who are likely to die of progressive heart failure and those with class I heart failure whose risk of sudden cardiac death is relatively low (Myerburg *et al.* 1997). MADIT II (Moss *et al.* 2002) supports implanting an ICD In all patients with an ischaemic cardiomyopathy (Fig. 44.4, Group A and B) and an ejection fraction ≤.30. However this approach carries some risk and would be extremely costly. Also, MADIT II does not address the large numbers of patients with ejection fraction between .30 and .40. TWA may be a more specific risk stratifier than non-sustained ventricular tachycardia or ejection fraction alone, and therefore a more suitable marker of arrhythmia vulnerability because, unlike non-sustained VT, it is highly reproducible over time and less dependant on clinical circumstances. Therefore, for the patients in Fig. 44.4, group A, we have used a positive TWA test as an indication for further evaluation by EPS. If, as it has been suggested by initial studies[33,42], TWA is comparable or better than EPS as a risk stratifier, it is conceivable that in the future we may be able to implant ICDs based on TWA positivity alone. Extrapolating the clinical data known about TWA, and applying them to a population of patients fitting the MADIT II entry criteria, one would be able to risk stratify patient for sudden cardiac death in a much more efficient and cost effective manner (Fig. 44.5).

In patients with an ischaemic cardiomyopathy with ejection fraction ≤0.40, non-sustained ventricular tachycardia and a positive EPS (Fig.

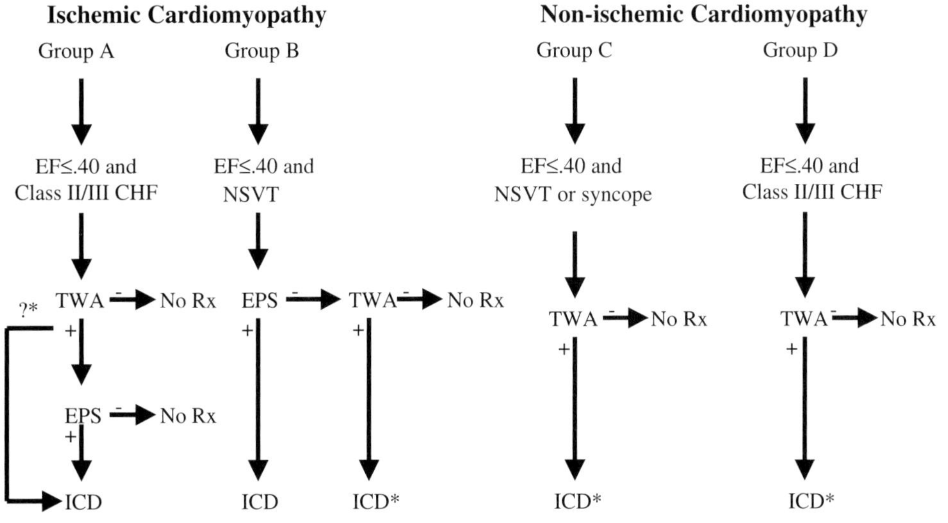

Fig. 44.4 Possible clinical applications of T wave alternans (TWA) for the primary prevention of sudden cardiac death. See text for discussion. EF, ejection fraction; NSVT, non-sustained ventricular tachycardia; CHF, congestive heart failure; ICD, implantable cardioverter defibrillator; EPS, electrophysiological study; *, currently not an approved indication for ICD implant.

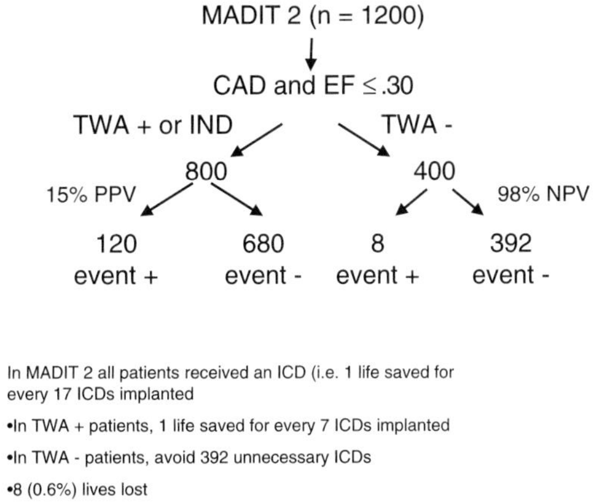

Fig. 44.5 Proposed primary prevention paradigm using T wave alternans (TWA). Extrapolating available clinical data on TWA and applying it to a MADIT 2-like population, sudden cardiac death prevention would become more efficient and less costly. MADIT 2, Multicentre Automatic Defibrillator Trial 2 (Moss *et al.* 2002) CAD, coronary artery disease; EF, ejection fraction; IND, indeterminate; PPV, positive predictive value; NPV, negative predictive value; ICD, implantable cardioverter defibrillator.

44.4, Group B), MADIT (Moss *et al.* 1996) and MUSTT (Buxton *et al.* 1999) support the practice of implanting defibrillators. Based on the MUSTT trial, however, the risk of sudden death in the patients with a negative EPS remains significant and these patients may benefit from a TWA study instead (or in addition to the EPS) to assess the risk further, with the possible implant of an ICD if the TWA test is positive. The hypothesis that TWA may be as good or better a risk stratifier for ventricular tachyarrhythmic events than EPS is being tested in the ongoing multicentre Alternans Before Cardioverter Defibrillator Trial (ABCD) where patients with MADIT and MUSTT entry criteria are being implanted with ICDs if either the EPS or the TWA test or both are positive.

Finally, for patients with a nonischaemic cardiomyopathy, TWA may become the risk stratifier of choice, given the inadequacy of non-sustained ventricular tachycardia and EPS in predicting sudden cardiac death in this population. For example, in patients with nonischaemic cardiomyopathy, a positive TWA test may prompt the decision of implanting an ICD with or without the presence of non-sustained ventricular tachycardia and regardless of the results of an EPS. In Fig. 44.4 we divided the nonischaemic patients in two groups: group C, patients with non-sustained ventricular tachycardia that are likely to present to the cardiologist's office for consultation, and group D, patients with congestive heart failure symptoms alone that at the present time are usually not risk stratified for sudden death in any way. Large multi-centre trials like the Sudden Cardiac Death in Heart Failure Trial (SCDHeFT) and the Defibrillator in Non-ischaemic Cardiomyopathy Treatment Evaluation (DEFINITE) will hopefully provide guidance in the clinical management of these patients in the future. Currently, for the patients in group C who have come to our attention, we have used TWA positivity, in combination with other risk stratifiers (inducible arrhythmias by EPS, non-sustained ventricular tachycardia, syncope) as an indication for ICD implant. The patients in group D constitute a large population who is often fairly young and functional. At this time, though we know that their risk of dying suddenly is significant, this group remains largely unscreened. The value of TWA as a risk stratifier for sudden cardiac death is proven. Further large, prospective clinical studies (some ongoing) are needed to link TWA guided ICD therapy to improved survival. Hopefully, with the aid of TWA, we will be able to more clearly identify and treat the large population of heretofore unrecognized patients at risk for sudden cardiac death.

References

Adachi, K., Ohnishi, Y., Shima, T. *et al.* (1999) Determinants of microvolt-level T wave alternans in patients with dilated cardiomyopathy. *Journal of the American College of Cardiology*, **34**, 374–380.

Armoundas, A.A., Rosenbaum, D.S., Ruskin, J.N. *et al.* (1998) Prognostic significance of electrical alternans vs. signal averaged electrocardiography in predicting the outcome of electrophysiological testing and arrhythmia free survival. *Heart*, **80**, 251–256.

Antiarrhythmics vs. Implantable Defibrillators (AVID) Investigators (1997) A comparison of antiarrhythmic drug therapy with implantable defibrillators in patients resuscitated from near-fatal ventricular arrhythmias. *New England Journal of Medicine*, **337**, 1576–1583.

Bigger, J.T., Fleiss, J.L., Kleiger, R. *et al.* (1984) The relationship among ventricular arrhythmias left ventricular dysfunction, and mortality in two years post myocardial infarction. *Circulation*, **69**, 250–258

Bloomfield, D.M., Hohnloser, S.H. & Cohen, R.J. (2002) Interpretation and classification of microvolt T wave alternans tests. *Journal of Cardiovascular Electrophysiology*, **13**, 502–512.

Buxton, A.E., Lee, K.L., Fisher, J.D. *et al.* (1999) A randomized study of the prevention of sudden death in patients with coronary artery disease. *New England Journal of Medicine*, **341**, 1882–1990.

Buxton, A.E., Lee, K.L., DiCarlo, L. *et al.* (2000) Electrophysiological testing to identify patients with coronary artery disease at risk for sudden death. MUSTT Investigators. *New England Journal of Medicine*, **342**, 1937–1945.

Cain, M.E., Anderson, J.L., Arnsdorf, M.F. *et al.* (1996) ACC Expert Consensus Document: signal averaged electrocardiography. *Journal of the American College of Cardiology*, **27**, 238–249.

Das, S.K., Morady, F., DiCarlo, L.J. *et al.* (1986) Prognostic usefulness of programmed electrical stimulation in idiopathic dilated cardiomyopathy without ventricular arrhythmias. *American Journal of Cardiology*, **58**, 998–1000.

Estes, N.A., Michaud, G., Zipes, D.P. *et al.* (1997) Electrical alternans during rest and exercise as predictors of vulnerability to ventricular arrhythmias. *American Journal of Cardiology*, **80**, 1314–1318.

Gold, M.R., Bloomfield, D.M., Anderson, K.P. *et al.* (2000) A comparison of T wave alternans, signal averaged electrocardiography, and programmed ventricular stimulation for arrhythmia risk stratification. *Journal of the American College of Cardiology*, **36**, 2247–2253.

Groh, W.J., Shinn, T.S., Eigelstein, E.E. *et al.* (1999) Amiodarone reduces the prevalence of T wave alternans in a population with ventricular tachyarrhythmias. *Journal of Cardiovascular Electrophysiology*, **10**, 1335–1339

Hering, H.E. (1909) Experimentelle Studien an Saugethieren Über das Elektrocardiogram. *Zeitschrift fuer Experimentelle Pathologie und Therapie*, **7**, 363.

Hohnloser, S.H., Klingenheben, T., Zabel, M. *et al.* (1997) T wave alternans during exercise and atrial pacing in humans. *Journal of Cardiovascular Electrophysiology*, **8**, 987–993.

Hohnloser, S.H., Klingenheben, T., Li, Y.G. *et al.* (1998) T wave alternans as a predictor of recurrent ventricular tachyarrhythmias in ICD recipients. *Journal of Cardiovascular Electrophysiology*, **9**, 1258–1268.

Huikuri, H.V., Castellanos, A. & Myerburg, R.J. (2001) Sudden death due to cardiac arrhythmias. *New England Journal of Medicine*, **345**, 1473–1482.

Ikeda, T., Saito, H., Tanno, K. *et al.* (2002) T wave alternans as a predictor for sudden cardiac death after myocardial infarction. *American Journal of Cardiology*, **89**, 79–82.

Kalter, H.H. & Schwartz, M.L. (1948) Electrical alternans. *New York State Journal of Medicine*, **1**, 1164–1166.

Kaufman, E.S., Mackall, J.A., Julka, B. *et al.* (2000) Influence of heart rate and sympathetic stimulation on arrhythmogenic T wave alternans. *American Journal of Physiology (Heart Circulation Physiology)*, **279**, H1248–H1255.

Klingenheben, T., Zabel, M., D'Agostino, R.B. *et al.* (2000) Predictive value of T wave alternans for arrhythmic events in patients with congestive heart failure. *Lancet*, **356**, 651–652.

Kuroda, N., Ohnishi, Y., Yoshida, A. *et al.* (2002) Clinical significance of TWA in hypertrophic cardiomyopathy. *Circulation*, **66**, 457–462.

La Rovere, M.T., Bigger, J.T., Marcus, F.I. *et al.* (1998) Baroreflex sensitivity and heart rate variability in prediction of total cardiac mortality after myocardial infarction: the Autonomic Tone and Reflexes After Myocardial Infarction (ATRAMI) Investigators. *Lancet*, **351**, 478–484.

Lewis, T. (1910) Notes upon alternation of the heart. *Quarterly Journal of Medicine*, **4**, 141–144.

Liu, D.-W. & Antzelevitch, C. (1995) Characteristics of the delayed rectifier current in canine ventricular epicardial, midmyocardial, and endocardial myocytes: a weaker *Iks* contributes to the longer action potential of the M cell. *Circulation Research*, **76**, 351–365.

Momiyama, Y., Hartikainen, J., Nagayoshi, H. *et al.* (1997) Exercise induced T wave alternans as a marker of high risk in patients with hypertrophic cardiomyopathy. *Japanese Circulation Journal*, **61**, 8–15.

Moss, A.J., Hall, W.J., Cannom, D.S. *et al.* (1996) Improved survival with an implanted defibrillator in patients with prior myocardial infarction, low ejection fraction, and asymptomatic non-sustained ventricular tachycardia: the Multicentre Automatic Defibrillator Trial (MADIT). *New England Journal of Medicine*, **335**, 1933–1940.

Moss, A.J., Zareba, W., Hall, W.J. *et al.* (2002) Prophylactic implantation of a defibrillator in patients with myocardial infarction and reduced ejection fraction. *New England Journal of Medicine*, **346**, 877–883.

Myerburg, R.J., Interian, A. Jr, Mitrani, R.M. *et al.* (1997) Frequency of sudden death and profiles of risk. *American Journal of Cardiology*, **80**, 10F–19F.

Pastore, J.M., Girouard, S.D., Laurita, K.R. *et al.* (1999) Mechanism linking T wave alternans to the genesis of cardiac fibrillation. *Circulation*, **99**, 1385–1394.

Pastore, J.M. & Rosenbaum, D.S. (2000) Role of structural barriers in the mechanism of alternans-induced reentry. *Circulation Research*, **87**, 1157–1163.

Platt, S.B., Vijgen, J.M., Albrecht, P. *et al.* (1996) Occult T wave alternans in long QT syndrome. *Journal of Cardiovascular Electrophysiology*, **7**, 144–148.

Poll, D.S., Marchlinski, F.S., Buxton, A.E. *et al.* (1986) Usefulness of programmed ventricular stimulation in idiopathic dilated cardiomyopathy. *American Journal of Cardiology*, **98**, 992–997.

Rashba, E.J., Cooklin, M., MacMurdy, K. *et al.* (2002a). Effects of selective autonomic blockade on T wave alternans in humans. *Circulation*, **105**, 837–842.

Rashba, E.J., Osman, A.F., MacMurdy, K. *et al.* (2002b) Influence of QRS duration on the prognostic value of T wave alternans. *Journal of Cardiovascular Electrophysiology*, **13**, 770–775.

Rosenbaum, D.S., Jackson, L.E., Smith, J.M. *et al.* (1994) Electrical alternans and vulnerability to ventricular arrhythmias. *New England Journal of Medicine*, **330**, 235–241.

Saitoh, H., Bailey, J. & Surawicz, B. (1989) Action potential duration alternans in dog Purkinje and ventricular muscle fibres. *Circulation*, **80**, 1421–1431.

Schwartz, P.J. & Malliani, A. (1975) Electrical alternation of the T wave: clinical and experimental evidence of its relationship to the sympathetic nervous system and with the long QT syndrome. *American Heart Journal*, **89**, 45–50

Smith, J.M. & Cohen, R.J. (1984) Simple finite-element model accounts for wide range of ventricular dysrhythmias. *Proceedings of the National Academy of Sciences USA*, **81**, 233–237.

Smith, J.M., Clancy, E.A., Valeri, C.R. *et al.* (1988) Electrical alternans and cardiac electrical instability. *Circulation*, **77**, 110–121.

Walker, M.H. & Rosenbaum, D.S. (2003) Repolarization alternans: implications for the mechanism and prevention of sudden cardiac death. *Cardiovascular Research*, **57**, 599–614.

Winkle, R.A. (1980) Ambulatory electrocardiography and the diagnosis, evaluation, and treatment of chronic ventricular arrhythmias. *Progress in Cardiovascular Diseases*, **23**, 99–128.

Zareba, W., Moss, A.J., Le Cessie, S. *et al.* (1994) T wave alternans in idiopathic long QT syndrome. *Journal of the American College of Cardiology*, **23**, 1541–1546.

CHAPTER 45

T Wave Alternans in Ischaemic Heart Disease

Stefan H. Hohnloser

Although the implantable cardioverter defibrillator (ICD) is an extremely effective therapeutic means for the prevention of sudden arrhythmogenic death (AVID Investigators, 1997; Connolly *et al.* 2000; Kuck *et al.* 2000; Moss *et al.* 2002), selection of patients at high risk for arrhythmogenic mortality deriving maximum benefit from ICD therapy is currently limited by the lack of risk stratification methods which could identify individuals at risk (Bigger 2002). Most victims of sudden death suffer from coronary artery disease as the underlying structural heart disease with the majority of these patients having a history of prior myocardial infarction. Accordingly, there is a continued need to develop new risk stratification techniques in order to noninvasively assess arrhythmogenic risk with high clinical precision in patients prone to sudden death.

Determination of microvolt level T wave alternans (MTWA) has recently been proposed to assess abnormalities in ventricular repolarization favouring the occurrence of re-entrant arrhythmias (Adam *et al.* 1984; Pastore *et al.* 1999). After experimental validation of the methodology, the first clinical study was conducted by Rosenbaum and coworkers (1994). They demonstrated that MTWA is closely related to arrhythmia induction in the electrophysiology laboratory as well as to the occurrence of spontaneous ventricular tachyarrhythmias during follow-up (Rosenbaum *et al.* 1994). Subsequently, the methodology to determine TWA has been improved and a number of clinical studies has examined its clinical applicability (Estes *et al.* 1997; Hohnloser *et al.* 1997, 1998; Gold *et al.* 2000). The present review summarizes the current knowledge on MTWA in ischaemic heart disease with particular emphasis on its potential use as a risk stratification method.

T wave alternans and ischaemic heart disease

Electrical alternans can affect any part of the ECG and is defined as beat-to-beat changes in the amplitude or width of the ECG signal. Alteration of the T wave is defined as a variation in the T wave amplitude on an every other beat basis which – when visible in the surface ECG – has been termed 'macroscopic' TWA. Early on, such electrical alternans has been associated with cardiac mortality (Kalter & Schwartz 1948) under various clinical conditions. Among them, the congenital long QT syndrome (Schwartz & Malliani 1975) and similarly important, various manifestations of ischaemic heart disease have been described. For instance, there are several reports on patients with Prinzmetal´s angina which have described an association between TWA and increased electrical instability in this condition (Kleinfeld & Rozanski, 1977; Rozanski & Kleinfeld, 1982). Salerno and colleagues (1986) and Turitto & El-Sherif (1988) demonstrated that the presence of alternans was statistically correlated with the onset of ventricular arrhythmias. Similarly, alternans has been observed during angioplasty (Nearing *et al.* 1994; Sochanski *et al.* 1992) and bypass graft occlusion (Sutton *et al.* 1991).

On the other hand, macroscopic TWA is a rarely observed phenomenon in clinical practice. Accordingly, sophisticated new computer processing techniques were developed to detect subtle alterations in T wave amplitude which were not visually seen upon inspection of the ECG. Spectral analytic techniques were first used by Adam, Smith and coworkers to detect (Adam *et al.* 1981, 1984) microvolt level TWA in a series of carefully designed experimental studies. Similarly, Nearing *et al.* (1991) used complex demodulation techniques to detect MTWA. Specifically, these authors observed in a study in anaesthetized dogs that during myocardial ischaemia and subsequent reperfusion there were marked increases in the degree of MTWA that paralleled the established time course of changes in electrical vulnerability (Nearing *et al.* 1991). It seems important to point out that there is significant evidence that alternans induced in the presence or absence of acute ischaemia have substantially different mechanisms. Acute ischaemia is associated more often with alternation of the ST segment, and to a lesser extent the T wave whereas pacing-induced MTWA is confined exclusively to the T wave. Moreover, the appearance of alternans during ischaemia is often transient and accompanied by depressed contractility (Abe *et al.* 1989; Murphy *et al.* 1996). Finally, MTWA, which is closely linked to enhanced arrhythmia susceptibility, is in no way dependent on the development or documentation of acute myocardial ischaemia.

More recent experimental findings have improved our understanding of the electrophysiological mechanisms underlying the genesis of MTWA in the presence of a underlying pathological substrate such as the myocardium in patients with chronic ischaemic heart disease.

Mechanisms underlying T wave alternans

Recently, experimental studies using high-resolution optical mapping with voltage-sensitive dyes showed that alternations in action potential duration induced by rapid pacing are not uniform across the myocardium (Pastore *et al.* 1999). Significant parts of the ventricular myocardium show sequential lengthening and shortening of the action potential with fluctuations in some regions being 180 degrees out of phase with those in other regions, constituting a phenomenon known as discordant alternans. The resulting spatial gradients in transmembrane potential alternate in magnitude and direction from beat to beat providing the basis for MTWA in the surface ECG. As shown by Pastore *et al.* (1999), discordant alternans can result in sufficiently steep spatial repolarization gradients as to produce unidirectional conduction block and functional re-entry, giving rise to VF. Studies utilizing computer simulations of 2-dimensional sheets of cardiac tissue (Qu *et al.* 2000) have produced results which are in agreement with these experimental findings (Pastore *et al.* 1999). Subsequent studies from the same laboratory examined the effects of cell-to-cell uncoupling, such as those produced by insulating structural barriers seen in structural heart disease (Pastore & Rosenbaum, 2000). In the presence of such barriers, neighbouring regions of cells can more easily manifest their underlying ionic differences because they are no longer under electrotonic influence of one another. Accordingly, the presence of structural barriers led to a significant reduction in the critical heart rate at which discordant alternans appeared. Moreover, it also served as a anchor for stable re-entry enabling the more readily induction of monomorphic VT rather than VF. As pointed out by Berger (2000), these new findings suggest that a common mechanism may link the presence of discordant repolarization alternans to the genesis of diverse re-entrant arrhythmias, depending on the anatomic substrate. Thus, under chronotropic or metabolic stress, discordant alternans leads to sufficiently large repolarization gradients to produce unidirectional block and re-entry. Without a structural barrier, re-entry is functional and manifests as VF or polymorphic VT. In the presence of structural barriers, re-entry can become anatomically fixed resulting in monomorphic VT. These findings strongly support the notion that MTWA arises at the cellular level. Although the primary alterations in ionic currents or those due to abnormalities in intracellular calcium handling remain to be unravelled, there is significant evidence in support of alternations in intracellular calcium handling as an important if not the primary step in the genesis of MTWA (Walker & Rosenbaum 2003).

Current technology to assess MTWA in the clinical setting

Since MTWA is heart rate dependent, it is necessary in the clinical setting to increase heart rate by either atrial stimulation or noninvasively by exercise testing for its assessment. The methodology of determination of MTWA has recently been described in detail (Rosenbaum *et al.* 1996). Briefly, sequential ECG cycles are aligned to their QRS complex and the amplitude of the T waves at a predefined point. Subsequently this beat-to-beat series of amplitude fluctuations are subjected to spectral analysis using fast Fourier transformation. MTWA manifests itself as a pronounced peak which is visible in the spectrum at 0.5 cycles/beat. To reduce background noise, special multicontact electrodes are applied. Other factors that can interfere with the measurement are the patient's respiration rate, the pedalling rate of the ergometer, and frequent premature beats (Rosenbaum *et al.* 1996). A significant MTWA is defined if the alternans voltage exceeds 1.9 μV and if the alternans ratio K (indicator of the significance of the measurement) is >3. Since both, atrial pacing and bicycle exercise have been shown to yield comparable efficacy for increasing heart rate, noninvasive assessment of MTWA has become possible in the majority of patients.

Prevalence and prognostic significance of TWA following myocardial infarction

Recent years have seen an increasing number of studies dealing with MTWA in the setting of coronary artery disease and previous myocardial infarction (Hohnloser *et al.* 1999; Ikeda *et al.* 2000, 2002a; Schwab *et al.* 2001; Tapanainen *et al.* 2001). In a large pilot study, 448 patients after myocardial infarction were tested for the presence or absence of MTWA 5–21 days after the heart attack. At a target heart rate of 110 beats/min, MTWA was positive in 18%, negative in 55%, indeterminate in 9% and incomplete in 17% of patients. At 28–56 days follow-up, MTWA was repeated in 184 patients showing a concordance between determinate TWA tests of 67% (Hohnloser *et al.* 1999). This observation indicates that MTWA evolves substantially during the immediate post infarction period (Berger 2000).

Subsequently, several reports from prospective post infarction studies evaluating the predictive value of MTWA for future events have been published. In a study by Ikeda *et al.* (2000), MTWA and late potentials from the SAECG were assessed in 102 infarct survivors. Primary percutaneous coronary intervention was performed in 98% of patients but only 31% were treated with beta blocking agents. The prevalence of a positive MTWA was high (50/102 patients; 49%). During a follow-up period of 13 ± 6 months, 14 patients (15%) had an episode of sustained ventricular tachycardia or ventricular fibrillation with all but one of these patients having tested positive for MTWA. The positive predictive value with respect to arrhythmic events was 28% for MTWA alone, and 50% for the combination of positive MTWA and SAECG (Ikeda *et al.* 2000). Of particular note, there was a high negative predictive value of this test (98%).

In another prospective follow-up study, Tapanainen *et al.* assessed MTWA and other risk markers in 379 consecutive infarct survivors (Tapanainen *et al.* 2001). Of these, 133 (35%) had an incomplete test (inability to perform exercise in 56, and target heart rate below 105 beats/min in 77 patients). A positive MTWA was found in 14.7% of patients, a negative test result in 38% ($n = 144$), and the test was indeterminate in 12% ($n = 46$). Of note, 97% of patients were treated with beta blocker and 2% with amiodarone at the time of MTWA testing. A positive MTWA was not a predictor of all-cause mortality in contrast to autonomic risk markers such as baroreflex sensitivity, and heart rate variability. However, an incomplete TWA test was the most significant predictor of cardiac death in that study (Tapanainen *et al.* 2001). A major limitation of this study, however, is the choice of the primary study outcome (total mortality). MTWA can only predict future tachyarrhythmic events but not death from heart failure or other causes.

In the largest post infarction study published at this point, Ikeda *et al.* studied 850 consecutive patients who underwent assessment of MTWA and SAECG during the late phase after myocardial infarction (Ikeda *et al.* 2002a). Specifically, 82% of patients underwent MTWA assessment 2–10 weeks after the index event, and 18% were tested months or years later. The primary study endpoint was sudden cardiac death or resuscitated VF, the secondary endpoint was defined as sustained VT. A positive MTWA was present in 36%, a negative result in 52% of patients. MTWA (hazard ratio 11.4; 95% CI, 3.4–37.9) and LVEF (hazard ratio 6.6; 95% CI, 3.0–14.6) were significant predictors for both endpoints. Combining MTWA and LVEF improved the accuracy of predicting the primary endpoint (Ikeda *et al.* 2002a).

In a spring-off study of this large study (Ikeda *et al.* 2002b), the same authors reported preliminary data on a subset of 82 infarct survivors with a LVEF of 30% thus resembling the patients enrolled in the MADIT II study (Moss *et al.* 2002). These 82 subjects were followed for 720 ± 490 days for primary outcome events consisting of resuscitated VF, sudden death or sustained VT. Presence of positive MTWA findings carried a hazard ratio of 9.3 (95% CI 1.2–70.3; P = 0.031) for the primary endpoint. Of note, however, there was again a particularly high negative predictive value of 97% indicating that MTWA negative patients were at extremely low risk for subsequent ventricular tachyarrhythmic events.

These findings are in line with data reported by Klingenheben *et al.* who conducted a prospective study in 107 consecutive patients with CHF (NYHA class II or III, LVEF < 0.46) of whom 67 patients suffered from ischaemic cardiomyopathy (Klingenheben *et al.* 2000). During 18 months of follow-up, seven patients died suddenly, five had sustained VT, and one was resuscitated from VF whereas three patients died from intractable heart failure. MTWA analysis was positive in 49%, negative in 31%, and indeterminate in 21%. Multivariate Cox regression analysis revealed that from all risk stratifiers assessed only MTWA was an independent significant risk predictor of arrhythmic events. Perhaps equally important, patients testing negative on MTWA had an extremely low risk of suffering VT, VF or SCD during the observation period. Results remained statistically significant when the analysis was run only for the subgroup of 67 patients with proven coronary artery disease (Klingenheben *et al.* 2000).

Conclusions

Assessment of MTWA has matured into an established clinical risk assessment method in patients with coronary disease and prior myocardial infarction. There is conclusive evidence from several controlled studies that MTWA holds promise for the prediction of future ventricular tachyarrhythmic events including sudden arrhythmogenic death. MTWA can nowadays be determined completely noninvasively by using bicycling or treadmill exercise testing. Of note, MTWA seems to evolve during the first week after an acute myocardial infarction. Accordingly, the test should be performed several weeks after the index infarct in order to yield maximum prognostic information. There are several limitations of this method which need to be taken into consideration. Currently, MTWA assessment can not be performed in individuals with persistent or permanent atrial fibrillation or frequent extrasystoles. Some patients will not be able to reach a target heart rate of 100 beats/min which is mandatory for provoking MTWA. Accordingly, the test should be repeated in such individuals after withholding rate slowing medications, particularly beta blocker, for 1 or 2 days. Doing so will enable to achieve determinate test results in the majority of patients subjected to MTWA assessment.

References

Abe, S., Nagamoto, Y., Fukuchi, Y. *et al.* (1989) Relationship of alternans of monophasic action potential and conduction delay inside the ischaemic border zone to serious ventricular arrhythmia during acute myocardial ischaemia in dogs. *American Heart Journal*, **117**, 1223–1233.

Adam, D.R., Akselrod, S. & Cohen, R.J. (1981) Estimation of ventricular vulnerability to fibrillation through T wave time series analysis. *Comput Cardiol* **8**, 307–310.

Adam, D.R., Smith, J.M., Akselrod, S. *et al.* (1984) Fluctuations in T wave morphology and susceptibility to ventricular fibrillation. *Journal of Electrocardiology*, **17**, 209–218.

AVID (Antiarrhythmics Vs. Implantable Defibrillators Investigators) (1997) A comparison of antiarrhythmic drug therapy with implantable defibrillators in patients resuscitated from near-fatal ventricular arrhythmias. *New England Journal of Medicine*, **337**, 1576–1583.

Berger, R.D. (2000) Repolarization alternans. Toward a unifying theory of re-entrant arrhythmia induction. *Circulation Research*, **87**,1083–1084.

Bigger, J.T. (2002) Expanding indications for implantable cardiac defibrillators. *New England Journal of Medicine*, **346**, 931–933.

Connolly, S.J, Gent, M., Roberts, R.S. *et al.* (2000)

Canadian Implantable Defibrillator study (CIDS): a randomized trial of the implantable defibrillator against amiodarone. *Circulation*, **101**, 1297–1302.

Estes, M.N.A., Michaud, G., Zipes, D.P. *et al.* (1997) Electrical alternans during rest and exercise as predictors of vulnerability to ventricular arrhythmias. *American Journal of Cardiology*, **80**, 1314–1318.

Gold, M.R., Bloomfield, D.M., Anderson, K.P. *et al.* (2000) A comparison of T wave alternans, signal-averaged electrocardiography and programmed ventricular stimulation for arrhythmia risk stratification. *Journal of the American College of Cardiology*, **36**, 2247–2253.

Hohnloser, S.H., Huikuri, H., Schwartz, P.J. *et al.* (1999) T wave alternans in post myocardial infarction patients (ACES Pilot Study). *Journal of the American College of Cardiology*, **33**, 144A (abstract).

Hohnloser, S.H., Klingenheben, T., Li, Y.G. *et al.* (1998) T wave alternans as a tool for risk stratification in patients with malignant arrhythmias: prospective comparison with conventional risk markers. *Journal of Cardiovascular Electrophysiology*, **9**, 1258–1268.

Hohnloser, S.H., Klingenheben, T., Zabel, M. *et al.* (1997) T wave alternans during exercise and atrial pacing in humans. *Journal of Cardiovascular Electrophysiology*, **8**, 987–993.

Ikeda, T., Saito, H., Tanno, K. *et al.* (2002a) T wave alternans as a predictor for sudden cardiac death after myocardial infarction. *American Journal of Cardiology*, **89**, 79–82.

Ikeda, T., Sakata, T., Takami, M. *et al.* (2000) Combined assessment of T wave alternans and late potentials used to predict arrhythmic events after myocardial infarction. *Journal of the American College of Cardiology*, **35**, 722–730.

Ikeda, T., Tanno, K., Shimizu, H. *et al.* (2002b) Usefulness of T wave alternans for effective prophylactic therapy in patients with prior myocardial infarction and reduced left ventricular ejection fraction. *Circulation*, **106**, II-372 (abstract).

Kalter, H.H. & Schwartz, M.L. (1948) Electrical alternans. *New York State Journal of Medicine* **1**, 1164–1166.

Kleinfeld, M.J., Rozanski, J.J. (1977) Alternans of the ST segment in Prinzmetal's angina. *Circulation*, **55**, 574–577.

Klingenheben, T., Zabel, M., D'Agostino, R.B. *et al.* (2000) Predictive value of T wave alternans for arrhythmic events in patients with congestive heart failure. *Lancet*, **356**, 651–652.

Kuck, K.H., Cappato, R., Siebels, J. *et al.* (2000) A randomized comparison of antiarrhythmic drug therapy with implantable defibrillators resuscitated from cardiac arrest: the Cardiac Arrest Study Hamburg (CASH). *Circulation*, **102**, 748–754.

Moss, A.J., Zarebra, W., Jackson, W. *et al.* (2002) Prophylactic implantation of a defibrillator in patients with myocardial infarction and reduced ejection fraction. *New England Journal of Medicine*, **346**, 877–883.

Murphy, C.F., Horner, S.M., Dick, D.J. *et al.* (1996) Electrical alternans and the onset of rate-induced pulsus alternans during acute regional ischaemia in the anesthetised pig heart. *Cardiovascular Research*, **32**, 138–147.

Nearing, B., Huang, H.A. & Verrier, R.L. (1991) Dynamic tracking of cardiac vulnerability by complex demodulation of the T wave. *Science*, **252**, 437–440.

Nearing, B.D., Oesterle, S.N. & Verrier, R.L. (1994) Quantification of ischaemia-induced vulnerability by precordial T wave alternans analysis in dog and human. *Cardiovascular Research*, **28**, 1440–1449.

Pastore, J.M., Girouard, S.D., Laurita, K.R. *et al.* (1999) Mechanism linking T wave alternans to the genesis of cardiac fibrillation. *Circulation*, **99**, 1385–1394.

Pastore, J.M., Rosenbaum, D.S. (2000) Role of structural barriers in the mechanism of alternans-induced re-entry. *Circulation Research*, **87**, 1157–1163.

Qu, Z., Garfinkel, A., Chen, P.-S. *et al.* (2000) Mechanism of discordant alternans and induction of re-entry in simulated cardiac tissue. *Circulation*, **102**, 1664–1670.

Rosenbaum, D.S., Albrecht, P. & Cohen, R.J. (1996) Predicting sudden cardiac death from T wave alternans of the surface electrocardiogram: promise and pitfalls. *Journal of Cardiovascular Electrophysiology*, **7**, 1095–1111.

Rosenbaum, D.S., Jackson, L.E., Smith, J.M. *et al.* (1994) Electrical alternans and vulnerability to ventricular arrhythmias. *New England Journal of Medicine*, **330**, 235–241.

Rozanski, J.J. & Kleinfeld, M.J. (1982) Alternans of the ST segment and T wave. A sign of electrical instability in Prinzmetal's angina. *PACE (Pacing and Clinical Electrophysiology)*, **5**, 359–365.

Salerno, J.A., Previtali, M., Panciroli, C. *et al.* (1986) Ventricular arrhythmias during acute myocardial ischaemia in man. The role and significance of R-ST–T alternans and the prevention of ischaemic sudden death by medical treatment. *European Heart Journal*, **7**, 63–75.

Schwab, J.O., Weber, S., Schmitt, H. *et al.* (2001) Incidence of T wave alternation after acute myocardial infarction and correlation with other prognostic parameters: results of a prospective study. *PACE* **24**, 957–961.

Schwartz, P.J., Malliani, A. (1975) Electrical alternation of the T wave: clinical and experimental evidence of its relationship with the sympathetic nervous system and with the long-QT syndrome. *American Heart Journal*, **89**, 45–50.

Sochanski, M., Feldman, T., Chua, K.G. *et al.* (1992) ST segment alternans during coronary angioplasty. *Catheterization and Cardiovascular Diagnosis*, **27**, 45–48.

Sutton, P.M.I., Taggart, P., Lab, M. *et al.* (1991) Alternans of epicardial repolarization as a localised phenomenon in man. *European Heart Journal*, **12**, 70–78.

Tapanainen, J.M., Still, A.M., Airaksinen, K.E.J. *et al.* (2001) Prognostic significance of risk stratifiers of mortality, including T wave alternans, after acute myocardial infarction: results of a prospective follow-up study. *Journal of Cardiovascular Electrophysiology*, **12**, 645–652.

Turitto, G. & El-Sherif, N. (1988) Alternans of the ST segment in variant angina. *Chest*, **93**, 587–591.

Walker, M.L. & Rosenbaum, D.S. (2003) Repolarization alternans: implications for the mechanism and prevention of sudden cardiac death. *Cardiovascular Research*, **57**, 599–614.

CHAPTER 46

Dynamic Repolarization Changes and Arrhythmia Risk Assessment in Nonischaemic Heart Disease

Richard L. Verrier and Aneesh Tolat

Abstract

The classification 'nonischaemic heart disease' encompasses a diverse group of pathologic entities that have in common markedly elevated risk for malignant ventricular arrhythmias and sudden cardiac death. The main conditions include idiopathic dilated and hypertrophic cardiomyopathy, left ventricular hypertrophy, congenital structural heart disease, right ventricular dysplasia, and the long QT syndrome. The electrophysiological mechanisms responsible for risk are not well understood because of the complexity of the various conditions and the absence of suitable large animal models. Available evidence suggests that the substrate predisposes to conduction abnormalities and spatial–temporal unevenness of repolarization. Enhanced adrenergic stimulation is implicated in the cardiomyopathies, the long QT syndrome, and hypertensive left ventricular hypertrophy. Another proarrhythmic characteristic of nonischaemic heart disease is disturbed calcium handling.

Risk stratification has proved to be a difficult challenge. Encouraging, however, is the growing body of literature indicating that measures of repolarization, particularly T wave alternans, may prove useful in risk assessment in the cardiomyopathies, left ventricular hypertrophy, and the long QT syndrome. Larger trials will be required to validate this evidence. Should the results be positive, the opportunity to measure T wave alternans magnitude not only during routine exercise treadmill testing but also during ambulatory ECG monitoring could improve repolarization-based risk assessment in nonischaemic heart disease.

Introduction

The category 'nonischaemic heart disease' generally refers to a cardiac condition that is unexplained by or out of proportion to the extent of a patient's coronary disease. Often, the aetiology is unknown, while at other times the development of disease may be multifactorial and result from a systemic process. Regardless of aetiology, patients with nonischaemic heart disease, including idiopathic dilated cardiomyopathy, hypertrophic cardiomyopathy, left ventricular hypertrophy, and congenital structural heart disease, are at increased risk for ventricular arrhythmias and sudden death. Patients with cardiomyopathy constitute the second largest group of sudden cardiac death victims, after those with ischaemic heart disease (Zipes & Wellens 1998). While risk assessment of patients with congenital arrhythmogenic right ventricular dysplasia and the long QT syndrome (Zipes & Wellens 1998) is expected to be enhanced by genetic testing, noninvasive risk parameters may also prove helpful in identifying those patients with heightened potential for sudden death.

The goals of this review are twofold. The first is to discuss the basic mechanisms responsible for abnormal repolarization leading to ventricular arrhythmias and sudden death in nonischaemic heart disease. The second objective is to review contemporary approaches to risk stratification. We will focus on the more prevalent conditions that have recently been studied using newer noninvasive risk stratification techniques.

Basic electrophysiological mechanisms of arrhythmia

The electrophysiological mechanisms responsible for enhanced susceptibility to life-threatening arrhythmias in patients with nonischaemic heart disease are not well understood. This deficiency relates to both the diversity of cardiac conditions subsumed under this classification of disease and to the absence of suitable large animal models to emulate derangements in cardiac substrate. Koumi and colleagues (1995) demonstrated that ventricular myocytes from patients with idiopathic dilated cardiomyopathy had a longer duration and slower repolarization phase 3 of the action potential than those from ischaemic hearts and suggested differences in the inward rectifying K^+ channel. Hsia and coworkers (2002) provided evidence that abnormal tissue either from scar or fatty tissue infiltration may lead to abnormal conduction and subsequent heterogeneity of repolarization in patients with idiopathic dilated cardiomyopathy or arrhythmogenic right ventricular dysplasia. Kawara and associates (2001) provided histological evidence that the architecture of fibrosis in both dilated and idiopathic cardiomyopathy contributes to activation delay, a correlate of sudden cardiac death. In hypertrophic cardiomyopathy, disarray of myocardial fibres has been implicated in arrhythmogenesis (Maron *et al.* 1981). There is also an apparent interaction with enhanced sensitivity to catecholamines, corresponding to hypertrophic changes in the myocardium (Lefroy *et al.* 1993; Li *et al.* 2000). Finally, disturbances in calcium handling have been implicated in both dilated and hypertrophic cardiomyopathy (Pieske *et al.* 1996; Bottinelli *et al.* 1998; Sen *et al.* 2000).

Although unproven, it is probable that the vulnerable substrate of patients with nonischaemic disease may be susceptible to transient factors such as alterations in neural activity and electrolyte imbalance in the initiation of disturbances in cardiac repolarization and ventricular arrhythmogenesis (Zipes & Wellens 1998). It has long been appreciated in the long QT syndrome that sympathetic nerve activity is an arrhythmogenic factor (Schwartz & Malliani 1975). This may also be the case in cardiomyopathies, in which enhanced adrenergic activity is an adaptive response to compensate for depression in myocardial contractility, with the potential for adverse consequences in terms of vulnerability to arrhythmias.

Risk assessment in nonischaemic heart disease

Intense interest has been focused on potential markers of electrical instability, but currently no single approach to risk assessment for nonischaemic heart disease is generally accepted. Baroreflex sensitivity and heart rate variability, measures of autonomic tone, and signal averaged ECG (SAECG), which indicates nonuniform activation across the myocardium, have been investigated as markers of susceptibility to ventricular arrhythmias. T wave alternans and *QT* interval dispersion measure changes in repolarization, the vulnerable period of the cardiac cycle, from which ventricular tachycardia/ fibrillation emerges (Bilitch *et al.* 1967; Verrier *et al.* 1978). *QT* interval dispersion, by which *QT* length is compared simultaneously across several leads, may in fact not constitute a true measure of dispersion of repolarization as currently implemented (Malik *et al.* 2000). Improvements in analysis of T wave morphology may provide additional means to measure spatial heterogeneity of repolarization (Nearing & Verrier 2003).

Electrophysiological basis for T wave alternans as a marker of risk

T wave alternans has achieved significant risk stratification in most studies of patients with nonischaemic heart disease (Table 46.1). Although the precise electrophysiological basis for the apparent predictive ability of TWA in these patients is unknown, it probably relates to the ability of TWA to provide a quantitative measure of temporal and spatial unevenness of repolarization (Nearing *et al.* 1991, 1994; Pastore *et al.* 1999; Armoundas *et al.* 2002; Nearing & Verrier 2002), factors that have been implicated in electrical instability and vulnerability to ventricular tachyarrhythmias. In patients with hypertrophic cardiomyopathy,

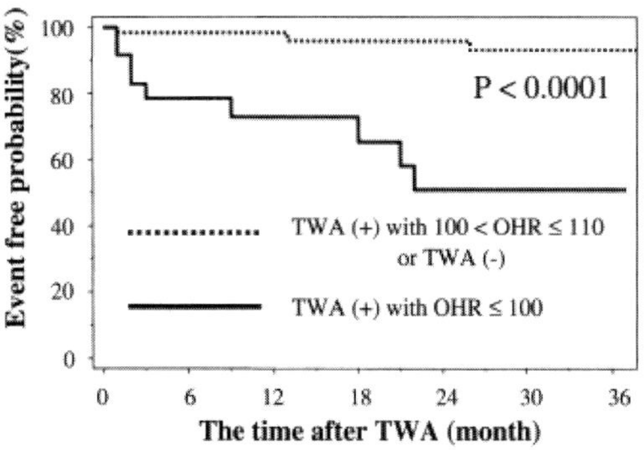

Fig. 46.1 T wave alternans (TWA) in the prediction of arrhythmia-free survival in 83 dilated cardiomyopathy patients whose symptoms were of low to moderate severity. The onset of TWA at heart rates ″ 100 beats/min identified patients at highest risk of sudden cardiac death and ventricular tachycardia and fibrillation (Reproduced from Kitamura *et al.* 2002, with permission from the American College of Cardiology.)

guiding implantable cardioverter defibrillator (ICD) therapy. They determined that the onset of TWA at heart rates ″ 100 beats/min and LVEF ″ 35% were significant predictors of sudden cardiac death and ventricular tachyarrhythmias (Fig. 46.1).

Arrhythmia risk stratification is expected to help address the important clinical question of identifying markers capable of guiding ICD implantation. Hohnloser and colleagues (2003) reported initial findings that TWA stratified arrhythmia risk in DCM patients. However, patients with ICDs for prior arrhythmias were enrolled in the study. TWA was not proved able to identify patients with an elevated risk of primary tachyarrhythmias, perhaps because the study was not sufficiently powered statistically due to limited enrolment of patients without prior events (Verrier *et al.* 2003a). In the 5-year prospective Marburg Cardiomyopathy Study, T wave alternans is being investigated in 221 dilated cardiomyopathy patients along with conventional measures and heart rate variability, QT dispersion, SAECG, baroreflex sensitivity, to determine whether any of these parameters or combinations of parameters is suitable to guide ICD implantation in dilated cardiomyopathy patients. The study endpoints are total mortality and major arrhythmia, namely VT or VF or sudden cardiac death. The patients are at relatively low risk of arrhythmia, as those on antiarrhythmic medications and those with a history of VT or VF are excluded. Initial findings indicate that T wave alternans is more common in dilated cardiomyopathy patients with LVEF < 30% as compared to patients with LVEF ≥30% (Grimm *et al.* 1998b).

Left ventricular hypertrophy

Once diagnosed, left ventricular hypertrophy constitutes a strong independent risk factor for SCD in patients with longstanding hypertension (McLenachan *et al.* 1987; Siegel *et al.* 1990; Zipes & Wellens 1998). Heart rate variability is depressed in hypertensive patients (Singh *et al.* 1998; Sevre *et al.* 2001), indicating autonomic dysregulation, and in those in whom hypertension has progressed to left ventricular hypertrophy (Mandawat *et al.* 1995). However, heart rate variability has not been shown capable of identifying patients who are at elevated arrhythmic risk. Hennersdorf and colleagues (2001) found that hypertensive patients who also manifested left ventricular hypertrophy were more likely to exhibit T wave alternans, and that TWA correlated with wall thickness, muscle mass index, and inducibility at electrophysiological study. In addition, the presence of T wave alternans identified hypertensive patients with a previous arrhythmic event.

Hypertrophic cardiomyopathy

The overall prevalence of hypertrophic dilated cardiomyopathy is low, 0.02 to 0.2% of the population, and the annual adult mortality is 1%. Their demise is most often sudden arrhythmic death. High-risk patients may exhibit sustained and nonsustained VT, recurrent syncope, and left ventricular hypertrophy > 3.5 cm (Spirito *et al.* 1997). Genetic mechanisms, particularly of mutations in the cardiac contractile protein genes, are suggested by characteristic family history of sudden cardiac death. Disordered calcium handling (Bottinelli *et al.* 1998) and sensitivity to catecholamines (Lefroy *et al.* 1993; Li *et al.* 2000) are also typical and may constitute important arrhythmogenic mechanisms. Momiyama and colleagues (1997) first discovered that T wave alternans was positive in a large proportion (71% or five of seven) of patients with hypertrophic cardiomyopathy known to be at high risk, based on documented nonsustained VT, syncope, and familial occurrence of sudden cardiac death.

There is evidence to suggest that the aetiology and pathogenesis for ventricular arrhythmias and positive T wave alternans test results in patients with left ventricular hypertrophy and hypertrophic cardiomyopathy may be related not to increased ventricular mass but to disarray in the orientation of myocardial fibres. Kon-No and colleagues (2001) compared the incidence of T wave alternans in patients with hypertrophic cardiomyopathy, left ventricular hypertrophy of equivalent mass, and normal volunteers. They found that T wave alternans was almost twice as prevalent in patients with hypertrophic cardiomyopathy than in those with left ventricular hypertrophy (61% vs. 31%), despite a nearly identical left ventricular mass index, and determined that at exercise heart rates between 100 and 110 beats/min, T wave alternans was more common in patients with ventricular tachyarrhythmias. Severity of myocardial disarray and fibrosis identified from biopsy correlated with T wave alternans, suggesting a possible mechanistic link. This finding has been corroborated by others (Kuroda *et al.* 2002). Importantly, severity of disorganization in myocardial fibres has been found to characterize hypertrophic cardiomyopathy patients who had died suddenly (Maron *et al.* 1981).

Conclusions and future directions

Nonischaemic heart diseases comprise a diverse group of pathologic conditions that are responsible for a significant number of ventricular arrhythmias and sudden death. Combinations of noninvasive markers as well as established clinical parameters are expected to improve risk assessment in this population (Adachi *et al.* 2001; Kondo *et al.* 2001). However, studies have been limited in size and generally restricted to single centres. Of the noninvasive markers currently being investigated for their potential to determine which patients are at heightened risk for ventricular arrhythmias, T wave alternans has most frequently been found to provide significant risk stratification (Table 46.1). Sensitivity of 63% to 92% for ventricular tachyarrhythmias in this patient population suggests its utility for initial screening. The importance of calcium handling in these diseases (Pieske *et al.* 1996; Bottinelli *et al.* 1998; Sen *et al.* 2000) and T wave alternans' sensitivity to calcium (Saitoh *et al.* 1989; Nearing *et al.* 1996; Diaz *et al.* 2002) may provide a mechanistic basis for this parameter's suitability in risk stratification.

Progress in terms of T wave alternans is likely to be accelerated by the recent development of methods for its assessment during routine AECG monitoring (Verrier *et al.* 2002, 2003b) and routine exercise treadmill testing (Nearing *et al.* 2000). The success of T wave alternans testing by bicycle ergometry has been limited by indeterminate test results, which have occurred in 10% to 23% of cardiomyopathy patients tested (Momiyama *et al.* 1997; Adachi *et al.* 1999; Grimm *et al.* 2000; Kondo *et al.* 2000; Kuroda *et al.* 2001, 2002; Sakabe *et al.* 2001a; Kitamura *et al.* 2002). Indeterminacy has been attributed both to atrial fibrillation and to low exercise tolerance. The latter shortcoming can be addressed by assessing TWA during daily activities, which encompass both physiological as well as behavioural stresses that challenge the myocardial substrate, to optimize the opportunity to uncover latent cardiac electrical instability (Verrier & Stone 1997).

In the future, risk stratification may also aid in evaluating the efficacy of therapy. Although most study protocols required removal of antiarrhythmic therapy for T wave alternans testing, this may not be necessary (Sakabe *et al.* 2001b). A forefront issue under current consideration is whether any of these risk factors has the potential to guide ICD implantation (Grimm *et al.* 1998a, 2000; Kitamura *et al.* 2002).

References

Adachi, K., Ohnishi, Y., Shima, T. *et al.* (1999) Determinant of microvolt-level T wave alternans in patients with dilated cardiomyopathy. *Journal of the American College of Cardiology*, **34**, 374–380.

Adachi, K., Ohnishi, Y. & Yokoyama, M. (2001) Risk stratification for sudden cardiac death in dilated cardiomyopathy using microvolt-level T wave alternans. *Japanese Circulation Journal*, **65**, 76–80.

Armoundas, A.A., Tomaselli, G.F. & Esperer, H.D. (2002) Pathophysiological basis and clinical application of T wave alternans. *Journal of the American College of Cardiology*, **40**, 207–217.

Bilitch, M., Cosby, R.S. & Cafferky, E.A. (1967) Ventricular fibrillation and competitive pacing. *New England Journal of Medicine*, **276**, 598–604.

Bottinelli, R., Coviello, D.A., Redwood, C.S. *et al.* (1998) A mutant tropomyosin that causes hypertrophic cardiomyopathy is expressed *in vivo* and associated with increased calcium sensitivity. *Circulation Research*, **82**, 106–115.

Chen, X., Shenasa, M., Borggrefe, M. *et al.* (1994) Role of programmed ventricular stimulation in patients with idiopathic dilated cardiomyopathy and documented sustained ventricular tachyarrhythmias: inducibility and prognostic value in 102 patients. *European Heart Journal*, **15**, 76–82.

Diaz, M.D., Eisner, D.A. & O'Neill, S.C. (2002) Depressed ryanodine receptor activity increases variability and duration of the systolic Ca^{2+} transient in rat ventricular myocytes. *Circulation Research*, **91**, 585–593.

Eisner, D.A., Choi, H.S., Diaz, M.E., O'Neill, S.C. & Trafford, A.W. (2000) Integrative analysis of calcium cycling in cardiac muscle. *Circulation Research*, **87**, 1087–1094.

Fauchier, L., Babuty, D., Cosnay, P., Poret, P., Rouesnel, P. & Fauchier, J.P. (2000) Long-term prognostic value of time domain analysis of signal-averaged electrocardiography in idiopathic dilated cardiomyopathy. *American Journal of Cardiology*, **85**, 618–623.

Fei, L., Goldman, J.H., Prasad, K. *et al.* (1996) QT dispersion and *RR* variations on 12-lead ECGs in patients with congestive heart failure secondary to idiopathic dilated cardiomyopathy. *European Heart Journal*, **17**, 258–263.

Greenwood, J.P., Scott, E.M., Stocker, J.B. & Mary, D.A. (2001) Hypertensive left ventricular hypertrophy: relation to peripheral sympathetic drive. *Journal of the American College of Cardiology*, **38**, 1711–1717.

Grimm, W., Steder, U., Menz, V., Hoffmann, J., Grote, F. & Maisch, B. (1996) Clinical significance of increased QT dispersion in the 12-lead standard ECG for arrhythmia risk prediction in dilated cardiomyopathy. *PACE (Pacing and Clinical Electrophysiology)*, **19**, 1886–1889.

Grimm, W., Glaveris, C., Hoffmann, J. *et al.* (1998a) Noninvasive arrhythmia risk stratification in idiopathic dilated cardiomyopathy: design and first results of the Marburg Cardiomyopathy Study. *PACE (Pacing and Clinical Electrophysiology)*, **21**, 2551–2556.

Grimm, W., Hoffmann, J., Menz, V., Luck, K. & Maisch, B. (1998b) Programmed ventricular stimulation for arrhythmia risk prediction in patients with idiopathic dilated cardiomyopathy and nonsustained ventricular tachycardia. *Journal of the American College of Cardiology*, **32**, 739–745.

Grimm, W., Hoffmann, J., Menz, V. & Maisch, B. (2000) Relation between microvolt level T wave alternans and other potential noninvasive predictors of arrhythmic risk in the Marburg Cardiomyopathy Study. *PACE (Pacing and Clinical Electrophysiology)*, **23**(11 Pt 2), 1960–1964.

Hennersdorf, M.G., Perings, C., Niebch, V., Vester, E.G. & Strauer, B.-E. (2000) T wave alternans as a risk predictor in patients with cardiomyopathy and mild-to-moderate heart failure. *PACE (Pacing and Clinical Electrophysiology)*, **23**, 1386–1391.

Hennersdorf, M.G., Neibch, V., Perings, C. & Strauer, B.-E. (2001) T wave alternans and ventricular arrhythmias in arterial hypertension. *Hypertension*, **37**, 199–203.

Hohnloser, S.H., Klingenheben, T., Blookfield, D. *et al.* (2003) Usefulness of microvolt T-wave alternans for prediction of ventricular tachyarrhythmic events in patients with dilated cardiomyopathy: results from a prospective observational study. *Journal of the American College of Cardiology*, **41**, 2220–2224.

Hsia, H.H. & Marchlinski, F.E. (2002) Characterization of the electroanatomic substrate for monomorphic ventricular tachycardia in patients with nonischaemic cardiomyopathy. *PACE (Pacing and Clinical Electrophysiology)*, **25**, 1114–1127.

Kawara, T., Derksen, R., de Groot, J. *et al.* (2001) Activation delay after premature stimulation in chronically diseased human myocardium relates to the architecture of interstitial fibrosis. *Circulation*, **104**, 3069–3075.

Kitamura, H., Ohnishi, Y., Okajima, K. *et al.* (2002) Onset heart rate of microvolt-level T wave alternans provides clinical and prognostic value in nonischaemic dilated cardiomyopathy. *Journal of the American College of Cardiology*, **39**, 295–300.

Klingenheben, T., Gronefeld, G., Li, Y.G. & Hohnloser, S.H. (2001) Effect of metoprolol and d,l-sotalol on microvolt-level T wave alternans. Results of a prospective, double-blind, randomized study. *Journal of the American College of Cardiology*, **38**, 2013–2019.

Kondo, N., Ikeda, T., Kawase, A. *et al.* (2001) Clinical usefulness of the combination of T wave alternans and late potentials for identifying high-risk patients with moderately or severely impaired left ventricular function. *Japanese Circulation Journal*, **65**, 649–653.

Kon-No, Y., Watanabe, J., Koseki, Y. *et al.* (2001) Microvolt T wave alternans in human cardiac hypertrophy: electrical instability and abnormal myocardial arrangement. *Journal of Cardiovascular Electrophysiology*, **12**, 764–765.

Koumi, S., Backer, C.L. & Arentzen, C.E. (1995) Characterization of inwardly rectifying K^+ channel in human cardiac myocytes. Alterations in channel behaviour in myocytes isolated from patients with idiopathic dilated cardiomyopathy. *Circulation* **92**, 164–174.

Kovach, J.A., Nearing, B.D. & Verrier, R.L. (2001) An

angerlike behavioural state potentiates myocardial ischaemia-induced T wave alternans in canines. *Journal of the American College of Cardiology*, **37**, 1719–1725.

Kuroda, N., Ohnishi, Y., Adachi, K. & Yokoyama, M. (2001) Relationship between the *QT* indices and the microvolt-level T wave alternans in cardiomyopathy. *Japanese Circulation Journal*, **65**, 974–978.

Kuroda, N., Ohnishi, Y., Yoshida, A., Kimura, A. & Yokoyama, M. (2002) Clinical significance of T wave alternans in hypertrophic cardiomyopathy. *Japanese Circulation Journal*, **66**, 457–462.

Lee, H.-C., Mohabir, R., Smith, N., Franz, M.R. & Clusin, W.T. (1988) Effect of ischaemia on calcium-dependent fluorescence transients in rabbit hearts containing indo 1. Correlation with monophasic action potentials and contraction. *Circulation* **78**, 1047–1059.

Lefroy, D.C., de Silva, R., Choudhury, L. *et al.* (1993) Diffuse reduction of myocardial beta-adrenoceptors in hypertrophic cardiomyopathy: a study with positron emission tomography. *Journal of the American College of Cardiology*, **22**, 1653–1660.

Li, S.T., Tack, C.J., Fananapazir, L. & Goldstein, D.S. (2000) Myocardial perfusion and sympathetic innervation in patients with hypertrophic cardiomyopathy. *Journal of the American College of Cardiology*, **35**, 1867–1873.

Malik, M., Acar, B., Gang, Y., Yap, Y.G., Hnatkova, K. & Camm, A.J. (2000) QT dispersion does not represent electrocardiographic interlead heterogeneity of ventricular repolarization. *Journal of Cardiovascular Electrophysiology*, **11**, 835–843.

Mandawat, M.K., Wallbridge, D.R., Pringle, S.D. *et al.* (1995) Heart rate variability in left ventricular hypertrophy. *British Heart Journal*, **73**, 139–144.

Maron, B.J., Anan, T.J. & Roberts, W.C. (1981) Quantitative analysis of the distribution of cardiac muscle cell disorganization in patients with hypertrophic cardiomyopathy. *Circulation*, **63**, 882–894.

McLenachan, J.M., Henderson, E., Morris, K.I. & Dargie, H.J. (1987) Ventricular arrhythmias in patients with hypertensive left ventricular hypertrophy. *New England Journal of Medicine*, **317**, 787–792.

Momiyama, Y., Hartikainen, J., Nagayoshi, H. *et al.* (1997) Exercise-induced T wave alternans as a marker of high risk in patients with hypertrophic cardiomyopathy. *Japanese Circulation Journal*, **61**, 650–656.

Nearing, B.D., Huang, A.H. & Verrier, R.L. (1991) Dynamic tracking of cardiac vulnerability by complex demodulation of the T wave. *Science*, **252**, 437–440.

Nearing, B.D., Oesterle, S.N. & Verrier, R.L. (1994) Quantification of ischaemia-induced vulnerability by precordial T wave alternans analysis in dog and human. *Cardiovascular Research*, **28**, 1440–1449.

Nearing, B.D., Hutter, J.J. & Verrier, R.L. (1996) Potent antifibrillatory effect of combined blockade of calcium channels and 5-HT_2 receptors with nexopamil during myocardial ischaemia and reperfusion in canines: comparison to diltiazem. *Journal of Cardiovascular Pharmacology*, **27**, 777–787.

Nearing, B.D., Stone, P.H., MacCallum, G., Clark, M.E., Karam, C. & Verrier, R.L. for the Vascular Basis Study Group (2000) New median beat analysis method for T wave alternans detection in standard treadmill testing of patients with stable coronary disease. *PACE (Pacing and Clinical Electrophysiology)*, **23**, 593 (abstract).

Nearing, B.D. & Verrier, R.L. (2002) Progressive increases in complexity of T wave oscillations herald ischaemia-induced VF. *Circulation Research*, **91**, 727–732.

Nearing, B.D. & Verrier, R.L. (2003) Tracking states of heightened cardiac electrical instability by computing interlead heterogeneity of T-wave morphology using second central moment analysis. *Journal of Applied Physiology*, **95**, 2265–2272.

O'Rourke, B., Ramza, B.M. & Marban, E. (1994) Oscillations of membrane current and excitability driven by metabolic oscillations in heart cells. *Science*, **265**, 962–966.

Pastore, J.M., Girouard, S.D., Laurita, K.R., Akar, F.G. & Rosenbaum, D.S. (1999) Mechanism linking T wave alternans to the genesis of cardiac fibrillation. *Circulation*, **99**, 1385–1394.

Pieske, B., Sutterlin, M., Schmidt-Schweda, S. *et al.* (1996) Diminished post-rest potentiation of contractile force in human dilated cardiomyopathy. Functional evidence for alterations in intracellular Ca^{2+} handling. *Journal of Clinical Investigation*, **98**, 764–776.

Qian, Y.W., Clusin, W.T., Lin, S.F., Han, J. & Sung, R.J. (2001) Spatial heterogeneity of calcium transient alternans during the early phase of myocardial ischaemia in the blood-perfused rabbit heart. *Circulation*, **104**, 2082–2087.

Rashba, E.J., Cooklin, M., MacMurdy, K. *et al.* (2002) Effects of selective autonomic blockade on T wave alternans in humans. *Circulation*, **105**, 837–842.

Saitoh, H., Bailey, J.C. & Surawicz, B. (1989) Action potential duration alternans in dog Purkinje and ventricular muscle fibres. Further evidence in support of two different mechanisms. *Circulation*, **80**, 1421–1431.

Sakabe, K., Ikeda, T., Sakata, T. *et al.* (2001a) Comparison of T wave alternans and *QT* interval dispersion to predict ventricular tachyarrhythmia in patients with dilated cardiomyopathy and without antiarrhythmic drugs: a prospective study. *Japanese Heart Journal*, **42**, 451–457.

Sakabe, K., Ikeda, T., Sakata, T. *et al.* (2001b) Predicting the recurrence of ventricular tachyarrhythmias from T wave alternans assessed on antiarrhythmic pharmacotherapy: a prospective study in patients with dilated cardiomyopathy. *Annals of Noninvasive Electrocardiology*, **6**, 203–208.

Schwartz, P.J. & Malliani, A. (1975) Electrical alternation

of the T wave: Clinical and experimental evidence of its relationship with the sympathetic nervous system and with the long QT syndrome. *American Heart Journal*, **89**, 45–50.

Sen, L., Cui, G., Fonarow, G.C. & Laks, H. (2000) Differences in mechanisms of SR dysfunction in ischaemic vs. idiopathic dilated cardiomyopathy. *American Journal of Physiology (Heart Circulatory Physiology)* **279**, H709-H718.

Sevre, K., Lefrandt, J.C., Nordby, G. *et al.* (2001) Autonomic function in hypertensive and normotensive subjects: the importance of gender. *Hypertension*, **37**, 1351–1356.

Siegel, D., Cheitlin, M.D., Black, D.M., Seeley, D., Hearst, N. & Hulley, S.B. (1990) Risk of ventricular arrhythmias in hypertensive men with left ventricular hypertrophy. *American Journal of Cardiology*, **65**, 742–747.

Singh, J.P., Larson, M.G., Tsuji, H., Evans, J.C., O'Donnell, C.J. & Levy, D. (1998) Reduced heart rate variability and new-onset hypertension: insights into pathogenesis of hypertension: the Framingham Heart Study. *Hypertension*, **32**, 293–297.

Spirito, P., Seidman, C.E., McKenna, W.J. & Maron, B.J. (1997) The management of hypertrophic cardiomyopathy. *New England Journal of Medicine*, **336**, 775–785.

Verrier, R.L., Brooks, W.W. & Lown, B. (1978) Protective zone and the determination of vulnerability to ventricular fibrillation. *American Journal of Physiology*, **234**, H592–H596.

Verrier, R.L. & Stone, P.H. (1997) Exercise stress testing for T wave alternans to expose latent electrical instability. *Journal of Cardiovascular Electrophysiology*, **8**, 994–997 (editorial).

Verrier, R.L., Nearing, B.D., La Rovere, M.T. *et al.* for the ATRAMI Investigators (2000) Median beat analysis of T wave alternans to predict arrhythmic death after myocardial infarction: Results from the autonomic tone and reflexes after myocardial infarction study. *Circulation*, **102**, II-713 (abstract).

Verrier, R.L., Nearing, B.D. & Stone, P.H. (2002) Optimizing ambulatory ECG monitoring of T wave alternans for arrhythmic risk assessment. In: Malik, M., (ed) *Cardiac Electrophysiology Review*. Kluwer Academic Publishers, Boston, **6**, 329–333.

Verrier, R.L., Tolat, A.V. & Josephson, M.E. (2003a) T-wave alternans for arrhythmia risk stratification in patients with idiopathic dilated cardiomyopathy [invited editorial]. *Journal of the American College of Cardiology*, **41**, 2225–2227.

Verrier, R.L., Nearing, B.D., La Rovere, M.T. *et al.* (2003b) Ambulatory ECG-based tracking of T-wave alternans in post-myocardial infarction patients to assess risk of cardiac arrest or arrhythmic death. *Journal of Cardiovascular Electrophysiology*, **14**, 705–711.

Wu, Y. & Clusin, W.T. (1997) Calcium transient alternans in blood-perfused ischaemic hearts: observations with fluorescent indicator fura red. *American Journal of Physiology*, **273**, H2161–H2169.

Zipes, D.P. & Wellens, H.H. (1998) Sudden cardiac death. *Circulation*, **98**, 2334–2351.

SECTION V
Atrial Fibrillation

CHAPTER 47

Pathophysiology of the Atrial Fibrillation Electrogram

Ulrich Schotten and Maurits A. Allessie

Historic remarks

The first description of atrial fibrillation (AF) has been given by McWilliam in 1887. He described patients with a 'conspicuously irregular arterial pulse' which he attributed to 'delirium of the heart' (McWilliam 1887). On examination, these patients suffered from palpitations, exercise intolerance, easy exhaustion, and a general feeling of ill-being. The radial pulse revealed a totally disordered rhythm. The heart action was rapid and irregular, strong pulsations taking turns with runs of almost imperceptible beats, and the intervals between the beats varying markedly.

Although by that time it was already known that cardiac contractions are caused by electrical impulses (Sanderson 1879), the electrophysiology of the heart could not be properly investigated until 1903, when Einthoven invented the string galvanometer (Einthoven 1903). The first clinical electrocardiogram of atrial fibrillation (AF) was published in 1906 (Einthoven 1906). A few years later Rothberger, Winterberg (Rothberger & Winterberg, 1909) and Lewis (Lewis 1909) established uniform criteria for the diagnosis of AF: total irregularity of the ventricular cycle length (*RR* intervals), absence of discrete atrial activation (P waves), and irregular fast oscillations of the baseline (Fig. 47.1).

Lewis supported the view that AF was caused by numerous electrical impulses in the atrial wall (Lewis 1909). Initially, he regarded it as a state in which many stimuli were generated at separate points, the incoordination of the contraction of the atria being the result of multiple impulses that block locally. Although the known causes of ectopic impulses, like increased cardiac pressure, fibrosis, and ischaemia, showed no consistent relationship with atrial fibrillation, nevertheless Lewis regarded the arrhythmia initially as extrasystolic in nature. Later he changed his mind, after Mines demonstrated that under certain conditions, a continuous circus movement of the electrical impulse could be initiated in myocardial rings (Mines 1913, 1914).

> . . . But if, on the other hand, the wave is slower and shorter (and it is made slower and shorter by the conditions which produce fibrillation) the excited state will have passed off at the region where the excitation started . . . Under these circumstances, the wave of excitation may spread a second time over the same tract of tissue; once started in this way it will continue unless interfered by some external stimulus . . .'

Mines argued that the rate of beating is than controlled by three factors: the conduction velocity and the duration of the refractory period on the one hand, and the size of the circuit on the other (Mines 1914). However, because of the irregular activity during AF it was difficult to prove any of the proposed mechanisms at that time, and it was not until 50 years later that Moe introduced his multiple wavelet hypothesis. Moe postulated that both ectopic activity and circus movement played a role in clinical atrial fibrillation. He assumed that if the spread of recovery is inhomogeneous, some fibres would already be excitable while nearby fibres would still be refractory (Moe 1962). Therefore,

> 'a second early premature response must spread . . . irregularly, along a more serrated wavefront, and . . . closely adjacent fibres may be thrown completely out of phase. . . . Once a fibre fails to respond to an impulse, its refractory period following a subsequent response will be increased; if it responds twice in a quick succession its refractory period will decrease accordingly.'

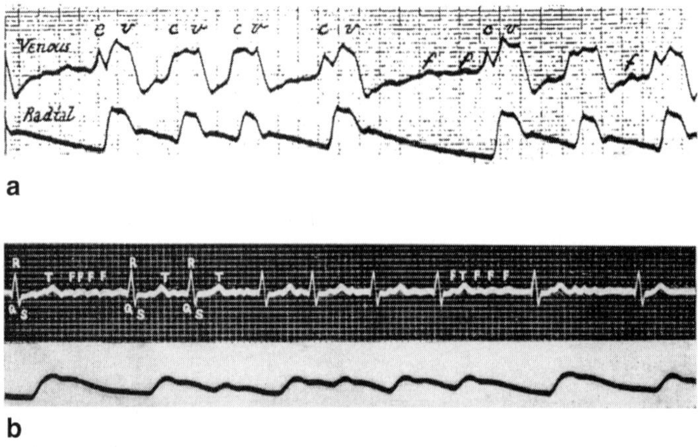

Fig. 47.1 (a) Venous and radialis pressures in a patient with atrial fibrillation. Undulations (f) of the venous pressure during diastole reflect fibrillatory contractions of the right atrium. Radialis curve with severe irregularity of the pulse. (Reproduced from Lewis 1909, with permission.) (b) ECG and radialis pulse in a patient with chronic AF. The ECG displays: (1) total irregularity of the *RR* interval, (2) absence of discrete P waves; (3) fast oscillations of the baseline. The irregularity of the ventricular rhythm is easily recognized in the radialis pressure curve (Reproduced from Boden 1939, with permission.)

As a result 'a grossly irregular wavefront becomes fractionated as it divides about islets or strands of refractory tissue and each of the daughter wavelets may now be considered as independent offspring.' Perpetuation of AF would then depend on the number of wavelets simultaneously present in the atria.

Experimental evaluation of the multiple wavelet hypothesis became possible by the development of computer technology, enabling to reconstruct the activation patterns during AF by high density mapping. In experimental studies in isolated Langendorff perfused canine hearts episodes of atrial flutter and atrial fibrillation were induced by infusion of acetylcholine and rapid pacing (Allessie *et al.* 1984, 1985). Endocardial mapping of both atria showed that during flutter a single fixed intra-atrial circuit existed, whereas during AF multiple wandering and reentering wavefronts were present. From these studies it was concluded that multiple reentering wavelets played an important role in the genesis of AF.

Analysis of atrial fibrillation electrograms

The first attempt to describe and classify atrial electrograms recorded during AF was undertaken by Wells *et al.* in 1991 (Wells *et al.* 1978). The nature of local atrial activation during AF was characterized in 34 patients following open heart surgery. The recorded *bipolar* atrial electrograms (interelectrode distance 0.5–1 cm) showed a high intra- and interindividual variation both in morphology, amplitude, polarity, and beat-to-beat interval. Four types of AF were distinguished (Fig. 47.2). In type I AF the fibrillation electrogram showed discrete complexes of varying morphology separated by a clear isoelectric baseline. Type II fibrillation was also characterized by discrete atrial complexes but now the baseline also showed perturbations of varying degree. During type III AF highly fragmented atrial electrograms were recorded and the less discrete complexes were no longer separated by an isoelectric segment. Type IV fibrillation was characterized by temporal alternations between type I, II, and III. The average atrial cycle length ranged from 179 ms during type I to 151 ms during type II fibrillation. Because of the chaotic nature of the bipolar electrogram, the exact atrial rate during type III AF could not be determined. This points to an important limitation of widely spaced bipolar electrograms for the characterization of AF. Due to the dissociation of wavefronts each of the pair of electrodes will frequently record from different fibrillation waves rather than that they record a differential signal of a single depolarization wave. From such a

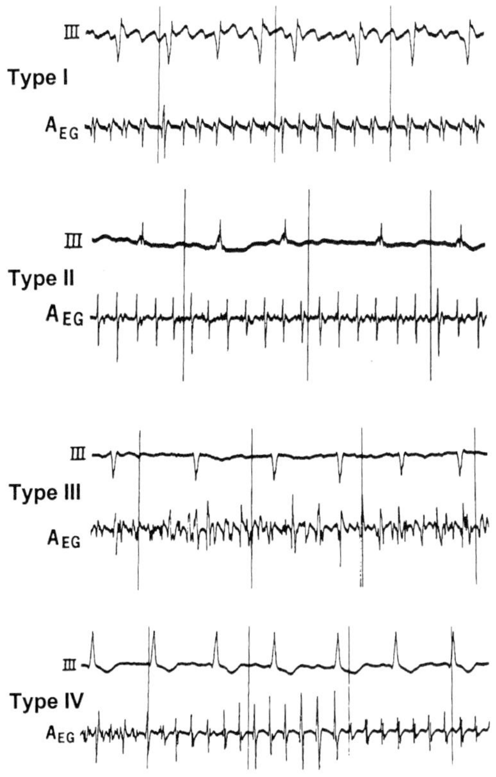

Fig. 47.2 Classification of AF based on morphology of the bipolar atrial electrogram. Four types of AF are distinguished (type I, II, III, and IV). The ECG (lead III) and a simultaneously recorded bipolar atrial electrogram (A_{EG}) are shown for each type of AF. (Reproduced from Wells *et al.* 1978, with permission.)

'mixed' signal the rate of atrial fibrillation can not be measured reliably. Therefore, the use of unipolar or closely spaced bipolar electrodes (<1 mm) is preferable for the recording of fibrillation electrograms.

The first mapping study of human AF was performed in 1991 by Cox *et al.* in patients with the Wolff–Parkinson–White syndrome undergoing cardiac surgery for interruption of the accessory atrio-ventricular pathway (Cox *et al.* 1991). AF was induced by burst pacing and the right and left atria were mapped using several epicardial templates containing a total of 160 bipolar electrodes (spatial resolution 0.5–1.0 cm). The data of this first human mapping study were consistent with previous experimental studies and supported re-entry as the basic underlying mechanism. All patients demonstrated non-uniform conduction around regions of bi-directional block resulting in multiple discrete wavefronts. In some re-entry circuits an anatomical obstacle like the orifice of the caval or pulmonary veins was involved. However, the majority of the atrial re-entrant circuits during AF was functional in nature. Sometimes, conduction block occurred at specific atrial structures such as the crista terminalis. In six of 13 patients, a re-entrant circuit could be identified in the right atrium around the sulcus terminalis. Although in all patients multiple wavefronts and lines of block were found both in the right and the left atrium, re-entrant circuits were more difficult to document in the left atrium and seemed to be more fleetingly. A major limitation of this first clinical mapping study of AF was that only single maps were analysed and that the temporal beat-to-beat changes in atrial activation was not studied.

In a second clinical study performed by Konings *et al.* (1994) the free wall of the right and left atria were mapped with a high density spoon-shaped electrode containing 244 unipolar electrodes (diameter 3.6 cm; interelectrode distance 2.25 mm). During acute AF, induced by rapid atrial pacing, both the atrial rate and degree of complexity of activation were quite variable. Uniform propagation of single broad wavefronts as well as highly disorganized activation by multiple wavelets of various size were observed. In an attempt to quantify the varying degree in complexity of atrial activation, the fibrillation maps were classified into three categories (Fig. 47.3). In type I, single broad fibrillation waves propagated through the atrial wall without any significant conduction delay or intra-atrial block. Some short lines of block or slow conduction could be present, but these did not disturb the main course of the fibrillation waves. Type II fibrillation was characterized by fibrillation waves with a higher degree of local conduction disturbances, or by the presence of two dissociated wavefronts in the free wall of the right or left atrium. During type III AF three or more wavelets propagated under the mapping electrode and multiple lines of conduction block and/or areas of slow conduction were present. The incidence of type I, II, and III AF was 40, 32, and 28% respectively. The type of fibrillation was correlated with the atrial fibrillation cycle length. In type I the median AF interval was 174 ± 20 ms, whereas in types II and III AF, the median fibrillation interval was 150 ± 14 and 136 ± 16 ms

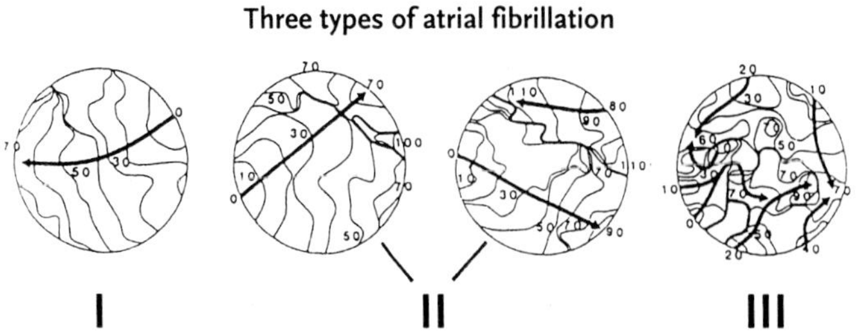

Fig. 47.3 Representative isochrone maps of the free wall of the human right atrium for the classification of AF (diameter 4 cm). In type I, single broad fibrillation waves propagated uniformly across the atrial wall. During type II AF, single fibrillation waves propagate with a considerable degree of conduction delay or intra-atrial conduction block, or the right atrium is activated by two separate fibrillation waves. During type III AF, the right atrial free wall is activated in a complex pattern by three or more dissociated wavelets. (Reproduced from Konings *et al.* 1994, with permission.)

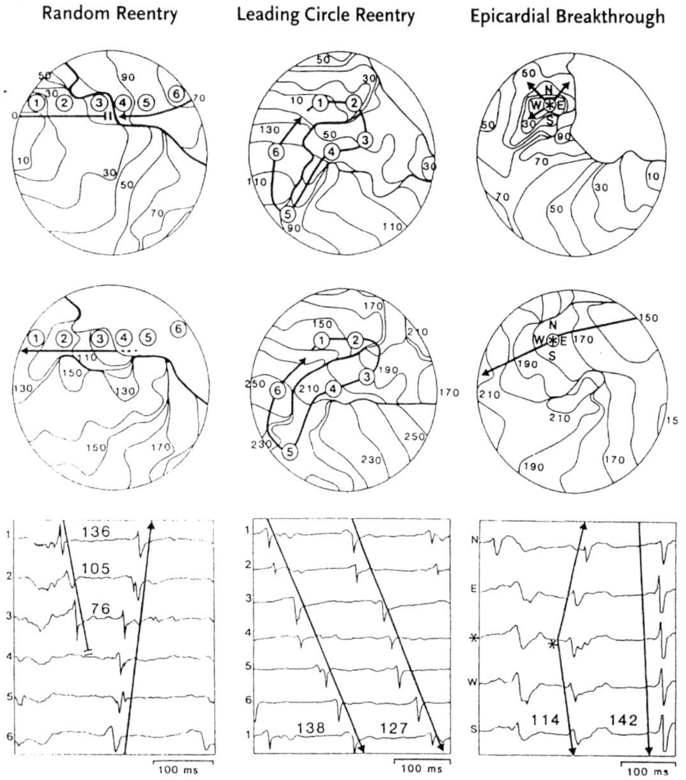

Fig. 47.4 Different types of re-entry during AF. During random re-entry (left) a fibrillation wave re-excites atrial tissue which shortly before was excited by another fibrillation wave. During leading circle re-entry (mid panels) closed loop re-entry around a shifting arc of functional conduction block is present. Occasionally, a 'focal' conduction pattern (right) was observed. The electrogram at the 'focus' showed a small R wave (*) indicating that the site of recording was not the origin of a new fibrillation wave. (Reproduced from Konings *et al.* 1994, with permission.)

respectively. In most patients a high temporal variation in the type of fibrillation was observed and propagation of single broad wavefronts (type I) alternated with more complex patterns of propagation (type II or III). This emphasizes that the three types of fibrillation should not be regarded as clinical or pathophysiological entities. Rather, they represent a continuous spectrum of different complexities and degree of disorganization of electrical activation during AF.

Two kinds of re-entry were observed in the free wall of the right atrium. During *random re-entry* a propagating fibrillation wave re-excited a part of the atrium which was shortly before activated by another wavelet. An example is shown in Fig. 47.4 (left). One fibrillatory wave is entering the mapping area from the left (t = 0) and propagated to the right in 70 ms. This fibrillation wave was blocked towards the upper third part of the mapping electrode, between electrodes 3 and 4 (Fig. 47.4, thick line). When this wave propagated away from the mapping area, another fibrillation wave entered from an opposite direction at electrode 6 ($t = 70$). This second fibrillation wave not only activated the upper part of the map which was left unexcited by the first wave, but actually activated the whole mapping area (from electrode 6 to 1 in Fig. 47.4, lower map). This was owing to re-entry of the tail of the first fibrillation wave at electrode 3 where a very short local fibrillation interval of 76 ms was recorded. An example of *leading circle re-entry* is illustrated in the mid panels of Fig. 47.4. The atrial impulse circulated in a clockwise direction around a functional arc of conduction block from electrodes 1–6. The cycle length was slightly irregular (138 and 127 ms in this case) and also the morphology of the unipolar electrograms showed some beat-to-beat variation. Stable re-entrant circuits were not observed in the free wall of the right atrium and after a few cycles, the functionally determined circuits usually terminated or shifted away from the mapping area. The incidence of *random-* and *leading circle re-entry* increased with the complexity of AF. In type I AF both forms of re-entry were rare, whereas in type III random re-entry was observed in 33%, and leading circle re-entry in 66% of the fibrillation maps.

Incidentally, a focal pattern of activation was recorded in the free wall of the right atrium (Fig. 47.4 right panel). These patterns of focal activation were only found as solitary events and did not occur repetitively. The electrograms recorded from the site of earliest activation (asterisks) still showed a small R wave preceding the negative deflection, indicating that these 'focal' activation patterns most probably were due to *epicardial breakthrough* of an endocardial fibrillation wave propagating through one of the pectinate muscles. In 1997 Holm *et al.* studied the activation pattern during *chronic* AF in the free right atrial wall in 16 patients during cardiac surgery (Holm *et al.* 1997). Using a mapping array of 56 bipolar electrodes the occurrence of three types of AF was confirmed. The major new finding was that in patients with chronic AF, the incidence of focal activation was much higher than in acutely induced AF. Also runs of repetitive focal activation of the right atrium were frequently observed. The site of 'focal' atrial activity was located preferentially at the right atrial appendage and was consistent with the explanation that it was due to epicardial breakthrough of fibrillation waves in the pectinate muscles. The higher incidence of epicardial breakthrough during chronic AF indicates that in diseased and dilated atria the activation during AF is a 3-dimensional process.

In acutely induced human AF, Konings *et al.* (1997) also studied the relationship between the morphology of the unipolar fibrillation electrograms and the different underlying spatial patterns of activation. The unipolar fibrillation electrograms were classified into four categories: (1) single potentials, (2) short-double potentials, (3) long-double potentials, (4) fragmented potentials. Single potentials were characterized by a single rapid negative deflection preceded by an R wave and smoothly returning to the baseline. Double potentials were defined as two clearly separated negative deflections, the amplitude of the smallest being at least 25% of the amplitude of the largest. Short-double potentials consisted of two deflections separated by <10 ms, whereas in long-double potentials the two components showed a time interval between 10 and 50 ms. Fragmented potentials were defined as electrograms exhibiting more than two negative deflections within a time period of 50 ms.

In Fig. 47.5 the relationship between the morphology of unipolar fibrillation electrograms and the spatial patterns of activation is illustrated. In Fig. 47.5(a) four wavelets are entering the mapping area from different directions (arrows). The four fibrillation waves collided along the dashed lines. The open squares on the map indicate atrial sites where short-double potentials were recorded during this cycle. Almost all short-double potentials were recorded along the lines of collision. Some examples are given around the map. Figure 47.5(b) shows an example of a fibrillation map with a long line of functional conduction block (thick line). The filled squares indicate electrodes from which long-double potentials were recorded (only some examples are shown). Long-double complexes were found almost exclusively along lines of conduction block. In Fig. 47.5(c) a map is shown in which

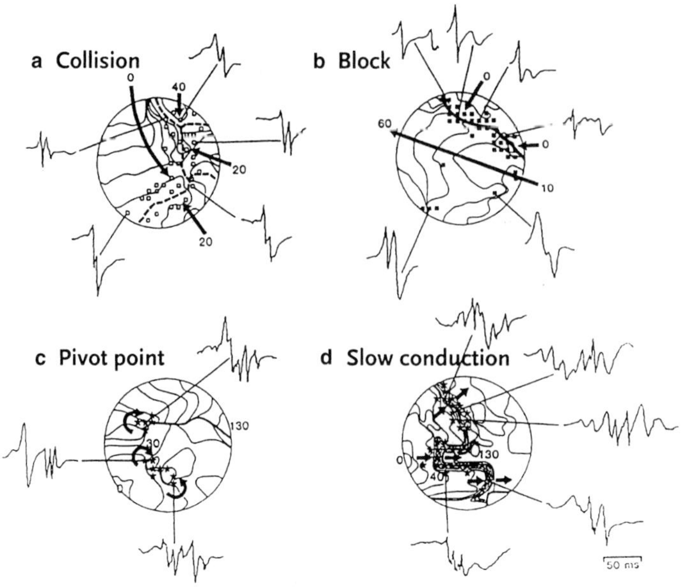

Fig. 47.5 Relation between unipolar electrogram morphology and activation pattern during atrial fibrillation. (a) Short-double potentials were observed at sites where fibrillation waves collided (dashed lines; open squares). (b) Long-double potentials were recorded at lines of conduction block (thick line; closed squares). The interval between the two deflections depended on the time delay between the two wavefronts at each side of the line of block. (c) and (d) Fractionated electrograms were recorded at pivot points of fibrillation waves and from zones of slow conduction. Isochrones are drawn at 10 ms intervals (Reproduced from Konings *et al.* 1997, with permission.)

three wavelets turn around the end of an arc of functional conduction block (arrows). The asterisks at these pivot points indicate electrodes from which fragmented potentials were recorded. Examples of fragmented electrograms of each of the pivot points are shown around the map. In Fig. 47.5(d) a broad fibrillation wave propagated from left to right with a high degree of local conduction delay. In the mid portion of the mapping area the fibrillation wave was delayed (crowding of isochrones) and it took as long as 130 ms to reach the right part of the map. Along the whole zone of slow conduction (asterisks), long fragmented complexes were recorded.

In Fig. 47.6 the fragmented unipolar fibrillation electrograms are shown in greater detail. In the left panel, a portion of the electrode array (5 × 5 electrodes; 6.25 × 6.25 mm) is selected where one of the fibrillation waves made a clockwise 180° turn around the end of a line of functional conduction block. The arrow indicates the pathway of the turning fibrillation wave. The horizontal thick line in the right middle part of the map indicates the end of the line of conduction block. The electrograms recorded around the pivot point are plotted at their respective sites of recording. The right lower corner of the map was activated early and in this area large single potentials were recorded. The electrograms at the right upper corner (above the line of block) were activated late and also showed large single potentials. At the tip of the line of block (right middle electrogram) a long double potential was recorded. The time delay between the two components reflected the difference in activation time at either side of the line of block. The three electrograms in the middle of the map were located at the centre of the pivoting wavefront. These electrograms, recorded at the area with the highest wavefront curvature, all showed clearly fractionated potentials. The completely functional nature of this fragmentation is illustrated by a longer tracing of one of the fractionated electrograms displayed below the map. The second complex (indicated by a dot) corresponds to the electrogram on the map of the pivoting fibrillation wave. The two complexes recorded

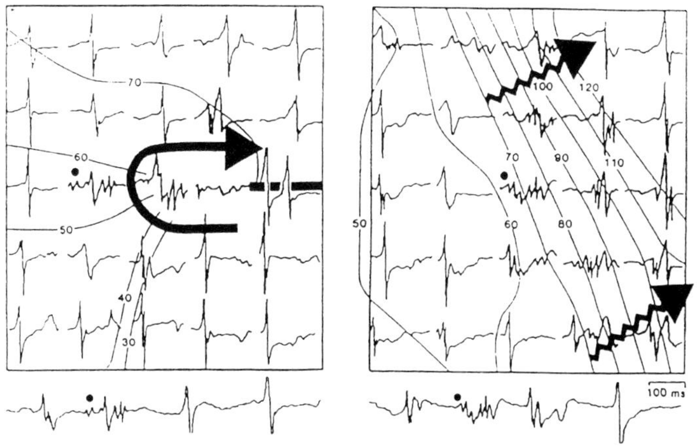

Fig. 47.6 Functional fractionation of unipolar electrograms during pivoting and slow conduction of fibrillation waves. The panels represent a selected area of 5 × 5 electrodes (9 × 9 mm) from the total map (diameter 4 cm) of the free wall of the right atrium during acutely induced atrial fibrillation. The electrograms are plotted at the relative sites of recording. At the bottom of the maps, a longer period of the fractionated electrogram (black dot) covering four fibrillation cycles is displayed. Fractionation proofs to be completely functional (owing to pivoting or slow conduction) because it is not present during AF cycles in which pivoting or slow conduction is absent (Reproduced from Konings *et al.*1997, with permission.)

immediately after the fractionated complex were both of high amplitude and showed no sign of fractionation. The maps of these two fibrillation cycles showed that the pivot area was now activated by a single uniformly conduction wavefront (maps not shown). The fractionation recorded during acute AF, thus was not the result of structural abnormalities of the atrium, but was caused by the high local curvature of the turning fibrillation wave. The same holds true for fractionation due to local slow conducting of fibrillation waves (Fig. 47.6 right panel). In this example fractionated electrograms were associated with slow propagation of a planar fibrillation wave (crowding of parallel isochrones). Again, fractionation promptly disappeared when the next fibrillation waves conducted normally (last complex of the electrogram below the map).

Fibrillation electrograms as a marker of structural conduction defects

Using small electrodes (diameter 0.3 mm) and recording unipolar electrograms, in normal human atria the incidence of fractionated potentials during acutely induced AF is quite low. Mapping of the whole free wall of the right atrium during acutely induced AF revealed an incidence of long double potentials of only 9%. The incidence of fractionated potentials was as low as 5% (Konings *et al.* 1997). Most (86%) fibrillation electrograms in normal human atria thus was of high amplitude and single in nature. This high predominance of non-fractionated fibrillation potentials in normal myocardium is important, because it opens the possibility to develop diagnostic tools for the diagnosis of structural atrial conduction defects based on the analysis of atrial fibrillation electrograms. The basis for our understanding of the relationship between fractionated electrograms and the architecture of the underlying atrial myocardium is given by the work of Spach and his coworkers (Spach & Dolber 1986). They studied the extracellular potential waveforms in isolated right atrial appendages of humans of different age groups. In older subjects extensive collagenous septa were present, dividing the atrial myocardium in small groups of fibres. Muscle bundles that were encircled by collagenous septa had lost their electrical coupling with adjacent pectinate muscles. This atrial architecture was associated with enhanced non-uniform anisotropy in conduction and a prominent zigzag course of the activation wave. Under these cir-

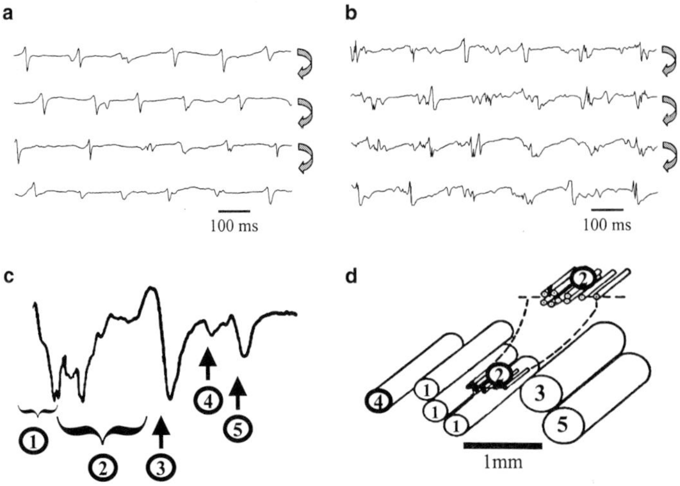

Fig. 47.7 Unipolar fibrillation electrograms from the free wall of the right (a) and left atrium (b) in a patient with chronic AF and mitral valve disease. In the dilated left atrium, the degree of fractionation was higher than in the non-dilated right atrium. At the bottom, a fractionated extracellular potential recorded with a very small endocardial electrode (diameter 50 μm) from the isolated right atrial appendage of a 62-year-old patient is shown together with the underlying atrial structure (d). (Reproduced from Spach & Dolber, 1986 , with permission.). The numbers on (c) and (d) link the components in the fractionated electrogram with the electrically dissociated atrial bundles (Reproduced from Spach & Dolber, 1986, with permission.)

cumstances very small unipolar electrodes (diameter 50 μm) could record highly complex extracellular waveforms.

In Fig. 47.7 unipolar fibrillation electrograms are shown recorded during chronic atrial fibrillation in a patient with mitral valve disease. The electrogram in Fig. 47.7(a) was recorded from the right atrium. In this relatively normal part of the atria, the fibrillation electrogram was only slightly fractionated and most of the fibrillation complexes were discrete and of high amplitude. The electrogram in Fig. 47.7(b) was recorded from the dilated left atrium. Here the degree of fractionation was more marked and single potentials were recorded only rarely. At the bottom (Fig. 47.7c) an example is shown of a fractionated electrogram recorded by Spach *et al.* (1986) from a 62-year-old male, together with the underlying atrial bundle structure (Fig. 47.7d). The numbers in Fig. 47.7(c,d) show the correspondence between each of the deflections in the fractionated electrogram and the respective bundles from which the deflections originated. Loss of side-to-side electrical coupling between these bundles by proliferation of connective tissue with advancing age, thus may produce complex pathways of 3Dl propagation at a microscopic level. It is likely that the higher degree of fractionation of fibrillation electrograms in the left atrium of patients with mitral valve disease (Fig. 47.7b), likewise is due to electrical dissociation of adjacent muscle bundles by stretch-induced fibrosis and disruption of side-to-side electrical connections.

Fragmentation mapping

The complexity of endocardial atrial activity during electrically induced AF was analysed by Jais *et al.* (1996) using a multipolar catheter (14 bipolar electrodes, 3 mm inter-electrode distance). The study population consisted of 25 patients with paroxysmal AF. The complex electrical activity time was defined as the ratio of the total duration of electrograms with fibrillation intervals smaller than 100 ms and the total recording time. Atrial activity was more complex in the left than in the right atrium. In the right atrium, disorganized atrial activity at the postero-septal area abruptly changed to more organized activity in the anterior and lateral wall. This transition occurred at the crista terminalis. In the left atrium, atrial activity in the septum and the area between the pulmonary

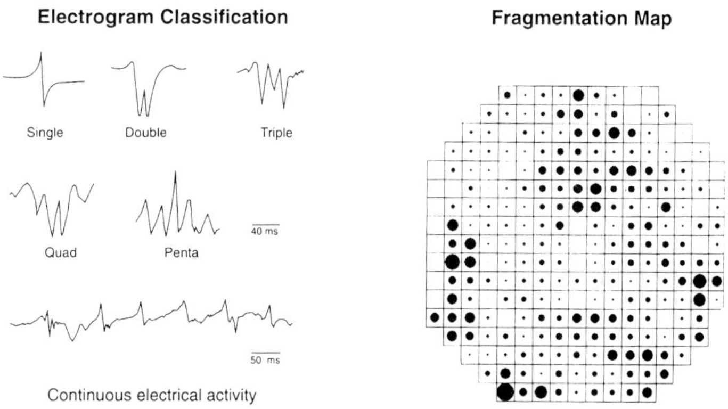

Fig. 47.8 Left: Classification of fractionation of unipolar fibrillation electrograms. Right: a fragmentation map of the free wall of the right atrium in a patient with chronic atrial fibrillation and mitral valve disease. The size of the dots represent the relative incidence of fragmented electrograms during 4 s of atrial fibrillation (Reproduced from de Groot *et al.* 2001, with permission.)

veins was more disorganized than in the appendage and the anterior left atrium. Thus, paradoxically, *organized* atrial activity appeared to be confined to the *trabeculated* parts of the right and left atria. The major limitation of this study was that only a relatively small number of atrial sites were analysed (four in the right and three in the left atrium).

Kuck *et al.* (1998) used an electro-anatomical mapping system (CARTO) to analyse bipolar fibrillation electrograms in patients with paroxysmal AF. Fibrillation electrograms were recorded during 45 s at multiple (36 ± 12) sites in the left atrium. Electrograms were classified as either type A (regular activation separated by a clear isoelectrical baseline), type B (irregular activation with perturbations of baseline and/or highly fragmented electrograms) or type C (alternation between type A and type B). Type B and C electrograms were equally present throughout the left atrium whereas the incidence of type A electrograms was higher in the upper left pulmonary vein (Kuck *et al.* 1998).

In a still ongoing study, the degree and nature of fragmentation of unipolar electrograms is studied by mapping of the right and left atrium in patients with chronic AF undergoing cardiac surgery. In Fig. 47.8 a right atrial fragmentation map (diameter 4 cm) of chronic AF is shown in a patient with mitral valve disease. In the left panel the different degrees of fragmentation (single, double, triple, quad, penta, continuous electrical activity) of fibrillation electrograms is illustrated. In Fig. 47.8, the right panel indicates the incidence of fragmented electrograms at each recording site. Fractionated electrograms were recorded at almost all electrodes. However, clear spatial differences in fractionation were present, some parts of the atrial wall showing a much higher prevalence of fragmentation than others. It is yet unknown whether these spatial differences in fragmentation of fibrillation electrograms are due to natural variations in atrial architecture or whether they express the degree of local atrial disease. It is a great challenge for the future to elucidate whether fragmentation mapping of chronic AF can be used to diagnose the underlying electropathological substrate. If so, mapping guided selective ablation of the most severely diseased parts of the atria, might be considered as an alternative approach for treatment of atrial fibrillation.

References

Allessie, M.A., Lammers, W.J., Bonke, I.M. *et al.* (1984) Intra-atrial re-entry as a mechanism for atrial flutter induced by acetylcholine and rapid pacing in the dog. *Circulation*, **70**, 123–135.

Allessie, M.A., Lammers, W.J.E.P., Bonke, F.I.M. *et al.* (1985) Experimental evaluation of Moe's multiple wavelet hypothesis of atrial fibrillation. In: *Cardiac Arrhythmias* (eds D. P. Zipes & J. Jalife), pp. 265–276. Grune & Stratton, New York.

Boden, E. (1939) Vorhofflimmern In: *Elektrokardiographie für die ärztliche Praxis* (ed. E. Boden), pp. 104–144. Steinkopff, Dresden.

Cox, J.L., Canavan, T.E., Schuessler, R.B. *et al.* (1991) The surgical treatment of atrial fibrillation. II. Intraoperative electrophysiological mapping and description of the electrophysiological basis of atrial flutter and atrial fibrillation. *Journal of Thoracic Cardiovascular Surgery*, **101**, 406–426.

Einthoven, W. (1903) Ein neues Galvanometer. *Ann Physik*, **4**, 1059–1061.

Einthoven, W. (1906) Le telecardiogramme. *Archives of International Physiology*, **4**, 132–164.

de Groot, M.S. & Allessie, M.A. (2001) Mapping of atrial fibrillation. *Annals of the first Super Sanita*, **37**, 383–392.

Holm, M., Johansson, R., Brandt, J. *et al.* (1997) Epicardial right atrial free wall mapping in chronic atrial fibrillation. Documentation of repetitive activation with a focal spread – a hitherto unrecognized phenomenon in man. *European Heart Journal*, **18**, 290–310.

Jais, P., Haissaguerre, M., Shah, D.C. *et al.* (1996) Regional disparities of endocardial atrial activation in paroxysmal atrial fibrillation. *PACE (Pacing and Clinical Electrophysiology)*, **19**, 1998–2003.

Konings, K.T., Kirchhof, C.J., Smeets, J.R. *et al.* (1994) High-density mapping of electrically induced atrial fibrillation in humans. *Circulation*, **89**, 1665–1680.

Konings, K.T., Smeets, J.L., Penn, O.C. *et al.* (1997) Configuration of unipolar atrial electrograms during electrically induced atrial fibrillation in humans. *Circulation*, **95**, 1231–1241.

Kuck, K.H., Ernst, S., Cappato, R. *et al.* (1998) Nonfluoroscopic endocardial catheter mapping of atrial fibrillation. *Journal of Cardiovascular Electrophysiology*, **9**, 57–62.

Lewis, T. (1909) Auricular fibrillation and its relationship to clinical irregularity of the heart. *Heart*, **1**, 306–372.

McWilliam, J. (1887) Fibrillar contraction of the heart. *Journal of Physiology*, **8**, 296–310.

Mines, G. (1913) On dynamic equilibrium in the heart. *Journal of Physiology*, **46**, 349–383.

Mines, G. (1914) On circulating excitation in heart muscles and their possible relation to tachycardia and fibrillation. *Transactions of the Royal Society of Canada*, **8**, 43–52.

Moe, G. (1962) On the multiple wavelet hypothesis of atrial fibrillation. *Archives Internationale de Pharmacodynamie et de Therapie*, **140**, 183–188.

Rothberger, C, Winterberg H. (1909) Vorhofflimmern und arrhythmia perpetua. *Wiener Klinische Wochenschrift*, **22**, 839–844.

Sanderson (1879) On the time-relations of the excitatory process in the ventricle of the heart of the frog. *Journal of Physiology*, **2**, 384–435.

Spach, M.S. & Dolber, P.C. (1986) Relating extracellular potentials and their derivatives to anisotropic propagation at a microscopic level in human cardiac muscle. Evidence for electrical uncoupling of side-to-side fibre connections with increasing age. *Circulation Research*, **58**, 356–371.

Wells, J.L., Jr, Karp, R.B., Kouchoukos, N.T. *et al.* (1978) Characterization of atrial fibrillation in man: studies following open heart surgery. *PACE (Pacing and Clinical Electrophysiology)*, **1**, 426–438.

CHAPTER 48

P Wave Abnormalities before AF Episodes

Polychronis E. Dilaveris

Atrial fibrillation (AF) is the most common of the serious cardiac rhythm disturbances and is responsible for substantial morbidity and mortality in the general population. Its prevalence doubles with each advancing decade of age, from 0.5% at age 50–59 years to almost 9% at age 80–89 years (Kannel *et al.* 1998). This statistically significant increase is demonstrated for both paroxysmal and chronic AF and after adjustment for age and sex (Kannel *et al.* 1998). Abnormalities in atrial conduction and refractoriness are associated with the occurrence of AF (Prystowsky & Katz 1998). The prolongation of P wave duration is considered an established indicator of an interatrial conduction disturbance (Josephson *et al.* 1977), and prolonged P wave duration is commonly used to predict paroxysmal AF (Dilaveris 2001). Therefore, numerous studies have focused in the evaluation of P wave abnormalities before AF episodes in an attempt to noninvasively identify those patients who are at risk of developing AF.

The idea of analysing P wave inscriptions to discriminate between patients with different diseases is not new. For more than a decade, different groups have tried to find easily definable P wave characteristics that can be used (Dilaveris 2001). The one most often used is the duration of the P wave on the standard 12-lead electrocardiogram (ECG), or its vector magnitude, $\sqrt{(X^2 + Y^2 + Z^2)}$ (Hofmann *et al.* 1996; Yamada *et al.* 2000). Another approach is to compute the P wave duration in each lead and to calculate P wave dispersion which is defined as the difference between the longest and the shortest P wave duration recorded from multiple different surface ECG leads (Dilaveris 2001). Analysis of the frequency content of the P wave has also been accomplished (Yamada *et al.* 1992), while lately there is an increasing interest for the P wave morphology (Dilaveris & Gialafos 2002).

12-lead surface electrocardiogram

Standard 12-lead electrocardiography remains a significant diagnostic tool for the prediction of AF because of its simplicity and wide-spread availability, although it is seriously hampered by a questionable accuracy and reproducibility (Dilaveris *et al.* 1999b). The prolongation of P wave duration has long been used for the prediction of paroxysmal AF in many studies (Buxton & Josephson 1981; Dilaveris *et al.* 1998; Kloter Weber *et al.* 1998; Dilaveris *et al.* 1999c; Ciaroni *et al.* 2000; Dilaveris *et al.* 2000). The role of prolonged P wave duration as a significant predictor of paroxysmal AF has been disputed in some studies and particularly in those measuring P wave duration in only one ECG lead (Steinberg *et al.* 1993; Klein *et al.* 1995). Recent studies measuring P wave duration from all the 12 surface ECG leads have shown promising results concerning the ability of maximum P wave duration to predict paroxysmal AF (Dilaveris *et al.* 1998, 1999c, 2000; Ciaroni *et al.* 2000; Özer *et al.* 2000; Tsikouris *et al.* 2001). Modern computer-assisted ECG systems have offered the opportunity to calculate P wave duration from the averaged complexes of all 12 leads and to define more accurately the start and the end of the P wave (Dilaveris *et al.* 1999a, 2000). Previous studies using standard paper printed ECGs and measuring P wave duration from only a selected number of ECG leads failed to show a significantly prolonged P wave duration in patients with paroxysmal AF compared to healthy controls (Stafford *et al.* 1997). Filtered P wave duration derived from signal-averaging ECG techniques showed better results (Stafford *et al.* 1997).

P-wave signal-averaged electrocardiogram

Similar to the ventricular signal-averaged ECG, the atrial signal-averaged ECG is an averaging of a high number of consecutive P waves that match the template created earlier. From the raw ECG data recorded in common Frank leads and after the appropriate filtering and averaging a vector magnitude of the P wave is constructed. Signal-averaged P wave duration has been shown to be significantly prolonged in patients with history of paroxysmal AF compared to controls (Fig. 48.1). Different cut-off values of filtered P wave duration have been utilized to identify patients at risk for paroxysmal AF with moderate to good sensitivity and specificity (Table 48.1).

To overcome the problem of fusion between the filtered P wave and QRS complex in patients with history of paroxysmal AF, frequency analysis was supplemented to the time-domain analysis of the P wave on the P wave-triggered signal-averaged ECG (Fukunami *et al.* 1991). The Fast Fourier Transform analysis was applied to the total signal-averaged P wave and the high frequency components in the range of 20–50 Hz were found to be significantly decreased in patients with clinical history of paroxysmal AF compared to controls (Hiraki *et al.* 1998). The summation of the absolute power found in frequency bands between 20 and 150 Hz was reported to be significantly increased in patients with paroxysmal AF compared to controls (Stafford *et al.* 1995a). Moreover, frequency domain analysis of the terminal part of the P wave alone failed to demonstrate significant differences between patients with paroxysmal AF and healthy subjects (Stafford *et al.* 1995a).

P wave dispersion

In a previous publication, a new ECG marker, P wave dispersion, was introduced as a simple ECG predictor of paroxysmal lone AF (Dilaveris *et al.* 1998). The authors of that study tested the hypothesis that the inhomogeneous propagation of sinus impulses found in patients with a history of paroxysmal lone AF could possibly result in a highly variable P wave duration measured from the differently oriented surface ECG leads. As an index of this interlead variation in P wave duration measurements they evaluated P wave dis-

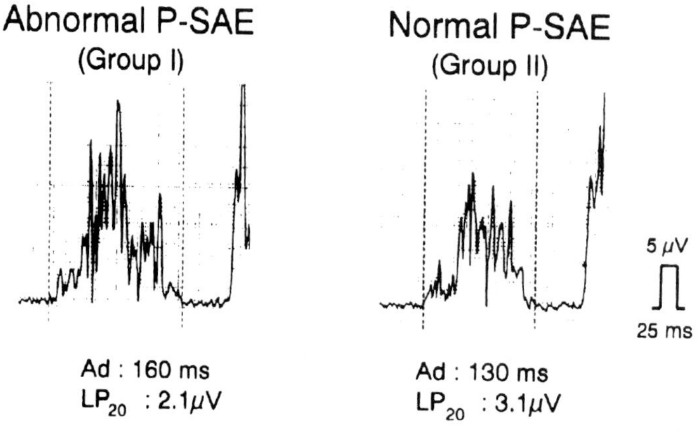

Fig. 48.1 Representative tracings of P-SAE (P-wave signal-averaged electrocardiogram) in a patient who developed paroxysmal atrial fibrillation (left, group I) and a patient who did not develop paroxysmal atrial fibrillation (right, group II) during the follow-up period. Note that the signal-averaged P-wave duration is longer and the terminal portion of the signal-averaged P wave is lower in the group I patients than in the group II patients. The abnormality of the P-wave signal-averaged electrocardiogram was Ad > 132 ms and LP_{20} < 2.3 μV (positive in group I; negative in group II). (Reproduced from the American College of Cardiology Foundation *Journal of the American College of Cardiology*, (2000) **35** (2), 405–413, with permission.)

Table 48.1 P wave signal-averaging in predicting the risk for atrial fibrillation

		Filtered P-wave			
Study	*Heart disease*	*Trigger*	*Cut-off (ms)*	*Sensitivity (%)*	*Specificity (%)*
Fukunami *et al.* 1991	HD	P	120	95	48
Guidera & Steinberg 1993		QRS	155	80	93
Steinberg *et al.* 1993	HD	QRS	140	77	55
Stafford *et al.* 1995b	HD	QRS	141	71	61
Maia *et al.* 1995	WPW	QRS	135	82	91
Klein *et al.* 1995	CAD-CABG	P	155	69	79
Montereggi *et al.* 1996	Hyperthyroidism	QRS	130	79	85
Stafford *et al.* 1997	CAD-CABG	QRS	141	73	48
Cecchi *et al.* 1997	HCM	QRS	140	56	83
Abe *et al.* 1997	HD	P	145	86	71
Hiraki *et al.* 1998	No	P	120	82	58
Dimmer *et al.* 1998	CAD-CABG	QRS	134	75	57
Aytemir *et al.* 1999a	CAD-CABG	QRS	122	68	88
Aytemir *et al.* 1999b	Post-cardioversion	QRS	128	70	76
Raitt *et al.* 2000	Post-cardioversion	QRS	130	81	89
Yamada *et al.* 2000	CHF	P	132	90	69
Zaman *et al.* 2000	CAD-CABG	P	155	63	74
Tuzcu *et al.* 2000	Post-Fontan operation	QRS	135	71	81

CABG, coronary artery bypass graft; CAD, coronary artery disease; CHF, congestive heart failure; HCM, hypertrophic cardiomyopathy; HD, organic heart disease; WPW, Wolff–Parkinson–White syndrome.

persion, which was derived from common 12-lead surface ECG and defined as the difference between the shortest and the longest P wave duration in any of the 12 ECG leads (Fig. 48.2). In the same study, P wave dispersion was found to be significantly higher in patients with paroxysmal lone AF than in healthy controls. A P dispersion value of 40 ms was found able to identify patients at risk for AF with a sensitivity of 83%, a specificity of 85%, and a positive predictive accuracy of 89% (Dilaveris *et al.* 1998).

Several studies have investigated the ability of P wave dispersion to predict AF in patients with coronary artery disease (Dilaveris *et al.* 1999a), in hypertensive subjects (Dilaveris *et al.* 1999c; Ciaroni *et al.* 2000; Ozer *et al.* 2000), in patients undergoing coronary artery bypass surgery (Kloter Weber *et al.* 1998; Fan *et al.* 2000; Gilligan *et al.* 2000; Tsikouris *et al.* 2001), in patients with mitral stenosis undergoing mitral balloon valvuloplasty (Turban *et al.* 2002), or in other groups of patients prone to AF (Yamada *et al.* 1999; Kubara *et al.* 1999; Dilaveris *et al.* 2000). The methodology used to date to obtain the interlead variation in the P wave duration differed between the various studies. Thermal (Dilaveris *et al.* 1998; Kloter Weber *et al.* 1998; Ciaroni *et al.* 2000; Fan *et al.* 2000; Gilligan *et al.* 2000; Özer *et al.* 2000; Tsikouris *et al.* 2001; Turban *et al.* 2002), digital (Dilaveris *et al.* 1999a,b,c, 2000), and signal-averaging ECG systems (Kubara *et al.* 1999; Yamada *et al.* 1999) have been used to evaluate P wave dispersion which was measured manually either on paper or on a high-resolution computer screen from 3–16, mainly 12, ECG leads. However, P wave dispersion has shown consistent clinically relevant differences between patients with history of paroxysmal AF and healthy controls irrespective of the method used for P wave measurement (Dilaveris *et al.* 1999b). The effect of Valsalva manoeuvre on P wave dispersion was evaluated in a previous study (Tukek *et al.* 2000), while another study assessed the effect of left atrial size and function on the same index (Tukek *et al.* 2001). The effects of overdrive atrial pacing on P wave dispersion have been evaluated in three studies (Fan *et al.* 2000; Gilligan *et al.* 2000; Yamada *et al.* 2001). Fan and colleagues showed that biatrial pacing, which was more effective in

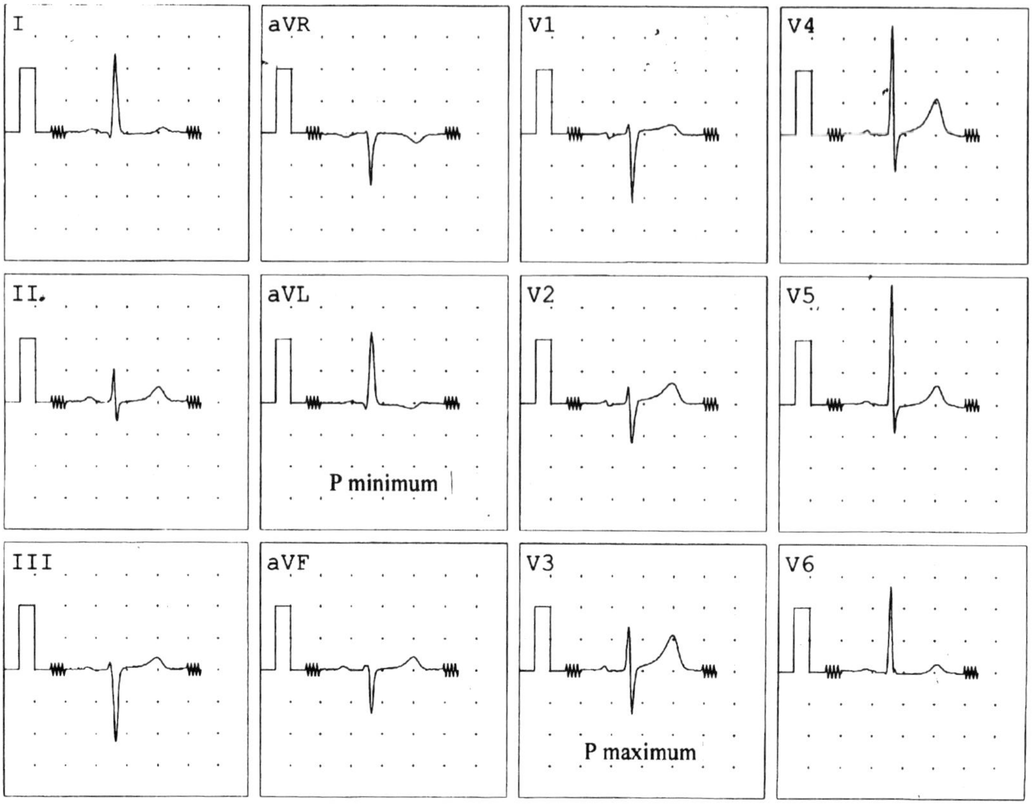

Fig. 48.2 Twelve-lead surface ECG from a 66-year-old woman with a previous history of paroxysmal atrial fibrillation. Maximum P wave duration (P maximum) and minimum P wave duration (P minimum) were found to be 125 ms in lead V3 and 75 ms in lead aVL, respectively. P wave dispersion was 50 ms.

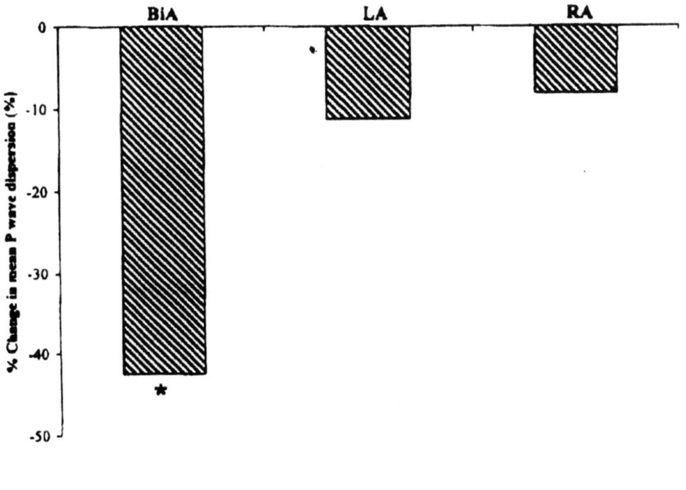

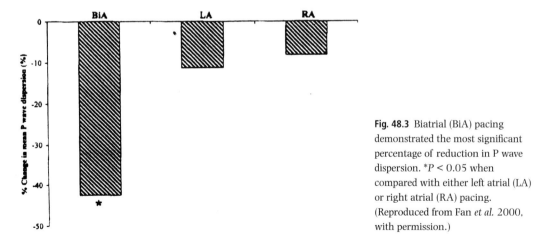

Fig. 48.3 Biatrial (BiA) pacing demonstrated the most significant percentage of reduction in P wave dispersion. $^*P < 0.05$ when compared with either left atrial (LA) or right atrial (RA) pacing. (Reproduced from Fan *et al.* 2000, with permission.)

the prevention of post-bypass AF than single-site atrial pacing, resulted in the most significant reduction in mean P wave dispersion when compared with single-site atrial pacing (Fig. 48.3). Furthermore, P wave dispersion was only reduced in those patients whose AF was prevented by pacing therapy (Fan *et al.* 2000).

The dispersion of the signal-averaged P wave duration on the precordial body surface constitutes an alternative approach to the standard 12-

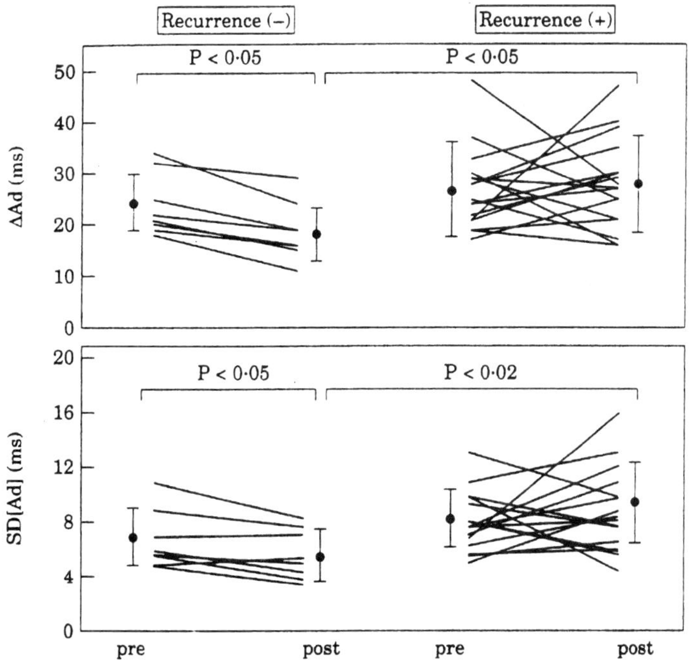

Fig. 48.4 Individual changes in signal-averaged P wave dispersion duration before (pre) and 1 h after (post) the single dose of pilsicainide in patients with and without the recurrence of paroxysmal atrial fibrillation (Paf). ΔAd, subtraction of the minimum from the maximum of the signal-averaged P wave duration; SD[Ad], the standard deviation of signal-averaged P wave duration in all 16 leads. In patients without paroxysmal atrial fibrillation recurrence, ΔAd and SD[Ad] significantly decreased after the administration of pilsicainide, while no significant change in ΔAd or SD[Ad] was observed in those with paroxysmal atrial fibrillation recurrence. Although there were no significant differences in ΔAd or SD[Ad] before the administration of pilsicainide between the two groups, the patients without paroxysmal atrial fibrillation recurrence had significantly smaller ΔAd and SD[Ad] after the administration than those with paroxysmal atrial fibrillation recurrence. (Reproduced from Yamada *et al.* 1999, with permission.)

lead ECG for the estimation of the regional differences in atrial activation and conduction (Kubara *et al.* 1999; Yamada *et al.* 1999). The dispersion of the filtered P wave duration has been calculated in two studies as the difference between the longest and the shortest filtered P wave recorded from 16 different precordial unipolar leads (Kubara *et al.* 1999; Yamada *et al.* 1999). In the same studies the dispersion of filtered P wave duration was shown to be significantly increased in patients with history of paroxysmal AF and it was used to assess the efficacy of the class I antiarrhythmic drugs pilsicainide and disopyramide. It was found that the dispersion of the filtered P wave decreases in patients in whom the antiarrhythmic drugs are effective in the suppression of AF attacks and increases in patients showing multiple recurrences of AF (Fig. 48.4).

P wave morphology analysis

Whereas standard approaches deal mainly with an analysis of the duration of the P wave, there is an increasing interest for the P wave morphology (Platonov *et al.* 2000; Carlson *et al.* 2001). Irregularities in the morphology of orthogonal P wave have been detected in patients with paroxysmal lone AF and were considered as markers of local interatrial conduction delay (Platonov *et al.* 2000). While a single-peaked P wave with a negative polarity in lead Z was characteristic of healthy subjects, a double-peaked P wave with a dominant positive phase in lead Z was characteristic of patients with paroxysmal lone AF (Fig. 48.5). More recently, a more advanced analysis of the P wave morphology based on impulse response analysis of the P wave was able to discriminate between patients with history of

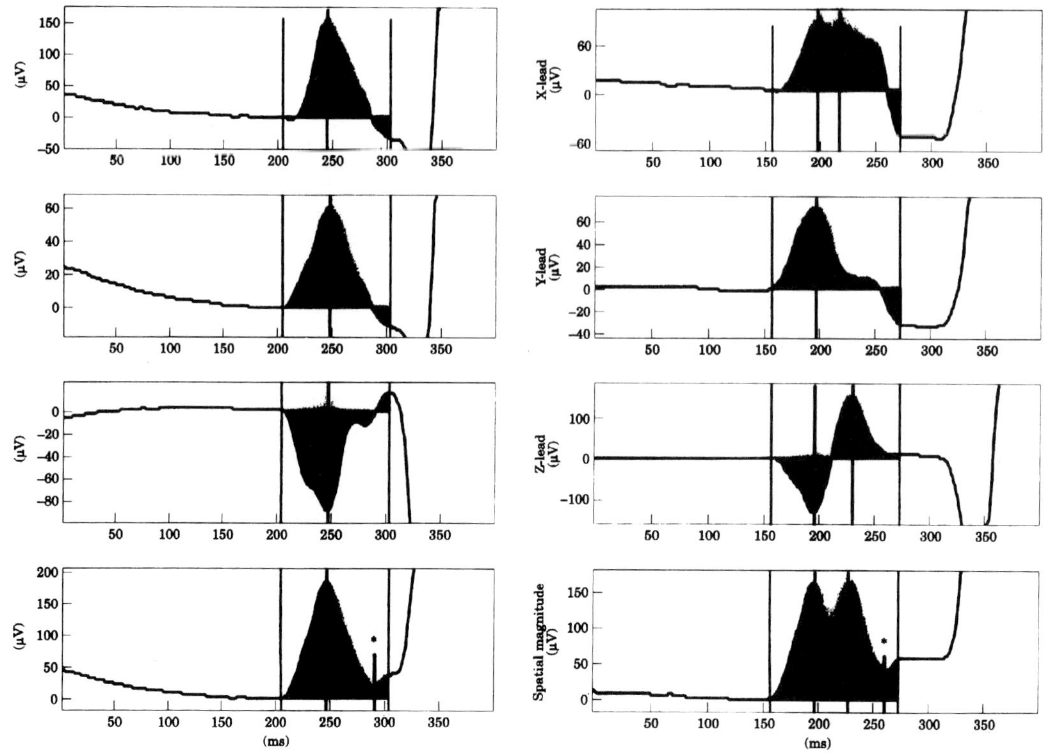

Fig. 48.5 Variations in the 'common' type of unfiltered P wave morphology. The nadir (*) is a result of the individual leads crossing the baseline at different times. Single-peaked spatial magnitude morphology with a mostly negative polarity in the Z lead was characteristic of the control group. A double-peaked spatial magnitude morphology with a dominating positive phase in the Z lead was characteristic of patients with lone paroxysmal atrial fibrillation. (Reproduced from Platonov *et al.* 2000, with permission.)

paroxysmal AF and healthy subjects (Carlson *et al.* 2001). Two types of P waves were identified with the most visible morphology differences in the Z lead. These different forms of P waves represent the presence or absence of an underlying pathophysiological condition in patients prone to attacks of AF (Carlson *et al.* 2001).

However, the well-known lability in P wave features may limit the use of P wave morphology analysis for the discrimination between different patient groups. The lability of P wave characteristics in normal subjects has been reported previously (Forfang & Erikseen 1978). Changes in P wave amplitude during physical daily activities such as positional changes, respiration, or exercise have already been demonstrated (Shandling *et al.* 1990; Ross *et al.* 1991). The presence of a significant circadian behaviour of P wave characteristics and of their dynamic adaptation to heart rate changes has been reported recently (Dilaveris *et al.* 2001).

The spatial characteristics of the 3-dimensional P wave loop might offer a more accurate than the scalar ECG description of the atrial electrical activity. However, such published data are still very sparse. We have recently calculated, from derived vectorcardiograms, the amplitude of the maximum spatial P wave vector and the squared ratio of the shorter to the longer axis of the P wave loop, which was defined as P eigenvalue and used as an index of the symmetry and the form of the P wave loop. By using these vector cardiographic indices we found lower spatial P amplitudes and higher P eigenvalues in patients with history of paroxysmal AF than in healthy subjects (P. Dilaveris *et al.* unpublished observations, 2001). Therefore, shorter and more rounded P wave loops may be charac-

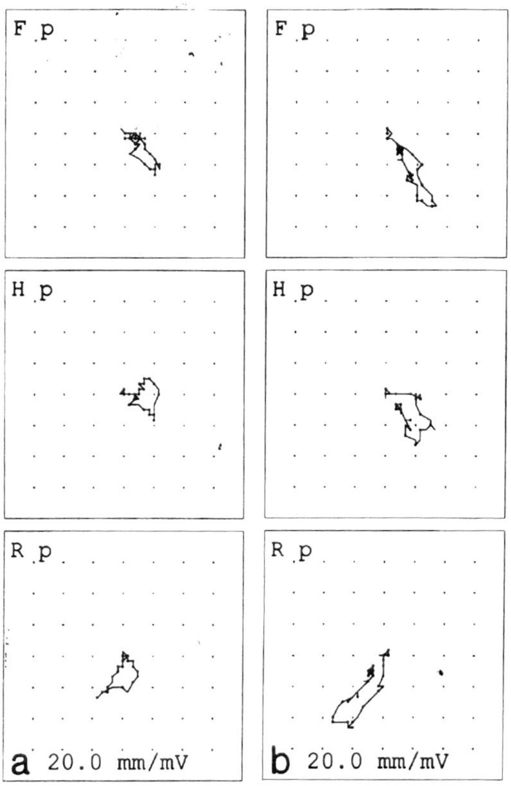

Fig. 48.6 P loop projections in the frontal (F), horizontal (H), and right saggital (R) planes from: (a) a 65-year-old woman with a previous history of paroxysmal atrial fibrillation, and (b) a 60-year-old woman without any history of paroxysmal atrial fibrillation. P wave loops are shorter and more rounded in patients with history of paroxysmal atrial fibrillation as compared to healthy controls.

teristic of patients with history of paroxysmal AF (Fig. 48.6).

Analysis of premature P wave patterns

Recent evidence has shown that AF may be induced by specific triggers: ectopic beats originating in the pulmonary veins (Haissaguerre *et al.* 1998; Chen *et al.* 1999). Most importantly these foci are amenable to focal ablation. The proportion of patients with AF triggered by this mechanism is not known, but there are accumulated data that it represents an important subset (Haissaguerre *et al.* 1998; Chen *et al.* 1999). The predominant distribution of atrial ectopic foci in the pulmonary veins indicates that premature P wave patterns may help to identify the source of firing (Haissaguerre *et al.* 1998). Prediction of the location of arrhythmogenic pulmonary vein before endocavitary exploration on the basis of surface ECG could facilitate and shorten the ablation procedure.

In previous studies, the P wave polarity and morphology on the 12-lead ECG and the P wave loop on the vectorcardiogram were examined during right atrial and left atrial pacing primarily in an attempt to differentiate left-sided from right-sided ectopic foci, but with conflicting results (Mirowski 1966; Leon *et al.* 1970; Josephson 1993). Alternatively, it has been suggested that the use of multichannel ECG recordings would offer improved resolution to localize ectopic atrial foci (Kawano & Hiraoka 1995; SippensGroenewegen *et al.* 1998).

In a previous study using simultaneous catheter mapping of initiating ectopics in right and left atrial regions, it was demonstrated that the P wave morphology on the surface ECG did not correlate with the site of origin in specific atrial regions (Saksena *et al.* 1999). However, it was lately shown that selective pacing at each of the four pulmonary veins produced distinct P wave characteristics that could be used to identify the pulmonary vein of origin of pacing with an accuracy of 79% (Yamane *et al.* 2001) (Fig. 48.7). Left pulmonary vein pacing produced low P wave amplitude (flat P wave) in lead I, negative polarity in lead aVL, similar amplitudes in both leads II and III, a notched morphology in lead II, and longer duration of positivity in lead V1. Conversely, right pulmonary vein origin was suggested by a positive P wave in lead I $\geq 50\,\mu V$, a relatively flat P wave in lead aVL, and a low amplitude ratio of lead III/II (less than 0.8). In addition, a clearly positive P wave in lead aVL was a specific marker of right pulmonary vein origin (Yamane *et al.* 2001). It is obvious that identification of the arrhythmogenic pulmonary vein could facilitate and shorten the ablation procedure.

However, it is sometimes difficult to locate the source of AF during selective pulmonary vein pacing owing to unpredictable firing, multiple sources and frequent induction of sustained AF. Rapid localization of arrhythmogenic pulmonary vein on a single initiating ectopy may be facilitated by P wave analysis (Yamane *et al.*

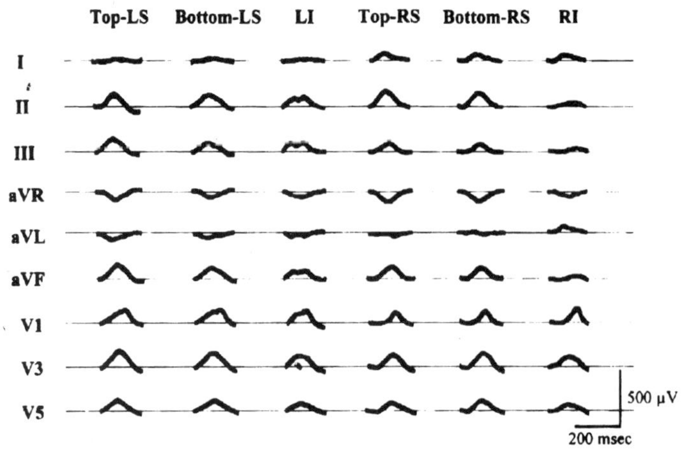

Fig. 48.7 Surface electrocardiogram P waves in one patient with atrial fibrillation (45-year-old man) during pacing at six sites in four pulmonary veins (PVs) are shown. Pacing in left PVs produced P waves with characteristic features of low amplitude in lead I, negativity in lead aVL, similar amplitude in both leads II and III, notched shape in lead II (most evident during left inferior [LI] pacing in this case), and long positive phase in lead V1. In contrast, P waves during right PV pacing were clearly positive in lead I, relatively flat in lead aVL, and had a low amplitude ratio of lead III/II (<0.8). The P waves during superior PV pacing are taller than those of inferior PV pacing in inferior limb leads. A positive P-wave in lead aVL, seen during RI pacing in this case, is a specific marker of right PV origin of pacing. Bottom-LS, bottom of the left superior PV; Bottom-RS, bottom of the right superior PV; RI, right inferior PV; Top-LS, top of the left superior PV; Top-RS, top of the right superior PV. (Reproduced from the American College of Cardiology Foundation *Journal of the American College of Cardiology* (2001), **38** (5), 1505–1510, with permission.)

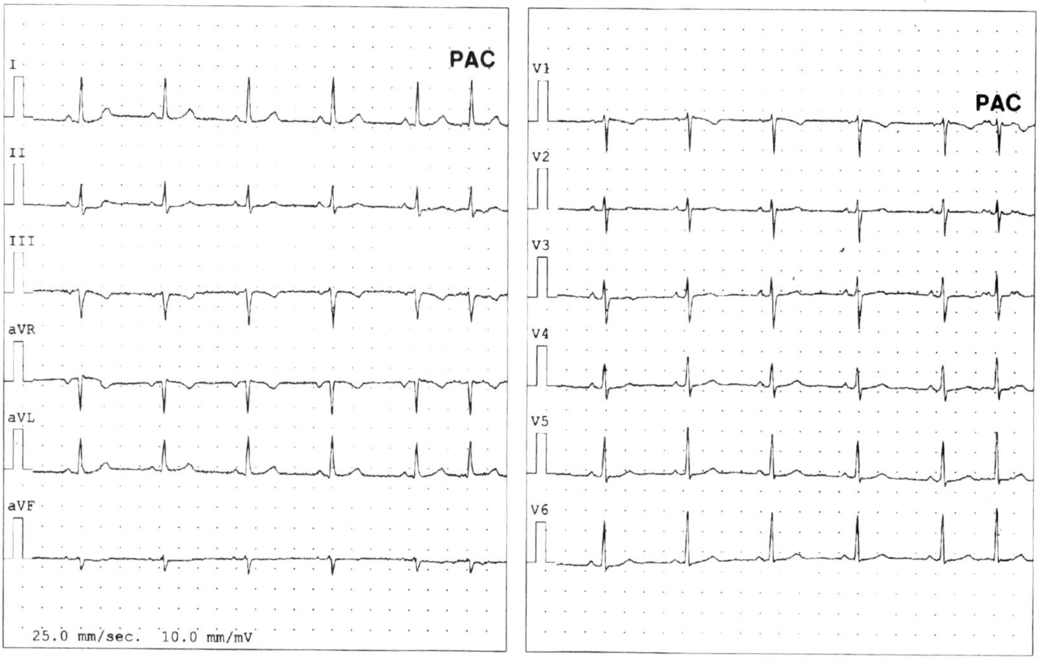

Fig. 48.8 Twelve-lead ECG strip from a patient with a history of paroxysmal atrial fibrillation showing a spontaneous premature atrial complex (PAC) with a coupling interval of 557 ms. Note the different morphology of the premature P wave compared to the previous sinus complexes, which is more evident in lead V1 (positive polarity in lead V1).

2001). The evaluation of the morphology of isolated spontaneous premature P waves from 12-lead raw ECG data may help localize the ectopic foci (Fig. 48.8). Unfortunately, the coupling interval of the premature P waves is often very short, thus overlapping with the T wave of the preceding sinus complex (Lu *et al.* 2001). To analyse P waves superimposed on T waves during spontaneous ectopics, an automatic QRST subtraction algorithm should be used. Methods reported in the literature to cancel ventricular activity from the ECG signal involve either direct suppression of the QRST, or subtraction of a fixed or adaptive template representing the QRST complex, or subtraction of an estimation of the QRST, obtained by transfer function identification between two ECG leads, or atrial activity enhancement by Wiener filtering using a dynamic time delay neural network (Dilaveris & Gialafos 2002). Future clinical application of these algorithms may enable improved ECG localization of focal triggers of paroxysmal AF, atrial tachycardia, and the atrial insertion of accessory pathways.

Conclusions

The ability of the surface ECG to identify patients at risk of developing AF is strengthened by analysing the P wave abnormalities before AF episodes. The simple 12-lead ECG and the P wave signal-averaged electrocardiogram provide much useful information, while more sophisticated techniques are currently under development. Detailed analysis of the low voltage P wave will require a hardware set-up that enables high-quality signal acquisition with low noise interference in combination with an ECG subtraction technique.

References

Abe, Y., Fukunami, M., Yamada, T. *et al.* (1997) Prediction of transition to chronic atrial fibrillation in patients with paroxysmal atrial fibrillation by signal-averaged electrocardiography: a prospective study. *Circulation*, **96**, 2612–2616.

Aytemir, K., Aksoyek, S., Ozer , N., Aslamaci, S. & Oto, A. (1999a) Atrial fibrillation after coronary artery bypass surgery: P wave signal averaged ECG, clinical and angiographic variables in risk assessment. *International Journal of Cardiology*, **69**, 49–56.

Aytemir, K., Aksoyek, S., Yildirir, A., Ozer, N. & Oto, A. (1999b) Prediction of atrial fibrillation recurrence after cardioversion by P wave signal-averaged electrocardiography. *International Journal of Cardiology*, **70**, 15–21.

Buxton, A.E. & Josephson, M.E. (1981) The role of P wave duration as a predictor of postoperative atrial arrhythmias. *Chest*, **80**, 68–73.

Carlson, J., Johansson, R. & Olsson, S.B. (2001) Classification of electrocardiographic P-wave morphology. *IEEE (Institute of Electrical and Electronic Engineers) Transactions on Biomedical Encineering*, **48**, 401–405.

Cecchi, F., Montereggi, A., Olivotto, I., Marconi, P., Dolara, A. & Maron, B.J. (1997) Risk for atrial fibrillation in patients with hypertrophic cardiomyopathy assessed by signal averaged P wave duration. *Heart* **78**, 44–49.

Chen, S.-A., Hsieh, M.-H., Tai, C.-T. *et al.* (1999) Initiation of atrial fibrillation by ectopic beats originating from the pulmonary veins. Electrophysiological characteristics, pharmacological responses, and effects of radiofrequency ablation. *Circulation*, **100**, 1879–1886.

Ciaroni, S., Cuenoud, L. & Bloch, A. (2000) Clinical study to investigate the predictive parameters for the onset of atrial fibrillation in patients with essential hypertension. *American Heart Journal*, **139**, 814–819.

Dilaveris, P.E. (2001) Noninvasive methods in atrial fibrillation. *Cardiac Electrophysiology Review*, **5**, 177–182.

Dilaveris, P.E., Andrikopoulos GK, Metaxas G *et al.* (1999a) Effects of ischaemia on P wave dispersion and maximum P wave duration during spontaneous anginal episodes. *PACE (Pacing and Clinical Electrophysiology)*, **22**, 1640–1647.

Dilaveris, P.E. & Gialafos, E.J. (2002) Future concepts in P wave morphological analyses. *Cardiac Electrophysiology Review* **6**, 221–224.

Dilaveris, P., Batchvarov, V., Gialafos, J. & Malik, M. (1999b) Comparison of different methods for manual P wave duration measurement in 12-lead electrocardiograms. *PACE (Pacing and Clinical Electrophysiology)*, **22**, 1532–1538.

Dilaveris, P.E., Färbom P, Batchvarov V, Ghuran A, Malik M. (2001) Circadian behaviour of P-wave duration, P-wave area, and PR interval in healthy subjects. *Annals of Noninvasive Electrocardiology* **6**, 92–97.

Dilaveris, P.E., Gialafos, E.J., Andrikopoulos GK *et al.* (2000) Clinical and electrocardiographic predictors of recurrent atrial fibrillation. *PACE (Pacing and Clinical Electrophysiology)*, **23**, 352–358.

Dilaveris, P.E., Gialafos, E.J., Chrissos D *et al.* (1999c) Detection of hypertensive patients at risk for paroxysmal atrial fibrillation during sinus rhythm by computer-assisted P wave analysis. *Journal of Hypertension*, **17**, 1463–1470.

Dilaveris, P.E., Gialafos, E.J., Sideris SK *et al.* (1998) Simple electrocardiographic markers for the prediction of paroxysmal idiopathic atrial fibrillation. *American Heart Journal*, **135**, 733–738.

Dimmer, C., Jordaens, L., Gorgov, N. *et al.* (1998) Analysis of the P wave with signal averaging to assess the risk of atrial fibrillation after coronary artery bypass surgery. *Cardiology*, **89**, 19–24.

Fan, K., Lee, K.L., Chiu, C. *et al.* (2000) Effects of biatrial pacing in prevention of postoperative atrial fibrillation after coronary artery bypass surgery. *Circulation*, **102**, 755–760.

Forfang, K. & Erikseen, J. (1978) Significance of P wave terminal force in presumably healthy men. *American Heart Journal*, **96**, 739–743.

Fukunami, M., Yamada, T., Ohmori, M. *et al.* (1991) Detection of patients at risk for paroxysmal atrial fibrillation during sinus rhythm by P wave-triggered signal-averaged electrocardiogram. *Circulation*, **83**, 162–169.

Gilligan, D.M., Fuller, I.A., Clemo, H.F. *et al.* (2000) The acute effects of biatrial pacing on atrial depolarization and repolarization. *PACE (Pacing and Clinical Electrophysiology)*, **23**, 1113–1120.

Guidera, S.A. & Steinberg, J.S. (1993) The signal-averaged P wave duration: a rapid and noninvasive marker or risk of atrial fibrillation. *Journal of the American College of Cardiology*, **21**, 1645–1651.

Haissaguerre, M., Jais, P., Shah, D.C. *et al.* (1998) Spontaneous initiation of atrial fibrillation by ectopic beats originating in the pulmonary veins. *New England Journal of Medicine*, **339**, 659–666.

Hiraki, T., Ikeda, H., Ohga, M. *et al.* (1998) Frequency- and time-domain analysis of P wave in patients with paroxysmal atrial fibrillation. *PACE (Pacing and Clinical Electrophysiology)*, **21** (Pt I), 56–64.

Hofmann, M., Goedel-Meinen, L., Beckhoff, A., Rehbach, K. & Schomig, A. (1996) Analysis of the P-wave in the signal-averaged electrocardiogram: Normal values and reproducibility. *PACE (Pacing and Clinical Electrophysiology)*, **19**, 1928–1932.

Josephson, M.E. (1993) Ectopic rhythms and premature depolarizations. In: *Clinical Cardiac Electrophysiology: Techniques and Interpretations* (ed. M. E. Josephson), pp. 167–180. Lea & Febiger, Malvern, PA.

Josephson, M.E., Kastor, A. & Morganroth, J. (1977) Electrocardiographic left atrial enlargement. Electrophysiologic, echocardiographic and hemodynamic correlated. *American Journal of Cardiology*, **39**, 68–73.

Kannel, W.B., Wolf, P.A., Benjamin, E.J. & Levy, D. (1998) Prevalence, incidence, prognosis, and predisposing conditions for atrial fibrillation: Population-based estimates. *American Journal of Cardiology*, **82**, 2N–9N.

Kawano, S. & Hiraoka, M. (1995) P wave mapping in ectopic atrial rhythm. In: *Advances in Body Surface Mapping and High Resolution ECG* (eds S. Yasui, J. A. Abildskov, K. Yamada & K. Harumi), pp. 47–56. Life Medicom, Nagoya, Japan.

Klein, M., Evans, S.J.L., Blumberg, S., Cataldo, L. & Bodenheimer, M.M. (1995) Use of P-wave-triggered, P-wave signal-averaged electrocardiogram to predict atrial fibrillation after coronary artery bypass surgery. *American Heart Journal*, **129**, 895–901.

Kloter Weber, U., Osswald, S., Huber, M. *et al.* (1998) Selective vs. non-selective antiarrhythmic approach for prevention of atrial fibrillation after coronary surgery: is there a need for pre-operative risk stratification? A prospective placebo-controlled study using low-dose sotalol. *European Heart Journal*, **19**, 794–800.

Kubara, I., Ikeda, H., Hiraki, T., Yoshida, T., Ohga, M. & Imaizumi, T. (1999) Dispersion of filtered P wave duration by P wave signal-averaged ECG mapping system: its usefulness for determining efficacy of disopyramide on paroxysmal atrial fibrillation. *Journal of Cardiovascular Electrophysiology*, **10**, 670–679.

Leon, D.F., Lancaster, J.F., Shaver, J.A., Kroetz, F.W. & Leonard, J.J. (1970) Right atrial ectopic rhythms: experimental production in man. *American Journal of Cardiology*, **25**, 6–10.

Lu, T.-M., Tai, C.-T., Hsieh, M.-H. *et al.* (2001) Electrophysiological characteristics in initiation of paroxysmal atrial fibrillation from a focal area. *Journal of the American College of Cardiology*, **37**, 1658–1664.

Maia, I.G., Cruz Filho, F.E., Fagundes, M.L. *et al.* (1995) Signal-averaged P wave in patients with Wolff–Parkinson–White syndrome after successful radiofrequency catheter ablation. *Journal of the American College of Cardiology*, **26**, 1310–1314.

Mirowski, M. (1966) Left atrial rhythm, diagnostic criteria and differentiation from nodal arrhythmias. *American Journal of Cardiology*, **17**, 203–210.

Montereggi, A., Marconi, P., Olivotto, I. *et al.* (1996) Signal-averaged P-wave duration and risk of paroxysmal atrial fibrillation in hyperthyroidism. *American Journal of Cardiology*, **77**, 266–269.

Özer, N., Aytemir, K., Atalar, E. *et al.* (2000) P wave dispersion in hypertensive patients with paroxysmal atrial fibrillation. *PACE (Pacing and Clinical Electrophysiology)*, **23** (Pt II), 1859–1862.

Platonov, P.G., Carlson, J., Ingemansson, M.P. *et al.* (2000) Detection of inter-atrial conduction defects with unfiltered signal-averaged P-wave ECG in patients with lone atrial fibrillation. *Europace*, **2**, 32–41.

Prystowsky, E.N. & Katz, A. (1998) Atrial fibrillation. In: *Textbook of Cardiovascular Medicine* (ed. E. J. Topol), pp. 1661–1693. Lippincott–Raven Publishers, Philadelphia.

Raitt, M.H., Ingram, K.D. & Thurman, S.M. (2000) Signal-averaged P wave duration predicts early recurrence of atrial fibrillation after cardioversion. *PACE (Pacing and Clinical Electrophysiology)*, **23**, 259–265.

Ross, B.A., Zeigler, V., Zinner, A., Woodall, P. & Gillette, P.C. (1991) The effect of exercise on the atrial electrogram voltage in young patients. *PACE (Pacing and Clinical Electrophysiology)*, **14**, 2092–2097.

Saksena, S., Prakash, A., Krol, R.B. & Shankar, A. (1999) Regional endocardial mapping of spontaneous and induced atrial fibrillation in patients with heart disease and refractory atrial fibrillation. *American Journal of Cardiology*, **84**, 880–889.

Shandling, A.H., Florio, J., Castellanet, M.J. *et al.* (1990) Physical determinants of the endocardial P wave. *PACE (Pacing and Clinical Electrophysiology)*, **13**, 1585–1589.

SippensGroenewegen, A., Peeters, H.A.P., Jessurun, E.R. *et al.* (1998) Body surface mapping during pacing at multiple sites in the human atrium. P-wave morphology of ectopic right atrial activation. *Circulation*, **97**, 369–380.

Stafford, P., Denbigh, P. & Vincent, R. (1995a) Frequency analysis of the P wave: comparative techniques. *PACE (Pacing and Clinical Electrophysiology)*, **18**, 261–270.

Stafford, P.J., Kolvekar, S., Cooper, J. *et al.* (1997) Signal averaged P wave compared with standard electrocardiography or echocardiography for prediction of atrial fibrillation after coronary bypass grafting. *Heart*, **77**, 417–422.

Stafford, P.J., Robinson, D. & Vincent, R. (1995b) Optimal analysis of the signal averaged P wave in patients with paroxysmal atrial fibrillation. *British Heart Journal*, **74**, 413–418.

Steinberg, J.S., Zelenkofske, S., Wong, S.C., Gelernt, M., Sciacca, R. & Menchavez, E. (1993) Value of the P-wave signal-averaged ECG for predicting atrial fibrillation after cardiac surgery. *Circulation*, **88**, 2618–2622.

Tsikouris, J.P., Kluger, J., Song, J. & White, C.M. (2001) Changes in P-wave dispersion and P-wave duration after open heart surgery are associated with the peak incidence of atrial fibrillation. *Heart & Lung*, **30**, 466–471.

Tükek, T., Akkaya, V., Demirel, S. *et al.* (2000) Effect of Valsalva manoeuver on surface electrocardiographic P wave dispersion in paroxysmal atrial fibrillation. *American Journal of Cardiology*, **85**, 896–899.

Tükek, T., Akkaya, V., Atilgan, D. *et al.* (2001) Effect of atrial size and function on P-wave dispersion: a study in patients with paroxysmal atrial fibrillation. *Clinical Cardiology*, **24**, 676–680.

Turban, H., Yetkin, E., Senen, K. *et al.* (2002) Effects of percutaneous mitral balloon valvuloplasty on P-wave dispersion in patients with mitral stenosis. *American Journal of Cardiology*, **89**, 607–609.

Tuzcu, V., Ozkan, B., Sullivan, N., Karpawich, P. & Epstein, M.L. (2000) P wave signal-averaged electrocardiogram as a new marker for atrial tachyarrhythmias in postoperative Fontan patients. *Journal of the American College of Cardiology*, **36**, 602–607.

Yamada, T., Fukunami, M., Ohmori, M. *et al.* (1992) Characteristics of frequency content of atrial signal-averaged electrocardiograms during sinus rhythm in patients with paroxysmal atrial fibrillation. *Journal of the American College of Cardiology*, **19**, 559–563.

Yamada, T., Fukunami, M., Shimonagata, T. *et al.* (1999) Dispersion of signal-averaged P wave duration on precordial body surface in patients with paroxysmal atrial fibrillation. *European Heart Journal*, **20**, 211–220.

Yamada, T., Fukunami, M., Shimonagata, T. *et al.* (2000) Prediction of paroxysmal atrial fibrillation in patients with congestive heart failure: A prospective study. *Journal of the American College of Cardiology*, **35**, 405–513.

Yamada, T., Fukunami, M., Shimonagata, T. *et al.* (2001) Effect of atrial septal pacing on P-wave duration dispersion and atrial late potentials in patients with paroxysmal atrial fibrillation. *American Journal of Cardiology*, **88**, 795–798.

Yamane, T., Shah, D.C., Peng, J.-T. *et al.* (2001) Morphological characteristics of P waves during selective pulmonary vein pacing. *Journal of the American College of Cardiology*, **38**, 1505–1510.

Zaman, A.G., Archbold, R.A., Helft, G., Paul, E.A., Curzen, N.P. & Mills, P.G. (2000) Atrial fibrillation after coronary artery bypass surgery: a model for postoperative risk stratification. *Circulation*, **101**, 1403–1408.

CHAPTER 49

Dynamics of atrial electrogram in AF

Bertil S. Olsson, Carl J. Meurling, Leif Sörnmo and Martin Stridh

Introduction

Atrial fibrillation (AF) is characterized by a continuously ongoing and spatially changing atrial myocardial excitation caused by multiple, interacting and variable electrical wavelets. Re-excitation occurs during the repolarization phase of the preceding electrical wave, implying that local excitation almost always occurs without any obvious latency beyond the refractory period. Therefore, the inherent nature of the arrhythmia implies that the average atrial fibrillatory rate is likely to reflect the averaged refractoriness at any part of the tissue involved. This assumption has been independently verified in both animal experiments and in patients (Lammers *et al.* 1986; Capucci *et al.* 1995; Kim *et al.* 1996). There is thus a significant relation between the duration of the fibrillatory cycle and measures of tissue refractoriness.

Hence, the length of the averaged atrial fibrillatory cycle can be used as an index of the averaged atrial myocardial refractoriness. Furthermore, a variability of the averaged fibrillatory cycle length can be supposed to reflect changes of the state of atrial myocardial refractoriness. Prompted by the probable usefulness of a noninvasive technique that assesses the average fibrillatory cycle length in the exploration of the pathophysiology of AF, the FAF-ECG (frequency analysis of fibrillation), was independently developed by two research groups (Holm *et al.* 1996, 1998; Bollmann *et al.* 1998). In short, the method disregards the electrical activity of the ventricles by a cancelling technique and uses fast Fourier transform (FFT) to identify the frequency content of the fibrillating atria.

In this chapter we describe the FAF-techniques, present findings from available studies exploring the temporal dynamics of atrial fibrillatory rate in patients with different types of AF and evaluate the clinical importance of these findings.

Methodological aspects

Using a digital recording technique, traditional ECG signals are obtained. After identification of QRST complexes, they are averaged and subtracted from the original signal, allowing a power/frequency analysis of the remaining atrial fibrillatory signal (Fig. 49.1). Originally, a fixed averaged QRST-complex was used for cancellation in individual leads. Further development of the method allowed an improved cancellation of the QRST complex by taking changes in QRS morphology owing to alterations in the electrical axis of the heart into account (Stridh & Sörnmo 2001). Furthermore, our studies of different interventions prompted a method for presenting the time–frequency relation with different time resolutions (Stridh *et al.* 2001).

Following QRST cancellation, a power spectrum is obtained, typically having a distinct peak which represents the most common fibrillatory cycle length of nearby endocardial sites (Holm *et al.* 1998; Bollmann *et al.* 1998). Although the gross appearance of the power/frequency relation is markedly influenced by the window length and interval overlap of the Welsh periodogram used to estimate the spectrum, the frequency value of the power maximum is unaffected (Holm *et al.* 1998). Therefore, in spite of the fact that different modes of calculating the spectrum

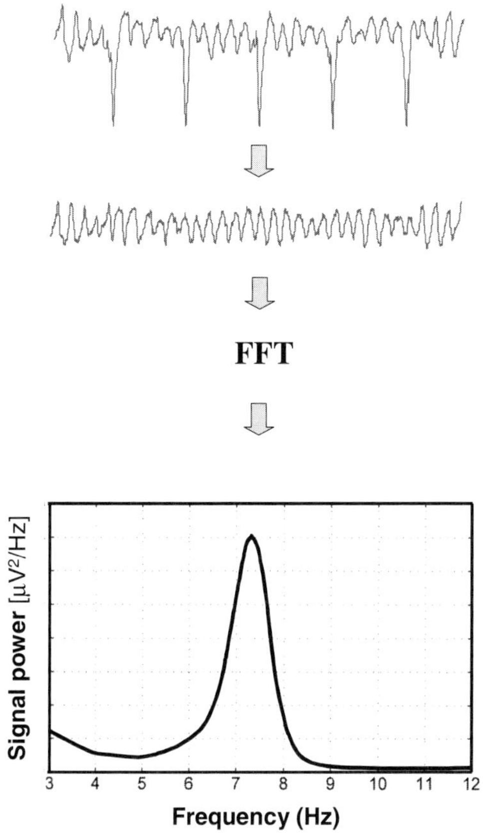

Fig. 49.1 The principle of the FAF-ECG. After identification and cancellation of QRST complexes, fast Fourier transform (FFT) is applied to the signal, yielding a power spectrum with a dominating peak within the frequency range 4–10 Hz.

have been used in the literature, the frequency values of the power maxima can still be directly compared. This maximum may be described by its frequency value (Hz), by the corresponding figure of atrial rate (beats/min) or by the corresponding cycle length (ms). Believing that the latter expression favours the integration of results from the FAF-ECG method with hitherto available information on atrial refractoriness, we have suggested that the frequency at which the largest peak is located is named the dominant atrial cycle length (DACL). In order to allow comparison with literature data, results from other modes of presenting the peak values from power-frequency analysis of fibrillation signals have sometimes been recalculated and expressed as DACL in the present paper. When the calculation is done from time periods less than one min however, the power/frequency maximum is instead described by its frequency value. Figure 49.2 illustrates the relation between cycle length (ms), frequency (Hz) and rate (beats/min), allowing also an easy recalculation between these different modes of expressing the repetitive electrical activity of the atria.

Method validation

A direct comparison between endocardially recorded electrograms and body surface recordings clearly evidences the validity of the DACL as an index of the average fibrillation cycle. The DACL calculated from lead V1 thus substitutes the right atrial free wall fibrillation rate (Bollmann *et al.* 1998; Holm *et al.* 1998) whilst the value obtained from an oesophageal lead reflects atrial septal and left atrial activity (Holm *et al.* 1998). Figure 49.3 illustrates the agreement between DACL values from simultaneously recorded intracavitary and precordial electrocardiograms.

Although the gross atrial fibrillatory pattern, studied by multiple simultaneous epicardial recordings, is reproducible already in repeated measurements of only 8 s duration (Holm *et al.* 1997), calculation of DACL during steady-state conditions from even longer time intervals discloses a true variability. Thus, increasingly longer recording times of up to 30 min result in a successive decrease of this variability. The reproducibility of the method is thus enhanced by prolonging the recording time during steady-state conditions, which allows integration of atrial fibrillatory activity over longer periods. For practical reasons, steady-state recordings may be restricted to 5 min, yielding a DACL variation coefficient of 2.1% (Holm *et al.* 1998).

Most literature reports which evaluate the atrial fibrillatory rate with the FAF-method have extracted information from resting ECG recordings. The method has however also been applied on ambulatory ECG recordings, using conventional ambulatory ECG leads (Bollmann *et al.* 1999, 2000; Cosson *et al.* 2000; Meurling *et al.* 2001). In these studies, the analysis of atrial fibrillatory cycle length has been done at predefined times, using parts of the entire recording of up to five minutes duration.

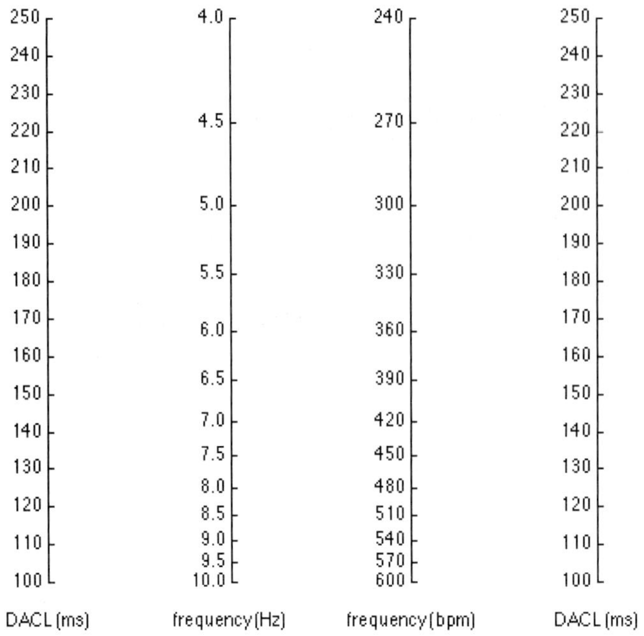

Fig. 49.2 Nomogram for recalculation between dominating atrial cycle length (DACL), frequency (Hz) and beats/min (beats/min), identified by FAF-ECG in patients with atrial fibrillation.

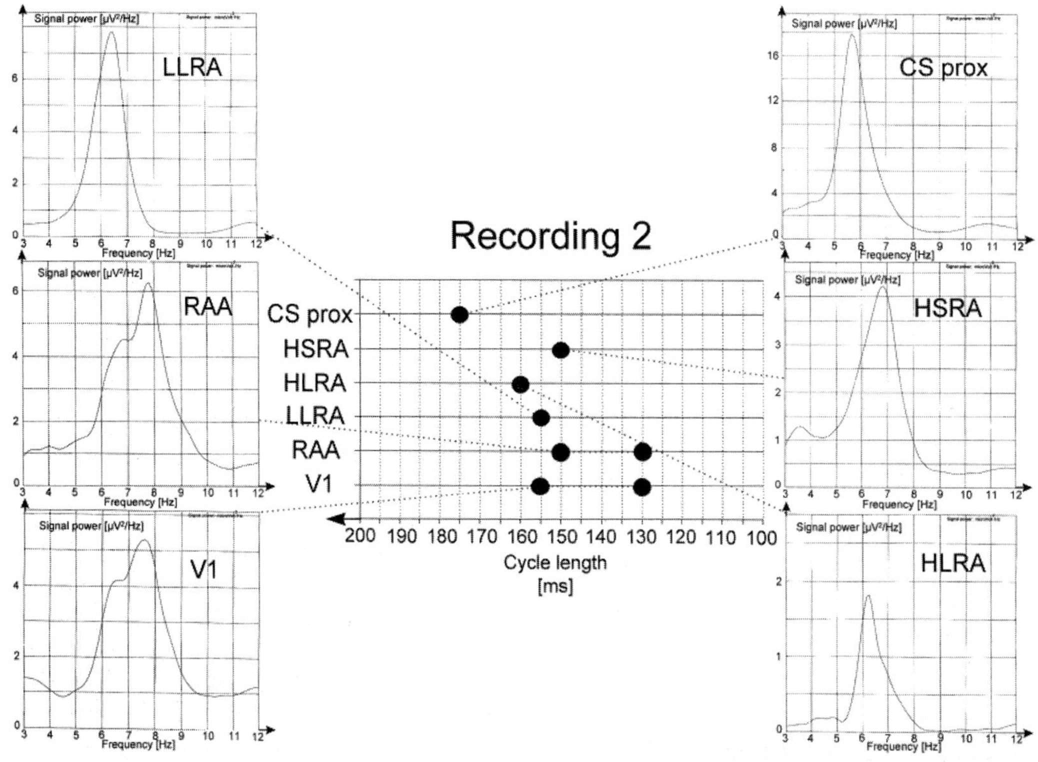

Fig. 49.3 Results of FAF-ECG recordings applied on signals recorded from different endocardial positions and the body surface. Note the similarities between right atrial free wall recording and lead V1 as well as between an oesophageal and a coronary sinus recordings.

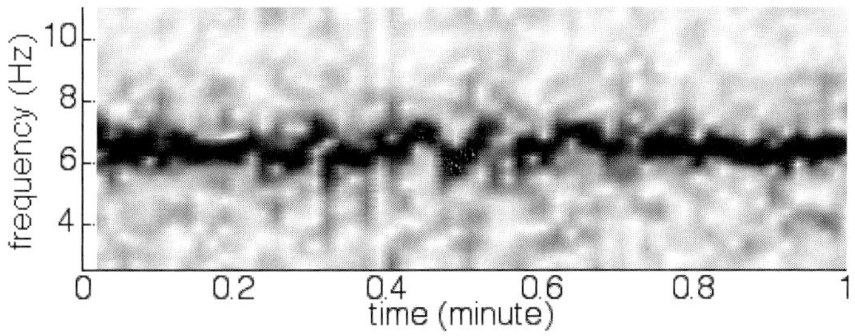

Fig. 49.4 Spontaneous variability of atrial fibrillatory rate in lead V1, estimated by the FAF-ECG method, applied during rest over one minute in a patient with permanent atrial fibrillation. The solid black colour indicates the maximum power of actual fibrillatory rate. Note that the power maximum is centred around 6 Hz and varies between 5 and 7 Hz.

Short-term spontaneous variability of fibrillatory rate

The diagnosis of AF in traditional resting 12-lead ECG is based upon lack of P-waves and instead the identification of a continuously changing electrical activity of an amplitude mostly less than that of a P-wave including rapid phases, indicating excitation phenomena – f-waves. This pattern of continuous electrical activity shifts in a seemingly unpredictable way, but occasionally resembles that of atrial flutter. Therefore, if the calculation of the frequency with maximal power is done within shorter time periods than a few seconds, it will be possible to follow even short-term changes of the atrial fibrillatory rate.

The second-to-second variability of atrial fibrillatory rate in patients with permanent AF and during resting conditions, studied in this way, is marked (Stridh *et al.* 2001). In a given example, the AF frequency is centred around 6 Hz, but with a considerable variation within the interval 5–7 Hz. Figure 49.4 illustrates DACL variability in a one min recording. In another patient, a 10 second episode of stable rate at 5.3 Hz interrupted the basic pattern with frequency changes between 5–7 Hz. This regular pattern may suggest either a flutter-like type of re-entry or a focal origin of the impulse. Interestingly, periodic activity is more often seen in left atrial recordings, possibly indicating a source of the fibrillation (Imai *et al.* 2001).

Circadian variability of DACL

Repeated daily estimation of DACL at identical medication and at the same time of the day discloses an insignificant variability with a mean variation of 2 ms with the absolute values differing by 2–11 ms (Meurling *et al.* 2001).

The circadian variability of atrial fibrillatory rate has been explored in several studies (Bollmann *et al.* 2000; Cosson *et al.* 2000; Meurling *et al.* 2001). There was a clear and uniform circadian pattern in the studies by Cosson *et al.* (2000) and Meurling *et al.* (2001). Thus, the DACL during daytime was 150 ± 17 ms (range 124–179) and 151 ± 12 ms (range126–171) respectively whilst during night, the DACL values were significantly higher, 157 ± 22 (range 125–195) and 156 ± 14 (range 129–177). Both these studies report a significantly increased day-to-night difference in patients with higher daytime DACL values. The patients included in these studies were allowed to take digitalis but not any other drug known to affect atrial myocardial refractoriness.

The third study reports a slightly different pattern (Bollmann *et al.* 2000). Thus, in agreement with the earlier cited studies, a significant increase of the atrial fibrillatory cycle occurred during night-time in the majority of the patients. In six out of 30 individuals however, the dominant nocturnal fibrillatory cycle decreased, concomitantly with a different effect on ventricular rate, in comparison with the 24 patients.

Circadian changes in atrial fibrillatory cycle length are believed to reflect changes in the discharge of the two limbs of the autonomous nervous system. The effect on atrial fibrillatory rate in patients with AF following vagal as well as sympathetic stimulation has been studied during experimental conditions. Thus, carotid sinus massage, supposed to mainly induce vagal

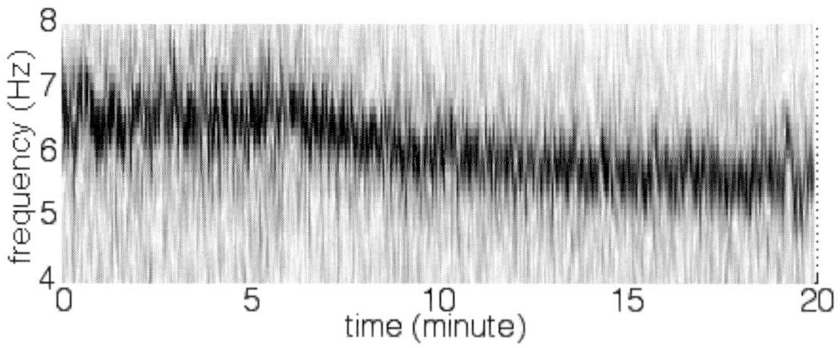

Fig. 49.5 Atrial fibrillatory rate, evidenced by the FAF-ECG method in a patient with atrial fibrillation, following intravenous infusion of dl-sotalol. The solid black colour indicates the maximum power of actual fibrillatory rate. Initially, the atrial rate is at the level of 6.5 Hz (= DACL 154 ms), but decreases successively to the level of 5.5 Hz (= DACL 182 ms).

stimulation, resulted in a variable effect on atrial fibrillation rate (Bollmann *et al.* 2001). An average decrease of atrial fibrillatory rate, compatible with a prolongation of DACL from 154 to 164 ms was noted in nine individuals, whilst a corresponding shortening from 156 to 141 ms was noted in eight and no change was observed in two.

The effect of stimulation of the adrenergic branch of the autonomous nervous system via head-up tilting on DACL was studied in 14 patients with long-lasting AF (Ingemansson *et al.* 1998). In the 12 patients, who followed the study design completely, the head-up tilt reduced DACL significantly, from 160 to 150 ms. The reduction of DACL was however not observed in all patients, two of them instead reacting with a prolongation by 2 ms.

In summary, although most patients with AF have a shorter DACL during daytime than during night-time, as well as following sympathetic stimulation, this reaction is not unanimous. Furthermore, vagal stimulation induces individual and contra-directional DACL changes. These findings clearly verify the complexity of the effect of the autonomous nervous system on atrial electrophysiology.

Temporal effects of antiarrhythmic drugs

The onset of action of intravenously administered drugs, acting on atrial repolarization or conduction is well fit to be explored by the FAF-ECG technique. Both mechanisms will result in a prolongation of the local fibrillatory interval, evidenced as a prolongation of the DACL. The method was applied in the study of the effect of i.v. ibutilide in patients with AF (Bollmann *et al.* 1998). Following drug infusion, atrial fibrillatory rate decreased by 114 ± 42 beats/min.

A continuous change of atrial fibrillatory rate was observed following i.v. dl-sotalol injection (Stridh *et al.* 2001). In the given example, the fibrillatory frequency was initially centred around 6.35 Hz (DACL = 158 ms). A successive decrease of the fibrillatory frequency could be identified during 10 min, reaching a post-drug value around 6.0 Hz (DACL = 167 ms). Figure 49.5 illustrates the effect of dl-sotalol on DACL following iv injection.

It is obvious that the time-dependant changes following iv injections of drugs which have a direct effect on atrial fibrillatory rate can be followed by a concomitant ECG-recording, using the FAF method with an appropriate temporal resolution. The study of the effect of orally administered drugs demands longer recording times and are therefore more easily done by a FAF-ECG analysis of ambulatory recordings. Examples of such studies include the exploration of effects of verapamil (Meurling *et al.* 1999) and Class I antiarrhythmic drugs (Fujiki *et al.* 2001).

Cardioversion of AF

Temporal changes of atrial fibrillatory rate, caused by the rate-induced remodelling, take place over several weeks time in the experimental situation (Wijffels *et al.* 1995). FAF-ECG recordings in patients with long-lasting, permanent AF verify a marked span of DACL, ranging between 115 (Pehrson *et al.* 1998) and 195 ms (Meurling *et al.* 2001). Interestingly, short DACL values, indicating a marked shortening of atrial refractoriness and a pronounced remodelling, are less influenced by different interventions in comparison with initially longer values (Meurling *et al.* 1999, 2001; Cosson *et al.* 2000)

The DACL value carries prognostic information regarding likelihood of maintaining sinus rhythm after cardioversion, with (Meurling 2000) or without (Bollmann *et al.* 2002) additional information from left atrial size. These observations are in agreement with earlier observations from patients with recent onset AF, receiving i.v. ibutilide (Bollmann *et al.*1998). Thus, conversion to sinus rhythm was significantly linked to the initial DACL value of the fibrillation frequency. All patients with an initial DACL exceeding 167 ms converted to sinus rhythm, in contrast to only 29% of those who had a lower initial DACL value. The FAF-ECG method may thus be used to identify treatment-responders as well in the setting of recent onset AF as in more long-lasting AF.

An interesting possible application of the method is linked to the energy demand necessary for conversion of AF. A well organized AF, i.e. of lower rate or longer DACL, seems to demand less energy for successful cardioversion (Everett *et al.* 2001), a finding of possible importance for the further development of automatic internal atrial defibrillators.

References

Bollman, A., Kanuru, N.K., McTeague, K.K., Walter, P.F., DeLurgio, D.B. & Langberg, J.J. (1998) Frequency analysis of human atrial fibrillation using the surface electrocardiogram and its response to ibutilide. *American Journal of Cardiology*, **81**, 1439–1445.

Bollman, A., Mende, M., Neugebauer, A. & Pfeiffer, D. (2002) Atrial fibrillatory frequency predicts atrial defibrillation threshold and early arrhythmia recurrence in patients undergoing internal cardioversion of persistent atrial fibrillation. *PACE (Pacing and Clinical Electrophysiology)*, **25** (8), 1179–1184.

Bollman, A., Sonne, K., Esperer, H.D., Toepffer, I. & Klein, H.U. (2000) Circadian variations in atrial fibrillatory frequency in persistent human atrial fibrillation. *PACE (Pacing and Clinical Electrophysiology)*, **23**, 1867–1871.

Bollman, A., Sonne, K., Esperer, H-D., Toepffer, I., Langberg, J.J. & Klein, H.U. (1999) Noninvasive assessment of fibrillatory activity in patients with paroxysmal and persistent atrial fibrillation using the Holter ECG. *Cardiovascular Research*, **44**, 60–66.

Bollman, A., Wodarz, K., Esperer, H.D., Toepffer, I. & Klein, H.U. (2001) Response of atrial fibrillatory activity to carotid sinus massage in patients with atrial fibrillation. *PACE (Pacing and Clinical Electrophysiology)*, **24**, 1363–1368.

Capucci, A., Biffi, M., Boriani, G. *et al.* (1995) Dynamic electrophysiological behaviour of human atria during paroxysmal atrial fibrillation. *Circulation*, **92**, 1193–1202.

Cosson, S., Maison-Blanche, P., Olsson, S.B., Leenhardt, A., Badilini, F. & Coumel, P. (2000) Circadian modulation of atrial cycle length in human chronic permanent atrial fibrillation: a noninvasive assessment using long-term surface ECG. *Annals of Noninvasive Electrocardiography*, **5**, 270–278.

Everett, T.H., 4th, Moorman, J.R., Kok, L.C., Akar, J.G., Haines, D.E. (2001) Assessment of global atrial fibrillation organization to optimise timing of atrial defibrillation. *Circulation*, **103**, 2857–2861.

Fujiki, A., Nagasawa, H., Sakabe, M. *et al.* (2001) Spectral characteristics of human atrial fibrillation waves of the right atrial free wall with respect to the duration of atrial fibrillation and effect of class I antiarrhythmic drugs. *Japanese Circulation Journal*, **65**, 1047–1051.

Holm, M., Johansson, R., Brandt, J., Lührs, C. & Olsson, S.B. (1997) Epicardial right atrial free wall mapping in chronic atrial fibrillation. Documentation of repetitive activation with a focal spread – a hitherto unrecognized phenomenon in man. *European Heart Journal*, **18**, 290–310.

Holm, M., Olsson, S.B., Johansson, R. *et al.* (1996) Non-invasive assessment of the atrial cycle length during chronic atrial fibrillation in man. *Circulation*, **94**, 1–69.

Holm, M., Pehrson, S., Ingemansson, M. *et al.* (1998) Non-invasive assessment of the atrial cycle length during atrial fibrillation in man: introducing, validating and illustrating a new ECG method. *Cardiovascular Research*, **38**, 69–81.

Imai, K., Sueda, T., Orihashi, K., Ishii, O. & Matsuura, Y. (2001) Electrophysiological analysis of chronic atrial fibrillation associated with mitral valve disease by using spectral analysis. *Hiroshima Journal of Medical Science*, **50**, 27–35.

Ingemansson, M.P., Holm, M. & Olsson, S.B. (1998) Autonomic modulation of atrial cycle length by the head-up tilt test. Noninvasive evaluation in patients with chronic atrial fibrillation. *Heart*, **80**, 71–76.

Kim, K-B., Rodefeld, M.D., Schuessler, R.B., Cox, J.L. & Boineau, J.P. (1996) Relationship between local atrial fibrillation interval and refractory period in the isolated canine atrium. *Circulation*, **94**, 2961–2967.

Lammers, W.J.E.P., Allessie, M.A., Rensma, P.L. & Schalij, M.J. (1986) The use of fibrillation cycle length to determine spatial dispersion in electrophysiological properties and to characterize the underlying mechanism of fibrillation. *New Trends in Arrhythmias*, **II** (1), 109–112.

Meurling, C. J. (2000) *Atrial fibrillation. Modulation of the atrial fibrillatory frequency. A noninvasive approach*. PhD thesis, Lund University.

Meurling, C.J., Ingemansson, M.P., Roijer, A. *et al.* (1999) Attenuation of electrical remodelling in chronic atrial fibrillation following oral treatment with verapamil. *Europace*, **1**, 234–241.

Meurling, C.J., Waktare, J.E.P, Holmqvist, F. *et al.* (2001) Diurnal fluctuation of the dominant atrial cycle length of chronic atrial fibrillation. *American Journal of Physiology*, **280** (1), 401–406.

Pehrson, S., Holm, M., Meurling, C. *et al.* (1998) Non-invasive assessment of magnitude and dispersion of atrial cycle length during chronic atrial fibrillation in man. *European Heart Journal*, **19**, 1836–1844.

Stridh, M., Sörnmo, L. (2001a) Spatiotemporal QRST cancellation techniques for analysis of atrial fibrillation. *IEEE (Institute of Electrical and Electronic Engineers) Transactions on Biomedical Engineering*, **48**, 105–111.

Stridh, M., Sörnmo, L., Meurling, C.J. & Olsson, S.B. (2001b) Characterization of atrial fibrillation using the surface ECG: time-dependent spectral properties. *IEEE (Institute of Electrical and Electronic Engineers) Transactions on Biomedical Engineering*, **48**, 19–27.

Wijffels, M.C.E.F., Kirchhof, C.J.H.J., Dorland, R. & Allessie, M.A. (1995) Atrial fibrillation begets atrial fibrillation. A study in awake chronically instrumented goats. *Circulation*, **92**, 1954–1968.

CHAPTER 50

Detection of Paroxysmal Atrial Fibrillation Episodes

Rahul Mehra and David Ritscher

Introduction

The prevalence of atrial fibrillation is increasing worldwide and it is estimated that in the United States it will more than double over the next 50 years (Go *et al.* 2001). Atrial fibrillation (AF) significantly reduces the quality of life of these patients and is associated with an increase in mortality and stroke. The goal for management of patients with AF is to improve these clinical outcomes by either maintaining patients in sinus rhythm, i.e. 'rhythm control' or by controlling the ventricular rate during AF, i.e. 'rate control.' Presently, the most common method of rhythm and rate control is the use of drugs, although ablative techniques and implantable devices are increasingly being used. In the presence of AF and clinical risk factors, patients must also be anticoagulated to prevent the risk of stroke. When drugs are used, the efficacy of rhythm and rate control and the need for anticoagulation is typically monitored by evaluating the patient's symptoms and with ECG recordings taken during infrequent clinic visits, external event monitors, and 24-h Holter monitors. These provide limited information and can lead to inadequate management of the arrhythmia. Optimal maintenance of rhythm or rate control is critically dependent on obtaining comprehensive information regarding the patient's episodes of AF and the associated ventricular rhythm.

Several external and implantable systems have been developed which detect atrial tachyarrhythmia (ATachy). The performance requirement of their detection algorithms is dependent on how the information is to be utilized and in which patient population. If the patient has an implantable device to terminate their episodes of ATachy with an automatic defibrillation shock, the detection algorithm needs to have high specificity to avoid delivery of inappropriate shocks and be highly sensitive to detect all episodes of AF. On the other hand, if the implantable device provides diagnostic information for management of rhythm control, rate control and anticoagulant therapy, the performance requirements may be slightly less stringent as the therapy is manually delivered and is based on several pieces of information including this diagnostic information provided by the monitoring system. An external monitoring system would have similar performance requirements. It is also important to distinguish AF from atrial flutter, as their methods of management can be different. Patients with flutter are usually ablated or their arrhythmias pace terminated by delivering rapid pacing through implantable devices. Discrimination between the two is less important for rate control and anticoagulant therapy. Atrial fibrillation and flutter can also coexist in the same patient.

Devices can provide useful diagnostic information to facilitate rhythm and rate control. Rhythm control is defined as maintenance of sinus rhythm (Fuster *et al.* 2001); and ATachy burden (i.e. the per cent of time a patient is in ATachy) is a measure of rhythm control. Two other parameters used to quantify the episodes of ATachy are their frequency and duration. ATachy frequency is measured by detecting the number of episodes over a certain follow-up period. Measurement of frequency and duration require accurate detection of onset as well as termination of the tachyarrhythmia. Typically, the tachyarrhythmias should last about 30 s to be classified as an episode (Fuster *et al.* 2001). The definition of when a tachyarrhythmia terminates is more controversial. For example, should two 48-h episodes separated by one or two sinus beats be classified as two or one episode? The ATachy burden metric is not affected by this definition, and is a more robust measurement. Which rhythm control metric is important from a clinical perspective and is the best surrogate of clinical outcome is not known. Optimal diagnostic information for management of anticoagulation is also not known as yet, although both ATachy burden and episode durations have been proposed.

Optimal rate control during ATachy is defined as a ventricular rate below 60–80 beats/min during rest and 90–115 beats/min during moderate exercise (Fuster *et al.* 2001). To provide this information, ATachy must be appropriately detected and the associated ventricular rate computed. This can be displayed as a histogram of ventricular rates vs. per cent of time spent in ATachy or as daily measurement of ventricular rate (mean, max, etc.) during ATachy over a long period of time.

Figure 50.1 shows ATachy diagnostic information from an AT500 pacemaker (Medtronic Inc.). The daily atrial tachyarrhythmia (AT/AF) burden and frequency over a 7–8 month period is displayed, where each vertical line represents one day's data. The patient can also mark an episode as 'symptomatic' (AT/AF patient check) with an external small unit and the physician can mark the time of drug changes, cardioversion (CV) or ablation. This provides a quick overview of the progression of a patient's disease. To be clinically useful, the data should be accurate and verifiable so that it can be trusted. Detailed episode information can help verify the algorithm performance. Figure 50.2 shows a list of episodes, with detailed information about each (date/time of the episode, atrial cycle length, duration, etc.). For the selected episode, an electrogram (EGM) is shown, along with the atrial (*AA*) and ventricular (*VV*) intervals and detection classification of each beat. Once it has been verified that episodes are being detected appropriately, overview statistics such as burden, frequency and duration metrics can then be used to guide patient treatment.

Automatic detection of ATachy is dependent on two criteria: accurate sensing/classification of an electrical activity as atrial in origin and appropriate classification of a number of such beats as a tachyarrhythmia, based on a unique algorithm. Detection of ATachy varies between various implantable systems and in external systems. Each of these will be discussed separately.

External systems

There are two types of external monitoring systems currently available: external Holter monitoring systems with offline analysis and systems with real time analysis. Almost all of the algorithms use the *RR* interval stream with or without QRS morphology to distinguish AF from sinus rhythm. Those that only use *RR* intervals rely on a high variability of these intervals during AF. Although the proprietary algorithms incorporated in the commercial systems are not known, variability metrics such as Lorentz plots,

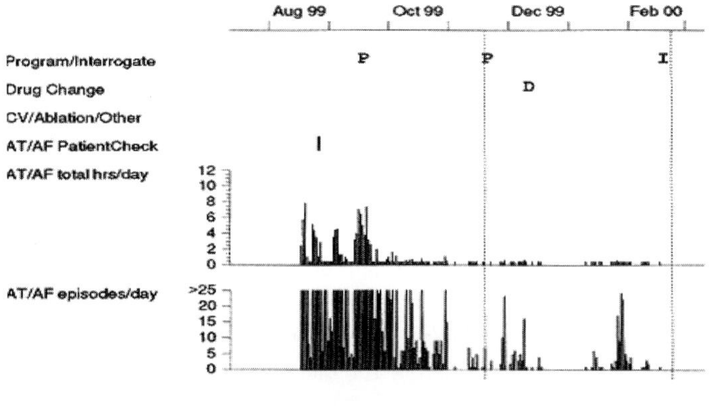

Fig. 50.1 Atrial tachyarrhythmia diagnostic information from an AT500 pacemaker.

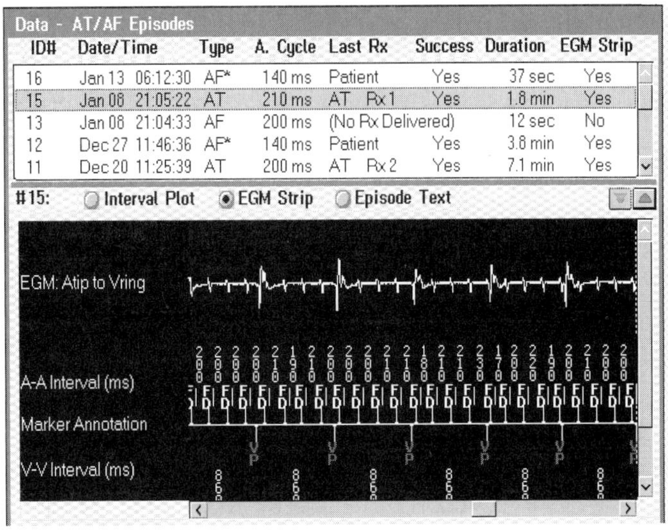

Fig. 50.2 Episode list and selected episode with EGM, Marker Channel, and detection classification.

Markov models, and neural networks have been used for detection of AF (Tateno & Glass 2001). These algorithms have a high sensitivity and specificity for distinguishing sinus rhythm from AF except during high sympathetic activity when the ventricular rate is very high and regular as a result of rapid AV conduction. These algorithms are also likely to provide false negative detections for rapid and regular supraventricular arrhythmias like 2:1 atrial flutter and AV nodal tachycardia (Duverney *et al.* 2002). In order to distinguish AF from these rapid and regular supraventricular tachyarrhythmias, morphological analyses of QRS complexes and neural network systems have been incorporated (Cubanski *et al.* 1994), achieving a sensitivity of 82% and a specificity of 96%.

Some investigators have also subtracted the QRS complexes and analysed the frequency content of the residual signal to detect AF as well as compute its cycle length (Slocum *et al.* 1992; Bollman *et al.* 1999; Holm *et al.* 1998). Suppression of QRST complexes is done by subtracting a time-averaged complex from each beat. A limitation of this technique is that exclusive suppression of the ECG complex is dependent on atrial and ventricular activity being completely unsynchronized (i.e. without 2:1 flutter) and it assumes that the QRST morphology is stable with time. In one study, a sensitivity of 88% and specificity of 68% for detection of AF was achieved (Slocum *et al.* 1992).

There are a few commercial external systems available today for detection of AF e.g. the King of Hearts Express AF Auto-Trigger recorder by Instromedix Inc, Quinton *Q*Track II Holter System and the Telemtry@Home system by Cardiac Telecom. No published information is available regarding their algorithms and performance.

Implantable systems

There are three types of implantable systems that require detection of ATachy: (a) atrial tachyarrhythmia management devices that are capable of delivering appropriate therapies for termination of atrial and ventricular tachyarrhythmias; (b) dual chamber pacemakers that detect ATachy to prevent inappropriate ventricular tracking during high atrial rates i.e. mode switching systems and (c) ventricular defibrillators that withhold inappropriate ventricular therapy if the rhythm is classified as a rapidly conducting atrial tachyarrhythmia. All these systems have significantly different performance requirements. The systems that terminate atrial arrhythmias need the highest sensitivity and specificity of ATachy detection whereas the ventricular defibrillators need to have high sensitivity for VT/VF detection even if the specificity is slightly compromised. Each of these three systems is discussed below.

Atrial tachyarrhythmia management devices that provide atrial therapies

The goal of these devices is to maintain rhythm control by reducing ATachy burden and thereby improve morbidity and mortality associated with the atrial tachyarrhythmia. Currently there are several implantable devices, which give therapies to terminate ATachy (Medtronic GEM® III AT, Jewel™ AF ICDs and AT500 pacemaker, Guidant Ventak® prizm™ AVT ICD, and the Biotronik Tachos DR® ICD). The implantable cardioverter-defibrillators (ICDs) can deliver antitachycardia pacing (ATP) and shocks whereas the AT500 only delivers ATP. With the Jewel AF, antitachycardia pacing has been shown to be effective in terminating about 48% of episodes lasting longer than 1 min (Adler *et al.* 2001). Automatic atrial cardioversion has been shown to be safe and effective (Schoels *et al.* 2001) and a combination of ATP and cardioversion shocks help maintain rhythm control by reducing ATachy burden (Friedman *et al.* 2001).

Detection of atrial tachyarrhythmias

Implantable systems should be able to sense all rapid atrial activity and, when it lasts for a certain number of beats or duration of time, classify it as an atrial tachyarrhythmia. Atrial activity is detected by amplifying and filtering the signal and when it reaches a certain threshold, classifying it as atrial activity. For accurate detection, noise such as far-field QRS signals must be rejected. Far-field signals have frequently been observed in the atrium, especially with widely spaced tip-ring electrodes, and when the lead is placed closer to the ventricle. Also, as the goal is only to treat pathologic ATachy, the algorithms should reject 1:1 rhythms such as sinus tachycardia.

Different implantable devices use different techniques to classify a string of sensed atrial signals as an 'atrial tachyarrhythmia.' The Medtronic devices (Jewel AF, Gem III AT and AT500) use an 'evidence counter' which increments or decrements at each *RR* interval. In order to reject sustained 1:1 rhythms, it increments if there are two or more atrial detections per *RR* interval and when the signal is not due to far-field, and decrements with 1:1 rhythms. The algorithm classifies the signal as a far-field if there is a short–long interval pattern of atrial activations. When the evidence counter reaches 32, and the atrial rate is faster than the programmable rate criteria, an ATachy is declared. A sensitivity of 100% and positive predictive value of 95% was observed with this algorithm in 293 patients (Schoels *et al.* 2001).

The Guidant Ventak Prizm AVT uses an 'X of Y' counter to remove noise in the detection process. The rhythm is classified as an ATachy when 32 out of 40 atrial intervals are within the programmed detection zone and if the mean atrial rate is ≥20 bpm faster than the mean ventricular rate. Requiring a higher atrial rate ensures that the detected rhythm is not 1:1 e.g. a sinus tachycardia. Up to 7 of 40 intervals can be incorrectly identified as fast atrial intervals without causing inappropriate detection even when they are far-field R-waves. The counter is based primarily on rate, followed by a confirmation of rhythm i.e > 1:1 AV relationship. The approach is similar in the Biotronik Tachos DR which uses an 'AT sample count' counter to track the number of averaged atrial intervals that fall within the ATachy rate zones. The 'Early far-field tolerance' algorithm is designed to reject far-field signals. Published performance data for these algorithms is not available to date.

Classification of atrial tachyarrhythmias

Apart from accurate detection of all ATachy, these systems need to be able to classify a rhythm as AT or AF so that different techniques can be used for their termination. Slow and/or regular atrial tachycardias (AT) are more likely to be terminated with atrial ATP whereas AF typically requires more aggressive therapies such as cardioversion. Atrial flutter is usually very regular and is therefore classified as an AT. The devices allow programming of different set of therapies for AT and AF.

Figure 50.3 shows the approach used for clas-

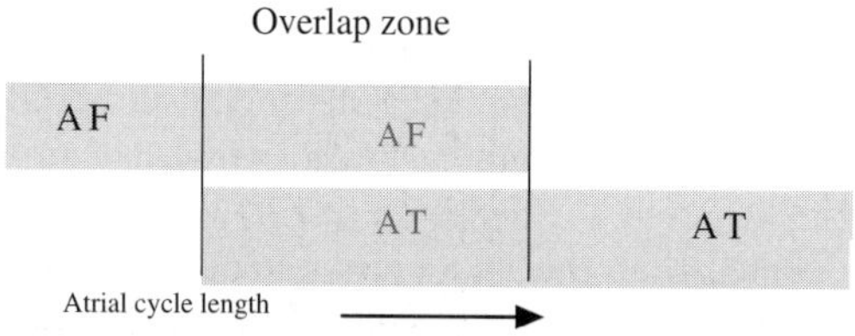

Fig. 50.3 Atrial tachyarrhythmia and atrial fibrillation detection zones.

sification of AF and AT in the Jewel AF, Gem III AT, and AT500 devices. If the atrial rhythm is fast, it is defined as AF; if it is slow, it is defined as AT. If the rate is in between in the 'overlap zone,' an additional criterion of regularity is used to classify it as AF or AT. A 'regular' rhythm is called AT and irregular rhythm as AF. It is important to note that the device-based classification of AF and AT may not reflect an electrocardiographic classification of AF and tachycardia as all detection is done from a single recording site in the right atrium. One of the surprises of the clinical trials with the Jewel AF has been that about 63% of the ATachy that lasted more than 1 min were AT (Adler *et al.* 2001).

The Ventak® Prizm™ AVT also uses two zones; for the AF zone, a rate and regularity classifier is used to differentiate between AF and AT therapy delivery.

The Biotronik Tachos DR has three rather than two zones: AF, AT-1 (lower-rate AT), and AT-2 (higher rate AT) and different therapies can be programmed for each zone. An important goal for devices that provide ATP is the ability to differentiate rhythms that can be effectively treated with ATP from those that cannot be treated. Most of the current algorithms are limited in their ability to distinguish this. In the future, morphological analysis may provide better discrimination. Since most of the algorithms use fixed rate zone definitions as the basis for the detection decision, rhythms that lie near the boundary can cross back and forth, resulting in unnecessary detections or terminations and creating problems with therapy delivery and diagnostics. Algorithms need to be refined to avoid such issues in the future.

Episode termination

It is important that an arrhythmia be appropriately classified as 'terminated' or undesirable therapies may be delivered. An episode falsely called 'terminated' will usually be redetected quickly resulting in additional therapy deliver for this 'new episode.' These therapies would not have been delivered had it been correctly identified as one episode. Appropriate classification of 'termination' also impacts device declaration of therapy success and the diagnostic information by increasing reported episode frequency and decreasing reported episode durations. Robustness of the termination rule is, therefore, very important. Different rules are used in the different devices to declare the end of an AT/AF episode.

The Medtronic Gem III AT, Jewel AF and the AT 500 use a rhythm-based approach, requiring either 5 sinus rhythm beats (1:1 beats with antegrade conduction) or for the evidence counter to decrement below a threshold. The Ventak Prizm AVT uses the same criteria for termination as for detection (less than 32 of 40 atrial intervals within the programmed rate and atrial rate not faster than ventricular rate by 20 bpm). The Biotronik Tachos DR uses a rate-based termination approach as with detection. Termination is declared when a programmed number of beats are within the sinus rate zone.

Dual chamber pacemakers with mode switching

Automatic mode switching algorithms are an important feature in dual chamber pacemakers and ICDs. Without this feature, an ATachy would result in fast ventricular pacing, since the device would attempt to track the rapid atrial rate in pacing the ventricle. To prevent rapid ventricular pacing, the sensitivity of 'mode switch' algorithms to detect even brief-duration ATachy must be very high. Upon detection of an atrial tachyarrhythmia, the Automatic Mode Switch (AMS) algorithm initiates a non-tracking pacing mode and when the arrhythmia terminates, the previous mode resumes. To avoid an abrupt rate change, the pacing algorithm typically transitions gradually.

Although there are several types of algorithms, they generally fall into two categories. One counts the number of atrial sensed events below a programmed interval and when this reaches a threshold, mode switch occurs. This type of algorithm responds quickly to atrial arrhythmia but may produce more intermittent tracking during AF or flutter if there is significant undersensing of atrial activations. The second type of algorithm computes a mean inter-atrial interval which is decremented or incremented by different values when the inter-atrial interval is more than or less than a programmed tachycardia detection interval. For example, the mean atrial interval may be decremented by 24 ms if the inter-atrial interval is less than tachycardia detection interval and incremented by 8 ms if it is longer. This helps maintain mode switching during periods of atrial undersensing. Such algorithms may be slower to activate and inactivate but provide less variation in ventricular pacing during AF. Typically, patients prefer algorithms that mode switch rapidly, i.e. in less than 5 rapid atrial beats. A major performance limitation of many mode switching algorithms systems is due to undersensing of ATachy as a result of the blanking periods. Many devices have atrial blanking throughout the AV delay and post ventricular atrial blanking (PVAB), allowing for no sensing throughout this long period. This can result in failure to mode switch or in intermittent mode switching. Although several partial solutions have been used to alleviate this problem, the most desirable is to eliminate blanking periods or reduce them to extremely short durations. This has been achieved in several implantable devices e.g. the AT500.

In addition to its therapeutic use, mode switch is also used to provide atrial diagnostic information. Mode switch frequency and duration are used for management of atrial arrhythmias (Lau *et al.* 2002a,b). Both underdetection of rapid atrial activations, as well as repeated redetection of the same episode can lower the reliability of the mode switch frequency counter and duration as an accurate measurement of AF/flutter. The ATachy burden can be inaccurate if there are long blanking periods. Therefore, there is need in such devices to be able to display stored electrograms to verify the detected mode switch episodes. It is important to note that since no automatic atrial therapy is delivered, the accuracy of the diagnostic information has been typically low. In the future, it is important to improve the accuracy of this information so that physicians can trust the device diagnostics for appropriate patient management.

Ventricular ICDs with VT/SVT discrimination

In all ICDs, detection and treatment of malignant ventricular tachyarrhythmias must take precedence over ATachy. Therefore, these devices need to be highly sensitive to detection of ventricular arrhythmias and reject supraventricular tachyarrhythmias (SVT) that do not need to be treated in the ventricle. Clearly, an SVT such as sinus tachycardia would not respond to ventricular therapies. When a high ventricular rate is observed, the algorithm first needs to determine whether it is a VT/VF or SVT. If there is a 1:1 association between the atrial and ventricular events, the discrimination between SVT and ventricular tachycardia is based on the timing between the atrial and ventricular events. Different devices use dual chamber data and various algorithms to differentiate VT from SVT (Mangrum *et al.* 2001). Only if a ventricular tachyarrhythmia is not detected, the device evaluates the presence of an ATachy using the methods discussed previously.

Conclusions

Detection of ATachy through implantable systems is presently used to deliver atrial therapies, obtain accurate diagnostic information, initiate a mode switch and reduce the incidence of inappropriate ventricular therapies during rapid ventricular rates. Although the requirements are slightly different for each of these functions, the performance of algorithms for detection of ATachy is the highest in dual chamber systems that deliver automatic atrial therapies. If important clinical decisions regarding rhythm, rate control, or anticoagulation are going to be made based on the diagnostic information provided by these devices, these advanced algorithms will need to be replicated in all implantable systems and further improved in the future. One factor that significantly compromises detection in many other implantable systems is the presence of long blanking periods. These need to be minimized significantly.

The accuracy of detection in external monitoring systems has not been evaluated extensively and is probably lower as it only relies on ventricular sensing in most systems. This will also need to be improved significantly if it is to be used for effective patient management.

References

Adler, S.W., 2nd, Wolpert, C., Warman, E.N. *et al.* (2001) Efficacy of pacing therapies for treating atrial tachyarrhythmias in patients with ventricular arrhythmias receiving a dual-chamber implantable cardioverter defibrillator. *Circulation*, **104**, 887–892.

Bollman, A., Sonne, K., Esperer, H.D. *et al.* (1999) Noninvasive assessment of fibrillatory activity in patients with paroxysmal and persistent atrial fibrillation using the Holter ECG. *Cardiovascular Research*, **44**, 60–66.

Cubanski, D., Cyganski, D., Antman, E.M. *et al.* (1994) A neural network system for detection of atrial fibrillation in ambulatory electrocardiograms. *Journal of Cardiovascular Electrophysiology*, **5**, 602–608.

Duverney, D., Gaspoz, J.M., Pichot, V. *et al.* (2002) High accuracy of automatic detection of atrial fibrillation using wavelet transform of heart rate interval. *PACE (Pacing and Clinical Electrophysiology)*, **25**, 457–462.

Friedman, P.A., Dijkman, B., Warman, E. *et al.* (2001) Atrial therapies reduce atrial arrhythmia burden in defibrillator patients. *Circulation*, **104**, 1023–1028.

Fuster, F.V., Ryden, L.E., Asinger, R.W. *et al.* (2001) ACC/AHA/ESC guidelines for management of patients with atrial fibrillation: a report of the ACC/AHA task force on practice guidelines and the ESC committee for practice guidelines and policy conferences. *Journal of the American College of Cardiology*, **38**, 1231–1266

Go, A.S., Hylek, E.M., Phillips, K.A. *et al.* (2001) Prevalence of diagnosed atrial fibrillation in adults: national implications for rhythm management and stroke prevention: the anticoagulation and risk factors in atrial fibrillation (ATRIA) Study. *JAMA (Journal of the American Medical Association)*, **285**, 2370–2375.

Holm, M., Pehrson, S., Ingemansson, M. *et al.* (1998) Non-invasive assessment of the atrial cycle length during atrial fibrillation in man: introducing, validating and illustrating a new ECG method. *Cardiovascular Research*, **38**, 69–81.

Lau, C.P., Leung, S.K., Tse, H.F. *et al.* (2002) Automatic mode switching of implantable pacemakers: I. Principles of instrumentation, clinical and hemodynamic considerations. *PACE (Pacing and Clinical Electrophysiology)*, **25**, 967–983.

Lau, C.P., Leung, S.K., Tse, H.F. *et al.* (2002) Automatic mode switching of implantable pacemakers: II. Clinical performance of current algorithms and their programming. *PACE (Pacing and Clinical Electrophysiology)*, **25**, 1094–1113.

Mangrum, J.M., Mounsey, J.P., DiMarco, J.P. (2001) Management of frequent or refractory supraventricular tachyarrhythmias in the dual chamber era. *Cardiac Electrophysiology Review*, **5**, 80–84.

Schoels, W., Swerdlow, C.D., Jung, W. *et al.* for the worldwide Jewel AF Investigators (2001) Worldwide clinical experience with a new dual-chamber implantable cardioverter defibrillator system. *Journal of Cardiovascular Electrophysiology*, **12**, 521–528.

Slocum J, Sahakian A, Swiryn S. (1992) Diagnosis of atrial fibrillation from surface electrocardiogram based on computer detected atrial activity. *Journal of Electrocardiography*, **25**, 568–576.

Tateno K, Glass L. (2001) Automatic detection of atrial fibrillation using the coefficient of variation and density histograms of RR and delta RR intervals. *Medical & Biological Engineering & Computing*, **39**, 664–671.

CHAPTER 51

Circadian Pattern of AF Paroxysms

Antonio Michelucci, Paolo Pieragnoli, Andrea Colella, Gianfranco Gensini and Luigi Padeletti

Atrial fibrillation (AF) is the most common arrhythmia in the general population. Epidemiological data demonstrate that AF is, in considerable measure, a disease of aging (Kannel *et al.* 1982; Feinberg *et al.* 1995; Khran *et al.* 1995), that about half the people in the United States with AF are >75 years old (Feinberg *et al.* 1995) and that there are very few instances (<5%) of so-called lone AF in the elderly (Furberg *et al.* 1994). Data also indicate that about 10% people in their 80s has AF, and about 1/3 patients in their 80s who present with a stroke also has AF, which further emphasizes the enormity of the public health problem associated with AF (Kannel *et al.* 1982; Wolf *et al.* 1991; Feinberg *et al.* 1995; Khran *et al.* 1995).

AF has been defined paroxysmal when it terminates spontaneously after a certain period of time. The classic AF paroxysmal form should be self-terminating in less than 48 h, otherwise is commonly termed persistent (Brugada 2002). A complementary system to classify paroxysmal AF considers its clinical aspects and includes the number of episodes and severity of symptoms (Levy *et al.* 1995). This classification underscores the existence of asymptomatic episodes which are known to be relatively more frequent than symptomatic ones (Savelieva & Camm 2000). The definition of paroxysmal AF must also be based on the cause since different aetiologies can result in different mechanisms of arrhythmia (Brugada 2002). There are therefore various clinical presentations and underlying mechanisms of paroxysmal AF and thus probably different relationships between triggers of arrhythmia and anatomical substrate. In fact, origin of extrasystoles (e.g. focal in the pulmonary veins), behaviour of the autonomic nervous system (age, existence of cardiopathy with or without heart failure) and abnormalities in the atria (enlargement, inflammation, hypertrophy, elevated pressure) can all manifest themselves in different ways. In summary, the occurrence of paroxysmal AF may depend not only on arrhythmic factors intrinsic to the atrium but also on extrinsic rhythmic factors including neurohumoral and hemodynamic factors. Even lifestyle can contribute to the appearance of the arrhythmia. Thus it can be reasonably affirmed that the number of episodes and the time of appearance of the arrhythmia during the day can vary according to underlying pathophysiological conditions and to environmental conditions.

All these aspects should be considered when attempting to describe circadian patterns of paroxysmal AF. Thus circadian variation probably represents a 'population rhythm', which is composed of many 'subpopulation rhythms'. The evaluation of circadian pattern of paroxysmal AF is difficult as atrial fibrillation events are random and frequently occur in clusters. Very few patients with sustained tachyarrhythmias have episodes daily and some patients may have weeks without an episode that are then followed by a cluster of events (Rose *et al.* 1999; Kaemmerer *et al.* 2001).

Clinical results

The study of circadian patterns of paroxysmal AF using only symptomatic episodes has produced contrasting results. Although some authors did not observe a circadian pattern (Clair *et al.* 1993; Rostagno *et al.* 1993), others have observed a double peak, one peak occurring in the morning and another late in the evening (Kupari *et al.* 1990; Viskin *et al.* 1999). The absence of evaluation of asymptomatic episodes could explain the different results. By contrast, other authors used Holter recordings, rather than presentation with symptoms, to assess the behaviour of paroxysmal AF. Yamashita *et al.* (1997) in a first report did not observe a circadian pattern for the onset of the arrhythmia, although they reported a nadir at 11.00 hours both for total duration and termination of the arrhythmia. In a second report (Yamashita *et al.* 1998), the same authors indicated the existence of a remarkable age dependence. The most obvious age dependence was observed in the circadian variation of onset of AF. In the younger group, there were triple peaks, with the highest one at night, whereas the older group exhibited a single peak in the daytime. By contrast, the probabilities of maintenance and termination showed similar circadian patterns between the groups, although their amplitudes were significantly reduced in the older group. On this basis, the authors suggested a prevalent vagal arrhythmogenic mechanism in the younger patients and a role of sympathetic tone in the older patients. It should be noted that in their reports these authors evaluated the number of patients with AF and not the number of arrhythmia episodes, thus not permitting a comparison with previously published results. Similar results regarding the influence of age on the maintenance of atrial fibrillation have been reported by Hnatkova *et al.* (1998).

The advent of pulse generators with enhanced data storage features in association with sensitive and reliable arrhythmia detection features has provided the opportunity to evaluate the natural history of AF in pacemaker patients. The use of a pulse generator as an implantable event recorder is a valuable tool for this study because many patients may not experience symptoms during AF (J. Gillis 2002). Furthermore, the ability to retrieve information on the duration of AF provides valuable information about the total AF burden over time. Only recently, data-logging capabilities of atrial pacemakers provided an insight into the patterns of atrial arrhythmias over extended periods (A. M. Gillis *et al.* 1999; Kaemmerer *et al.* 2001). The large quantities of information available from these devices allow for a more thorough evaluation of temporal patterns of atrial arrhythmias than was previously possible. Thus more appropriate and accurate conclusions can be derived from analysing the study of A. M. Gillis *et al.* (2001), who used pacemakers with diagnostic features that permit the detection and storage of information about the date, time of onset, and duration of multiple, sequential episodes of atrial tachyarrhythmias. These data confirmed the presence of a circadian variation of AF with a distinct bimodal distribution. AF initiation peaks in the night-time during sleep and also in the late afternoon and early evening. Note, however, that in this study the bimodal distribution of AF initiation was observed in patients with atrial rate-adaptive pacing and not in the no-pacing group. Atrial pacing is associated with an evening peak in initiation of AF, whereas this phenomenon was not so marked in the no-pacing group. Although vagal tone may have contributed to the initiation of AF at night, this pattern was not altered by atrial pacing at a lower rate of 70 beats/min, which was selected to eliminate relative bradycardia as a trigger for AF. Thus the authors suggested that if vagal modulation contributes to the electrophysiological substrate for AF, this mechanism is at least partially independent of significant bradycardia. Beta-adrenergic blocking agents, including amiodarone, eliminated the circadian variation of AF. It seems that beta-adrenergic blocking agents were able to reduce the number of AF episodes thus allowing therapeutic intervention. The circadian variation of AF also seems to be related to duration of the arrhythmia because longer episodes tended not to have a marked evening peak in initiation. The disease burden (i.e. the frequency and duration of AF as well as the presence or absence of structural heart disease) might have also influenced the time course of AF termination and recurrence.

Recent research by Frost *et al.* (2002) sheds additional light on the temporal pattern of atrial fibrillation and its seasonal variation. Their results showed a winter peak and a summer trough in the incidence of atrial fibrillation. The relative incidence of atrial fibrillation during winter compared with summer, estimated as the ratio of the incidence in the month of the peak relative to the incidence in the month of the trough, was small (relative risk 1.20; 95% CI 1.12–1.29). Stratification by sex, age, and the presence or absence of diabetes and underlying cardiovascular diseases did not affect the seasonal pattern. An inverse relation between mean outdoor temperature and incidence of atrial fibrillation was also reported.

Circadian pattern of the contributing factors

A relationship between autonomic tone and the onset and duration of paroxysmal AF has been described (Sopher *et al.* 1998; Zimmermann & Kalusche 2001). Moreover it has been reported that the occurrence of sustained atrial arrhythmias in patients who have frequent ectopy related to an arrhythmogenic focus in the pulmonary veins is highly dependent on variations in autonomic tone (Tai 2001; Zimmermann & Kalusche 2001). These results show that the knowledge of the circadian behaviour of autonomic tone is important when attempting to evaluate circadian patterns of paroxysmal AF. The behaviour of the autonomic nervous system has been analysed by using heart rate variability, which should be considered as a measure of vagal or sympathetic modulation, not as a marker of basic autonomic tone (Malik & Camm 1993). In fact, *RR* interval variation is determined by a complex interplay among autonomic modulation, central influences, and humoral regulation. Heart rate variability has a diurnal rhythm (Lombardi *et al.* 1992; Yamasaki *et al.* 1996) that can reflect the sympathetic–parasympathetic autonomic balance (Massin *et al.* 2000). In general, indices of heart rate variability decrease significantly during the daytime and increase during the night-time (Lombardi *et al.* 1992; Yamasaki *et al.* 1996; Massin *et al.* 2000). The ratio of LF to HF (the ratio of spectral power in the low frequency band to the spectral power in the high frequency band), which is believed to reflect the sympatho-vagal balance, has an inverse rhythm, with a higher level during the daytime and a lower value during the night-time. The origin of circadian variation of heart rate variability seems more likely to be sympathetic withdrawal rather than a parasympathetic effect because the amplitude of the cycle was maintained in the presence of vagal neuropathy (Malpas & Purdie 1990; Massin *et al.* 2000). Note that the circadian rhythm of catecholamines has been described with a trough at 04.00 hours (Barnes *et al.* 1980). Circadian rhythm of heart rate variability is affected by age and gender. A decrease with age of heart rate variability has been reported (Yeregani *et al.* 1997). In a study published by Yamasaki *et al.* (1996), the low-frequency component of heart rate variability showed high values during 08.00–12.00 hours in male subjects and during 1200–2400 hours in female subjects. Even some pathophysiological conditions can condition and/or change circadian pattern of heart rate variability. Lombardi *et al.* (1992) investigated a group of patients with a myocardial infarction, and found that, compared to healthy subjects, the circadian rhythm of heart rate variability indices of myocardial infarction patients were significantly different, with lower median values and amplitude, and with earlier or later peaks. Korpelainen *et al.* (1997) reported that, in patients with acute stroke, circadian rhythm of heart rate variability indices were reversibly abolished, even though a circadian rhythm of stroke onset among patients with AF, with a significantly higher number of strokes occurring between 06.00 and 18.00 hours had been reported (Lip *et al.* 2001). Finally circadian rhythmicity of heart rate variability was present preoperatively only in patients remaining in sinus rhythm after coronary artery bypass surgery (Jideus *et al.* 2001).

A circadian pattern for sinus node function and for atrial refractoriness and an interrelationship between them and autonomic tone has also been described. It has been found that sinus node function changes follow the circadian rhythm of autonomic nervous system (Mitsuoka *et al.* 1990). Sinus node recovery time, the main index of sinus node function, follows a circadian rhythm with a peak between 24.00 and 07.00 hours. Coefficients of variation of sinus node recovery time over 24-h may be as high as 10% (Cinca *et al.* 1986; Mitsuoka *et al.* 1990). Between 24:00 and 08:00, a significant lengthening of the sinus node rate and of sinus recovery time was also found (Cinca *et al.* 1986). Moreover a significant prolongation of atrial effective refractory period (between 23:00 and 08:00 hours) has been reported (Cinca *et al.*

1986, 1990). Coefficients of variation were 3–8% over 24 h. Finally, even P wave duration and its area showed a circadian behaviour (Dilaveris *et al.* 2001).

Methodological aspects

Actual data indicate that the underlying mechanism for circadian rhythm in the cardiovascular system is not yet completely clear. Although most studies confirmed the existence of these circadian variations, it has not been determined whether these changes are associated with the 'clock' itself. Most authors believe that circadian phenomena are primarily linked to the time schedule of life, but not to the clock *per se*. Thus, it is reasonable to believe that circadian rhythms of noninvasive electrophysiological indices may be also linked to wake time or activity levels. Consistent with this hypothesis, it has been shown that there are a series of changes in the body soon after waking and commencing activity that may include a surge in heart rate, blood pressure, plasma catecholamine levels and renin activity (Mulchahy & Quyyumi 1996).

Clinical implications

Clinically, we should consider the circadian properties of some cardiac electrophysiological measurements when we try to decide whether or not a result is normal and/or whether it has been changed by an intervention. For example, we often monitor *QT* and *QT*c intervals in patients treated with amiodarone to detect the prolongation of this index. In these cases, it would not be reliable to compare measurements taken at 0.007 and 17.00 hours, as even in normal subjects the *QT* values can differ by 30% at different times of the day (Romano *et al.* 1988). Also, it would be not valid to compare a measurement of short-term heart rate variability taken at 10:00 hours one day with another taken at 17:00 hours on another day. Similarly, the same patient could theoretically be inducible in the early morning and not inducible in an electrophysiological study performed in the late afternoon. In a high-risk population, a negative electrophysiological test might not demonstrate that this patient is at low risk if the test is performed during a relative 'safe' period of the day. It has become clear that we must consider 'time' as an important factor when we treat patients. For example, antiarrhythmic medication should cover the early morning hours when there is a higher prevalence of arrhythmic events and sudden cardiac death. Also, it is important to conduct prospective studies of circadian rhythm in electrophysiology to determine which results may be affected by the 'clock.' Until that time, we must keep in mind that 'everything is changing all the time,' and try to make test–retest results as comparable as possible by obtaining them at the same time of day.

Final remarks

Currently no definitive conclusions have been reported about the circadian behaviour of AF paroxysms. To better assess this problem, it is important to standardize and refine analytical methods. The mathematical technique of Halberg and coworkers (1973), for example, seems particularly useful for illustrating the characteristics of circadian rhythms and for making comparisons between patient groups. Moreover it is necessary to accumulate experience in different pathophysiological conditions. Analyses should not be performed, as has often been the case in the past, on cumulative data obtained from different cardiac diseases that probably have different effects on the autonomic nervous system. In the future, the data-logging capability of pacemakers could probably not only permit better characterization of the different pathophysiological conditions, but also increase our understanding of how therapy (drugs, ablation, pacing) can influence the predisposing factors of AF.

References

Barnes, P., Fitzgerald, G., Brown, M. & Dollery, C. (1980) Nocturnal asthma and changes in circulating epinephrine, histamine, and cortisol. *New England Journal of Medicine*, **303**, 263–267.

Brugada, J. (2002) Relevance of atrial fibrillation classification in clinical practice. *Journal of Cardiovascular Electrophysiology*, **13**, S27–S30.

Cinca, J., Moya, A., Bardaji, A., Rius, J. & Soler-Soler, J. (1990) Circadian variations of electrical properties of the heart. *Annals of the New York Academy of Sciences*, **601** (1), 222–233.

Cinca, J., Moya, A., Figueras, J., Roma, F. & Rius, J. (1986) Circadian variations in the electrical properties of the human heart assessed by sequential bedside electrophysiological testing. *American Heart Journal*, **112**, 315–321.

Clair, W.K., Wilkinson, W.E., McCarthy, E.A., Page, R.L. & Pritchett, E.L.C. (1993) Spontaneous occurrence of symptomatic paroxysmal atrial fibrillation and paroxysmal supraventricular tachycardia in untreated patients. *Circulation*, **87**, 1114–1122.

Dilaveris, P.E., Färbom, P., Batchvarov, V., Ghuran, A. & Malik, M. (2001) Circadian behaviour of P-wave duration, P-wave area, and PR interval in healthy subjects. *Annals of Noninvasive Electrocardiology*, **6** (2), 92–97.

Feinberg, W.M., Blackshear, J.L., Laupacis, A., Kronmal, R. & Hart, R.G. (1995) Prevalence, age distribution, and gender of patients with atrial fibrillation. Analysis and implications. *Archives of Internal Medicine*, **155**, 459–473.

Frost, L., Johnsen, S.P., Pedersen, L. *et al.* (2002) Seasonal variation in hospital discharge diagnosis of atrial fibrillation: a population-based study. *Epidemiology*, **13** (2), 211–215.

Furberg, C.D., Psaty, B.M., Manolio, T.A., Gardin, J.M., Smith, V.E. & Rautaharju, P.M. (1994) Prevalence of atrial fibrillation in elderly subjects (The Cardiovascular Health Study). *American Journal of Cardiology*, **74**, 236–241.

Gillis, A.M., Connolly, S.J., Dubuc, M. *et al.* (2001) Circadian variation of paroxysmal atrial fibrillation. *American Journal of Cardiology*, **87**, 794–798.

Gillis, A.M., Wyse, D.G., Connolly, S.T. *et al.* (1999) Atrial pacing periablation for prevention of paroxysmal atrial fibrillation. *Circulation*, **99**, 2553–2558.

Gillis, J. (2002) Modeling temporal patterns of atrial tachyarrhythmias: A new surrogate outcome measure for clinical stusdies? *Journal of Cardiovascular Electrophysiology*, **13**, 310–311.

Halberg, F., Johnson, E.A., Nelson, W., Runge, W. & Sothern, R. (1973) Autorhythmometry procedures for physiological self-measurements and their analysis. *Physiology Teacher*, **1**, 1–11.

Hnatkova, K., Waktare, J.E., Murgatroyd, F.D., Guo, X., Camm, A.J. & Malik, M. (1998) Age and gender influences on the rate and duration of paroxysmal atrial fibrillation. *Pacing and Clinical Electrophysiology*, **21**, 2455–2458.

Jideus, L., Ericson, M., Stridsberg, M., Nilsson, L., Blomstrom, P. & Blomstrom-Lundqvist, C. (2001) Diminished circadian variation in heart rate variability before surgery in patients developing postoperative atrial fibrillation. *Scandinavian Cardiovascular Journal*, **35** (4), 238–244.

Kaemmerer, W.F., Rose, S. & Mehra, R. (2001) Distribution of patients' paroxysmal atrial tachyarrhythmias episodes: implications for detection of treatment efficacy. *Journal of Cardiovascular Electrophysiology*, **12**, 121–130.

Kannel, W.B., Abbott, R.D., Savage, D.D. & McNamara, P.M. (1982) Epidemiologic features of chronic atrial fibrillation: The Framingham Study. *New England Journal of Medicine*, **306**, 1018–1022.

Korpelainen, J.T., Sotaniemi, K.A., Huiluri, H.V. & Myllyla, V.V. (1997) Circadian rhythm of heart rate variability is reversibly abolished in ischaemic stroke. *Stroke*, **28**, 2150–2154.

Krahn, A.D., Manfreda, J., Tate, R.B., Mathewson, F.A. & Cuddy, T.E. (1995) The natural history of atrial fibrillation: incidence, risk factors, and prognosis in the Manitoba Follow-up Study. *American Journal of Medicine*, **98**, 476–484.

Kupari, M., Koskinen, P. & Lenonen, H. (1990) Double-peaking circadian variation in the occurrence of sustained supraventricular tachyarrhythmias. *American Heart Journal*, **120**, 1364–1369.

Levy, S., Novella, P., Ricard, P. & Paganelli, F. (1995) Paroxysmal atrial fibrillation: a need for classification. *Journal Cardiovascular Electrophysiology* **6**, 69–74.

Lip, G.Y.H., Lau, C.K.Y. & Kamath, S. (2001) Diurnal variation in stroke onset in atrial fibrillation. *Stroke*, **32** (6), 1443–1448.

Lombardi, F., Sandrone, G. & Mortara A, (1992) Circadian variation of spectral indices of heart rate variability after myocardial infarction. *American Heart Journal*, **123**, 1521–1529.

Malik, M. & Camm, A.J. (1993) Components of heart rate variability: What they really mean and what we really measure. *American Journal of Cardiology*, **72**, 821–822.

Malpas, S.C. & Purdie, G.L. (1990) Circadian variation of heart rate variability. *Cardiovascular Research*, **24**, 210–213.

Massin, M.M, Maeyns, K., Withofs, N., Ravet, F. & Gerard, P. (2000) Circadian rhythm of heart rate and heart rate variability. *Archives of Disease in Childhood*, **83**, 179–182.

Mitsuoka, T., Ueyama, C., Matsumoto, Y. & Hashiba, K. (1990) Influences of autonomic changes on the sinus node recovery time in patients with sick sinus syndrome. *Japanese Heart Journal*, **31**, 645–660.

Mulchahy, D.A. & Quyyumi, A.A. (1996) Clinical implications of circadian rhythms detected by ambulatory monitoring techniques. In:, *Noninvasive electrocardiology – clinical aspects of Holter monitoring* (eds A. J. Moss, & S. Stern), pp. 493–508. W. B. Saunders, London.

Romano, M., Clarizia, M., Onofrio, E. *et al.* (1988) Heart rate, PR, and *Q–T* intervals in normal children: a 24-h Holter monitoring study. *Clinical Cardiology*, **11**, 839–842.

Rose, M.S., Gillis, A.M. & Sheldon, R.S. (1999) Evaluation of the bias in using the time to the first event when the inter-event intervals have a Weibull distribution. *Statistics in Medicine*, **18**, 139–154.

Rostagno, C., Taddei, T., Paladini, B., Modesti, P.A., Utari, P. & Bertini, G. (1993) The onset of symptomatic atrial fibrillation and paroxysmal supraventricular tachycardia is characterized by different circadian rhythms. *American Journal of Cardiology*, **71**, 453–455.

Savelieva, I. & Camm, A.J. (2000) Clinical relevance of silent atrial fibrillation: prevalence, prognosis, quality of life, and management. *Journal of Interventional Cardiac Electrophysiology*, **4**, 369–382.

Sopher, S.M., Hnatkova, K., Waktare, J.E.P., Murgatroyd, F.D., Camm, A.J. & Malik, M. (1998) Circadian variation in atrial fibrillation in patients with frequent paroxysms. *PACE (Pacing and Clinical Electrophysiology)*, **21** (Pt II), 2445–2449.

Tai, C.-T. (2001) Role of autonomic influences in the initiation and perpetuation of focal atrial fibrillation. *Journal of Cardiovascular Electrophysiology*, **12** (3), 292–293.

Viskin, S., Golovner, M., Malov, N. *et al.* (1999) Circadian variation of symptomatic paroxysmal atrial fibrillation. Data from almost 10,000 episodes. *European Heart Journal*, **20**, 1429–1434.

Wolf, P.A., Abbott, R.D. & Kannel, W.B. (1991) Atrial fibrillation as an independent risk factor for stroke: the Framingham Study. *Stroke*, **22**, 983–988.

Yamasaki, Y., Kodama, M. & Matsuhisa, M. (1996) Diurnal heart rate variability in healthy subjects: effects of aging and sex difference. *American Journal of Physiology*, **271**, H303–H310.

Yamashita, T., Murakawa, Y., Hayami, N. *et al.* (1998) Relation between aging and circadian variation of paroxysmal atrial fibrillation. *American Journal of Cardiology*, **82**, 1364–1367.

Yamashita, T., Murakawa, Y., Sezaki, K. *et al.* (1997) Circadian variation of paroxysmal atrial fibrillation. *Circulation*, **96**, 1537–1541.

Yeregani, V.K., Sobolewski, E., Kai, J., Janpala, V.C. & Igel, G. (1997) Effect of age on long-term heart rate variability. *Cardiovascular Research*, **35** (1), 35–42.

Zimmermann, M. & Kalusche, D. (2001) Fluctuation in autonomic tone is a major determinant of sustained atrial arrhythmias in patients with focal ectopy originating from the pulmonary veins. *Journal of Cardiovascular Electrophysiology*, **12** (3), 285–291.

CHAPTER 52

Monitoring After Cardioversion of Atrial Fibrillation

Samuel Lévy

Introduction

Atrial fibrillation (AF) is a common clinical problem, and its incidence increases with age and with the presence of organic heart disease. Epidemiological studies have shown an incidence of 3–5% in subjects over 65 years of age (Kannel *et al.* 1982; Cairns & Connolly, 1991) and this incidence will increase as the population is ageing. Atrial fibrillation may be associated with hemodynamic impairment, symptoms occasionally disabling and a decrease in life expectancy. The most important concern with AF relates to the risk of frightening embolic complications which in three-quarters of cases are represented by cerebrovascular accidents (Petersen & Godtfredsen, 1986; Cabin *et al.* 1990). Atrial fibrillation may occur in the presence or absence of detectable heart disease and in the presence or absence of related symptoms.

Recently, a classification system was reported in the ACC/AHA/ESC Guidelines (Fuster *et al.* 2001) based on the clinical presentation of the arrhythmia. They distinguished three clinical subsets of AF (first detected episode of AF, paroxysmal AF and persistent AF), and permanent AF. A paroxysmal episode of AF was defined as a self-terminating episode and persistent episode of AF as a non-self terminating episode. The first detected episode of AF either self-terminating or not, was isolated as it represents a reference point and as it may not require antiarrhythmic drug prevention of recurrences as we do not know if recurrence will happen or when. The permanent form of AF is *accepted AF* either because cardioversion failed or was not attempted. The three types of AF may evolve eventually to permanent AF. Both paroxysmal and persistent AF can be symptomatic and asymptomatic and may occur over time in the same patient. Paroxysmal AF was arbitrarily defined as attacks of arrhythmia lasting <7 days with most episodes lasting <24 h.

Restoration of sinus rhythm using pharmacological or electrical cardioversion represents a desirable endpoint of therapy in persistent AF, as it could restore normal hemodynamics and likely decrease the risk of emboli. Atrial fibrillation sometimes deeply affects the quality of life of the patients due to its abrupt onset and frequent recurrences. The recurrences of AF following cardioversion may be symptomatic or asymptomatic. Furthermore, even in a patient with initially symptomatic persistent AF the recurrences may take the form of paroxysmal asymptomatic AF emphasizing the need for frequent or if possible continuous electrocardiographic monitoring

Classification of recurrences after electrical cardioversion of persistent atrial fibrillation

Restoration of sinus rhythm after successful cardioversion of AF is often followed by recurrences of AF. Some recurrences called immediate recurrences may occur within 1 or 2 min after restoration of sinus P waves. The recent advent of atrial defibrillators has emphasized the high prevalence of immediate recurrences which occur in about 25% of cases following cardioversion of AF using a physician-activated atrialimplantable defibrillator (Lau & Tse, 2001).

Van Gelder *et al.* (1995) and Tieleman *et al.*

(1998) have subdivided recurrences of AF after electrical cardioversion of AF into three types: immediate recurrences as defined above, subacute recurrences starting the day of cardioversion and continuing for 1–2 weeks, and late recurrences occurring from 2 weeks to 1 year. Pretreatment with antiarrhythmic agents (class I or class III agents) before cardioversion may prevent immediate and subacute recurrences. Long-term prophylactic antiarrhythmic therapy may also prevent late recurrences. In the absence of prevention with antiarrhythmic therapy about 25% of patients only will remain in sinus rhythm whereas with prophylactic antiarrhythmic therapy about 50% of patients will be in sinus rhythm at 1 year.

Technical aspects of electrocardiographic monitoring

Monitoring of patients to detect recurrences of AF following electrical cardioversion of AF spontaneous, pharmacological or electrical may be achieved using different techniques.

In-hospital telemetry monitoring may be a research tool to study the recurrences of AF following cardioversion in hospitalized patients and the effect of various pharmacological agents aimed at preventing immediate and subacute recurrences in coronary care or intensive care units or in appropriately equipped wards. However, as AF is not a life threatening arrhythmia in most patients, electrical cardioversion is usually performed in appropriately anticoagulated patients as an outpatient technique in many centres. Therefore, for most patients, in-hospital telemetry may not be the technique of choice for detecting subacute recurrences of AF.

Ambulatory electrocardiographic Holter monitoring

Continuous electrocardiographic monitoring of patients who underwent cardioversion of AF using 24 h or 48 h ambulatory recording may be used to detect AF (Kennedy & Wiens 1987) provided the episodes are frequent enough to be recorded within a 24 h period. Tape recordings or solid-state recordings offering a 24-h ECG recording printout may be helpful in detecting AF recurrences. However, the usefulness and the cost-effectiveness of such approaches have not been evaluated on a large scale. A recent study found that frequent premature atrial complexes (>10/h) in the 24-h Holter recording after electrical cardioversion was associated with a higher risk of recurrences (Maounis *et al.* 2001).

Transtelephonic monitoring

Transmission of an ECG as an audio signal through transtelephonic devices has been used to monitor the cardiac rhythm following cardioversion of AF (Antman *et al.* 1986). This transmission can be continuous or episodic. The recording device is carried by the patient who can record when he has symptomatic arrhythmia or at regular intervals preset by the physician. Recording can be achieved by applying the device directly on the precordial area or through continuously attached electrodes. Some devices use recording through the index and thumb of both hands and can record only one lead. Transmission of the ECG recording may be direct or indirect as the device has a memory of several minutes (Brown *et al.* 1987; Krahn *et al.* 2001). The advantage of such a technique is that the device can be kept by the patient for long periods of time, which allows long periods of cardiac rhythm to be monitored. However it requires a base station with a demodulator and a recorder or transmission to a facsimile machine.

Monitoring through implantable devices

Implantable loop recorder

The implantable loop recorder is under evaluation in the diagnosis of syncope of unknown origin (Brown *et al.* 1987; Simantirakis *et al.* 2000). To our knowledge they have not been used so far for monitoring recurrences of arrhythmia in patients with AF.

Pacemakers and defibrillators

Pacemakers and defibrillators with Holter capabilities indicated for AF prevention and termination have provided important information on AF (Sopher & Camm, 2000).

Pacemakers for AF prevention. Modern pacemakers for AF prevention have a pacemaker memory, which gives a better understanding of the mode of initiation and termination of atrial arrhythmias and which allows the measurement of AF burden. Data from these devices have shown that AF episodes may be induced by premature atrial contractions (PACs) in most cases, but other mechanisms such as bradycardia or tachycardia together with PACs may also play a role in their initiation. These pacemakers could be used to monitor the recurrences of AF following cardioversion of AF, but progress is needed in the technology for providing cardiac electrograms or ECG-like tracings that will permit differentiation of true AF from artefacts.

Atrial defibrillators

The Metrix system. The initial results of the clinical evaluation of the Metrix system have been reported by Wellens *et al.* (1998). In all patients, the device was activated by the physician in this initial phase of evaluation, which was aimed at assessing its safety and efficacy. Out of 3719 shocks delivered, for treatment or testing, no ventricular proarrhythmia was observed. The device has proved also to be effective in detecting AF episodes with a specificity of 100% and terminating 96% of them successfully. Initial experience has used the physician-activated mode only in patients without significant organic heart disease. The experience using the patient-activated mode confirmed the results of the physician-activated mode. Early recurrences of AF occurred in 27% of episodes with 51% of patients requiring repeat cardioversion through device activation sometimes resulting in secondary shock failure.

Double chamber defibrillators. Only experience with the Medtronic 7250 has been to our knowledge reported so far. The initial experience of the Worldwide Jewel AF Investigators was reported by Gold *et al.* (2001) in 144 patients with drug-refractory AF followed with an average follow-up of 12 ± 6 months. The report showed a positive predictive accuracy for atrial arrhythmia detection of 99% and arrhythmia termination in 40% of episodes using atrial pacing and in 87% of episodes using shocks. Adler *et al.* (2001) reported the efficacy of pacing therapies for the Worldwide Jewel AF Investigators experience, which includes 537 patients followed for a mean of 11.4 ± 8.2 months. In all patients, a clinical indication for the implantation of a ventricular ICD was present. Pacing therapies successfully terminated 59% of 1500 episodes of spontaneous AT episodes in 127 patients and 30% of 880 episodes of AF in 101 patients. The latter is explained by the fact that in 30% of patients AF is initiated by an organized atria arrhythmia which can be terminated by rapid atrial pacing. The overall efficacy of pacing for AT/AF episodes was 48% with a median time of 1.1 min. Immediate recurrences (within 1 min) occurred in 25% of cases. Using data from patients of the Worldwide Jewel AF Investigators, Friedman *et al.* (2001) analysed the effect of atrial therapies on the arrhythmia burden of 52 of 269 patients who had atrial tachyarrhythmias during a follow-up of ≥30 days. Pacing and shock therapies reduced arrhythmia burden from 58.5 to 7.8 h per month, which was highly significant. Of interest, the reduction of arrhythmia burden persisted when only pacing therapies were considered.

Home monitoring system. Home monitoring is a recent concept under evaluation in patients with implanted pacemakers or defibrillators (Stellbrink *et al.* 2001; Santini, 2002). It consists of capturing data from an implanted device, allowing physician review and timely intervention. The system proposed by Biotronik includes a message from the pacemaker data transmitted through the GSM network to a service centre which in turn transmits a report by fax (called Cardio Report) to the attending physician. The interval between two interrogations can be programmed by the attending physician. In addition the patient may activate a message by applying a magnet over the pacemaker pocket. The report contains patient information, data on heart rate, atrial rhythm, ventricular rhythm, AV conduction, and therapy delivered in patients with implantable cardioverter defibrillators and technical data such as battery and lead status. This ingenious system presents some limitations: only a small number of units are equipped with this system; transmission depends of the GSM network; the system does not so far transmit ECG or electrogram recordings and ignores patient status, which can only be evaluated at follow-up visits. Despite these limitations, home monitoring systems open the way to a new field of surveillance for patients with AF or prone to AF that are using implanted devices. Home monitoring may help the early detection and treatment of AF and possibly reduce the incidence of permanent AF and embolic complications in pacemaker patients.

Clinical implications and perspectives of monitoring post-cardioversion of atrial fibrillation

Monitoring of AF using external devices or implanted devices is currently underused. The incidence of paroxysmal asymptomatic AF is underestimated, particularly after cardioversion of persistent AF (Timmermans *et al.* 2000). The possibility of asymptomatic episodes makes it hazardous to interrupt anticoagulation therapy even in patients who apparently remain in sinus rhythm. Similarly in patients with paroxysmal AF, the high prevalence of asymptomatic AF does not allow evaluation of therapy solely using patient symptoms. Recent pacemakers and atrial defibrillators with Holter monitoring capabilities will allow a better understanding of the AF mechanism and its evolution. Furthermore, by allowing the constant monitoring of patient rhythm they provide a fantastic tool for evaluating pharmacological and non-pharmacological therapy. In the AF Therapy Study, Camm *et al.* (2001) in a prospective randomized trial compared conventional pacing to pacing using four algorithms for AF prevention using the Selection 900 (Vitatron®, Nederlands) and found that the later significantly ($P < 0.01$) decreased AF burden (pace-conditioning, premature atrial contraction suppression, post-premature atrial contraction response, post-exercise response) by 30.4%. Such study would not have been possible without a device allowing event storage. A study using the patient-activated atrial defibrillator showed that there were significantly ($P < 0.05$) more episodes untreated than episodes treated (971 untreated vs. 190 treated) suggesting that the untreated episodes were asymptomatic or not symptomatic enough to warrant treatment for the patient (Timmermans *et al.* 2000). In a recent review, Mehra (2002) emphasized the role of implanted devices memory in the evaluation of therapy.

Conclusion

Proper evaluation of AF therapies cannot be achieved without careful monitoring. Recent techniques including home monitoring through implanted devices and device memory are likely to represent an advance in that direction. As the possibility of recording intracardiac electrograms (as in the Metrix system, a device no longer available), or ECG-like tracings (as in some ventricular ICDs), we will be able to increase pharmacological or non-pharmacological therapies used alone or in combination – the so-called hybrid therapy.

References

Adler, S.W., Wolpert, C., Warman, E.N. *et al.* (2001) Efficacy of pacing therapies for treating atrial tachyarrhythmias in patients with ventricular arrhythmias receiving a dual-chamber defibrillator. *Circulation*, **104**, 887–892.

Antman, E.M., Ludmer, P.L., MacGowan, N. *et al.* (1986) Transtelephonic electrocardiographic transmission for management of cardiac arrhythmias. *American Journal of Cardiology*, **58**, 1021–1024.

Brown, A.P., Dawkins, K.D. & Davies, J.G. (1987) Detection of arrhythmias: use of a patient-activated ambulatory electrocardiogram device with a solid state memory loop. *British Heart Journal*, **58**, 251–253.

Cabin, H.S., Clubb, K.S., Hall, C. *et al.* (1990) Risk for systemic embolization of atrial fibrillation without mitral stenosis. *American Journal of Cardiology*, **61**, 714–717.

Cairns, J.A. & Connolly, S.J. (1991) No rheumatic atrial fibrillation: risk of stroke and role of antithrombotic therapy. *Circulation*, **84**, 46–79.

Camm, A.J. for participating centres of the AF Therapy Study (2001) *The Atrial Fibrillation Therapy Study*. Presented at the Hotline session of the European Society of Cardiology, Stockholm.

Friedman, P.A., Dijkman, B., Warman, E.N. *et al.* (2001) Atrial therapies reduce arrhythmia burden in defibrillator patients. *Circulation*, **104**, 1023–1028.

Fuster, V., Ryden, L., Asinger, R.W. *et al.* (2001) ACC/AHA/ESC guidelines for the management of patients with atrial fibrillation. A Report of the American College of Cardiology/American Heart Association Task Force on Practice Guidelines and the European Society of Cardiology for Practice Guidelines and Policy Conferences. *European Heart Journal*, **22**, 1852–1923.

Gold, M.R., Sulke, N., Schwartzman, D.S. *et al.* (2001) Clinical experience with a dual-chamber defibrillator to treat atrial tachyarrhythmias. *Journal of Cardiovascular Electrophysiology*, **12**, 1247–1252.

Kannel, W.B., Abbot, R.D., Savage, D.D. *et al.* (1982) Epidemiologic features of chronic atrial fibrillation: the Framingham study. *New England Journal of Medicine*, **306**, 1018–1022.

Kennedy, H.L. & Wiens, R.D. (1987) Ambulatory (Holter) electrocardiography using real time analysis. *American Journal of Cardiology*, **59**, 1190–1195.

Krahn AD, Klein GJ, Yee R *et al.* (2001) Randomized assessment of syncope trial: conventional diagnostic testing vs. a prolonged monitoring strategy. *Circulation*, **104**, 46–51.

Lau, C.P. & Tse, H.F. (2001) Early reinitiation of atrial fibrillation after electrical defibrillation: a new electrophysiological phenomenon. *PACE (Pacing and Clinical Electrophysiology)*, **24**,1581–1584.

Maounis, T., Kyrozi, E., Katsaros, K. *et al.* (2001) The prognostic significance of atrial arrhythmias recorded early after cardioversion of atrial fibrillation. *PACE (Pacing and Clinical Electrophysiology)*, **24**,1076–1081.

Mehra, R. (2002) Monitoring of atrial arrhythmias. *Cardiac Electrophysiology Review*, **6**, 225–232.

Petersen, P. & Godtfredsen, J. (1986) Embolic complications in paroxysmal atrial fibrillation. Stroke **17**, 622–626.

Santini M. (2002) Home monitoring for the management of patients with atrial arrhythmias. An international multicentre trial. *Progress in Biomedical Research*, **7**, 258–264.

Simantirakis, E.N., Chrysostomakis, S.I., Manios, E.G. *et al.* (2000) Insertable loop recorder in unmasking the cause of syncope. *PACE (Pacing and Clinical Electrophysiology)*, **23**, 1573–1575.

Sopher, M.S. & Camm, A.J. (2000) Atrial pacing to prevent atrial fibrillation. *Journal of Interventional Cardiac Electrophysiology*, **4**, 149–153.

Stellbrink, C., Filzmaier, K., Mischke, K. *et al.* (2001) Potential applications of home monitoring in pacemaker therapy-A review with emphasis on atrial fibrillation and congestive heart failure. *Progress in Biomedical Research*, **6**, 107–114.

Tieleman, R.G., van Gelder, I.C., Crijns, H.J.G.M. *et al.* (1998) Early recurrences of atrial fibrillation after electrical cardioversion: a result of fibrillation-induced electrical remodeling of the atria? *Journal of the American College of Cardiology*, **31**, 167–173.

Timmermans, C., Levy, S., Ayers, G.M. *et al.* (2000) Spontaneous episodes of atrial fibrillation after implantation of the Metrix Atrioverter: observations on treated and nontreated episodes. Metrix Investigators. *Journal of the American College of Cardiology*, **35**, 1428–1433

Van Gelder, I.C., Crijns, H.J.G.M., Hillege, H. *et al.* (1995) Value and limitations of DC electrical cardioversion of chronic atrial fibrillation. *PACE (Pacing and Clinical Electrophysiology)*, **18**, 798.

Wellens, H.J.J., Lau, C.P., Lüderitz, B. *et al.* for the Metrix Investigators (1998) Atrioverter: an implantable device for the treatment of atrial fibrillation. *Circulation*, **98**, 1651–1656.

CHAPTER 53

Heart Rate Profile in Chronic Atrial Fibrillation

Alessandro Capucci, Giovanni Quinto Villani and Massimo Piepoli

Introduction

The study of the heart rate profile in chronic atrial fibrillation (AF) has been mainly associated with the evaluation of the adverse haemodynamic changes occurring during the arrhythmia. An uncontrolled and fast ventricular response may develop alterations in ventricular function and structure, also called tachycardia-related cardiomyopathy (Schumaker *et al.* 1998; Redfiel *et al.* 2000). Furthermore the irregular sequence of *RR* intervals typical of AF may induce adverse haemodynamic consequences which are not strictly dependent on heart rate *per se* (Daoud *et al.* 1996; Clark *et al.* 1997).

More recently *RR* intervals variations have been studied from an electrophysiological point of view. In fact, the heart rate evaluated by 24-h ECG monitoring has allowed the identification of patients with atrio-ventricular (AV) nodal duality (Olsson *et al.* 1986; Raeder, 1990), which may benefit from modification of the AV node (Feld *et al.* 1994; Morady *et al.* 1997). Heart rate profile is also affected by the modulation of the autonomic nervous system and provides a prognostic marker in different heart diseases.

The most recent acquisitions concerning the experimental and clinical use of heart rate profile evaluation during chronic AF are reviewed in this chapter.

Determinants of ventricular rate during atrial fibrillation: experimental findings

Traditionally, AV node conduction properties have been considered a main factor for determining ventricular rate during AF. The length of nodal refractoriness after a premature impulse, which underlies the concept of concealed conduction, provided the most common explanation for the variability of ventricular rhythm during AF based on the hypothesis of the elimination-by-block of the vast number of AF impulses (Watanabe, 1994). More recently, the electrotonic modulation of AV node excitability by repetitive atrial impulses has been proposed as a more viable explanation for the characteristics of the ventricular response in patients with AF (Maijler *et al.* 1996).

After the introduction of ablative techniques in clinical practice (Feld *et al.* 1994; Krahn *et al.* 1997; Morady *et al.* 1997), the problem of conduction of atrial activity during AF has been proposed with a more global approach. Recent observations suggested that ventricular rate during AF is a consequence of a more complex interaction between electrophysiological, anatomical and neural factors.

The relationship between atrial electrophysiology and the anatomy of the AV junction has been shown to be the main factor influencing AV conduction during AF.

In a rabbit model of AF, Garrigue *et al.* (1999a, b) evaluated the mechanism predicting the success of the postero-septal (slow-pathway) ablation of the AV node. The approach was based on the cooling of the posterior and/or the anterior AV node and had nonspecific effects on the slow and fast pathway portions of the AV node curve. In contrast, postero-septal surgical cuts resulted in a slowing of the AV node bombardment rate associated with a longer mean *HH* interval. These results suggested that a posterior intra-atrial block rather than slow-pathway elimination was associated with a ventricular rate slowing in AF. Subsequently Garrigue *et al.* (1999) studied the relationship between the site of the activation and the rate of atrial engagement of the AV node inputs and the resulting ventricular rate. In a rabbit heart, they observed that the alternations in the sequence of activation of posterior and anterior AV input resulted in a substantial changes of the organization of intranodal cellular responses: consequently the ventricular rate was shown to be significantly dependent on differential bombardment of the AV node inputs and on the site of initiation of the atrial wavefronts.

Capucci and coworkers confirmed the importance of the site of AV node stimulation (Igel *et al.* 1999). In a human model of AF, they investigated the effect on the ventricular rate of the atrial pacing near the AV node. In induced AF, excitable gaps were measured at the anterior and the posterior regions, and during atrial pacing, the ventricular cycle durations at the longest and at the shortest excitable gap cycle length were compared. During posterior pacing, the increase in the cycle length determined a lengthening of the ventricular cycle, while anterior pacing showed an opposite effect (Fig. 53.1), suggesting that atrial impulses from the posterior region are more likely to be conducted to the ventricle than the impulses from the anterior region as the cycle length of activation is decreased.

Recently, novel insights have been reported from an optical map showing the anatomical–electrophysiological correlations in AV conduction (Mazgalev *et al.* 2001; Wu *et al.* 2001). Mazgalev *et al.* (2001) observed that atrio-nodal electrical excitation occurred in multiple layers (from the surface to deeper structures) and asymmetrically. The atrial wavefront engaging the central nodal region was curved in a such way that the earliest depolarization took place in the anterior regions, followed by the intermediate and posterior extensions of the node. However the AV wavefront seemed to be functionally single, albeit very inhomogeneous, while no distinct spatial boundaries were observed. It suggested that the superficial envelope of transitional cells, with a predominant superior entrance into the AV node, may support the fast wavefront, whereas the deeper structures of the posterior nodal extension are associated with the slow wavefront pathway.

These findings are consistent with the concept that AV node conduction should be considered a complex process, influenced not only by the electrophysiological properties (slow–fast pathways), but also by the site of activation, and by the anatomical structure of the AV node. The correct management of AV node modification, ventricular rate slowing and maintenance of normal anterograde conduction are critically dependent on the exact knowledge of all the different mechanisms mentioned above.

The possibility of changing the filtering prop-

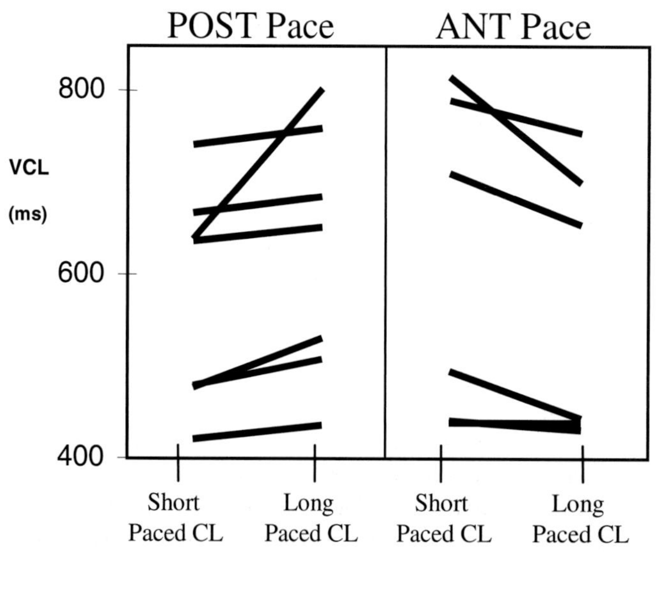

Fig. 53.1 Behaviour of ventricular cycle length (VLC) during anterior (ANT) and posterior (POST) pacing.

erties of the AV node by manipulation of its own chemical environment by selective vagal nerve stimulation has been reported recently. Experimental studies have demonstrated the existence of (1) a high density of vagal nerve terminals in the compact area of AV node and (2) a selective projection of vagal fibres from an epicardial fat pad, located near the inferior vena cava–left atrium junction, into the AV nodal region. The stimulation of these fibres (directly from the epicardium or via an endocardial approach) resulted in a highly selective depression of conduction and in slowing of the ventricular rate during AF (Schauerte *et al.* 1999; Wallick *et al.* 2001).

Mazgalev *et al.* (1999) reported that postganglionic vagal stimulation of a short burst of subthreshold current determined acetylcholine release from myocardial nerve terminals. During AF, this stimulation produced a reduction in ventricular rate secondary to depression in AV node conduction.

In a canine model of AF, Zhuang *et al.* (2002) compared the haemodynamic parameters during heart rate controlled either by selective AV nodal stimulation or by AV junctional ablation. They observed that the AV nodal vagal stimulation was haemodynamically superior to AV node ablation, indicating that the benefits of preserving the physiological antegrade ventricular activation sequence outweigh the detrimental effect of irregularity.

In view of a possible clinical application in selected groups of postoperative AF patients, further studies are necessary to assess the long-term effect and tolerability of this approach.

Heart rate profile during AF: clinical observations

More recently, experimental electrophysiological data have been used to explain the clinical observations derived from the analysis of the behaviour of atrial and ventricular activity evaluated by 24-h ECG monitoring during AF.

Distribution of *RR* intervals during chronic atrial fibrillation

Studies from the 1980s have suggested that a bimodal distribution of *RR* intervals during AF may indicate the presence of dual AV nodal physiology. Olsson *et al.* (1986) firstly evaluated a population of AF patients, without evidence of AV node paroxysmal tachycardia, by 24-h ambulatory monitoring: they reported the presence of bitrimodal *RR*-distribution in 70% of cases, suggesting that the presence of two separate atrionodal pathways may be a ubiquitous phenomenon.

These observations had no clinical impact until radiofrequency (RF) modification of the AV node was introduced as a therapeutic option for AF patients with uncontrolled rapid ventricular response despite medical therapy, but with a limited and an unpredictable success rate (Morady *et al.* 1997).

Recently several authors have focused their attention on the *RR* interval pattern, trying to evaluate a possible correlation between *RR* distribution, existence of 'dual' node physiology and outcome of RF procedure. Rokas *et al.* (1999) proposed and validated a noninvasive method for the detection of the dual atrioventricular node physiology in chronic AF. They compared the *RR* interval distribution measured by 24-h ECG monitoring during AF with the electrophysiological results obtained after sinus rhythm restoration. The distribution pattern of *RR* intervals (unimodal vs. bimodal) showed 88% sensitivity and 80% specificity for detecting dual AV node physiology, with positive and negative predictive values of 79% and 89%, respectively.

Later several authors tried to correlate the results from the 24-h ECG Holter monitoring with the clinical success in the RF modification procedure of AV node. Weismuller *et al.* (2000) evaluated the prevalence of two or more peaks on 24-h ECG *RR* interval histograms in a population of patients with permanent AF. The authors reported the presence of two or more peaks in 39% of the population and concluded that the ablation of all supernumerary AV nodal pathways (with a presumed shorter refractory period) resulted in clinically significant reductions in heart rate in a subgroup of these AF patients.

Tebbenjohanns *et al.* (2000) evaluated a population of patients with drug-refractory chronic AF and uncontrolled ventricular rate who underwent RF ablation to decrease the ventricular response, prospectively subdivided according to

RR histogram of 24-h Holter monitoring. The patients of group A showed a bimodal *RR* histogram with predominantly two peaks (with a predominant left peak) suggesting dual AV nodal physiology. Group B patients had a unimodal distribution pattern of their *RR* intervals and thus no evidence for dual AV nodal pathway. These assumptions were further verified by electrophysiological evaluation of AV nodal properties after internal cardioversion before RF ablation. Before ablation, evidence for dual AV nodal physiology was found in 77% of group A patients and in 13% patients of group B. After ablation of posterior atrionodal input, the mean ventricular rate decreased by 32%, and the *RR* bimodal interval histogram pattern changed to a unimodal distribution in all group A patients. Patients who presented late recurrence of symptomatic tachyarrhythmic AF showed restoration of bimodal *RR* pattern (which was previously converted to a unimodal pattern by RF ablation) (Fig. 53.2).

More recently, Rokas *et al.* (2001) performed a RF modification of AV node in a population of patients with chronic AF who underwent to 24-h Holter monitoring before ablation. In patients with a bimodal distribution of *RR* intervals, the short-term success rate of AV modification reached 94%, with no recurrence of procedural AV block, with a small number of ablative attempts, mainly located in the posterior and the midseptal regions of the tricuspid annulus.

In conclusion, the analysis of the *RR* interval distribution pattern in patients with chronic AF and rapid ventricular response may help to identify the candidates more suitable to be treated by safe and successful RF modification of the AV node.

However limitations must be considered in the clinical application of these results. The prevalence of bimodal *RR* interval histograms among AF patients depends on the criteria used to define the presence this pattern. Previous studies have reported that marked bimodality exists in nearly 25% of unselected patients with AF while a subtle bimodality may be present in a larger percentage of AF patients (Olsson *et al.* 1994). Furthermore the *RR* interval distribution analysis does not provide 100% accuracy in the detection of dual AV node physiology and an unimodal pattern may be associated with dual AV pathways in nearly 10% of patient (Rokas *et al.* 1999).

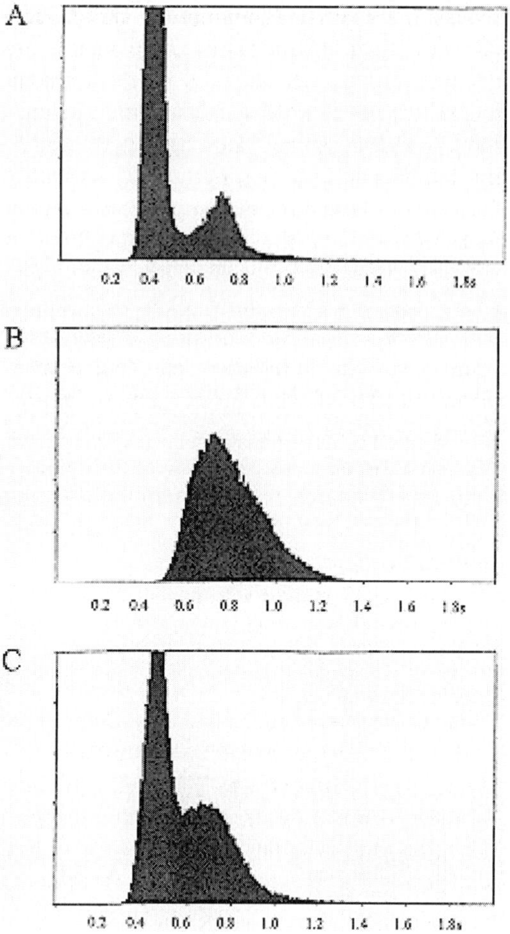

Fig. 53.2 Circadian variations in the average RR interval and measures of the Lorenz plot in a patient with chronic AF without CHF. Thick solid lines indicate the least-square cosine curves fitted to the circadian variation of individual variables. The time resolution is 5 min for all plots. (Modified from Stein *et al.*, 1994, with permission.)

Circadian variation of atrial and ventricular rate in chronic atrial fibrillation

The analysis of long-term ambulatory monitoring during AF evidenced the presence of a circadian pattern of variation both of the atrial and the ventricular activities. This behaviour has been related to the influence of autonomic neural modulation on the electrophysiological properties of atria and AV node.

Bolman *et al.* (2000) first noninvasively investigated the diurnal fluctuation of atrial fibrillatory frequency in persistent human AF and determined the relationship between changes in ventricular rate and the fibrillatory frequency. Using 24-h ECG Holter monitoring and comparing maximal diurnal vs. nocturnal fibrillatory frequencies, they distinguished the presence of two fibrillatory patterns of differing frequency. In 80% of patients a nocturnal decrease in fibrillatory frequency was found with a moderate positive correlation between relative changes in ventricular rate and fibrillatory frequency, whereas in 20% of patients an increase in nocturnal fibrillatory frequency with inverse correlation with ventricular rate occurred. These data suggested possible circadian changes in AF pattern in the same patient which may influence ventricular rate changes.

Hayano *et al.* (1998) analysed the circadian variation in atrioventricular conduction properties during AF and their relation with ventricular rate by a technique based on the Lorenz plot of successive ventricular response, derived by 24-h Holter monitoring, providing information about the AV node refractoriness and concealed AV conduction. They evaluated a population of patients with or without cardiac heart failure and chronic AF, in medical therapy with digoxin or calcium channel antagonists or both. They observed that both AV node refractoriness and the degree of concealed AV conduction during AF may show a circadian rhythm, with a nocturnal acrophase (time of peak estimated rhythm between 23.30 to 00.45 hours). Furthermore the circadian rhythm of these properties may contribute independently to the circadian variation of the ventricular rate, which shows a similar behaviour.

Despite of the lack of clear direct evidence, these observations suggest that circadian variations are most probably mediated by autonomic neural modulation, according to the results of the experimental studies mentioned above, with possible clinical implications. It is accepted that a reduction in heart rate variability is associated with a worse prognosis in patients with ischaemic heart disease or heart failure. Less data are available about patients with chronic AF and underlying heart disease.

Stein *et al.* (1994) reported that reduction of circadian variation in the ventricular rate inter-

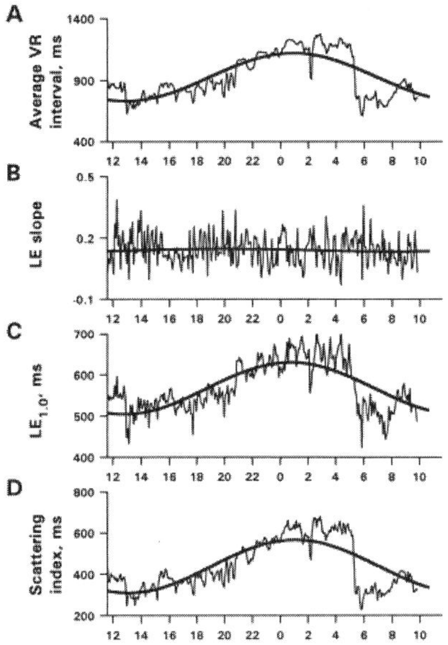

Fig. 53.3 Circadian variations in the average RR interval and measures of the Lorenz plot in a patient with chronic AF without CHF. Thick solid lines indicate the least square cosine curves fitted to the circadian variation of individual variables. The time resolution is 5 min for all plots (modified from Hayano et al, 1998)

val was associated with a combined risk of death and the need for valvular surgery during a follow-up period of 9.1 years in patients with AF and nonischaemic mitral regurgitation. Frey *et al.* (1995) observed an association between decreased ventricular rate circadian variation and 12-month deterioration (death or need of heart transplantation) in patients with AF and advanced heart failure. Hayano *et al.* (1998) reported an attenuation in the circadian ventricular rate rhythm without direct prognostic implication in their patients with heart failure compared to control patients.

These findings indicate that the analysis of ambulatory ECG recordings may provide a useful probe into the autonomic mechanisms underlying circadian variation of ventricular rate in AF patients with or without heart disease. However this direct clinical application needs further studies on larger patient populations.

Conclusions

Heart rate during AF is related to different mechanisms, such as atrial and AV node properties, anatomical and physiological structures of the

AV node, neurohumoral modulation, and possibly more to be established. According to the underlying heart disease, autonomic balance, exercise and daily activity, their interactions may contribute differently to the origin of heart rate pattern. At present, 24-h ECG Holter monitoring is the only method for evaluating this aspect of AF patients.

The final goal is to provide a patient with the most valuable pharmacological and nonpharmacological support to maintain the best profile of quality of life without being negatively deeply influenced by the persistence of AF.

References

Bolmann, A., Sonne, K., Esperer, H.D. *et al.* (2000) Circadian variations in atrial fibrillatory frequency in persistent human atrial fibrillation. *PACE (Pacing and Clinical Electrophysiology)*, **23**, 1867–1871.

Clark, D.M., Plumb, V.J., Epstein, A.E. *et al.* (1997) Hemodynamic effects of an irregular sequence of ventricular cycle lengths during atrial fibrillation. *Journal of the American College of Cardiology*, **30**, 1039–1045.

Daoud, E.G., Weiss, R., Bahu, M. *et al.* (1996) Effect of an irregular rhythm on cardiac output. *American Journal of Cardiology*, **78**, 1433–1436.

Feld, G., Fleck, P., Fujimura, O. *et al.* (1994) Control of rapid ventricular response by radiofrequency catheter modification of the atrioventricular node in patients with medically refractory atrial fibrillation. *Circulation*, **90**, 2299–2307.

Frey, B., Heinz, G., Binder, T. *et al.* (1995) Diurnal variation of ventricular response to atrial fibrillation in patients with advanced heart failure. *American Heart Journal*, **129**, 58–65.

Garrigue, S., Mowrey, K.A., Fahy, G. *et al.* (1999) Atrioventricular nodal conduction during atrial fibrillation: role of atrial input modification. *Circulation*, **99**, 2323–2333.

Garrigue, S., Tchou, P.J. & Mazgalev, T.N. (1999) Role to differential bombardment of atrial inputs to the atrioventricular node as a factor influencing ventricular rate during high atrial rate. *Cardiovascular Research*, **44**, 249–251.

Hayano, J., Sakata, S., Okada, A. *et al.* (1998) Circadian rhythms of atrioventricular conduction properties in chronic atrial fibrillation with and without heart failure. *Journal of the American College of Cardiology*, **31**, 158–166.

Igel, D.A., Villani, G.Q., Marotta, T. *et al.* (1999) Effects of atrial pacing cycle length on ventricular cycle length during atrial fibrillation. *PACE (Pacing and Clinical Electrophysiology)*, **22**, 6 (abstract).

Krahn, A., Klein, G., Yee, R. *et al.* (1997) Progressive anterior ablation in the coronary sinus region: evidence to support the presence of 'slow-pathway' input in normal patients? *Circulation*, **96**, 3477–3483.

Mazgalev, T.N., Garrigue, S., Mowrey, K.A. *et al.* (1999) Autonomic modification of the atrioventricular node during atrial fibrillation. *Circulation*, **99**, 2806–2814.

Mazgalev, T.N., Ho, S.Y. & Anderson, R.H. (2001) Anatomic–electrophysiological correlation concerning the pathways for atrioventricular conduction. *Circulation*, **103**, 2660–2667.

Meijler, F.L., Jalife, J. & Vaidya, D. (1996) AV nodal function during atrial fibrillation: the role of electrotonic modulation of propagation. *Journal of Cardiovascular Electrophysiology*, **7**, 843–861.

Morady, F., Hasse, C., Strickberger, S. *et al.* (1997) Long-term follow-up after radiofrequency modification of the atrioventricular node in patients with atrial fibrillation. *Journal of the American College of Cardiology*, **27**, 113–121.

Olsson, S.B., Cai, N., Donhal, M. *et al.* (1986) Noninvasive support for and characterization of multiple intranodal pathways in patients with mitral valve disease and atrial fibrillation. *European Heart Journal*, **7**, 320–333.

Olsson, S.B., Cai, N., Donhal, M. (1994) Prerequisites for nodal AV re-entry during atrial fibrillation. In: *Atrial Fibrillation: Mechanisms and Therapeutic Strategies* (eds S. B. Olsson, M. A. Allessie & R. W. F. Campbell), pp. 141–156. Futura Publishing, Armonk, NY.

Raeder, E.A. (1990) Circadian fluctuation in ventricular response to atrial fibrillation. *American Journal of Cardiology*, **66**, 1013–1060.

Redfiel, M.M., Kay, G.N., Jenkins, L.S. *et al.* (2000) Tachycardia-related cardiomyopathy: a common cause of ventricular dysfunction in patients with atrial fibrillation referred to atrioventricular ablation. *Mayo Clinic Proceedings*, **75**, 790–795.

Rokas, S., Gaitanidou, S., Chatzidou, S. *et al.* (1999) A noninvasive method for detection of dual atrioventricular node physiology in chronic atrial fibrillation. *American Journal of Cardiology*, **84**, 1442–1445.

Rokas, S., Gaitanidou, S., Chatzidou, S. *et al.* (2001) Atrioventricular node modification in patients with chronic atrial fibrillation. Role of morphology of *R–R* interval variation. *Circulation*, **103**, 2942–2948.

Schauerte, P., Scherlag, B.J., Scherlag, M.A.S. *et al.* (1999) Ventricular rate control during atrial fibrillation by cardiac parasympathetic nerve stimulation: a transvenous approach. *Journal of the American College of Cardiology*, **34**, 2043–2050.

Schumaker, B., Luderitz, B. *et al.* (1998) Rate issue in atrial fibrillation: consequences of tachycardia and therapy for rate control. *American Journal of Cardiology*, **82**, 29N–36N.

Stein, K.M., Borer, J.S., Hocreiter, C. *et al.* (1994) Variability of the ventricular response in atrial fibrillation and prognosis in chronic nonischaemic mitral regurgitation. *American Journal of Cardiology*, **74**, 906–911.

Tebbenjohanns, J., Schumacher, B., Korte, T. *et al.* (2000) Bimodal *RR* interval distribution in chronic atrial fibrillation: impact of dual atrioventricular nodal physiology on long-term rate control after catheter ablation of the posterior atrionodal input. *Journal of Cardiovascular Electrophysiology*, **11**, 497–503.

Wallick, D.W., Zhang, Y., Tabata, T. *et al.* (2001) Selective AV nodal vagal stimulation improves hemodynamics during acute atrial fibrillation in dogs. *American Journal of Physiology*, **281**, H1490–H1497.

Watanabe, Y. (1994) Impulse formation and conduction of excitation in the atrioventricular node. *Journal of Cardiovascular Electrophysiology*, **5**, 517–531.

Weismuller, P., Braunss, C., Ranke, C. *et al.* (2000) Multiple AV nodal pathways with multiple peaks in the *RR* interval histograms of the Holter monitoring ECG during atrial fibrillation. *PACE (Pacing and Clinical Electrophysiology)*, **23**, 1921–1924.

Wu, J., Olgin, J., Miller, J.M. *et al.* (2001) Mechanisms underlying the re-entrant circuit of atrioventricular nodal re-entrant tachycardia in isolated canine atrioventricular nodal preparation using optical mapping. *Circulation Research*, **88**, 1189–1195.

Zhuang, S., Zhang, Y., Mowrey, K.A. *et al.* (2002) Ventricular rate control by selective vagal stimulation is superior to rhythm regularization by atrioventricular nodal ablation and pacing during atrial fibrillation. *Circulation*, **106**, 1853–1858.

CHAPTER 54

Monitoring of Heart Rate Control in Atrial Fibrillation

Shamil Yusuf and A. John Camm

Introduction

The control of ventricular rate is an essential aspect of the management of atrial fibrillation (AF) be it acute, paroxysmal, persistent or permanent (Gallagher & Camm 1998). In an acute setting rapid ventricular rates may be associated with symptomatic hypotension, congestive cardiac failure or angina. In established AF tachycardia induced cardiomyopathy may result (Engel *et al.* 1974; Scheinman *et al.* 1974; Gallagher 1985; Grogan *et al.* 1992; Redfield *et al.* 2000). This may also hold true also for paroxysmal AF with frequent occurrences and where rate control is more difficult (Rodriguez *et al.* 1993). Like all forms of ventricular dysfunction tachycardia induced cardiomyopathy has prognostic implications. However, unlike the other forms, tachycardiomyopathy is reversible (McLaran *et al.* 1985; Packer *et al.* 1986) either with restoration of sinus rhythm (Peters & Kienzle, 1988), or with medical attainment of optimum ventricular rate (Brignole *et al.* 1998) or with invasive AV node ablation and permanent pacing (Lemery *et al.* 1987; Edner *et al.* 1995; Dupuis *et al.* 1997; Geelen *et al.* 1997). Recently a number of studies have advocated ventricular rate control and anticoagulation as acceptable management of recurrent persistent AF (Hohnloser *et al.* 2000; Wyse *et al.* 2002). Yet the issue of what constitutes adequate ventricular rate control is not universally agreed. Neither is there consensus on what methods need to be employed for effective assessment of ventricular rates. This chapter therefore deals with the clinical and electrocardiographic evaluation of ventricular rates in AF. It also highlights those values that are the most useful and relevant in the overall clinical management of the patient.

Optimum heart rate in atrial fibrillation

Before discussing the monitoring of ventricular rate in AF it is important to know and understand the basis of optimum heart rate in AF. This can be defined as the rate at which the cardiac output would be equivalent to that in sinus rhythm under similar conditions of observation, provided that symptomatic status is not compromised and without any long-term detrimental consequences. Based on the acceptance that normal heart rate in sinus rhythm is 70 beats/min, conventionally heart rates of 50–90 beats/min or 60–80 beats/min have been recommended for patients in AF at rest. Rates of 90–115 beats/min are advocated during exertion. Such assumptions are deeply flawed for a number of reasons. First, atrial contraction, absent in AF, contributes between 20 and 30% of the total stroke volume depending on left ventricular functional characteristics (Rahimtoola *et al.* 1975; DeMaria *et al.* 1976). A marked decrease in cardiac output may occur with the loss of atrial contraction, especially in patients with impaired diastolic filling, hypertension, mitral stenosis, hypertrophic or restrictive cardiomyopathy. Secondly, increased ventricular rates in AF lead to decreased diastolic filling, stroke volume and cardiac output (Raeder 1990). Hence, although rapid ventricular rates in AF can be detrimental they cannot be too low either. In fact they need to be slightly higher than that in sinus rhythm to maintain a similar cardiac output. Thirdly, the mere presence of irregular *RR* intervals in AF also impairs ventricular haemodynamic function irrespective of rate (Daoud *et al.* 1996). In a canine model with complete heart block, a decrease in cardiac output of approximately 9% was noted during irregular ventricular pacing at the same mean cycle length as a regularly paced rhythm (Naito *et al.* 1983). Cardiac cycle irregularity during AF can also decrease cardiac output in human subjects (Clark *et al.* 1997). In fact, myocardial contractility is not constant during AF. When left ventricular volumes and pressures were measured continuously in six patients, cycle–cycle changes in myocardial contractility were observed in AF because of the force interval relationships associated with cycle length (Brookes *et al.* 1998).

Using Doppler ultrasound to measure cardiac output at different ventricular rates, Rawles (1990) demonstrated that rates of up to 90 beats/min maintain good cardiac output for patients in AF at rest. He also demonstrated that ventricular rates of between 90 and 140 beats/min may be necessary during exercise to maintain cardiac outputs similar to those of patients in sinus rhythm.

With respect to long-term detrimental consequences, Packer *et al.* showed that ventricular rates needed to be persistently ≥130 beats/min to run the risk of tachycardiomyopathy (Packer *et al.* 1986). Although it seems that this affords some leeway for optimal ventricular rates before the risk of ventricular dysfunction ensues, such high rates need only be present for 10–15% of the day to significantly increase this risk (Fenelon *et al.* 1996). Furthermore, animal studies have demonstrated that the higher the heart rate in any particular species, the lower the life expectancy (Levine 1997) and initial changes in the ventricular myocardium have been reported at rates as low as 100 beats/min in the canine model (Redfield *et al.* 1993). In humans several cohorts have demonstrated a firm mortality benefit from lower heart rates: for example, in post myocardial infarction (ISIS Collaborative Group 1986; Gottlieb *et al.* 1998), in congestive cardiac failure (ANZHFR Collaborative Group 1995; MDC Trial Study Group 1998; CIBIS-II Investigators and Committees 1999) and in hypertension. One could thus conclude from these observations that the aim in AF should be to target the lowest possible heart rate without comprising patient symptoms.

In summary, generally the ventricular rate in AF can be assumed to be controlled at <90 beats/min at rest; uncontrolled at >140 beats/min during exercise and although rates of 90–115 beats/min are recommended during daily activity, up to 140 beats/min may be necessary for more strenuous exertion. Rates should never be allowed to run persistently above 130 beats/mean.

Clinical assessment of heart rate

Like any clinical assessment, the monitoring of the ventricular rate begins with a careful history and examination of the patient. Cardiovascular symptoms such as dyspnoea at rest or on exertion, rapid palpitations and fatigue may be the first and most important indicators that ventricular rate control may be suboptimal (Ostermaier & von Essen 1997). This may be confirmed initially by radial pulse examination but this is rather unsatisfactory. At best, rates are usually underestimated due to non-transmitted ventricular contractions and at worst, the arrhythmia may be missed altogether in slow AF. Apical rate assessment is better but this can be difficult owing to the absence of the second heart sound in mechanically ineffective beats and in the presence of murmurs, obstructive airways disease, pleural or pericardial effusions. For these reasons electrocardiography is the gold standard in the clinical assessment of ventricular rates both at rest and during exercise.

Electrocardiographic assessment of heart rate

Despite the routine and widespread use of electrocardiography in clinical cardiology, its application for the assessment of heart rates in AF remains a challenge. The three main reasons for this are *RR* interval variation; circadian heart rate variation and variability of heart rate during exercise.

RR interval variation

A variable *RR* interval is the hallmark of AF (Hering 1903). This concept denoting oscillations in the interval between consecutive heart beats or cardiac cycles needs to be distinguished from 'heart rate variability' and 'heart period variability' (Malik 1996) where autonomic influences upon the sinus node, atrial myocytes and the atrioventricular nodes of patients in sinus rhythm give rise to variable cycle lengths. Numerous studies have demonstrated unfavourable prognostic implications of reduced heart rate variability associated with various underlying conditions (Malik & Camm 1994). In AF however, the variable *RR* interval is not entirely due to autonomic influence; it characteristically diminishes and stabilizes with both time and conditions (Bootsma *et al.* 1970; van den Berg *et al.* 1995b; Piot, 1999); and its decrease has been shown to have prognostic implications only in advanced heart failure (Frey *et al.* 1995) and severe, non- ischaemic mitral regurgitation settings (Stein *et al.* 1994).

The electrophysiological basis for the variation in *RR* intervals in AF has been much debated. It appears to be the result of a combination of three factors: (1) the irregular, chaotic and rapid bombardment of the atrioventricular (AV) node with fibrillatory potentials from atrial myocytes at rates of between 350 and 600 beats/min (van den Berg *et al.* 1995a); (2) the inhomogeneous structure and transmission characteristics of the AV node; (3) the autonomic modulation of the AV node (Nagayoshi *et al.* 1997). The AV node is a complex and sophisticated structure with most of its anatomical characteristics having been derived by studying the rabbit heart, because of its strong structural and functional similarities to the human heart (Rubart & Zipes 2001). In the rabbit, the normal AV junctional area can be divided into an outer transitional cell zone (or nodal approaches), a compact portion (or the AV node) and a penetrating part of the AV bundle (His bundle). The transitional cells are elongated and smaller than atrial cells, and are separated by numerous strands of connective tissue. They merge at the entrance of the compact portion where the cells are small and spherical, not separated by muscle or connective tissue and have very few nexi. In humans, there are two distinct inputs to the AV node, one directed posteriorly via the crista terminalis and the other anteriorly via the interatrial septum. On the basis of electrophysiological characteristics, the AV node is divided into an AN, N and NH regions. The AN region corresponds to the transitional cell groups of the posterior portion of the node in the rabbit, the NH region to the anterior portion of the bundle of lower nodal cells and the N region to the small enclosed node where the transitional cells merge with mid-nodal cells. Propagation of impulses through the AV node to the bundle of His depends in part on the relative timing of the anterior and posterior septal activation inputs to the AV node (Mazgalev *et al.* 1982). Rapid irregular bombardment of the AV node with impulses from the atria results in different periods of refractoriness within the AV nodal cells giving rise to the concept of concealed conduction (Moe & Abildskov 1964; Lagendorf *et al.* 1965). This denotes atrial impulses traversing part of the AV node but not conducting to the ventricle. It plays a major part in determining the ventricular rate during AF (Page *et al.* 1996). In a significant proportion of patients with AF there seem to be multiple AV nodal pathways with different refractory periods that also influence heart rate. Frequency histogram analysis of *RR* interval distribution from 24-h Holter monitors for patients in sinus rhythm show a bell-shaped curve with a single peak. The majority of patients with AF also exhibit similar but much more broadly based unimodal distributions. However, up to 40% of patients with AF exhibit two, three or four peaks in their *RR* interval distribution (Fig. 54.1) (Weismuller *et al.* 2000). This denotes the presence of multiple AV nodal pathways usually associated with faster and more refractory ventricular rates and may arguably help identify those patients in AF with poor rate control who may be suitable for AV node modification rather then AV node ablation (Rokas *et al.* 1999). Conventional 24-h Holter monitors do not provide specific *RR* interval data and special software is usually required to obtain this information. Finally, autonomic influences upon the AV node also determine *RR* intervals (Page *et al.* 1991, 1996; van den Berg *et al.* 1994). Increased parasympathetic and decreased sympathetic tone exert negative dromotropic effects on AV nodal conduction; the opposite is true in states of decreased parasympathetic and increased sympathetic tone. Vagal tone also enhances the negative dromotropic effects of concealed conduction in the AV node (van den Berg *et al.* 1994; Page *et al.* 1996).

The variation of the *RR* interval and the lack

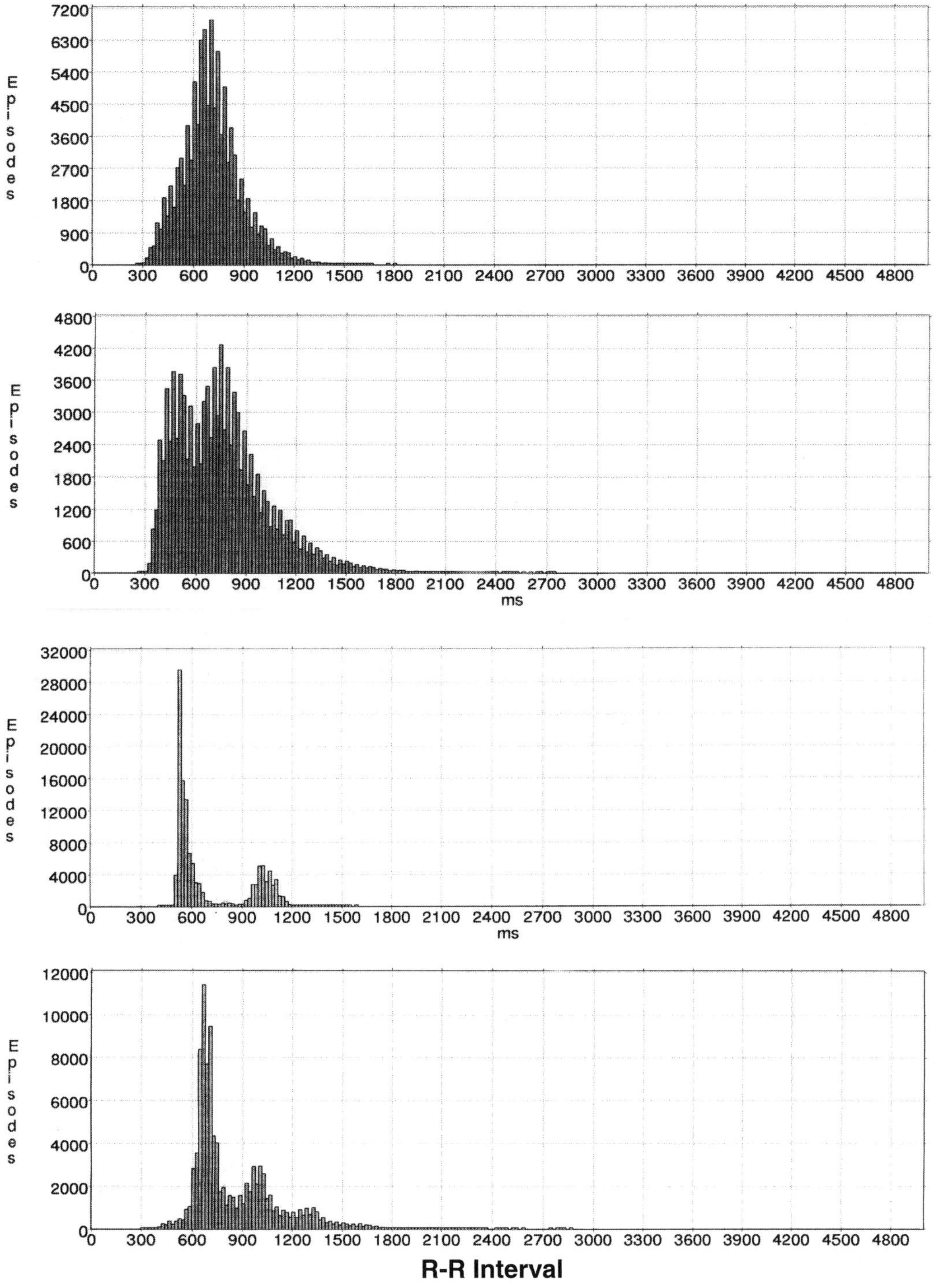

Fig. 54.1 Examples of *RR* interval histograms derived from Holter monitor recordings of patients in atrial fibrillation. Upper left graph shows one peak and hence one AV nodal pathway; upper right graph show two peaks (two pathways); bottom left shows three peaks (three pathways); bottom right shows four peaks (four pathways). (Reproduced from Weismuller *et al.* 2000, with permission.)

of pattern to the ventricular rate in AF raise the issue of optimal sampling intervals. Clearly, the smaller the sampling interval during AF the greater the yield of variability from true heart rates. Watt *et al.* (1984) demonstrated that at rest the average heart rate derived from a 20 second sample of AF approximates (±5%) the true value in an estimated 92.5% of patients. On the other hand, a two minute sample is required to approximate the shortest *RR* interval within 5% of the true value in 90% of patients. Atwood *et al.* (1989) addressing this same issue found that during exertion a one second sampling interval could be expected, on average, to fall within a range of 33 beats and increasing the sampling interval to 20 s yielded an error of 2.4 beats. What constitutes an acceptable error in heart rate measurement is not universally agreed and needs to be addressed in individual cases. Atwood *et al.* (1989) conclude that accurate estimates of ventricular rate at rest and during exercise are obtained using at least 6-s intervals among patients in AF and because of the high variability from sample to sample two measurements improve the precision of this measurement.

Circadian variation

The phenomenon of diurnal heart rate variation in humans with sinus rhythm is physiological and has been well documented with a nadir between midnight and 07.00 hours and a late peak in the morning around 11.00 hours. The autonomic influence upon the sinus node plays a major part in this phenomenon (Mitsuoka *et al.* 1990) and all aspects of the cardiac cycle measurable through conventional electrophysiological parameters (sinus node recovery time (SNRT); ventriculoatrial (VA) effective refractory period (ERP); AV nodal ERP; AH interval; HV interval; atrial ERP; right ventricular ERP; *QT* interval; VA interval; and the retrograde Kent bundle ERP) are subject to diurnal variability (Cinca *et al.* 1986). Similarly to sinus node refractory time, AV node refractory time and myocardial refractoriness also demonstrate an acrophase between 24.00 and 07.00 hours (Bexton *et al.* 1986; Cinca *et al.* 1986). Not surprisingly, therefore, the *RR* interval and the ventricular rate in AF also exhibit diurnal variability which closely mirrors that of sinus rhythm, although overall rates are higher in AF (Raeder, 1990). This variability results from autonomic modulation of the AV node (Raeder 1990). The demonstration by Farshi *et al.* (1999), using cosinar analysis of 24-h Holter recordings of patients in AF, that only a combination of digoxin and atenolol clinically eliminated this cyclical pattern in AF implies a role for both the sympathetic and parasympathetic systems for this phenomenon. How important it is to maintain diurnal rate variation when controlling ventricular rate in the presence of AF is unknown. Studies on ventricular rates during permanent pacing indicate that a loss of nocturnal bradycardia may be associated with ventricular dysfunction (see later) and therefore it is likely to be significant. However there is no evidence to suggest that preserving diurnal variability improves the patient's symptomatic status.

Twenty-four hour Holter recordings are an important investigation in the monitoring of ventricular rates in AF. Such recordings provide *RR* interval analysis over a 24 h period, information relating to diurnal ventricular rate variation, mean values over a 24 h period and documentation of maximum and minimum ventricular rates during normal activity (Fig. 54.2). Furthermore long pauses (i.e. >3 s) on 24-h Holter recordings especially during the day may indicate overzealous treatment and/or underlying conducting tissue disease. Djordjevich *et al.* (1989) in a quest to investigate optimal pacing rates for patients with permanent pacemakers used a study group of subjects in sinus rhythm divided into six age groups, 25 subjects each, ranging from 20–29 years to 60–69 years. They showed that the minimum heart rate during the night was <65 beats/min for all groups. Furthermore, Chew *et al.* studying patients with dual chamber permanent pacemakers, showed pacing at 80 ppm during the night impairs systolic and diastolic ventricular function compared to 50 ppm (Chew *et al.* 1996). On the basis of these observations we would advocate using two means to optimize ventricular rates in AF based on 24-h Holter recordings – a nocturnal mean of 60–70 beats/min but without any pauses >3.5 s and a diurnal mean of 90–115 beats/mean. Transient increases in rates of up to 140 beats/min would be acceptable if they were associated

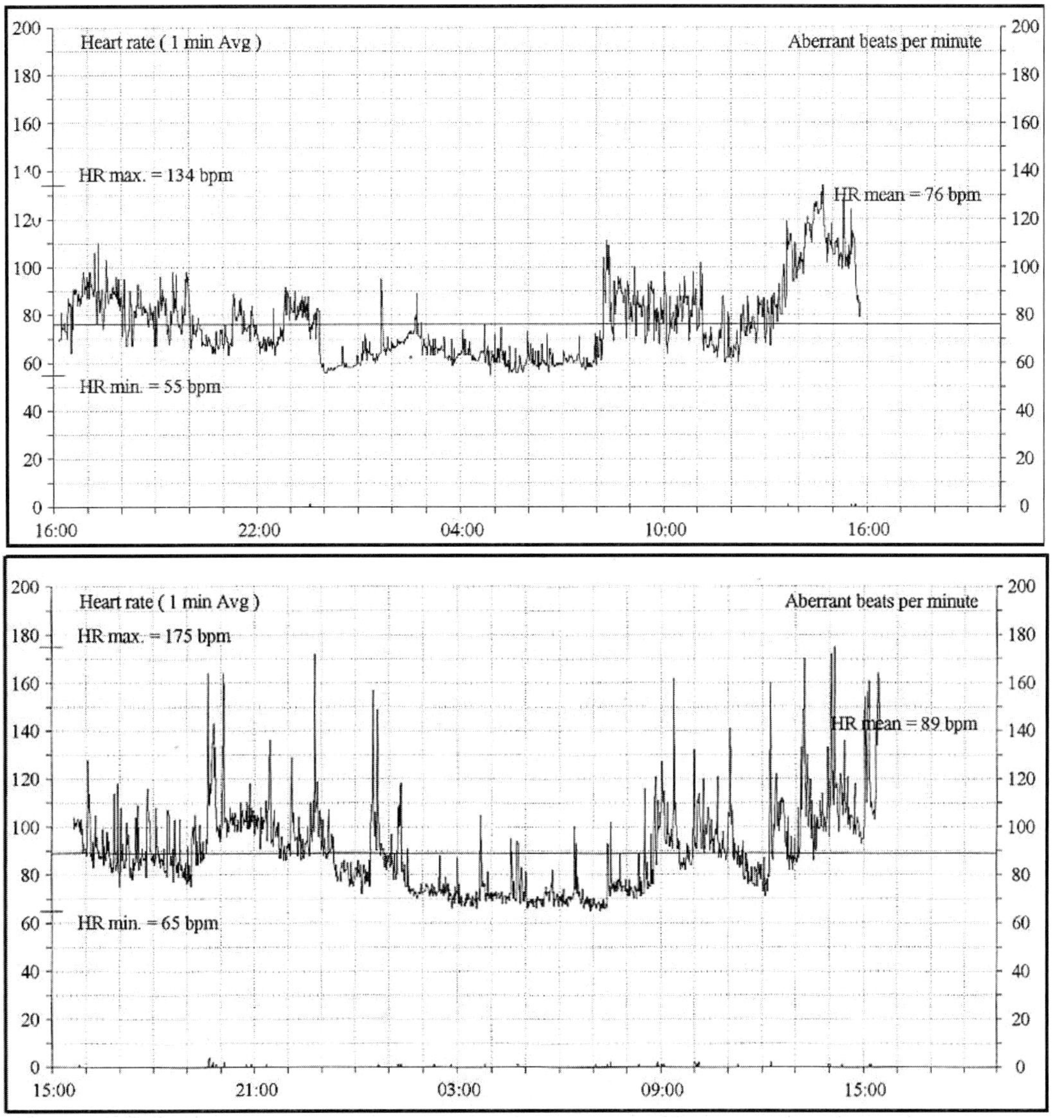

Fig. 54.2 Twenty-four-hour Holter recording demonstrating: (a) excellent ventricular rate control with preservation of diurnal variation; mean diurnal heart rate, 80–90 beats/min; mean nocturnal heart rate, 60–70 beats/min; (b) poor ventricular rate control with rates frequently exceeding 140 beats/min; mean diurnal heart rate, 110–120 bpm; mean nocturnal heart rate, 80–90 beats/min.

with more strenuous exertion. Thus meticulous diary keeping by the patient forms an important part of ventricular rate monitoring, and formal exercise tolerance testing may provide further essential information about rates during strenuous exertion.

Exercise-induced heart rate changes

The chronotropic response to exercise of the heart in AF has been of concern to clinicians since it was first described in 1924 (Blumgart 1924), and since 1972 numerous trials have demonstrated that adequate ventricular rate control at rest does not translate into effective control during activity, especially with digoxin monotherapy (Fig. 54.3) (Aberg *et al.* 1972a,b; Beasley *et al.* 1985; Farshi *et al.* 1999; Segal *et al.* 2000). Pioneering work on ventricular rate response to exercise in patients with AF was undertaken by Knox in 1949 using the step test

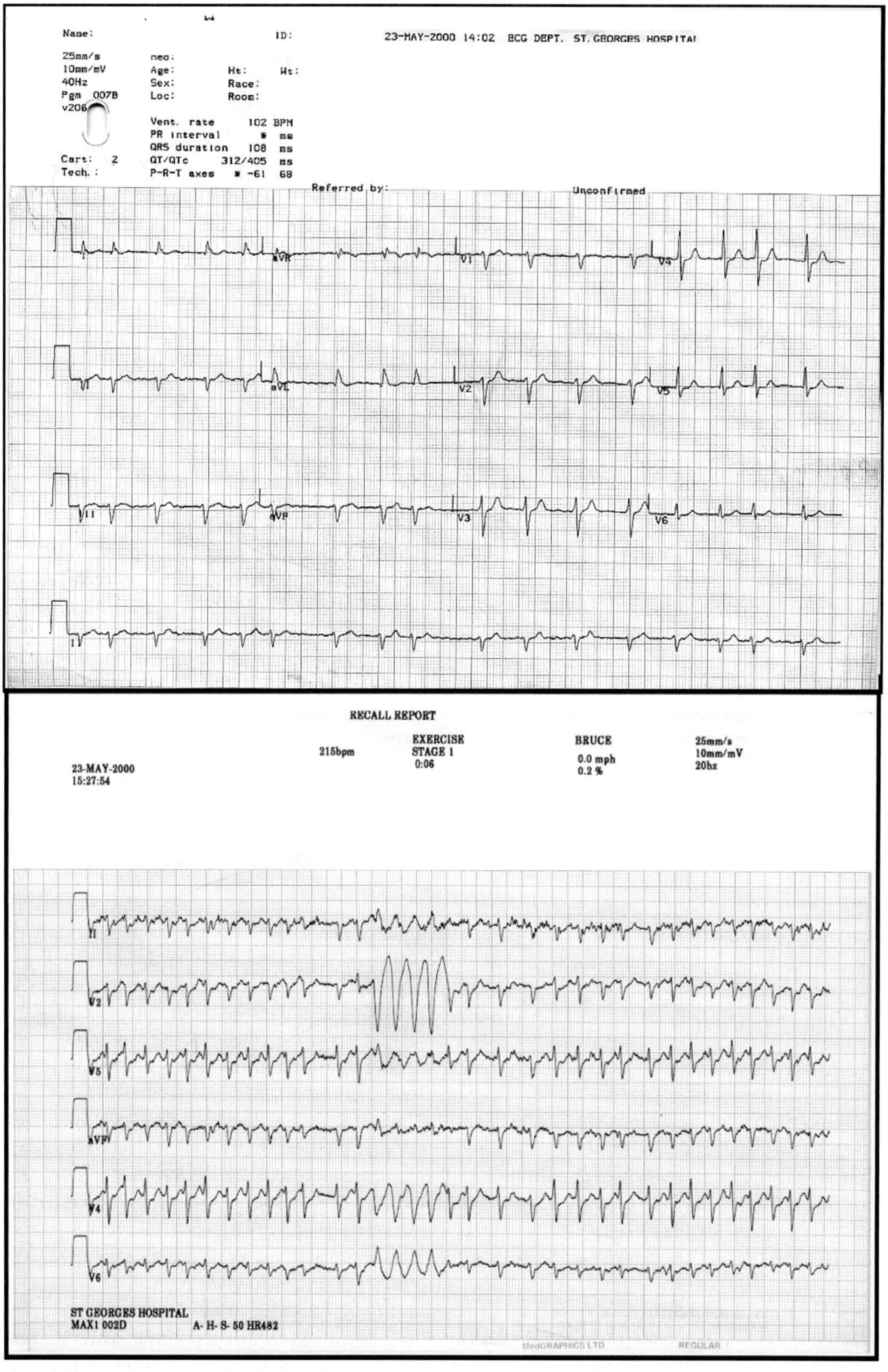

Fig. 54.3 Electrocardiograms showing poor rate control on minimum exertion in a patient on digoxin monotherapy.

(Knox 1949). He demonstrated a delayed acceleration in the first phase of exercise followed by an exaggerated heart rate response with prolonged tachycardia in the recovery period. However, patients in AF not only respond differently to exercise compared to patients in sinus rhythm, but they form a heterogeneous and complicated group with at least three different exercise response patterns (an inappropriate bradycardia, an inappropriate tachycardia, or an early bradycardia followed by an inappropriate tachycardia) (Corbelli *et al.* 1990). Furthermore, as in patients with sinus rhythm, any underlying organic heart disease also influences heart rate (Hornsten & Bruce 1968). Additionally patients in AF may demonstrate erratic transient tachycardic responses irrespective of the stage of the exercise. Corbelli *et al.* (1990) demonstrated that approximately 16% of patients with AF in fact exceed 115% of their predicted maximum heart rate at some point during the test and 42% failed to achieve 85% of their predicted maximum heart rate. Hence the normal criteria used to assess chronotropic response during exercise tests for patients in sinus rhythm cannot easily be applied to patients in AF. Formal criteria to interpret exercise tests in patients with AF do not exist. A combined approach can be advocated when assessing ventricular rates during exercise in patients with AF. The criteria applied to patients in sinus rhythm should be borne in mind but three additional principles need to be applied. First, identifying an early, late or overall tachycardic response denotes inadequate rate control and consideration should be given to terminating the exercise test once the 100% predicted heart rate has been reached. Secondly, a bradycardic response to exercise suggests too vigorous rate control therapy or the presence of conducting tissue disease where patients may benefit from pacing therapy. The exercise test should be terminated only if there is a demonstrable drop in the systolic blood pressure of at least 20 mmHg or more, or of course if the patients reports any significant symptoms, or requests cessation of the test. This should ensure that any patients with a late tachycardic response are not missed. Finally, a careful recording of any transient tachycardic response should be made together with a note of its duration and any symptoms reported by the patient. This will help determine whether these transient tachycardic episodes require special attention and management.

It may be possible to combine all of the above tests into one during the clinical assessment of ventricular rates in patients with AF by adopting simple manoeuvres. Wassmer *et al.* (2001) using a cohort of 18 patients with permanent AF demonstrated that a combination of ventricular rate assessment after 5 min of rest, after a 50 yard walk and after 1 min of stair stepping exercise could be correlated with 24-h Holter recordings. They found that the ventricular rate at rest during the clinic visit was significantly less than the mean Holter ventricular rate but correlated well with the minimum heart rate if a subtraction factor of 20 was included. The mean of the ventricular heart rate at rest and after a 50 yard walk was similar to the average ventricular rate recorded from a 24-h Holter monitor. The heart rate after 1 min of stair stepping was similar to the maximum ventricular rate recorded on 24-h Holter. However these findings need further verification.

The account given above provides a comprehensive review of the methods that can be used for effective monitoring of ventricular rates in AF. These methods would allow not only judgement of adequate rate control but also establish the paroxysmal or persistent nature of AF and enable evaluation of the trigger mechanisms which may be responsible. However no such account would be complete without a mention of long-term heart rate monitoring techniques. A significant proportion of patients with AF present with intermittent symptoms which may be the result of infrequent paroxysms of AF, infrequent pauses or even other arrhythmias which may not necessarily be identified with a conventional 24-h Holter monitor recording, or even during an exercise tolerance test. In such cases either cardiomemo devices or implantable Reveal devices are an invaluable option. Cardiomemo devices are small credit card like gadgets which patients apply to their chest at the occurrence of palpitations or other cardiovascular symptoms and press a button to record the underlying cardiac rhythm. Such devices can be very useful in relating an underlying arrhythmia to patient symptoms but are of little help in asymptomatic patients with a strong suspicion of

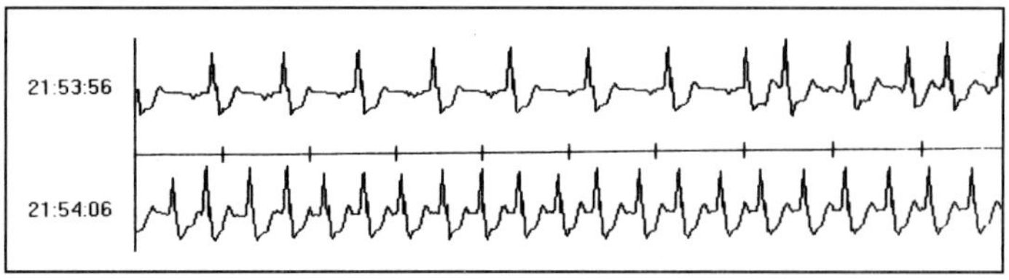

Fig. 54.4 REVEAL device recording demonstrating atrial fibrillation triggered by an atrial ectopic beat.

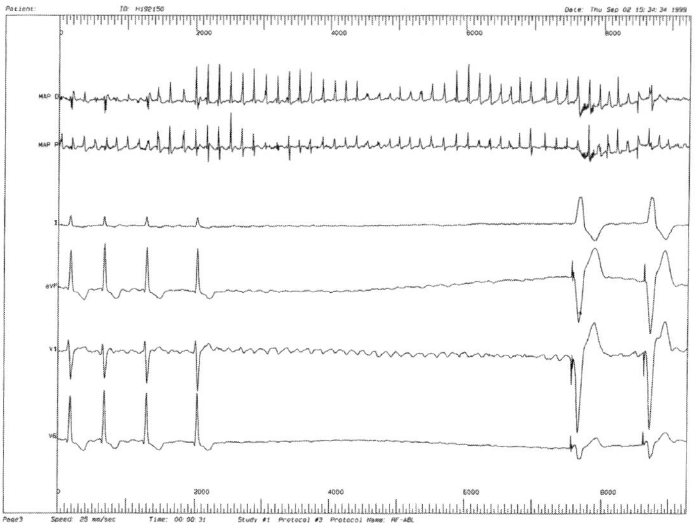

Fig. 54.5 A rhythm strip from a patient undergoing AV node ablation and permanent pacing. This strategy was adopted due to inadequate ventricular rate control despite the use of multiple AV nodal blocking agents.

underlying arrhythmia. Reveal devices are small recorders the size of fountain pen cartridges which can be implanted subcutaneously and can remain in situ for up to 14 months, recording any arrhythmias that may occur which can then be related to patients symptoms (Figure 54.4). At present such devices only record a maximum of three electrocardiogram leads but this suffices for most cases. In certain cases however, especially those in which the nature of the trigger mechanism is desirable, a 12-lead recording is much more useful. It is only a matter of time before these devices will be able to provide such information and probably a whole lot more.

Conclusion

1 Electrocardiography remains the gold standard means of monitoring ventricular rates in AF but all three modes of data acquisition, namely static 12-lead electrocardiography, 24-h Holter monitoring and exercise tolerance testing, need to be used for a thorough and complete assessment.

2 Ventricular rates in AF can be assumed to be controlled at <90 beats/min at rest; uncontrolled at >140 beats/min during exercise and although rates of 90–115 beats/min are recommended during daily activity, rates of up to 140 beats/min may be necessary for more strenuous exertion. Rates should never persistently be allowed to run above 130 beats/min.

3 At least 6-s sampling intervals of ECG recordings should be adopted to provide an accurate reflection of the ventricular rate in AF. The high variability of ventricular rate from sample to sample warrants at least two measurements of a given sample and will improve the precision of heart rate measurement.

4 Twenty-four-hour Holter recordings can provide a whole variety of information from *RR* interval data to diurnal ventricular rate variation, mean ventricular rate readings over a 24 h period, and maximum and minimum ventricular rate values. For normal daily activity two separate ventricular rate means should be adopted. A diurnal mean of 90–100 beats/min and a nocturnal mean of 60–70 beats/min should be aimed for. Any pause of >3 s, especially diurnal pauses, should trigger extreme caution.

5 In patients with ongoing cardiovascular symptoms despite what seems to be adequate rate control as assessed by conventional methods, exercise tolerance testing helps identify individuals with atypical atypical ventricular rate responses and/or over-zealous rate control. They also help identify patients where symptoms may be owing to other cardiovascular pathologies such as coronary artery disease.

6 Simple manoeuvres can be adopted to provide a reasonably thorough assessment of ventricular rate control in clinical settings.

References

Aberg, H., Strom, G. & Werner, I. (1972a) The effect of digitalis on the heart rate during exercise in patients with atrial fibrillation. *Acta Medica Scandinavica*, **191**, 441–445.

Aberg, H., Strom, G. & Werner, I. (1972b) Heart rate during exercise in patients with atrial fibrillation. *Acta Medica Scandinavica*, **191**, 315–320.

Atwood, J.E., Myers, J., Sandhu, S. *et al.* (1989) Optimal sampling interval to estimate heart rate at rest and during exercise in atrial fibrillation. *American Journal of Cardiology*, **63**, 45–48.

ANZHFR (Australia and New Zealand Heart Failure Research) Collaborative Group (1995) Effects of carvedilol, a vasodilator-beta blocker, in patients with congestive heart failure due to ischaemic heart disease. *Circulation*, **92**, 212–218.

Beasley, R., Smith, D.A. & McHaffie, D.J. (1985) Exercise heart rates at different serum digoxin concentrations in patients with atrial fibrillation. *British Medical Journal (Clinical Research Edition)*, **290**, 9–11.

van den Berg, M.P., Crijns, H.J., Haaksma, J., Brouwer, J. & Lie, K.I. (1994) Analysis of vagal effects on ventricular rhythm in patients with atrial fibrillation. *Clinical Science (London)*, **86**, 531–535.

van den Berg, M.P., de Langen, C.D., Haaksma, J. *et al.* (1995a) Analysis of randomness of atrial and ventricular rhythm in atrial fibrillation. *European Heart Journal*, **16**, 971–976.

van den Berg, M.P., Haaksma, J., Brouwer, J., Crijns, H.J. & Lie, K.I. (1995b) Analysis of heart rate variability in a patient with paroxysmal atrial fibrillation. *European Heart Journal*, **16**, 2011–2012.

Bexton, R.S., Vallin, H.O. & Camm, A.J. (1986) Diurnal variation of the *QT* interval–influence of the autonomic nervous system. *British Heart Journal*, **55**, 253–258.

Blumgart, H. (1924) The reaction to exercise of the heart affected by auricular fibrillation. *Heart*, **11**, 49.

Bootsma, B.K., Hoelsen, A.J., Strackee, J. & Meijler, F.L. (1970) Analysis of RR intervals in patients with atrial fibrillation at rest and during exercise. *Circulation*, **41**, 783–794.

Brignole, M., Menozzi, C., Gianfranchi, L. *et al.* (1998) Assessment of atrioventricular junction ablation and VVIR pacemaker vs. pharmacological treatment in patients with heart failure and chronic atrial fibrillation: a randomized, controlled study. *Circulation*, **98**, 953–960.

Brookes, C.I., White, P.A., Staples, M. *et al.* (1998) Myocardial contractility is not constant during spontaneous atrial fibrillation in patients. *Circulation*, **98**, 1762–1768.

Chew, P.H., Bush, D.E., Engel, B.T., Talan, M.I. & Abell, R.T. (1996) Overnight heart rate and cardiac function in patients with dual chamber pacemakers. *PACE (Pacing and Clinical Electrophysiology)*, **19**, 822–828.

CIBIS-II Investigators and Committees (1999) The Cardiac Insufficiency Bisoprolol Study II (CIBIS-II): a randomised trial. *Lancet*, **353**, 9–13.

Cinca, J., Moya, A., Figueras, J., Roma, F. & Rius, J. (1986) Circadian variations in the electrical properties of the human heart assessed by sequential bedside electrophysiological testing. *American Heart Journal*, **112**, 315–321.

Clark, D.M., Plumb, V.J., Epstein, A.E. & Kay, G.N. (1997) Hemodynamic effects of an irregular sequence of ventricular cycle lengths during atrial fibrillation. *Journal of the American College of Cardiology*, **30**, 1039–1045.

Corbelli, R., Masterson, M. & Wilkoff, B.L. (1990) Chronotropic response to exercise in patients with atrial fibrillation. *PACE (Pacing and Clinical Electrophysiology)*, **13**, 179–187.

Daoud, E.G., Weiss, R., Bahu, M. *et al.* (1996) Effect of an irregular ventricular rhythm on cardiac output. *American Journal of Cardiology*, **78**, 1433–1436.

DeMaria, A.N., Miller, R.R., Amsterdam, E.A., Markson, W. & D.T., M. (1976) Mitral valve early diastolic closing velocity: relation to sequential diastolic flow and ventricular compliance. *American Journal of Cardiology*, **37**, 693–700.

Djordjevic, M., Kocovic, D., Pavlovic, S., Velimirovic, D. & Kostic, D. (1989) Circadian variations of heart rate and stim-T interval: adaptation for night-time pacing. *PACE (Pacing and Clinical Electrophysiology)*, **12**, 1757–1762.

Dupuis, J.M., Victor, J., Le Davay, M., Asfar, P., Pezard, P. & Tadei, A. (1997) [Results of radiofrequency ablation of the atrioventricular junction in patients with refractory atrial arrhythmia and severe impairment of the left ventricular systolic function.] *Archives des Maladies du Coeur et des Vaisseaux*, **90**, 1255–1262 [in French].

Edner, M., Caidahl, K., Bergfeldt, L., Darpo, B., Edvardsson, N. & Rosenqvist, M. (1995) Prospective study of left ventricular function after radiofrequency ablation of atrioventricular junction in patients with atrial fibrillation. *British Heart Journal*, **74**, 261–267.

Engel, T.R., Bush, C.A. & Schaal, S.F. (1974) Tachycardia-aggravated heart disease. *Annals of Internal Medicine*, **80**, 384–388.

Farshi, R., Kistner, D., Sarma, J.S., Longmate, J.A. & Singh, B.N. (1999) Ventricular rate control in chronic atrial fibrillation during daily activity and programmed exercise: a crossover open-label study of five drug regimens. *Journal of the American College of Cardiology*, **33**, 304–310.

Fenelon, G., Wijns, W., Andries, E. & Brugada, P. (1996) Tachycardiomyopathy: mechanisms and clinical implications. *PACE (Pacing and Clinical Electrophysiology)*, **19**, 95–106.

Frey, B., Heinz, G., Binder, T. *et al.* (1995) Diurnal variation of ventricular response to atrial fibrillation in patients with advanced heart failure. *American Heart Journal*, **129**, 58–65.

Gallagher, J.J. (1985) Tachycardia and cardiomyopathy: the chicken–egg dilemma revisited. *Journal of the American College of Cardiology*, **6**, 1172–1173.

Gallagher, M. & Camm, A. (1998) Classification of atrial fibrillation. *American Journal of Cardiology*, 82 (8A), 1998.

Geelen, P., Goethals, M., de Bruyne, B. & Brugada, P. (1997) A prospective hemodynamic evaluation of patients with chronic atrial fibrillation undergoing radiofrequency catheter ablation of the atrioventricular junction. *American Journal of Cardiology*, **80**, 1606–1609.

Gottlieb, S.S., McCarter, R.J. & Vogel, R.A. (1998) Effect of beta-blockade on mortality among high-risk and low-risk patients after myocardial infarction. *New England Journal of Medicine*, **339**, 489–497.

Grogan, M., Smith, H.C., Gersh, B.J. & Wood, D.L. (1992) Left ventricular dysfunction due to atrial fibrillation in patients initially believed to have idiopathic dilated cardiomyopathy. *American Journal of Cardiology*, **69**, 1570–1573.

Hering, H.E. (1903) Analyse des pulses irregularis perpetuus. *Prager Medizinische Wochenschrift*, **28**, 377–381.

Hohnloser, S.H., Kuck, K.H. & Lilienthal, J. (2000) Rhythm or rate control in atrial fibrillation – Pharmacological Intervention in Atrial Fibrillation (PIAF): a randomised trial. *Lancet*, **356**, 1789–1794.

Hornsten, T.R. & Bruce, R.A. (1968) Effects of atrial fibrillation on exercise performance in patients with cardiac disease. *Circulation*, **37**, 543–548.

ISIS (International Study of Infarct Survival) Collaborative Group (1986) Randomised trial of intravenous atenolol among 16 027 cases of suspected acute myocardial infarction: ISIS-1. *Lancet*, **2**, 57–66.

Knox, J.A. C. (1949) The heart rate with exercise in patients with auricular fibrillation. *British Heart Journal*, **11**, 119.

Lagendorf, R., Pick, A. & Katz, L. (1965) Ventricular response in atrial fibrillation: role of concealed conduction in the AV junction. *Circulation*, **32**, 69–75.

Lemery, R., Brugada, P., Cheriex, E. & Wellens, H.J. (1987) Reversibility of tachycardia-induced left ventricular dysfunction after closed-chest catheter ablation of the atrioventricular junction for intractable atrial fibrillation. *American Journal of Cardiology*, **60**, 1406–1408.

Levine, H.J. (1997) Rest heart rate and life expectancy. *Journal of the American College of Cardiology*, **30**, 1104–1106.

Malik, M. (1996) Heart rate variability. Standards of measurement, physiological interpretation, and clinical use. Task Force of the European Society of Cardiology and the North American Society of Pacing and Electrophysiology. *European Heart Journal*, **17**, 354–381.

Malik, M. & Camm, A.J. (1994) Heart rate variability and clinical cardiology. *British Heart Journal*, **71**, 3–6.

McLaran, C.J., Gersh, B.J., Sugrue, D.D., Hammill, S.C., Seward, J.B. & Holmes, D.R., Jr (1985) Tachycardia induced myocardial dysfunction. A reversible phenomenon? *British Heart Journal*, **53**, 323–327.

Mazgalev, T., Dreifus, L.S., Bianchi, J. & Michelson, E.L. (1982) Atrioventricular nodal conduction during atrial fibrillation in rabbit heart. *American Journal of Physiology*, **243**, H754–H760.

MDC (Metoprololin Dilated Cardiomyopathy) Trial Study Group (1998) 3-Year follow-up of patients randomised in the Metoprolol in Dilated Cardiomyopathy Trial. *Lancet*, **351**, 1180–1181.

Mitsuoka, T., Ueyama, C., Matsumoto, Y. & Hashiba, K. (1990) Influences of autonomic changes on the sinus node recovery time in patients with sick sinus syndrome. *Jpn Heart J*, **31**, 645–660.

Moe, G. & Abildskov, J. (1964) Observations on the ventricular dysrhythmia associated with atrial fibrillation in the dog heart. *Circulation Research*, **4**, 447–460.

Nagayoshi, H., Janota, T., Hnatkova, K., Camm, A.J. & Malik, M. (1997) Autonomic modulation of ventricular rate in atrial fibrillation. *American Journal of Physiology*, **272**, H1643–H1649.

Naito, M., David, D., Michelson, E.L., Schaffenburg, M. & Dreifus, L.S. (1983) The hemodynamic consequences of cardiac arrhythmias: evaluation of the relative roles of abnormal atrioventricular sequencing, irregularity of ventricular rhythm and atrial fibrillation in a canine model. *American Heart Journal*, **106**, 284–291.

Ostermaier, R. & von Essen, R. (1997) [Heart frequency control in chronic and paroxysmal atrial fibrillation.

Critical evaluation of traditional therapy concepts.] *Fortschritte der Medizin*, **115**, 26–28, 30, 32, passim.

Packer, D.L., Bardy, G.H., Worley, S.J. *et al.* (1986) Tachycardia-induced cardiomyopathy: a reversible form of left ventricular dysfunction. *American Journal of Cardiology*, **57**, 563–570.

Page, R.L., Tang, A.S. & Prystowsky, E.N. (1991) Effect of continuous enhanced vagal tone on atrioventricular nodal and sinoatrial nodal function in humans. *Circulation Research*, **68**, 1614–1620.

Page, R.L., Wharton, J.M. & Prystowsky, E.N. (1996) Effect of continuous vagal enhancement on concealed conduction and refractoriness within the atrioventricular node. *American Journal of Cardiology*, **77**, 260–265.

Peters, K.G. & Kienzle, M.G. (1988) Severe cardiomyopathy due to chronic rapidly conducted atrial fibrillation: complete recovery after restoration of sinus rhythm. *Am J Med*, **85**, 242–244.

Piot, O. (1999) Heart rate variability is decreasing during paroxysmal atrail fibrillation. *Annals of Noninvasive Electrocardiography*, **4**, 144–151.

Raeder, E.A. (1990) Circadian fluctuations in ventricular response to atrial fibrillation. *American Journal of Cardiology*, **66**, 1013–1016.

Rahimtoola, S.H., Ehsani, A., Sinno, M.Z., Loeb, H.S., Rosen, K.M. & Gunnar, R.M. (1975) Left atrial transport function in myocardial infarction. *American Journal of Medicine*, **59**, 686–694.

Rawles, J.M. (1990) What is meant by a 'controlled' ventricular rate in atrial fibrillation? *British Heart Journal*, **63**, 157–161.

Redfield, M.M., Aarhus, L.L., Wright, R.S. And Burnett, J.C., Jr (1993) Cardiorenal and neurohumoral function in a canine model of early left ventricular dysfunction. *Circulation*, **87**, 2016–2022.

Redfield, M.M., Kay, G.N., Jenkins, L.S., Mianulli, M., Jensen, D.N. & Ellenbogen, K.A. (2000) Tachycardia-related cardiomyopathy: a common cause of ventricular dysfunction in patients with atrial fibrillation referred for atrioventricular ablation. *Mayo Clinical Proceedings*, **75**, 790–795.

Rodriguez, L.M., Smeets, J.L., Xie, B. *et al.* (1993) Improvement in left ventricular function by ablation of atrioventricular nodal conduction in selected patients with lone atrial fibrillation. *American Journal of Cardiology*, **72**, 1137–1141.

Rokas, S., Gaitanidou, S., Chatzidou, S., Agrios, N. & Stamatelopoulos, S. (1999) A noninvasive method for the detection of dual atrioventricular node physiology in chronic atrial fibrillation. *American Journal of Cardiology*, **84**, 1442–1445, A8.

Rubart, M. & Zipes, D. (2001) Genesis of cardiac arrhythmias: electrophysiological considerations. In: *Braunwalds Heart Disease – A Textbook of Cardiovascular Medicine* (eds Braunwald, D. Zipes & Libby), 6th edn, pp. 659–664. W. B. Saunders, Philadelphia.

Scheinman, M.M., Basu, D. & Hollenberg, M. (1974) Electrophysiological studies in patients with persistent atrial tachycardia. *Circulation*, **50**, 266–273.

Segal, J.B., McNamara, R.L., Miller, M.R. *et al.* (2000) The evidence regarding the drugs used for ventricular rate control. *Journal of Family Practice*, **49**, 47–59.

Stein, K.M., Borer, J.S., Hochreiter, C., Devereux, R.B. & Kligfield, P. (1994) Variability of the ventricular response in atrial fibrillation and prognosis in chronic nonischaemic mitral regurgitation. *American Journal of Cardiology*, **74**, 906–911.

Wasmer, K., Oral, H., Sticherling, C. *et al.* (2001) Assessment of ventricular rate in patients with chronic atrial fibrillation. *Journal of the American College of Cardiology*, **37** (Suppl. A), 93a (abstract).

Watt, J.H., Donner, A.P., McKinney, C.M. & Klein, G.J. (1984) Atrial fibrillation: minimal sampling interval to estimate average rate. *Journal of Electrocardiology*, **17**, 153–156.

Weismuller, P., Braunss, C., Ranke, C. & Trappe, H.J. (2000) Multiple AV nodal pathways with multiple peaks in the *RR* interval histogram of the holter monitoring ECG during atrial fibrillation. *PACE (Pacing and Clinical Electrophysiology)*, **23**, 1921–1924.

Wyse, D.G., Waldo, A.L., DiMarco, J.P. *et al.* (2002) A comparison of rate control and rhythm control in patients with atrial fibrillation. *New England Journal of Medicine*, **347**, 1825–1833.

CHAPTER 55

Autonomic Influence of Atrial Fibrillation

Philippe Coumel

Introduction

Two ingredients are necessary to any arrhythmia genesis: a substrate and its modulating factors. They can always be found combined at any level, but precisely characterizing their role and weighting their respective influence in clinical tachyarrhythmia is impossible in practice. Invasive electrophysiological investigations are well adapted for exploring the substrate in terms of location and mechanism provided it can be manipulated by programmed electrical stimulation. Ambulatory monitoring by the Holter technique, on the other hand, is the only tool available for studying spontaneous arrhythmia behaviour in the clinical situation (Coumel 1987). These two approaches are technically very different, and usually investigators have their preferred tool, but this means that their investigation addresses only one aspect of the problem. In the case of atrial fibrillation (AF), both approaches are easily available, and an increasing number of studies aim at exploring the precisely located substrate as well as its largely predominating if not exclusive modulating factor formed by the autonomic nervous system (ANS).

Electrophysiology and the autonomic nervous system

The now well-admitted predominance of arrhythmogenic foci located in the left atrium or the pulmonary veins probably makes the situation homogeneous in atrial tachyarrhythmias (Haïssaguère *et al.* 1998). Substrates are in essence of the same nature among patients, and they are also stable over time because structural changes are unlikely in tissues of supposedly embryonic origin that are not exposed to active pathological process. However, the respective role of this substrate and its modulation in arrhythmia genesis needs to be evaluated to explain the large variation in clinical pattern between patients. From Fig. 55.1, it is possible to envisage that the severity of the arrhythmias may be owing either to substrate activity or to its sensitivity to the ANS: the proportion each contributes is necessarily different between substrates and between patients. The largely predominant activity of a substrate can be close to 100%, thus being responsible for an almost permanent tachyarrhythmia, whereas a somewhat inactive substrate only fires when particularly favourable conditions of its environment are operating, as result of abnormal conditions of the ANS or of an abnormal sensitivity of the focus to their influence.

Many factors contribute to make the analysis of the ANS and its influence on electrophysiological mechanism of arrhythmias difficult (Levy 1990). The anatomical distribution of the neural fibres is different for vagal and sympathetic innervation, the latency time and duration of the physiological response also differs, so that the combination of inhomogeneity of the autonomic effects in space and time may have deleterious effects, although these are difficult to dissociate and analyse. Sympathetic and parasympathetic terminals lie in close proximity to one another, and both are close to the target cells, but they do not have an identical distribution (Ninomyia 1966). Stimulation of the sympathetic system may affect vagal function and vice versa. For example, acetylcholine released from vagal nerve endings diminishes noradrenaline release from

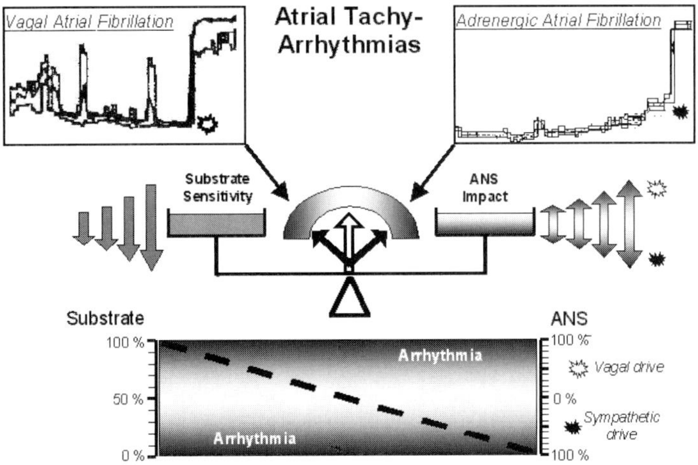

Fig. 55.1 Role of the substrate and the autonomic nervous system in arrhythmia genesis. Upper panels, trends of heart rate preceding the onset of a vagally mediated AF (left panel, progressive slowing) and an adrenergic AF (right panel, heart rate acceleration). Middle diagram, the balance between the ANS impact and the substrate sensitivity: either of them may attain the maximal 100% level, but the ANS impact may concern either the sympathetic and the vagal drive, both of them being potentially arrhythmogenic. Lower panel, the quantification of the role of the substrate in the arrhythmia genesis ranges from 0% to 100%. The ANS impact may also range from 0% to 100%, but either branch of the system can be operative.

neighbouring sympathetic nerve endings. The functional responses to cholinergic stimulation occurs within a few milliseconds, while those to adrenergic stimulation require seconds for target activation (Levy *et al.* 1993). This temporal difference, which has important clinical implications for heart rate variability, certainly also applies to atrial vulnerability (Allessi *et al.* 1958). Isoproterenol reduces the action potential but not duration of the refractory period, whereas acetylcholine shortens both and provokes a cellular hyperpolarization. There are consistent arguments to suggest that atrial vulnerability to vagal stimulation mainly depends on the shortening of the wavelength of the atrial impulse which then favours the formation of macro-re-entrant circuits such as flutter. Recently, Schauerte and co-workers have shown that modification of the transvascular atrial parasympathetic nerve system by radiofrequency catheter ablation could abolish vagally mediated AF, thus proving the major role played by parasympathetic tone on the induction and/or maintenance of AF (Schauerte *et al.* 2000). It is not clear whether these agents have different effects on conduction velocity, and overall whether normal and diseased atria react in the same way. Comparing data from different studies is difficult because the conditions of experiments are rarely strictly comparable, and apparently negligible differences may in fact be crucial. Finally, the spatial dispersion of refractoriness can be increased by various manipulations including acetylcholine as well as complete autonomic blockade (Rensma *et al.* 1990). Although some effects such as action potential shortening may apparently coincide with the vagal and sympathetic actions, there are indeed many contrasts between atrial vulnerability resulting from vagal or sympathetic activity. Micro-re-entries, automatic and triggered activities are more likely to occur as a consequence of a predominant sympathetic stimulation. Another important factor that is frequently neglected is the rate-dependence of any electrophysiological parameter (refractoriness, conduction speed) and of some arrhythmogenic mechanisms: the bradycardia-dependence of the early afterdepolarizations contrasts with the tachycardia-dependence of delayed afterdepolarizations, and therefore the ANS-induced heart rate changes in the sinus node do have an indirect influence on the arrhythmogenesis.

Finally, there is a predominance of vagal influences in normal atria, and vagal withdrawal is an early characteristic of diseased hearts that precedes even the increase of the sympathetic drive. Thus much remains to be determined, but the clinician can speculate that if either limb of the ANS may produce arrhythmogenic effects, these are more likely to occur through the vagal limb in normal tissues, and the sympathetic arm in diseased tissues.

Clinical considerations on paroxysmal atrial fibrillation

Studying patients with frequent attacks of paroxysmal AF recorded at Holter, we observed that according to the trend of sinus rate preceding the arrhythmia onset on a short- or mid-term basis, and taking into account the conditions of occurrence of the attacks, two opposite patterns and mechanisms could be distinguished. What we qualified at the time of 'vagal' and 'adrenergic' paroxysmal AF are rather easy to identify provided the clinical history of the patient is closely examined and attention paid to changes in heart rate before arrhythmia onset (Coumel *et al.* 1982; Coumel 1992).

Vagally mediated AF typically is more frequent in men than in women, and the patients usually have no structural cardiac disease ('lone' AF). The age at first symptom is relatively young, between 30 and 50 years. The usual history is that of weekly episodes, lasting a few hours and predominantly occurring at night. The morning period is the commonest time for spontaneous conversion into sinus rhythm. There are definitely no attacks during the day between breakfast and lunch, during which sympathetic predominance probably protects against the potentially deleterious effect of vagal influences. Neither physical exertion nor emotional stress triggers the arrhythmia. However, the relaxed period that follows effort or emotional stress may be the time of an attack. Rest, post-prandial state, particularly after dinner, and alcohol are also precipitating factors. In fact, a necessary condition for the diagnosis is the trend of heart rate preceding the attacks, which usually consistently shows a progressive decrease over time that may range from hours (Fig. 55.1 left panel) to a few minutes.

In contrast, paroxysmal AF that are adrenergically mediated occur preferentially at daytime, during activity or even exercise. They can be observed in the absence of heart disease, but this is less frequent than in vagally mediated AF. Exceptional diseases like phaeochromocytoma can be occasionally identified. Hyperthyroidism must be looked for attentively, particularly in women: not unusually, AF attacks may precede the clinical or even biological evidence of hyperthyroidism. Finally, if truly 'idiopathic' forms indeed exist, in valvular or myocardial diseases the role of sympathetic influences at the onset of the arrhythmia is predominant when systematically studied at Holter. A trend of heart rate acceleration is very often present and precedes the arrhythmia by a few hours or just a few minutes (see Fig. 55.1 right panel).

Correlations of electrophysiology and clinical data

As long as an episode of paroxysmal AF was not recorded in a given patient whose history is known, one cannot accurately conclude whether and how the ANS conditions the AF onset. We observed several patients with nocturnal attacks thus suggesting a vagally mediated AF, but the recording revealed an adrenergic mechanism. On the other hand, vagal AF are frequent at daytime, but they often appear as a rebound to adrenergic stimulation. The two limbs of the ANS form an unstable balance making it difficult to distinguish the actual role of action and reaction in arrhythmia genesis. In Fig. 55.2 demonstrates an example: clearly an adrenergic stimulation generated a vagal reaction but qualifying the AF as 'vagal' or 'adrenergic' would not be justified although there is no doubt that ANS changes were indeed responsible for the arrhythmia on a very short-term basis.

The clinical symptoms of AF, particularly palpitations, may be lacking during the attacks, as mentioned by Savelieva & Camm (2000) and confirmed by our experience. Symptoms may be lacking in paroxysmal AF in up to 25% of the cases (Lévy *et al.* 1999), although this is less often than in sustained forms of AF. Even though the reasons for the presence or absence of symptoms are unclear, our clinical experience with vagal or adrenergic paroxysmal AF indicates that the tolerance to arrhythmia is related to the autonomic nervous system; in practice vagally

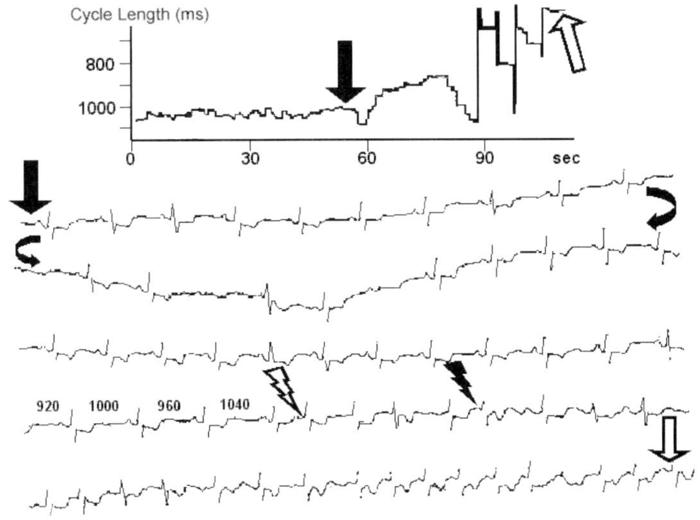

Fig. 55.2 The onset of a paroxysmal AF. Upper panel, the heart rate on a cycle-by-cycle basis, the last 30 s show a sudden unstable situation that is clearly at the origin of the arrhythmia onset. A sinus rate acceleration of sympathetic origin (perhaps in reaction to an initial transient slowing) is followed by a dramatic vagal rebound: it is not possible to define which of these opposite ANS shifts triggers the AF. The arrows point to the atrial premature beat (open arrow) and to the AF onset (solid arrow), respectively.

mediated paroxysmal AF are less symptomatic than adrenergic AF.

In general, our experience is that vagally-mediated paroxysmal AF form about one-third of the cases, adrenergically mediated AF 10–15%, with the rest remaining undetermined. We recognize that these proportions may be arbitrary, and that studies are conflicting on this particular point. For instance, Hnatkova *et al.* (1988) did not find any significant differences in the heart rate of various groups of patients before AF onset. Mixing patients with opposite trends tends to mask the presence of different groups, and classifying patients strictly depends on the predefined conditions of the analysis. Defining the limits of heart rate is obviously necessary for methodological reasons, but when defining a gradient of heart rate, there are absolutely no reasons for preferring increments or decrements of 10 or 5 rather than 2 beats/min over a certain period of time, or for choosing to consider the heart rate over 10 or 30 min rather than 1 or 24 h.

The trend of heart rate may not be the best tool to explore the role of the ANS in these patients, although it strictly correlates with heart rate variability (HRV) when the ratio of low- and high-frequency variations in the spectral analysis (Coumel *et al.* 1994) are considered. A number of studies using HRV aimed to penetrate deeper in the comprehension of ANS changes, and to help differentiate and to quantify the vagal and sympathetic influences on the sinus rhythm, but conflicting results have been reported (Coccagna *et al.* 1997; Dimmer *et al.* 1998; Herweg *et al.* 1998; Wen *et al.* 1998; Klingenheben *et al.* 1999). A shift towards vagal predominance was observed essentially in patients with paroxysmal AF and a structurally normal heart (Fioranelli *et al.* 1999; Klingenheben *et al.* 1999), especially in young patients with nocturnal AF (Herweg *et al.* 1998) or in patients with paroxysmal AF related to pulmonary vein foci (Zimmermann & Kalusche, 2001). Several observations suggest that most patients with lone paroxysmal AF are vagally dependent, with a heightened susceptibility to vasovagal cardiovascular response, whereas most patients with organic paroxysmal AF are more dependent on sympathetics (Coumel 1993; Herweg *et al.* 1998; Huang *et al.* 1998; Lok & Lau 1998). On the other hand some authors have suggested that there is an increase in sympathetic tone (or a loss of vagal tone) before the onset of paroxysmal AF in certain subsets of patients (Dimmer *et al.* 1998; Wen *et al.* 1998; Fioranelli *et al.* 1999; Tai *et al.* 2000).

Bettoni & Zimmermann recently published the most documented study involving the largest group of patients and using a careful HRV analysis. They considered spectral and time-domain parameters during periods of 24 and 1 h, and four successive periods of 5 min preceding 147 episodes of AF in 77 patients. In two-thirds of the patients the history was not suggestive of any ANS precipitating influence, and a vagal factor was more frequent (24%) than adrenergic influences (10%) in the others. A surprisingly homogeneous pattern of HRV was found among the various groups, including a primary increase in adrenergic drive occurring over at least 20 min before onset of paroxysmal AF, followed by a shift in the autonomic tone towards more vagal predominance immediately before onset of paroxysmal AF. There were no significant differences between patients with lone AF and those with structural heart disease, episodes observed at daytime or at night, the latter having however more vagal influences. The authors conclude that there was 'a primary increase in adrenergic drive occurring over at least 20 min before onset of paroxysmal AF followed by a shift in the autonomic tone towards more vagal predominance immediately before onset of paroxysmal AF'. Their observations are very much in favour of a global effect of the ANS with a complex and permanent interaction between both branches of the system, thus making somewhat artificial the Manichean distinction between the adrenergic and the vagal drive. Conceivably, and knowing the relative lack of reliability of the clinical history, it may be that the symptoms may predominate clinically without necessarily including a close correlation with the actual physiology of the ANS. Conceivably, the presence or absence of structural heart disease (including a higher mean 24-h heart rate in the former), the diurnal or nocturnal occurrence of the attacks may play an important role.

There is an additional important theoretical limitation in the interpretation of these findings, with particular reference to Levy's (1995) comments on the significance of the conditions of experiments and observations. Figure 55.3 illustrates a particular situation in the respective role of the substrate and the ANS for substrate *sensitivity* rather than for the *power* of the ANS influences on this substrate. If the arrhythmia fires at the peak of an exercise-induced sinus tachycardia (Fig. 55.3 right panel), then there is no doubt that the tachyarrhythmia is adrenergically dependent. If, on the other hand, a much less marked trend of acceleration precedes the tachyarrhythmia in another patient (Fig. 55.3 left panel), then the role of adrenergic stimulation seems much less marked, although the contrary may well apply. In this latter case, it is possible that the arrhythmia substrate was indeed very

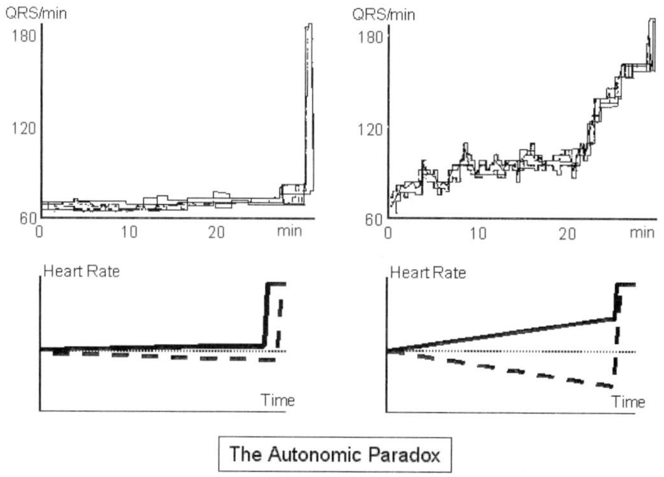

Fig. 55.3 The autonomic paradox. The upper panels display two examples of tachyarrhythmias following a heart rate acceleration. The adrenergic stimulation obviously is more marked on the right panel compared to the left one, and the trends are diagrammatically represented in the lower panels. Taking substrate *sensitivity* to the ANS rather *intensity* of adrenergic stimulation into account, it becomes clear that the role of the ANS on arrhythmia genesis is more important in the case shown on the compared to the one on the right. This illustrates the concept of the adrenergic paradox, that logically has its equivalence in the vagal domain, as shown by the dashed lines of heart rate slowing in the lower panels.

sensitive to a limited adrenergic stimulation, that is, with reference Fig. 55.1, the difference between the two cases is simply formed by a much greater impact of the ANS in the left, compared to the right panels of the figure. Of course, what applies to adrenergic influences can also apply to the vagal ones, as represented on the diagrams in dashed lines showing the heart rate trends. What we proposed to call the adrenergic paradox (Coumel 1987, 1993) is a concept that should actually be extended to the notion of autonomic paradox. The autonomic paradox is just a corollary of Levy's (1971) accentuated vagal antagonism. This concept supposes that the stronger the adrenergic stimulation, the stronger the vagal counter-reaction it induces, and this is just what we observed in the situation of Fig. 55.2.

The practical consequence of the concept of the autonomic paradox is that the analysis and interpretation of the HRV behaviour must be approached with extreme cautioun as it is possible that the more visible a phenomenon, the less important the real consequences of its influence. In other words, the significance of the quantitative analysis of HRV as well as the heart rate may well be biased by the inverted importance of the physiological influences in terms of sensitivity rather than direct impact of the ANS.

Conclusion

At variance from the situation at the ventricular level where the sympathetic influences are largely predominant, paroxysmal atrial tachyarrhythmias form the best model we have for studying the role of the arrhythmogenic substrate and its dependence on the actions of either limb of the autonomic nervous system. However, there are still important technical limitations to the exploration of the various factors involved, but this may not be the most important obstacle to the progression of our knowledge. We must be aware that knowing the pharmacological effect of adrenaline or acetylcholine on the action potential duration is undoubtedly insufficient if the *in situ* pathophysiology of the ANS is imperfectly known, and if its somewhat unexpected or even paradoxical effects are ignored. Both technical and theoretical progress are still necessary.

References

Allessi, R., Nusynowitz, M., Abildskov, J.A. *et al.* (1958) Nonuniform distribution of vagal effects on the atrial refractory period. *American Journal of Physiology*, **194**, 406–410.

Bettoni, M. & Zimmermann, M. (2002) Autonomic tone variations before the onset of paroxysmal atrial fibrillation. *Circulation*, **105**, 2753–2759.

Coccagna, G., Capucci, A., Bauleo, S. *et al.* (1997) Paroxysmal atrial fibrillation in sleep. *Sleep*, **20**, 396–398.

Coumel, P.H. (1992) Neural aspects of paroxysmal atrial fibrillation. In: *Atrial Fibrillation: Mechanisms and Management* (eds R. H. Falk & P. J. Podrid), pp. 109–125. Raven Press, New York.

Coumel, P., Maison-Blanche, P. & Catuli, D. (1994) Heart rate and heart rate variability in normal young adults. *Journal of Cardiovascular Electrophysiology*, **5**, 899–911.

Coumel, P. (1993) Cardiac arrhythmias and the autonomic nervous system. *Journal of Cardiovascular Electrophysiology*, **4**, 338–355.

Coumel, P. (1987) The management of clinical arrhythmias. An overview on invasive vs. noninvasive electrophysiology. *European Heart Journal*, **8**, 92–99.

Coumel, P.H., Attuel, P., Leclercq, J.F. *et al.* (1982) Arythmies auriculaires d'origine vagale ou catécholergique. Effets comparés du traitement bêta-bloquant et phénomène d'échappement. *Archives des Maladies du Coeur et des Vaisseaux*, **75**, 373–388.

Dimmer, C., Tavernier, R., Gjorgov, N. *et al.* (1998) Variations of autonomic tone preceding onset of atrial fibrillation after coronary artery bypass grafting. *American Journal of Cardiology*, **82**, 22–25.

Fioranelli, M., Piccoli, M., Mileto, G.M. *et al.* (1999) Analysis of heart rate variability five min before the onset of paroxysmal atrial fibrillation. *PACE (Pacing and Clinical Electrophysiolgy)*, **22**, 743–749.

Haïssaguère, M., Jaïs, P., Shah, D.C. *et al.* (1998) Spontaneous initiation of atrial fibrillation by ectopic beats originating in the pulmonary veins. *New England Journal of Medicine*, **339**, 659–666.

Herweg, B., Dalal, P., Nagy, B. *et al.* (1998) Power spectral analysis of heart period variability of preceding sinus rhythm before initiation of paroxysmal atrial fibrillation. *American Journal of Cardiology*, **82**, 869–874.

Hnatkova, K., Waktare, J.E.P., Murgatroyd, F.D. *et al.* (1988) Analysis of the cardiac rhythm preceding episodes of paroxysmal atrial fibrillation. *American Heart Journal*, **135**, 1010–1019.

Huang, J.L., Wen, Z.C., Lee, W.L. *et al.* (1998) Changes in autonomic tone before the onset of paroxysmal atrial fibrillation. *International Journal of Cardiology*, **66**, 275–283.

Klingenheben, T., Grönefeld, G., Li, Y.G. *et al.* (1999) Heart rate variability to assess changes in cardiac vagal modulation before the onset of paroxysmal atrial fibrillation in patients with and without structural heart disease. *Annals of Noninvasive Electrocardiography*, **4**, 19–26.

Levy, M.N. (1971) Sympathetic–parasympathetic actions in the heart. *Circulation Research*, **29**, 437–445.

Levy, M.N. (1995) Neural control of the heart: the importance of being ignorant. *Journal of Cardiovascular Electrophysiology*, **6**, 283–293.

Levy, M.N. (1990) Autonomic interactions in cardiac control. In: Coumel, P., Garfein, O.B. (eds) Electrocardiography: past and future. *Annals of the New York Academy of Sciences*, **601**, 209–221.

Levy, M.N., Yang, T. & Wallik, D.W. (1993) Assessment of beat-by-beat control of heart rate by the autonomic nervous system: molecular biology techniques are necessary, but not sufficient. *Journal of Cardiovascular Electrophysiology*, **4**, 183–190.

Lévy, S., Maarek, M., Coumel, P. *et al.* (1999) Characterization of different subsets of atrial fibrillation in general practice in France: the ALFA Study. *Circulation*, **99**, 3028–3035.

Lok, N.S. & Lau, C.P. (1998) Abnormal vasovagal reaction, autonomic function, and heart rate variability in patients with paroxysmal atrial fibrillation. *PACE (Pacing and Clinical Electrophysiolgy)*, **21**, 386–395.

Ninomyia, I. (1966) Direct evidence of nonuniform distribution of vagal effects on dog atria. *Circulation Research*, **19**, 576–583.

Rensma, P.L., Allessie, M.A., Lammers, W.J.E.P. *et al.* (1990) Length of excitation wave and susceptibility to re-entrant atrial arrhythmias in normal conscious dogs. *Circulation Research*, **62**, 395–400.

Savelieva, I. & Camm, A.J. (2000). Clinical relevance of silent atrial fibrillation: prevalence, prognosis, quality of life, and management. *Journal of Interventional Cardiac Electrophysiology*, **4**, 369–382.

Schauerte, P., Scherlag, B.J., Pitha, J. *et al.* (2000) Catheter ablation of cardiac autonomic nerves for prevention of vagal atrial fibrillation. *Circulation*, **102**, 2774–2780.

Tai CT, Chiou CW, Wen ZC *et al.* (2000) Effect of phenylephrine on focal atrial fibrillation originating in the pulmonary veins and superior vena cava. *Journal of the American College of Cardiology*, **36**, 788–793.

Wen, Z.C., Chen, S.A., Tai, C.T. *et al.* (1998) Role of autonomic tone in facilitating spontaneous onset of typical atrial flutter. *Journal of the American College of Cardiology*, **31**, 602–607.

Zimmermann, M. & Kalusche, D. (2001) Fluctuation in autonomic tone is a major determinant of sustained atrial arrhythmias in patients with focal ectopy originating from the pulmonary veins. *Journal of Cardiovascular Electrophysiology*, **12**, 285–291.

CHAPTER 56

Long Time Monitoring of Cardiac Rhythm in Patients with Atrial Fibrillation

Milos Kesek and Mårten Rosenqvist

Why monitor patients with atrial fibrillation?

More than 5% of all individuals older than 65 years suffer from atrial fibrillation. The range of symptoms varies from none to severely disabling. The disease carries a significant comorbidity and associated mortality. For reviews of atrial fibrillation see Falk (2001) and Carlsson *et al.* (2000).

Any therapy aims at treating the symptoms and/or reducing the comorbidity. These two goals can be in conflict with each other. Pharmacological treatment of arrhythmias aiming at reduction of symptoms can in some instances increase the risk for the patient.

Rhythm monitoring in clinical practice can:

- link symptomatology to objective findings such as heart rate or irregularity;
- detect asymptomatic periods of high or low heart rate in persistent arrhythmia and asymptomatic episodes of arrhythmia in paroxysmal atrial fibrillation;
- help to evaluate treatment;
- detect conditions treatable by catheter ablation or cardiac pacemaker, that can mimic atrial fibrillation.

In some cases of AV-nodal re-entry and concealed WPW-syndrome the initial regular tachycardia rapidly progresses to atrial fibrillation. Sinus node disease, a frequent cause of pacemaker implantation, is sometimes found in patients with paroxysmal atrial fibrillation. In these cases the atrial fibrillation can mask a condition for which specific treatment is available. Patients with atrial fibrillation also exhibit fast organized atrial activity (Israel *et al.* 2001b). This could be an expression of a coexisting atrial flutter. It has also been shown that the activity in atrial fibrillation is more organized when recorded from the atrial wall as compared to recordings from some distance within the atrial cavity (Baerman *et al.* 1990) (see below).

Paroxysmal atrial fibrillation

In patients with paroxysmal atrial fibrillation, the incidence of asymptomatic atrial fibrillation events is 3 -12 times higher than the incidence of symptomatic episodes (Page *et al.* 1994; Montenero *et al.* 2002). The burden of asymptomatic arrhythmias (percentage time spent in asymptomatic arrhythmia) is however unknown.

Why only some episodes are symptomatic is an unresolved issue. In a study of patients with implanted atrial cardioverter for paroxysmal atrial fibrillation, only 55% of the episodes caused the patients to seek for cardioversion. These episodes had significantly longer duration and higher maximal heart rate compared to the episodes that didn't prompt the patient to seek medical help (Frykman *et al.* 2002). In patients with atrial fibrillation and a conventional pacing indication, implantation of a DDDRP-pacemaker lead to a significant improvement in quality of life that was unrelated to the atrial fibrillation burden (Grönefeld *et al.* 2002).

Paroxysmal atrial fibrillation probably poses a similar risk of stroke as persistent atrial fibrillation (Hart *et al.* 2000). Detection of asymptomatic episodes of paroxysmal atrial fibrillation is clinically warranted if it can be shown that decreasing the burden of asymptomatic arrhythmia decreases the comorbidity. A surgical maze procedure diminishes the risk for stroke in patients with atrial fibrillation (paroxysmal or permanent) at high risk for thromboembolic complications (Cox *et al.* 1999). Emerging data indicate that catheter intervention in paroxysmal atrial fibrillation has a similar effect (Scavée *et al.* 2002).

Persistent and permanent atrial fibrillation

The patients experience discomfort to a various degree; 20–30% of the patients are asymptomatic (Savelieva & Camm, 2000). Monitoring can link a patient's symptoms to fast heart rate and strengthen the indication for an invasive procedure. Generally, the relation between symptomatology and objective findings is unclear. A Holter study on patients with persistent atrial fibrillation showed that approximately one third of the patients were asymptomatic during the monitoring. Presence of valvular heart disease was associated with symptoms while no difference was found between the asymptomatic and symptomatic patients with respect to heart rate, its irregularity or left ventricular function (Frykman *et al.* 2001). Further research in this area is necessary.

Development of monitoring devices

Technical progress during the last decade has resulted in small devices that offer monitoring possibilities during considerably longer periods than conventional Holter recordings. The technology has been incorporated in external ECG loop recorders capable of monitoring the heart activity during weeks. Implantable monitoring devices have more recently obtained similar capability, thus extending the possible duration of monitoring to years. These insertable loop recorders have been shown to be useful in the diagnosis of infrequent syncope of unknown origin (Krahn *et al.* 1999). The devices can record arrhythmias but do not yet have the capacity for automatic differentiation between various supraventricular tachycardias.

The evolution in the monitoring area has gained considerably from the development in the field of nonpharmacological therapies for arrhythmias. The ability of implantable devices to record measured data, rate histograms and events was developed for monitoring the activity of the device itself and optimizing the therapies. In DDD-pacing it has become desirable to prevent ventricular tracking of atrial tachycardias. General techniques for arrhythmia detection and storage of signal have emerged in the ICD-field. In order to minimize inappropriate ICD-therapies, there has also appeared a more specific need for automatic recognition of atrial tachycardias. The role of pacemakers and ICD-devices has thereby evolved from the domain of pure therapy towards collection of diagnostic data that can later be retrieved by the operator and used for decisions about the therapy strategy.

Due to technical limitations, some kind of selection and destructive compression of the information has to be applied in the storage process. The diagnostic capacity of the implantable devices was initially limited to cumulative counters and frequency histograms of intracardiac events. Any algorithmic classification that reduces the electrogram to counts is a source of error. Even with a correct classification, data from cumulative counters are crude as tools for evaluating arrhythmia episodes. A few, clinically highly significant arrhythmia episodes of 5 min duration will in the counter data be diluted into statistical insignificance by the 100 000 normal heart beats/day. When the data processing power of the devices increased, the storage was extended to counters of more complex sequences of intracardiac events, time based diagnostics in the form of histograms for repeated shorter periods of time (Defaye *et al.* 1998) and individual marker chains during selected events (Machado *et al.* 1996).

More recently it became feasible to store electrograms. This feature allows for a retrospective comparison of the automatic classification by the device with the underlying events. It should be noted that the amplification and filtering of the signal used for detection and classification may differ from the processing of the electrogram stored at the same time (Nowak 1999).

Signal acquisition

A far-field electrogram can be recorded between an electrode located in the heart (or possibly, in the central vessels) and the device can. The ventricular signal contains morphology information that can be useful for differentiating between supraventricular and ventricular tachyarrhythmias. A ventricular electrogram that exhibits the same morphology during arrhythmia as during sinus rhythm indicates a supraventricular rhythm. A wide, aberrant electrogram can result either from a ventricular rhythm or from a supraventricular rhythm with a conduction disturbance. Morphology features have little use in direct monitoring of atrial electrogram.

Devices connected to electrodes placed inside the heart can obtain bipolar electrograms. The signal is suitable for time measurements but less useful for morphology discrimination. Decreasing of the tip to ring distance in a bipolar electrode construction to a certain degree increases the amplitude of the signal and improves the detection of the atrial electrogram (Pignalberi *et al.* 2002). The relation of the distance between the two recording poles and the amplitudes of the local and far-field electrograms is however complex. Recordings from the atrial wall show a much higher amplitude and a more discrete electrogram with greater apparent organization than recordings from within the cavity (Baerman *et al.* 1990). The amplitude is higher with close bipolar spacing in recordings from the wall while the wider bipole spacing gives a somewhat higher electrogram amplitude in the cavity.

Some pacemakers can record cross-channel electrograms between atrial and ventricular electrodes.

Implantable electrodeless monitoring devices can collect a far-field subcutaneous electrogram suitable for arrhythmia analysis (Theres *et al.* 1998; Mazur *et al.* 2001). Direct detection of atrial fibrillation as fibrillatory waves in the low amplitude atrial far-field signal obtained by an electrodeless device will however remain a technical challenge. In a series of insertable looprecorders, P-waves were identified in less than half of the patients (Krahn *et al.* 1999). As opposed to devices with electrodes, the future algorithms for diagnosis of atrial fibrillation by the electrodeless devices will probably have to rely on a combination of indirect measures, such as variations in *RR* intervals (Fotuhi *et al.* 2001), absence of detectable P-waves and possibly a normal morphology of the ventricular electrogram.

Sensing, far-field R

Even during sinus rhythm the atrial signal occasionally has a low and variable amplitude, specially when recorded by a floating bipolar electrode in a VDD-pacemaker (Israel & Bockenforde, 1998). During atrial fibrillation the amplitude of the bipolar atrial signal is somewhat lower than during sinus rhythm and exhibits much greater variations (Leung *et al.* 1998).

Intermittent undersensing of the atrial electrogram will cause underdetection of arrhythmia. It will introduce an error in calculations of derived parameters that depend critically on adequate atrial sensing such as AV-synchrony and prevalence of premature ventricular complexes. In a dual chamber device (Israel *et al.* 2001), atrial undersensing can lead to a false positive diagnosis of ventricular arrhythmia. In several pacemakers currently in use, paradoxical undersensing of atrial tachyarrhythmias has been shown to occur: A programming to high sensitivity can give rise to a repeated artefact that causes blanking and undersensing, possibly resulting in underdetection, inappropriate modeswitching or even detection of a bradycardia during a true tachycardia (Willems *et al.* 2001). Automatic atrial sensitivity adjustment can be useful for improving the detection of atrial arrhythmias (Lam *et al.* 1999).

The far-field R-wave amplitude in bipolar atrial electrograms is around 0.2–0.5 mV (Cools *et al.* 2002; Brandt & Worzewski 2000). For sensed ventricular complexes it can occur up to 20 ms before the native R-wave is sensed in the ventricular channel, i.e. technically in the AV-interval. The amplitude of the far-field R is not constant in a given patient. It causes seldom clinical problems in modern pacemaker treatment of bradycardia. It however confounds the automatic tachycardia diagnostics and can in atrial anti tachycardia devices lead to delivery of inappropriate therapies. The operator can be reasonably confident to avoid oversensing after measuring the far-field R-wave sensing threshold in the acute setting and programming the atrial sensitivity at least 0.3 mV above this threshold (Cools *et al.* 2002). A mechanism has been designed for avoiding far-field R-oversense, namely the post ventricular atrial blanking period. It can however cause underdetection of atrial flutter when every second flutter wave occurs within the blanking period (Seidl *et al.* 1998; Lau *et al.* 2002a; Israel, 2002).

Occasionally, a biphasic atrial electrogram during sinus rhythm can cause double counting (near-field P-wave oversense).

Storage

Continuous long-term recording of the signal is technically still not within reach. When this approach becomes technically feasible it will generate an immense amount of data. Therefore, criteria for selection of relevant episodes will always have to be applied before the recording or analysis. This introduces a bias in the data available for the operator.

The compression of the signal in the storage process can remove relevant information. For discussion of sampling frequency, compression process, storage capacity and limitations inherent in counter data in current devices see Nowak (2002) and Israel & Barold (2001).

The storage can be symptom triggered when the patient activates the storing of the signal when he experiences an episode with some clinical symptom of arrhythmia. This is done by pushing a button or applying a magnet over the device. The stored data can afterwards be compared to a description in a patient diary. Alternatively, an arrhythmia can activate an automatic signal triggered storage.

Automatic detection of atrial arrhythmia

The detection algorithms are most often sensitive to the rate of the atrial electrogram.

With adequate sensing the atrial rate can differentiate sinus rhythm from tachyarrhythmia and initiate storage of markers and electrograms for later retrieval and evaluation. In a pacemaker the detection of atrial arrhythmias often implies a modeswitch. Several reviews of algorithms used for detection of atrial tachyarrhythmias and modeswitching in pacemakers have recently been published (Lau *et al.* 2002a, b; Israel, 2002). Mode-switch counter data have been used for evaluating the number of attacks of paroxysmal atrial fibrillation.

With a detection criterion set at 200 atrial complexes and a sensitivity of 0.5 mV, Fitts *et al.* found that only 3% of 1636 detected episodes of paroxysmal atrial fibrillation were classified as false positive in a population of patients with pacemakers implanted before AV-nodal ablation (Fitts *et al.* 2000). The evidence is indirect, as the classification was done by comparing the stored tachograms with typical patterns of sensed and paced events in far-field R-sense and near-field P-sense. No verification with stored electrograms was possible and the study doesn't give an estimation of underdetected episodes.

The counts are subject to errors due to underdetection as well as overdetection of arrhythmia. Reliable detection of atrial tachyarrhythmia and mode-switching depend on adequately programmed atrial sensitivity and atrial refractory periods. The variations in electrogram amplitude during atrial fibrillation often result in intermittent undersensing. A programming to high sensitivity, short refractory periods and low arrhythmia detection frequency on the other hand increases the problem with oversensing of a far-field R-wave. Both behaviours lead to inappropriate modeswitching and irrelevant number of modeswitch counts. In a validation study of the atrial high rate diagnostics in the same pacemaker model as above against Holter monitoring in patients with paroxysmal atrial fibrillation (Seidl *et al.* 1998), the authors observed 26% falsely negative episodes, mainly consisting of short runs of atrial fibrillation. The two long episodes consisted of 2:1 undersensed atrial flutter. A false positive detection was seen in 11% of episodes, corresponding to 11% of the arrhythmia burden as measured by the pacemaker.

In a study relating pacemaker-detected episodes of atrial tachycardia to recorded snapshots of the electrogram, 62% of all detected episodes were not true atrial tachycardias (Pollak *et al.* 2001). An episode with high atrial rate and long duration was more likely to be a true atrial tachyarrhythmia. Similar results emerged from an analysis of patients with dual-chamber or atrial ICD (Swerdlow *et al.* 2000). Far-field R-wave oversensing, frequent supraventricular extrasystole, supraventricular bigeminy and sinus tachycardia were the common pitfalls.

A comparison between Holter recordings and

pacemaker diagnostics of atrial fibrillation has found overdetection as well as underdetection of the arrhythmia (Plummer *et al.* 2001). The overdetection was mainly due to far-field R-wave oversensing. The underdetection was a smaller problem that was seen only during very short arrhythmia episodes. Examination of automatically stored electrograms from single lead VDD pacemaker systems revealed that only 35% of modeswitch episodes were adequate. The rest was due to atrial oversensing, mainly of a far-field R-wave (Israel *et al.* 2000).

Modeswitching is a fast but crude process and the parameters derived from event counters should be viewed with some caution. This is even more the case with the automatically generated diagnostic statements concerning physiological and pathological function that some devices generate on the basis of counter data. An estimate of arrhythmia burden i.e. proportion of time spent in arrhythmia is a more reliable measure than counter based data. Stored electrograms during arrhythmia episodes are desirable for verification of arrhythmia detections. A separate diagnostic unit that is more accurate than the mode switch unit is desirable for differential diagnosis of an atrial tachyarrhythmia that may be followed by device therapy, as well as for reliable diagnostic data. Future technical development may accommodate for several useful methods outlined below that are currently unsuitable for use in implantable devices due to the need for computational power and energy demand.

Onset recording

Storage of onset of the triggering episode helps the operator to resolve many disputable episodes of automatically stored rhythm (McMeekin *et al.* 2002). The loop recorders, some ICDs and pacemakers employ an endless loop technique for storing information immediately before the start of an assumed episode. The signal is recorded in a circular buffer, continuously overwriting the previously collected information. When a storage trigger is activated, the most recent information recorded in the buffer is 'frozen' and stored. Stored onsets of atrial arrhythmias are useful for investigation of the events immediately preceding the start of atrial fibrillation. It has been shown that in the initiation of atrial fibrillation, the 'long-short-long' sequence is a rare pattern (Copperman *et al.* 2002).

Analysis of *AA* intervals during atrial fibrillation

An analysis of mean atrial cycle length, its standard deviation and coefficient of variation was able to separate between patients with sinus rhythm, ongoing atrial fibrillation and atrial flutter (Jung *et al.* 1998). For atrial fibrillation, such straightforward rate calculations are however dependent on recording conditions and physical properties of the electrode, which limits their usefulness for precise automatic detection of atrial fibrillation. A global electrogram overestimates the frequency of atrial fibrillation in comparison to the frequency of the local activity (Baerman *et al.* 1990). There is no simple answer to the question of what the atrial frequency is during atrial fibrillation. Analyses of the frequency content of atrial fibrillation in surface ECG, oesophageal ECG and intracardiac recordings have shown the median and mean peak frequencies to be in the range of 5–6.5 cycles/s (Baerman *et al.* 1990; Pehrson *et al.* 1998).

Analysis of *RR* intervals

In ICD-therapy, stability of consecutive *RR*-cycle lengths is often used as an additional criterion for differentiating between atrial fibrillation and ventricular tachycardia. In atrial fibrillation with high ventricular rate (>170 bpm) the variations in *RR*-cycle length are however too small for an acceptable discrimination by a simpler stability algorithm (Kettering *et al.* 2001). More complex algorithms have been developed that analyse the *RR*-variability in frequency domain. These diagnose atrial fibrillation with a sensitivity and specificity of 95–100% for episodes down to duration of less than 100 heart beats when applied to Holter recordings (Duverney *et al.* 2002).

Monitoring of heart rate variability

Paroxysmal atrial fibrillation has links with the autonomic nervous system (Gillis *et al.* 2001;

Lombardi & Tundo 2002; Zimmermann & Bettoni 2002). Symptoms from paroxysmal atrial fibrillation may be related to autonomic dysfunction. Impaired autonomic function predicts dizziness at onset of atrial fibrillation (van den Berg, 2001). Patients with lone paroxysmal atrial fibrillation exhibit impaired quality of life (at level with patients suffering from angina) (van den Berg *et al.* 2001). One predictor for this impairment is depressed autonomic function.

RR intervals stored in an ICD before an arrhythmic event have already been used for a retrospective computation of heart rate variability. An exciting possibility is automatic continuous monitoring of autonomic balance by implanted devices that compute the heart rate variability. Such a procedure cannot be applied in patients that are largely pacemaker dependent or exhibit frequent arrhythmias. Some time domain measures of heart rate variability are however relatively insensitive to ectopic beats and could be useful in an automated processing of a signal containing arrhythmias (Malik *et al.* 1999).

Continuous monitoring of heart rate variability could also be investigated in patients with ongoing atrial fibrillation. The variations of *RR* intervals during atrial fibrillation are related to vagal tone (van den Berg, 1997). In a study of patients with permanent atrial fibrillation, cardiac death was associated with a low heart rate variability measured by conventional measures and a low *RR* irregularity measured by approximate entropy (a relative measure useful for comparison of regularity between multiple series of measurements) (Yamada *et al.* 2000). In a small group of patients with severe mitral insufficiency and permanent atrial fibrillation, depressed heart rate variability was found to correlate to the need for mitral surgery but not to mortality during follow-up (Stein *et al.* 1994). The authors anticipated that the autonomous influence on the AV-node is comparable to that to the sinus node and should affect the function along the same direction. Heart rate variability during atrial fibrillation has however by far not the same distinct interpretation and prognostic impact as during sinus rhythm. An investigation of *AA* intervals and *RR* intervals during induced atrial fibrillation indicated that the input to the AV-node during atrial fibrillation has random frequency. During atrial fibrillation, the autonomous influence would thus not be reflected in the *RR* interval variability.

Signal-averaged P wave

Signal-averaged P wave parameters acquired from surface ECG discriminate between patients with paroxysmal atrial fibrillation and controls (Ishimoto *et al.* 2000). The method requires a sampling rate about 10 times higher than the sampling rate used in current implantable devices (Nowak 2002). It has, however, been applied to Holter recordings that usually use much lower sampling rates (Kasamaki *et al.* 2002). In monitoring devices it could be used for predicting exacerbations in patients with paroxysmal atrial fibrillation.

The patients with atrial fibrillation have often associated morbidity with risk of malignant ventricular arrhythmias. The drugs used for treatment are potentially proarrhythmic. A possible role for the monitoring in atrial fibrillation might therefore be detection of markers for ventricular arrhythmias. This development will probably be powered by the strong commercial interests in the ICD-field. Some pacemakers have features for diagnosis of ventricular arrhythmias. The current algorithms seem however unreliable and ventricular oversensing (Israel *et al.* 2000) or atrial undersensing can lead to false positive diagnosis of ventricular arrhythmia.

Approximately 10–13% of a mixed population implanted with a DDD-pacemaker have paroxysmal atrial fibrillation (Lamas *et al.* 1995) or will within 2 years develop atrial fibrillation (Gross *et al.* 1990). In the future nearly all pacemakers can be expected to contain advanced diagnostic features able to reliably track asymptomatic events. This capacity in excess of the clinical needs in large populations could be employed in epidemiological studies using hard endpoints with a relatively low incidence in populations with asymptomatic atrial tachyarrhythmia.

Problems

The monitoring devices collect a huge amount of information but a lot of the data have not a clear meaning within our current knowledge. New facets of cardiac physiology are exposed by the possibilities; we do not know what is normal and what implications the findings have.

The information stored in a device is dependent on the setting of the sensing parameters and detection algorithms. These differ between the available products. The signal collection and condensing of information is done differently in the various systems. A comparison between various devices or even between similar devices with different programming is unreliable. The different algorithms must thus be individually validated. Their performance should also ideally not be dependent on a too complex individual programming.

There is not much room left for devices constructed by independent scientists. The technical development is in the hands of commercial interests that decide or largely influence the choice of hardware and algorithms. These in turn determine the data on which we base our knowledge.

References

Baerman, J.M., Ropella, K.M., Sahakian, A.V. *et al.* (1990) Effect of bipole configuration on atrial electrograms during atrial fibrillation. *PACE (Pacing and Clinical Electrophysiology)*, **13**, 78–87.

Brandt, J. & Worzewski, W. (2000) Far-field QRS complex sensing: prevalence and timing with bipolar atrial leads. *PACE (Pacing and Clinical Electrophysiology)*, **23**, 315–320.

Carlsson, J., Neuzner, J. & Rosenberg, Y.D. (2000) Therapy of atrial fibrillation: rhythm control vs. rate control. *PACE (Pacing and Clinical Electrophysiology)*, **23**, 891–903.

Cools, F.J.C., Backers, J., van Twembeke, R. *et al.* (2002) Failure of acute threshold testing to prevent far field R wave sensing. *Europace*, **3** (abstract).

Copperman, Y., Glick, A., Hochenberg, M. *et al.* (2002) Onset pattern analysis of paroxysmal atrial fibrillation based on a DDRP pacemaker with extended diagnostics. *Europace*, **3**, 127 (abstract).

Cox, J.L., Ad, N. & Palazzo, T. (1999) Impact of the maze procedure on the stroke rate in patients with atrial fibrillation. *Journal of Thoracic Cardiovascular Surgery*, **118**, 833–840.

Defaye, P., Dournaux, F. & Mouton, E. (1998) Prevalence of supraventricular arrhythmias from the automated analysis of data stored in the DDD pacemakers of 617 patients: the AIDA study. The AIDA Multicentre Study Group. Automatic Interpretation for Diagnosis Assistance. *PACE (Pacing and Clinical Electrophysiology)*, **21**, 250–255.

Duverney, D., Gaspoz, J.M., Pichot, V. *et al.* (2002) High accuracy of automatic detection of atrial fibrillation using wavelet transform of heart rate intervals. *PACE (Pacing and Clinical Electrophysiology)*, **25**, 457–462.

Falk, R.H. (2001) Atrial fibrillation. *New England Journal of Medicine*, **344**, 1067–1078.

Fitts, S.M., Hill, M.R., Mehra, R. *et al.* (2000) High rate atrial tachyarrhythmia detections in implantable pulse generators: low incidence of false-positive detections. The PA Clinical Trial Investigators. *PACE (Pacing and Clinical Electrophysiology)*, **23**, 1080–1086.

Fotuhi, P., Combs, W., Condie, C. *et al.* (2001) R-wave detection by subcutaneous ECG. Possible use for analyzing *RR* variability. *Annals of Noninvasive Electrocardiology*, **6**, 18–23.

Frykman, V., Ayers, G.M., Darpö, B. & Rosenqvist, M. (2003) What characterizes episodes of atrial fibrillation requiring cardioversion? Experience from patients with an implantable atrial cardioverter. *American Heart Journal*, **145** (4), 670–675.

Frykman, V., Frick, M., Jensen-Urstad, M. *et al.* (2001) Asymptomatic vs. symptomatic persistent atrial fibrillation: clinical and noninvasive characteristics. *Journal of Internal Medicine*, **250**, 390–397.

Gillis, A.M., Connolly, S.J., Dubuc, M. *et al.* (2001) Circadian variation of paroxysmal atrial fibrillation. PA3 Investigators. Atrial Pacing Peri-ablation for Prevention of Atrial Fibrillation Trial. *American Journal of Cardiology*, **87**, 794–798.

Grönefeld, G., Ehrlich, A., Israel, C.W. *et al.* (2002) Pacing therapy in patients with paroxysmal atrial fibrillation: correlation between atrial tachycardia burden and quality of life. *Europace*, **3**, 35 (abstract).

Gross, J., Moser, S., Benedek, Z.M. *et al.* (1990) Clinical predictors and natural history of atrial fibrillation in patients with DDD pacemakers. *PACE (Pacing and Clinical Electrophysiology)*, **13**, 1828–1831.

Hart, R.G., Pearce, L.A., Rothbart, R.M. *et al.* (2000) Stroke with intermittent atrial fibrillation: incidence and predictors during aspirin therapy. Stroke Prevention in Atrial Fibrillation Investigators. *Journal of the American College of Cardiology*, **35**, 183–187.

Ishimoto, N., Ito, M. & Kinoshita, M. (2000) Signal-averaged P-wave abnormalities and atrial size in patients with and without idiopathic paroxysmal atrial fibrillation. *American Heart Journal*, **139**, 684–689.

Israel, C.W. (2002) Analysis of mode switching algorithms in dual chamber pacemakers. *PACE (Pacing and Clinical Electrophysiology)*, **25**, 380–393.

Israel, C.W. & Barold, S.S. (2001) Pacemaker systems as implantable cardiac rhythm monitors. *American Journal of Cardiology*, **88**, 442–445.

Israel, C.W. & Bockenforde, J.B. (1998) Pacemaker event counters: possible sources of error in calculation of AV synchrony in VDD single lead systems as an example for present limitations. *PACE (Pacing and Clinical Electrophysiology)*, **21**, 489–493.

Israel, C.W., Gascon, D., Nowak, B. *et al.* (2000) Diagnostic value of stored electrograms in single-lead VDD systems. *PACE (Pacing and Clinical Electrophysiology)*, **23**, 1801–1803.

Israel, C.W., Grönefeld, G., Iscolo, N. *et al.* (2001a) Discrimination between ventricular and supraventricular tachycardia by dual chamber cardioverter defibrillators: importance of the atrial sensing function. *PACE (Pacing and Clinical Electrophysiology)*, **24**, 183–190.

Israel, C.W., Hugl, B., Unterberg, C. *et al.* (2001b) Pace-termination and pacing for prevention of atrial tachyarrhythmias: results from a multicentre study with an implantable device for atrial therapy. *Journal of Cardiovascular Electrophysiology*, **12**, 1121–1128.

Jung, J., Hohenberg, G., Heisel, A. *et al.* (1998) Discrimination of sinus rhythm, atrial flutter, and atrial fibrillation using bipolar endocardial signals. *Journal of Cardiovascular Electrophysiology*, **9**, 689–695.

Kasamaki, Y., Jiazina, T., Yanagawa, S. *et al.* (2002) P-wave SAECG using Holter monitoring in patients with paroxysmal atrial fibrillation. *Europace*, **3**, 68 (abstract).

Kettering, K., Dornberger, V., Lang, R. *et al.* (2001) Enhanced detection criteria in implantable cardioverter defibrillators: sensitivity and specificity of the stability algorithm at different heart rates. *PACE (Pacing and Clinical Electrophysiology)*, **24**, 1325–1333.

Krahn, A.D., Klein, G.J., Yee, R. *et al.* (1999) Use of an extended monitoring strategy in patients with problematic syncope. Reveal Investigators. *Circulation*, **99**, 406–410.

Lam, C.T., Lau, C.P., Leung, S.K. *et al.* (1999) Improved efficacy of mode switching during atrial fibrillation using automatic atrial sensitivity adjustment. *PACE (Pacing and Clinical Electrophysiology)*, **22**, 17–25.

Lamas, G.A., Pashos, C.L., Normand, S.L. *et al.* (1995) Permanent pacemaker selection and subsequent survival in elderly Medicare pacemaker recipients. *Circulation*, **91**, 1063–1069.

Lau, C.P., Leung, S.K., Tse, H.F. *et al.* (2002a) Automatic mode switching of implantable pacemakers: I. Principles of instrumentation, clinical, and hemodynamic considerations. *PACE (Pacing and Clinical Electrophysiology)*, **25**, 967–983.

Lau, C.P., Leung, S.K., Tse, H.F. *et al.* (2002b) Automatic mode switching of implantable pacemakers: II. Clinical performance of current algorithms and their programming. *PACE (Pacing and Clinical Electrophysiology)*, **25**, 1094–1113.

Leung, S.K., Lau, C.P., Lam, C.T. *et al.* (1998) Programmed atrial sensitivity: a critical determinant in atrial fibrillation detection and optimal automatic mode switching. *PACE (Pacing and Clinical Electrophysiology)*, **21**, 2214–2219.

Lombardi, F. & Tundo, F. (2002) Heart rate variability in atrial fibrillation. *Europace*, **3**, 25 (abstract).

Machado, C., Johnson, D., Thacker, J.R. *et al.* (1996) Pacemaker patient-triggered event recording: accuracy, utility, and cost for the pacemaker follow-up clinic. *PACE (Pacing and Clinical Electrophysiology)*, **19**, 1813–1818.

Malik, M., Padmanabhan, V. & Olson, W.H. (1999) Automatic measurement of long-term heart rate variability by implanted single-chamber devices. *Medical & Biological Engineering & Computing*, **37**, 585–594.

Mazur, A., Wang, L., Anderson, M.E. *et al.* (2001) Functional similarity between electrograms recorded from an implantable cardioverter defibrillator emulator and the surface electrocardiogram. *PACE (Pacing and Clinical Electrophysiology)*, **24**, 34–40.

McMeekin, J., Nowak, B., Coutu, B. *et al.* (2002) Onset-recordings and markers improve diagnostic value of electrograms in pacemakers. *Europace*, **3**, 127 (abstract).

Montenero, A.S., Quayyum, A., Franciosa, P. *et al.* (2002) Atrial fibrillation: Role of the loop recorder to identify the initiating mechanism and monitor patients. *Europace*, **3**, 163.

Nowak, B. (1999) Taking advantage of sophisticated pacemaker diagnostics. *American Journal of Cardiology*, **83**, 172D–179D.

Nowak, B. (2002) Pacemaker stored electrograms: teaching us what is really going on in our patients. *PACE (Pacing and Clinical Electrophysiology)*, **25**, 838–849.

Page, R.L., Wilkinson, W.E., Clair, W.K. *et al.* (1994) Asymptomatic arrhythmias in patients with symptomatic paroxysmal atrial fibrillation and paroxysmal supraventricular tachycardia. *Circulation*, **89**, 224–227.

Pehrson, S., Holm, M., Meurling, C. *et al.* (1998) Noninvasive assessment of magnitude and dispersion of atrial cycle length during chronic atrial fibrillation in man. *European Heart Journal*, **19**, 1836–1844.

Pignalberi, C., Ricci, R., Santini, L. *et al.* (2002) Role of the tip to ring spacing as a determinant of a better sensing in a new pacing lead. *Europace*, **3**, 48 (abstract).

Plummer, C.J., Henderson, S., Gardener, L. *et al.* (2001) The use of permanent pacemakers in the detection of cardiac arrhythmias. *Europace*, **3**, 229–232.

Pollak, W.M., Simmons, J.D., Interian, A., Jr *et al.* (2001) Clinical utility of intraatrial pacemaker stored electrograms to diagnose atrial fibrillation and flutter. *PACE (Pacing and Clinical Electrophysiology)*, **24**, 424–449.

Savelieva, I. & Camm, A.J. (2000) Clinical relevance of silent atrial fibrillation: prevalence, prognosis, quality of life, and management. *Journal of Interventional Cardiac Electrophysiology*, **4**, 369–382.

Scavée, C., Jais, P., Weerasooriya, R. *et al.* (2002) Reduced thromboembolism risk following atrial fibrillation ablation. *Europace*, **3**, 193 (abstract).

Seidl, K., Meisel, E., VanAgt, E. *et al.* (1998) Is the atrial high rate episode diagnostic feature reliable in detecting paroxysmal episodes of atrial tachyarrhythmias? *PACE (Pacing and Clinical Electrophysiology)*, **21**, 694–700.

Stein, K.M., Borer, J.S., Hochreiter, C. *et al.* (1994) Variability of the ventricular response in atrial fibrillation and prognosis in chronic nonischaemic mitral regurgitation. *American Journal of Cardiology*, **74**, 906–911.

Swerdlow, C.D., Schsls, W., Dijkman, B. *et al.* (2000) Detection of atrial fibrillation and flutter by a dual-chamber implantable cardioverter-defibrillator. For the Worldwide Jewel AF Investigators. *Circulation*, **101**, 878–885.

Theres, H., Combs, W., Fotuhi, P. *et al.* (1998) Electrogram signals recorded from acute and chronic pacemaker implantation sites in pacemaker patients. *PACE (Pacing and Clinical Electrophysiology)*, **21**, 11–17.

van den Berg, M.P., Haaksma, J., Brouwer, J. *et al.* (1997) Heart rate variability in patients with atrial fibrillation is related to vagal tone. *Circulation*, **96**, 1209–1216.

van den Berg, M.P., Hassink, R.J., Tuinenburg, A.E. *et al.* (2001) Quality of life in patients with paroxysmal atrial fibrillation and its predictors: importance of the autonomic nervous system. *European Heart Journal*, **22**, 247–253.

Willems, R., Holemans, P., Ector, H. *et al.* (2001) Paradoxical undersensing at a high sensitivity in dual chamber pacemakers. *PACE (Pacing and Clinical Electrophysiology)*, **24**, 308–315.

Yamada, A., Hayano, J., Sakata, S. *et al.* (2000) Reduced ventricular response irregularity is associated with increased mortality in patients with chronic atrial fibrillation. *Circulation*, **102**, 300–306.

Zimmermann, M. & Bettoni, M. (2002) Fluctuations of autonomic tone before onset of paroxysmal atrial fibrillation. *Europace*, **3**, 41 (abstract).

SECTION VI
Ventricular Arrhythmias

CHAPTER 57

Monitoring Ectopic Activity

Bogdan G. Ionescu, Xavier Vinolas, Iwona Cygankiewicz, Antoni Bayes Genis and Antoni Bayes de Luna

Introduction

The surface electrocardiogram (ECG) is of limited value for detecting the presence of arrhythmias because it represents a short period of time. Various studies have demonstrated the advantage of longer recordings, especially using Holter technology, to better detect the incidence of cardiac arrhythmias in health and disease.

In this chapter we will comment on the different techniques for monitoring ventricular arrhythmias and their advantages and disadvantages.

Methods of monitoring

Electrocardiogram

The simplest way to get information about heart rate and rhythm is to perform a 12-lead routine ECG. The conventional ECG strip shows rhythm and conduction abnormalities.

Surface ECG in a population of males, survivors of a myocardial infarction (MI), highlights the predictive power of recording of a simple premature ventricular complex (PVC). The presence of one PVC in 1 min of ECG recording predicts huge numbers of PVC in 24-h recordings and correlates highly with cardiac mortality during a 3 year follow-up (CDP Research Group 1973).

Different surface techniques have been used to predict the occurrence of malignant arrhythmias. The time-domain signal-averaging technique gives us information about the risk of sudden death (SD), but unfortunately with a low positive predictive value (Breithardt *et al.* 1991). In Fig. 57.1, signal-averaged ECGs from a normal subject, and a patient with arrhythmogenic right ventricular dysplasia that met all the criteria for the presence of late potentials, are shown.

In the past few years, measurement of alternans of ECG waves, especially repolarization-microvolt T wave alternans have increased in importance as a marker of fatal ventricular arrhythmias (Rosenbaum *et al.* 1994).

Exercise stress testing

Exercise stress testing gives us information on heart rate and rhythm during a standardized exercise test, usually a treadmill exercise lasting 5–15 min.

Continuous ECG monitoring is performed during the whole duration of exercise. Normally, a progressive increase in heart rate occurs as a marker of chronotropic competence of the heart. The usefulness of exercise stress testing resides in its sensitivity to detect ischaemia-related changes of ventricular repolarization (Tavel 2001).

The appearance or any increase in the number of PVCs during exercise testing has proved to be a suggestive marker of future cardiovascular events. Nevertheless, it has recently been demonstrated that descent of the ST segment in PVCs is more reliable for detecting ischaemia than changes in the sinusal complexes (Rasouli *et al.* 2001).

Holter electrocardiography

Since Norman J. Holter introduced the basis of continuous electric monitoring of the heart in 1957 and since the first device became commercially available in 1960, new avenues have opened in the field of arrhythmia diagnosis and management.

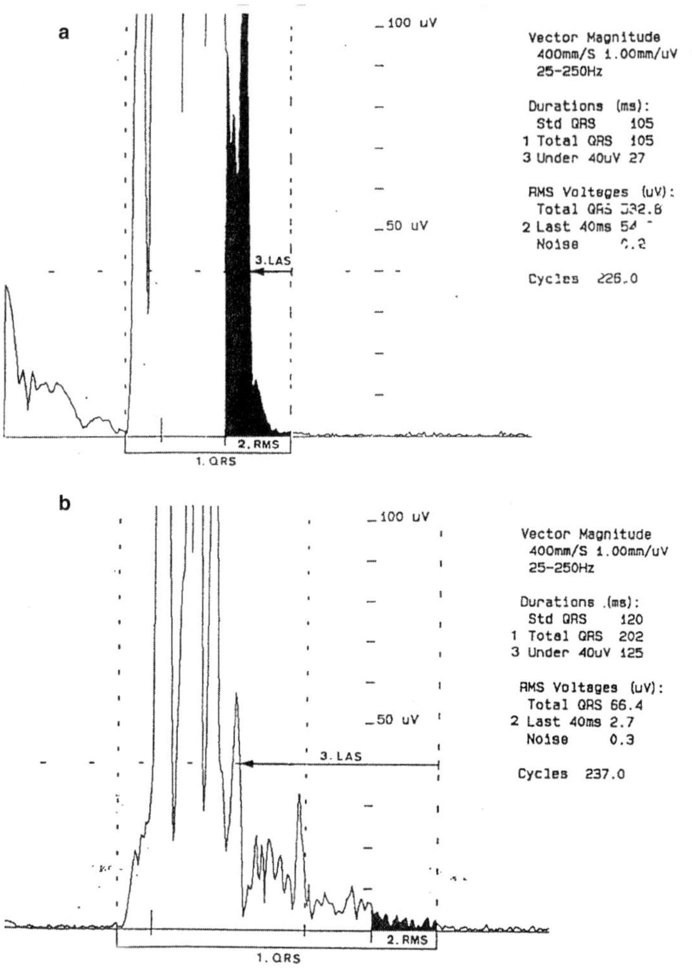

Fig. 57.1 Recording of late potentials in a normal subject (a) and in a patient with right ventricular dysplasia (a).

Holter ECG recordings, whose duration may vary from a few hours to one or even several days, provide the clinical electrophysiologist with a wide spectrum of data. Usually most devices record three orthogonal ECG tracings, or even 12-lead ECG. Introduction of long-term electric monitoring of the heart was a step forward in the diagnosis of heart rhythm and rate disturbances.

Usually, Holter reports comprise a full count of normal and premature beats, or runs of premature beats. Analysis of *RR* sequences permits calculation of the heart rate. Moreover, now we can record heart rate variability, dynamics of *QT* (Laguna *et al.* 1990; Bayes de Luna & Vinolas 1996; Homs *et al.* 1997; Caminal *et al.* 1998), and late potentials. Therefore we have information not only about the presence of ventricular arrhythmia, but also about the risk to present arrhythmias in the future.

It is difficult to know how many hours of Holter ECG recording are necessary to ensure that the results obtained are true evidence of the presence of disease, with prognostic significance, and may repeat in future recordings. Ruberman *et al.* (1981a), studied 1 h of recording and Bigger *et al.* (1986), and Moss *et al.* (1987), 24 h of continuous recordings. Nevertheless, according to Morganroth *et al.* (1978) if the length of recording is 24 h, a reduction of 83% of PVCs is required to be sure that this reduction is the result of treatment. For a recording of 72 h, a reduction of 65% in the number of PVCs is sufficient.

Normal individuals

In normal individuals without any history of manifest cardiac disease, Holter monitoring shows the normal occurrence of PVCs and their

Table 57.1 Holter recordings in apparently normal subjects (Bayes de Luna 1983)

Study	*Sample*	*Hours of registration*	*Prevalence of PVCs*
Kleiger *et al.* (1974a)	51, ages 35–65	10	45
Engel *et al.* (1975)*	35, ages 24 ± 4	7.5	29
Clarke *et al.* (1976)	86, ages 16–65	48	73
Raftery *et al.* (1976)	52, ages 20–79	24	15
Verbaan *et al.* (1977)	74, ages 20–80	24	76
Kennedy *et al.* (1977)	23, ages 35–66	24	30
Goulding (1977)	100, ages 25–74	24	27
Brodsky *et al.* (1977)	50, ages 23–27	24	50
Federman *et al.* (1978)	21, ages 40–66	24	48
Djiane *et al.* (1979)	50, ages 22–57	24	22
Kostis *et al.* (1979)	100, ages 16–68	24	46
Bayes de Luna *et al.* (1980a, b)	27, cases		
	18, ages 18–23	24	16.5
	9, ages 17–22	10	44
Bethge *et al.* (1980)	121, ages 18–70	10	31

* Cited by Brodsky *et al.* (1977).

Table 57.2 Prevalence of PVCs in post-MI patients (Bayes de Luna 1983)

Study	*No. of patients*	*Time of registration*	*% with PVCs*
CDP (1973)	2035	1 min	11.5
Moss *et al.* (1971)	100	6 h	72
Kotler *et al.* (1973)	160	10–12 h	43
Kleiger *et al.* (1974b)	141	10–24 h	91
Myburgh *et al.* (1974)	84	6–7 h	73
Moss *et al.* (1975)	193	6 h	51
Vismara *et al.* (1975)	56	10 h	73
Wenger *et al.* (1975)	100	22 h	88
Tuna *et al.**	104	24 h	36
Bayes de Luna *et al.* (1980c)	449	24 h	65

* Cited by Bayes de Luna 1983.

benign prognostic significance (Table 57.1) (Bayes de Luna 1983)

Post-myocardial infarction patients

The incidence of PVCs shortly after myocardial infarction is much higher in 6–24 h recordings than in a standard 12-lead ECG (Table 57.2). In some series, patients with >10 PVCs/h had a mortality rate 2.5–4.0 times higher compared with patients with a lower incidence of PVCs. Moreover, increased prevalence of pairs or short runs of PVCs was associated with a high risk of death, independent of that of isolated PVCs (Ruberman *et al.* 1981b; Bigger *et al.* 1986; Moss *et al.* 1987). The prognosis was worse particularly when ventricular function was diminished (Figs 57.2 and 57.3).

The risk of post-MI patients is related to the presence of different markers, especially those related to electrical instability, left ventricular dysfunction, and residual ischaemia (Fig. 57.4).

Heart failure

Patients with heart failure of different aetiologies, present PVCs and/or runs of complex ventricular arrhythmias (Table 57.3). Nevertheless, there is no clear relation between the presence of ventricular arrhythmia and sudden death (Table

In mitral valve prolapse, life-threatening ventricular arrhythmia is rare. However, the presence of a long QT or an electrolyte imbalance may add a supplementary risk.

Sudden cardiac death

Final arrhythmia. Sudden cardiac death (SCD) is defined as naturally occurring death of cardiac origin (excluding accidents, suicides, poisoning and so on) that completes within 1 h after the onset of the symptoms of death (Bayes de Luna 1983). Unwitnessed SD is so defined if the subject was seen alive in the 24 h preceding the event. The final events before SD vary in different subsets of patients (Fig. 57.5), in early phases of acute coronary syndromes (ACS) (Adgey *et al.* 1982) and in ambulatory patients (Bayes de Luna *et al.* 1989). In patients with end-stage heart failure, a lower incidence of ventricular tachyarrhythmias was found, and the most frequent cause of death in these patients was a bradyarrhythmia (Luu *et al.* 1989).

Markers of sudden death. We have commented about the importance of different markers of sudden death, especially in post-MI patients (Figs 57.2–57.4). Patients with coronary artery disease, left ventricular dysfunction (LVEF < 40%), and asymptomatic unsustained ventricular tachycardia, in whom sustained ventricular tachycardia was inducible have a higher probability to suffer sudden death or cardiac arrest, and a higher mortality than noninducible patients (Buxton *et al.* 2000).

Moss *et al.* (1996) suggested that in coronary patients with nonsustained ventricular tachycardia and electrophysiological inducible sustained ventricular tachycardia (VT), implantable cardioverter defibrillator (ICD) therapy reduces the incidence of death. Moreover, MADIT II trial demonstrated that in post-MI patients with lower LVEF (<30%), implantation of ICD significantly reduces global mortality and might be a prophylactic therapeutic alternative (Moss *et al.* 2002).

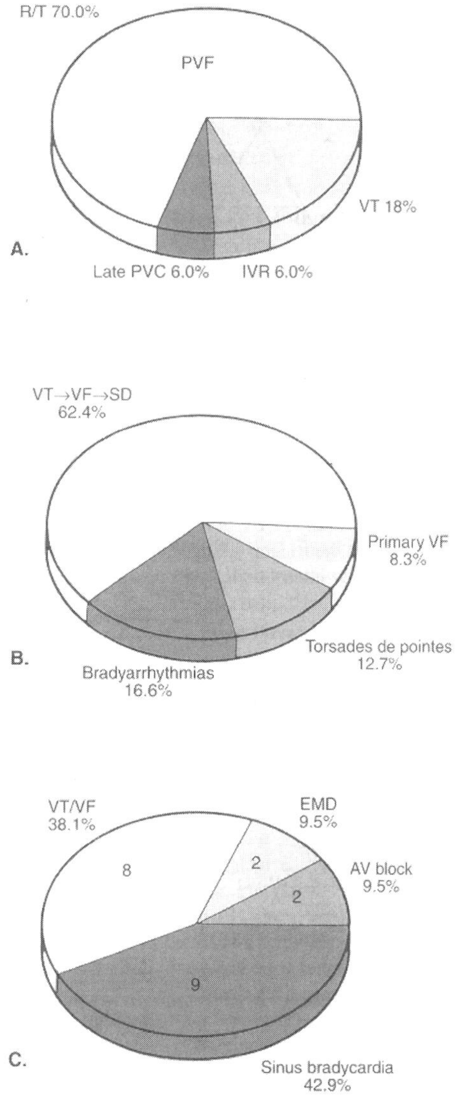

Fig. 57.5 A. The proportions of final arrhythmia in patients with cardiac arrest during the acute phase of MI; B. Causes of ambulatory sudden death recorded by Holter electrocardiography; C. Incidence of final events in patients with advanced heart failure who died suddenly (R/T, R-on-T phenomenon; PVF, primary ventricular fibrillation; PVC, premature ventricular contractions; IVR, idioventricular rhythm; VT, ventricular tachycardia; PVF, primary ventricular fibrillation, VF, ventricular fibrillation; EMD, electromechanical dissociation; AV, atrioventricular).

Holter monitoring and treatment of arrhythmia

The efficacy of antiarrhythmic drug treatment in cardiac disease patients was assessed by Morganroth *et al.* (1978), Sami *et al.* (1980) by the diminution of PVC in Holter recordings

Table 57.5 Reduction of PVCs after therapeutic intervention

Time of monitoring	No. of periods		% reduction		
Hours	*Control*	*Test*	*PVC*	*Pairs*	*VT*
Morganroth et al. (1978)					
12	1	1	89	87	71
24	1	1	83	75	66
24	3	3	65	55	45
24	7	7	49	41	32
Sami et al. (1980)					
% of PVC per h in 24 monitoring	1	1	% Reduction		
2.2–3	1	1	100		
3–5	1	1	80–90		
5.5–11	1	1	70–80		
11–20	1	1	68–70		
20–30	1	1	65–68		
30 or more	1	1	65		

Table 57.6 Arrhythmia-induced therapy in carriers of ICDs (Marchlinski *et al.* 1993)

Diagnosis	*EGM morphology same as baseline**	*Mean CL (ms)*	*Cycle length variability†*
Probable VT	No	>260	No
Rapid VT/VF	No	≤260	No/yes
Probable regular SVT	Yes	>260	No
AF	Yes	>260	Yes

* During some VT the electrogram morphology may be very similar to the baseline rhythm: development of the bundle branch block ipsilateral to the side of the recording, leads to a change of the electrogram morphology during the supraventricular tachycardias.

† Cycle length variability is present if there is greater than 60 ms difference in cycle length for 3/10 intervals.

before and after treatment, and was previously commented on in this chapter (Table 57.5).

Patients with implantable cardioverter defibrillation
Sensing circuits incorporated in the device have made it possible to save intracavitary registries before arrhythmic episodes. Therapy (intracavitary rapid pacing or internal shock) is delivered as the sensing circuit detects a sustained sequence of short *RR* intervals. The mechanism of initiation of ventricular tachycardias can be analysed, as well as the outcome after the therapy delivery.

Various attempts have been made to enable software to distinguish between ventricular and supraventricular tachycardias by the pattern of QRS (amplitude of R wave, QRS area), to avoid inappropriate shocks in tachyarrhythmias not of ventricular origin. New dual chamber devices allow simultaneous analysis of atrial and ventricular activity to better discriminate ventricular vs. supraventricular arrhythmias.

As heart rate exceeds a certain programmed limit and falls within one of the tachycardia zones previously defined by the operator, Holter recording starts, providing a posteriori the full picture of the arrhythmic episode. Therapy may then be further adjusted.

Marchlinski *et al.* (1993) synthesized the rhythms that may trigger therapy in carriers of ICD, as shown in Table 57.6.

Table 57.7 Comparison between various techniques in different pathological settings (Bayes de Luna 1983)

Arrhythmia	*Holter*	*Exercise stress testing*	*Events recorder*
Sporadic arrhythmias	+	–	++
Exercise induced arrhythmia	+	++	+
Frequent arrhythmia	++	+	+

Patients with pacemaker

In patients in whom an antibradycardia device has been implanted, external ECG monitoring is useful in detecting isolated failure of capture, owing to the failure of electric circuits. Holter functions of the device provide information about periods of pacing or sensing, as heart rate falls below or above the ranges imposed by the operator. In physiological devices, changes of pacing mode may also reflect variations in heart rate particularly as a result of a supraventricular arrhythmia.

Event recorders

Instantaneous monitoring of isolated arrhythmic events can be achieved by events recording systems that allow ambulatory patients to activate the system as many times as symptoms occur. Furthermore, these systems allow remote transmission of ECG data to a medical centre for processing by medical specialists. Event recorders provide an excellent correlation between a wide spectrum of clinical manifestations such as palpitations, dizziness, presyncope, and even syncope and concomitant ECG data on a large time base.

Recently introduced loop recording implantable devices (Brignole *et al.* 2001) allow patients to self-activate monitoring as symptoms occur. Loops of one- or two-channel ECG tracings are continuously generated and subsequently stored in the memory of the device as the patient activates the system by pressing a remote control button. The full picture of the ECG before and after the clinical event thus becomes available. Also, the device may activate automatically as heart rate enters the ranges previously defined by the clinician. The implantable devices are small and have batteries that last up to 14 months. The operator must clear the memory after every cycle of clinical events and subsequent activation to ensure that free space is available for subsequent events. A complete picture of arrhythmic events facilitates diagnosis of arrhythmia in difficult clinical cases, permitting clinical decision making such as the start of medical therapy, and implantation of antitachycardia or antibradycardia devices.

The comparison between different methods

The usefulness of various techniques of monitoring ventricular electric activity in various clinical settings is displayed in Table 57.7. From the table it can be seen that event and loop recorders are the best options for sporadic arrhythmia and syncope, exercise testing is best for arrhythmia induced by exercise, and Holter the technique of choice of monitoring for frequent arrhythmias.

References

Adgey, A.A., Devlin, J.E., Webb, S.W. & Mulholland H.C. (1982) Initiation of ventricular fibrillation outside the hospital in patients with ischaemic heart disease. *British Heart Journal*, **47**, 55–61.

Bayes de Luna, A. (ed.) (1983) Electrocardiografía de Holter – Enfoque Práctico, Ed científico-médica.

Bayes de Luna, A., Coumel, P. & Leclerq, J.F. (1989) Ambulatory sudden death: mechanisms of production of fatal arrhythmias on the basis of data from 157 cases. *American Heart Journal*, **117**, 151–159.

Bayes de Luna, A., Serra Grima, J.R., Julia, J., Riba, J. & Sadurni, J. (1980c) Prevalence, prognosis, and treatment of ventricular premature complex. *Revista Espanola de Cardiologia*, **33**, 425–441.

Bayes de Luna, A., Trilla, E., Turull, J. *et al.* (1980a) Arrhythmias and alterations of repolarization in the young healthy adult. In: *VIII European Congress of Cardiology Paris, P.* 180, abstract.

Bayes de Luna, A., Trilla, E., Turull, J. *et al.* (1980b) Seminario Nuove Frontiere delle aritmie Ed Furlanello (abstract).

Bayes de Luna, A. & Vinolas, X. (1996) QT dispersion and heart rate variability. *European Heart Journal*, **17** (2), 165–166.

Bethge, K.P., Meiners, G. & Lichtlen, P.R. (1980) Incidence of ventricular dysrrhythmia in normal. In: *VIII European Congress of Cardiology Paris*, 1980.

Bigger, J.T., Fleiss, J.L., Kleiger, R., Miller, J.P., Rolnitzky, L.M. and the Multicentre Post-Infarction Research Group (1984) The relationship between ventricular arrhythmia, left ventricular dysfunction and mortality in the 2 years after myocardial infarction. *Circulation*, 69, 250–258.

Bigger, J.T., Jr, Fleiss, J.L. & Rolnitzky, L.M. (1986), Prevalence, characteristics and significance of ventricular tachycardia detected by 24-h continuous electrocardiographic recordings in the late hospital phase of acute myocardial infarction, *American Journal of Cardiology*, **58** (13), 1151–1160.

Breithardt, G., Cain, M.E., el-Sherif, N. *et al.* (1991) Standards for analysis of ventricular late potentials using high resolution or signal-averaged electrocardiography. A Statement by a Task Force Committee between the European Society of Cardiology, The American Heart Association and the American College of Cardiology, European Society of Cardiology, Rotterdam, the Netherlands. *Circulation*, **83** (4), 1481–1488.

Brignole, M., Menozzi, C, Moya, A. & Garcia-Civera, R. (2001) Implantable loop recorder: towards a gold standard for diagnosis of syncope? *Heart*, **85** (6), 610–612.

Brodsky, M., Wu, D., Denes, P., Kanakis, C. & Rosen, K.M. (1977) Arrhythmias detected by 24 h continuous ECG monitoring in 50 male medical students without apparent heart disease. *American Journal of Cardiology*, **39**, 390.

Buxton, A.E., Lee, K.L., DiCarlo, L. *et al.* (2000) Eletrophysiological testing to identify patients with coronary artery disease who are at risk for sudden death. Multicentric Unsustained Tachycardia Trial Investigators. *New England Journal of Medicine*, **342** (26), 1937–1945.

Caminal, P., Blasi, A., Valverdu, M. *et al.* (1998) New algorthythm for QT dispersion analysis in XYZ-lead Holter ECG. Performance and applications. *IEEE (Institute of Electrical and Electronic Engineers) Computing in Cardiology*, 709–712.

Chakko, C.S. & Gheorghiade, M. (1985) Ventricular arrhythmias in severe heart failure: Incidence, significance, and effectiveness of antiarrhythmic therapy. *American Heart Journal*, **109**, 497.

Clarke, J.M., Hamer, V., Shelton, J.R., Taylor, S. & Venning, G.R. (1976) The rhythm of the normal human heart. *Lancet*, **1** (7084), 508–512.

Cleland, J.G.F., Chattopadhyay, A.K., Khand, A., Houghton, T. & Kaye, G.C. (2002) Prevalence and incidence of arrhythmias and sudden death in heart failure. *Heart Failure Reviews*, **7** (3), 229–242.

CDP (Coronary Drug Project) Research Group (1973) Prognostic importance of premature beats following myocardial infarction. *JAMA (Journal of the American Medical Association)*, **223** (10), 1116–1124.

Djiane, P., Egre, A., Bory, M., Savin, B., Mostefa, S. & Serradimigmi, A. (1979) L'enregistrement ECG chez les sujets normaux. *Archives des Maladies du Coeur et des Vaisseaux*, **72** (6), 655–661.

Federman, J., Withford, J.A., Anderson, S.T. & Pitt, A. (1978) Incidence of ventricular arrhythmias in the first year after myocardial infarction. *British Heart Journal*, **40** (11), 1243–1250.

Fletcher, R.D., Cintron, G.B., Johnson, G., Orndorff, J., Carson, P., Cohn, J.N. for the V-HeFT II VA Cooperative Studies Group (1993) Enalapril decreases prevalence of ventricular tachycardia in patients with chronic congestive heart failure. *Circulation*, **87**, VI49–V155.

Francis, G.S. (1986) Development of arrhythmias in the patient with congestive heart failure: Pathophysiology, prevalence and prognosis. *American Journal of Cardiology*, **57** (3), 3B–7B.

Goulding, L. (1977) *24 h Ambulatory ECG Recording from Normal Urban and Rural Population*, pp. 13–22. Harrow (England).

Guindo, J., Bayés Genis, A., Dominguez de Rozas, J.M., Fiol, M., Vinolas, X. & Bayes de Luna, A. (1996) Sudden death in heart failure. *Heart Failure Reviews*, **1**, 249–260.

Holter, N.J. (1957) Radioelectrocardiography: a new method technique for cardiovascular studies. *Annals of the New York Academy of Sciences*, **65**, 913.

Holter, N.J. (1961) New method for heart studies. *Science*, **134**, 1214.

Holmes, J., Kubo, S.H., Cody, R.J. & Kligfield, P. (1985) Arrhythmias in ischaemic and nonischaemic dilated cardiomyopathy: prediction of mortality by ambulatory electrocardiography. *American Journal of Cardiology*, **55** (1), 146–151.

Homs, E., Marti, V., Guindo, J. *et al.* (1997) Automatic measurement of corrected *QT* interval in Holter recordings: comparison of its dynamic behaviour in patients after myocardial infarction with and without life-threatening arrhythmias. *American Heart Journal*, **134** (2 Pt 1), 181–187.

Huang, S.K., Messer, J.V. & Denes, P. (1983) Significance of ventricular tachycardia in idiopathic dilated cardiomyopathy; observations in 35 patients. *American Journal of Cardiology*, **51** (3), 507–512.

Kennedy, H.L., Caralis, D.G., Kahn, M.A., Poblete, P.F. & Pescarmona, J.E. (1977) Ventricular arrhythmias 24 h before and after maximal treadmill testing. *American Heart Journal*, **94** (6), 718–724.

Kleiger, R.E. & Senior, R.M. (1974a) Long term ECG monitoring of ambulatory patients with chronic airway obstruction. *Chest*, **65** (5), 483–487.

Kleiger, R.E., Martin, T.F., Miller, S.P. & Oliver, G.C. (1974b) Ventricular tachycardia and ventricular extrasystoles during the late recovery phase and myocardial infarction. *American Journal of Cardiology*, **33**, 194.

Kotler. M, Tabatznik, B., Mower, M.M. & Tominage, S. (1973) Prognostic significance of ventricular ectopic beats with respect to sudden death in the late postinfarction period. *Circulation*, **47** (5), 959–966.

Kostis, J.B., Moreyra, A.E., Natarajen, N. *et al.* (1979) Ambulatory ECG. What is normal? *American Journal of Cardiology*, **43**, 420 (abstract).

Laguna, P., Thakor, N.V., Caminal, P. *et al.* (1990) New algorithm for *QT* interval analysis in 24-h Holter ECG: performance and applications. *Medical & Biological Engineering & Computing*, **28** (1), 67–73.

Luu, M., Stevenson, W.G., Stevenson, L.W., Baron, K., Walden, J. (1989) Diverse mechanisms of unexpected sudden death in advanced heart failure. *Circulation*, (80) **6**, 1675–1670.

Marchlinski, F.E., Gottlieb, C.D., Sarter, B. *et al.* (1993) ICD data storage: value in arrhythmic management. *PACE (Pacing and Clinical Electrophysiolgy)*, **16** (3 Pt 2), **527**, 24.

Maron, B.J., Savage, D.D., Wolfson, J.K. & Epstein, S.E. (1981) Prognostic significance of 24 h ambulatory electrocardiographic monitoring in patients with hypertrophic cardiomyopathy: a prospective study. *American Journal of Cardiology*, **48** (2), 252–257.

Maskin, C.S., Siskind, S.J. & LeJemtel, T.H. (1984) High prevalence of nonsustained ventricular tachycardia in severe congestive heart failure. *American Heart Journal*, **107** (5 Pt 1), 896–901.

McKenna W.J. & Iglesias L. M. (2000), Identification y tratamiento de los pacientes con miocardiopatía hipertrófica y riesgo de muerte súbita. *Revista Espanola de Cardiologia*, **53**, 123–130.

Meinertz, T., Hofman, T., Kasper, W. *et al.* (1984) Significance of ventricular arrhythmias in idiopathic dilated cardiomyopathy. *American Journal of Cardiology*, **53** (7), 902–907.

Morganroth, J., Michelson, E.L., Horowitz, L.N., Josephson, M.E., Pearlman, A.S. & Dunkman, W.B. (1978) Limitations of routine long-term electrocardiographic monitoring to assess ventricular ectopic frequency. *Circulation*, **58** (3), 408–414.

Moss, A.J., Schnitzler, R., Green, R. & Decamilla, J. (1971) Ventricular arrhythmias three weeks after acute myocardial infarction. *Annals of Internal Medicine* **75** (6), 837–841.

Moss, A.J., DeCamilla, J., Mietlowski, W., Greene, V.A., Goldstein, S. & Locksley, R. (1975) Prognostic grading and significance of PBV after recovery from myocardial infarction. *Circulation*, **51** (6 Suppl), 204–210.

Moss, A.J., Bigger, J.T., Jr & Odoroff, C.L. (1987) Postinfarct risk stratification. *Progress in Cardiovascular Diseases*, **29** (6), 389–412.

Moss, A.J., Hall, W.J., Cannom, D.S. *et al.* (1996) Improved survival with an implanted defibrillator in patients with coronary artery disease at high risk for ventricular arrhythmia. Multicentric Automatic Defibrillator Implantation Trial Investigators. *New England Journal of Medicine*, **335** (26), 1933–1940.

Moss, A.J., Zareba, W., Hall, W.J. *et al.* (2002) Prophylactic implantation of a defibrillator in patients with myocardial infarction and reduced ejection fraction. *New England Journal of Medicine*, **346** (12), 877–883.

Mukharji, J., Rude, R.E., Poole, K. and the MILIS Investigators (1984) Risk factors for sudden death after acute myocardial infarction: two years of follow-up. *American Journal of Cardiology*, **54** (1), 31–36.

Myburgh, D.P. & Ven Gelder, A.L. (1974) The nature of ventricular ectopic beats in chronic ischaemic heart disease. *South African Medical Journal*, **48** (25), 1067–1071.

Packer, M. (1992) Lack of correlation between ventricular arrhythmias and sudden death in patients with chronic heart failure. *Circulation*, **85** (1 Suppl.), 150–156.

Raftery, E.B. & Cashman, P.M. (1976) Longterm recording of the ECG in normal population. *Postgraduate Medical Journal*, **52** (Suppl. 7), 32–38.

Rasouli, M.L. & Ellestad, M.H. (2001) Usefulness of ST depression in ventricular premature complexes to predict myocardial ischemia. *American Journal of Cardiology*, **87**, 891–894.

Rosenbaum, D.S., Jackson, L.E., Smith, J.M., Garan, H., Ruskin, J.N. & Cohen, R.J. (1994) Electrical alternans and vulnerability to ventricular arrhythmias. *New England Journal of Medicine*, **330** (4), 235–241.

Ruberman, W., Weinblatt, E., Goldberg, J.D., Frank, C.W. & Shapiro, S. (1977) Ventricular premature beats and mortality after myocardial infarction. *New England Journal of Medicine*, **297** (14), 750–757.

Ruberman, W., Weinblatt, E., Frank, C.W., Goldberg, J.D. & Shapiro, S. (1981a) Repeated 1 h electrocardiographic monitoring of survivors of myocardial infarction at 6 months intervals: arrhythmia detection and relation to prognosis. *American Journal of Cardiology*, **47** (6), 1197–1204.

Ruberman, W., Weinblatt, E., Goldberg, J.D., Frank, C.W., Chaudhary, B.S. & Shapiro, S. (1981b) Ventricular premature complexes and sudden death after myocardial infarction. *Circulation*, **64** (2), 297–305.

Sami, M., Kraemer, H., Harrison, D.C., Houston, N., Shimasaki, C. & DeBusk, R.F. (1980) A new method for evaluating antiarrhythmic drug efficacy. *Circulation*, **62** (6), 1172–1179.

Singh, B.N. (2002) Significance and control of cardiac arrhythmias in patients with congestive heart failure. *Heart Failure Reviews*, **7** (3), 285–300.

Tavel, M.E. (2001) Stress testing in cardiac evaluation: current concepts with emphasis on the ECG. *Chest*, **119** (3), 907–925.

Unverferth, D.V., Magorien, R.D., Moechsberger, M.L., Baker, P.B., Fetters, J.K. & Leier, C.V. (1984) Factors influencing one-year mortality of dilated cardiomyopathy. *American Journal of Cardiology*, **54** (1), 147–152.

Verbaan, C.J., Pool, J. & Vanroy, J.V. (1977) Incidence of cardiac arrhythmias in a presumed healthy population. In: *International Symposium on Holter Monitoring*, pp. 1–3. Harrow (England).

Vismara, L.A., Anderson, E.A. & Mason, D.T. (1975) Relation of ventricular arrhythmia in the late hospital phase of acute myocardial infarction to sudden death after hospital discharge. *American Journal of Medicne*, **59** (1), 6–12.

Von Olshausen, K., Schafer, A., Mehmel, H.C., Schwartz, F., Senges, J. & Kubler, W. (1984) Ventricular arrhythmias in idiopathic dilated cardiomyopathy. *British Heart Journal*, **51** (2), 195–201.

Wenger, T.L., Bigger, J.T. & Merrill, G.S. (1975) Ventricular arrhythmias in the late phase of acute myocardial infarction. *Circulation*, **52** (Suppl. II), 110.

Wilson, J.R., Schwartz, J.S., Sutton, MS-J. *et al.* (1983) Prognosis in severe heart failure: relation to hemodynamic measurements and ventricular ectopic activity. *Journal of the American College of Cardiology*, **2** (3), 403–410.

CHAPTER 58

Circadian Pattern of Arrhythmic Episodes

Yi-Fang Guo and Phyllis K. Stein

Many functions of living organisms exhibit predictable variations, called biological rhythms. Biological rhythms can be divided into three types based on their cycle lengths: circadian (or diurnal) rhythms with a period of about 24 h; ultradian rhythms, with a period significantly shorter than 24 h (hours, minutes or even seconds); and infradian rhythms, with a period longer than 24 h (days, months or longer). Circadian rhythms in the functioning of the cardiovascular system are well known. Most cardiovascular physiological parameters (heart rate, blood pressure, cardiac output, ECG measurements, etc.) and pathophysiological events (myocardial ischaemia, arrhythmias, and sudden cardiac death) show this feature (Saitoh 2000). It has been well established that diurnal changes in the cardiovascular system are clinically significant and should be considered in diagnosis and treatment.

Circadian patterns in the onset of arrhythmic events have been the focus of considerable interest. The introduction of dynamic electrocardiographic techniques made it possible to monitor the diurnal distribution of most kinds of arrhythmias. Furthermore, the implantable cardioverter-defibrillator (ICD) had greatly advanced our understanding of circadian changes in ventricular tachyarrhythmias. The distribution of most ventricular and supraventricular arrhythmias have been proved to follow circadian patterns. Both atrial premature beats and atrial tachycardias are more common during the daytime. Moreover, it has been shown that abnormal atrial foci are under long-term autonomic regulation in the same manner as is normal pacemaker tissue (Huikuri *et al.* 1999). However, in the case of paroxysmal atrial fibrillation, the circadian character is different, with a nadir in prevalence occurring at about 11.00 hours (Yamashita *et al.* 1997). Because of their relatively benign nature, atrial arrhythmias will not be reviewed in any greater detail here, and the remainder of the chapter will focus on ventricular arrhythmias.

Circadian pattern of ventricular arrhythmias

Ventricular tachyarrhythmias are the primary cause of sudden cardiac death, and their circadian rhythm has been extensively studied (Tofler *et al.* 1995; Goldstein *et al.* 1996). Regardless of whether they have been studied using Holter monitoring or stored implantable defibrillator waveforms, the peak frequency of ventricular tachycardias and fibrillations has been found to be in the daytime and the trough during the night, similar to findings for most other cardiovascular physiological variables or pathological events (Auricchio & Klein 1997). However, unlike heart rate, blood pressure and some other cardiovascular indices that show a clear peak in the morning hours, the crest of ventricular tachyarrhythmias has variously been reported to occur during the morning or the afternoon (Tofler *et al.* 1995, Goldstein *et al.* 1996).

Auricchio & Klein (1997) used data stored by ICDs to evaluate the circadian distribution of ventricular tachyarrhythmias in 30 survivors of cardiac arrest. A circadian variation in episodes of ventricular tachyarrhythmias was evident. The incidence of ventricular arrhythmias sharply increased at 06.00 hours, and reached a maximum 4 h later, after which there was a decline and then a small peak between 15.00

and 17.00 hours. In the study conducted by Tofler *et al.* (1995), diurnal variation of ventricular tachyarrhythmias was investigated in 483 patients based on cardioverter/defibrillator recordings. Similar to the results of Auricchio & Klein (1997), a circadian rhythm was found, with a higher proportion of both rapid and less rapid ventricular tachyarrhythmias in the morning compared with other times of the day. However, an earlier study had slightly different results. Canada *et al.* (1983) analysed series of three 24-h electrocardiographic recordings from 164 untreated patients. A clear circadian pattern of ventricular arrhythmias was found, but with the highest frequency during noon to 16.00 hours, rather than in the morning, and the lowest between 01.00 and 05.00 hours.

Because of their lesser clinical significance, the circadian character of ventricular premature beats has not been widely studied. Surprisingly, since ventricular arrhythmias are initiated by a ventricular premature beat, the chronobiological features of this subtype are, according to the available reports, somewhat different compared with other types of ventricular arrhythmias (i.e. ventricular tachycardia and fibrillation). While the latter have almost always been demonstrated 'typical' circadian distributions, results regarding the circadian rhythm of ventricular premature beats have been less consistent. In the cohort reported by Tammaro *et al.* (1986), 30 subjects aged over 65 years with no clinical or instrumental signs of heart disease were studied, and 30 young healthy adults were included as controls. Results showed premature ventricular beats present in all subjects and occurring mostly during the day, but a significant circadian rhythm was present only in the patients with 30–150 PVCs/h. In another study reported by de Leonardis *et al.* (1987), chronobiological analysis of the circadian variations of heart rate, ventricular and atrial ectopies, was carried out on 11 patients with previous myocardial infarction matched with 11 controls. They failed to demonstrate a significant group rhythm in ectopies, but a trend for a higher frequency of arrhythmias during the activity span was detected. The author concluded that these results do not allow postulating a circadian pattern of arrhythmias common to all subjects examined, and the individual circadian behaviour of premature ventricular beats should be recognized for monitoring antiarrhythmic therapy. Similar findings have been reported by Cafiero *et al.* (1986). In this study, 24-h Holter ECGs were recorded on 34 subjects (17 cardiopathic and 17 normal, mean age 56 ± 14 vs. 41 ± 18) with, on average, over 30 PVCs/h. No statistically significant difference in mean PVCs/h was recorded between the two groups. Single cosinor analysis demonstrated a statistically significant circadian rhythm in 11 cardiopathic (64.7%) and 13 normal subjects (76.4%). Again, the cosinor analysis of the population means failed to demonstrate a significant global rhythm in either group. Results suggest that individual circadian rhythms of ventricular arrhythmias should be studied to identify the most appropriate antiarrhythmic treatment. The mechanisms and clinical significance of the different circadian properties of ventricular premature beats, ventricular tachycardia and flutter/fibrillation are still unclear, and require further investigation, although differences in their electrophysiological properties may be part of the explanation.

Potential mechanisms and mediating factors

The mechanisms underlying biological rhythm are not yet completely clear. There is accumulating evidence that the period and phase of rhythms are coordinated by pacemaker clocks located at various levels of biological organization, with those located in the brain believed to be the most important (Hastings 1998). It has been suggested that the suprachiasmatic nucleus–pineal gland axis acts as the heart of the internal 'biological clock', and that melatonin, synthesized and secreted from the pineal gland, plays a key role in the regulation of endogenous rhythms. Recent studies suggest that the running of the biological clock is under the regulation of periodic expressions of genes, providing insight into biological rhythm at the molecular level (Glass 2001). Exogenous factors too, however, have considerable effects on circadian rhythms (Hastings 1998).

Diurnal fluctuations in the activity of autonomic nervous function are believed to be an important moderator of the circadian pattern of arrhythmic events (Janssen *et al.* 1995). The peak frequency of arrhythmic events almost always occurs during times of high sympathetic activity, and the trough during times of higher parasympathetic activity (i.e. sleep hours). Heart rate variability studies (which reflect the sympathetic-parasympathetic autonomic balance) strongly support this viewpoint: Indices of heart rate variability decrease significantly during the daytime and increase during the night-time, the same pattern as the circadian rhythm of arrhythmic events (Janssen *et al.* 1995; Yamasaki *et al.* 1996; Massin *et al.* 2000). Circadian hormonal changes could be another key factor in the pattern of events. Adrenaline and noradrenaline peak between 06.00 and 12.00 hours, while end-organ responsiveness to noradrenaline are exaggerated during the same time period (Venditti *et al.* 1996). These changes may facilitate the genesis of ventricular arrhythmias during the vulnerable phase. Ultimately, however, ventricular arrhythmias are the result the complex interrelationship of many factors such as heart rate, blood pressure, left ventricular function,adrenaline/noradrenaline, ischaemic episode, etc, which are all affected by circadian factors.

Age has a significant association with the circadian character of ventricular arrhythmias. Massin *et al.* (2000) demonstrated a circadian variation of premature ventricular beats in children, although with a variable time of highest frequency, but no such phenomenon was found in infants. In studies of adults, diurnal changes in peak ventricular arrhythmia frequency have almost always been concordant (Tofler *et al.* 1995; Auricchio & Klein 1997; Saitoh 2000). These results may reflect the effect of the maturation of autonomic nervous system function.

Left ventricular function is another factor that affects the diurnal properties of ventricular arrhythmias. Gillis *et al.* (1992) evaluated 132 patients with frequent VPCs and reduced LV function after myocardial infarction. Patients were prospectively divided in two groups based on LV ejection fraction (EF). Median hourly VPC frequencies and heart rates were compared between the two groups. In patients with LVEF > 30%, a distinct circadian pattern of VPCs with the expected morning increase in VPC frequency was present. In contrast, a distinct circadian variation of VPCs was absent in patients with LVEF ″ 0.30.

Beta-adrenoceptor blocking agents may blunt the diurnal changes in patterns of ventricular arrhythmias. In the Gillis's study (1992) mentioned above, treatment with beta-adrenoceptor blocking agents was associated with a loss of the circadian variation of VPC frequency. However, this effect has not been demonstrated in most other antiarrhythmic drugs. Behrens *et al.* (1997) investigated a subgroup in the Congestive Heart Failure-Survival Trial of Antiarrhythmic Therapy (CHF-STAT) to determine the circadian pattern of deaths and compare the distribution of sudden cardiac death between the amiodarone and the placebo arms. A similar morning peak of sudden cardiac death was found in both the amiodarone and the placebo groups, and the overall circadian pattern did not differ between them, which suggested that amiodarone does not influence the circadian pattern of sudden death. Similarly, none of the other antiarrhythmic agents, such as propafenone, quinidine, disopyramide, or flecainide, have been shown to change the circadian pattern of VAs (Paisana *et al.* 1993).

The aetiology of ventricular arrhythmias is probably not a determinant of the presentation of circadian variation. Paisana *et al.* (1993) studied a cohort of patients with ventricular arrhythmias, 65 patients with ischaemic cardiopathy and 37 who were free of any structural abnormality. Results showed no difference in the diurnal distribution of ventricular arrhythmias in patients with or without structural abnormalities. Englund *et al.* (1999) also examined the circadian variation of ventricular arrhythmias in patients with and without ischaemic heart disease. They found the typical pattern of morning and afternoon peaks in both groups of patients and no significant differences between groups. Results suggest that the origin of circadian properties of ventricular arrhythmias is not in the heart itself, but in the higher level(s) of the body.

Heart rate and sleep–wake cycles could affect diurnal patterns of ventricular arrhythmias to some extent (Gillis *et al.* 1989). However, at least in one study, (Biffi *et al.* 1987), the peak frequency time of events was not associated with physical activity. Further studies are needed to support the hypothesis that intrinsic, rather than extrinsic, factors are the primary determinant of the circadian pattern of ventricular arrhythmias.

The types of ventricular arrhythmias can also affect their diurnal properties. In one ICD study, ventricular tachycardia and ventricular fibrillation with a cycle length ″350 ms demonstrated a circadian rhythm, but ventricular tachycardia with a cycle length of <350 ms or spontaneously terminating before device discharge had a more even distribution throughout the day. These results clearly show the existence of different circadian rhythms in the occurrence of ventricular tachyarrhythmias (Auricchio & Klein 1997).

Clinical implications

A large proportion of sudden cardiac deaths is attributable to the excess morning incidence of severe ventricular arrhythmias. Chronobiological studies of ventricular arrhythmias provide us with clues to the triggers of and influences on the origination of events, as described above, leading to insights into the underlying pathology. Recognition of the circadian variation of the onset of ventricular arrhythmias reinforces the need for pharmacological protection of patients during vulnerable periods. Also, Wood *et al.* (1995) have suggested that different diurnal patterns of ventricular arrhythmias may be associated with different prognoses. However, no relationship was found between the circadian rhythm of ventricular ectopic beats and the time of subsequent death in an analysis of the CAST (Cardiac Arrhythmia Suppression Trial) data (Goldstein 1996). Traditionally, risk stratification systems pay attention to the average number or frequency of events, without considering their chronobiological characteristics. This may cause the loss of important prognostic information. Investigations of circadian properties and identification of atypical rhythmic pattern may improve risk stratification. Further research on circadian patterns of ventricular arrhythmias could, therefore, significantly influence diagnosis and management of cardiac arrhythmic events.

References

Auricchio, A. & Klein, H. (1997) Circadian variations of ventricular tachyarrhythmias detected by the implantable cardioverter-defibrillator. *Giornale Italiano di Cardiologia*, **27** (2), 113–122.

Behrens, S., Ney, G., Fisher, S.G., Fletcher, R.D., Franz, M.R. & Singh, S.N. (1997) Effects of amiodarone on the circadian pattern of sudden cardiac death. *American Journal of Cardiology*, **80** (1), 45–48.

Biffi, A., Cugini, P., Pelliccia, A., Spataro, A., Caselli, G. & Piovano, G. (1987) Chronobiologic study of the dynamic electrocardiogram in healthy athletes with frequent ventricular ectopic beats. *Giornale Italiano di Cardiologia*, **17** (7), 563–568.

Cafiero, M., Scalzone, A.M., Borgia, M., Costantino, N.F., Fiorenza, B. & Eramo, A.N. (1986) Dynamic electrocardiographic evaluation of the circadian rhythms of the ectopic ventricular beats in healthy and cardiopathic subjects. *Minerva Medica*, **77** (28–29), 1377–1380.

Canada, W.B., Woodward, W., Lee, G. *et al.* (1983) Circadian rhythm of hourly ventricular arrhythmias frequency in man. *Angiology*, **34** (4), 274–282.

Englund, A., Behrens, S., Wegscheider, K. & Rowland, E. (1999) Circadian variation of malignant ventricular arrhythmias in patients with ischaemic and nonischaemic heart disease after cardioverter defibrillator implantation. *Journal of the American College of Cardiology*, **34** (5), 1560–1568.

Gillis, A.M., Guilleminault, C., Partinen, M., Connolly, S.J. & Winkle, R.A. (1989) The diurnal variability of ventricular premature depolarizations: influence of heart rate, sleep, and wakefulness. *Sleep*, **12** (5), 391–399.

Gillis, A.M., Peters, R.W., Mitchell, L.B., Duff, H.J., McDonald, M. & Wyse, D.G. (1992) Effects of left ventricular dysfunction on the circadian variation of ventricular complexes in healed myocardial infarction. *American Journal of Cardiology*, **69** (12), 1009–1014.

Glass, L. (2001) Synchronization and rhythmic processes in physiology. *Nature (London)*, **410**, 277–284.

Goldstein, S., Zoble, R.G., Akiyama, T. *et al.* (1996) Relation of circadian ventricular ectopic activity to cardiac mortality. CAST Investigators. *American Journal of Cardiology*, **78**, 881–885.

Hastings, M. (1998) The brain, circadian rhythms, and clock genes. *British Medical Journal*, **317**, 1704–1707.

Huikuri, H.V., Poutiainen, A.M., Makikallio, T.H. *et al.* (1999) Dynamic behaviour and autonomic regulation of ectopic atrial pacemakers. *Circulation*, **100**, 1416–1422.

Janssen, M.J., Swenne, C.A., Manger, C.A., van Bemmel, J.H. & Bruschke, A.V. (1995) Autonomic, ischaemic, circadian and rhythmic factors as causes of the spontaneous variability of ventricular arrhythmias. *European Heart Journal*, **16** (5), 674–681.

de Leonardis, V., de Scalzi, M., Vergassola, R., Romano, S., Becucci, A. & Cinelli, P. (1987) Circadian variations of heart rate and premature beats in healthy subjects and in patients with previous myocardial infarction. *Chronobiology International*, **4** (2), 283–289.

Massin, M.M., Maeyns, K., Withofs, N., Ravet, F. & Gerard, P. (2000) Circadian rhythm of heart rate and heart rate variability. *Archives of Disease in Childhood*, **83**, 179–182.

Paisana, J.P., Gomes, F., Cruz, J. *et al.* (1993) The circadian profile of ventricular extrasystole. *Revista Portuguesa de Cardiologia*, **12** (1), 7–8.

Saitoh, H. (2000) Biorhythms in ischaemic heart disease, cardiac sudden death, and arrhythmias. *Asian Med J*, 43 (5), 199–206.

Tammaro, A.E., Casale, G. & de Nicola, P. (1986) Circadian rhythms of heart rate and premature ventricular beats in aged. *Age & Ageing*, **15** (2), 93–98.

Tofler, G.H., Gebara, O.C., Mittleman, M.A. *et al.* (1995) Morning peak in ventricular tachyarrhythmias detected by time of implantable cardioverter/defibrillator therapy. *Circulation*, **92**, 1203–1208.

Venditti, F.J., John, R.M., Hull, M., Tofler, G.H., Shahian, D.M. & Martin, D.T. (1996) Arrhythmias/pacing: circadian variation in defibrillation energy requirements. *Circulation*, **94** (7), 1607–1612.

Wood, M.A., Simpson, P.M., London, W.B. *et al.* (1995) Circadian pattern of ventricular tachyarrhythmias in patients with implantable cardioverter-defibrillators. *Journal of the American College of Cardiology*, **25** (4), 901–907.

Yamasaki, Y., Kodama, M., Matsuhisa, M. *et al.* (1996) Diurnal heart rate variability in healthy subjects: effects of aging and sex difference. *American Journal of Physiology*, **271**, H303–H310.

Yamashita, T., Murakawa, Y., Sezaki, K. *et al.* (1997) Circadian variation of paroxysmal atrial fibrillation. *Circulation*, **96**, 1537–1541.

CHAPTER 59

Holter Monitor-Guided Antiarrhythmic Therapy

Kelley P. Anderson

Guidelines developed by a committee of the American Heart Association and American College of Cardiology (AHA/ACC) recommends ambulatory electrocardiography 'to assess antirrhythmic drug response in individuals in whom baseline frequency of arrhythmia has been well characterized as reproducible and of sufficient frequency to permit analysis' (Crawford *et al.* 1999). The Class I assignment indicates that there is evidence and/or general agreement that ambulatory electrocardiography, usually in the form of Holter monitoring (HM) is useful and effective for guiding antiarrhythmic drug therapy. Guidelines are created to improve patient care but clinicians are not bound to follow them and should not follow a guideline that does not serve their patients' interests. However, guidelines have legal and regulatory implications that may have consequences for professional activity beyond the care of individual patients (Schwartz *et al.* 1999). Therefore, clinicians must be cognizant not only of the guidelines that apply to their practice, but they must understand the limitations and when appropriate, clinicians must be able to provide a rationale for deviating from the standard of care.

The AHA/ACC Committee's recommendations and the current status of HM-guided antiarrhythmic therapy to prevent sustained ventricular tachyarrhythmias (VTA) and arrhythmic death can be understood only in the context of observations and experiments that began when Hoffa & Ludwig (1850) reported that faradic and galvanic stimulation produce ventricular fibrillation (VF). The significance of the induced arrhythmia was recognized by MacWilliam (1889) who proposed that VF, rather than cardiac standstill, was the mechanism of sudden death. Observations of accidental events and deliberate experiments performed by several teams of investigators between 1900 and 1940 led Wiggers (1940) to conclude that brief, localized electrical stimuli could initiate VTA when they occurred late in systole or on the T wave during an interval that he called the 'vulnerable phase'. Smirk (1949) noted that R waves appearing on the downslope of T waves (R-on-T) were observed in experimental studies and clinical cases to precede the onset of VTA and were associated with sudden death. Smirk surmised that the R-on-T phenomenon might be a predictor of a poor prognosis and suggested that patients with R-on-T premature ventricular complexes (PVCs) be treated with quinidine based on his observation that quinidine eliminated early cycle PVCs. The assumptions underlying HM-guided antiarrhythmic therapy were implicit: 1) VTAs were responsible for sudden death, 2) appropriately timed PVCs trigger VTAs, and 3) suppression of PVCs by antiarrhythmic drugs can eliminate the PVC-triggers and prevent sudden death.

Although suggested earlier by Smirk (1949), Lown and colleagues (1967) provided the most persistent influence that promulgated the use of HM for guiding antiarrhythmic therapy. Electrocardiographic monitoring became a standard in the care of patients at high risk for VTA as coronary care units spread in the 1960s. The original rationale was to reduce mortality in patients with acute myocardial infarction (MI) by prompt recognition and treatment of life-threatening tachy- and bradyarrhythmias. Lown and coworkers (1967) asserted that VTA could be prevented by prophylactic treatment using antiarrhythmic drugs administered in response to 'warning' arrhythmias. They cited animal experiments that demonstrated the arrhythmogenic potential of R-on-T stimuli and experiments in which death resulted from VTA after coronary ligation. In the latter experiments, the terminal arrhythmia was observed to be preceded by salvos of PVCs. Lown and colleagues proposed that certain characteristics of PVCs were harbingers of life-threatening VTA: 1) R-on-T PVCs (QR'/QT <0.85), 2) ≥2 consecutive PVCs, 3) multiform PVCs, 4) >5 PVCs/min. They developed a treatment algorithm that included administration of antiarrhythmic drugs in increasing doses until the warning arrhythmias were suppressed. If lidocaine failed, procainamide in increasing doses was administered. Lown *et al.*, reported that none of the 130 patients with MI admitted to their CCU developed primary VF (1967). Five patients developed rapid VTA and were successfully cardioverted. The investigators compared their observations to past series in which primary VF occurred in 14% to 21% of patients with acute MI and concluded that suppression of specific configurations of PVCs with antiarrhythmic drugs effectively prevented primary VF in patients with acute MI.

Based on their observations in patients with acute MI, Lown & Wolf (1971) adapted their approach to prevention of out-of-hospital sudden death. They cited animal experiments, observations in the coronary care unit and anecdotal evidence to support the assumption that out-of-hospital sudden death is due to VTAs. To support the assumption that PVCs are essential to arrhythmogenesis, they cited epidemiological studies that showed that PVCs recorded on a routine electrocardiogram was associated with a high risk of cardiac death (including a proportion of sudden death). To support the assumption that the control of PVCs by antiarrhythmic drugs will prevent VF in the ambulatory patient, Lown and Wolf (1971) cited animal studies that demonstrated that antiarrhythmic drugs prevented VF after acute coronary ligation and release in dogs. Lown and Wolf indicated that they were uncertain 'whether VF which follows occlusion or reperfusion is the better model for sudden death in man,' but they observed that antiarrhythmic drugs suppressed arrhythmias resulting from either manipulation.

Lown and colleagues reported the results of their approach in a series of studies. The approach, results and conclusions changed over time. In 1982 they reported their experience with 123 patients with malignant VTA (Graboys *et al.* 1982). In the 98 patients in whom antiarrhythmic drugs abolished nonsustained ventricular tachycardia (NSVT, Lown grade 4B) and R-on-T PVCs (grade 5) there were 6 sudden deaths. In the 25 patients in whom suppression was not achieved, there were 17 sudden deaths. The investigators concluded that suppression of certain grades of PVCs can protect against recurrence of VTA. They also noted that among patients with left ventricular dysfunction, control of ventricular premature beats was a critical element predicting survival.

In 1988, the investigators published observations from a series of 161 patients who presented with malignant VTAs (Lampert *et al.* 1988). All patients underwent 48 h of ambulatory ECG monitoring and an exercise stress test. Patients were required to exhibit Lown grade 2 PVCs (>1 PVC/min or 30 PVC/h) for >50% of the hours and grade 4B arrhythmia for at least 3 h per day or at least 2 PVCs per min provoked by exercise. PVCs had to be reproducible from one 24-h period to the next. The presence R-on-T (grade 5) PVCs were not reported and were not a therapeutic target in this study. If the criteria for the noninvasive approach were not met (43 patients), serial electrophysiological studies (EPS) were used to guide antiarrhythmic therapy. In patients who were eligible for the HM-guided approach, several antiarrhythmic drugs were tested using a short-term protocol in which a single large oral dose of an antiarrhythmic agent was administered after monitoring a 30-min control period. Hourly PVC counts and hourly exercise on a bicycle ergometer was performed. The objective of therapy was elimination of grades 4A (PVC pairs) and NSVT and reduction by 50% of frequent PVCs. Drugs that appeared effective in phase I or drugs that could not be tested with the short protocol due to long half-lives were administered using a dosing scheme to simulate long-term therapy. The effects of drugs were tested by HM and treadmill stress testing. An effective response required total elimination of NSVT, >90% reduction of grade 4A, >50% reduction in the total number of PVCs on both the HM and during the stress test. If a single drug failed to control the arrhythmia, two partially effecting drugs were combined and re-evaluated. For added protection, patients with recurrent VF were generally treated with two antiarrhythmic drugs even if one was predicted to be effective. Sixty-one of the 118 patients guided by HM were considered to be controlled (up to two runs NSVT <6 beats was permitted). Independent predictors of sudden death included râles during the initial physical examination, the number of runs of NSVT on the discharge (i.e. on drug) exercise test, a history of heart failure and the number of hours of grade 2 PVCs on the discharge HM. The cumulative sudden death rates in the controlled and uncontrolled groups were 5% and 19%, respectively, at 1 year and 29 and 48% at 5 years, respectively ($P = 0.02$ overall). Compared to the 1982 publication, the difference in outcome between controlled and uncontrolled groups appeared to decline. Moreover, the investigators noted that arrhythmia suppression occurred more often in the patients with left ventricular ejection fractions (EF) >30%. Furthermore, in apparent contrast to the 1982 findings, arrhythmia suppression in patients with a low EF did not predict protection from sudden death. The investigators concluded that their results supported the concept that suppression of repetitive arrhythmic on HM and exercise testing is a marker for improved survival among patients with malignant VTA. Thus, they acknowledged the possibility that antiarrhythmic drug-mediated suppression of PVCs did not affect outcome, but merely identified patients with a better prognosis (Lampert *et al.* 1988).

Although it was expected that the Cardiac Arrhythmia Suppression Trial (CAST) would support the PVC-suppression theory, it represents the clearest repudiation of the HM-guided approach to antiarrhythmic therapy. CAST was a randomized placebo-controlled trial involving patients after MI with no history of VTA (Echt *et al.* 1991). Patients with recent MI (<90 days) and EF 55% or greater were recruited. Or patients could be enrolled 90 days after MI or longer with an EF of 40% or less and frequent PVCs (>5 per h) or NSVT. Open-label drug titration was performed to determine if one or more of three drugs (encainide, flecainide and moricizine) resulted in suppression of PVCs by 80% and NSVT by 90%. Patients who demonstrated suppression were randomized to receive a placebo or a drug that had been shown to suppress PVCs. Despite PVC reduction, patients in the active drug limbs of the study had an increased risk of arrhythmic death or cardiac arrest (relative risk [RR] 2.6). The risk of all-cause death or cardiac arrest was also higher in the drug-treated group (RR 2.4). The possibility that the CAST findings resulted from reduced effectiveness of PVC suppression in patients with reduced EF was unlikely because a subgroup analysis showed that the increased risk of cardiac arrest or sudden death was also observed in the treatment subgroups of patients with EF <30% (RR 2.0) and EF 30% or more (RR 3.4).

Although CAST clearly did not support the PVC-suppression theory it did not disprove it because the adverse effects observed in the treatment group may have resulted from toxicity of the drugs selected for the trial. It also remained possible that selection of patients at higher risk of arrhythmic death would improve the balance of risk and benefit associated with antiarrhythmic drugs. These possibilities were indirectly addressed by the Survival Trial of Antiarrhythmic Therapy in patients with Congestive Heart Failure (STAT-CHF) (Singh *et al.* 1995). Patients with congestive heart failure, EF 40% or higher and at least 10 PVCs per h were randomized to receive amiodarone or placebo. The high risk nature of the study population was reflected in the high mortality, 29% at 2 years by actuarial analysis in the placebo group, 52% of which was classified as sudden. PVC frequency in the placebo group was 279 ± 387/h and did not change significantly thereafter. In contrast, in the amiodarone-treated patients PVC frequency was reduced from 254 ± 370/h at baseline to 66±156/h after 2 weeks ($P < 0.001$) and 44 ± 145/h at 3 months ($P < 0.001$). Despite these changes in PVC frequency, amiodarone had no significant effect on all-cause mortality or sudden death. In addition, symptomatic VT developed in 18 patients in the amiodarone arm and 20 patients in the placebo arm (*P* not significant). In the subgroup of patients with NSVT at baseline, amiodarone had no effect on mortality.

Furthermore, among the patients treated with amiodarone, survival did not differ between the 159 patients in whom PVCs were reduced by ≥80% and the 71 patients with less or no reduction. Also, there was no significant difference in mortality between the 111 amiodarone-treated patients in whom NSVT was eliminated at two weeks and the 65 patients who continued to exhibit runs of NSVT. Unlike CAST, randomization in STAT-CHF was not based on the response of PVC frequency to the antiarrhythmic drug treatment. Nevertheless, in this trial of high risk patients in whom antiarrhythmic therapy demonstrated no significant life-threatening toxicity, there was no discernable benefit for PVC suppression.

The beneficial effects of HM-guided antiarrhythmic drug therapy reported by Lown and colleagues included patients with malignant VTA who would have been ineligible for CAST and STAT-CHF (Lampert *et al.* 1988). However, the risk of sudden death in such individuals was considered so high that trials with placebo-controls were considered unethical (CASCADE 1993). The Electrophysiological Study Vs. Electrocardiographic Monitoring (ESVEM) trial compared HM-guided therapy modelled on the approach advocated by Lown and colleagues to EPS-guided antiarrhythmic drug selection in patients with documented VTA, aborted sudden death or unmonitored syncope (Mason 1993). To be eligible, patients also had to have at least 10 PVCs per h on two 24-h HM and inducible VTA at EPS. Subjects were randomized to one of the guidance approaches and each received an antiarrhythmic drug selected from a predefined set in random order followed by serial testing according to the assigned limb. Drug efficacy in the HM limb required a at least 70% reduction in PVC frequency, at least 80% reduction in PVC pairs, at least 90% reduction in NSVT episodes and no VT episodes longer than 15 beats. If these criteria were satisfied the patient underwent a treadmill exercise test to exclude exercise-provoked VT lasting >15 beats. Drug efficacy in the EP limb was based on standard criteria. The investigators who represented institutions who primarily used EPS to guide drug selection, were very surprised by the results which showed that there was no significant difference between the two guidance methods with respect to the accuracy of prediction for the primary endpoint of arrhythmia recurrence. The trial was not powered to compare mortality, however, there also were no significant differences between the groups with respect to all-cause, cardiac or arrhythmic deaths. In fact, the ESVEM trial suggested that HM-guided antiarrhythmic therapy was superior to EPS-guidance because efficacy criteria were more often met (77% in the HM limb vs. 45% in the EPS limb) and the testing period was shorter (actuarial median time 10 days in HM limb vs. 25 days in EPS limb). Although this could be seen as argument in favour of the HM-guided approach, it ignores the most important revelation of the ESVEM trial, i.e. that the recurrence rate was extremely high despite either form of guidance, 66% at 4 years (Anderson & Schloss 1995).

The Cardiac Arrest In Seattle Conventional vs. Amiodarone Drug Evaluation (CASCADE) included another very high risk group: non-Q wave MI VF survivors (CASCADE 1993). Eligible subjects were randomized to treatment with antiarrhythmic drug therapy guided by EPS or HM (n = 115) or to unguided amiodarone treatment (n = 113). Patients had to have VTA induced at EPS or complex arrhythmias on HM. Patients underwent HM-guided therapy only if a VTA was not induced or EPS was not performed (n = 45). Criteria for success in the HM limb included reduction of PVC frequency by 70% or more and reduction of NSVT events by at least 90%. Survival free of cardiac death, resuscitated VF or syncopal defibrillator shock at 2, 4 and 6 years was 82%, 66% and 53% in the amiodarone group and 69%, 52% and 40% in the EPS/HM-guided limb. HM-guided therapy was attempted in 45 patients and PVCs and NSVT were suppressed in 25. Outcome did not differ among patients whose arrhythmias were not induced during drug therapy. The outcome variables were confounded by the use of implantable defibrillators that was not randomized or stratified. Clinicians were free to implant defibrillators in patients who arrhythmias were inadequately controlled. Later in the course of the study, all patients were encouraged to undergo defibrillator implantation. The investigators concluded that unguided therapy with amiodarone was more effective than therapy with other drugs guided by HM or EPS.

Physiological basis for HM-guided antiarrhythmic therapy

More than 50 years after Smirk proposed that sudden death could be prevented by using drugs to suppress R-on-T PVCs, the theoretical underpinnings of this approach remain unproved. The first postulate, that sudden death is due to VTAs, lacks demonstrative electrocardiographic recordings in a representative sample of the most common events, i.e. unexpected sudden death without survival. Nevertheless, this assumption has been strongly supported by evidence obtained from several sources: fortuitous electrocardiographic recordings, stored electrograms from implanted defibrillators and autopsy studies. Importantly, there has been no contradictory evidence. Critical evidence needed to prove the postulate that PVCs trigger VTA in the most frequent form of arrhythmic death is also lacking. There has been some support from animal experiments, computer simulations and clinical sources. However, analysis of electrocardiographic recordings of spontaneous VTA suggest that a large proportion of events are not initiated by PVCs (Anderson *et al.* 1995). Furthermore, recordings obtained in patients who demonstrate apparent PVC-triggered VTA demonstrate frequent PVCs whereas VTA are very rare. This indicates that other factors are essential to the initiation of VTA. Analysis of heart rate and heart rate variability signals indicate that changing sympathetic activity beginning hours before the onset of the spontaneous VTA may be an important contributor (Anderson *et al.* 1999). The alternative possibility is that PVCs represent single-beat runs of VTA. If this were the case then PVC-suppression could represent disablement of the VTA source. However, this also lacks support in most patients (Anderson *et al.* 1990). The third postulate, that antiarrhythmic drugs suppress PVCs that are causally related to VTA, has little if any supportive evidence.

Conclusions

The original proposition by Smirk (1949) that antiarrhythmic drugs could be used to prevent sudden death by suppressing R-on-T was based on animal experiments and limited clinical observations. As is often the case in medical science, patients were treated without a proven mechanistic basis. Most of the support for this approach has come from uncontrolled observations involving relatively few patients. Although the ESVEM trial showed that HM-guided drug therapy was as accurate as EPS-guided treatment, both methods were associated with very high recurrence rates. The CASCADE trial suggested unguided amiodarone treatment was superior to treatment guided by EPS or HM. Randomized controlled trials have indicated that implantable defibrillator therapy is superior to unguided amiodarone treatment in patients at high risk for VTA (AVID Investigators 1997). However, the risk of implantable defibrillators has not been shown to outweigh the benefit in lower risk populations. Moreover, defibrillators remain an exclusive form of therapy owing to the high cost. Therefore, there are groups of patients for whom drug therapy might be indicated and for whom HM-guided antiarrhythmic therapy is an option. The evidence that supports the use of HM-guidance could be explained by a marker effect, i.e. that drug-related PVC suppression identifies patients with a better long-term outcome. In addition, there is evidence that drug-associated worsening of PVC frequency may identify patients with a worse long-term outcome (Wyse *et al.* 1994). However, the balance of evidence does not support the PVC-suppression theory. Rather, there is evidence to suggest the risk of sudden death may be increased with antiarrhythmic drug selected by HM. Nevertheless, it must be acknowledged that substantial gaps remain in the knowledge needed to satisfactorily guide preventive therapy particularly for patients at risk for sudden death who are not candidates for defibrillators or for whom defibrillators are not available.

References

Anderson, K.P., Lux, R.L. & Dustman, T. (1990) Comparison of QRS morphologies of spontaneous premature ventricular complexes and ventricular tachycardia induced by programmed stimulation. *American Heart Journal*, **119**, 1302–1311.

Anderson, K.P. & Schloss, E.J. (1995) ESVEM tells us what we don't know. *Circulation*, **92**, 3144

Anderson, K.P., Shusterman, V., Aysin, B. *et al.* (1999)

Distinctive *RR* dynamics preceding two modes of onset of spontaneous sustained ventricular tachycardia. *Journal of Cardiovascular Electrophysiology*, **10**, 897–904.

Anderson, K.P., Walker, R., Dustman, T. *et al.* (1995) Spontaneous sustained ventricular tachycardia in the Electrophysiological Study Vs. Electrocardiographic Monitoring (ESVEM) trial. *Journal of the American College of Cardiology*, **26**, 489–496.

AVID (Antiarrhythmics Vs. Implantable Defibrillators) Investigators (1997) A comparison of antiarrhythmic-drug therapy with implantable defibrillators in patients resuscitated from near-fatal ventricular arrhythmias. *New England Journal of Medicine*, **337**, 1576–1583.

CASCADE Investigators (1993). Randomized antiarrhythmic drug therapy in survivors of cardiac arrest (the CASCADE Study). The CASCADE Investigators. *American Journal of Cardiology*, **72**, 280–287.

Crawford, M., Bernstein, S., Deedwania, P. *et al.* (1999) ACC/AHA Guidelines for Ambulatory Electrocardiography – a report of the American College of Cardiology/American Heart Association Task Force on practice guidelines. *Journal of the American College of Cardiology*, **34**, 912–945.

Echt, D.S., Liebson, P.R., Mitchell, L.B. *et al.* (1991) Mortality and morbidity in patients receiving encainide, flecainide, or placebo: the Cardiac Arrhythmia Suppression Trial. *New England Journal of Medicine*, **324**, 781–788.

Graboys, T.B., Lown B., Podrid, P.J. & DeSilva, R (1982). Long-term survival of patients with malignant ventricular arrhythmia treated with antiarrhythmic drugs. *American Journal of Cardiology*, **50**, 437–43.

Hoffa, M. & Ludwig, C. (1850). Einige neue Versuche über Herzbewegung. *Zeitschrift fuer Naturwissenschaftlich-Medicinische*, **9**, 107.

Lampert, S., Lown, B., Graboys, T.B. *et al.* (1988) Determinants of survival in patients with malignant ventricular arrhythmia associated with coronary artery disease. *American Journal of Cardiology*, **61**, 791–797.

Lown, B., Fakhro, A.M., Hood, W.B., Jr & Thorn, G.W. (1967) The coronary care unit: new perspectives and directions. *JAMA (Journal of the American Medical Association)*, **199**, 156–166.

Lown, B. & Wolf, M. (1971) Approaches to sudden death from coronary heart disease. *Circulation* **44**, 130–142.

MacWilliam, J. (1889) Cardiac failure and sudden death. *British Medical Journal*, **1**, 6–8.

Mason, J.W. (1993) A comparison of electrophysiological testing with Holter monitoring to predict antiarrhythmic-drug efficacy for ventricular tachyarrhythmias: Electrophysiological Study Vs. Electrocardiographic Monitoring Investigators. *New England Journal of Medicine*, **329**, 445–451.

Schwartz, P.J., Breithardt, G., Howard, A.J. *et al.* (1999). Task Force Report: the legal implications of medical guidelines – a Task Force of the European Society of Cardiology. *European Heart Journal*, **20**, 1152–1157.

Singh, S.N., Fletcher, R.D., Fisher, S.G. *et al.* (1995) Amiodarone in patients with congestive heart failure and asymptomatic ventricular arrhythmia: Survival Trial of Antiarrhythmic Therapy in Congestive Heart Failure. *New England Journal of Medicine*, **333**, 77–82.

Smirk, F.H. (1949) R waves interrupting T waves. *British Heart Journal*, **11**, 23.

Wiggers, C.J. (1940) The mechanism and nature of ventricular fibrillation. *American Heart Journal*, **20**, 399–412.

Wyse, D.G., Morganroth, J., Ledingham, R. *et al.* (1994) New insights into the definition and meaning of proarrhythmia during initiation of antiarrhythmic drug therapy from the Cardiac Arrhythmia Suppression Trial and its pilot study: the CAST and CAPS Investigators. *Journal of the American College of Cardiology*, **23**, 1130–1140.

CHAPTER 60

Dynamics of Heart Rate Before Arrhythmias

Polychronis E. Dilaveris and John E. Gialafos

Introduction

The idea that the dynamics of cardiac cycles may reveal hidden instabilities that precede the onset of arrhythmias is not new (Goldberger *et al.* 1984). Ambulatory electrocardiographic (ECG) or implantable cardioverter defibrillator (ICD) recordings have been used to study the factors that may serve as triggers or contribute to initiation of spontaneously occurring malignant ventricular arrhythmias (Fig. 60.1) (Zimmermann *et al.* 1986). Because autonomic activity is thought to be an important trigger of ventricular arrhythmias and because cardiac cycle lengths are modulated by autonomic tone, it has been assumed that the analysis of the changes in cardiac cycle length could predict the timing as well as the triggers of ventricular arrhythmias (Shusterman *et al.* 1998). Previous studies have focused on the characteristics of premature ventricular contractions (PVCs) initiating ventricular tachycardias and changes in basic heart rate preceding spontaneous episodes of ventricular tachycardia (Zimmermann *et al.* 1986). Advances in heart rate variability (HRV) analysis have provided powerful methods for assessing autonomic nervous system activity before ventricular arrhythmias (Huikuri *et al.* 1993; Leclercq *et al.* 1996; Shusterman *et al.* 1998; Pruvot *et al.* 2000).

Heart rate dynamics before premature ventricular contractions

A multiple of factors, either alone or in combination may facilitate the genesis of cardiac arrhythmias. Heart rate, in particular, may be related to the development of ventricular arrhythmias (Winkle 1982). Winkle first used an algorithm in which the number of PVCs is tabulated for each min during the 24-h ECG monitoring period by averaging all the *RR* intervals occurring during each minute. The graphs were then inspected to estimate the relationship between the frequency of PVCs and heart rate in each patient. Winkle (1982) found that most patients showed an increase in the incidence of PVCs at a high heart rate. Coumel (1989) showed that patients with PVCs often have lower and upper thresholds that form the limits of the heart rate window of arrhythmias. This dependence on rate is affected by the autonomic nervous system and, following these limits throughout the 24-h period, they shift toward higher values with adrenergic influences. Pitzalis *et al.* (1997) analysed the distribution of ventricular ectopic beats according to the immediately preceding sinus *RR* interval (rate enhanced method). Patients were classified into three groups: tachycardia-enhanced, indifferent and bradycardia-enhanced PVCs dependent on whether the distribution showed a decrease, no definite change or an increase in the incidence of PVCs as a function of the preceding *RR* interval (Fig. 60.2). The patients with a reproducible tachycardia-enhanced pattern had the highest incidence of cardiac disease, with a significantly higher incidence of ventricular tachycardia than the patients with a bradycardia-enhanced pattern (Pitzalis *et al.* 1997). They also found that the patients with a tachycardia-enhanced pattern had the highest incidence of PVCs during the daytime and the lowest incidence of night-time PVCs per h compared to the other two groups. The coupling interval of the patients with a tachycardia-enhanced pattern was

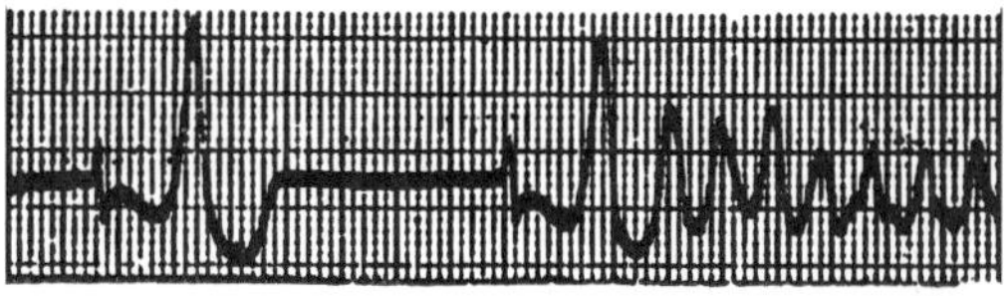

Fig. 60.1 Electrocardiographic strip showing ventricular bigeminy preceding an episode of sustained ventricular tachyarrhythmia in a 62-year old female patient with history of coronary artery disease.

always significantly shorter than that of the patients of the other two groups (Pitzalis *et al.* 1997). In another study, the dynamic behaviour of sinus *RR* intervals before PVCs was estimated from the dynamic changes of the last five *RR* intervals before the PVC rather than to the preceding single *RR* interval (Sapoznikov *et al.* 1999). By use of this methodology, patients with frequent PVCs were also classified into three

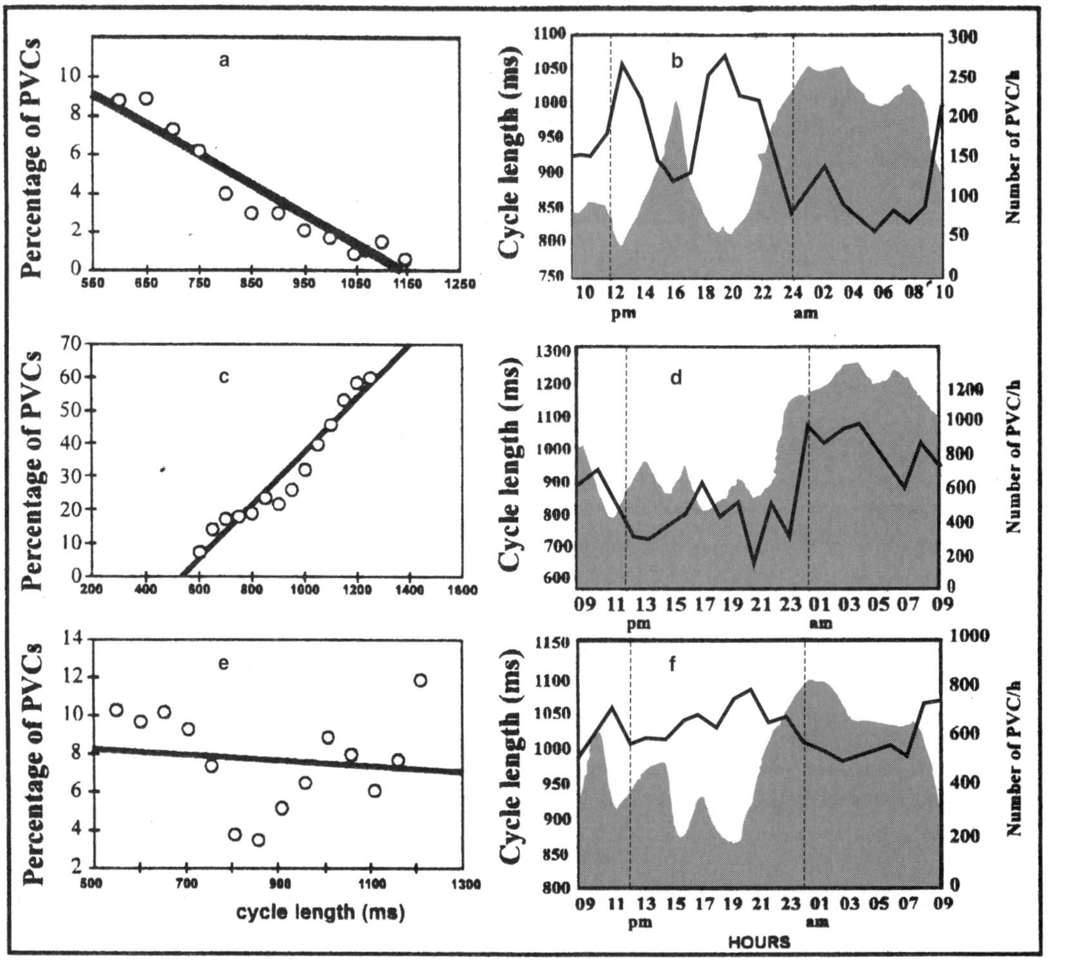

Fig. 60.2 Three types of arrhythmic patterns and their respective trends of cardiac cycle lengths and premature ventricular contractions (PVCs) throughout 24-h electrocardiographic (ECG) monitoring periods. (a), (c), (e) *x*-axis, sinus cycle length; *y*-axis, percentage of cycles followed by PVC; circles, percentage incidence of such cycles; line connecting the percentage at each sinus length reflects linear regression analysis. (b), (d), (f) *x*-axis, different daytime and night-time h; *y*1-axis, sinus cycle length; *y*2-axis, number of PVCs per h; shaded area, prevalence of different cardiac cycle lengths throughout the 24-h period; line, trend of PVCs throughout same period. (a) Tachycardia-enhanced pattern and (b) trend of cardiac cycle lengths and PVCs throughout 24-h ECG monitoring periods in same patient. (c) Bradycardia-enhanced pattern and (d) trend of cardiac cycle lengths and PVCs throughout the 24-h ECG monitoring periods in same patient. (e) Indifferent pattern and (f) trend of cardiac cycle lengths and PVCs throughout 24-h ECG monitoring periods in same patient. (Reproduced from Pitzalis *et al.* 1997, with permission.)

groups: bradycardia-enhanced patients who were younger with a high proportion of males and longer, more variable coupling intervals; tachycardia-enhanced patients who exhibited sleep suppression of PVCs and had shorter, less variable coupling intervals; and patients with predominantly no change in the *RR* intervals preceding the PVCs who were significantly older, with greater prevalence of cardiovascular disease and reduced sinus *RR* variability, indicating decreased autonomic nervous system activity (Sapoznikov *et al.* 1999). Ischaemia-induced reflex sympathoexcitation during the recovery period of maximal treadmill exercise testing when PVCs are more prevalent has also been reported previously (Dilaveris *et al.* 1998).

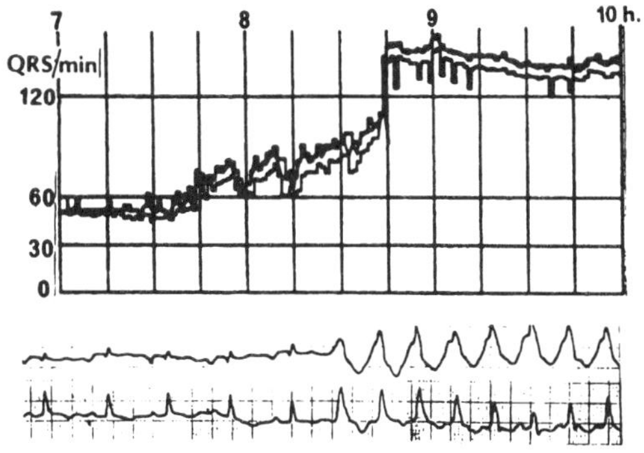

Fig. 60.3 Typical example of the first sustained ventricular tachycardia episode recorded in a young patient who had nondiagnosed episodes of palpitation. The sustained ventricular tachycardia is preceded by a progressive and continuous increase in sinus rate during morning physical activities (top) and is initiated directly from sinus rhythm without previous significant premature ventricular complexes or morphologic changes of the first ventricular tachycardia beats (bottom). (Reproduced from the American College of Cardiology Foundation *Journal of the American College of Cardiology* (1996), 28 (3), 720–724, with permission.)

Heart rate dynamics before ventricular tachycardia

The proarrhythmic role of increased sympathetic and reduced vagal activity directed to the heart is supported by several observations (Lombardi *et al.* 1983; Schwartz *et al.* 1992). Lately, measuring HRV has facilitated the clinical appraisal of alteration in neural modulation of the sinus node (ESC/NASPE Task Force 1996) and identification of patients with increased cardiac mortality (Kleiger *et al.* 1987; ESC/NASPE Task Force 1996). Low HRV has been recognized as an independent risk factor of cardiac events after myocardial infarction (Kleiger *et al.* 1987; ESC/NASPE Task Force 1996), and it has also been used to assess changes in the dynamics before the onset of ventricular tachyarrhythmias (Kleiger *et al.* 1987; La Rovere *et al.* 1998; Shusterman *et al.* 1998; Anderson *et al.* 1999). Controversy exists regarding heart rate increases and the implications for changes in autonomic activity before the onset of spontaneous ventricular tachyarrhythmias. Increases in heart rate preceding the onset of sustained ventricular tachyarrhythmias have been observed in a number of studies (Huikuri *et al.* 1993; Leclercq *et al.* 1996), but not in others (Gomes *et al.* 1989; Bardy & Olson 1990). Increased heart rate and shortening of the coupling intervals of the first cycles before the onset of sustained ventricular tachycardia was present in a series of patients with arrhythmogenic right ventricular dysplasia (Leclercq *et al.* 1996). It seems that increased sympathetic stimulation is the main determinant of spontaneous initiation of ventricular tachycardia in arrhythmogenic right ventricular dysplasia, allowing the necessary change in electrophysiological ventricular tachycardia substrate (Fig. 60.3). Although heart rate increases before ventricular tachyarrhythmias have been interpreted by several investigators as indicating an increase in sympathetic tone (Huikuri *et al.* 1993; Leclercq *et al.* 1996), heart rate is relatively nonspecific sign in isolation.

Several investigators have used time domain HRV analysis to assess changes before sustained ventricular arrhythmias. Pozzati *et al.* (1996) reported reductions in SDNN before sustained ventricular arrhythmias, but these were preceded by ST segment shifts owing to acute myocardial ischaemia. In a previous publication, the Poincaré plot analyses have shown abnormal patterns of beat-to-beat *RR*-interval dynamics in the patients with a propensity for spontaneous onset of ventricular tachycardia (Huikuri *et al.* 1996). However, the last as well as many other studies failed to find changes in time domain indices of HRV before ventricular tachycardia

(Huikuri *et al.* 1996; Shusterman *et al.* 1998; Diaz *et al.* 2001).

Frequency domain HRV variables provide more specific information about autonomic activity (ESC/NASPE Task Force 1996). Although the published experience is limited in this area, several studies report significant reductions in frequency domain indices before episodes of sustained ventricular tachycardia. Huikuri *et al.* (1993) found that all HRV frequency components were lower before ventricular tachycardia compared to non-sustained ventricular tachycardia and all frequency components demonstrated reduced power compared to the 24-h average values in patients with both sustained and non-sustained ventricular tachycardia. In the same study, the ratio between low-frequency and high-frequency components of HRV increased substantially before both non-sustained and sustained episodes of ventricular tachycardia. Shusterman *et al.* (1998) also found lower HRV frequency components before episodes of ventricular tachycardia (Fig. 60.4) including the ratio between low-frequency and high-frequency HRV components. On the contrary, a significant increase in the ratio between low-frequency and high-frequency HRV components before episodes of ventricular tachycardia was demonstrated in another study (Lombardi *et al.* 2000). With the use of heart rate recording retrieved from ICD memory, a state of sympathoexcitation was also observed as expressed by the reduction in HRV frequency components before the onset of episodes of ventricular tachycardia (Pruvot *et al.* 2000). In the same study the use of beta blockers and dl-sotalol enhanced HRV. Nevertheless, HRV declined before the onset of ventricular tachyarrhythmias regardless of the antiarrhythmic drug regimen (Pruvot *et al.* 2000). However, in other reports, the investigators failed to find significant differences in the frequency domain measures of HRV before sus-

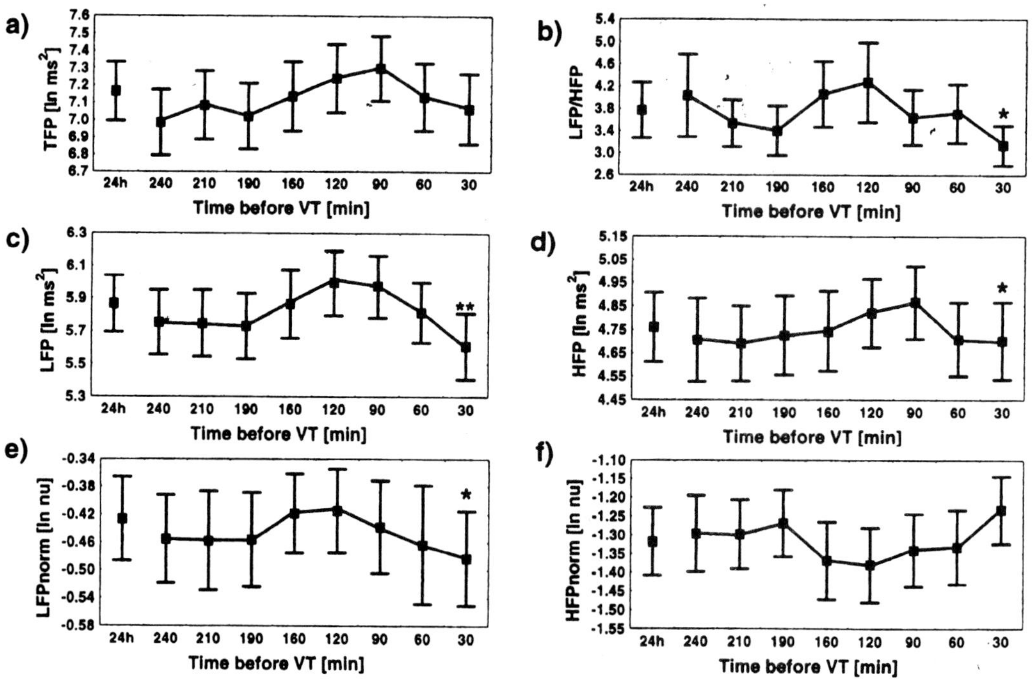

Fig. 60.4 Frequency components of the heart rate variability signal, 24-h average and at 30-min intervals before the onset of sustained ventricular tachycardia: (a) total power (TFP); (b) ratio of low to high frequency power (LFP/HFP); (c) low frequency power; (d) high frequency power; (e) normalized low frequency power; (f) normalized high frequency power. *$P < 0.05$ for comparison 30-min vs. 24-h average; ** $P < 0.01$ compared to the 24-h average; nu, normalized units. Significance of changes during 24-h period before ventricular tachycardia was assessed by analysis of variance and is discussed in the text. (Reproduced from the American College of Cardiology Foundation *Journal of the American College of Cardiology* (1998), **32** (7), 1891–1899, with permission.)

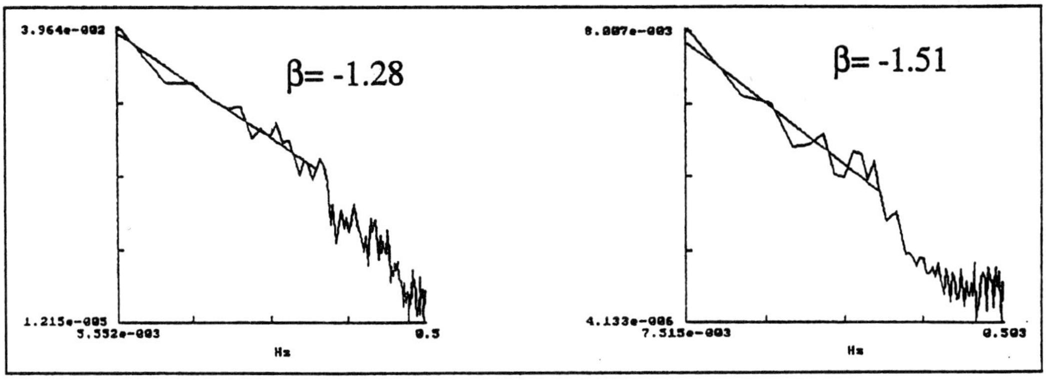

Fig. 60.5 Power-law behaviour of the stored time series recorded during control conditions (right) and before ventricular tachycardia (VT) (left). A more negative scaling index characterizes the min before VT onset. (Reproduced from the American College of Cardiology Foundation *American Journal of Cardiology* (2000), 86 (9), 959–963, with permission.)

tained ventricular arrhythmias (Valkama *et al.* 1995; Huikuri *et al.* 1996). These inconsistencies may be related to low statistical power due to the small number of the enrolled subjects, or to clinical differences among the different study cohorts.

Lately, analysis of fractal correlation properties of *RR* interval dynamics has been proven superior to time- and frequency-domain parameters of HRV in identifying patients with increased cardiac and arrhythmic mortality after myocardial infarction (Huikuri *et al.* 2000). Negative values of the scaling exponent $\beta < -1$ were demonstrated in patients with coronary artery disease and left ventricular dysfunction at the control period, whereas more negative values were noticed before the onset of ventricular tachycardia (Fig. 60.5), indicating further loss of complexity of the variability signal (Lombardi *et al.* 2000). Such a more negative slope was considered indicative of a diminished long-range correlation of cardiac cycles (Lombardi *et al.* 2000).

However, the high complexity of the interacting physiological influences and the violation of statistical assumptions that underlie traditional HRV techniques may result in failure of HRV descriptors to predict the timing of ventricular tachyarrhythmias onset (Ivanov *et al.* 1999). In addition, the attempts to summarize highly nonstationary and individually variable cardiac cycle length dynamics in a few indices may result in non-uniform data compression and frequent oversight of individual changes that precede the onset of ventricular tachyarrhythmias (Shusterman *et al.* 2000). To overcome these problems, an adaptive technique has been developed, referred to as the modified Karhunen–Loeve transform (MKLT), that identifies an individual characteristic ('core') pattern of cardiac cycles and then tracks the changes in the pattern by projecting the signal onto characteristic eigenvectors (Shusterman *et al.* 2001). Disturbances in the core pattern were found in 82% of the recordings before the onset of impending ventricular tachyarrhythmia, and their dimensionality, defined as the number of unstable orthogonal projections, increased gradually several hours before the onset (Fig. 60.6) (Shusterman *et al.* 2001). The multidimensional disturbances in the individual pattern of cardiac cycles provided more sensitive (70%) and specific (93%) prediction of the onset time of ventricular tachyarrhythmias than any of the traditional linear or non-linear methods (Shusterman *et al.* 2001).

Heart rate dynamics before ventricular fibrillation

The risk of life-threatening arrhythmias after acute myocardial infarction has been shown to be increased in patients with reduced HRV (Farrell *et al.* 1991). However, controversial information has been available on possible abnormalities in heart rate dynamics before the

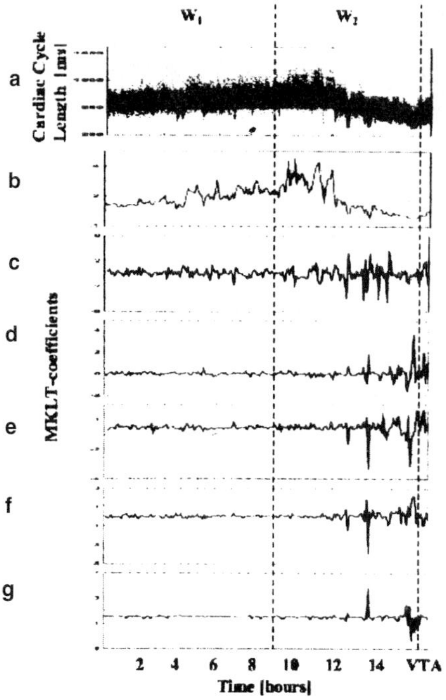

Fig. 60.6 Cardiac cycle dynamics during 16 h before onset of a sustained ventricular tachyarrhythmia (VTA). (a) Black dots, original, unfiltered cardiac cycle series; grey dots, series filtered to eliminate ectopic beats, pauses, and outliers, as described in Shusterman *et al.* (2001: materials and methods). (b–g) MKLT coefficients c_1 to c_6 (arbitrary units). Data are separated into two windows, W_1 and W_2, as described in the online supplement available at http://www.circresaha.org. In the first window, the core pattern of cardiac cycles is at steady state, which is indicated by low variations in MKLT coefficients. None of the coefficients exceeds the 3σ thresholds. In W_2, there is a fivefold increase in variations of c_1 to c_6 compared with W_1, and five of six coefficients (c_2 to c_6) in both filtered and unfiltered series exceed the 3σ thresholds, indicating simultaneous instabilities in the five orthogonal projections of the signal. VTA starts at the end of W_2 after 7 h of multidimensional ($Dm = 5$) disturbances in the core pattern of cardiac cycles. (Reproduced from Shusterman *et al.* 2001, with permission.)

spontaneous onset of ventricular fibrillation (Kimura *et al.* 1986; Lindsay *et al.* 1990; Vybiral *et al.* 1993). Vybiral *et al.* (1993) have shown that the conventional analysis of HRV fails to predict imminent ventricular fibrillation, whereas Skinner *et al.* (1993) observed changes in the non-linear correlation dimension of *RR* intervals several hours before the onset of ventricular fibrillation. Altered beat to beat *RR* interval dynamics were also found by Mäkikallio *et al.* (1999) to precede the onset of ventricular fibrillation, using analysis of fractal scaling based on detrended fluctuation analysis and 1/f scaling analysis. Apart from the altered beat to beat dynamics, the long-range correlation properties of *RR* intervals were also altered before the onset of ventricular fibrillation. The computed slope of the power-law relation of HRV was more negative in patients with ventricular fibrillation, despite the absence of differences in the low-frequency spectral components between patients with and those without ventricular fibrillation (Fig. 60.7) (Mäkikallio *et al.* 1999). Similar qualitative alterations in heart rate regulation were also found to be present before the onset of ventricular fibrillation in patients with Chagas heart disease (Diaz *et al.* 2001).

Heart rate dynamics before torsades de pointes

Torsades de pointes is a rapid polymorphic ventricular tachycardia with a distinctive, twisting configuration, typically associated with prolonged repolarization, either congenital or acquired (Locati *et al.* 1995). Torsades de pointes is variable in duration and often stops spontaneously (Fig. 60.8), although runs may degenerate into ventricular fibrillation, thus provoking sudden cardiac death (Locati *et al.* 1995). The role of torsades de pointes in the genesis of sudden death should be clearly individualized. The two major determinants, bradycardia and long-short *RR* sequence contribute to the prolongation and to the inhomogeneity of the ventricular refractory period (Leclercq *et al.* 1988).

In pause-dependent torsades, an escalating sequence of events, referred to as cascade phenomenon, has been well described (Locati *et al.* 1995): (1) A premature depolarization generates a post-extrasystolic pause; (2) the sinus complex that follows the pause shows marked post-extrasystolic TU changes from which a subsequent ventricular extrasystole originates; (3) this extrasystole generates a new pause, which in turn is followed by more bizarre TU changes from which progressively longer and faster runs of polymorphic ventricular tachycardia originate (Locati *et al.* 1995). It has been demonstrated that, as the amplitude of the oscillatory initiat-

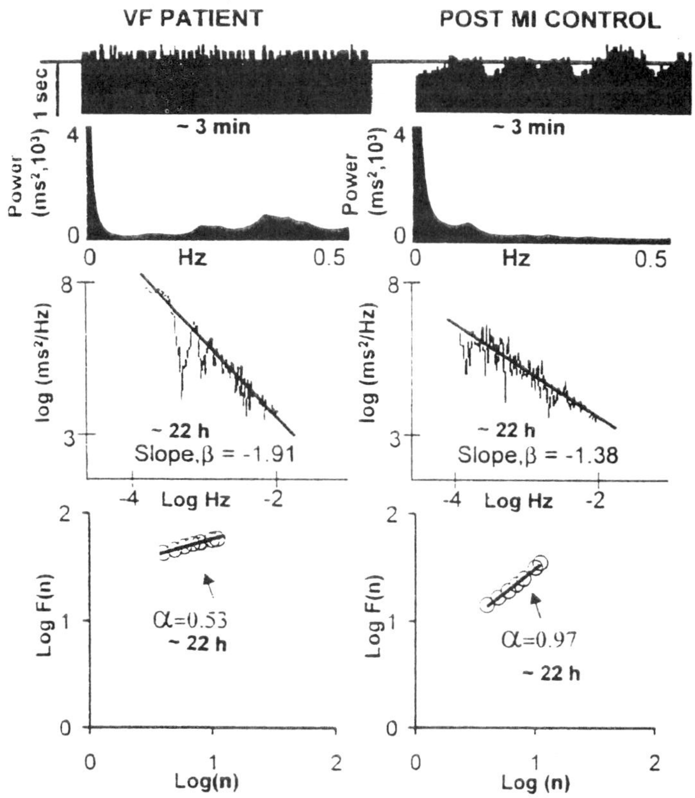

Fig. 60.7 Examples of *RR* interval tachograms (upper panels), power spectrums (upper middle panels), power-law slopes (middle lower panels) of *RR* intervals, and detrended fluctuation analyses (lower panels) preceding the spontaneous ventricular fibrillation of 1 patient (left column). This patient shows a widened high-frequency spectral band, a steeper power-law slope, and a reduced short-term scaling exponent (α ~ 0.5). A representative postinfarction control patient without arrhythmia during the recording or during a follow-up of 2 years afterwards shows fractal short-term exponent value α ~ 1.0 (right column). α, short-term scaling exponent; β, power-law scaling slope; MI, myocardial infarction. (Reproduced from the American College of Cardiology Foundation *American Journal of Cardiology* (1999), 83 (6), 880–884, with permission.)

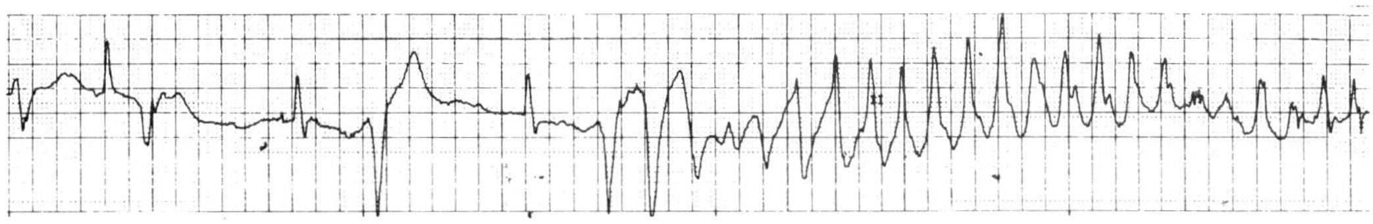

Fig. 60.8 Electrocardiographic strip from a 74-year-old patient showing third-degree atrioventricular block and bradycardia accompanied by a short-long-short sequence which initiates a self-terminating episode of torsades de pointes.

ing sequences increases, with shorter short intervals followed by longer post-extrasystolic pauses, the probability of observing torsades de pointes also increases (Locati *et al.* 1995). The role of long *RR* cycles, name the post-extrasystolic pause is important: they are implicated in all torsades de pointes and 50% of the cases of ventricular tachycardia/ventricular fibrillation (Leclercq *et al.* 1988). By contrast, a progressive increase in heart rate, reflecting changes in the vago-sympathetic balance, seems to be needed to start a sustained ventricular tachycardia in the absence of long–short cycle sequences (Fig. 60.9) (Leclercq *et al.* 1988). The short-coupled variant of torsades de pointes forms an ECG entity that may be responsible for sudden cardiac death in the absence of any evidence of structural heart disease and acute illness (Leenhardt *et al.* 1994).

Conclusions

Ambulatory ECG or ICD recordings are currently in use to study the factors that may serve as triggers or contribute to the initiation of spontaneously occurring malignant ventricular arrhythmias. Tachycardia-enhanced, indifferent and bradycardia-enhanced PVCs are reported in

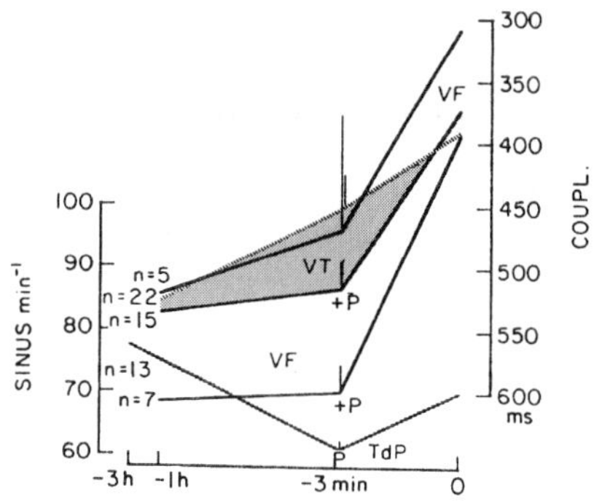

Fig. 60.9 In both ventricular tachycardia (VT)/ventricular fibrillation (VF), the preceding heart rate is higher and increases more during the last h when the arrhythmia is not triggered by a pause (P). In torsades de pointes (TdP), the pause is constant. (Reproduced from *European Heart Journal* (1988), **9**, 1276–1283, Leclercq, J.F., Maison-Blanche, P., Cauchemez, B. & Coumel, P., Respective role of sympathetic tone and of cardiac pauses in the genesis of 62 cases of ventricular fibrillation recorded during Holter monitoring, by permission of the publisher W. B. Saunders.)

the literature, while increased heart rate has been reported before the onset of ventricular tachycardia in most but not all the previous publications. Reduced HRV spectral components were demonstrated before episodes of ventricular tachycardia, while more negative values of the scaling exponent β were noticed before the onset of ventricular tachycardia or ventricular fibrillation. On the other hand, bradycardia and long–short *RR* sequences are found before most episodes of torsades de pointes. Modern, sophisticated parameters assessing the heart rate complexity will offer in the future, a more comprehensive approach in the evaluation of heart rate dynamicity before imminent ventricular tachyarrhythmias and may further improve arrhythmia diagnosis and management.

References

Anderson, K.P., Shusterman, V., Aysin, B. *et al.* for the ESVEM Investigators (1999) Distinctive *RR* dynamics preceding two modes of onset of spontaneous sustained ventricular tachycardia. *Journal of Cardiovascular Electrophysiology*, **19**, 897–904.

Bardy, G.H. & Olson, W.H. (1990) Clinical characteristics of spontaneous-onset sustained ventricular tachycardia and ventricular fibrillation in survivors of cardiac arrest. In: *Cardiac Electrophysiology: From Cell to Bedside* (eds D. P. Zipes & J. Jalife), pp. 778–790. W. B. Saunders, Philadelphia.

Coumel, P. (1989) Rate-dependence and adrenergic-dependence of arrhythmias. *American Journal of Cardiology*, **64**, 41J–45J.

Diaz, J., Mäkikallio, T., Huikuri, H. *et al.* (2001) Heart rate dynamics before the spontaneous onset of ventricular tachyarrhythmias in Chagas' heart disease. *American Journal of Cardiology*, **87**, 1123–1125.

Dilaveris, P., Zervopoulos, G., Michaelides, A. *et al.* (1998) Ischaemia-induced reflex sympathoexcitation during the recovery period after maximal treadmill exercise testing. *Clinical Cardiology*, **21**, 585–590.

ESC/NASPE (European Society of Cardiology/ North American Society of Pacing and Electrophysiology) Task Force (1996) Heart rate variability. Standards of measurement, physiological interpretation, and clinical use. *Circulation*, **93**, 1043–1065.

Farrell, T.G., Bashir, Y., Cripps, T. *et al.* (1991) Risk stratification for arrhythmic events in postinfarction patients based on heart rate variability, ambulatory electrocardiographic variables and the signal-averaged electrocardiogram. *Journal of the American College of Cardiology*, **18**, 687–697.

Goldberger, A.L., Findley, L.J., Blackburn, M.R. & Mandell, A.J. (1984) Nonlinear dynamics in heart failure: implications of long-wavelength cardiopulmonary oscillations. *American Heart Journal*, **107**, 612–615.

Gomes, J.A., Alexopoulos, D., Winters, S.L., Deshmuckh, P., Fuster, V. & Suh, K. (1989) The role of silent ischaemia, the arrhythmic substrate and the short-long sequence in the genesis of sudden cardiac death. *Journal of the American College of Cardiology*, **14**, 1618–1625.

Huikuri, H., Valkama, J., Airaksinen, J. *et al.* (1993) Frequency domain measures of heart rate variability before the onset of nonsustained and sustained ventricular tachycardia in patients with coronary artery disease. *Circulation*, **87**, 1220–1228.

Huikuri, H., Seppänen, T., Koistinen, M.-J. *et al.* (1996) Abnormalities in beat-to-beat dynamics of heart rate before the spontaneous onset of life-threatening ventricular tachyarrhythmias in patients with prior myocardial infarction. *Circulation*, **93**, 1836–1844.

Huikuri, H.V., Makikallio, T.H., Peng, C.K., Goldberger, A.L., Hintze, U. & Moller, M. for the DIAMOND Study Group (2000) Fractal correlation properties of RR interval dynamics and mortality in patients with depressed left ventricular function after an acute myocardial infarction. *Circulation*, **101**, 47–53.

Ivanov, P.C., Amaral, L.A.N., Goldberger, A.L. *et al.* (1999) Multifractality in human heartbeat dynamics. *Nature (London)* **399**, 461–465.

Kimura, S., Bassett, A.L., Kohya, T., Kozlovskis, P.L. & Myerburg, R.J. (1986) Simultaneous recording of action potentials from endocardium and epicardium during ischaemia in the isolated cat ventricle: relation of temporal electrophysiological heterogeneities to arrhythmias. *Circulation*, **74**, 401–409.

Kleiger, R.E., Miller, J.P., Bigger, J.T. & Moss, A.R. for the Multicentre Post-Infarction Research Group (1987) Decreased heart rate variability and its association with increased mortality after acute myocardial infarction. *American Journal of Cardiology*, **59**, 256–262.

La Rovere, M.T., Bigger, J.T., Jr, Marcus, F.I. *et al.* (1998) Baroreflex sensitivity and heart-rate variability in prediction of total cardiac mortality after myocardial infarction: ATRAMI (Autonomic Tone and Reflexes After Myocardial Infarction) Investigators. *Lancet* **351**, 478–484.

Leclercq, J., Maison-Blanche, P., Cauchemez, B. & Coumel, P. (1988) Respective role of sympathetic tone and of cardiac pauses in the genesis of 62 cases of ventricular fibrillation recorded during Holter monitoring. *European Heart Journal*, **9**, 1276–1283.

Leclercq, J.-F., Potenza, S., Maison-Blanche, P., Chastang, C. & Coumel, P. (1996) Determinants of spontaneous occurrence of sustained monomorphic ventricular tachycardia in right ventricular dysplasia. *Journal of the American College of Cardiology*, **28**, 720–724.

Leenhardt, A., Glaser, E., Burguera, M., Nürnberg, M., Maison-Blanche, P. & Coumel, P. (1994) Short-coupled variant of torsades de pointes. A new electrocardiographic entity in the spectrum of idiopathic ventricular tachyarrhythmias. *Circulation*, **89**, 206–215.

Lindsay, B.D., Ambos, H.D., Schechtman, N.B., Arthur, R.M. & Cain, M.E. (1990) Noninvasive detection of patients with ischaemic and nonischaemic heart disease prone to ventricular fibrillation. *Journal of the American College of Cardiology*, **16**, 1656–1664.

Locati, E., Maison-Blanche, P., Dejode, P., Cauchemez, B. & Coumel, P. (1995) Spontaneous sequences of torsades de pointes in patients with acquired prolonged repolarization: Quantitative analysis of Holter recordings. *Journal of the American College of Cardiology*, **25**, 1564–1575.

Lombardi, F., Verrier, R.L. & Lown, B. (1983) Relationship between sympathetic neural activity, coronary dynamics, and vulnerability to ventricular fibrillation during myocardial ischaemia and reperfusion. *American Heart Journal*, **105**, 958–965.

Lombardi, F., Porta, A., Marzegalli, M. *et al.* (2000) Heart rate variability patterns before ventricular tachycardia onset in patients with an implantable cardioverter defibrillator. *American Journal of Cardiology*, **86**, 959–963.

Mäkikallio, T., Koistinen, J., Jordaens, L. *et al.* (1999) Heart rate dynamics before spontaneous onset of ventricular fibrillation in patients with healed myocardial infarcts. *American Journal of Cardiology*, **83**, 880–884.

Pitzalis, M.-V., Mastropasqua, F., Massari, F. *et al.* (1997) Dependency of premature ventricular contractions on heart rate. *American Heart Journal*, **133**, 153–161.

Pozzati, A., Pancaldi, L., Di Pasquale, G., Pinelli, G. & Bugiardini, R. (1996) Transient sympatho-vagal imbalance triggers 'ischaemic' sudden death in patients undergoing electrocardiographic Holter monitoring. *Journal of the American College of Cardiology*, **27**, 847–852.

Pruvot, E., Thonet, G., Vesin, J.-M. *et al.* (2000) Heart rate dynamics at the onset of ventricular tachyarrhythmias as retrieved from implantable cardioverter-defibrillators in patients with coronary artery disease. *Circulation*, **101**, 2398–2404.

Sapoznikov, D., Luria, M. & Gotsman, M. (1999) Changes in sinus *RR* interval patterns preceding ventricular ectopic beats: assessment with heart rate enhancement and dynamic heart rate trends. *International Journal of Cardiology*, **68**, 217–224.

Schwartz, P.J., La Rovere, M.T. & Vanoli, E. (1992) Autonomic nervous system and sudden cardiac death: experimental basis and clinical observations for post-myocardial infarction risk stratification. *Circulation*, **85**, 177–191.

Shusterman, V., Aysin, B., Gottipaty, V. *et al.* (1998) Autonomic nervous system activity and the spontaneous initiation of ventricular tachycardia. *Journal of the American College of Cardiology*, **32**, 1891–1899.

Shusterman, V., Aysin, B., Weiss, R. *et al.* (2000) Dynamics of the low frequency *RR*-interval oscillations preceding spontaneous ventricular tachycardia. *American Heart Journal*, **139**, 126–133.

Shusterman, V., Aysin, B., Anderson, K. & Beigel, A. (2001) Multidimensional rhythm disturbances as a precursor of sustained ventricular tachyarrhythmias. *Circulation Research*, **88**, 705–712.

Skinner, J.E., Pratt, C.M. & Vybiral, T. (1993) A reduction in the correlation dimension of heartbeat intervals precedes imminent ventricular arrhythmias. *American Heart Journal*, **125**, 731–743.

Valkama, J.O., Huikuri, H.V., Koistinen, M.J., Yli-Macyry, S., Airaksinen, K.E.J. & Myerburg, R.J. (1995) Relation between heart rate variability and spontaneous and induced ventricular arrhythmias in patients with coronary artery disease. *Journal of the American College of Cardiology*, **25**, 437–443.

Vybiral, T., Glaeser, D.H., Goldberger, A.L. *et al.* (1993) Conventional heart rate variability analysis of ambulatory electrocardiographic recordings fails to predict imminent ventricular fibrillation. *Journal of the American College of Cardiology*, **22**, 557–565.

Winkle, R.A. (1982) The relationship between ventricular ectopic beat frequency and heart rate. *Circulation*, **66**, 439–446.

Zimmermann, M., Maison-Blanche, P., Cauchemez, B., Leclercq, J.-F. & Coumel, P. (1986) Determinants of the spontaneous ectopic activity in repetitive monomorphic idiopathic ventricular tachycardia. *Journal of the American College of Cardiology*, **7**, 1219–1227.

SECTION VII

Electrocardiogram of an Implanted Device

CHAPTER 61

Electrocardiographic Monitoring with Implantable Devices

Richard Houben and Fred Lindemans

Introduction

The first implantable cardiac pacemaker was developed by Dr Rune Elmqvist and used in a patient in 1958 by Dr Ake Senning (Elmqvist & Senning 2002). It paced the ventricle asynchronously, not having the capability of electrogram sensing which was introduced in 1963 to synchronize ventricular stimuli to spontaneous atrial activation. Since that time, clinical, surgical and technological developments have proceeded at a remarkable rate, providing us with the highly reliable, extensive therapeutic and diagnostic implantable device functions that we know today. A modern pulse generator system contains a power source, timing circuitry, sense amplifiers and stimulation output stages for either one, two or three channels connected to the electrodes, memory circuits and a transceiver enabling telemetric communication between the implanted device and the physician using a dedicated programming device. The most significant improvements have included reduction of device size, extended longevity, added device functionality, sensor driven pacing rate, and extensive programmability.

The use of electrocardiographic signals in implantable devices started in pacemakers when the cardiac electrogram recorded from the pacing electrode was used to either inhibit or trigger stimuli. The ability to analyse the electrogram as it was recorded by the pacemaker in real time was introduced with the development of electrogram telemetry. Using the programmer, atrial or ventricular electrograms could be displayed for the purpose of troubleshooting and assessing lead function. With the introduction of the implantable automatic defibrillator in 1980 (Mirowski *et al.* 1980) the clinical need was recognized to reconstruct the arrhythmic events causing defibrillation therapy. As arrhythmia detection was based on interval criteria applied to the cardiac electrogram, storage of electrogram episodes pre- and post therapy was a logical and practical approach. Initially, just a few seconds of the electrogram, sampled at about 128 samples/s from one channel and one arrhythmia episode could be stored. Nowadays, up to 20-min recordings of atrial and ventricular electrograms, using programmable electrode combinations as source, representing several arrhythmia episodes with date and time annotation can be stored in defibrillator memory. The information can later be retrieved and displayed using the device programmer but it is also possible to transmit the electrogram information in real time to a modified Holter recorder for detailed analysis of device functions. When the clinical utility of continuous arrhythmia monitoring as developed for implantable cardioverter defibrillators was recognized, electrogram storage was also incorporated in implantable pacemakers where it helped understand the reason for high rate episodes as well as documented the incidence of non-sustained tachyarrhythmia and the success or failure of drug therapy for AF. Finally storage of a subcutaneously recorded pseudo-ECG signals using pacemaker technology was introduced in 1997 with

The authors thank Jaak Minten, Veronique Mahaux and Brian Lee for their kind support providing us with episodes of electrograms obtained from Medtronic GemDR® and Reveal®Plus.

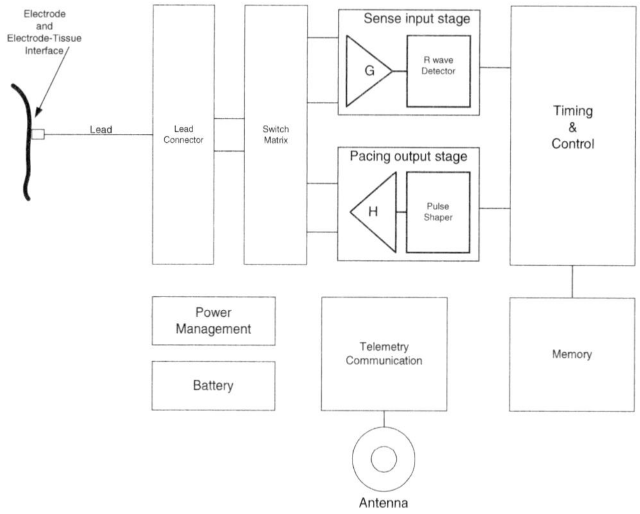

Fig. 61.1 Representation of the main functions included in an implantable cardiac pacemaker system. The switch matrix ensures mutually exclusive connection of the sensing input stage or the pacing output stage to the electrode system. The timing and control block includes functions for interpretation of the sensed events controlling the execution of pacing algorithms. The telemetric communication channel allows parameter adjustments and retrieval of diagnostic information from the implanted device.

the purpose of documenting rarely occurring arrhythmias that escaped the external Holter approach (Krahn *et al.* 1997a,b, 1999).

This chapter will deal with some of the technological challenges encountered in recording cardiac electrograms or pseudo ECGs with implanted devices.

Implantable cardiac pacemakers

The block schematic of Fig. 61.1 shows the system functions of an implantable single chamber pulse generator (IPG) with the signal path from and to the heart and various support functions that include power management, telemetric communication and memory.

The lead system

The connection between the heart and the implanted pulse generator is provided by an implantable electrode catheter called 'lead'. A unipolar lead system has a single isolated conductor with an electrode located at the tip. A bipolar lead has two separate and isolated conductors connecting the two electrodes, i.e. the anode and cathode, usually not more than 15 mm apart. Cathode refers to the electrode serving as the negative pole for delivering the stimulation pulse, anode to the positive pole. For unipolar pacing-sensing systems, the distance between anode and cathode easily exceeds 10 cm. Its cathode is typically located at the lead tip while the pulse generator housing, usually located in the pectoral region is used as anode. Several types of bipolar leads exist, including the coaxial lead allowing a diameter in the range of 4 to 5 F, which is comparable to state-of-the-art unipolar leads. Sensing behaviour of bipolar lead systems outperform their unipolar counterparts by providing a better signal to noise ratio. Bipolar leads are less sensitive to electromagnetic interference (EMI) sources and skeletal muscle potentials. However, owing to their construction, bipolar leads are stiffer and more complex from a mechanical construction point of view.

Electrode–tissue interface and sensing preamplifier

Many analytical models have been developed to describe the complex electrochemical reactions that take place at the interface between tissue and electrode surface. These models have been used to characterize the sense amplifier input source as well as the load 'seen' by the stimulator output circuit. These models can become quite complicated, and are often over-determined making them inconclusive in finding values for the individual components in the model. A simple but frequently adequate model is shown in Fig. 61.2, which includes a voltage source V_p modelling the half-cell potential, a series resistor R_s and a capacitor C_H connected in parallel to a resistor R_F. The series resistor R_s describes the ohmic impedance of the tissue surrounding the

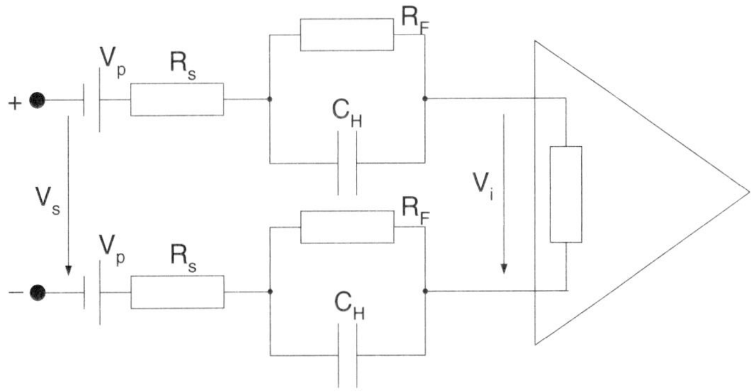

Fig. 61.2 A simple but practical impedance network is shown modelling the tissue–electrode interface. The signal generated by the bioelectrical source V_s enters the network at the left two terminals. The voltage source V_p is included to model the electrode half-cell potential. A capacitor C_H connected in parallel to a resistor R_F represents the impedance and polarization associated with the electrode-electrolyte interface. A series resistor R_s associated with the geometric area of the electrode, the conductivity of the tissue, and the resistance of the electrode materials and conductors. The impedance network connected to the sense amplifier with an input resistance R_i creates a transfer function which enables the calculation of the voltage presented at the input terminals of the amplifier given the source potential V_s.

electrode. Its magnitude is largely determined by the geometric properties of the electrode surface. The parallel resistor R_F and capacitor C_H describe the electrochemical processes occurring at the electrode tissue interface such as the formation of an electric double layer and electrochemical reactions such as the discharge of positively charged ions at the cathode. The combined effect of these components on the transfer of the cardiac electrogram to the circuitry of the device depends on signal frequency and, of course, the input impedance of the amplifier representing the first stage of the sensing circuitry. The half-cell potential V_p is important for diagnostic applications recording the electrogram. When the electrode-tissue interface is mechanically disturbed, e.g. by patient movement, this will cause the magnitude of V_p to change abruptly, generating signal artefacts. Furthermore, it should be realized that each of the two electrodes necessary to form a sensing or stimulation circuit has its own electrode-tissue interface with potentially different model components depending on electrode size, material and surface finish. Even two electrodes that are manufactured as identical may have slightly different component properties depending on the surface at the microscopic level. (Neuman 2000).

Although AC-coupling of the electrode system to the input amplifier will filter out the DC-components caused by the half-cell potentials, sudden changes at the electrode-tissue interface may still cause DC-swings in the electrogram, also well known in surface electrocardiograms owing to motion artefacts (Ferguson 1997).

It is clear that the transfer function of an electrode–amplifier interface is frequency dependent. At low frequencies, the impedance is dominated by the series resistor R_s and R_F, whereas at higher frequencies C_H bypasses the effect of R_F leaving the effect of R_s. In an electrode system that is used for stimulation and sensing, challenges are posed by the disturbance of the electrode-tissue interface caused by every stimulus charging or discharging the interface and modifying the half-cell potential. (Kindermann *et al.* 1992). In practice, this means that sensing has to be deactivated for a brief period during and after each stimulus in order to resolve the electrode polarization effects of the stimulus and to allow the amplifier and filters to settle after the stimulus artefact. In pacemakers, these totally or partially blind periods are called blanking and refractory periods respectively. In applications where shortening the blanking period is crucial, e.g. those where sensing of the T wave is required, the use of a tri-phasic pulse as proposed by Vonk & van Oort (1998) has proven to be successful in minimizing residual charge resulting from polarization.

Detection and sensing circuitry

The dynamic ranges of atrial and ventricular electrograms to be handled by the sense circuitry typically are in the range between 0.5–7 and 3–20 mV, respectively. Slew rates range between 0.1 and 4 V/s. For the QRS complex, spectral power concentrates in the band from 10 to 30 Hz. The T wave is a slower signal component with a reduced amount of power in a band not exceeding 10 Hz. While enhancing intrinsic cardiac signals, the circuit needs to be robust against artefacts generated from non-cardiac sources located outside or inside the patient. Since the introduction of electronic article surveillance systems (EAS), concerns have existed with regard to the possible interaction between emitting field sources and the sense amplifiers of medical implantable devices like pacemakers (Harthorne 2001), implantable cardioverter defibrillators and insertable loop recorders (de Cock *et al.* 2000). Other sources of electromagnetic inference (EMI) include cellular phones, metal detector gates, high voltage power lines (Dawson *et al.* 2000, 2002), electrocautery devices and MRI equipment (Lauck *et al.* 1995). The more sensitive atrial sensing channel of bradyarrhythmia devices is most prone to detection of EMI. Any type of EMI having sufficient amplitude could cause the pacemaker to react in a clinically undesirable way, either inhibiting or triggering stimuli. Noise reversion algorithms and circuits, however, most often provide reliable discrimination between EMI and intrinsic cardiac activity.

Once the electrogram enters the sensing circuit, carefully tuned band-pass filters isolate those cardiac components most clearly representing cardiac depolarization while attenuating noise sources. The detection circuit following the sense amplifier facilitates robust discrimination of P, T and R waves based on the slew rate of the signal. A comparator relating the filtered signal against a reference voltage generates a logical signal if the instantaneous signal exceeds the reference voltage. The sensing threshold is a representation of the minimum slew rate of the wave to be detected. Modulation of the sensitivity during the cardiac cycle increasing sensitivity towards the end of the cycle is implemented either by changing the reference voltage or the amplifier gain. This avoids oversensing of the T wave while allowing high sensitivity after the T wave. Amplifier gain control will change the sensing threshold at a constant reference voltage. Optimal settings need to be found to prevent oversensing of myopotentials while assuring an adequate sensitivity floor. Implantable cardioverter defibrillators (ICD) are presented with an extended range of R wave amplitudes because the electrogram amplitude may drop substantially during fibrillation. At the same time detection of P and T waves must be prevented as they might cause overestimation of heart rate causing inappropriate therapy (shock delivery). Automatic threshold control (ATC) algorithms are used to adjust sensitivity based on electrogram qualities such as R wave amplitude. As an alternative, automatic gain control (AGC) is used by some manufacturers. Threshold modulation functions now are shifted from the R wave detector to the preamplifier (Fig. 61.1) The amplifier gain is changed as a function of time starting from the moment of expiration of the sensed refractory period (Niehaus *et al.* 2002). Although AGC is electronically different it is functionally equal to ATC (Brewer *et al.* 1996).

So far in this chapter, electrogram sensing has been described for the purpose of detecting cardiac activation in order to determine the need for stimulation or defibrillation therapy.

Implantable cardioverter defibrillators

All of the above considerations are also important when looking at the properties of devices that store cardiac electrograms or subcutaneous electrocardiograms for diagnostic purposes. Initially, the capability to look at pacemaker electrograms was developed to better monitor pacemaker function and to diagnose sensing problems.

Standard pacemaker diagnostic capabilities include long-term assessment of battery status, energy consumption, and lead impedance. Counters allow quantitative assessment of sense circuitry performance for both the atrial and the ventricular channel separately (Waktare & Malik 1997). Pacemakers were equipped with circuitry to transmit electrograms and diagnostic information via telemetry to the pacemaker programmer.

The capability to automatically store electrograms in a device was first developed for implantable cardioverter defibrillators (ICDs) in order to allow evaluation of cardiac rhythms that had triggered device intervention. Initially, device memory was limited and only a few seconds of electrogram could be stored into the device for later retrieval by the programmer (Fig. 61.1). More recent ICD models are equipped with more elaborate functions like the capability of automatic storage of both atrial and ventricular electrograms for several minutes. Reliable sensing, detection and classification of atrial and ventricular arrhythmias enabled effective use of the available memory making relevant episodes available to the physician by telemetric communication. Various combinations of implanted electrodes can be selected as a source for the electrograms further enhancing the interpretation of the arrhythmias. Electrograms stored in ICD digital memory have a wider bandwidth and dynamic range than electrograms used for event detection. Entering the digital, discrete time domain requires conversion of the electrogram. Although it is generally accepted that the frequency content of the recorded electrogram does not exceed 100 Hz, measures must be taken to prevent aliasing effects. Anti-aliasing circuits need to be included reducing input signal bandwidth below a maximum related to the frequency where the sample and hold circuits operate. Both analogue and digital anti-aliasing filters may be considered. The analogue approach is straightforward. Constant group-delay filters are preferred since they prevent the introduction of harmonic distortion in the electrogram. Since a steep filter is required at a low cut-off frequency, the design will contain relative large capacitors taking up precious device volume. As an alternative, digital handling of the aliasing problem may be considered by including a delta-sigma analogue to digital converter (ADC), over-sampling the electrogram generating a single bit pulse-code modulated sequence. Over-sampling ADCs typically sample the electrogram at a rate of 16 or 32 times the bandwidth of the electrogram. Because of this high sampling rate, aliasing problems are minimized at this stage and therefore lacking the need for rigorous analogue filtering. A digital filter removes the high frequency quantization noise introduced by the modulator and decimates the data sequence to the required sampling frequency and digital word length required. Most of the aliasing problem now has been shifted from the analogue to the digital domain handled by the digital decimating filter. This enables a higher degree of integration saving device space occupied by analogue filters. Another advantage is the flexibility of trading sampling rate against resolution depending on the decimating filter used. Without changing the structure of the circuits, sample rate can be increased while word length (or resolution, number of bits) is decreased and vice versa. This enables digitization of the electrogram specific for cardiac event detection as well as for storage in the device memory.

The minimum required resolution is determined by the dynamic range of the signal to be covered in the digital domain. If a signal range of $\pm$ 20 mV and a resolution of 20 μV have to be maintained (60 dB), a minimum ADC resolution of 10 bits is required.

Although electrogram storage capabilities in ICDs were originally developed for better interpretation of the appropriateness of device intervention, physicians quickly recognized the value of these stored electrograms for rhythm and arrhythmia evaluation (Fig. 61.3).

Along with other diagnostic data a patient information base can be compiled which allows for monitoring of disease progression and therapy efficacy including pharmacological treatment e.g. for atrial fibrillation (Wijffels *et al.* 1995).

Implantable diagnostic and Holter devices

Supported by the availability of even more dense, low-power digital memories and microcomputers, automatically triggered recording of arrhythmias developed for ICDs has been implemented in implantable devices specifically developed for capturing arrhythmias that could not be diagnosed with traditional Holter monitoring due to their rare occurrence (Nowak 2002). Specifically, Insertable Loop Recorders (ILRs) like the Medtronic Reveal®Plus (Medtronic Inc., Minneapolis MN, USA), are indicated for patients who experience transient symptoms like unexplained cardiac syncope (Simantirakis *et al.*

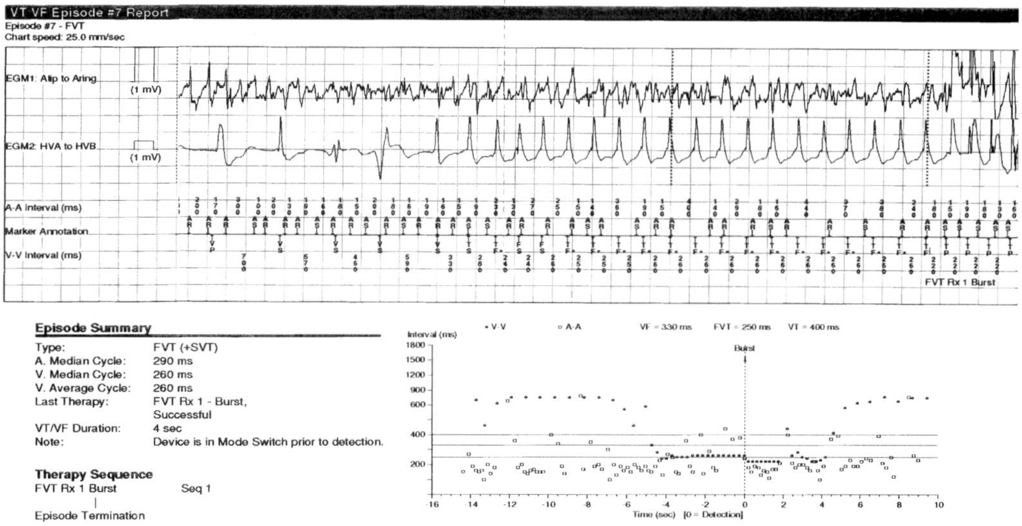

Fig. 61.3 Shows a selected strip including an episode summary and an interval plot of a double tachycardia obtained from a Medtronic GemDR 7221. A fast VT is initiated by a premature beat when AF is already ongoing. The strip displays atrial (EGM1: Atip–Aring) and ventricular electrograms (EGM2: HVA–HVB) together with the associated marker channel. The episode summary gives the double tachycardia classification information. The interval plot (lower right panel) displays the atrial and ventricular intervals before and after ventricular arrhythmia detection and therapy. AR, atrial refractory; Atip, atrial electrode tip; Aring, atrial electrode ring; HVA, high voltage electrode A; HVB, high voltage electrode B; VP, ventricular pace.

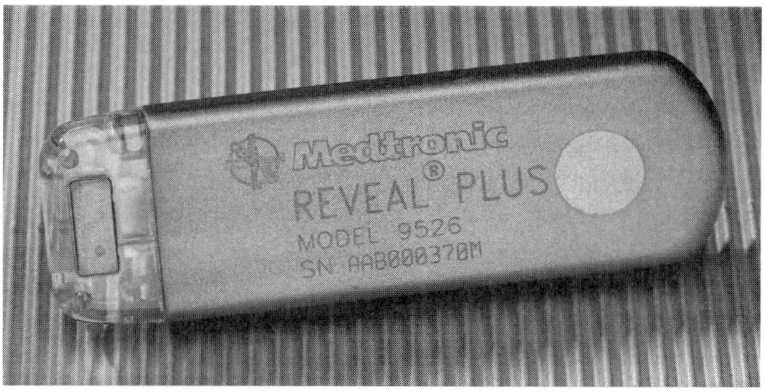

Fig. 61.4 Medtronic Reveal®Plus insertable loop recorder. Recording electrodes are shown at the left (rectangular shape) and right (round shape) with an interelectrode distance of 47 mm.

2000) that may suggest cardiac arrhythmias or dizziness (Fig. 61.4).

Such insertable loop recorders use subcutaneous (SubQ) electrodes to measure a pseudo ECG signal for diagnostic purposes. SubQ electrodes located on the ILR provide a small, direction sensitive recording dipole (Fig. 61.4). The advantage of this lead-less approach is the minimally invasive implant procedure that does not require placement of a lead in the heart. It is recognized that optimal ECG quality, i.e. large QRS amplitude, visible P-wave and pacemaker spikes, is found by left parasternal implantation, preferably with the electrodes directed away from pectoral muscles (Krahn *et al.* 1997a,b; Himmrich *et al.* 2000). Figure 61.5 shows two examples of automatic detection by the Reveal Plus insertable loop recorder.

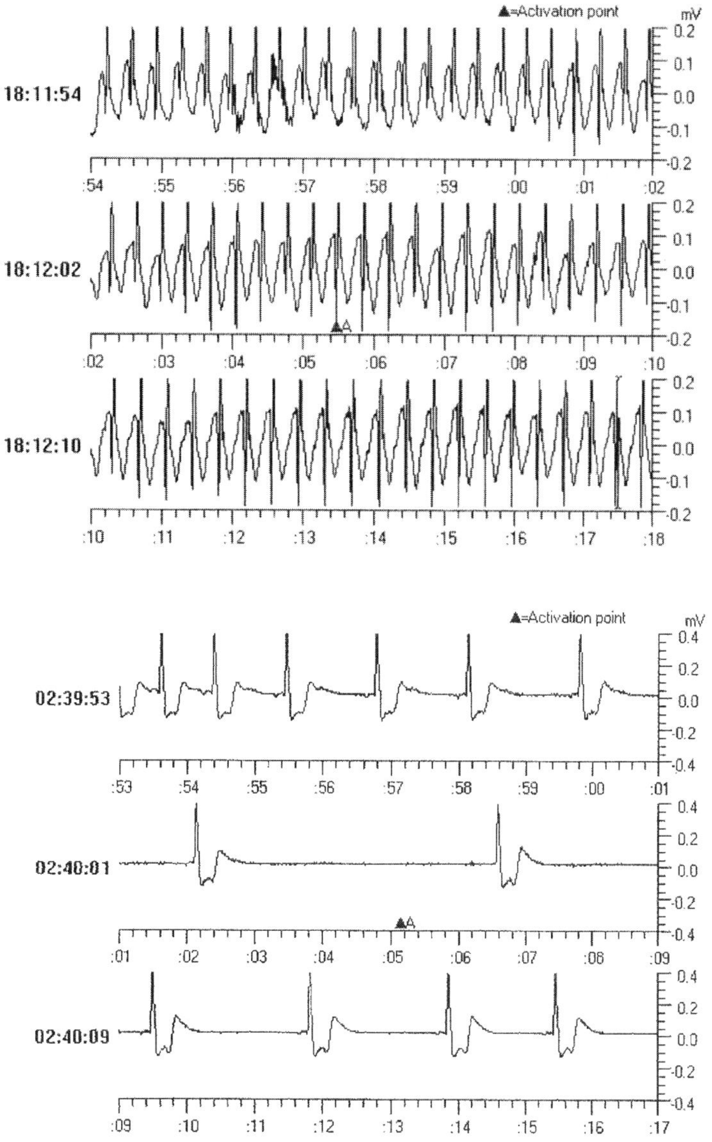

Fig. 61.5 Two examples of automatic detection by Reveal®Plus insertable loop recorder (ILR). Top, detection of a ventricular tachycardia; triangle marked with an 'A', activation point triggering the ILR for storage of the event. Bottom, a rhythm strip of an asystole captured by Reveal®Plus ILR.

Patient movements or pectoral muscle exercise may induce pressure variations at the electrode-skin interface. Referring to the electrode-tissue model (Fig. 61.2), pressure variations change polarization potentials (V_p) and contact resistance, generating an input bias current to the amplifier. AC coupling of the signal to the input of the amplifier solves the problem to some extent, at the expense of loosing low frequency signal content but does not eliminate voltage swings at the input due to sudden changes in the interface potential. Removal of spectral components and nonlinear phase behaviour of the filter around the cut-off frequency will induce harmonic distortion and the ILR is presently unsuitable for analysis of *ST* segment for this reason.

Novel techniques like Static and Dynamic TransLinear circuits (STL, DTL) (Serdijn 2001) allow design and implementation of high dynamic range amplifiers that may be better capable to handle the full range of input signals as a preamplifier preceding digitization. Having the electrogram available in digital format using such circuits, various digital QRS detection algorithms have been described in literature (Pan &

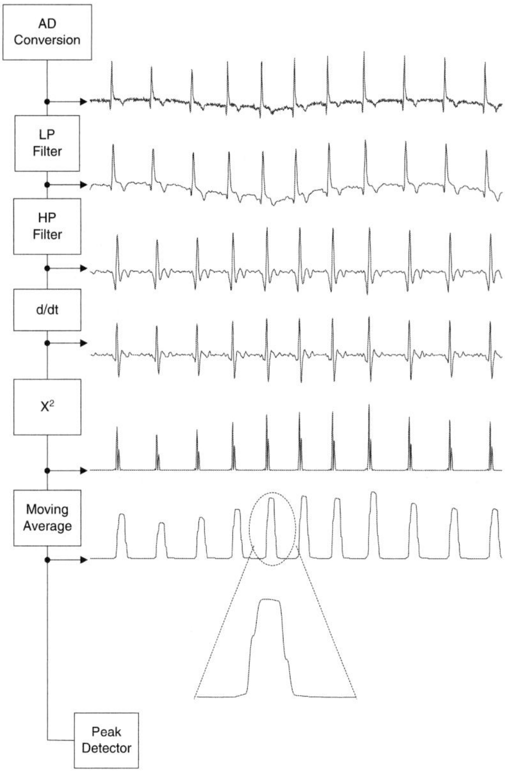

Fig. 61.6 Digital signal processing chain of functions implementing pre-filtering steps prior peak detection. A pseudo ECG signal (top trace), recorded from electrodes (47 mm interelectrode distance) positioned at the left parasternal position, enters the cascade of functions at the top starting with band-pass filtering implemented as a low-pass (LP) filtering step followed by a high pass (HP) filter. Subsequent results of the filtering steps are shown on the right. Next this result is differentiated using a five-point differentiator. The squaring function performs nonlinear amplification of the output of the derivative. Moving window integration is used to obtain waveform feature information related to the slope of the R wave.

Tompkins 1985) that rely on detection of the maximum negative slope in the signal, by several digital filtering stages preceding a peak detector. Digital filtering mainly involves multiply-accumulate operations taking input samples and filter coefficients as arguments. Quantization noise introduced because of word length effects is minimized by using integer filter coefficients. For efficient implementation, filter coefficients are preferably powers of two and have small variation. Classically a cascade of signal processing functions include a linear filter, with a pass-band between 5 and 11 Hz followed by a differentiator, a square or absolute value function and a moving average filter generating a peak feature signal to detect the maximum negative slope of the R wave (Hamilton & Tompkins 1986). Next, detection of the R wave is accomplished by comparing the feature signal against a predefined threshold (Fig. 61.6). The threshold may be adapted to feature signal variations, e.g. rhythm or respiration effects observed in the amplitude of the R-peak increasing detection sensitivity (Kohler *et al.* 2002). Although such a detector is suited for real-time applications, group delay characteristics of the filter stage generating the feature signal as well as the peak detector induce a fixed delay which makes this method less suited for closed loop control applications that require immediate feedback.

Detection of the electrogram fiducial points may be used to generate long series of *RR* intervals for rate monitoring and high rate detection or as a midpoint reference for extraction of beats for morphology analysis. Analysis of such data can trigger storage of relevant episodes of electrogram data inside or outside the device.

Novel biomedical signal processing methods

To ensure efficient use of the memory available in the implantable device, the incidence of false positives, erroneously triggering automatic storage, should be minimized. For ILRs, promoting factors include a low amplitude electrogram signal as a result of the limited vector available for pseudo ECG measurement, the presence of muscle EMG and mechanical disturbance of the electrode tissue interface. Therefore, signal analysis methods that improve discrimination of signals from noise are of great importance. Frequently however signal and noise components share the same spectral bands limiting the performance of simple filtering.

Signal analysis methods derived from wavelet analysis (Daubechies 1992) carry large potential to support a wide range of biomedical signal processing applications including noise reduction (Mallat 1999; Jansen 2001), feature recognition (Donoho & Johnstone 1994) and signal compression. Wavelets allow analysis of the electrogram focusing on the signal at various levels of detail in analogy with inspection of a sample with a microscope at various levels of magnification. At very fine scales, details of the electrogram are revealed while unimpaired by the overall structure of the signal. At coarse scales the overall structure of the electrogram can be studied while overlooking the details. Analysing the structure of the electrogram over multiple scales allows discrimination of electrogram features pertaining over all scales from those only seen at fine or coarse scales. Based on such observation, the presence or absence of certain electrogram features, e.g. related to proximal or distal electrophysiological phenomena, can be discriminated. An algorithm based on wavelet analysis that compares morphologies of baseline and tachycardia electrograms based on differences between corresponding coefficients of their wavelet transforms has been found highly sensitive for VT detection (Wilkoff *et al.* 2001; Swerdlow *et al.* 2002).

Whereas smoothing attenuates spectral components in the stop band of the linear filter used, wavelet-denoising attempts to remove noise and retain whatever signal is present in the electrogram. Moreover, wavelet methods allow efficient implementation in the digital domain (Strang & Nguyen 1996) using multi-rate filter banks and analogue domain taking advantage of Dynamic TransLinear (DTL) circuit technology (Haddad *et al.* 2002a,b).

It remains to be demonstrated in clinical practice that these novel signal analysis methods will contribute to the further development and application of dynamical electrocardiography. It is clear however that implantable devices can document arrhythmias that typically escape more conventional means of diagnosis. If they should be a method of last resort or if they should be applied early in the diagnostic chain deserves further clinical research including cost effectiveness considerations.

References

Brewer, J.E., Perttu, J.S., Kroll, M.W. & Donohoo, A.M. (1996) Dual level sensing significantly improves automatic threshold control for R wave sensing in implantable defibrillators. The Angeion Corporation. *PACE (Pacing and Clinical Electrophysiology)*, **19** (12 Pt 1), 2051–2059.

de Cock, C.C., Spruijt, H.J., van Campen, L.M., Plu, A.W. & Visser, C.A. (2000) Electromagnetic interference of an implantable loop recorder by commonly encountered electronic devices. *PACE (Pacing and Clinical Electrophysiology)*, **23** (10 Pt 1), 1516–1518.

Daubechies I. (1992) *Ten Lectures on Wavelets.* Society for Industrial and Applied Mathematics, Philadelpha, PA.

Dawson, T.W., Caputa, K., Stuchly, M.A. & Kavet, R. (2002) Pacemaker interference by 60-Hz contact currents. *IEEE (Institute of Electrical and Electronic Engineers) Transactions on Biomedical Engineering*, **49** (8), 878–886.

Dawson, T.W., Stuchly, M.A., Caputa, K., Sastre, A., Shepard, R.B. & Kavet, R. (2000) Pacemaker interference and low-frequency electric induction in humans by external fields and electrodes. *IEEE (Institute of Electrical and Electronic Engineers) Transactions on Biomedical Engineering*, **47** (9), 1211–1218.

Donoho, D. & Johnstone, I. M. (1994) Adapting to unknown smoothness via wavelet shrinkage. *Journal of the American Statistical Association*, **90** (432), 1200–1224.

Elmqvist R. & Senning, A. (2002) *An Implantable Pacemaker for the Heart* (ed. C. N. Smyth), pp. 253–254. Tliffe, London.

Ferguson, T.B., Jr (1997) Pacemakers. *Current Problems in Surgery*, **34** (1), 1–108.

Haddad S, Gieltjes S, Houben R. & Serdijn W.A. (2002a) An ultra low power dynamic translinear cardiac sense amplifier for pacemakers. In: *Proceedings of IEEE International Symposium on Circuits and Systems, Bangkok, Thailand*, pp. V39–V40.

Haddad S, Houben R. & Serdijn W.A. (2002) First derivative Gaussian wavelet function employing dynamic translinear circuits for cardiac signal characterization. In: *Proceedings of the ProRISC/IEEE Workshop on Semiconductors, Circuits, Systems and Signal Processing*, pp. 288–291.

Hamilton, P.S. & Tompkins, W.J. (1986) Quantitative investigation of QRS detection rules using the MIT/BIH arrhythmia database. *IEEE (Institute of Electrical and Electronic Engineers) Transactions on Biomedical Engineering*, **33** (12), 1157–1165.

Harthorne, J.W. (2001) Pacemakers and store security devices. *Cardiology Review*, **9** (1), 10–17.

Himmrich, E., Zellerhoff, C., Nebeling, D. *et al.* (2000) [Where should the implantable ECG event recorder be placed?] *Zeitschrift fuer Kardiologie*, **89** (4), 289–294.

Jansen, M. (2001) *Noise Reduction by Wavelet Thresholding.* Springer Verlag, Berlin.

Kindermann, M., Schwerdt, H., Frohlig, G. & Schieffer, H. (1992) Threshold and polarization properties of modern active fixation atrial leads. *PACE (Pacing and Clinical Electrophysiology)*, **15** (11 Pt 2), 1971–1976.

Kohler, B.U., Hennig, C. & Orglmeister, R. (2002) The principles of software QRS detection. *IEEE Engineering in Medicine and Biology*, **21** (1), 42–57.

Krahn, A.D., Klein, G.J. & Yee, R. (1997) Recurrent syncope. Experience with an implantable loop recorder. *Cardiology Clinics*, **15** (2), 313–326.

Krahn, A.D., Klein, G.J., Yee, R. & Manda, V. (1999) The high cost of syncope: cost implications of a new insertable loop recorder in the investigation of recurrent syncope. *American Heart Journal*, **137** (5), 870–877.

Krahn, A.D., Klein, G.J., Yee, R. & Norris, C. (1997) Maturation of the sensed electrogram amplitude over time in a new subcutaneous implantable loop recorder. *PACE (Pacing and Clinical Electrophysiology)*, **20** (6), 1686–1690.

Lauck, G., von Smekal, A., Wolke, S. *et al.* (1995) Effects of nuclear magnetic resonance imaging on cardiac pacemakers. *PACE (Pacing and Clinical Electrophysiology)*, **18** (8), 1549–1555.

Mallat, S.G. (1999) *A Wavelet Tour of Signal Processing*, 2nd edn. Academic Press, San Diego, CA.

Mirowski, M., Reid, P.R., Mower, M.M. *et al.* (1980) Termination of malignant ventricular arrhythmias with an implanted automatic defibrillator in human beings. *New England Journal of Medicine*, **303** (6), 322–324.

Neuman M.R. (2000) Biopotential electrodes. In: *The Biomedical Engineering Handbook* (ed. J. D. Bronzino), pp. 48.1–48.4. CRC Press, Boca Raton, FL.

Niehaus, M., Neuzner, J., Vogt, J., Korte, T. & Tebbenjohanns, J. (2002) Adjustment of maximum automatic sensitivity (automatic gain control) reduces inappropriate therapies in patients with implantable cardioverter defibrillators. *PACE (Pacing and Clinical Electrophysiology)*, **25** (2), 151–155.

Nowak, B. (2002) Pacemaker stored electrograms: teaching us what is really going on in our patients. *PACE (Pacing and Clinical Electrophysiology)*, **25** (5), 838–849.

Pan, J. & Tompkins, W.J. (1985) A real-time QRS detection algorithm. *IEEE (Institute of Electrical and Electronic Engineers) Transactions on Biomedical Engineering*, **32** (3), 230–236.

Serdijn, W.A. (2001) Low voltage ultra-low-power analog IC design – dynamic translinear circuits. In: *IEEE International Symposium on Circuits and Systems, Sydney*, pp. 1.3.1–1.3.12. Institute of Electrical and Electronic Engineers, Sydney.

Simantirakis, E.N., Chrysostomakis, S.I., Manios, E.G. & Vardas, P.E. (2000) Insertable loop recorder in unmasking the cause of syncope. *PACE (Pacing and Clinical Electrophysiology)*, **23** (10 Pt 1), 1573–1575.

Strang, G. & Nguyen T. (1996) *Wavelets and Filter Banks*. Wellesley Cambridge Press.

Swerdlow, C.D., Brown, M.L., Lurie, K. *et al.* (2002) Discrimination of ventricular tachycardia from supraventricular tachycardia by a downloaded wavelet-transform morphology algorithm: a paradigm for development of implantable cardioverter defibrillator detection algorithms. *Journal of Cardiovascular Electrophysiology*, **13** (5), 432–441.

Vonk, B.F. & Van Oort, G. (1998) New method of atrial and ventricular capture detection. *PACE (Pacing and Clinical Electrophysiology)*, **21** (1 Pt 2), 217–222.

Waktare, J.E. & Malik, M. (1997) Holter, loop recorder, and event counter capabilities of implanted devices. *PACE (Pacing and Clinical Electrophysiology)*, **20** (10 Pt 2), 2658–2669.

Wijffels, M.C., Kirchhof, C.J., Dorland, R. & Allessie, M.A. (1995) Atrial fibrillation begets atrial fibrillation. A study in awake chronically instrumented goats. *Circulation*, **92** (7), 1954–1968.

Wilkoff, B.L., Kuhlkamp, V., Volosin, K. *et al.* (2001) Critical analysis of dual-chamber implantable cardioverter-defibrillator arrhythmia detection: results and technical considerations. *Circulation*, **103** (3), 381–386.

CHAPTER 62

Ischaemic Patterns

Andreas Grom, Christoph Bode and Manfred Zehender

Introduction

The impact of the surface ECG for detection of myocardial ischaemia has been well known for a long time. Typically the ST segment is used for detection of myocardial ischaemia (Bayley *et al.* 1944; Toyoshima *et al.* 1964; Horacek & Wagner 2002). Monitoring the ECG of implanted devices for the occurrence of ischaemic changes could lead to clarification of the substrate of arrhythmias, the origin of chest pain and to administration of anti-ischaemic therapies. Therefore the detection of ischaemic ECG changes is of special interest in ICDs. The implantable cardioverter-defibrillator is well established in the treatment of life-threatening ventricular tachyarrhythmias (Cannom & Prystowsky 1999; Connolly *et al.* 2000; Moss *et al.* 2002). Once implanted, the device will continuously monitor the patient for the occurrence of bradyarrhythmic and tachyarrhythmic complications. As a result, sudden cardiac death remain a rare event in patients with an implanted cardioverter-defibrillator (Cannom & Prystowsky 1999; Pires *et al.* 1999). With the option to effectively prevent sudden cardiac death, progression of the underlying heart disease becomes the prime determinant of the patients' prognosis. In the majority of ICD treated patients suffering from coronary artery disease, such progression will be characterized by new onset ischaemia, acute myocardial infarction and/or the development of ischaemic cardiomyopathy (Moise *et al.* 1985; Waters *et al.* 1993; Gill *et al.* 1996). Ischaemia monitored by the implanted device, therefore, would provide an interesting new diagnostic option in these patients. New onset ischaemia, any change in the frequency and severity of ischaemia episodes, as well as the patients' daily ischaemic burden would become routinely assessable whenever of interest. In addition, ischaemia monitoring in ICDs would further improve the overall and individual understanding of ischaemia and spontaneous ventricular tachyarrhythmias when fatally interacting with each other.

Technical considerations

However the electrocardiograms of implanted devices, such as pacemakers, implantable cardioverter/defibrillators or loop recorders, differ in some major points from the surface ECG:

• Filter properties and frequency response of implantable devices. Common filter properties of implantable devices contain a high pass filter with a cut at a frequency of 3 Hz. This filter is necessary to keep the input signal in a given range despite low frequency interferences such as breathing-dependent alterations with consecutive floating of the baseline. On the other hand, due to a usual sampling rate of 128 Hz and with respect to the sampling theorem, signals with frequencies higher than 64 Hz cannot be analysed. Signals of higher frequencies can even cause artefacts with changes in a low-frequency response. Thus, due to filter properties and due to the temporal resolution, signals in the range between 3 and 64 Hz can be analysed in present implantable devices. Deviations of the ST segment are usually analysed for detection of myocardial ischaemia. These signals consist of frequencies at about 1 Hz, and are therefore not assessable in implantable devices at the moment. The resolution of the amplitude of ST segment changes depends on the digitalization. In commonly-used 8 bit systems, resolution in 128 (or 256 depending on additional stored information, such as time components) steps within the analysed range is possible. This leads to a calculated amplitude resolution between 0.1 and 0.3 mV, depending on safety margins. When applying the criteria of significant ischaemia of the surface ECG (0.1 mV in the Einthoven and Goldberger leads and 0.2 mV in the chest leads), ischaemia should be also recognizable in the ECG in implanted devices (Wood *et al.* 2000).

• Recorded signals are often superimposed by local signals. Stored or analysed electrograms in implantable devices in pacemakers can be derived in unipolar systems only between the tip electrode of the pacemaker electrode and the pacemaker housing. Due to the direct contact of the tip electrode with the myocardial wall, the signal in such an ECG configuration is often superimposed by local signals with morphologies similar to local action potentials. (Wood *et al.* 2000). No criteria are known for the diagnosis of local ischaemia in these signals; furthermore it remains unclear whether ischaemia of more distant regions of the myocardium can be assessed. In bipolar present pacemaker systems, the ECG derived between the tip and the ring electrode is analysed. The considerations about the ECG in unipolar pacemakers can similarly be applied to these systems. But more sophisticated ECG systems for analysis of myocardial ischaemia could become available in bipolar systems: since the ring electrode usually is not directly adjacent to the myocardium, an ECG with farfield signals could be constructed in dual-chamber pacemakers between the ring electrodes of the atrial and ventricular electrode and the pacemaker housing. This ECG system should not be subject to superimposition by local signals. In principle, ECG leads could be constructed in single- and dual- chamber ICD-systems between all available electrodes: the tip and ring electrodes of the ventricular lead, the shock coils in the right ventricle and, if present, the shock coil in the superior cava vein and the ICD-housing. In dual-chamber ICDs, the tip and ring electrodes of an atrial electrode are additionally available. In the ICD again, one has to expect a superimposition of the ECG by local signals in all ECG leads involving the tip electrodes of the ventricular or atrial lead.

• The spatial vector in farfield ECGs in implantable devices is different from the standard surface ECG leads. As the spatial array of the available farfield ECGs in implantable devices differs from the standard surface ECG, the allocation between regional ischaemia and the affected intrathoracic ECG lead is new. Also, not all available ECG leads seem to be suitable for ischaemia detection, as the vector encompasses only a small myocardial area. E.g. one would not expect significant changes in an ECG lead between the right ventricular ring electrode and the right atrial ring electrode if myocardial ischaemia affects the left lateral myocardial wall. At present, only few data are available on the selection of the optimal lead configuration for detection of ischaemia. All these studies were performed with ICD-systems, not with pacemaker systems (see below).

• Alterations due to pacemaker stimulation. Due to ventricular pacing in many patients with implantable devices, the ECG is changed (often similar to a left bundle-branch block). Criteria for detection of myocardial ischaemia in these patients for the surface ECG are available, but these criteria are less well documented than the criteria for normal ECGs (Sgarbossa *et al.* 1996; Theres *et al.* 2000). Furthermore due to lasting electric electrode charge after pacing, the ECG derived via a pacing electrode can also be altered by afterpotentials.

• The processing of the ECG in implanted devices. Different options for processing the ECG in implantable devices with regard to detection of myocardial ischaemia are currently being discussed. The most sophisticated systems could offer continuous online analysis of the ECG in a device for the occurrence of ischaemic changes. In case of such changes an immediate patient alert would be possible to inform the patient (e.g. to stop exercising or to contact a physician), an online alert to a cardiology centre could be transmitted (e.g. via a connected cellular phone) or anti-ischaemic medication could be supplied automatically via a drug pump. Problems in realising such a system are of a technical nature: e.g. high energy consumption of the implantable systems for continuous ECG analysis, sensitivity and specificity of algorithms for detection of ischaemia. Less sophisticated systems could only store the ECG in the implanted device, e.g. for a

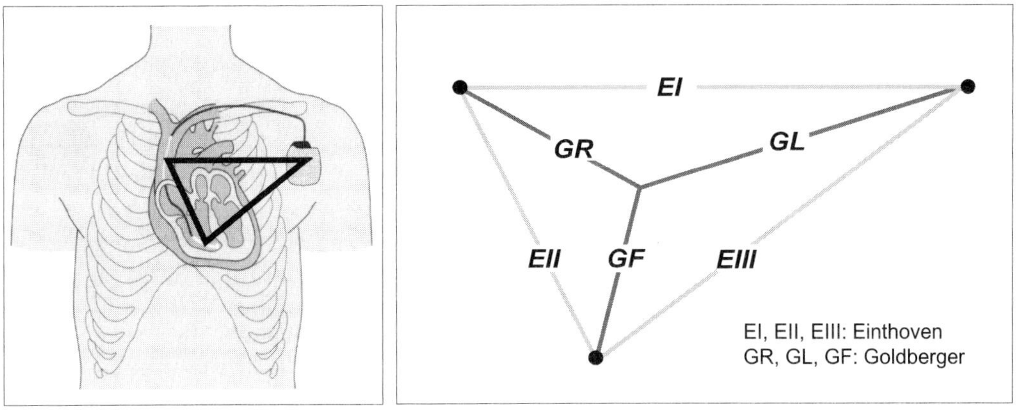

Fig. 62.1 Six ECG leads according to Einthoven and Goldberger derived from the ICD housing, and the two shock coils of the ICD electrode.

few seconds before the delivery of an ICD therapy, during sinus tachycardia or activated by the patient. After interrogating such a system, an offline analysis of the ECG in the device could be performed and ischaemic changes could give evidence of, for example, progression of an underlying coronary artery disease. An advantage of such a system would be lower energy consumption and less technical complexity. Therefore such a system could become available soon.

Current studies

In a study including 22 patients undergoing PTCA at 27 coronary vessel sites, a multipolar electrode catheter was positioned with two electrodes in the right ventricle and two electrodes in the vena cava superior to simulate an ICD-lead with its defibrillation coils in the right ventricle and a second coil in the vena cava superior (Grom *et al.* 1999a,b). Additionally, a cutaneous patch electrode was fixed at the usual ICD implantation site above the left pectoral muscle. Using this electrode system, six intrathoracic ECG leads were constructed according to Goldberger and Einthoven (Fig. 62.1) and registered during the PTCA. These ECGs were compared to the simultaneously recorded standard 12-channel surface ECG. Ischaemic ST segment changes were present already after 30 s of coronary occlusion in all patients in at least one intrathoracic lead compared to about 60% in the surface ECG (also at least one lead). After 120 s of coronary occlusion, these changes were still detectable in all patients in the intrathoracic ECG; whereas in only about 80% of cases ischaemic changes could be detected in the surface ECG at this point of time. An example of a registered intrathoracic ECG is given in Fig. 62.2. Therefore, it is concluded that myocardial ischaemia is detectable in the ICD-based intrathoracic ECG, independent of its localization. Furthermore ischaemic *ST*-changes were visible earlier after coronary occlusion compared to the surface ECG.

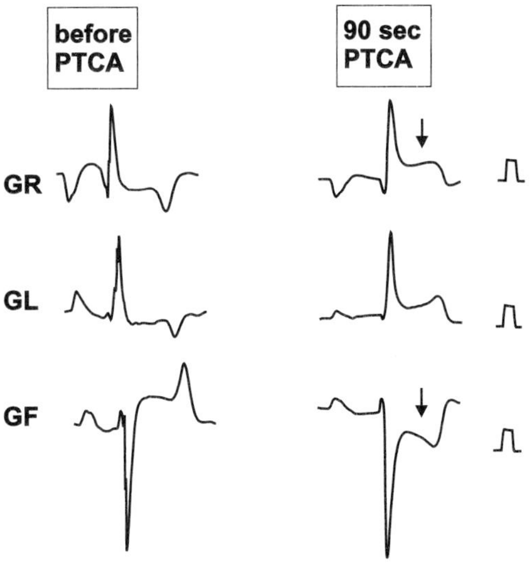

Fig. 62.2 Intrathoracic electrogram (Goldberger leads) before and after 90 s of coronary occlusion owing to PTCA (LAD). Arrows, leads with the highest degree of ST changes.

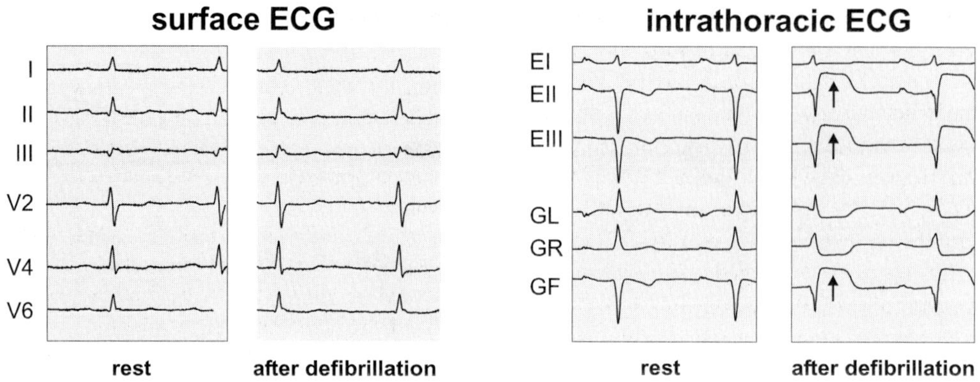

Fig. 62.3 Electrogram before and defibrillation for termination of induced ventricular fibrillation during ICD implantation. Arrows, leads with the highest degree of ST changes.

In another study, during the implantation of 32 ICD systems (Baron *et al.* 2001, personal communication), the intrathoracic ECG derived from a conventional ICD-electrode with two defibrillation coils and an ICD testhousing was digitally stored and analysed. Again, six intrathoracic leads according to Goldberger and Einthoven were reconstructed. In these patients *ST*-changes after defibrillation for termination of induced ventricular fibrillation were easily detectable in the intrathoracic ECG and more marked than in the standard surface ECG (Fig. 62.3).

ST-changes due to coronary artery occlusion detected in the intrathoracic Goldberger lead GF were also analysed in a swine model (Benser 2000) with implantation of a two-electrode (right ventricle, superior cava vein) defibrillation catheter and a left pectoral can electrode. In 11 swine, coronary occlusions at 40 coronary sites were created (each for 2 min) with the help of a balloon catheter. Before occlusion, ST levels were stable; upon occlusion ST levels were altered monotonically, so that ischaemic ST changes could be detected in 30/40 coronary occlusions. Additionally, the detection of absence of occlusion 6 min after arrhythmia-free reperfusion was studied. In 88% of cases the absence of occlusion with a regression of ST changes could be detected.

In an older study performed on 22 dogs (Siegel *et al.* 1982) intracavity catheters were introduced into the left ventricle, the right ventricle and the coronary sinus while graded stenoses of the circumflex and left anterior descending coronary arteries were created. This study was addressed to the detection of ECG changes due to low-grade stenoses and to detect early ECG changes caused by high-grade stenoses. In low-grade stenoses with only unspecific changes in the surface ECG, specific ischaemic changes were found in the intracardiac ECG in 100% of cases in the left ventricle, in 60% in the right ventricle and in 89% in the coronary sinus. In stenoses with no changes in the surface ECG, the figures were 29%, 10% and 19%. Furthermore, localized pacing-induced subendocardial ischaemia in humans could be detected by placement of a unipolar catheter directly at the endocardial surface of the ischaemic region. (Nabel *et al.* 1988).

These data emphasize that local signals from the right ventricle are not sufficient for detection of myocardial ischaemia in the ECG based on implantable devices. The spatial arrangement of intrathoracic electrogram must assure that changes in the whole left ventricle are also assessed. Based on these data and considerations, a system for assessment of relevant ischaemia based on an implantable device would have the following requirements: (1) no direct contact of the ECG lead with the endocardium; (2) spatial arrangement of far field ECG leads including all areas of the left ventricle; (3) avoidance of electrodes used for pacing at the same time. In such a system, myocardial ischaemia could be detected comparable to the surface ECG by changes of the ST segment. However, at the present time it remains unclear if individual reference ECGs are needed in intracardiac electrograms or if deflection of the ST segment from a constructed isoelectric neutral line is sufficient for the diagnosis of myocardial ischaemia. With respect to the feasibility in implantable devices with the limited computing and energy resources, an algorithm for real-time ST segment monitoring was developed and evaluated on ECG examples of the European ST–T-database (surface ECGs; Taddei *et al.* 1992). This algorithm is based on the measurement of the ST deviation at a rate-adapted time after the dominant peak of each QRS complex and subsequent filtering features. The performance of this algorithm seems comparable to other published electrogram algorithms that were validated on the same data set. Estimation of the computational burden suggests that this algorithm could process two electrogram channels continuously for >5 years with current ICD device technology (Stadler *et al.* 2001). A validation of this algorithm on electrograms derived from implantable systems is still missing.

No data are available on detection of myocardial ischaemia in pacemaker systems, albeit such a system seems conceivable. To meet the above-specified requirements, detection of myocardial ischaemia in pacemakers could be based on ECG leads derived from the ring electrodes of bipolar pacemaker electrodes and a left pectoral implanted pacemaker housing. Only unipolar pacemaker stimulation would be advisable in this system. The problem of ischaemia detection in the paced electrogram was addressed above. In one patient with known coronary artery disease, significant ST changes related to typical ischaemic chest pain could be recorded by an implanted event recorder (Vlay & Lawson 2000).

Detection of myocardial ischaemia with intrathoracic farfield ECGs based on ICD- or pacemaker technique seems a promising new feature. Such a system could be implemented in ICD systems, with the above mentioned special benefits for this patients group. In a second step, analogous to progress in engineering, ischaemia-detecting features could also be implemented in the smaller pacemaker devices with even less energy and computing resources compared to ICD devices.

References

Baron, T.W., Grom, A., Brunner, M., Pietsch, M., Faber, T.S. & Zehender, M. (2001) Intrathoracic 6-lead ECG in the ICD – a new diagnostic tool providing extended information like the standard ECG. *Circulation*, **104** (17 Suppl. II), 655.

Bayley, R. H., Ladue, J. S. & York, D. J. (1944) Electrocardiographic changes (local ventricular ischaemia and injury) produced in the dog by temporary occlusion of a coronary artery showing a new stage in the evolution of myocardial infarction. *American Heart Journal*, B, 164.

Benser, M.E., Walcott, G.P., Killingsworth, C.R., Girouard, S.D. & Ideker, R.E. (2000) Detection of regional myocardial ischaemia using an ICD lead set. *Journal of the American College of Cardiology*, 2000 (Suppl. A), 135A.

Cannom, D.S. & Prystowsky, E.N.(1999) Management of ventricular arrhythmias – detection, drugs and devices. *JAMA (Journal of the American Medical Association)*, **281**, 172–179.

Connolly, S.J., Hallstrom, A.P., Cappato, R. *et al.* (2000) Meta-analysis of the implantable cardioverter secondary prevention trials. *European Heart Journal*, **21**, 2071–2078.

Gill, J.B., Cairns, J.A., Roberts, R.S. (1996) Prognostic importance of myocardial ischaemia detected by ambulatory monitoring early after acute myocardial infarction. *New England Journal of Medicine*, **334** (2), 65–70.

Grom, A., Faber, T.S., Brunner, M., Baron, T. & Zehender, M. (1999a) Reconstructed 'farfield' ECG leads in the ICD vs. standard surface ECG: a new option to monitor myocardial ischaemia. *European Heart Journal*, **20** (Suppl.), 115 (abstract).

Grom, A., Faber, T.S., Macharzina, R., Baron, T.W. & Zehender, M. (1999b) Detection of localized myocardial ischaemia by ECG leads available in the implantable cardioverter-defibrillator *Circulation*, **100** (18 Suppl. I), 786.

Horacek, B. M. & Wagner G. S. (2002) Electrocardiographic ST segment changes during acute myocardial ischaemia. *Cardiac Electrophysiology*, **6** (3), 196–203.

Moise, A., Bourassa, M.G. & Theroux, P. (1985) Prognostic significance of progression of coronary artery disease. *American Journal of Cardiology*, **55**, 941–948.

Moss, A.J., Zareba, W., Hall, W.J. *et al.* (2002) Prophylactic implantation of a defibrillatior in patients with myocardial infarction and reduced ejection fraction. *New England Journal of Medicine*, **346**, 877–883.

Nabel, E.G., Shook, T.L., Meyerovitz, M., Ganz, P., Selwyn, A.P. & Friedman, P.L. (1988) Detection of pacing induced myocardial ischaemia by endocardial electrograms recorded during cardiac catheterisation. *Journal of the American College of Cardiology*, **11** (5), 983–992.

Pires, L.A., Lehmann, M.H., Steinman, R.T., Baga, J.J. & Schuger, C.D. (1999) Sudden death in implantable cardioverter-defibrillator recipients: Clinical context, arrhythmic events and device responses. *Journal of the American College of Cardiology*, **33**, 24–32.

Sgarbossa, E.B., Pinski, S.L., Barbagelata, A. *et al.* (1996) Electrocardiographic diagnosis of evolving acute myocardial infarction in the presence of left bundle-branch block. GUSTO-1 (Global Utilization of Streptokinase and Tissue Plasminogen Activator for Occluded Coronary Arteries) Investigators. *New England Journal of Medicine* 22, **334** (8), 481–487.

Siegel, S., Brodman, R., Fischer, J., Matos, J., Furman, S. (1982) Intracardiac electrode detection of early or subendocardial ischaemia. *Pacing and Clinical Electrophysiology*, **5**, 892–902.

Stadler, R.W., Lu, S.N., Nelson, S.D. & Stylos, L. (2001) A real-time ST segment monitoring algorithm for implantable devices. *Journal of Electrocardiology*, **34** (Suppl.), 119–126.

Taddei, A., Distante, G., Emdin, M. *et al.* (1992) The European *S–T*–T-database: standard for evaluating systems for the analysis of ST–T changes in ambulatory electrocardiography. *European Heart Journal*, **13**, 1164–1172.

Theres, H., Stylos, L., Stadler, R.W. *et al.* (2000) Comparison of subcutaneous electrode array, intracardiac electrogram, and ECG for detection of ischaemia during ventricular paced and normal sinus rhythm. *Europace*, **1** (Suppl.), D31.

Toyoshima, H., Ekmekci, A., Flamm, E. *et al.* (1964) Angina pectoris. VII. The nature of ST depression in acute myocardial ischaemia. *American Journal of Cardiology*, **13**, 498–509.

Vlay, S.C. & Lawson, W.E. (2000) Demonstration of myocardial ischaemia by an internal loop recorder. *PACE (Pacing and Clinical Electrophysiology)*, **23**, 1576–1578.

Waters, D., Craven, T.E. & Lesperance, J. (1993) Prognostic significance of progression of coronary atherosclerosis *Circulation*, **87**, 1067–1075.

Wood, M.A., Swerdlow, C. & Olson, W. H. (2000) Sensing and arrhythmia detection by implantable devices. In *Clinical Cardiac Pacing and Defibrillation* (eds K. A. Ellenbogen, G. N. Kay & G. N. Wilkoff), 2nd edn, pp. 68–82. W. B. Saunders, Philadelphia.

CHAPTER 63

State-of-the-Art Marker Channels

Walter H. Olson

ECG interpretation for pacemakers

During the 1960s and 1970s the ECGs of single chamber pacemakers were easy to interpret. Pacing outputs were large and often unipolar so pacing artefacts were prominent. The pacing rate was fixed so sensing for either VVI or AAI mode could be easily interfered by measuring back in time from the pacing spike by the interval corresponding to the lower pacing rate. Ventricular undersensing of intrinsic QRS complexes was apparent and ventricular oversensing resulted in inappropriate delay of pacing spikes. Loss of capture was obvious if the paced QRS morphology did not follow each pacing spike. Simple ECG ladder diagrams were sometimes used to aid this indirect timing analysis.

In the early 1980s when dual chamber pacemakers were introduced, the interpretation of pacemaker ECGs became difficult. There were separate atrial and ventricular pacing spikes, oversensing of pacing spikes from the opposite chamber (cross-talk), atrial oversensing of ventricular depolarizations (far-field R waves (FFRW)), and atrial sensing of retrograde conduction from the ventricle to the atrium could combine with the pacemaker A-V delay to produce pacemaker-mediated tachycardia (PMT). Pacemaker timing logic was added to mitigate these problems. Safety pacing prevents ventricular asystole in heart block patients due to ventricular oversensing from atrial pacing cross-talk. The pacemaker postventricular atrial refractory period (PVARP) prevents atrial tracking of oversensed FFRW. Automatic PVARP extension after premature ventricular contractions (PVC) prevents most PMTs. The knowledge required to interpret ECGs produced by pacemakers increased dramatically and has continued with rate smoothing, rate adaptive AV intervals, automatic mode switching, capture management, search AV, rate drop response, and tachyarrhythmia detection, termination and prevention features.

Marker channel development

In June 1979, during the design of dual chamber pacemakers, Toby Markowitz found that single channel real-time telemetered electrograms had limited value. Toby invented the marker channel™, which is a time series of events, such as sensing and pacing, that occur within the pacemaker when it interacts with the heart (US Patent 4,374,382). When an event occurred, the real-time telemetry sent an encoded signal that was displayed on an ECG recorder as a pulse that had an amplitude and polarity corresponding to the type of event. This original marker channel of baseline and pulses was recorded, without annotations, below the surface ECG on a two channel strip chart recording. The simultaneous display of the ECG from the heart and the marker channel from the pacemaker provided useful clinical information and was rapidly implemented by engineering.

A pacemaker timing event has two characteristics: (1) the instant in time when the event occurred with respect to other events; (2) the type of event that occurred, such as a ventricular pace (VP) or a ventricular sense (VS). The marker channel was a summary of the pacemaker logic and timing that showed how it was interacting with the heart. Clinicians could then visually align the marker channel pacemaker events with whatever waveforms appeared on the surface ECG. Markowitz (1982) described this new pacemaker feature as telling the physician 'what it is doing' and it is 'similar to having an oscilloscope probe inside the pacemaker at the time of clinical follow-up'. By measuring the time between atrial and ventricular events, one can easily monitor pacemaker rate and the pacemaker A-V interval. When unusual phenomena occur, such as cross-talk mediated safety pacing, the marker channel shows what the pacemaker did and the ECG shows how the heart responded (Kruse *et al.* 1983).

Soon marker channels on dual chamber pacemakers used both graphic symbols and annotations to describe each of the six types of events (Duffin 1984). From the marker channel baseline, upward markers described atrial events with triple amplitude pulse for atrial pace (AP), double amplitude pulse for atrial sense (AS) and single amplitude pulse for unused (refractory) atrial sense (~~AS~~). Similarly, downward markers were triple amplitude for ventricular pace (VP), double amplitude for ventricular sense (VS) and single amplitude for ventricular refractory sense (VR). Figure 63.1 illustrates the marker channel from a Medtronic Symbios® pacemaker plotted below the simultaneous recorded ECG. The fifth atrial event is an unused atrial sense that occurred in the atrial refractory period. This is normal pacemaker Wenckebach upper-rate limiting operation. Later, another unused atrial sense allowed normal A-V conduction to emerge resulting in complete inhibition of both pacemaker output pulses.

Direct confirmation of sensing with markers permitted definitive diagnoses of undersensing and oversensing caused by many phenomena. The exact timing of a sense marker corresponded to the instant when the intracardiac electrogram signal exceeded the sensing threshold of the sense amplifier for the programmed sensitivity. This occurred when the wavefront of depolarization passed the tip of the pacemaker lead. This pacemaker sensing from the endocardial electrogram can occur at any time during the corresponding waveform on the surface ECG because the ECG is a far-field representation of the cardiac depolarization. Therefore, the leading edge of sense markers often do not line up exactly with the onset of a depolarization on the surface ECG. If, however, the telemetered intracardiac electrogram from the same electrodes used by the sense amplifier is recorded next to the marker channel, then the part of the waveform that met the sense amplifier's criteria for sensing will be aligned with the sense marker. Small jitter of sense markers can occur in defibrillator systems that use auto-adjusting sensing thresholds because the threshold for sensing is affected by the amplitude and timing of the previous depolarization. Electronics and software processing time for any marker can cause small delays that are generally <10 ms for modern implantable devices. Marker channel events are dependent on the integrity of

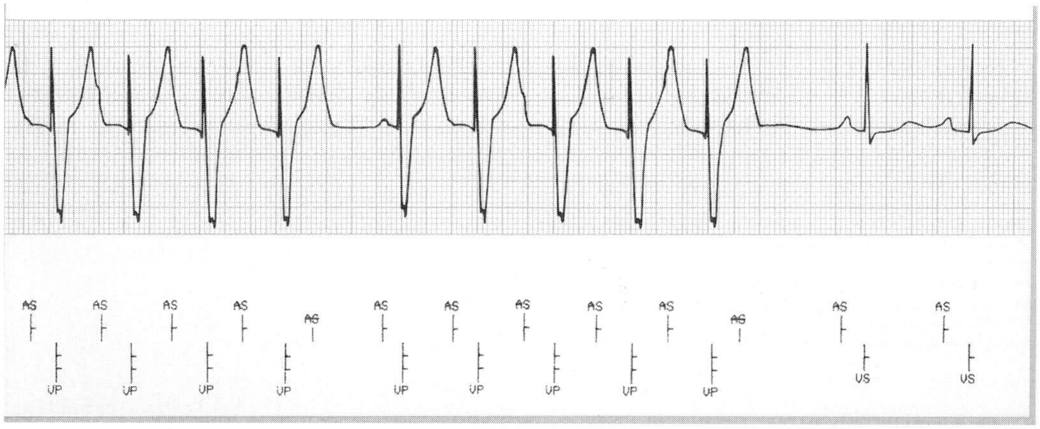

Fig. 63.1 Surface ECG and Marker Channel™ were recorded from a Symbios DDD pacemaker. As the atrial sensed (AS) events exceed the pacemaker ventricular upper rate limit of 100 beats/min, the ventricular paced (VP) events show pacemaker Wenckebach operation until the atrial rate slows near the end of the strip. The marker channel shows that some atrial sensed events are not used (~~AS~~).

the radio-frequency telemetry between the pacemaker and the programmer. Markers can be lost due to transient electrical noise or programmer head movement. Markers are sent as digital codes with error checking so it is nearly impossible for extraneous markers to appear.

Marker channel diagrams

In the early 1980s the introduction of dual chamber pacemakers led to many methods for combining marker channel events, current programmed parameters and knowledge of pacemaker logic to explain pacemaker operation.

Brownlee *et al.* (1982) described a symbolic representation for diagramming the pacemaker/heart interactions. Application of 16 symbols for manually diagramming rhythms required significant interpretation of both the ECG and marker events.

Bernstein & Parsonnet (1983) developed a set of notations and overlay diagrams for use in teaching of rhythm strip analysis that included pacing with capture, loss of capture and inhibited stimuli as well as sensed, undersensed, refractory sensed and noise sensed symbols. This manual system required extensive knowledge of the specific pacemaker and complete manual analysis of the ECG.

A diagramming system developed by Sutton *et al.* (1985) used A-V and V-A ladder diagramming to represent physiological conduction and how events in each chamber interact with pacemaker timing. This system also used a pacemaker ladder diagram to explain the pacemaker timing.

Lindemans (1985) diagram system was described in a book chapter that also reviewed all the other diagrams. His diagrams explicitly show the pacemaker lower rate counter and A-V counter for timing as well as refractory periods for both chambers and the ventricular upper-rate timing for every beat. This diagram shows only pacemaker timing. Lindemans went on to describe another diagramming technique that combined the strong point of previous diagrams. The lower rate counter and AV counter were combined into a central field with atrial functions above and ventricular functions below. An advantage of these diagrams was that only the timers that were actually used during a given rhythm were displayed.

A fully automated pacemaker timing diagram was described by Olson *et al.* (1985) that used actual telemetered marker inputs and employed all the timing rules for a specific pacemaker and its programmed parameter values. The measured timing of all events was compared to the pacemaker design specifications and there were 22 possible error messages to describe various faults that might occur in pacemaker timing. Unusual phenomenon such as ventricular safety pacing were explicitly explained and labelled. This system was tested clinically by Olson *et al.* (1987) and was distributed commercially for several generations of Medtronic pacemakers and was used in Technical Manuals to explain pacemaker operation. Teletronics used this same diagramming system for several pacemakers.

Malik & Camm (1988) developed a system for analysis of pacemaker ECG's that solved the pacemaker-inverse problem. This computer system used the ECG for a specific pacemaker to analyse all possible combinations of heart-

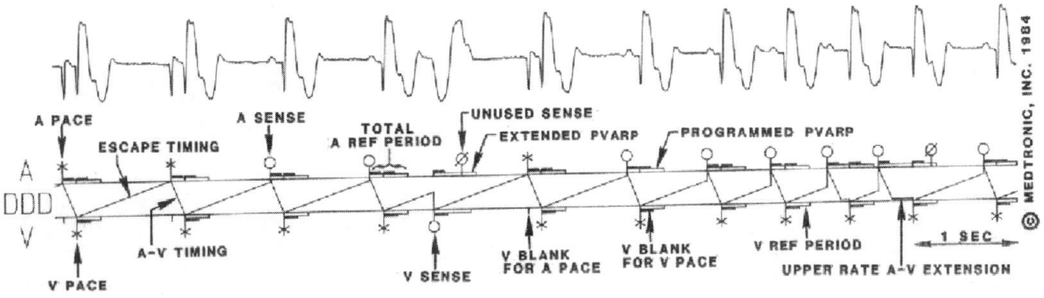

Fig. 63.2 Surface ECG and pacemaker diagnostic diagram for DDD pacing were recorded with increasing atrial rate, PVC, and Wenckebach upper rate limiting. Lower rate, 60 beats/min; AV delay, 125 ms; upper rate, 100 beats/min; postventricular atrial refractory period, 225 ms.

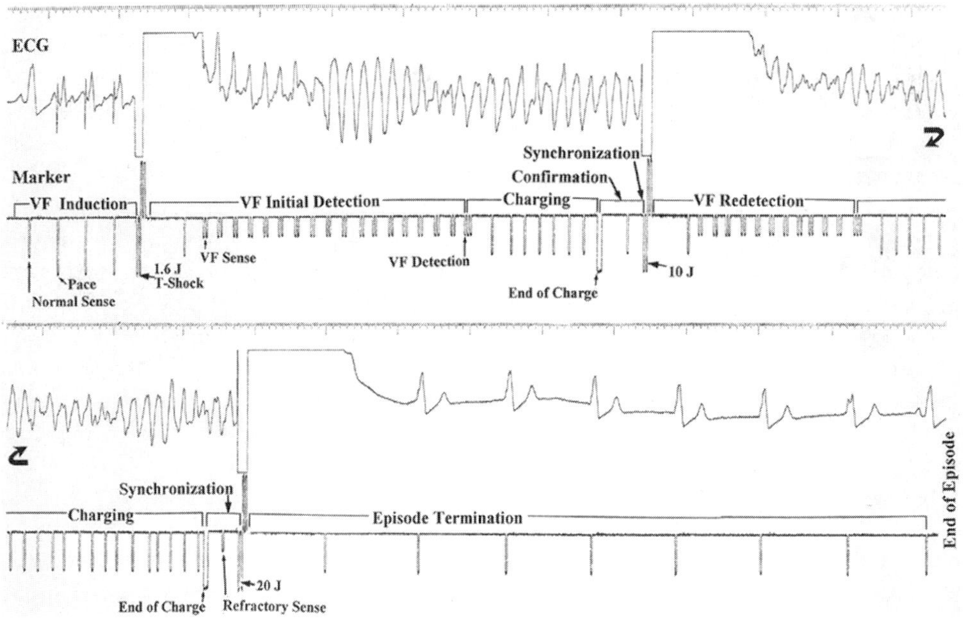

Fig. 63.3 ECG and marker channel from a single chamber ICD showing an induced episode of VF, initial detection, charging, confirmation, synchronization, failed 10 J shock, VF redetection, charging, synchronization, a successful 20 J shock, and episode termination.

pacemaker interactions and suggested probable explanations for a particular rhythm strip.

None of these pacemaker timing diagrams has stood the test of time (Levine & Love 2000). Significant new software and testing were required for each new model of pacemaker. Also, definitive clinically significant conclusions for a rhythm strip were difficult to reach because there were often several interpretations for many of the rhythm strips (Levine 1987). The main purpose served by these diagrams was to educate pacemaker clinicians on the complex patterns of normal pacemaker operation.

Single chamber defibrillators

Pacemaker operation is rarely affected by more than one or two preceding cardiac cycles. Implantable cardioverter-defibrillators (ICDs) have the added complexity of tachyarrhythmia detection algorithms and episodes of therapy sequences that can be quite lengthy. The marker channels required many more symbols as each *RR* interval was classified into one of several zones, and multi-event processes such as detection, charging, confirmation, synchronization, redetection and episode termination needed to be explained. Figure 63.3 illustrates most of these markers for single events and processes for a single chamber ICD. This is a real-time recording of induced VF at the time of ICD implant when the first shock failed and the second shock succeeded. Even with the marker channel, the user must know many details of ICD operation to understand fully the operation of the device. Special markers were needed to indicate when someone was programming device parameters during a real-time strip.

Stored electrogram marker channels

Infrequent occurrence of tachyarrhythmia episodes in ICD patients led to the need to save both the electrogram waveforms and the corresponding marker channel in the memory of the ICD. The marker channels were so similar to real-time markers that it was often difficult to determine if a rhythm strip was real-time or stored. To conserve ICD memory, stored recordings were sometimes suspended during charging or after shock therapy. Figure 63.4 shows an unusual stored electrogram from an electrician who was being

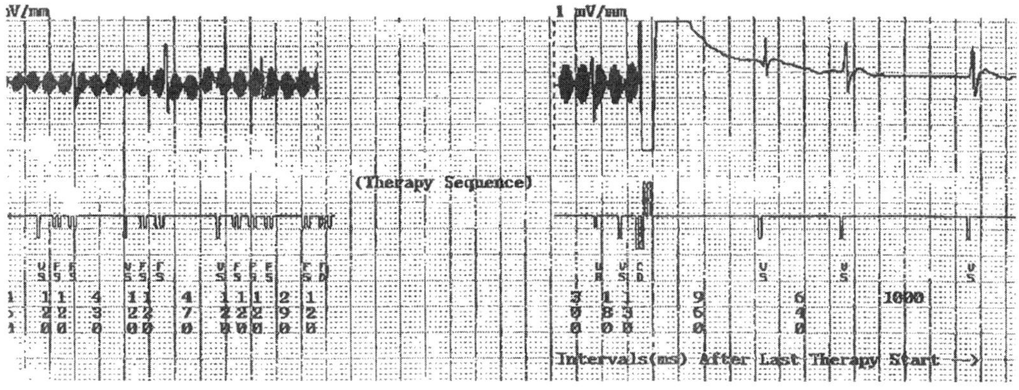

Fig. 63.4 Stored electrogram and marker channel showing an electrician being electrocuted by 60 Hz current shows the artefact on the electrogram that was inappropriately detected as VF. The shock knocked the patient loose from the electric power and restored sinus rhythm.

electrocuted when he mistakenly contacted electrical wiring. The electric current flowing through his body was sufficient to contract his skeletal muscles so he could not 'let go'. The 60 Hz electric current, shown by the heavily shaded area on the stored electrogram, caused sufficient oversensing by the ICD to deliver a shock. This inappropriate shock threw him off the electric wiring, and restored sinus rhythm. Note that during the oversensing, on the left side of the strip, the R waves of sinus rhythm are larger than the noise and raise the auto-adjusting sensing threshold above the noise level for a while resulting in the two long *RR* intervals labelled 430 ms and 470 ms.

Dual chamber defibrillator marker channels

Further complexity of marker channels was needed when atrial sensing and pacing were added to ICDs and atrial information was used for dual chamber tachyarrhythmia detection algorithms. Atrial blanking periods were reduced to improve detection of atrial tachyarrhythmias and atrial oversensing of far-field R waves became more common. The complexity of the dual chamber detection algorithms required higher-level rhythm annotation markers to explain ICD operation (Weretka *et al.* 2001; Nowak, 2002). Figures 63.5–63.7 illustrate dual chamber electrograms and the more complex marker channels needed to explain device operation to the user. Comparison of these three figures shows that industry has not heeded the request by Dr Seymour Furman (1990), in a *PACE* editorial 'for an industry standard ECG interpretation channel'. Figure 63.5 shows intermittent T wave oversensing that eventually caused an inappropriate shock from a Gem II DR ICD. Adequate low frequency response was helpful to clearly distinguish between R waves and T waves on this strip. Some of the T waves were not oversensed resulting in true 400 ms *RR* intervals. The 1 mV calibration pulse on the ventricular electrogram shows that the R waves were only 1–2 mV. When R waves are this small, the auto-adjusting sensing threshold after each R wave does not increase enough to avoid oversensing of the following T wave. Furthermore, when chronic R waves are <3 mV in sinus rhythm, experience has shown that ventricular fibrillation may be undersensed for nominal 0.3 mV programmed sensitivity. Therefore, the RV sensing lead probably needed to be repositioned.

Figure 63.6 shows an atrial arrhythmia episode recorded by a VENTAK PRIZM 2 DR ICD. The atrial electrogram, ventricular electrogram and the far-field shock electrogram are shown from top to bottom. The arrows show both atrial and ventricular events with annotations and intervals below each arrow. Atrial arrhythmia is indicated by ATR when the atrial rate exceeds the ventricular rate and mode switching prevents tracking of the high atrial rate.

Figure 63.7 shows an atrial arrhythmia episode with mode switching recorded by a

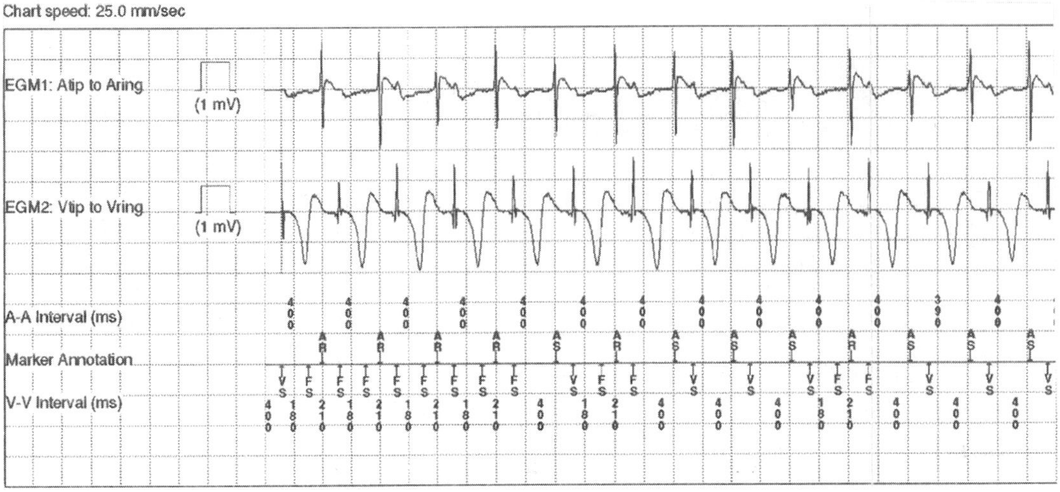

Fig. 63.5 Stored atrial electrogram, ventricular electrogram, and marker channel from a Gem II DR dual chamber ICD showing inappropriate intermittent ventricular oversensing of T waves because the amplitude of the R waves was only 1–2 mV.

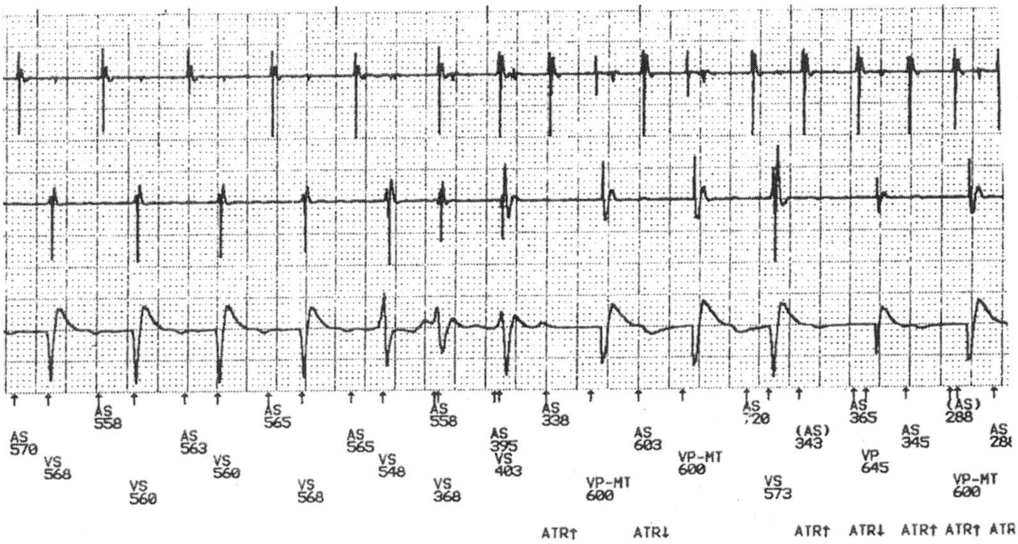

Fig. 63.6 Stored atrial electrogram, ventricular electrogram, shock electrogram and markers from a VENTAK PRIZM 2 DR ICD showing sinus rhythm with onset of an atrial tachyarrhythmia and automatic mode switching.

Photon DR ICD. All the marker information is displayed above the atrial and ventricular electrograms. Atrial markers are P for sensed and A for paced. Ventricular markers are R for sensed and V for paced. *AV* and *VA* intervals are shown in addition to the *AA* and *VV* intervals. During the atrial tachyarrhythmia all the *AA* intervals are shown but only every other P marker is displayed until the mode switch to DDI occurs.

Holter monitor marker channels

All Medtronic pacemakers and ICDs can be programmed to send uplink markers and supplemental markers for a fixed period of time, such as 24 h, without a magnet. The telemetry then automatically turns off to minimize battery drain that is only several days of device longevity for each day of continuous telemetry. This allows

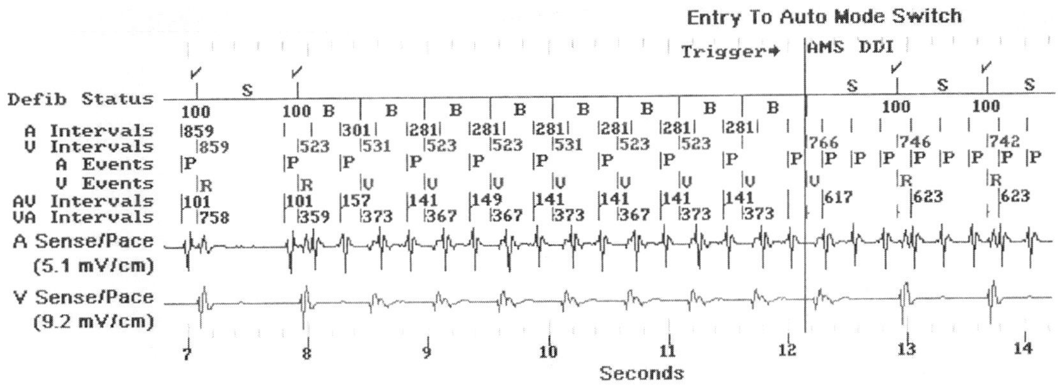

Fig. 63.7 Stored atrial electrogram, ventricular electrogram and markers from a Photon DR ICD showing onset of an atrial tachyarrhythmia with automatic mode switching to DDI mode.

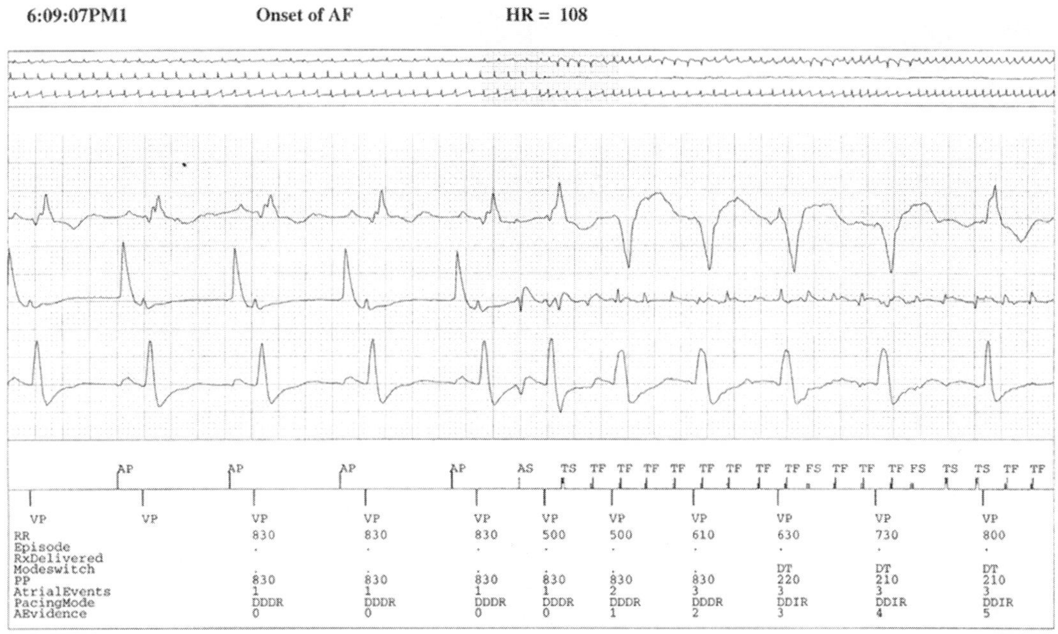

Fig. 63.8 Holter ECG, telemetered atrial electrogram, ventricular electrogram, marker channel and supplemental markers from a Gem III AT dual chamber antitachyarrhythmia ICD showing onset of an atrial tachyarrhythmia and automatic mode switching to DDIR mode.

special Holter monitors capable of receiving and recording telemetered electrograms and markers in addition to the ECG from surface electrodes (Feldman *et al.* 1993). Special Holter analysis software can process these data and scan for particular device markers or waveform morphologies on the electrograms or the surface ECG. These Holter tools have been helpful to study new pacemakers and ICDs during clinical studies and for troubleshooting intermittent sensing and pacing problems (Moak *et al.* 2002; Wiegand *et al.* 2002).

An example of a telemetered Holter recording with markers and supplemental markers is shown in Figure 63.8 for the Gem III AT dual chamber antitachycardia ICD. The spontaneous onset of atrial fibrillation is shown with mode switching to DDIR after three ventricular cycles of atrial tachyarrhythmia. The two atrial tachyarrhythmia zones are allowed to overlap so there are AT markers for the slow atrial rate zone, FS markers for the fibrillation zone, and TF markers for the overlap zone where *PP* interval variability is used to determine the type of detection. An example of a supplemental marker is the AF evidence counter (AEvidence) shown on the bottom of the strip. This counter begins incrementing in the middle of the strip and must reach 32 to detect a sustained atrial tachyarrhythmia.

Future – diagnostic systems, advanced telemetry and Internet

Marker channel systems are increasingly important as implantable pacemakers and ICDs be-come more complex. Implantable devices being designed today have over 100 marker codes for events. The addition of left ventricular sense amplifiers in biventricular systems will require presentation of at least three chambers of marker channels and electrograms. New implantable sensors may lead to four or more channels of signals and markers to explain device operation.

Diagnostic systems capable of clinical conclusions about sensing, pacing and lead performance status are being developed. Then, recommendations for corrective action become feasible, particularly using distributed computation and possible live human interaction using the Internet. Newer tachyarrhythmia detection algorithms need to generate better explanations for why an arrhythmia diagnosis was made, in context, on the stored electrogram. These performance summary statements for a particular episode need to use clinical language that is easily understood by clinicians.

Future wireless telemetry and Internet connectivity will permit 'silent alerts' for health care providers to monitor critical patient conditions and when feasible, patients will become more involved in their own care. Future implantable systems will use real-time analysis of signals and marker information to adaptively adjust device parameters within certain ranges automatically in order to optimize short-term and long-term patient outcomes.

References

Bernstein, A.D. & Parsonnet, V. (1983) Notation system and overlay diagrams for the analysis of paced electrocardiograms. *Pacing and Clinical Electrophysiology*, **6** (1), 73–80.

Brownlee, R.R., Shimmel-Golden, J.B., Del Marco, C.J. *et al.* (1982) A new symbolic language for diagramming pacemaker/heart interaction. *Pacing and Clinical Electrophysiology*, **5** (5), 700–709.

Duffin, E.G., (1984) The marker channel: a telemetric diagnostic aid. *Pacing and Clinical Electrophysiology*, **7** (6), 1165–1169.

Feldman, C.L., Olson, W.H., Hubbelbank, M. *et al.* (1993) Identification of an implantable defibrillator lead fracture with a new Holter system. *Pacing and Clinical Electrophysiology*, **16** (6), 1342–1344.

Furman, S. (1990) Editorial: The ECG interpretation channel. *Pacing and Clinical Electrophysiology*, **13**, 255.

Kruse, I.B., Markowitz, T. & Ryden, L. (1983) Timing markers showing pacemaker behaviour to aid in the follow-up of a physiological pacemaker. *Pacing and Clinical Electrophysiology*, **6** (4), 801–805.

Levine, P.A. (1987) The complementary role of electrogram, event marker, and measured data telemetry in the assessment of pacing system function. *Journal of Electrophysiology*, **1** (5), 404–416.

Levine, P.A. & Love, C.J. (2000) Pacemaker diagnostics and evaluation of pacing system malfunction. In: *Clinical Cardiac Pacing and Defibrillation* (eds K. A. Ellenbogen, G. N. Kay & B. L. Wilkoff), 2nd edn, pp. 827–875. W. B. Saunders, Philadelphia.

Lindemans, F.W. (1985) Diagramatic representation of pacemaker function. In: *Modern Cardiac Pacing* (ed. S.S. Barold), pp. 323–353. Futura Publishing, Mount Kisco, NY.

Malik, M., and Camm, A.J (1988) The pacemaker inverse problem – computer diagnosis of paced electrocardiograms. *Computers and Biomedical Research* **21**, 289–306.

Markowitz, H.T. (1982) The marker channel. *Medtronic Pacing Concept Paper*, No. 5, 1–2.

Moak, J.P., Gunderson, B. & Freedenberg, V. (2002) Pacemaker troubleshooting: Improved efficacy using a new diagnostic digital Holter recording system. *Europace*, **4**, 55–59.

Nowak, B. (2002) Review: Pacemaker stored electrograms: teaching us what is really going on in our patients. *Pacing and Clinical Electrophysiology*, **25** (5), 838–849.

Olson, W.H., Goldreyer, B.A. & Goldreyer, B.N. (1987) Computer-generated diagnostic diagrams for pacemaker rhythm analysis and pacing system evaluation. *Journal Electrophysiology*, **1** (5), 376–387.

Olson, W.H., McConnell, M.V., Sah, R.L. *et al.* (1985) Pacemaker diagnostic diagrams. *Pacing and Clinical Electrophysiology*, **8** (5), 691–700.

Sutton, R., Perrins, E.J. & Duffin, E. (1985) Interpretation of dual chamber pacemaker electrocardiograms. *Pacing and Clinical Electrophysiology*, **8** (1), 6–16.

Weretka, S., Becker, R., Hibel, T. *et al.* (2001) Far-field R wave oversensing in a dual chamber arrhythmia management device: predisposing factors and practical implications. *Pacing and Clinical Electrophysiology*, **24** (8), 1240–1246.

Wiegand, U.K.H., Bonnemeier, H., Bode, F. *et al.* (2002) Continuous Holter telemetry of atrial electrograms and marker annotations using a common Holter recording system: Impact on Holter electrocardiogram interpretation in patients with dual chamber pacemakers. *Pacing and Clinical Electrophysiology*, **25** (12), 1724–1730.

CHAPTER 64

Interpretation of Device Stored Rhythms and Electrocardiograms

Paul J. Erlinger and Gust H. Bardy

Introduction

In the latest generation of implantable cardioverter-defibrillator (ICD) devices, the stored electrocardiograms, *RR* intervals, physiological sensors and interpretation channels serve as powerful tools in diagnosing therapeutic episodes. Manufacturers have increased the amount of stored electrocardiograms, *RR* intervals and interpretation annotation, as memory chip manufacturing processes have evolved to higher densities and greater power efficiency. The trend to provide greater stored data will continue to grow, as physicians will want to observe patient's behaviour and monitor the appropriateness of each delivered therapy.

Over the years stored electrocardiograms have provided tremendous insight into the appropriateness of ICD therapy. The root cause of inappropriate therapy has been linked to failures in almost every major element of the ICD. Such elements include: mechanical integrity of the system such as loose setscrews and lead breakage; sense-related problems such as oversensing or undersensing; electromagnetic interference and muscle noise; programming problems, such as poor parameter settings, especially algorithm-related parameters. Stored electrocardiograms and annotation or marker channels have provided the evidence of these problematic episodes. Peer reviews and publication of these types of episodes have fed back to the ICD user community and to manufacturers, who in turn have provided a steady incremental improvement of the effectiveness of their devices. Before the development of stored episodic event data, determining appropriateness of each shock could only be accomplished by means of surface electrocardiogram (ECG) monitors.

Stored electrocardiograms tell a story for each episode about what the device senses, how the device interprets what it senses, and what actions the device takes based on the interpretation of what it senses. After all, modern ICDs are implantable computers making decisions based on the programming of the device. The most valuable tool for making an assessment of a tachyarrhythmia therapy and its appropriateness is the stored electrocardiogram.

Sensing

One of the best starting points for a full understanding of stored electrocardiograms is the concept of device sensing. Sensing is the mechanism by which the device detects physiological and nonphysiological electrical stimuli. The device senses through a pair of sense electrodes. The difference in voltage potential between one sense electrode and the other sense electrode is filtered, then digitally sampled and presented to the device's microprocessor.

Two types of ventricular ICD leads are common: integrated bipolar (Fig. 64.1) and dedicated bipolar (fig. 64.2) leads. With integrated bipolar sense leads, sensing occurs between the tip electrode and the distal shock electrode. With dedicated bipolar leads sensing occurs between the tip electrode and a dedicated distal sense electrode.

The intracardiac electrocardiogram has a greater slew rate than that of surface ECGs (Fig. 64.3). Like surface ECGs, the amplitude of intrac-

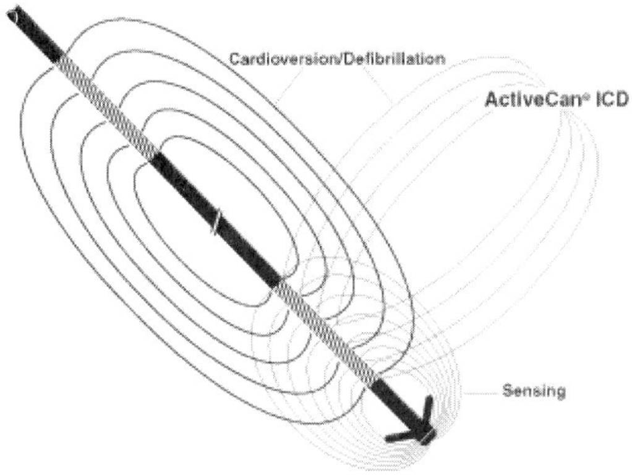

Fig. 64.1 Integrated bipolar sense leads.

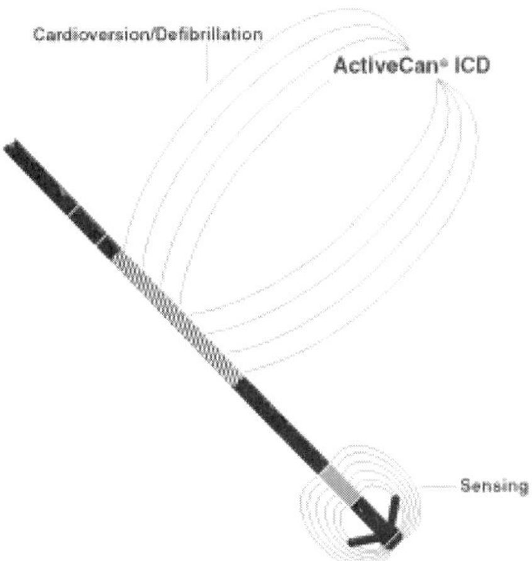

Fig. 64.2 Dedicated bipolar leads.

ardiac ECGs will vary depending on lead location, tissue health, and the vector of current flow.

Automatic sensing control

(Courtesy of Dr Paul A. Levine of St Jude Medical Inc.)

Implantable defibrillators have automatic sensing control. Most automatic sensing control methods set the sense threshold to a programmed percentage of the peak signal detected following each sensed event. The Photon®DR device (St Jude Medical) incorporates a feature called automatic sensitivity control (ASC) (Figs 64.4 and 64.5). It starts at a value that is percentage of the peak R wave amplitude as measured by the ICD on a beat-by-beat basis. The

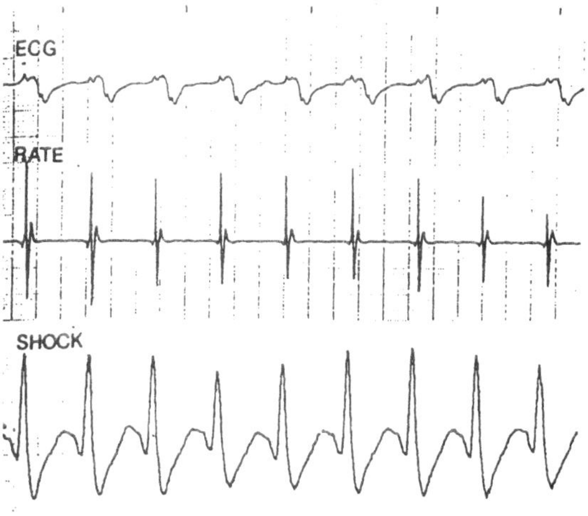

Fig. 64.3 Electrogram recordings from an implantable cardioverter defibrillator (ICD) during an episode of VT. Top trace, surface ECG; middle trace ('RATE'), bipolar sensing; bottom trace ('SHOCK'), between two shock coils. (Reproduced from Sarter *et al.* 1998, with permission.)

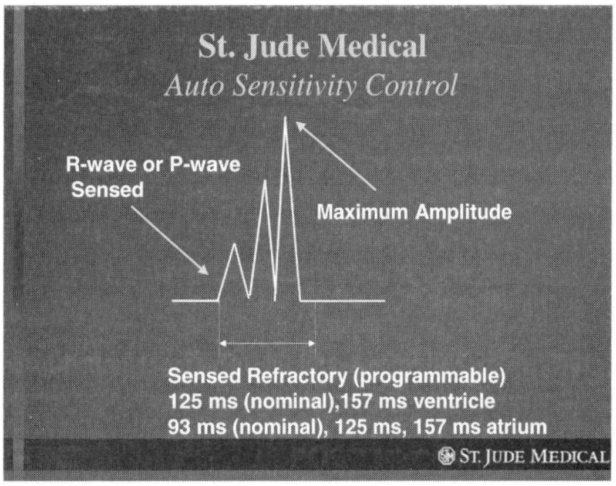

Fig. 64.4 Schematic diagram of an intracardiac signal. The processed signal is often splintered. Sensing may occur at the leading edge but the actual signal is significantly larger. Despite the normal refractory period that begins when the signal is first sensed, detection and measurement continue throughout the signal. The Threshold Start begins as a percentage of the largest component of the signal.

sensitivity progressively increases (becomes more sensitive) to assure detection of the potentially very small fibrillatory signals. While the sensitivity typically starts at a large value, it

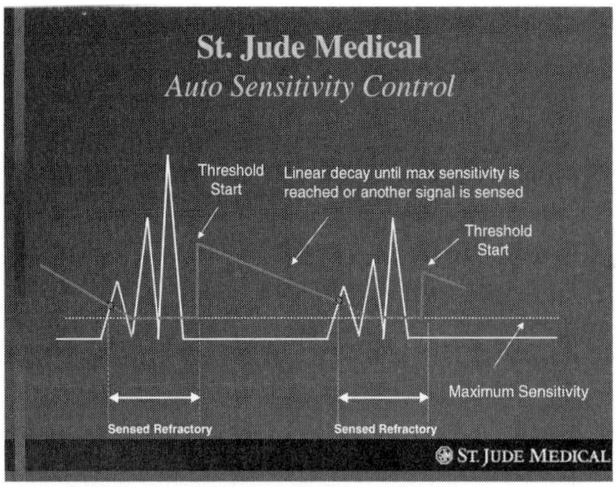

Fig. 64.5 This schematic shows consecutive processed signals with the second being significantly smaller than the first. Both are detected early but following the second, the Threshold Start begins at a more sensitive setting than with the first complex.

rapidly becomes more sensitive which can lead to T wave oversensing. This results in double-counting of the rhythm which can fulfil VF criteria with mild sinus tachycardias. There are four approaches to the management of this problem available in Photon and the subsequent family of ICDs from St Jude Medical.

1 Reduce the ventricular sensitivity. This could potentially compromise recognition of episodes of true ventricular fibrillation (VF).

2 Extend the ventricular refractory period as this is a programmable value. This could also compromise detection of VF.

3 Increase the Threshold Start so that rather than starting at 50% of the measured QRS amplitude, it starts at 75% or even 100%. As the system becomes progressively more sensitive, this may keep the system from becoming sufficiently sensitive to detect the T wave when the T wave is present and help prevent oversensing.

4 Enable a feature called Delay Decay such that the system does not begin to progressively increase its sensitivity until sometime after the QRS ends.

By using a combination of Decay Delay and Threshold Start, one maintains the maximal sensitivity for detection of ventricular fibrillation while avoiding detection of inappropriate signals such as T waves.

Algorithms

Rate-based algorithms

The detection algorithm determines how the device will interpret what it senses. The rate is classified as bradycardia, normal sinus rhythm, ventricular tachycardia (VT) and ventricular fibrillation. Enhanced rate algorithms are added to provide a reasonable specificity level for VT detection. Enhanced rate algorithms commonly include sudden onset and rate stability, AV association and morphology.

Sudden onset relies on an abrupt change in rate into a therapy zone for the rhythm to be considered treatable. This is primarily used as a means to differentiate sinus tachycardia from VT. Stability relies on a beat-to-beat variability below a certain limit to sort atrial fibrillation from other tachycardias (Sweesy *et al.* 2000).

Dual chamber algorithms (See Figs 64.6–64.8)

Electrocardiogram storage mechanism

Most electrocardiograms are stored in the ICD by way of a circular memory buffer (Fig. 64.9). The continuous stream of electrogram (EGM) data and associated markers pass through the memory buffer in a first-in first-out manner. When therapy detection occurs, the buffer fills to a predetermined state and then the contents of the memory buffer are transferred to a permanent memory space so the episode can be retrieved at a later date. Most devices allow the user to adjust the memory buffer by programming the amount of pre-shock and post-shock data that can be stored or by changing the buffer size. A device may also allow the user to adjust the EGM sampling rate, which if adjusted lower, will allow more real-time data to be stored at the expense of resolution. Each device model is different in the amount of memory that is available and the marker annotation. Most devices also allow storage of non-treated episodes such as spontaneous conversions, or snapshots of sustained high rates.

Case study: diagnosing and correcting T wave oversensing

(Courtesy of Dr Paul Levine, Erol Kosar and St Jude Medical)

This was a case where T wave oversensing trig-

Biotronik Phylax AV SMART ™ Algorithm

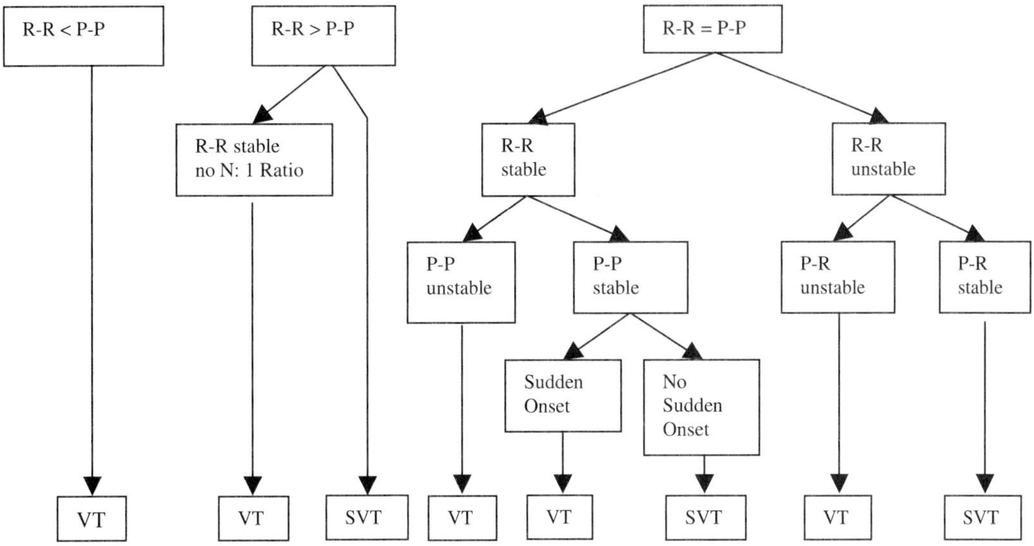

Fig. 64.6 Biotronik SMART™ algorithm. Once an *R-R* interval is detected in the ventricular tachycardia detection zone, the 'SMART' ™ dual chamber detection algorithm compares the mean atrial cycle length to the mean ventricular cycle length. *RR* stability, *PP* stability AV association and sudden onset classify the rhythm as VT or SVT. (Reproduced from Hintringer *et al.* 2001, with permission.)

ELA Defender IV Algorithm
(Courtesy of ELA Medical)

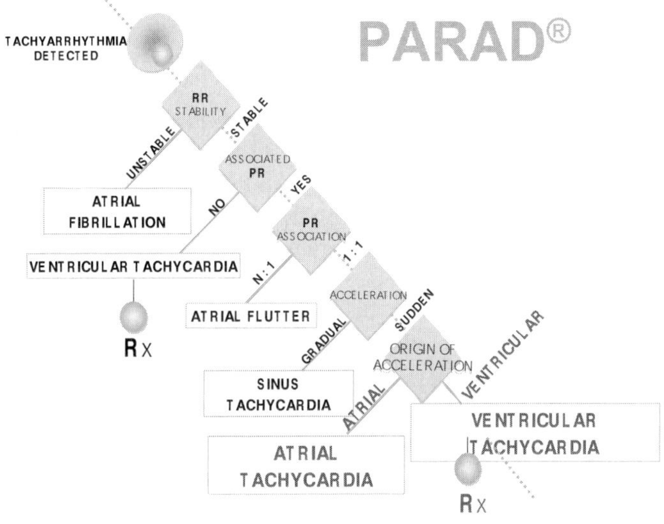

Fig. 64.7 ELA PARAD algorithm. PARAD® is a dual chamber detection algorithm that classifies a rhythm based on *RR* stability, *PR* association, onset, and origin of acceleration. ELA Defender IV Algorithm. (Courtesy of ELA Medical.)

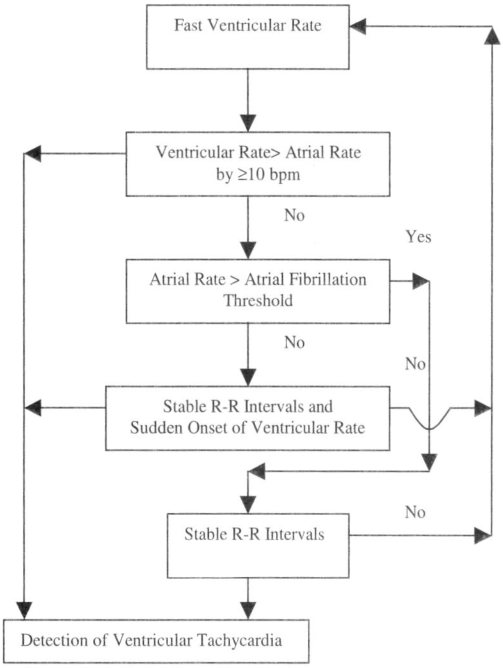

Fig. 64.8 Guidant Ventak AV Algorithm. If the ventricular rate exceeds the atrial rate by >10 beats/min, ventricular tachycardia is diagnosed. If not, the atrial fibrillation enhancement criterion is applied. If the atrial rate is greater than the atrial fibrillation threshold and the *R-R* intervals are not stable, the rhythm is classified as SVT. If the atrial rate is not greater than the atrial fibrillation threshold, then therapy can still be withheld despite stable *R-R* intervals if no sudden onset of the ventricular rate was detected. (Courtesy of Guidant.)

gered inappropriate therapy. The device was a Photon® from St Jude Medical. At the beginning of this stored EGM shown in Fig. 64.10, the magnet is in place over the ICD, which inhibits detection thus disabling ICD therapy. The top tracing is the atrial EGM, the bottom tracing is the ventricular EGM with annotated markers and electronic callipers displayed between the two EGMs. The numbers along the bottom reflect units of time in seconds. P and R refer to native atrial and ventricular sensed events. A and V refer to paced events in the atrium and ventricle, respectively.

There is also a diagnostic line. In Fig. 64.10, M refers to a magnet being applied to the ICD, to inhibit detection and disable tachy therapy. In this case the magnet slipped out of alignment and the rapid events equivalent to a rate >200 p.p.m. are recognized as fibrillation. After a diagnosis is made (identified by the trigger marker), the device starts to charge to the first shock level while the persistence of the rhythm is being reconfirmed. ('R' above the diagnosis/therapy line represents reconfirmation.) The high voltage (HV) shock is delivered. No attempt is made to employ sino-ventricular tachycardia (SVT) discrimination algorithms (morphology discrimination, rate stability, sudden onset, AV relationships) if the rate places the tachycardia in the fibrillation rate zone.

The continued EGM segment of Fig. 64.11 shows a small amplitude native signal with T wave detection associated with the progressive increase in sensitivity in accord with the automatic sensitivity control algorithm (ASC). Starting from a relative sensitive value and becoming more sensitive results in T wave sensing. Delaying the point at which the increase in sensitivity begins (Decay Delay) still allows the system to reach the most sensitive setting facilitating detection of VF while avoiding inappropriate detection of T waves.

Another interesting phenomenon was noted in this patient. Following a shock, there was a regular rhythm at a rate between 100 and 110 that the ICD labelled 'sinus' (Fig. 64.12). However, there is AV dissociation with the P wave following the QRS. This is not labelled as P wave as it also coincided with the PVARP, but the vertical marker identified this as a P wave (downward arrow- added, not part of the original printout) and calculated the atrial intervals. With sufficient separation between the P and R wave, the endogenous P wave conducts through the AV node and captures the ventricle. During sinus rhythm, the morphology of the QRS differs from that associated with AV dissociation further indicating that the dissociated complex is of idioventricular origin. Also, the T wave oversensing only occurs with the sinus conducted complexes and not the idioventricular complexes (double arrow).

Figure 64.13 indicates that this was a very significant problem with repeated inappropriate shocks. However, given the low amplitude R wave, reducing the sensitivity or extending the refractory period was not considered appropriate. Thus, the clinician took advantage of Decay

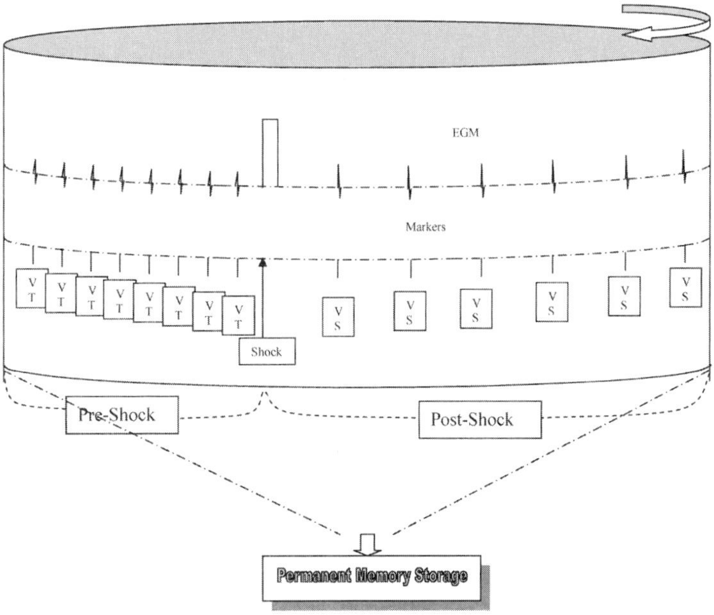

Fig. 64.9 Circular ECG buffer.

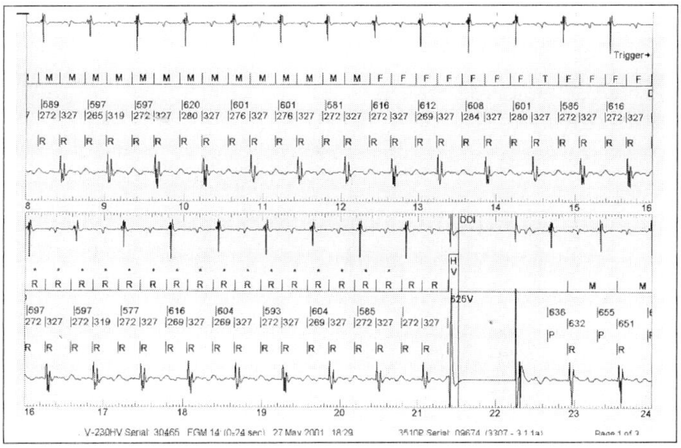

Fig. 64.10 Stored EGM of HV shock delivered for false indication of VF caused by T wave oversensing.

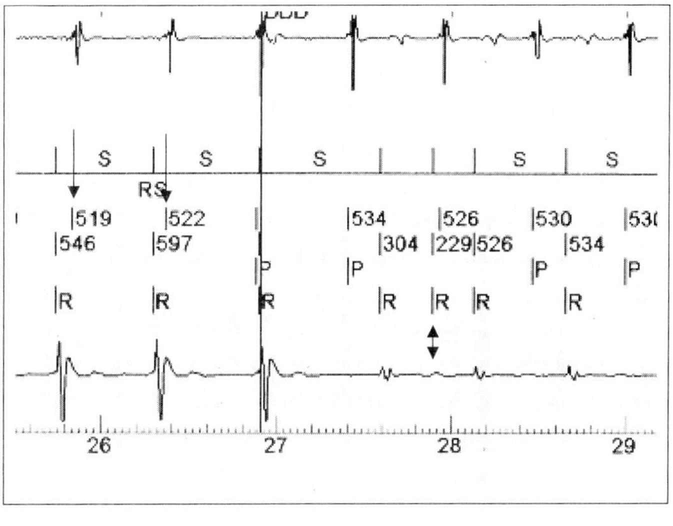

Fig. 64.11 Segment of Stored EGM with endogenous P wave and T wave oversensing of sinus conducted complexes.

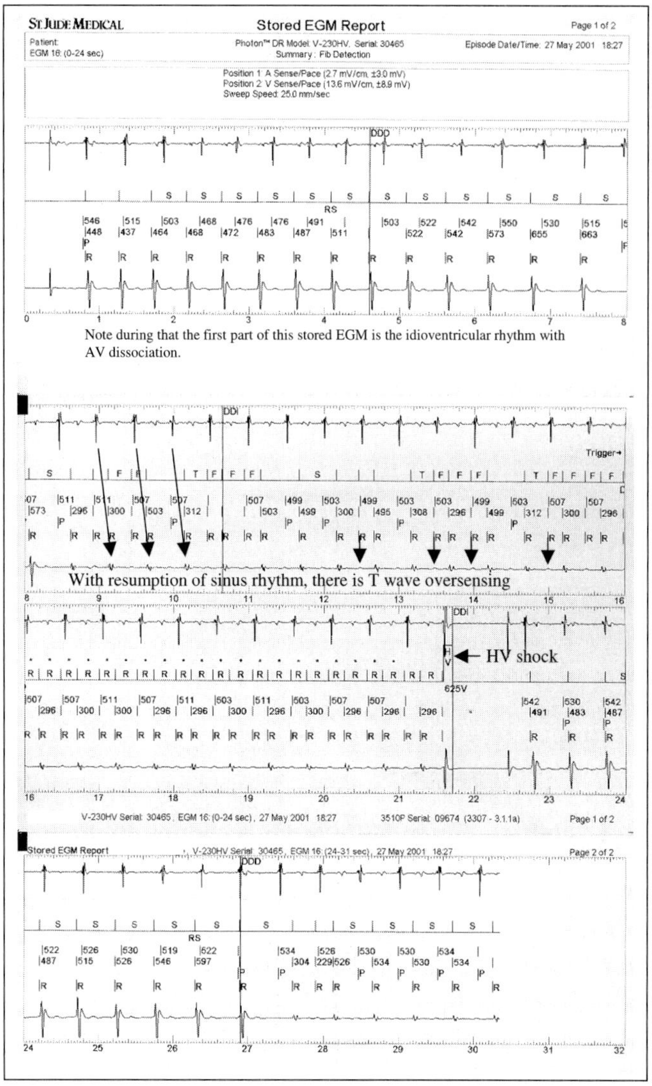

Fig. 64.12 After each shock, there is a brief period of the accelerated idioventricular rhythm followed by a resumption of sinus, repeat T wave oversensing and a presumptive diagnosis of fibrillation resulting in delivery of a shock.

Delay and increased Threshold Start to 100%. After that, it became necessary to confirm that this would not compromise detection of true ventricular fibrillation in this patient. Repeat DFT testing was performed and the corresponding stored EGM is shown in Fig. 64.14.

Case study: sinus tachycardia

(Courtesy of Medtronic)

Using PR Logic, the GEM II DR device discriminates sinus tachycardia from VT even in the presence of far-field R waves. The stored information (Fig. 64.15) can be evaluated to verify that therapy was appropriately withheld:

- AFib/AFlutter and Sinus Tach criterion are ON.
- V. Median Cycle length of 340 ms is greater than or equal to SVT Limit.
- A. Median Cycle length is 200 ms, implying an atrial arrhythmia.
- Pattern identified as Sinus Tach; duration of episode is 57 s.

A pattern for sinus tachycardia (ST) with far-field R waves (Fig. 64.16) allows the device to withhold therapy when the atrial channel consistently senses far-field R waves. ST has a good 1:1 AV conduction. A counter is kept for patterns recognized as ST; it is satisfied when the count

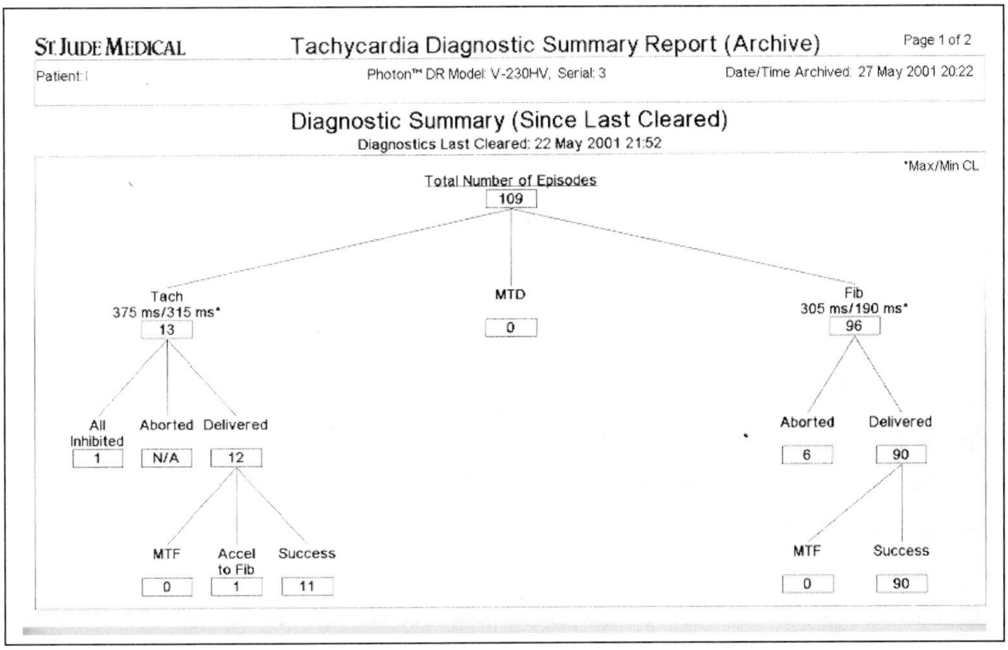

Fig. 64.13 Summaries of the tachycardia events and responses supplement the stored EGMs.

reaches 6. The device classifies the rhythm as sinus tachycardia and annotates 'ST'. The atrial channel shows clear indications of over-sensed far-field R waves (EGM strip and marker channel). The far-field R wave criterion reviews the last 12 *RR* intervals. Therapy is withheld.

The interval plot (Fig. 64.17) shows an atypical view of ST with far-field R wave oversensing on the atrial channel. Note that the gradual onset is typical of a ST episode.

Case study: double tachycardia

(Courtesy of Medtronic)

The episode presented in Fig. 64.18 has a fast, irregular atrial rate with an irregular ventricular response. The ventricular rate and pattern changes following a sudden onset of VT where regular ventricular rhythm develops. The episode report is as shown in Fig. 64.18.

The interval plot of this episode (Fig. 64.19) shows the sudden onset of the ventricular arrhythmia along with the fast and irregular atrial rhythm. A fast, regular ventricular rhythm is evident at the point of VT onset.

The ECG (Fig. 64.20) shows a spontaneous VT during AF (double tachycardia). One sequence of burst ATP is delivered and breaks the VT. The Atrial EGM shows a fast, irregular atrial rate through the entire episode. Initially the ventricular rate is irregular. Sudden onset of VT changes rhythm to fast and regular with EGM morphology change. Detection criteria are met and the arrhythmia is classified as FVT+SVT (double tachycardia). Therapy (burst ATP) is delivered.

After therapy, atrial rate remains fast and irregular; ventricular rate and morphology returns to pre-VT conditions (Fig. 64.21).

Case study: evaluation of multiple episodes in VT zone soon after implant

A 74 year-old male with ischaemic cardiomyopathy, prior myocardial infarction (MI), 28% ejection fraction (EF) and documented non-sustained ventricular tachycardia (VT) was implanted with a VENTAK PRIZM DR Model 1851 ICD several days ago. The patient was evaluated one day post-shock.

The device is capable of antitachycardia pacing (ATP) and programmable high energy shocks. The VT-1 zone was programmed from 160 beats/min to 179 beats/min; the VT zone was programmed from 180 beats/min to 209 beats/min; the VF zone was programmed for

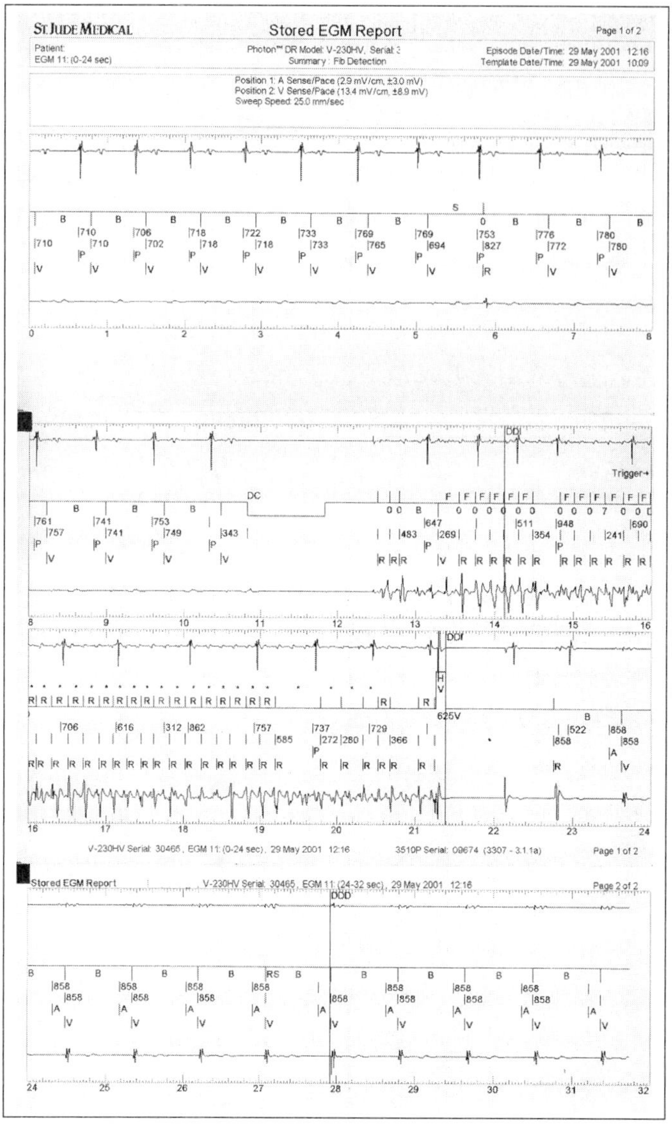

Fig. 64.14 Repeated DFT Test. In the tracing, VF was induced using the DC fibber. This is also fully annotated identified by the label 'DC'. VF is promptly recognized and labelled 'F'. Once the diagnosis is made, the ICD begins to charge and during this time, reconfirms the presence of VF (or VT) and labels these complexes with an 'R' placed above the diagnosis line.

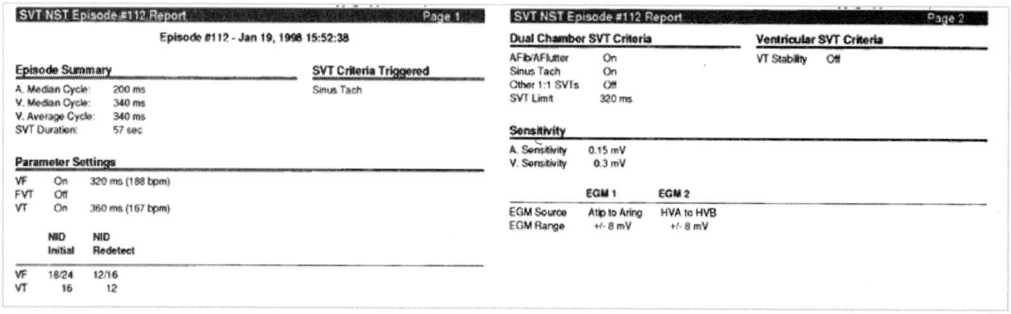

SVT NST Episode #112 Report — Page 1

Episode #112 - Jan 19, 1998 15:52:38

Episode Summary

A. Median Cycle:	200 ms
V. Median Cycle:	340 ms
V. Average Cycle:	340 ms
SVT Duration:	57 sec

SVT Criteria Triggered

Sinus Tach

Parameter Settings

VF	On	320 ms (188 bpm)
FVT	Off	
VT	On	360 ms (167 bpm)

	NID Initial	NID Redetect
VF	18/24	12/16
VT	16	12

SVT NST Episode #112 Report — Page 2

Dual Chamber SVT Criteria

AFib/AFlutter	On
Sinus Tach	On
Other 1:1 SVTs	Off
SVT Limit	320 ms

Ventricular SVT Criteria

VT Stability Off

Sensitivity

A. Sensitivity	0.15 mV
V. Sensitivity	0.3 mV

	EGM 1	EGM 2
EGM Source	Atip to Aring	HVA to HVB
EGM Range	+/- 8 mV	+/- 8 mV

Fig. 64.15 Sinus tachycardia episode report.

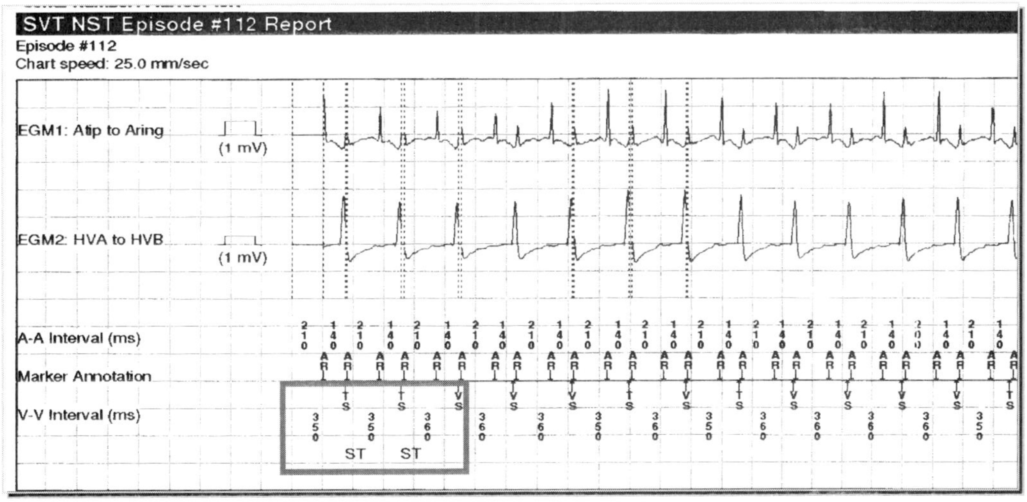

Fig. 64.16 Sinus tachycardia episode report, continued.

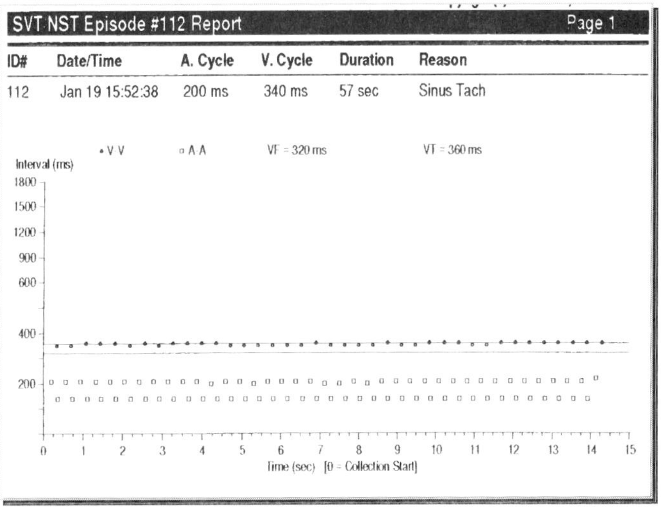

Fig. 64.17 Sinus tachycardia episode report, continued.

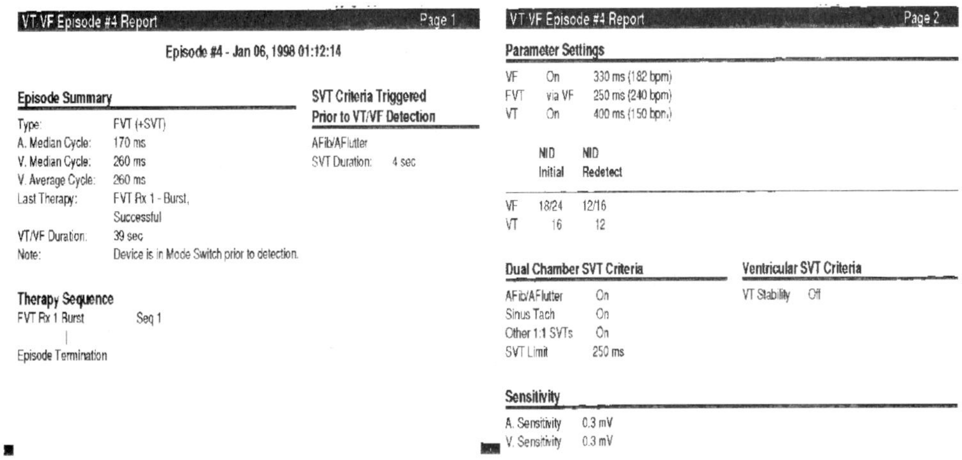

VT VF Episode #4 Report — Page 1

Episode #4 - Jan 06, 1998 01:12:14

Episode Summary

Type: FVT (+SVT)
A. Median Cycle: 170 ms
V. Median Cycle: 260 ms
V. Average Cycle: 260 ms
Last Therapy: FVT Rx 1 - Burst, Successful
VT/VF Duration: 39 sec
Note: Device is in Mode Switch prior to detection.

SVT Criteria Triggered Prior to VT/VF Detection

AFib/AFlutter
SVT Duration: 4 sec

Therapy Sequence

FVT Rx 1 Burst Seq 1
|
Episode Termination

VT VF Episode #4 Report — Page 2

Parameter Settings

VF	On	330 ms (182 bpm)
FVT	via VF	250 ms (240 bpm)
VT	On	400 ms (150 bpm)

	NID Initial	NID Redetect
VF	18/24	12/16
VT	16	12

Dual Chamber SVT Criteria

AFib/AFlutter On
Sinus Tach On
Other 1:1 SVTs On
SVT Limit 250 ms

Ventricular SVT Criteria

VT Stability Off

Sensitivity

A. Sensitivity 0.3 mV
V. Sensitivity 0.3 mV

Fig. 64.18 Double tachycardia episode report.

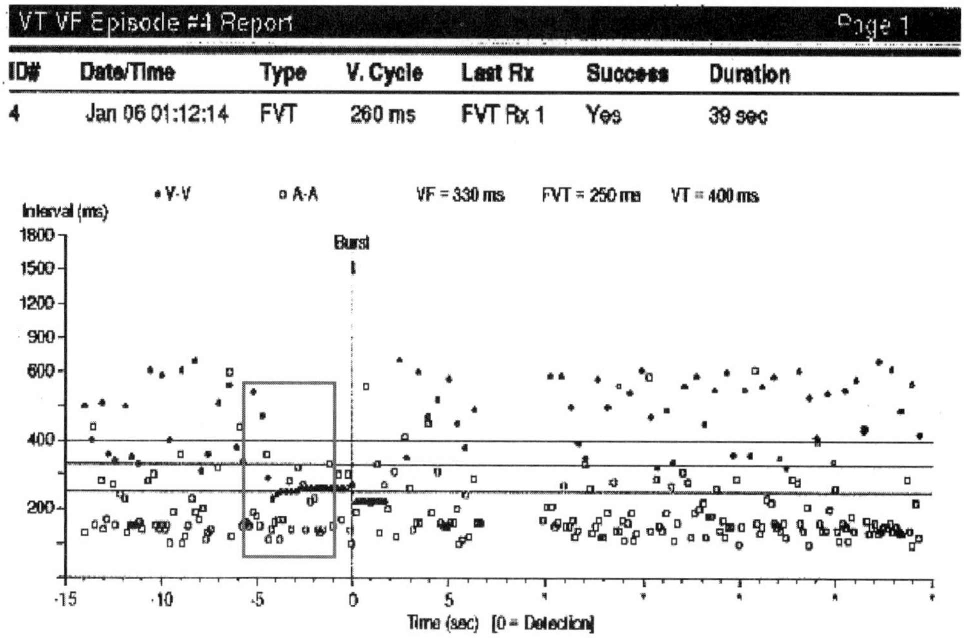

Fig. 64.19 Double tachycardia episode report, continued.

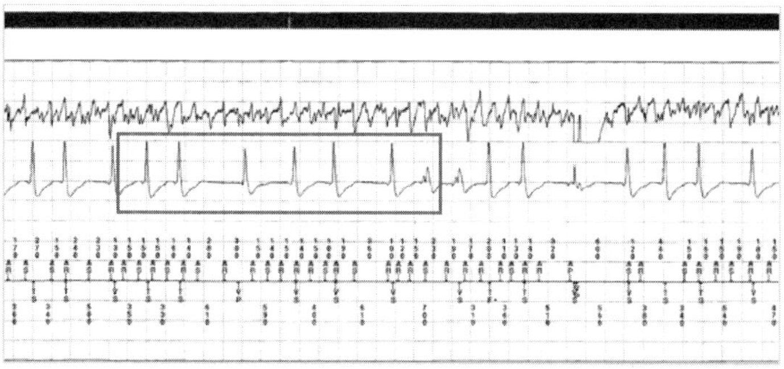

Fig. 64.20 Double tachycardia episode report, continued.

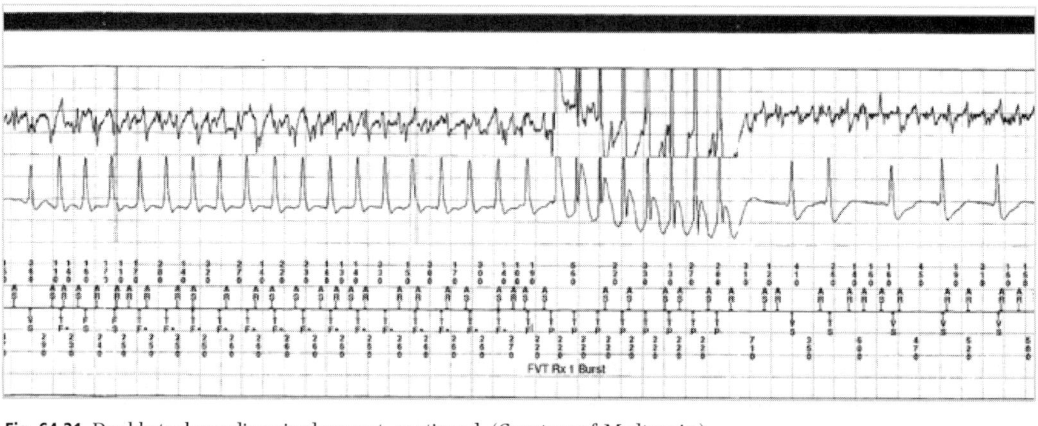

Fig. 64.21 Double tachycardia episode report, continued. (Courtesy of Medtronic.)

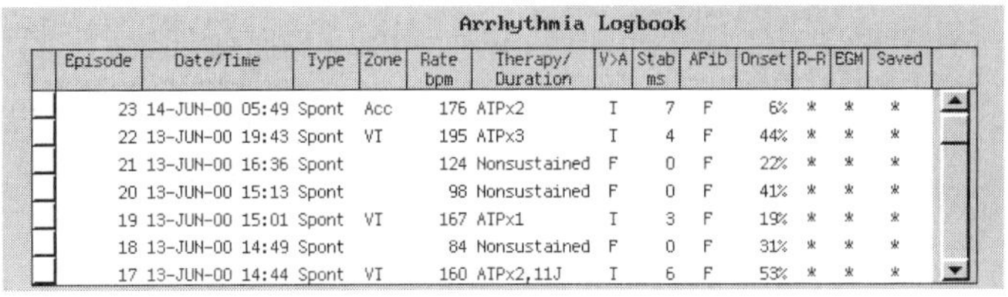

Arrhythmia Logbook

Episode	Date/Time	Type	Zone	Rate bpm	Therapy/ Duration	V>A	Stab ms	AFib	Onset	R-R	EGM	Saved
23	14-JUN-00 05:49	Spont	Acc	176	ATPx2	I	7	F	6%	*	*	*
22	13-JUN-00 19:43	Spont	VT	195	ATPx3	I	4	F	44%	*	*	*
21	13-JUN-00 16:36	Spont		124	Nonsustained	F	0	F	22%	*	*	*
20	13-JUN-00 15:13	Spont		98	Nonsustained	F	0	F	41%	*	*	*
19	13-JUN-00 15:01	Spont	VT	167	ATPx1	I	3	F	19%	*	*	*
18	13-JUN-00 14:49	Spont		84	Nonsustained	F	0	F	31%	*	*	*
17	13-JUN-00 14:44	Spont	VT	160	ATPx2,11J	I	6	F	53%	*	*	*

Fig. 64.22 Arrhythmia logbook.

rates greater than 210 beats/min. The Arrhythmia Logbook (Fig. 63.22) indicates each occurrence of a potentially treatable arrhythmia. Episode 17 indicates that the patient received an 11 J shock.

The EGM report shown in Fig. 64.23 is that of episode 23, the last stored episode, where two ATP therapies were delivered. The onset of the episode indicates that a sinus tachycardia at approximately 151 beats/min accelerates into the VT-1 detection zone in one cycle. After eight fast intervals an episode is declared. The EGM for pre-attempt 1 shows an average ventricular rate of 176 beats/min. The EGM for post attempt 1 indicates that an ATP therapy consisting of 1 burst of a ramp\scan sequence of pacing resulted in an accelerated rhythm of 202 beats/min. The EGM for post attempt 2 indicates that an ATP therapy consisting of 1 burst of a scan sequence of pacing resulted in termination of the episode followed by DDD pacing.

The counters (Fig. 64.24) and data in the Arrhythmia Logbook (Fig. 64.23), show frequent premature ventricular contractions (PVCs) and episodes of nonsustained VT and three sustained episodes. The device was reprogrammed to make the antitachycardia pacing (ATP) therapy in VT-1 zone less aggressive. The ATP therapy in VT zone was maintained as programmed due to efficacy in other VT episodes. The patient was placed on Amiodarone to manage ventricular arrhythmias. The prevalence of P-wave tracking–intrinsic AV conduction was promoted using AV Search Hysteresis.

Case study: far-field R wave oversensing in a dual chamber ICD

This first recording (Fig. 64.26a) is that of a 50-year-old man with two-vessel coronary artery disease (CAD) who received a Medtronic Jewel 7250 dual chamber defibrillator for drug refractory ventricular tachyarrhythmia with concomitant multifocal ATs (Weretka *et al.* 2001). Atrial sensitivity was set at 0.3 mV as the nominal value suggested by the manufacturer. Stored episode data showed paced and sensed events that could have reflected presence of frequent atrial extrasystolic beats and far-field R-Wave oversensing, falsely identified as AT. As a result, detection criteria for AF, a ramp of 16 decremental paced impulses was initiated. The first atrial therapy produced VT (Fig. 64.26b) that fulfilled device criteria for VF detection. Consequently, the first programmed VF therapy, a defibrillation shock of 27 J, was delivered and terminated the episode (Fig. 64.26c).

Case study: inappriopriate shock due to atrial fibrillation from a dual chamber ICD

Figure 64.27 is a stored electrocardiogram from a patient who had a Medtronic 7271 dual chamber ICD. Stability was set to 30 ms, P/R relation was on; SVT minimal interval 240 ms. The patient had 9 episodes of QRS complex far-field sensing in the atrial channel. The resulting therapy was 13 ATP; 1 delivered shock and 1 aborted shock. The solution to the inappropriate therapy was to reduce the atrial sensitivity to 0.9mV (Deisenhofer *et al.* 2001).

Case study: intermittent atrial undersense of atrial fibrillation (AF) with pseudoregular AV conduction leading to inaccurate detection of ventricular tachycardia (VT)

Figure 64.28 is a real-time electrocardiogram from a patient with a Medtronic 7250 dual chamber ICD. Stability was set to 40 ms, P/R relation was on; SVT minimal interval 240 ms. The patient had 24 episodes of AF with rapid AV conduction; intermittent atrial undersensing and atrial oversensing leading to malfunction of the P/R relation detection algorithm. The resulting therapy was 16 ATP; 15 shocks in the VT zone,

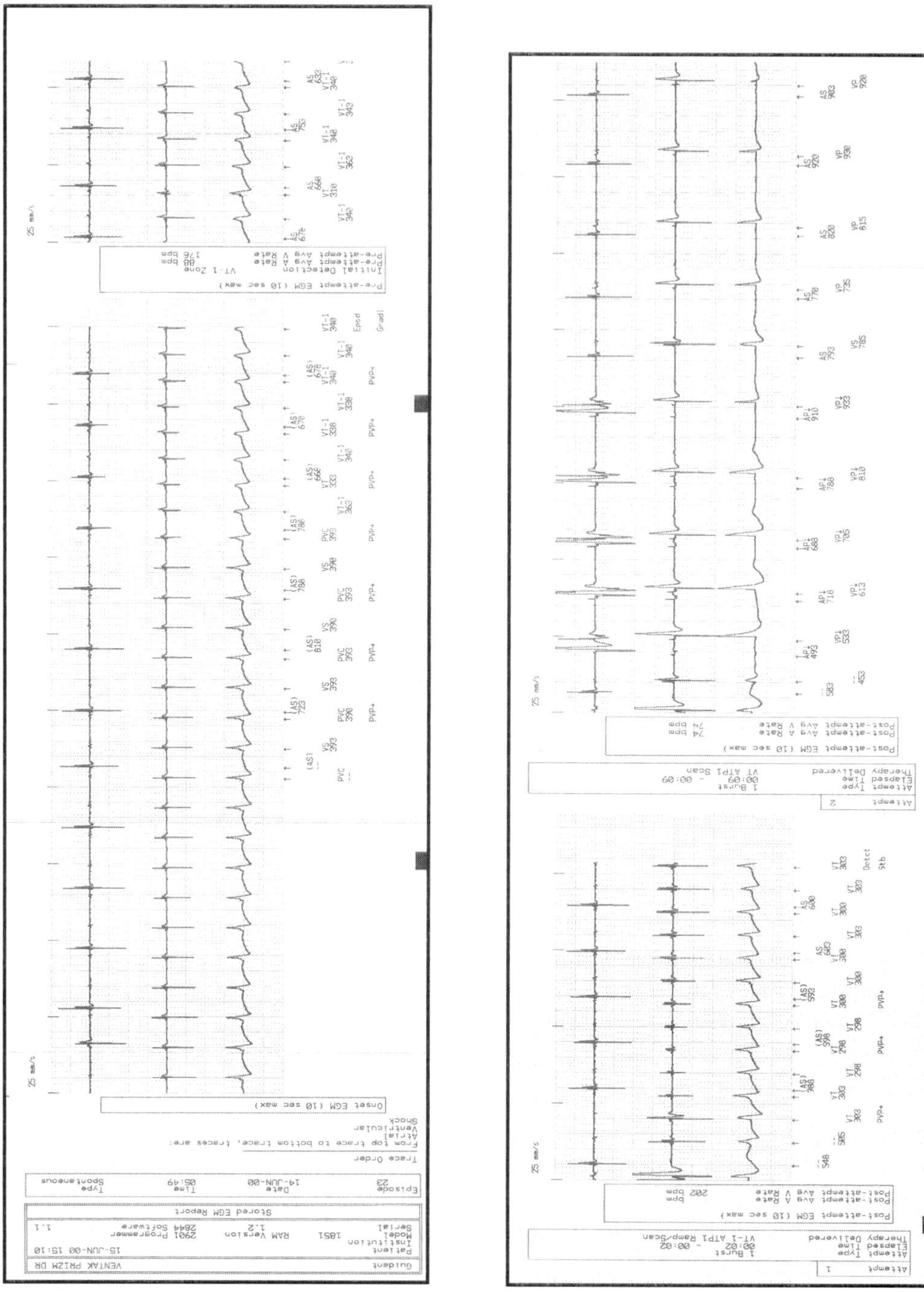

Fig. 64.23 Stored EGM report.

Counters (Tachy | Brady)

	Percent	Since Last Reset	Percent	Device Totals
Atrial				
Paced	27%	16.0K	11%	102.5K
Sensed	73%	44.2K	89%	828.1K
ATR Switches		0		0
Minimum Duration		00:00 m:s		00:00 m:s
Maximum Duration		00:00 m:s		00:00 m:s
Mode Switch Time		0%		0%
PMT		0		0
Ventricular				
Paced	63%	42.1K	52%	514.0K
Sensed	37%	24.4K	48%	481.8K
Single or Double PVCs		4.6K		49.6K
Three or More PVCs		13		53
Hysteresis				
Rate Hysteresis Searches		0		0
Successful Searches		0		0
AV Hysteresis Searches		46		1.7K
Successful Searches		46		1.7K
Rate Smoothing				
Atrial				
Up Smoothing		0		0
Down Smoothing		7.5K		104.2K
Ventricular				
Up Smoothing		61		923
Down Smoothing		6.5K		73.1K

10-JUN-00 to 14-JUN-00 | Reset...

Fig. 64.24 Counters.

3 shocks in VF zone. Reprogramming of atrial sensitivity was not successful. AV ablation was the required solution (Deisenhofer *et al.* 2001).

Present expectations

In today's environment it is important for the clinician to be an expert in assessing device performance and programming. This task has become increasingly more difficult as manufacturers have introduced more complicated devices without definitive randomized clinical trial evidence of improved clinical outcomes.

More than 200 000 patients have received ICDs in the past two decades (Pinsky *et al.* 1999; Deisenhofer *et al.* 2001). Clinical studies have demonstrated that inappropriate therapy occurs in 20–30% of patients with single chamber ICDs (VVI-ICD) (Grimm *et al.* 1992). The most common cause for inappropriate therapy in patients with an implanted VVI-ICD are SVT erroneously identified by the device as ventricular tachycardia (VT) or ventricular fibrillation (VF) (Deisenhofer *et al.* 2001).

In a recent study of 92 patients, 45 of whom had single chamber ICDs and 47 of whom had dual chamber ICDs, the data showed that the applied detection algorithms of dual chamber ICDs did not offer improved benefits in avoiding inappropriate therapies during SVT (Deisenhofer *et al.* 2001).

Other studies have shown that atrial undersensing during a tachycardia event or ventricular oversensing may alter the relationship of atrial and ventricular relationships and trigger inappropriate therapy (Lee & Chu-Pak Lau 1999). In addition, it has been reported in at least one case that P-wave amplitude variability, caused by exercise, can lead to lack of 1:1 PR association, causing Medtronic's P-R logic algorithm to erroneous classify a normal sinus rhythm as VT, leading to inappropriate shock (Sarter *et al.* 1998).

Future trends

The future trend appears to be that of more sophisticated dual chamber devices. More digital signal processing (DSP) functions seem to be migrating into these devices. New DSP algorithms under investigation include the ARGUS (Merkely *et al.* 2001) algorithm from Biotronik and wavelet transform morphology algorithms from Medtronic (Swerdlow *et al.* 2002).

A new type of ICD, with the potential to significantly change ICD therapy as it exists today, is the subcutaneous only implantable cardioverter/defibrillator (S-ICD®) from Cameron Health Inc. (Bardy *et al.* 2002). The S-ICD® does not require intravenous leads or any penetration into the thoracic cavity. The device and electrodes reside entirely between the skin and ribs, therefore, eliminating the need for X-ray systems for implantation. The device uses algorithms based on a combination of rate and far-field correlation waveform analysis, and in doing so eliminates the need for separate atrial and ventricle chamber sensing and the problems associated with such conventional approaches.

The value of the far-field signal seen from an

Case Study: Slow VT

(Courtesy of ELA)

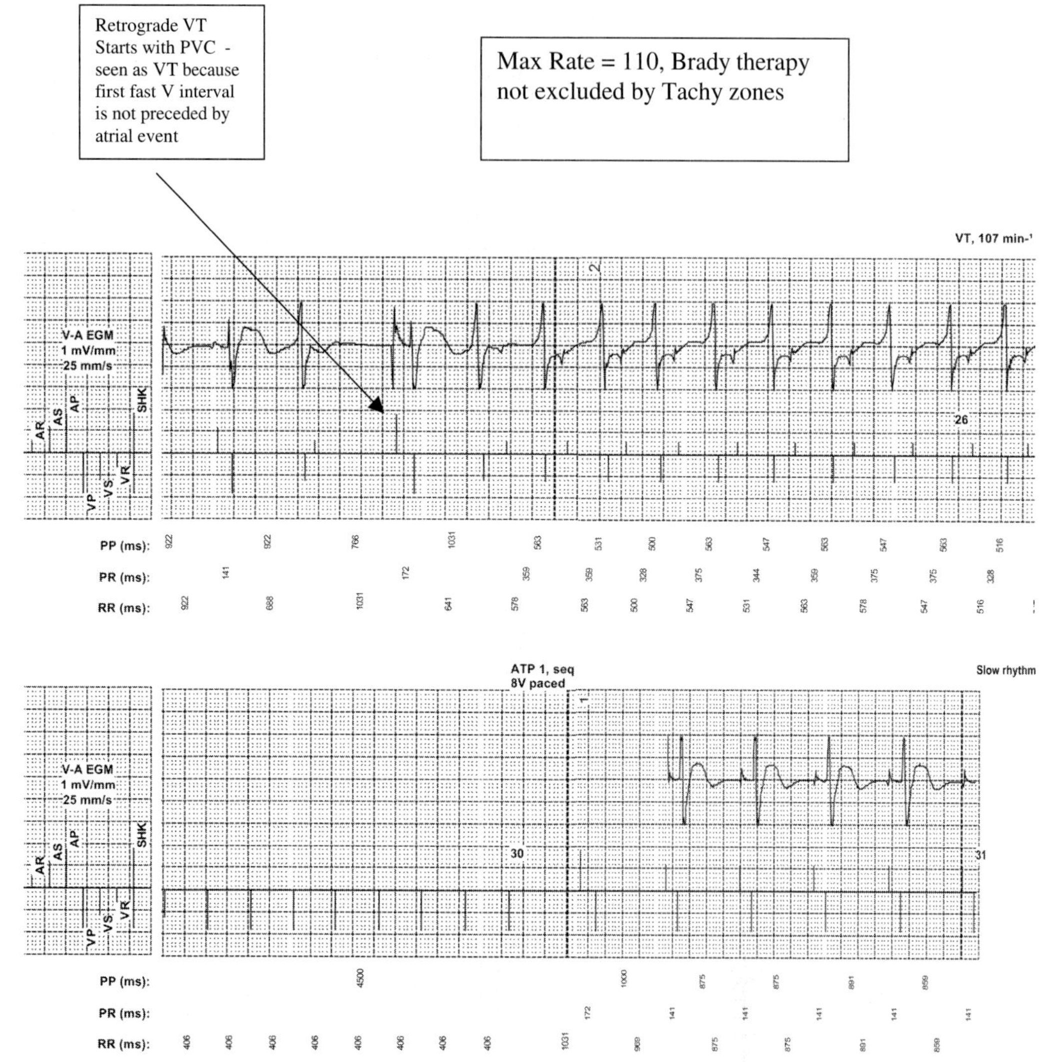

Fig. 64.25 An example of the PARARD algorithm and determination of slow VT. Retrograde VT starts with a PVC – seen as VT because first fast V interval is not preceded by atrial event. VT is converted with ATP burst. (Courtesy of ELA.)

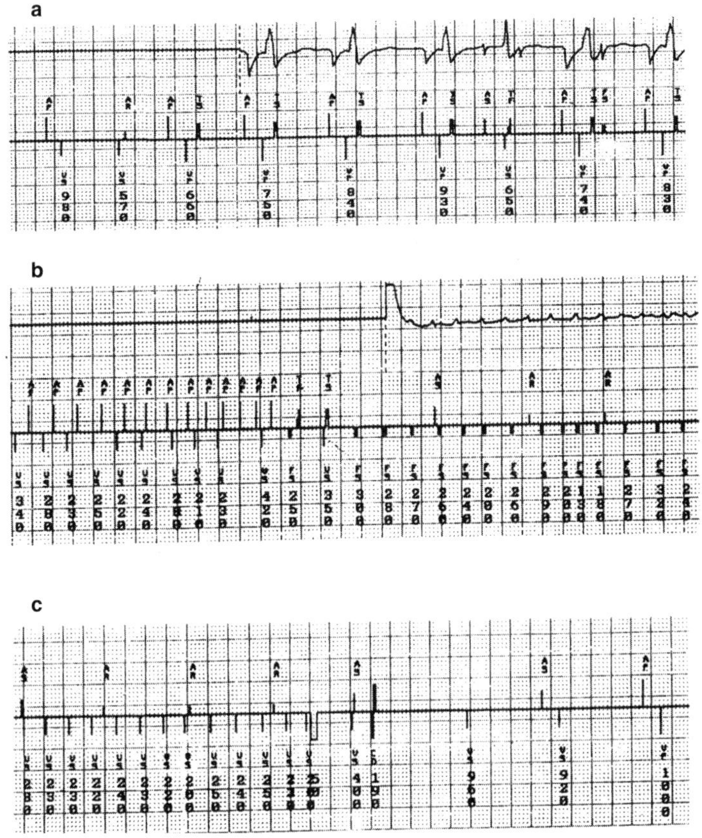

Fig. 64.26 Far-field R wave oversensing (TS, TF) following ventricular events (a). Atrial antitachycardia pacing (ramp) subsequent to oversensing of R wave in the atrium produces VT (b). Ongoing ventricular tachyarrhythmia initiated delivery of defibrillation shock which ultimately terminated the episode restoring stable ventricular rhythm (c).

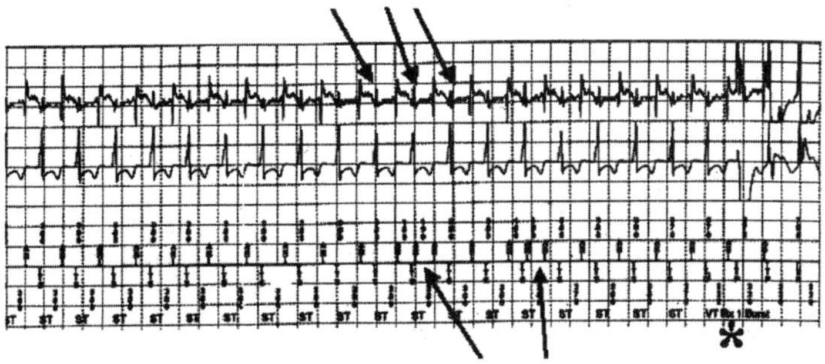

Fig. 64.27 Intermittent QRS far-field sense in the atrial channel during initially correctly detected sinus tachycardia ('ST' on the marker channel) leading to inappropriate ventricular tachycardia (VT) detection ('TD' on the marker channel). Due to intermittent QRS far-field sensing in the atrial channel (arrows on the ventricular far-field potential in the atrial channel and annotation in the marker channel), the device can no longer establish a clear relation (e.g., 1 1 conduction) between atrial and ventricular rhythm. As the VT zone detection rate is reached and the stability criterion fulfilled, VT is detected and inappropriately treated with ventricular antitachycardia pacing (* = on 'TP' annotation on the marker channel). From top to bottom are shown the bipolar atrial electrogram, ventricular electrogram, and marker annotation channel with PP and *RR* intervals.

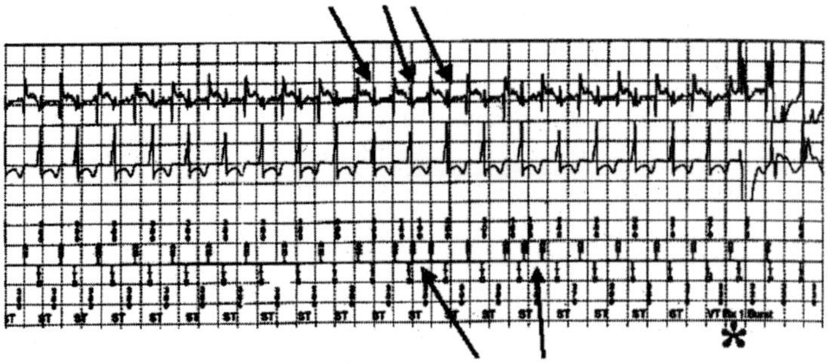

Fig. 64.28 Arrows point to AF wavelets in the bipolar atrial electrogram (EGM), which are not detected in the marker channel. Shown from the top to bottom are the surface ECG, bipolar atrial EGM, and the marker annotation channel with PP and *RR* intervals. Example recorded from patient during in-clinic control because of inappropriate therapy, with atrial sensitivity at 0.2mV and stability at 30 ms. P wave at implantation and at postoperative discharge test were 3.2 and 2.6 mV, respectively.

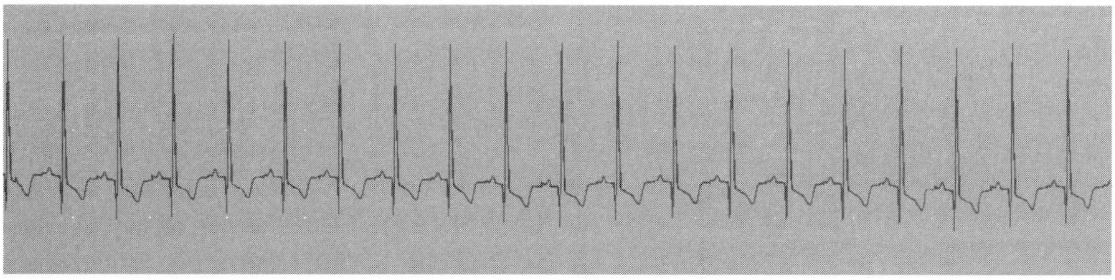

Fig. 64.29 ECG seen from the implanted subcutaneous only implantable cardioverter/defibrillator (S-ICD®) from Cameron Health Inc. Signal sensed between the lateral active can and parasternum sense/shock electrode. The *P*-wave, QRS complex and T wave are clearly seen.

S-ICD® is that it houses as much data as a surface ECG, giving a more global view of the heart during normal and abnormal rhythms.

This view may avoid some of the SVT-VT discrimination problems that occur with intracardiac electrodes that have only a near-field view of the heart. Such systems may serve to function more like AED detection algorithms unburdened by the need to provide tiered therapy.

References

Bardy, G.H., Cappato, R., Smith, W.M. *et al.* (2002) The totally subcutaneous ICD system (the S-ICD). In: *NASPE 23rd Annual Scientific Sessions.* Cameron Healthand Green Lane Hospital, Auckland, New Zealand.

Deisenhofer, I., Kolb, C., Ndrepepa, G. *et al.* (2001) Do current dual chamber cardioverter defibrillators have advantages over conventional single chamber cardioverter defibrillators in reducing inappropriate therapies? *Journal of Cardiovascular Electrophysiology*, **12**, 134–142.

Fan, K., Lee, K. & Lau, C.P. (1999) Dual chamber implantable cardioverter defibrillator-benefits and limitations. *Journal of Interventional Cardiac Electrophysiology*, **3**, 239–245.

Fogoros, R. N. (1999) *Practical Cardiac Diagnosis Series Electrophysiological Testing*, 3rd edn. Blackwell Scientific Publications, Oxford.

Furman, S., Hayes, D.L. & Holmes, D.R. (1993) *A Practice of Cardiac Pacing*, 3rd edn.: Futura Publishing, Armonk, NY.

Glotzer, T.V. *et al.* (1999) Variability of atrial sensing during exercise in a patient with a dual chamber ICD caused inappropriate ICD discharges. *PACE (Pacing and Clinical Electrophysiology)*, **22**, 1838–1841.

Grimm, W., Flores, B.F. & Marchlinski, F.E. (1992) Electrocardiographically documented unnecessary, spontaneous shocks in 241 patients with implantable carioverter defibrillators. *PACE (Pacing and Clinical Electrophysiology)*, **15**, 1667–1673.

Grimm, W., Menz, V., Hoffmann, J. & Maisch, B. (1998)

Failure of third-generation implantable cardioverter defibrillators to abort shock therapy for nonsustained ventricular tachycardia due to shortcomings of the vf confirmation algorithm. *PACE (Pacing and Clinical Electrophysiology)*, **21**(I), 722–727.

Hamer, M.E., Clair, W.K., Wilkinson, W.E., Greenfield, R.A., Pritchett, E.L.C. & Page R.L. (1994) Evaluation of outpatients experiencing implantable cardioverter defibrillator shocks associated with minimal symptoms. *PACE (Pacing and Clinical Electrophysiology)*, **17** (1).

Hintringer, F., Schwarzacher, S., Eibl, G. & Pachinger O. (2001) Inappropriate detection of supraventricular arrhythmias by implantable dual chamber defibrillators: a comparison of four different algorithms. *PACE (Pacing and Clinical Electrophysiology)*, **24**, 835–841.

Horton, R.P., Canby, R.C., Roman, C. A., Jessen, M.E., Schulte, T.J. & Page, R.L. (1995) Diagnosis of ICD lead failure using continuous event marker recording. *PACE (Pacing and Clinical Electrophysiology)*, **18**,1331–1334.

Kettering, K., Dornberger, V., Lang, R. *et al.* (2001) Enhanced detection criteria in implantable cardioverter defibrillators: sensitivity and specificity of the stability algorithm at different heart rates. *PACE (Pacing and Clinical Electrophysiology)*, **24**, 1325–1333.

Krishen, A., Shepard, R.K., Leffler, J.A., Wood, M.A. & Ellenboen, K.A. (2001) Implantable cardioverter defibrillator T wave oversensing caused by hyperglycemia. *PACE (Pacing and Clinical Electrophysiology)*, **24**, 1701–1703.

Lee, K. L. & Chu-Pak Lau (2001) Inappropriate defibrillator therapies: are dual chamber devices providing a remedy? *Journal of Cardiovascular Electrophysiology*, **12**, 143–144.

Mann, D.E, Kelly, P.A. & Reiter, M.J. (1998) Inappropriate shock therapy for nonsustained ventricular tachycardia in dual chamber pacemaker defibrillator. *PACE (Pacing and Clinical Electrophysiology)*, **21**, 2005–2006.

Mazur, A., Wang, L., Anderson, M.E. *et al.* (2001) Functional similarity between electrograms recorded from an implantable cardioverter defibrillator emulator and the surface electrocardiogram. *PACE (Pacing and Clinical Electrophysiology)*, **24**, 34–40.

Medtronic (1997) *Slide presentation of GEM II DR Dual Chamber ICD Systems. Advanced choices for arrhythmia management*. Medtronic, Minneapolis, MN.

Merkely, B., Zima, E., Geller, L., Lang, V. & Schaldach, M. (2001) A new detection algorithm for implantable cardioverter defibrillator. *Biomedizinische Technik*, **46**, 226–229.

Natale, A., Sra, J., Axtell, K. et al. (19960 Undetected ventricular fibrillation in transvenous implantable cardioverter-defibrillators. Prospective comparison of different lead system–device combinations. *Circulation*, **93**, 91–98.

Pfitzner, P. & Trappe, H. J. (1998) Oversensing in a cardioverter defibrillator system caused by interaction between two enocardial defibrillation leads in the right ventricle. *PACE (Pacing and Clinical Electrophysiology)*, **21**(I), 764–768.

Pinski, S.L. & Fahy, G.J. (1999) Implantable cardioverter-defibrillators. *American Journal of Medicine*, **106**, 446–458.

Sarter, B.H., Callans, D.J., Gottlieb, C.D., Schwartzman, D.S. & Marchlinski, F.E. (1998) Implantable defibrillator diagnostic storage capabilities: evolution, current status, and future utilization: *PACE (Pacing and Clinical Electrophysiology)*, **21**, 1287–1298.

Schmitt, C., Montero, M. & Melichercik, J. (1994) Significance of supraventricular tachyarrhythmias in patients with implanted pacing cardioverter defibrillators. *PACE (Pacing and Clinical Electrophysiology)*, **17** (1).

Stroobandt, R.X. (2002) Morphology discrimination of ventricular tachycardia from supraventricular tachycardia by implantable cardioverter defibrillators: are implantable cardioverter defibrillators really starting to look at arrhythmias with the eyes of a cardiologists. *Journal of Cardiovascular Electrophysiology*, **13**, 442–443.

Sweesy, M.W., Holland, J.L., Pirucki, R. & Redenbaugh, S. (2000) *Cardiac Device & Basic EP Self-Assessment*, pp. 390–430. Cardiac Device Consultants, Simpsonville, SC.

Swerdlow, C.D., Brown, M.L., Lurie, K. *et al.* (2002) Discrimination of ventricular tachycardia from supraventricular tachycardia by a download wavelet-transform morphology algorithm: a paradigm for development of implantable cardioverter defibrillator detection algorithms. *Journal of Cardiovascular Electrophysiology*, **13**, 432–441.

Weretka, S., Becker, R., Hilbel, T. *et al.* (2001) Far-field R wave oversensing in a dual chamber arrhythmia management device: predisposing factors and practical implications. *PACE (Pacing and Clinical Electrophysiology)* **24**, 1240–1246.

Index